Sports Injuries

Sports Injuries

Edited by

Dr Mike Hutson MA, MB BCHIR, DRCOG, DMSMED

Department of Musculo Skeletal Medicine, Royal London Hospital
for Integrated Medicine, London

and

Dr Cathy Speed BMED SCI, MA, DIP SPORTS MED, PHD, FRCP, FFSEM(I) (UK)

Department of Rheumatology, Addenbrookes Hospital, Cambridge University
Hospitals NHS Foundation Trust, Cambridge

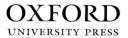

OXFORD

UNIVERSITY PRESS

OXFORD

UNIVERSITY PRESS

Great Clarendon Street, Oxford OX2 6DP

Oxford University Press is a department of the University of Oxford.
It furthers the University's objective of excellence in research, scholarship,
and education by publishing worldwide in

Oxford New York

Auckland Cape Town Dar es Salaam Hong Kong Karachi
Kuala Lumpur Madrid Melbourne Mexico City Nairobi
New Delhi Shanghai Taipei Toronto

With offices in

Argentina Austria Brazil Chile Czech Republic France Greece
Guatemala Hungary Italy Japan Poland Portugal Singapore
South Korea Switzerland Thailand Turkey Ukraine Vietnam

Oxford is a registered trade mark of Oxford University Press
in the UK and in certain other countries

Published in the United States
by Oxford University Press Inc., New York

British Library Cataloguing in Publication Data is available

Library of Congress Cataloging in Publication Data is available

Typeset in Minion
by Glyph International, Bangalore, India
Printed in China
on acid-free paper by Asia Pacific Offset

ISBN 978-0-19-953390-9

10 9 8 7 6 5 4 3 2 1

Oxford University Press makes no representation, express or implied, that the drug
dosages in this book are correct. Readers must therefore always check the product
information and clinical procedures with the most up-to-date published product
information and data sheets provided by the manufacturers and the most recent codes of
conduct and safety regulations. The authors and the publishers do not accept responsibility
or legal liability for any errors in the text or for the misuse or misapplication of material in
this work. Except where otherwise stated, drug dosages and recommendations are for the
non-pregnant adult who is not breast-feeding

Contents

Foreword

As a middle distance athlete, I have always recognized the challenge of prevention and treatment of sport related injuries. Even a minor 'niggle' can have serious consequences on sporting performance. All athletes—recreational or elite—should have access to expert medical care to allow prompt diagnosis and appropriate intervention to allow a safe and effective return to sport.

Since my athletic career, the delivery of medical care to athletes has progressed beyond recognition. In the past decade alone we in the UK have seen the recognition and development of Sport and Exercise Medicine as a medical specialty, the establishment of the Faculty of Sport & Exercise Medicine and the 2012 Olympic games being awarded to London. These events represent a major leap forward for sport in the UK, and the development of medical expertise should be seen as part of the legacy of the 2012 Olympic Games.

I congratulate Drs Speed and Hutson for their Textbook of Sports Injuries, with contributions from a number of authors who are true experts in their fields. The text is a thorough, highly illustrated and practical guide to expert management of sport injuries across a variety of sports. It takes the reader through basic and applied sciences, to in-depth but accessible sections on injuries and concludes with a section on sport specific complaints.

This textbook will undoubtedly make a significant contribution to the education of a range of professionals working in the field of Sport & Exercise Medicine. Specialty trainees, specialists, and allied practitioners alike will find it an enjoyable and informative read, and an invaluable reference.

Steve Cram
Chairman, English Institute of Sport
Middle distance runner
European, Commonwealth and World Champion and
Olympic Silver medalist

Preface

The evolution of Sports and Exercise Medicine (SEM) in the UK over the last century is well documented in the period after the foundation of BASM (British Association of Sports Medicine) in 1952. Prior to the 1950s, records of services to the injured are sketchy, though there is evidence of a Footballers' Hospital in Manchester at the turn of the nineteenth century, and the creation of the first official post of Medical Officer to the BOA (British Olympic Association) in 1928, the same year as the foundation of FIMS (International Federation of Sports Medicine). BASM (latterly renamed BASEM), was the spur to the formation of the ISM (Institute of Sports Medicine) in 1965, at much the same time as the creation of the English Sports Council. Finally, in February 2005, Sports and Exercise Medicine was established as a stand-alone specialty in the United Kingdom. The Faculty (FSEM) was created under the auspices of the Royal College of Surgeons of Edinburgh and the Royal College of Physicians of London (RCP) and was officially launched by its patron, the Princess Royal, at the RCP in September 2006.

The Faculty declares that the speciality is 'founded on the disease and wellness models of medicine. It is through the latter, in particular, that SEM physicians in the future can play a leading and vital role in helping determine the Health of the Nation'. The role of the specialist physician in SEM includes the promotion of exercise for health; the prescription of exercise programmes for needy subgroups of the population; management of soft tissue injuries with specific focus on exercise- and sport-related injuries; the provision of highly skilled services to elite athletes; rehabilitation of able and disabled sportsmen and women of all standards 'to expedite return to physical activity, work and increase participation in sport'.

This textbook is intended to provide guidance for all clinicians involved in sports medicine practice, including therapists, the enthusiastic doctor, the sub-specialist SEM doctor, and the specialist consultant in SEM, all of whom require appropriate skills set upon a sound knowledge base of injuries related to sport and exercise, thereby providing a high level of service to all exercising patients from diverse backgrounds who require help.

Michael Hutson
Cathy Speed

Contributors List

JOHN ALDRIDGE
(Formerly) University Hospitals Coventry and Warwickshire NHS Trust, Coventry, UK

ELI BARON
Cedars Sinai Institute for Spinal Disorders, Los Angeles, CA, USA

PHILIP BEARCROFT
Department of Radiology, Cambridge University Hospitals NHS Foundation Trust, Cambridge, UK

LAURENCE BERMAN
Department of Radiology, University of Cambridge, Cambridge, UK

EMMA BLAIN
Arthritis Research UK Biomechanics and Bioengineering Centre, Cardiff University, Cardiff, UK

LYNN BOOTH
Littleborough, Lancashire, UK

KEVIN BOYD
Department of Sports Medicine, University Hospitals of Leicester NHS Trust, Leicester, UK

RICHARD BUDGETT
British Olympic Association, London, UK

HENRY COLACO
Trauma & Orthopaedics, Eastbourne District General Hospital, Eastbourne, UK

SHARON DIXON
School of Sport and Health Sciences, University of Exeter, Exeter, UK

NICHOLAS DOWNING
University Hospitals of Nottingham NHS Trust, Nottingham, UK

VICTOR DUANCE
Arthritis Research UK Biomechanics and Bioengineering Centre, Cardiff University, Cardiff, UK

VIKTOR DVORAK
Musculoskeletal and Sport medicine, Bonaduz, Switzerland

PATRICK FARHART
Cricket New South Wales, Sydney, Australia

CRAIG FINLAYSON
Department of Orthopaedic Surgery, University of Illinois at Chicago, Chicago, IL, USA

JOHN FIRTH
Queens Medical Centre, University Hospital, Nottingham, UK

COLIN FULLER
Centre for Sports Medicine, University of Nottingham, UK

NICK GALLOWAY
University Hospital, Nottingham, UK

EZEQUIEL GHERSCOVICI
Cedars Sinai Institute for Spinal Disorders, Los Angeles, CA, USA

ANDREW GIBBONS
Oral & Maxillofacial Surgery Department, Peterborough NHS Foundation Hospital, Peterborough, UK

MARK GILLETT
English Insitute of Sport, Birmingham High Performance Centre, Birmingham, UK

DAMIAN GRIFFIN
University of Warwick and University Hospitals, Coventry and Warwickshire NHS Trust, Coventry, UK

ROGER HACKNEY
Department of Orthopaedics, Leeds General Infirmary, Leeds, UK

FARES HADDAD
University College Hospital, London, UK

BRUCE HAMILTON
ASPETAR, Qatar, Orthopaedic and Sports Medicine Hospital

WAYNE HOSKINS
Melbourne Medical School, University of Melbourne, Victoria, Australia

GLYN HOWATSON
School of Psychology and Sport Sciences, Northumbria University, Newcastle upon Tyne, UK

MARK HUTCHINSON
Department of Orthopaedic Surgery, University of Illinois at Chicago, Chicago, IL, USA

MIKE HUTSON
Department of Musculo Skeletal Medicine, Royal London Hospital for Integrated Medicine, London, UK

TREFOR JAMES
Cricket Australia, Jolimont, Victoria, Australia

ROD JAQUES
EIS High Performance Centre, University of Bath, Bath, UK

MICHAEL KJAER
Institute of Sports Medicine Copenhagen (ISMC), Bispebjerg Hospital, Faculty of Health Sciences, University of Copenhagen, Copenhagen, Denmark

ALEX KOUNTOURIS
La Trobe University, Bundoora, Victoria, Australia

MIKE LOOSEMORE
English Institute of Sport, UCLH, London, UK

NEIL MACKENZIE
Maxillofacial Unit, Queen Alexandra Hospital, Cosham

ABIGAIL MACKEY
Institute of Sports Medicine Copenhagen (ISMC), Bispebjerg Hospital, Faculty of Health Sciences, University of Copenhagen, Copenhagen, Denmark

NICOLA MAFFULLI
Centre for Sports and Exercize Medicine, Institute of Health Sciences Education, Barts and The London School of Medicine and Dentistry, London, UK

LYLE MICHELI
Division of Sports Medicine, Department of Orthopedics, Children's Hospital, Boston, MA, USA

GERARD MULLINS
Addenbrooke's Hospital, Cambridge University Hospitals NHS Foundation Trust, Cambridge, UK

JOHN ORCHARD
School of Public Health University of Sydney, Sydney, Australia

NICHOLAS PEIRCE
East Midlands English Institute of Sport, National Cricket Performance Centre/EIS Performance Centre, Loughborough University, Loughborough, UK

LAURA PURCELL
Division of Emergency Medicine, Department of Internal Medicine, Paediatrics, and Family Medicine, University of Western Ontario, London, Ontario, Canada

JULIAN RAY
Addenbrooke's Hospital, Cambridge University Hospitals NHS Foundation Trust, Cambridge, UK

JAE RHEE
Robert Jones & Agnes Hunt Orthopaedic and District Hospital NHS Trust, Oswestry, Shropshire, UK

BILL RIBBANS
Northampton General Hospital, Northampton, UK

GRAHAM RILEY
Rheumatology Research Unit, Addenbrooke's Hospital, Cambridge, UK

SALLY ROBERTS
Spinal Studies & Institute of Science and Technology in Medicine (Keele University), Robert Jones & Agnes Hunt Orthopaedic and District Hospital NHS Trust, Oswestry, Shropshire, UK

SIMON ROBERTS
Robert Jones & Agnes Hunt Orthopaedic and District Hospital NHS Trust, Oswestry, Shropshire, UK

SOPHIE ROBERTS (NÉE COX)
The Gait Lab, Parkside Hospital, London, UK

LEANNE SAXON
Royal Veterinary College, London, UK

MURALI SAYANA
Department of Trauma and Orthopaedics, Royal College of Surgeons in Ireland, Dublin, Ireland

HUGH SEWARD
Australian Football League Medical Officers Association Melbourne, Victoria, Australia

CHEZHIYAN SHANMUGAM
Department of Trauma and Orthopaedic Surgery, Weston General Hospital, Weston-Super-Mare, UK

NILAM SHERGILL
University Hospitals Coventry and Warwickshire NHS Trust, Coventry, UK

CATHY SPEED
Department of Rheumatology, Addenbrookes Hospital, Cambridge University Hospitals NHS Foundation Trust, Cambridge, UK

HANS SPRING
Clinic for Rehabilitation and Rheumatology Swiss Olympic Medical Center, Leukerbad, Switzerland

JAI TRIVEDI
Centre for Spinal Studies, Robert Jones & Agnes Hunt Orthopaedic and District Hospital NHS Trust, Oswestry, Shropshire, UK

STEPHEN TURNER
University Hospitals Coventry and Warwickshire NHS Trust, Coventry, UK

ALEXANDER VACCARO
Rothman Institute, Thomas Jefferson University, Philadelphia, PA, USA

KEN VAN SOMEREN
English Institute of Sport, Bisham Abbey National Sports Centre, Marlow, UK

ANDREW WALLACE
Shoulder Unit, Hospital of St John & St Elizabeth, London, UK

NICK WEBBORN
Sussex Centre for Sport and Exercise Medicine, University of Brighton, Brighton, UK

PATRICK WHEELER
East Midlands English Institute of Sport, Loughborough, UK University Hospitals of Leicester NHS Trust University of Bath

Figure acknowledgements

The following figures and tables are reproduced from Soft Tissue Rheumatology, edited by Hazelman, B., Riley, G., and Speed, C. (Oxford University Press, 2004).

Figures 1.1.1–1.1.19, 1.3.1, 1.4.2–1.4.4, 2.5.1, 3.5.1–3.5.20, 3.5.22, 3.5.23, 3.5.25, 3.5.27, 3.5.28, 3.6.1–3.6.10, 3.12, 3.8.1–3.8.8, 3.8.11–3.8.17, 3.8.21, 3.8.26–3.8.29,

3.11.1–3.11.10, 3.12.2, 3.12.4, 3.12.6(b), 3.12.7, 3.13.2–3.13.7, 3.13.12, 3.13.16, 3.14.1–3.14.10, 3.14.12, and 3.14.13.

Tables 3.5.2, 3.5.3, 3.5.6, 3.5.8–3.5.13, and 3.6.1.

We would also like to acknowledge Phil Ball and Greg Harding, Medical Illustration Department at Addenbrooke's Hospital, and Primal Pictures Ltd, who provided many of the figures reproduced from the above title. Additionally, we acknowledge the contribution of Dr Hany Elmadbouh, Consultant Musculosketal Radiologist, Peterborough Hospitals.

Abbreviations

ABC	airway–breathing–circulation		GDF	growth and development factor
ACL	anterior cruciate ligament		GTN	glyceryl trinitrate
ACPSM	Association of Chartered Physiotherapists in Sports Medicine		HGF	hepatocyte growth factor
			HU	Hounsfield unit
AF	annulus fibrosus		IGF	insulin-like growth factor
ALL	anterior longitudinal ligament		IL	interleukin
ANA	antinuclear antibodies		IP	interphalangeal
AP	anteroposterior		ITB	iliotibial band
APL	abductor pollicis longus		IU	international unit
AS	ankylosing spondylitis		IVD	intervertebral disc
ASIS	anterior superior iliac spine		LA	local anaesthetic
ATLS	Acute Trauma Life Support		LCL	lateral collateral ligament
BMC	bone mineral content		LED	light-emitting diode
BMD	bone mineral density		LHB	long head of the biceps
BMI	body mass index		LIUS	low-intensity ultrasound
BMP	bone morphogenic protein		MCL	medial collateral ligament
BMSF	bone marrow stromal fibroblast		MCP	metacarpophalangeal
CI	confidence interval		M-CSF	macrophage-colony stimulating factor
CK	creatine kinase		MDP	methylene diphosphonate
CNS	central nervous system		MRI	magnetic resonance imaging
COMP	cartilage oligomeric matrix protein		MSC	mesenchymal stem cell
COX	cyclo-oxygenase		MTP	metatarsophalangeal
CRP	C-reactive protein		MTPJ	metatarsophalangeal joint
CT	computed tomography		NMES	neuromuscular electrical stimulation
DOMS	delayed-onset muscle soreness		NP	nucleus pulposus
ECM	extracellular matrix		NSAIDs	non-steroidal anti-inflammatory drugs
EDL	extensor digitorum longus		OA	osteoarthritis
EHL	extensor hallucis longus		ODI	Oswestry Disability Index
EIMD	exercise-induced muscle damage		OPG	osteoprotegrin
EM	electromagnetic		PBL	problem-based learning
EMG	electromyography		PDGF	platelet-derived growth factor
ESR	erythrocyte sedimentation rate		PG	proteoglycan, prostaglandin
ESWT	extracorporeal shock wave therapy		PGE2	prostaglandin E2
FCU	flexor carpi ulnaris		PIPJ	proximal interphalangeal joint
FDA	US Food and Drug Administration		PLL	posterior longitudinal ligament
FDB	flexor digitorum brevis		PNF	proprioceptive neuromuscular facilitation
FDL	flexor digitorum longus		pQCT	peripheral quantitative computed tomography
FDP	flexor digitorum profundus		PRICES	protection, rest, ice, elevation, support
FDS	flexor digitorum superficialis		PSIS	posterior superior iliac spine
FGF	fibroblast growth factor		PTFJ	proximal tibiofibular joint
FHL	flexor hallucis longus		PTFL	posterior talofibular ligament

PTH	parathyroid hormone		TA	tibialis anterior
RCT	randomized controlled trial		TENS	transcutaneous electrical nerve stimulation
RF	rheumatoid factor		TFCC	triangular fibrocartilage complex
RICE	rest, ice, compression, elevation		TFL	tensor fascia lata
RoM	range of motion		TGF	transforming growth factor
ROS	reactive oxygen species		TIMP	tissue inhibitor of metalloproteinase
SAWS	sportsman's abdominal wall syndrome		TLHB	tendon of the long head of the biceps
SCIWORA	spinal cord injuries without obvious radiological abnormalities		TNF	tumour necrosis factor
			TOS	thoracic outlet syndrome
SCJ	sternoclavicular joint		TP	tibialis posterior
SEM	sports and exercise medicine		TTS	tarsal tunnel syndrome
SIJ	sacroiliac joint		US	ultrasonography, ultrasonic
SLAP	superior labrum from anterior to posterior		VAS	visual analogue scale
SPN	superficial peroneal nerve		VEGF	vascular endothelial growth factor
SPR	superior peroneal retinaculum		Vo2 max	maximum oxygen uptake
STIR	short inversion time inversion recovery		WADA	World Anti-Doping Agencycontributors

SECTION 1

Basic science

1.1

Tendon and ligament biochemistry and pathology

Graham Riley

Introduction

Tendon and ligament pathologies are often seen by general practitioners, rheumatologists, and specialists in musculoskeletal medicine and sports and exercise medicine. Increased participation in recreational exercise and sport, although beneficial for general health and well-being, has led to a substantial rise in their incidence. However, only belatedly are these conditions receiving the attention they deserve from the research community.

Tendons and ligaments are dense fibrous connective tissues, important for joint movement and stabilization, respectively. They have a similar composition and structure and are metabolically active and capable of responding to extrinsic factors such as mechanical load, exercise, and immobilization. Tendon and ligament are grouped together in this chapter so as to avoid repetition of common principles, although it is important to note that there are differences in the range of pathology affecting these tissues. Despite superficial similarities, there are differences in structure, composition, and function between tendon and ligament that make it unwise to extrapolate from one tissue to another.

The purpose of this chapter is to review what is known about the biochemistry and pathology of tendons and ligaments, focusing on conditions that are relevant to the practising clinician in sports and exercise medicine. The chapter begins with an overview of tendon and ligament biochemistry, which is fundamental to an understanding of the disease process.

Extracellular matrix components of tendon and ligament

Like all connective tissues, tendon and ligament are composite materials consisting of collagens, proteoglycans, and a variety of other non-collagenous proteins. Although the extracellular matrix (ECM) is predominantly collagen, many other components contribute to the strength, elasticity, and physiology of the tissue (Fig. 1.1.1). The relatively few cells in the mature tissue are responsible for the synthesis and organization of the ECM. These cells are also responsible for the degradation and replacement of ECM, an activity that is particularly important in tissue development, injury, and pathology. Degradation of the ECM is mediated largely by the resident fibroblasts and macrophages, either by phagocytosis or extracellular proteolysis. The maintenance of the normal tendon and ligament architecture is the result of a delicate balance between the synthesis

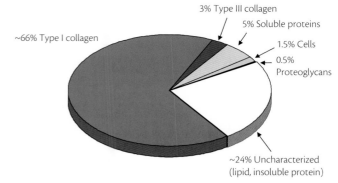

Fig. 1.1.1 Matrix (ECM) composition of tendon. Pie chart showing the approximate proportions of ECM components in a typical flexor tendon as a percentage of the tendon dry weight. The bulk of the tendon is collagen, predominantly type I with a small amount (up to 5 per cent) of type III collagen. The proportion of proteoglycan varies in different tendons and in different sites, representing 0.5–3.5 per cent of the matrix dry weight. A large proportion of the matrix is uncharacterized, thought to be insoluble protein and lipids. The composition of ligament is similar, although the proportion of type III collagen is greater—usually around 10 per cent but up to 40 per cent in some ligaments.

and degradation of ECM. Disruption of this balance leads to a loss of ECM organization and will ultimately lead to pathology.

Collagens

The collagen family of glycoproteins has been extensively reviewed elsewhere (Van der Rest and Garrone 1990; Prockop and Kivirikko 1995). Collagen has a unique triple helix structure that, once secreted into the ECM, spontaneously associates with other collagen molecules to form characteristic banded fibrils (Fig. 1.1.2). Since early descriptions of collagen as a single entity, it is now known that there are at least 27 different collagen types, each with a different structure, function, and tissue distribution (Tables 1.1.1 and 1.1.2). However, it is increasingly apparent that collagens, once thought to be restricted to specific tissues, are in fact distributed more widely, albeit as minor constituents of the ECM though no doubt important for the tissue structure and function.

Tendon and ligament are predominantly type I collagen, organized into fibril bundles and orientated with the long axis of the tissue. Collagen comprises between 50 and 85 per cent of the tendon dry

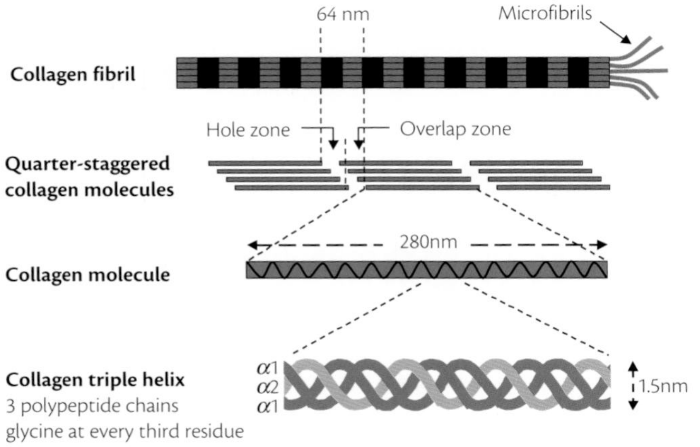

Fig. 1.1.2 Schematic representation of the prototypic collagen molecule. The collagen (type I) molecule consists of three polypeptide chains (designated α1 and α2), wound in a tight triple helix. This is made possible by the unusual amino acid content, with a high proportion of glycine, proline, and hydroxyproline in repeating triplets. Once secreted, each collagen molecule spontaneously associates end-to-end with other molecules, forming a quarter-staggered array. The 'hole zone' takes up electron-dense stains, which accounts for the striated appearance of the fibril under electron microscopy. (Reproduced (modified) from Cawston, T.E. (1998), fig. 1, p. 130, © 1998 with permission from Elsevier Science.)

weight depending on the tendon, species, and location (Elliott 1965). In studies of human tendon, collagen comprised on average 56 per cent of the dry weight in both the supraspinatus and the biceps brachii tendon, although there was considerable variation within each sample group (Riley *et al.* 1994).

In the tendon mid-substance, approximately 95 per cent of the collagen is type I, with the remainder consisting of types III, IV, V, VI, XII, and XIV. Type V collagen is thought to form the core of the collagen fibril and may comprise around 2 per cent of the total collagen (Niyibizi *et al.* 1994). Type III collagen is thought to represent up to 5 per cent of the total collagen (Niyibizi *et al.* 1994), although in studies of normal human supraspinatus tendon we found an average of just over 2 per cent type III collagen (Riley *et al.* 1994). Type III collagen is generally restricted to the endotenon or epitenon, the thin layers of connective tissue that surround the collagen fibre bundles (Duance *et al.* 1977). However many older supraspinatus tendons show distribution of type III collagen throughout the matrix, consistent with the formation of heterotypic fibre bundles (Kumagai *et al.* (1994) and Riley, G.P., unpublished observations). A similar distribution has been found in skin, with type I and type III collagens cross-linked together and found within the same fibrils (Lapiere *et al.* 1977). This interaction appears to have a role in conditioning the collagen fibre organization and ultimate fibre diameter. Type III collagen tends to form smaller diameter fibrils, and changes in the ratio of type III to type I collagen are correlated with the average fibril diameter (Birk and Mayne 1997). The resulting tissue may be more compliant and less resistant to mechanical strain. Although there have been suggestions that changes in the proportion of collagen types may be a consequence of ageing (Kumagai *et al.* 1994), this is not a feature of all tendons, which suggests that other factors such as mechanical strain and injury are implicated. In the supraspinatus tendon the increase in type III collagen is thought likely to represent a history of previous injury and matrix remodelling events in the tissue.

Changes in the proportion of collagen types I and III have been reported in other ruptured tendons (Holz 1980), consistent with some underlying process that weakens and predisposes the tendon to rupture. This is discussed in more detail below.

Type IV collagen is present in the basement membranes of tendon blood vessels, and type V collagen is encapsulated within the type I collagen fibrils (von der Mark 1981). Type VI collagen is found distributed throughout the matrix (Bray *et al.* 1993), and collagen types XII and XIV are associated with the collagen (type I) fibril surface (von der Mark 1981; Shaw and Olsen 1991). The precise roles of these so-called 'minor' collagens are uncertain, but they are thought to be important for both cell and matrix interactions.

Ligaments are essentially similar in collagen composition to tendon, although the proportion of type III collagen is generally higher, with reported values from 12 per cent to greater than 40 per cent in some ligaments (Amiel *et al.* 1984; Johnston *et al.* 1995). The amount of type III collagen is thought to account for the elasticity of the tissue, with higher levels in intrinsic ligaments of the wrist (41 per cent) compared to extrinsic ligaments (19 per cent), and these correlated with the strain to failure (Johnston *et al.* 1995). Type III collagen is relatively abundant in the epiligament, the equivalent of the epitenon, that surrounds the ligament fibre bundles (Amiel *et al.*1984). Type VI collagen in ligament is found in microfilaments stretching between the collagen fibrils in a network of electron-dense seams (Bray *et al.* 1993).

Site-specific variations in collagen composition

The collagen composition and organization varies at different sites within tendons and ligaments—they are not homogeneous tissues. At the insertion of bovine knee ligaments and Achilles tendons there are found collagen types II, IX, X, and XI in addition to collagen type I (Fukuta *et al.* 1998; Visconti *et al.* 1996). Type XIV collagen is more abundant at the insertion than elsewhere in the tendon/ligament (Niyibizi *et al.* 1994). Type X collagen is found at the Achilles insertion in the rodent, associated with the region of transition between calcified and non-calcified fibrocartilage (Fujioka *et al.* 1997). In the human Achilles at the bone insertion there are found collagen types I, II, III, V, and VI (Waggett *et al.* 1998). A higher concentration of type III is reported in the rotator cuff tendon at or near the insertion where it might contribute to the high incidence of tear at this site (Riley *et al.* 1994; Kumagai *et al.* 1994; Fan *et al.* 1997). Type II collagen is also found at regions of tendon fibrocartilage where tendon is compressed as it wraps around bone or passes through fibrous pulleys (Ralphs *et al.* 1991; Kumagai *et al.* 1994). In these regions the collagen has a different organization with a meshwork structure reminiscent of that of cartilage (Vogel and Koob 1989). The cells in these regions are rounded and chondrocyte-like, and express proteoglycans once thought to be restricted to cartilage (see below). Type VI collagen, which is normally associated with micro-fibillar networks between adjacent collagen fibres in the tendon mid-substance, is cell-associated in fibrocartilage, similar to the distribution seen in articular cartilage. Levels of matrix gene expression in the fibrocartilaginous regions of bovine tendon are higher than in the tension-bearing regions of the same tendon, demonstrating increased matrix turnover at these sites (Perez-Castro and Vogel 1999).

Collagen fibril organization and structure

The hierarchical structure of a typical tendon was described by Kastelic *et al.* (1978) as consisting of collagen molecules laid down

Table 1.1.1 Molecular composition and tissue distribution of collagens[a]

Collagen type	Molecular composition	Mature chain size[b] $Mr \times 10^{-3}$	Tissue distribution
Fibril-forming collagens			
I	$[\alpha1(I)_2\alpha2(I)]$	95	Most connective tissues
II	$[\alpha1(II)_3]$	95	Cartilage, vitreous
III	$[\alpha1(III)_3]$	95	Synovium, skin, tendon, ligament
V/XI	$[\alpha1(V)_2\alpha2(V)]$ $[\alpha1(V)\alpha2(V)\alpha3(V)]$ $[\alpha1(XI)\alpha2(XI)\alpha3(XI)]$ mixed molecules of V and XI	120–145	Heterotypic fibrils of type V with type I collagen, type XI with type II collagen, but mixed molecules possible
Network collagens			
IV	$[\alpha1(IV)_2\alpha2(IV)]$ also unknown combinations of $\alpha3(IV)$, $\alpha4(IV)$, $\alpha5(IV)$, $\alpha6(IV)$	150	Basement membrane
VIII	$[\alpha1(VIII)_2\alpha2(VIII)]$	70	Descemets membrane
X	$[\alpha1(X)_3]$	59	Growth plate
Filamentous collagen			
VI	$[\alpha1(VI)\alpha2(VI)\alpha3(VI)]$	$\alpha1/\alpha2 = 140$, $\alpha3 = 200–280$	Skin, cartilage, tendon, blood vessels
Fibril-associated collagens (FACITs)			
IX	$[\alpha1(IX)\alpha2(IX)\alpha3(IX)]$	$\alpha1 = 66$ (short form) or 84 (long form) $\alpha2 = 66$ (non-glycanated) or 66–115 (glycanated) $\alpha3 = 72$	Cartilage, vitreous
XII	$[\alpha1(XII)_3]$	220 (short form) 340 (long form) (long form can be glycanated)	Fetal tendon, skin
XIV	$[\alpha1(XIV)_3]$	220 (can be glycanated)	Fetal tendon, skin
XVI	$[\alpha1(XVI)_3]$	160	Fibroblasts, keratinocytes
XIX	$[\alpha1(XIX)_3]$	115	Rhabdosarcoma
Multiplexins			
XV	$[\alpha1(XV)_3]$	140	Fibroblasts
XVIII	$[\alpha1(XVIII)_3]$	130	Liver, lung
Orphans			
VII	$[\alpha1(VII)_3]$	270	Epithelial basement membrane
XIII	$[\alpha1(XIII)_3]$	60	Many connective tissues
XVII	$[\alpha1(XVII)_3]$	140	Epithelial hemidesmosomes

[a] Modified with permission from Aumailley, M. and Gayraud, B. (1998), table 1, p. 254 © 1998, Springer-Verlag.
[b] Mr, Relative molecular mass.

into fibrils, bundles of fibrils forming fibres, and fibre bundles surrounded by endotenon to form fascicles (Fig. 1.1.3). A similar structure is found in ligament.

The smallest basic structural unit is the collagen fibril, with diameters ranging from 10 to 500 nm depending on the age, location, and species from which the tendon/ligament is sampled (Dyer and Enna 1976). There is not a continuous spectrum of fibril sizes, but usually two or three distinct populations are present within a specific tendon or ligament (Dyer and Enna 1976; Greenlee and Ross 1967; Moore and De Beaux 1987). In the young animal, fibrils are predominantly of small average diameter, whilst in the adult there is a bimodal distribution, with large- and small-diameter fibrils (Moore and De Beaux 1987; Parry *et al.* 1978). In adult

human tendons, for example, there were two distinct populations with average diameters of 60 and 170 nm, respectively (Józsa and Kannus 1997). Since large-diameter fibrils are associated with greater tensile strength (Parry *et al.* 1978), the factors that control the ultimate diameter of developing fibrils are important in both development and injury. An important contribution is thought to be provided by the glycosaminoglycan/proteoglycan content of the tissue, with different molecular species exerting differential effects on the formation of collagen fibres, at least *in vitro* (Flint *et al.* 1984; Merrilees *et al.* 1987; Scott 1990).

Fibre bundles (fascicles) exhibit a planar zigzag or 'crimp', and the stretching out of crimped fibrils is thought to account for the 'toe' region of the tendon/ligament stress-strain curve, as described

Table 1.1.2 Schematic representation of the collagen superfamily[a]

Collagen type	Structure
I, II, III, V, XI	
IV	
VI	
VII	
VIII	
XII	
XV	
XVII	

[a] Each collagen contains at least some triple-helix structure (green) and variable amounts of globular (non-helical) domains (yellow). Some collagens form long rods (types I, II, III, V, and XI) with small globular domains at the ends. Other collagens have interrupted or short triple-helical regions resulting in a variety of different structures. (Modified with permission from Aumailley, M. and Gayraud, B. (1998), Fig. 1.1.1, p. 255 © 1998, Springer-Verlag.)

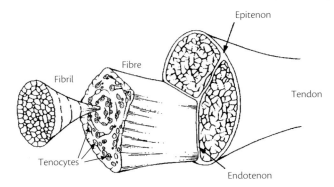

Fig. 1.1.3 Structural hierarchy of tendon and ligament. Collagen fibrils are arranged into fibres, and fibres are surrounded by a thin layer known as the endotenon. Bundles of fibres may form into fascicles, and the whole tendon is enveloped with a thin surface layer known as the epitenon. Fibroblasts (tenocytes) are dispersed throughout the fibre. The endotenon and epitenon contain a variety of different cell types and carry blood vessels, lymphatics, and nerves. The tendon is surrounded by paratenon, which at some sites is further specialized to form a sheath. (Reproduced from Kastelic et al. (1978). Copyright 1978 from *Connective Tissue Research* by Kastelic J, Galeski A, and Baer E. Reproduced by permission of Taylor & Francis, Inc., http://www.routledgeny.com.)

later (see Fig. 1.1.13) and outlined in more detail below (Butler *et al.* 1978). The angle of crimp can vary in different tendons and at different sites and has implications for the mechanical properties of tendon: collagen fibrils with smaller crimp angles will fail at a given strain before those with a larger crimp angle (Wilmink *et al.* 1998).

Bundles of fascicles are bound together and surrounded by the epitenon. The number of fibre bundles in a fascicle and the number of fascicles varies between tendons, and often within the same tendon (Józsa and Kannus 1997). Fibre bundles are predominantly aligned with the long axis of the tendon and responsible for the mechanical strength of the tissue. However, not all fibres run parallel along the course of the tendon. A proportion of fibres run transversely, and there are more complex fibre arrangements including spirals and even a plait-like formation (Józsa and Kannus 1997; Józsa *et al.* 1991). This complex ultrastructure is thought to provide resistance against transverse shear, and rotational force.

Many tendons also exhibit a complex macrostructure, with a spiralling rotation of the fibre bundles in some tendons and a multidirectional orientation with interdigitation of fibres in others. In the Achilles, for example, fibre bundles may spiral up to 90° laterally, with a wide variation between individuals depending on the site of the fusion between the gastrocnemius and soleus fibre bundles (Józsa and Kannus 1997). The concentration of stress where the two tendons join, between 2 and 5 cm from the calcaneus insertion, has been associated with the high frequency of pathology at this site. Further demonstration of the complexity of organization in some tendons is provided by the multilayered organization of the supraspinatus tendon, which was shown to comprise at least five distinct layers, each with a different orientation and organization of fibres (Clark and Harryman 1992). This structure has presumably developed to cope with the complex demands placed upon the supraspinatus in its role as a dynamic stabilizer of the shoulder joint. Pathology may be associated with the unequal distribution of load across the tendon, resulting in separation of adjacent layers within the tendon substance (Uhthoff and Sano 1997).

The size of the fibre bundles is proportional to the macroscopic size of the tendon, with small fascicles generally found in digital tendons and large bundles in big, weight-bearing tendons such as the Achilles (Józsa and Kannus 1997). The fascicular structure provides a fail-safe mechanism, so that failure of one or a few collagen fibre bundles does not compromise the strength of the whole tendon. Tendons are normally immensely strong under tension, able to withstand loads of up to 100 N m^{-2}, thought to be many times the functional requirements under normal conditions of loading (Elliott 1965). However, the physical properties of tendon can be severely compromised by repeated strain, resulting in fatigue failure of the fibres and deterioration in tendon quality (Schechtman and Bader 1997; Ker *et al.* 2000). This is the theoretical basis for tendon 'overuse injury' as discussed in more detail below.

Collagen cross-linking

Once synthesized and secreted into the matrix, collagen molecules associate together and these macromolecular assemblies are stabilized by the formation of stable cross-links (Eyre *et al.* 1984; Bailey *et al.* 1998). Cross-linking of collagen can occur by two different processes (Van der Rest and Garrone 1990): an enzyme-mediated process (Prockop and Kivirikko 1995); a non-enzymic reaction with plasma sugars known as glycation.

Cross-linking increases the stiffness of the collagen fibrils and is important for the mechanical properties of connective tissues. However, the process of glycation has deleterious effects on tissues, a problem particularly in diabetics as a result of elevated blood sugar levels.

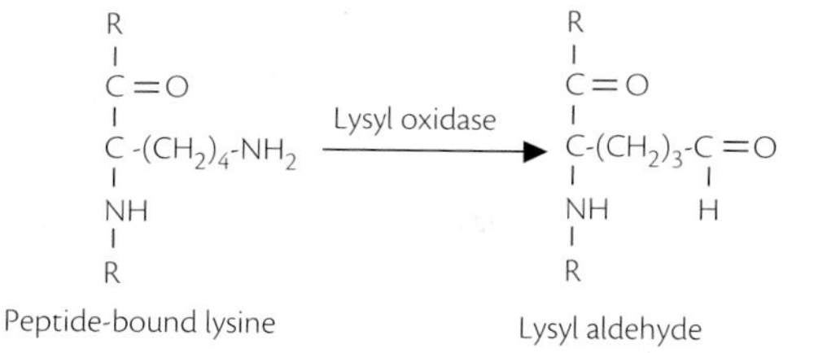

Fig. 1.1.4 Lysyl oxidase activity. The oxidative deamination of specific lysines (and hydroxylysines) is mediated by lysyl oxidase, forming aldehydes. Adjacent aldehydes then form reducible, covalent cross-links. Lysyl oxidase is the only enzyme required for cross-link formation in the matrix.

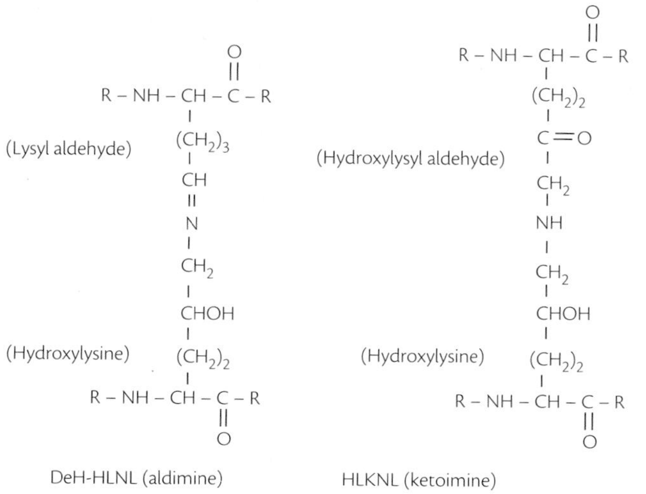

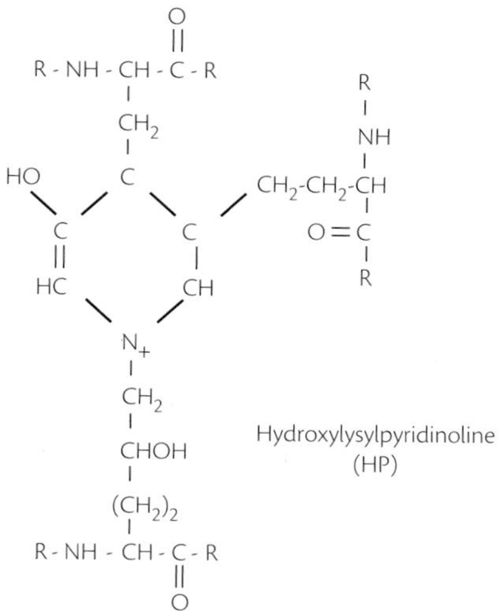

Fig. 1.1.6 Hydroxylysyl-pyridinoline (HP)—a mature collagen cross-link. Further condensation of the immature, di-functional cross-links with a third adjacent hydroxylysine residue results in the formation of mature, tri-functional cross-links such as hydroxylysyl-pyridinoline (HP). HP is the most abundant collagen cross-link in adult tendon and ligament.

Fig. 1.1.5 Immature collagen cross-links. The initial products of cross-linking, such as dehydro-hydroxylysino-norleucine (deH-HLNL) and hydroxylysino-5-ketonorleucine (HLKNL), are between two adjacent amino acids. deH-HLNL, an aldimine, is derived from a lysyl-aldehyde in the non-helical domain of one collagen molecule and a hydroxylysine in the triple helix of an adjacent molecule. HLKNL, a ketoimine, is derived from a hydroxylysyl aldehyde in the non-helical domain of one collagen molecule and a hydroxylysine in the triple helix of an adjacent molecule. Aldimine cross-links, deH-HLNL in particular, are predominant in skin and tendon. They are readily cleaved at acid pH and by hot water, accounting for the high solubility of collagen in immature skin and tendon. Ketoimines are more abundant in bone and cartilage and, since they are stable to heat and acid pH, account for the insolubility of collagen from immature tissues.

Enzyme-mediated cross-linking

Enzyme-mediated cross-linking is initiated in the ECM by the action of lysyl oxidase, generating aldehydes from specific lysine or hydroxylysine residues (see Fig. 1.1.4) (Eyre *et al.* 1984; Bailey *et al.* 1998). Lysyl oxidase is the only enzyme known to be involved in the process and all ensuing reactions are spontaneous. Immature aldimine and ketoimine cross-links form via the condensation of an aldehyde with an adjacent lysine or hydroxylysine residue (Fig. 1.1.5). In fibrillar collagens, aldehydes in the globular 'telopeptides' at each end of the molecule interact with lysines or hydroxylysines within the helical region of adjacent molecules. These di-functional cross-links are reducible, decrease in number with age, and are absent by the time of skeletal maturity. They are gradually replaced by tri-functional cross-links due to further reaction with adjacent aldehydes (Fig. 1.1.6). Although not all of

the mature cross-links have been identified, the best characterized are hydroxylysylpyridinoline (HP, otherwise known as pyridinoline), derived from three hydroxylysine residues, and lysylpyridinoline (LP, otherwise known as deoxypyridinoline), derived from two hydroxylysines and one lysine residue. LP is essentially restricted to bone and present only in small quantities in soft connective tissues.

The amount of HP in a given connective tissue is related to its mechanical function (Bailey *et al.* 1974). The highest concentration is reported in hyaline cartilage and intervertebral disc, with approximately two residues of HP per collagen molecule (Eyre *et al.* 1984). Flexor tendons have a high HP density compared to other type I collagen-containing tissues, although there are substantial variations between different tendons. Short head of biceps brachii tendons contained on average 0.25 residues of HP per collagen molecule compared to 0.8 residues of HP per collagen molecule in the supraspinatus (Bank *et al.* 1999). These differences presumably reflect the different functional demands placed on these tendons, with the supraspinatus experiencing substantial shear and compressive loads as a consequence of its anatomical position in the shoulder joint. A high HP content was also reported in the compressed region of the bovine flexor digitorum profundus, compared to regions of the tendon experiencing purely tensile loads (Vogel and Koob 1989). However since the levels of the HP cross-link do not change significantly with age post-maturity, they do not appear to contribute to the altered physicochemical properties with increasing age, such as the reduction in elasticity and decrease in solubility of the matrix.

Non-enzymic glycation of collagen

The second type of collagen cross-linking occurs by non-enzymic glycation (Sell and Monnier 1989; Reiser *et al.* 1992; Bailey *et al.* 1993). Glycation reactions are a major cause of tissue dysfunction in the elderly due to cross-linking, which stiffens the tissues and alters normal cell-matrix interactions. Reducing sugars (e.g. pentoses) in

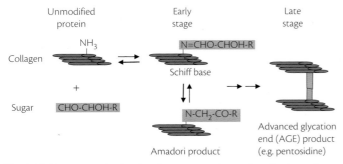

Fig. 1.1.7 Non-enzymatic glycation. Sugars accumulate on long-lived proteins such as collagen in a non-enzymatic and irreversible process known as glycation. Following a process of Amadori rearrangement, adjacent sugars become cross-linked to form various AGE cross-links such as pentosidine.

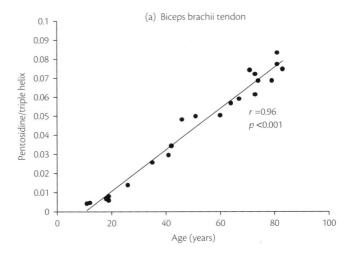

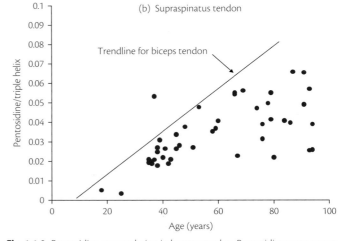

Fig. 1.1.8 Pentosidine accumulation in human tendon. Pentosidine content was measured by reversed-phase high-performance liquid chromatography (HPLC) and expressed relative to the collagen content. (a) Pentosidine accumulated in a linear fashion with age in a sample of biceps brachii tendons, demonstrating minimal collagen turnover over lifetime. (b) In supraspinatus tendons the pentosidine content did not increase in a linear fashion with age, consistent with relatively high levels of collagen turnover, presumably as a consequence of repeated injury and matrix remodelling. (Modified from Bank et al. (1999). Reproduced with permission from the BMJ publishing group.)

the plasma react with matrix proteins resulting in the formation of advanced glycation end products (AGEs) (Fig. 1.1.7).

Over time, these sugars form irreversible cross-links with adjacent molecules as a result of Amadori rearrangement, producing Maillard browning products that alter the physical and chemical characteristics of tissues (Sell and Monnier 1989; Bailey *et al.* 1993). These effects include a decrease in elasticity and a substantial decrease in solubility, even with chemical agents such as cyanogen bromide, making it difficult to assess the biochemical composition of ageing human tendon (Riley *et al.* 1994). Although there are a variety of AGEs, the best characterized is the naturally fluorescent cross-link pentosidine (Sell and Monnier 1989). Since the turnover of collagen in mature connective tissues is generally very low, it has been shown that AGEs such as pentosidine accumulate with age. Therefore pentosidine content serves as a marker of the age of the collagen network. We have found that pentosidine accumulates in a linear fashion with age in the human short head of biceps brachii tendon, consistent with very low levels of collagen turnover in this tissue (Fig. 1.1.8(a)) (Bank *et al.* 1999). However, pentosidine content was not correlated with age in the supraspinatus, consistent with significantly increased matrix (collagen) turnover at this site (Fig. 1.1.8(b)) (Bank *et al.* 1999). This turnover may have a number of implications for tendon pathology as discussed in more detail below.

Proteoglycans

Proteoglycan nomenclature, structure, and function have been extensively reviewed elsewhere (Hardingham and Fosang 1992; Iozzo 1998) and are also covered in Chapters 1.3, 1.4 and 1.5 on meniscus, intervertebral disc and articular cartilage, respectively. Briefly, proteoglycans are an extremely heterogeneous group of molecules, characterized by the presence of at least one chain of glycosaminoglycan (GAG) attached to the protein core (Table 1.1.3). There are five major classes of GAGs, each consisting of repeating disaccharides of hexosamine and a uronic acid, and those that bind to the proteoglycan core protein are sulfated. Their sulfate moiety and high uronic acid content mean that GAGs are highly anionic and therefore hydrophilic, in large part responsible for holding water within the tissues. The non-sulfated GAG hyaluronan forms huge multimolecular aggregates with large proteoglycans such as aggrecan, the major proteoglycan in articular cartilage. It has a core protein size of around 250 kDa, with three globular domains (G1, G2, and G3) and contains many GAG chains (chondroitin sulfate

and keratan sulfate) attached to specific sites throughout its length (Hardingham and Fosang 1992; Hardingham and Fosang 1995). Versican is a large proteoglycan identified in soft connective tissues, with a similar structure to aggrecan although lacking the G2 domain and containing less GAG (Margolis and Margolis 1994).

Small proteoglycans are found in most connective tissues. Decorin has a core protein of 45 kDa and one GAG chain, which may be chondroitin sulfate (in muscle and bone) or dermatan sulfate (in tendon and articular cartilage) (Heinegård *et al.* 1990). It is found attached to collagen fibres at specific sites and is thought to modulate collagen fibril formation (Hedbom and Heinegård 1993). Fibromodulin has a closely related core structure and carries a single keratan sulfate GAG chain. As its name implies, it is thought to influence the development and ultimate diameter of collagen fibres. Biglycan contains two GAG chains, either chondroitin sulfate or dermatan sulfate, and although it is widely

Table 1.1.3 Schematic representation of large and small proteoglycans[a]

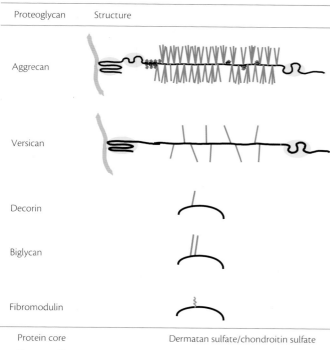

Proteoglycan	Structure
Aggrecan	
Versican	
Decorin	
Biglycan	
Fibromodulin	

Protein core

Keratan sulfate

Globular protein domain

Dermatan sulfate/chondroitin sulfate

[a] Proteoglycans are a heterogeneous group of molecules with a wide range of sizes and functions, although all possess at least one chain of glycosaminoglycan (GAG). The large proteoglycans, aggrecan and versican, are rich in chondroitin sulfate, although only aggrecan has keratan sulfate chains. Decorin carries a single chain of GAG, which is predominantly dermatan sulfate in tendon and ligament. Biglycan has two GAG chains, either chondroitin sulfate or dermatan sulfate. Fibromodulin has a single keratan sulfate chain. (Modified from Hardingham *et al.* 1992.)

distributed its function is unknown. However, like other small proteoglycans, it binds to growth factors such as transforming growth factor β (TGFβ) and may act to sequester cytokines within the ECM and modulate their activity on the resident cell population (Hildebrand *et al.* 1994).

Proteoglycans in tendon and ligament

In the tension-bearing regions of a bovine flexor tendon, proteoglycans comprise between 0.2 and 0.5 per cent of the tendon dry weight. The most abundant is the small proteoglycan decorin carrying dermatan sulfate GAG side chains, in addition to small amounts of biglycan (Vogel and Heinegard 1985). Small proteoglycans represent 88 per cent of the total and the remainder is large proteoglycan, thought to be a processed form of aggrecan rather than versican (Vogel *et al.* 1994).

In weight-bearing and compressed regions of bovine tendons, the proteoglycan content is around 3.5 per cent of the tendon dry weight, with a high content of aggrecan and biglycan (Vogel and Koob 1989; Koob and Vogel 1987). A similar proteoglycan composition has been described in fibrocartilaginous regions of rabbit and dog tendons (Okuda *et al.* 1987; Merrilees and Flint 1980). The accumulation of aggrecan at these sites occurs following weight bearing in the neonate, and the maintenance of synthesis is dependent on

compressive load (Gillard *et al.* 1979). The presence of fibrocartilage at these sites is a protective adaptation, with the aggrecan functioning to hold water within the tissue and resist shear and compression as it does in articular cartilage (Vogel and Koob 1989).

Regional differences in tendon morphology and composition have also been identified in human tendons (Waggett *et al.* 1998; Riley *et al.* 1994; Benjamin *et al.* 1995; Vogel *et al.* 1993). In Achilles tendons, decorin, biglycan, lumican, and fibromodulin have all been identified in both fibrocartilage and tension-bearing regions, at both the mRNA and protein level (Waggett *et al.* 1998). Versican was identified as the major large proteoglycan in the tendon mid-substance, with lesser amounts of aggrecan. In contrast, the fibrocartilage of the Achilles insertion contained mainly aggrecan with lesser amounts of versican. Site-specific variations in proteoglycan content are related to the mechanical history and function of the tendon. Short heads of biceps brachii tendons contain around 0.2 per cent proteoglycan, with the majority carrying dermatan sulfate GAG side chains (80 per cent) and the remainder chondroitin sulfate, consistent with a predominance of decorin in flexor tendons that experience mainly tensile loads (Riley *et al.* 1994). Substantially higher levels of proteoglycan are found in supraspinatus tendons, mainly chondroitin sulfate with lesser amounts of dermatan sulfate and keratan sulfate (Riley *et al.* 1994). These proteoglycans have since been characterized, confirming that aggrecan is the major large proteoglycan in the supraspinatus, in addition to significant amounts of biglycan (Berenson *et al.* 1996). This fibrocartilaginous composition is thought to be a result of adaptive metaplasia to the compressive load experienced by the tendon in the rotator cuff, which wraps around the head of humerus and may experience some impingement from the overlying bone and ligament. Similar fibrocartilaginous regions have also been described in human peroneus, tibialis, and extensor digitorum tendons (Benjamin *et al.* 1995; Vogel *et al.* 1993).

In normal ligaments, 80 per cent of the proteoglycan is decorin, with the remainder biglycan and a large proteoglycan thought to be similar or related to versican (Hey *et al.* 1990; Campbell *et al.* 1996). Ligaments also have fibrocartilaginous regions and the proteoglycan distribution is generally similar to that found in tendon (Vogel *et al.* 1993; Benjamin and Ralphs 1998), although there are differences between ligaments. In the collateral ligaments of the knee, for example, biglycan and decorin are found mainly between the collagen fibre bundles, whereas in cruciate ligaments these proteoglycans are largely cell-associated. Aggrecan is the major large proteoglycan in ligament fibrocartilage where the tissue is subject to compression, and versican is thought to be more characteristic of the fibrous, tensile-load-bearing regions.

Pathological significance of tendon and ligament fibrocartilage

The pathological significance of tendon (and ligament) fibrocartilage at insertions and other sites remains to be established. Fibrocartilage has an altered collagen composition and organization as well as an altered proteoglycan content (Vogel and Koob 1989). The region is generally less vascularized, or even avascular, and therefore may be vulnerable if damaged and less capable of repair. Some studies have suggested that there is indeed a differential repair potential, although whether this is linked to biochemical, cellular, or vascular differences is unclear (Nessler *et al.* 1992).

A lower elastic modulus was measured in the fibrocartilaginous region of the dog flexor digitorum profundus compared to the tensional region (Amadio *et al.* 1992). Pathology is frequently located in the fibrocartilaginous regions of tendons such as the supraspinatus, tibialis anterior, and tibialis posterior. There may be a causal relationship between the relative avascularity and the development of fibrocartilage. However, other common sites of tendon pathology, such as the Achilles tendon mid-substance, that are thought to be relatively avascular (although this is questioned by some studies) are not fibrocartilaginous. Consequently, the development of fibrocartilage does not necessarily represent a pathological process, although fibrocartilaginous change may represent a precursor of tendon pathology induced by excessive compression or shear forces.

Non-collagen components of tendon and ligament

The other non-collagen components of the tendon/ligament ECM have not been extensively investigated. In biochemical studies we found that around that 20–25 per cent of the tendon dry mass was not accounted for by the collagen and proteoglycan component (Fig. 1.1.1) (Riley *et al.* 1994; Riley *et al.* 1994). Apart from the cellular content, which is only 1–3 per cent of the dry weight (Józsa and Kannus 1997), the remaining mass consists of lipids, inorganic components, and non-collagen proteins such as elastin and various glycoproteins.

Elastin

Only a small proportion of the tendon ECM is elastin, with estimates in the literature of approximately 2 per cent of the tendon dry weight (Elliott 1965). Elastin is a very stable and extremely insoluble protein composed mainly of hydrophobic amino acids, with a high proportion of glycine and proline (Uitto 1979). Unlike collagen, it contains little hydroxyproline and no hydroxylysine and is rich in two unusual amino acids, desmosine and isodesmosine, that form covalent cross-links between the polypeptide chains (Eyre *et al.* 1984; Uitto 1979). Elastin is a major component of elastic fibres, which consist of a central core and microfilaments that are found distributed throughout the ECM. Elastic fibres are found in young and old tendons, at the insertion as well as the mid-substance, and may be increased in some pathological conditions such as Ehlers-Danlos syndrome and chronic uraemia (Józsa and Kannus 1997; Cooper and Misol 1970). The function of elastic fibres in tendon is unclear, but they may contribute to the recovery of the crimp in the collagen fibres after tendon is stretched (Butler *et al.* 1978).

Fibronectin

Fibronectin is a high molecular weight extracellular protein important in mediating interactions between the cell and the surrounding matrix (Labat-Rober *et al.* 1990). It is a multidomain protein, with specific domains involved in interactions with cells and molecules such as fibrin, actin, hyaluronan, collagen, heparin, and coagulation factors. It has a range of functions including cell adhesion, cell migration, control of differentiation, haemostasis, phagocytosis, and chemotaxis. Fibronectin has been detected in the matrix of tendons and ligaments, although there are site-specific variations, with a higher concentration in intrasynovial anterior cruciate ligaments (ACL) compared to extrasynovial medial collateral ligaments (MCL) and patellar tendon (Józsa *et al.* 1989; Amiel *et al.* 1989). It is not greatly abundant in normal tissues, comprising just 0.2 per cent of the ACL dry weight and less than 0.1 per cent of that of the patellar tendon (Józsa *et al.* 1989; Amiel *et al.* 1989). Fibronectin was primarily associated with synovial-like cells in the epitenon, which produce fibronectin in culture unlike cells from the centre of the tendon (Banes *et al.* 1988). However, in human Achilles tendons fibronectin was not detected in the normal tendon mid-substance or paratenon, but was restricted to the vascular walls and myotendinous junction (Józsa *et al.* 1989; Lehto *et al.* 1990). After tendon rupture, fibronectin was massively increased and found associated with tenocytes and collagen fibres in the vicinity of the rupture, in addition to cells in macroscopically normal regions of the tendon (Lehto *et al.* 1990). It is not known whether the increase in fibronectin expression precedes tendon rupture, although it is an important part of the early tendon response to injury, implicated in fibroblast adhesion, migration, and differentiation at the wound site (Banes *et al.* 1984; Gelberman *et al.* 1991).

Tenascin-C

Tenascin-C is a disulfide-linked hexameric protein with subunits of between 200 and 300 kDa in the human, created by alternative splicing of a signal gene transcript (Chiquet and Fambrough 1984; Gulcher *et al.* 1991). Tenascin-C was identified as a component of developing chick tendon, where it was particularly associated with the myotendinous junction, and consequently first described as myotendinous antigen (Chiquet and Fambrough 1984). Its distribution in mature tendon suggests at least two functional roles. In normal fibrous tendon, tenascin is associated with the collagen fibres, consistent with a role in collagen fibril organization, perhaps maintaining the interface between fibrils and adjacent structures (Riley *et al.* 1996). The greatest concentration is at the myotendinous junction and bone insertion, suggesting a role in the transmission of tensile loads (Kannus *et al.* 1998). In fibrocartilaginous regions of tendon, tenascin-C was found to be predominantly cell-associated, and its expression may be implicated in the development of fibrocartilage and the altered cell activity in response to compressive load (Riley *et al.* 1996; Mehr *et al.* 2000). An increase in tenascin-C expression was also associated with tendon and soft connective tissue injuries, where it has a restricted pattern of expression and a major role in the control of cell activities (Mackie *et al.* 1988; Whitby and Ferguson 1991). Tenascin is a poor adhesive substratum for cells, and its effects on cell behaviour may be mediated by effects on cell shape, such as cell rounding and the development of a chondrocytic phenotype (Mackie 1994). It is also strongly associated with connective tissue remodelling in development and disease, with increased expression in osteoarthritic cartilage (Chevalier *et al.* 1994). We have shown that the there is an increase in tenascin-C expression in degenerate tendon pathology, with a change from predominantly the 200 kDa isoform to a mixed expression of 200 and 300 kDa isoforms (Riley *et al.* 1996). Biochemical studies also showed evidence of enzymic degradation of tenascin-C in degenerate tendons, with the presence of multiple degradation products consistent with matrix metalloproteinase enzyme activity (Riley *et al.* 1996; Siri *et al.* 1995). It is not known whether changes in tenascin-C expression and structure occur before or after tendon rupture, although it is interesting to note that tenascin may have a direct stimulatory effect on matrix metalloproteinase (MMP) enzyme expression (Tremble *et al.* 1994).

Cartilage oligomeric matrix protein (COMP)

Despite its name COMP is not restricted to cartilage, but is found in other connective tissues and is a major component of tendon and ligament, representing up to 3 per cent of the tendon dry weight (DiCesare *et al.* 1994; Smith, *et al.* 1997). A member of the thrombospondin gene family, it is now also referred to as thrombospondin 5 (Oldberg *et al.* 1992). COMP is a large (524 kDa) oligomer, composed of five subunits connected by disulfide bonds (Oldberg *et al.* 1992). Its function is unclear, although its association with collagen fibre bundles suggests both a structural role and an interactive role with the cell population. There is a strong relationship with the loading pattern of tissues, with increased levels of COMP in flexor tendons compared to extensor tendons and ligaments, and it may function to signal cellular responses to mechanical load (Smith, *et al.* 1997). The structural importance of COMP is demonstrated by the discovery that a mutation in the COMP gene is responsible for pseudoachondroplasia, a rare genetic disorder characterized by short stature, lax joints, and early-onset osteoarthritis (Briggs *et al.* 1995). COMP levels increase as a function of age up to skeletal maturity in a variety of tissues, although only in weight-bearing tendons (Smith, *et al.* 1997). It also increases after injury as part of the healing response, possibly driven by mechanical forces across the granulation tissue. After skeletal maturity, levels of COMP in equine tendon decline, possibly by a combination of increased enzymic degradation and a decrease in the synthetic activity of mature tenocytes (Smith, *et al.* 1997). Thus it has been suggested that, in adult animals, strenuous exercise has deleterious effects on the biochemical composition of the tendon matrix, and that there is a window of opportunity for adaptive responses to exercise only in the immature animal (Smith *et al.* 1999). Fragments of COMP released into the synovial fluid and bloodstream may be useful indicators of tendon injury, assuming that COMP fragments derived from tendon can be differentiated from those derived from cartilage and other tissues (Smith *et al.* 1999).

Other matrix glycoproteins

Apart from serum proteins such as albumin, other glycoproteins in tendon/ligament include laminin, which is found as a major constituent of the blood vessel basement membranes, and link protein, which stabilizes large proteoglycan-hyaluronan interactions (Józsa and Kannus 1997; Hardingham and Fosang 1992; Oldberg *et al.* 1991). Other multidomain adhesive glycoproteins include members of the thrombospondin family, which like COMP, tenascin, and fibronectin mediate cell-matrix interactions in normal tissues as well as in repair and pathology (Sage and Bornstein 1991; Bornstein 1992; Miller and McDevitt 1991). Amongst other as yet unidentified proteins there are soluble proteins of 52, 54, and 55 kDa, respectively, that vary in distribution throughout the length of a tendon (Jones and Bee 1990).

Lipids

Cholesterol esters, thought to be derived from circulating plasma low-density lipoprotein, accumulate in tendons and fascia with increasing age (Adams and Bayliss 1973). There are also variable amounts of triglyceride, which are generally found between the collagen fibre bundles. Most lipid deposits are closely associated with GAGs, which act to entrap low-density lipoprotein similar to atherosclerotic plaques in arteries (Adams and Bayliss 1973). The GAG-rich tendon fibrocartilage is reported to contain more lipid deposits than normal tensile regions of tendon, and this may help the tissue withstand compression (Vogel and Koob 1989). The precise contribution of lipids to tendon pathology is unknown, although increased lipid deposits are found relatively frequently in ruptured and degenerate tendons where they have been described as 'tendolipomatosis' (Józsa *et al.* 1984; Jarvinen *et al.* 1997).

Amyloid

Amyloid deposits are derived from normally soluble proteins, which can form insoluble aggregates in a number of connective tissues including cartilage, fibrocartilage, meniscus, and joint capsule. Deposition of amyloid is age-related and in osteoarthritic cartilage is associated with degenerative changes in the matrix attributable to the change in GAG composition (Athanasou *et al.* 1995). Amyloid deposits were frequently found in ruptured supraspinatus tendons, localized to degenerate areas of the tendon where there was a high concentration of GAG (Cole *et al.* 2001). Once deposited, amyloid is insoluble and resistant to proteolytic degradation, and may contribute to the structural and functional failure of the tissue. However, the incidence of amyloid deposition in normal tendon is not known; consequently the pathological significance is uncertain.

Inorganic components

A variety of inorganic constituents have been identified in tendon, with sodium, potassium, calcium, phosphorus, and magnesium most abundant among the different elements represented (Ellis *et al.* 1969). Most are primarily associated with soluble proteins, although the most abundant element, calcium, is also present as insoluble mineral deposits in tendon (Ellis *et al.* 1969; Riley *et al.* 1996). The concentration of calcium was found to be similar in different tendons, accounting for around 0.1 per cent of the tendon dry weight in human supraspinatus and biceps brachii tendons (Riley *et al.* 1996). There was a small but significant increase in calcium with age, and this was accompanied by an increase in phosphorus content, consistent with the accumulation of mineral deposits in ageing organelles and necrotic cell debris. Although the age-related increase in calcium is unlikely on its own to have any significance for tendon pathology, a substantial increase in calcium salt deposition is a common pathological feature in some tendons, particular at insertion sites and especially in the supraspinatus (Urist *et al.* 1964; Józsa *et al.* 1980; Uhthoff and Loehr 1997). The increased deposition of calcific deposits in tendon pathology may be either degenerative ('dystrophic calcification') or a self-limiting and resolving condition ('calcific tendinitis') (Uhthoff 1975). This is discussed in more detail below.

Cell activity and matrix metabolism of tendon and ligament

Embryonic and neonatal tendon is a relatively cellular tissue, and there is a rapid fall in cell density during development and a gradual decrease in cellularity with increasing age post-maturity (Greenlee and Ross 1967; Squier and Magnes 1983). Although adult tendons and ligaments were once considered metabolically inactive structures (Neuberger *et al.* 1951; Peacock 1957), tenocytes do have a significant aerobic capacity, but substantially less than that of liver and skeletal muscle (Vailas *et al.* 1978).

Tendon and ligament cells contain enzymes for all three pathways of energy generation: aerobic; anaerobic; and pentose phosphate shunt pathways (Tipton *et al.* 1975; Birch et al. 1997). The metabolic activity changes with age, with a decline in aerobic and pentose phosphate shunt activity, and predominantly anaerobic metabolism at skeletal maturity (Floridi *et al.* 1981). Glycolytic activity is present even in old tendons, with similar levels of activity in young and old tendons (Floridi *et al.* 1981). Hypoxia has been suggested as a possible cause of tendon degeneration, although tendon cells are more resistant to hypoxia than other cell types (Birch et al. 1997; Webster and Burry 1982). Differences in lactate dehydrogenase activity, an indicator of anaerobic glycolysis, have been detected in tendons from different sites, although there was no apparent correlation with age, tendon size, and strength (Józsa and Kannus 1997; Vandor *et al.* 1982). Tendons normally have a relatively good vascular supply (see Chapter 1.2), although the diffusion of nutrients may be an important factor in tendon segments where the blood supply is limited or restricted (Lundborg and Rank 1978). Restriction of the tendon blood supply by compression, arterial occlusion, or in the face of high demand from the actively contracting muscle may be a significant factor in tendon pathology (MacNab 1973).

The ECM is synthesized and maintained by the activity of the resident fibroblasts (Greenlee and Ross 1967). In general, synthetic activity is high during development and diminishes with age, although activity may change dramatically in some pathological conditions. Normal tissue homeostasis requires a balance between the processes of synthesis and breakdown (Perez-Tamayo 1982; Stetler-Stevenson 1996). This balance can be modified in response to nutritional and hormonal stimuli as well as trauma and mechanical stress. Our own studies have shown that the collagen in some adult tendons, such as short head of biceps brachii, turns over very slowly if at all, as shown by the accumulation of pentosidine and the racemization of D-aspartate (Bank *et al.* 1999; Riley *et al.* 2002). In tendons exposed to high mechanical demands, however, such as the supraspinatus and Achilles, the rate of collagen turnover is much higher, consistent with either a history of repair or a constant maintenance function. This activity is mediated by a variety of enzymes including MMPs, as described in more detail below.

Cell populations

There are a number of different cell populations within tendon, with regional variations in cell morphology and activity (Banes *et al.* 1988; Riederer-Henderson *et al.* 1983; Gelberman *et al.* 1988). Synovial-like cells from the endotenon and epitenon have a greater proliferative potential than the cells of the tendon mid-substance, which are predominantly synthesizing matrix (Gelberman *et al.* 1991; Gelberman *et al.* 1988; Banes, *et al.* 1988). Similar cell populations are present in the epiligament. Cells from the epitenon (and perhaps also the endotenon) are more active in repair after injury, migrating to the site of the lesion and being responsible for the synthesis of new matrix (Gelberman *et al.* 1988; Garner *et al.* 1989). Since most tendon cells are terminally differentiated and relatively quiescent, repair activity has been ascribed to a resident subpopulation of mesenchymal 'stem' cells resident in the epitenon. Alternatively, cells from the surrounding tissues or derived from a circulating population of 'fibrocytes' may be involved in tendon/ligament repair (Chesney and Bucala 1997). The relative contribution of intrinsic and extrinsic cell populations may depend on the nature, site, and extent of the initial injury.

Epitenon-derived cells have a different matrix synthetic activity, producing fibronectin and type III collagen in culture, unlike the internal fibroblasts (Banes *et al.* 1988). However, studies comparing human tendon fibroblasts from internal and superficial regions have shown no difference in their proliferative response to serum, and no difference in their ability to respond to growth factors and synthesize matrix (Chard *et al.* (1987) and Riley, G.P., unpublished observations). Rounded, chondrocyte-like cells are a feature of the fibrocartilage at the insertion sites and in regions subject to compression (Vogel and Koob 1989; Cooper and Misol 1970). These cells have a very different pattern of matrix synthesis compared to that of tension-bearing regions of tendon, with higher levels of gene expression for matrix components such as type II collagen and aggrecan. These cells are responsive to the application of compressive load, and require continued dynamic compression for the maintenance of this synthetic activity *in vitro* (Koob *et al.* 1992). The cell populations at the myotendinous junction have not been characterized.

A number of studies have shown that tendon and ligament cells, either in explant culture or isolated cell populations, respond to exogenous agents and factors such as the application of mechanical strain (Spindler *et al.* 1995; Banes *et al.* 1995; Schmidt *et al.* 1995; Rees *et al.* 2000). These studies are useful for understanding basic cellular mechanisms, but may not have physiological or pathological relevance. Cellular activities in standard culture conditions do not remotely resemble the situation *in vivo* where cells are surrounded by matrix and other chemical and physical interactions that modify the cell response. Chapter 1.2, for example, described how tenocytes within the fibres of a normal tendon communicate via gap junctions and how these mediate the tendon response to mechanical load (McNeilly *et al.* 1996). Although some studies have shown differences in collagen expression between culture-derived cell populations from normal and diseased tendon (Maffulli *et al.* 2000), other studies have shown no significant difference (Riley, G.P., unpublished observations). Research into the cell biology of tendon and ligament is complicated by the absence of any cell-specific markers that can be used to discriminate between different fibroblast populations.

Matrix degradation

The remodelling of the matrix in tendon and ligament is important for maintaining the health of the tissue. Although some matrix turnover is probably taking place in normal adult flexor tendons, the process is extremely slow, as shown by studies of pentosidine content and D-aspartate accumulation in the biceps brachii tendon (Bank *et al.* 1999; Riley *et al.* 2002). Turnover is higher in tendons such as the supraspinatus and Achilles, and this is probably associated with the high levels of strain normally experienced by these tendons in every day use (Bank *et al.* 1999; Riley *et al.* 2002). Increased turnover is also found in compressed regions of tendon and ligament, presumably part of the adaptation process to protect the tissue from damage (Perez-Castro and Vogel 1999). After tissue injury, repair involves the limited destruction of matrix to weave new collagen into the existing structure. Scar tissue is also extensively remodelled during the maturation phase of wound healing. Inappropriate or excessive matrix degradation is

Table 1.1.4 The MMP superfamily—diversity in size and substrate specificity

MMP number	Enzyme name	Molecular weight (kDa)		Known substrates
		Latent	Active	
MMP-1	Collagenase-1	55	45	Collagens I, II, III, VII, VIII, X; gelatin; aggrecan; versican; link protein; casein; alpha-1 proteinase inhibitor; alpha2 macroglobulin (α2M); pregnancy zone protein; ovostatin; nidogen; myelin basic protein (MBP); pro-TNF; L-selectin; MMP-2; MMP-9
MMP-2	72 kDa gelatinase	72	66	Collagens I, IV, V, VII, X, XI, XIV; gelatin; elastin; fibronectin; aggrecan; versican, link protein; MBP; alpha-1 proteinase inhibitor; pro-TNF; MMP-9; MMP-13
MMP-3	Stromelysin-1	57	45	Collagens III, IV, IX, X; gelatin; aggrecan; versican, perlecan; link protein; nidogen; fibronectin; laminin; elastin; casein; fibrinogen; antithrombin-III; α2M; ovostatin; alpha-1 proteinase inhibitor; MBP; pro-TNF; MMP-1; MMP-7; MMP-8; MMP-9; MMP-13
MMP-7	Matrilysin (PUMP-1)	28	19	Collagens IV, X; gelatin; aggrecan; link protein; fibronectin; laminin; entactin; elastin; casein; transferrin; alpha-1 proteinase inhibitor; MBP; pro-TNF; MMP-1; MMP-2; MMP-9
MMP-8	Neutrophil collagenase	75	58	Collagens I, II, III, V, VII, VIII, X; gelatin; aggrecan; alpha-1 proteinase inhibitor; alpha-2 antiplasmin; fibronectin
MMP-9	92 kDa gelatinase	92	86	Collagens IV, V, VII, X, XIV; gelatin; elastin; aggrecan; versican; link protein; fibronectin; nidogen; alpha-1 proteinase inhibitor; MBP; pro-TNF
MMP-10	Stromelysin-2	57	44	Collagens III, IV, V; gelatin; casein; aggrecan; elastin; link protein; fibronectin; MMP-1; MMP-8
MMP-11	Stromelysin-3	51	44	alpha-1 proteinase inhibitor
MMP-12	Macrophage metalloelastase	54	45	Collagen IV; gelatin; elastin; alpha-1 proteinase inhibitor; fibronectin; vitronectin; laminin; pro-TNF; MBP
MMP-13	Collagenase-3	60	48	Collagens I, II, III, IV; gelatin; plasminogen activator inhibitor 2; aggrecan; perlecan; tenascin
MMP-14	MT1-MMP	66	56	Collagens I, II, III; gelatin; casein; elastin; fibronectin; laminin B chain; vitronectin; aggrecan; dermatan sulphate proteoglycan; pro-TNF; MMP-2; MMP-13
MMP-15	MT2-MMP	72	60	MMP-2; gelatin; fibronectin; tenascin; nidogen; laminin
MMP-16	MT3-MMP	64	52	MMP-2
MMP-17	MT4-MMP	57	53	
MMP-18	*Xenopus* collagenase	55	22	
MMP-19		54	45	Aggrecan
MMP-20	Enamelysin	54	22	Amelogenin
MMP-21	XMMP	70	53	
MMP-22	CMMP	52	43	Gelatin; casein
MMP-23		?	?	
MMP-24	MT5-MMP	63	45	MMP-2

a likely cause of matrix weakening in degenerative diseases. A failure of the remodelling process, such as in the injured ACL, may also account for the poor quality of repair at this site (Spindler *et al.* 1996).

Collagen degradation

The collagen (type I) fibres of tendon and ligament are highly resistant to degradation by most proteases. Some collagen is probably degraded by a phagocytic route, with fibroblasts and macrophages engulfing collagen molecules, which are then digested by lysosomal enzymes (Everts *et al.* 1996; Creemers *et al.* 1998). This is a major activity in the remodelling peridontal ligament, although few studies have investigated the relative importance of this route in tendon and ligament.

Several studies have shown release of collagen-degrading enzymes by tendon tissues in explant culture (Harper *et al.* 1988;

Piening and Riederer-Henderson 1989; Dalton *et al.* 1995). We have shown that collagenase-1, a member of the MMP superfamily, is the main mediator of collagen degradation in tendon explant culture, since levels of collagenase-1 (MMP-1) activity are closely associated with the release of collagen degradation products (Cawston *et al.* 1998). MMP-1 is one of the few enzymes capable of cleaving the intact type I collagen molecule, doing so at a specific locus in the triple helix, leaving three- and one-quarter length fragments that are in turn susceptible to other proteinases (Cawston 1995; Cawston 1995; Matrisian 1990; Matrisian 1992).

The MMPs are a family of related enzymes that are major mediators of connective tissue turnover in the extracellular environment. MMPs are active at neutral pH, contain a catalytic zinc ion, and require calcium for activity. There are at least 23 MMPs, which can be subdivided into collagenases, gelatinases, stromelysins, and membrane-type MMPs, based on their structures and substrate specificities (Table 1.1.4) (Cawston 1995; Matrisian 1992;

Table 1.1.5 Schematic representation of the domain structure of the MMP superfamily[a]

MMP type	Structure
Collagenase (MMP-1, MMP-8, MMP-13)	
Gelatinase (MMP-2, MMP-9)	
Stromelysin (MMP-3, MMP-10, MMP-11)	
Membrane-type (MMP-14, MMP-15, MMP-16, MMP-17, MMP-24)	
Matrilysin (PUMP) (MMP-7)	

= Signal peptide   = Pro-peptide   = Catalytic domain

= Gelatin-binding domain   = Zinc-binding domain   = Hinge region

= Hemopexin domain   = Transmembrane domain

[a] MMPs share common domains: a signal peptide that is cleaved prior to synthesis; a pro-peptide that renders the enzyme inactive until removed by proteolysis; a catalytic domain with zinc-binding site. The hemopexin domain confers substrate specificity. Gelatinases have an additional, gelatin-binding domain. Membrane-type MMPs have an additional transmembrane domain. Matrilysin (MMP-7) lacks the hemopexin domain. (Reproduced from *Extracellular matrix proteases and proteins technical guide*, Vol. 2, January 2002, with permission of Calbiochem.)

Nagase 1994). MMPs have a common domain structure, and most are secreted in an inactive form with a propeptide that is removed upon activation (Table 1.1.5).

The activity of MMPs is tightly controlled *in vivo*, with the regulation of transcription, translation, activation, and inhibition by specific inhibitors known as tissue inhibitors of metalloproteinases (TIMPs) (Cawston 1995; Murphy, *et al.* 1994; Murphy and Willenbrock 1995). There are four TIMPs that have been characterized, and these may be constitutively expressed (TIMP-2) or stimulated by growth factors such as TGFβ (TIMP-1, TIMP-3). Each TIMP will bind to active MMPs in a stoichiometric ratio (1:1), resulting in an inactive complex. In general, expression and activity of the MMPs is stimulated by pro-inflammatory cytokines such as interleukin-1 (IL-1) and tumour necrosis factor (TNF) and inhibited by growth factors such as TGFβ.

In normal flexor tendons such as the biceps brachii, the activity of MMPs is low, consistent with the low rate of collagen turnover in these tendons (Riley *et al.* 2002). MMP activity, particularly that of MMP-1, MMP-2, and MMP-3, is higher in normal supraspinatus tendons (Fig. 1.1.9). Similarly, high levels of MMP-3 are found in normal Achilles, suggesting an important role for MMPs in the maintenance of the tendon structure in tendons exposed to high levels of strain or repeated injury (Riley *et al.* 2002). Further evidence for the importance of MMPs in tendon physiology comes from the observation that a broad-spectrum matrix metalloproteinase inhibitor can induce painful tendon lesions (Millar *et al.* 1998). The cause of the tendon pain is still unknown, and may be related to inhibition of one or more MMPs, although related metalloproteinase enzymes such as the ADAMs (A disintegrin and metalloprotease) may also be implicated.

There are at least 40 ADAMs, the majority of which function as zinc binding proteases, although the natural substrates and inhibitors are known for relatively few, such as tumour necrosis factor (TNF) for ADAM17 (otherwise known as TNF-alpha converting enzyme or TACE) (Schlondorff and Blobel 1999). Their diverse range of activities, from cytokine processing to the control of matrix assembly, has made members of this group of enzymes an attractive target for therapeutic intervention in various pathologies. Inhibition of one or more of these proteases could account for the onset of tendon pain induced by inhibitors of metalloproteinases. The potential role of enzymes in chronic tendinopathy is discussed in more detail below.

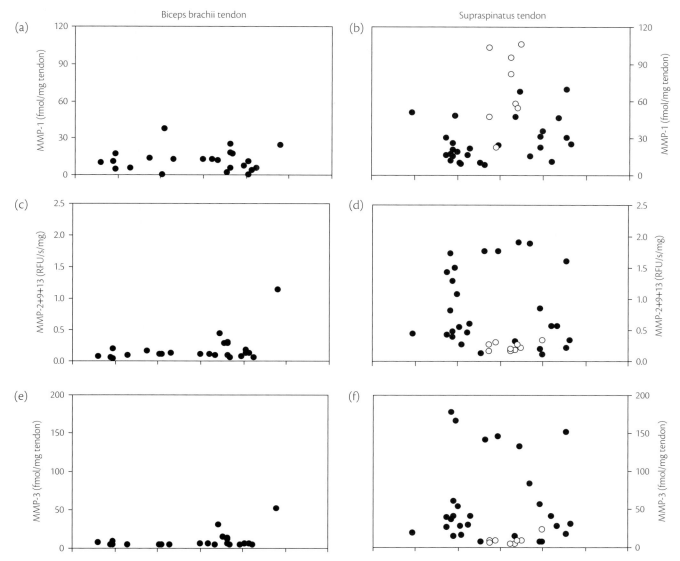

Fig. 1.1.9 MMP enzyme activities in tendon. MMPs were extracted from tendon and activities were measured using specific fluorogenic substrates. MMP-1 and MMP-3 activities were expressed as fentamoles per milligram tendon dry weight (fmol/mg tendon). Gelatinase activities (MMP-2, MMP-9, and MMP-13) were expressed as relative fluorescent units per second per milligram tendon dry weight (RFU/s/mg). Data for biceps brachii tendons are shown in (a), (c), and (e). Data for supraspinatus tendons are shown in (b), (d) and (f). Closed circles represent macroscopically normal 'control' tendons and open circles represent ruptured tendons. MMP-1, gelatinase (mostly MMP-2), and MMP-3 activities were significantly higher in control supraspinatus compared to biceps brachii tendons ($p < 0.01$ for each activity). Ruptured supraspinatus tendons had significantly higher levels of MMP-1 activity, but lower levels of gelatinase (mostly MMP-2) and MMP-3 compared to controls. (Data modified and reprinted from Riley *et al,*. (2002). © 2002 with permission from Elsevier Science.)

Proteoglycan degradation

Proteoglycans are turned over much more rapidly than the fibrillar collagens. Although some members of the MMP family such as MMP-3 (stromelysin) can degrade proteoglycans such as aggrecan, most activity *in vivo* is associated with a related but distinct group of enzymes known as 'aggrecanases' (Fig. 1.1.10).

Aggrecanases, of which there are at least three members, were recently identified as members of the ADAM-TS family, a subgroup of ADAMs with thrombospondin (TS) type I motifs (Kaushal and Shah 2000). ADAM-TS4 (aggrecanase 1) and ADAM-TS5 (aggrecanase 2) both cleave aggrecan at a specific locus, between residues Glu[373] and Ala[374] in the interglobular domain of the

core protein (Kaushal and Shah 2000; Tortorella *et al.* 1999; Abbaszade *et al.* 1999). ADAM-TS1 can also degrade aggrecan at the same locus, at least *in vitro* (Kuno *et al.* 2000). ADAM-TS4 also has activity against the brain-specific proteoglycan brevican (Nakamura *et al.* 2000). Little is known about the enzymes responsible for the degradation of other matrix proteoglycans.

Recent studies have demonstrated rapid catabolism and loss of proteoglycans from tendon and ligament explants maintained in culture (Rees *et al.* 2000; Campbell *et al.* 1996). Antibodies to aggrecan, biglycan, and decorin showed that catabolites of these proteoglycans were present in both young and mature tendon, consistent with constitutively high levels of proteoglycan turnover (Rees *et al.* 2000). Aggrecanase-generated fragments of aggrecan were found in

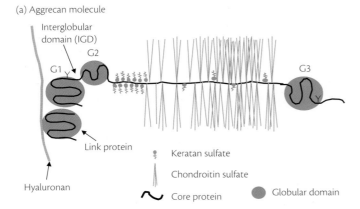

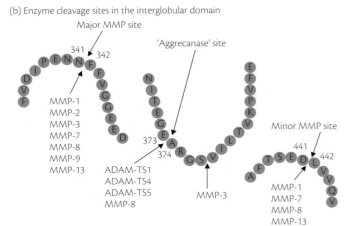

Fig. 1.1.10 Enzyme cleavage sites in aggrecan. (a) Aggrecan consists of three globular domains (G1 to G3) separated by linear core protein. The region between G2 and G3 is rich in sulfated glycosaminoglycans, which attract and hold water in the tissue. Aggrecan binds to hyaluronan via the G1 domain, stabilized by link protein, to form multimolecular aggregates. The interglobular domain (IGD) contains sequences susceptible to cleavage by several enzymes, (b) Although several MMPs can cleave aggrecan at multiple sites in the IGD, the predominant cleavage *in vivo* is made by aggrecanases, between specific glutamate and alanine residues (Glu[373] and Ala[374]). (Reproduced from Cawston, T.E. (1998), © 1998 with permission from Elsevier Science.)

both tensional and compressed regions, and the release of these fragments into the culture media was found both in control cultures and in cultures stimulated by IL-1 (Rees *et al.* 2000). There was no evidence of MMP-mediated proteoglycan turnover, although aggrecan turnover did not correlate with the expression of mRNA for either ADAM-TS1 or ADAM-TS2, at least in the compressed region of young tendon. Further work is required to determine which aggrecanases (and other proteoglycanases) are involved in tendon and ligament physiology and pathology.

Age-related changes of tendon and ligament matrix

Increasing age is associated with a number of significant changes in cell metabolism and in the structure, composition, and mechanical properties of the ECM. During development the cellularity decreases, collagen content increases, and there are changes in collagen fibre diameters and collagen cross-linking as described above. After maturity, there are additional changes including decreased solubility of the collagen and decreased GAG content (Riley *et al.*

1994; Riley *et al.* 1994; Ippolito *et al.* 1975; Ippolito *et al.* 1980). The total collagen content in human tendon remains constant over a wide age range, from 12 to 96 years (Riley *et al.* 1994). With ageing, however, collagen becomes stiffer, fibres shrink, and the tensile strength decreases (O'Brien 1992). The tensile modulus (stiffness) of canine tendons, calculated from the slope of the stress–strain curve, is not directly related to age, although it is positively correlated with the insoluble (cross-linked) collagen content (Haut *et al.* 1992). The increase in tensile modulus with age in equine superficial digital flexor tendon (SDFT) was positively correlated with an increase in HP cross-link content and negatively correlated with the cross-sectional area of the central tendon fascicles, which decreased with age (Gillis *et al.* 1997). There was a corresponding increase in the number of fascicles with increasing age. There are changes in the average diameter of the collagen fibres, which in the equine SDFT increased to a peak of 170 nm at the age of 1.5 years and then declined gradually (Patterson-Kane *et al.* 1997). The angle of crimp and crimp length declined with age but reached a plateau in the mature animal. Mechanical properties such as hysteresis, the energy lost during stress-relaxation, decline considerably during maturation as a result of cross-link formation but change little as a result of ageing, at least in rat tail tendon (Vogel 1983).

Age is strongly associated with the development of chronic tendon pathology, which tends to predominantly affect individuals in late middle-age. This is often thought to be associated with a lower cell activity and a reduction in tendon blood flow, implying a failure to repair or maintain the matrix. However, far from being senescent, tenocytes isolated from ageing individuals show proliferative potential similar to that of young tenocytes (Chard *et al.* 1987). It is therefore important to distinguish the effects of ageing from pathological degenerative changes, such as lipid deposits, calcification, and mucoid degeneration, that may accumulate as a function of age (Chard *et al.* 1989; Riley *et al.* 2001). Although these are more frequently found in older tendons, they are not found in all tendons and are therefore likely to be an indirect consequence of ageing (Riley *et al.* 2001). More work needs to be done to clarify the role of age in the tendon/ligament cell response to mechanical strain and injury.

Effect of exercise and immobilization on tendon and ligament

Tendons and ligaments are known to be capable of responding to changes in mechanical stresses and loading, although there are differences between tendons and more dramatic effects are seen in immature animals (Gillard *et al.* 1979; Birch et al. 1997; Woo *et al.* 1981; Woo *et al.* 1982). Atrophy induced by immobilization is relatively slow compared to that in muscle, although there is a significant loss of water, GAGs, collagen, and tensile strength after a period of 8–9 weeks (Fig. 1.1.11) (Vailas *et al.* 1978; Woo *et al.* 1982; Akeson *et al.* 1967; Vailas *et al.* 1985). The reduction in strength was attributed to increased collagen degradation, although apparently not mediated by collagenase, which decreased in immobilized ligaments and tendons (Harper *et al.* 1992). Collagen synthesis is also decreased and there is a reduction in both aerobic and anaerobic metabolism. Matrix properties return towards normal after the period of immobilization is ended, although there are site-specific variations, with a slower rate of recovery at the insertion compared to the tendon/ligament mid-substance (Woo *et al.* 1987). Rehabilitation of immobilized tendons and ligaments takes much more time than that

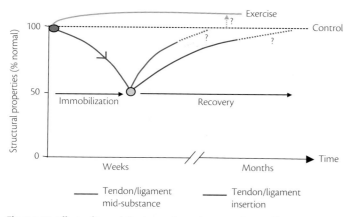

Fig. 1.1.11 Effects of immobilization and exercise on tendon and ligament. The structural properties of tendons and ligaments are considerably reduced following several weeks immobilization. There is a gradual recovery in the material properties after remobilization of the tissue, although it is questionable whether there is ever a full recovery. There are differences in the rate of recovery at different sites, with a more rapid rate in the mid-substance compared to the insertion. The effects of exercise on the structural properties are small (if any), greater in extensor tendons compared to flexors, and more pronounced in immature animals than in adults. (Modified and reproduced from Woo *et al* (1988), © 1988 with permission from the American Academy of Orthopaedic Surgeons.)

needed to cause the atrophy, and complete recovery of the original material properties of the ECM may never be reached.

Information on the functional adaptation of tendons/ligaments to exercise is limited and responses to training have been variable depending on anatomical site, species, and age. Exercise can produce an increase in collagen fibril size, ultimate strength, and stiffness, although the effects are small and more pronounced in (swine) extensor tendons compared to flexor tendons (Woo *et al.* 1981; Woo *et al.* 1982). Exercise can delay some of the changes with age such as the increase in maximum stress and stiffness (Nielsen *et al.* 1998). Most studies have been conducted on immature animal tendons, however, and the effects of exercise on adult tendon may be minimal and possibly damaging. Exercise can have deleterious effects on equine tendons, for example, although this would appear to be highly dependent on the type and level of physical activity and the age of the animal. Tendons in trained horses were shown to have a reduced average fibril diameter, which was interpreted as the effect of microtrauma (Patterson-Kane *et al.* 1997). Since the average diameter of fibrils is correlated with tendon mechanical strength, this change represents a deterioration in the quality of the tendon matrix. The crimp angle was also reduced in the core of the tendon (Patterson-Kane *et al.* 1997). A hypothesis has been presented suggesting that improvement in tendon properties is only possible in immature animals and that exercise can only be damaging in older animals (Smith *et al.* 1999). However, the flexor tendons of the equine athlete are operating close to their functional limits with very high levels of strain and this theory may not be applicable to the human, particular the non-athletic population.

Tendon and ligament pathology

The range of pathology affecting tendons and ligaments is different. Both tissues may be subject to acute injury as a result of trauma, overload, or direct mechanical insult resulting from crushing blows or penetrating objects. The repair response is thought to follow the same general pattern, with the important proviso that some

ligaments and tendons are apparently able to mount a more effective repair response than others. This has been linked to a number of factors, such as whether tendons are intrasynovial or extrasynovial, or whether ligaments are intraarticular or extraarticular. There is also evidence to suggest that the ability to repair is dependent on the quantity and quality of the vascular network at different sites. Repair may also be affected by the adaptive formation of fibrocartilage in response to compressive forces as described above.

Tendons are more prone to chronic, insidious forms of injury than ligaments. This pathology is often associated with repeated strain and repetitive microtrauma rather than a single traumatic episode. This form of soft tissue pathology, variously described as tendinitis, tendinosis, or tendinopathy, is commonly seen in rheumatology clinics and is one of the most difficult conditions to manage. Although more is now known about the biochemistry of this condition, there are still substantial gaps in our knowledge.

Acute tendon and ligament injuries

The cellular events occurring after traumatic injury to a tendon or ligament are thought to be broadly similar and common to all soft connective tissues (Gelberman *et al.* 1988; Andriacchi *et al.* 1988). The response is usually divided into three or four phases, more for convenience as the phases merge imperceptibly into each other and represent a continuum rather than discrete stages (Fig. 1.1.12). The timing of the different phases varies in different tissues and is influenced by nutrition, metabolic disorders (e.g. diabetes), age, and factors such as the location and extent of the tissue injury.

The first phase, occurring in the first 7 days after disruption of the tendon fibres, is characterized by inflammation. There is accumulation of serous fluid (oedema) and the infiltration of a variety of cell types attracted to the region by inflammatory mediators. Platelets and mast cells release histamine, a potent agent promoting vasodilatation and increasing blood vessel permeability. Serotonin, bradykinin, leukotrienes, and prostaglandins act together to recruit polymorphonuclear leucocytes and lymphocytes from the circulation. Growth factors released by platelets include platelet-derived growth factor (PDGF), TGFβ, and epidermal growth factor (EGF). Macrophages are present within 24 hours, phagocytosing tissue debris and releasing numerous inflammatory

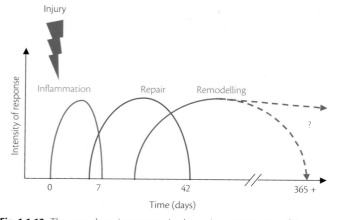

Fig. 1.1.12 The wound repair response. A schematic representation of the tissue response to injury, showing three overlapping phases of inflammation, repair (matrix synthesis), and remodelling. The time points shown are purely illustrative and vary according to tissue, site, age, etc. In tendons and ligaments the remodelling process may not be complete more than a year after injury.

mediators and growth factors including basic fibroblast growth factor (bFGF), transforming growth factor alpha (TGFa), TGFβ, and PDGF. These growth factors are chemotactic for fibroblasts and other cells, and generally act to stimulate matrix synthesis. Angiogenic factors such as bFGF and vascular endothelial growth factor (VEGF) stimulate capillary ingrowth into the fibrous clot. Toward the end of the inflammatory phase, which may last several days, fibroblasts become the predominant cell type.

The second phase, lasting up to 6 weeks after injury, is characterized by cell proliferation and new matrix synthesis by fibroblasts. This new matrix is different in both quality and quantity from the normal matrix. Described as granulation tissue, it consists of a disorganized matrix with an elevated cell density that fills the tissue defect. The DNA content of the healing rabbit MCL reaches twice normal levels during this period (Andriacchi et al. 1988).

The third phase, occurring 3–6 weeks after injury and lasting for at least a year, is a prolonged period of remodelling and maturation in which the matrix components and tissue cellularity revert gradually toward normal. During this stage many cells in the scar are contractile myofiboblasts, specialized cells important for the organization of the wound tissue, approaching 10 per cent of the cells after 12 weeks of healing in the rabbit MCL (Faryniarz et al. 1996).

Cell response to injury

The cellular response of tendons to injury has been extensively studied in sheathed animal flexor tendons following a surgical laceration (Lundborg and Rank 1978; Postacchini et al. 1978; Postacchini et al. 1980; Goldin et al. 1980; Lundborg et al. 1980; Gelberman et al. 1984). Some investigators have suggested that lacerated tendons are incapable of healing without the involvement of cells from the surrounding connective tissues (Potenza 1963). More recently, a number of studies have shown that the resident tenocytes have an intrinsic capacity to heal (Gelberman et al. 1984; Manske and Lesker 1984; Graham et al. 1984). The first changes are observed in the epitenon, with cellular proliferation and migration of cells into the tendon and the site of the lesion by the seventh day after injury. However, it is likely that extrinsic cell proliferation and infiltration may overwhelm the intrinsic cell response and the contribution of each cell type may depend on the site and type of the tendon injury (Gelberman et al. 1988). The cells from the outermost layers of the tendon (the epitenon) have been shown to synthesize both collagen types I and III, whereas the innermost cells produced only type I collagen (Riederer-Henderson et al. 1983). Some investigators have argued that the increase in type III collagen, observed in healing equine tendon, is a consequence of the activity of cells derived from the epitenon or peritendinous tissues (Williams et al. 1980). The cells most active in tendon/ligament repair may be a subpopulation of mesenchymal 'stem' cells, possibly present as vascular pericytes in the epitenon, although some authors have suggested that circulating 'fibrocytes' may be involved in the soft tissue repair response (Chesney and Bucala 1997).

Growth factors

Growth factors are signalling peptides that regulate many cellular activities in connective tissues including proliferation, matrix synthesis, matrix degradation, differentiation, and death (Dexter and White 1990; Haralson 1993). A variety of growth factors have been associated with wound repair(Gailit and Clark 1994), and some of these and their activities are summarized in Table 1.1.6. Growth factors are produced by most cell types and can act both locally and systemically. The expression and activity of growth factors can be regulated at the level of transcription, translation, and secretion. Once secreted, activity is affected by specific and non-specific interactions with the surrounding matrix and other molecules. Activity is also influenced by other growth factors, forming a complex network of influences on the cell population. The activity of growth factors is mediated by specific receptors on the cell surface. Different cell types express different receptors, and levels of receptor expression can also be modulated, so that the responses of specific cell types are influenced by a complex array of factors (Gailit and Clark 1994).

Despite the importance of growth factors as regulators of wound healing, relatively little is known about the timing of their expression in tendon and ligament injury. TGFβ, which directly or indirectly promotes cell recruitment, angiogenesis, and matrix synthesis and inhibits matrix breakdown, is found at low levels in normal tendon and is upregulated after injury (Chang et al. 1998; Duffy et al. 1995; Natsu-ume et al. 1997). Cells in the sheath and tendon mid-substance, including inflammatory cells infiltrating the lesion, showed increased levels of TGFβ1 expression just 1 day after injury, and these levels were maintained for up to 56 days (Chang et al. 1998). bFGF, a growth factor that also stimulates angiogenesis, is not abundant in normal tendon (Chang et al. 1998). After injury, bFGF is expressed in tenocytes concentrated along the epitenon and by infiltrating fibroblasts and inflammatory cells from the tendon sheath (Chang et al. 1998). PDGF and EGF have also been shown to increase in injured digital flexor tendons (Duffy et al. 1995).

Slightly more is known about growth factors expressed after ligament injury. PDGF, bFGF, and TGFβ1 were elevated in the rabbit MCL 3–7 days after injury, and their levels began to decrease after 14 days (Lee et al. 1998). The strong expression of PDGF, which has mitogenic and chemotactic properties, correlated with the increased cellularity of the tissue. In wounded ACL, expression of these growth factors was limited to the edge of the wound and levels were lower than in the MCL (Lee et al. 1998). Expression of genes for endothelin-1 (ET-1), TGFβ1, insulin-like growth factor-1 (IGF-1), and IGF-2 was increased up to five times control levels 3 weeks after injury, returning close to normal at 14 weeks (Sciore et al. 1998). The importance of growth factor receptor expression was recognized in studies from Panossian et al. since these are essential for the transmission of growth factor effects after ligand binding at the cell surface (Panossian et al. 1997). These authors showed that bFGF and EGF receptors were strongly expressed during the early inflammatory phase after ligament injury, peaking at 7 days after injury (Panossian et al. 1997). Expression of the IGF-2 receptor rose and fell in parallel with the expression of IGF-2. Thus it is clear that, if the addition of exogenous growth factors is to be used to promote tendon/ligament repair, delivery must be timed to coincide with receptor expression, or additional factors provided to stimulate the expression of the appropriate receptors.

Biochemical changes in tendon and ligament injury

Collagen synthesis is seen during the first week after injury, with the initial deposition of a random, disorganized fibre network. A large proportion of the newly synthesized collagen is type III collagen (Banes et al. 1984;Gelberman et al. 1988; Williams et al. 1980; Watkins et al. 1985). The concentration of immature, reducible

Table 1.1.6 Cytokines associated with wound repair and their effects[a]

Cytokine	Family	Action
PDGF-AB	PDGF	Stimulates proliferation of most mesenchymal cells including fibroblasts and smooth muscle cells
PDGF-BB		Stimulates chemotaxis
		Stimulates myofibroblast contraction
PDGF-AA	PDGF	Less potent than PDGF-AB: does not stimulate chemotaxis or myofibroblast contraction
VEGF	PDGF	Stimulates endothelial cell proliferation
		Increases vascular permeability
TGF-β1	TGF-β	Inhibits proliferation of most cells
TGF-β2		Stimulates fibroblast chemotaxis
TGF-β3		Stimulates matrix synthesis and protease inhibitor production
EGF	EGF	Stimulates proliferation of most epithelial cells, fibroblasts, and endothelial cells
		Stimulates keratinocyte migration
TGF-α	EGF	Similar to EGF, but more potent stimulator of angiogenesis
HB-EGF	EGF	Stimulates proliferation of keratinocytes, fibroblasts, and smooth muscle cells
Basic FGF	FGF	Stimulates proliferation of endothelial cells, keratinocytes, and fibroblasts
		Stimulates chemotaxis
		Stimulates protease synthesis
KGF	FGF	Stimulates epithelial cell proliferation
		Stimulates keratinocyte migration
IGF	Insulin	Stimulates proliferation of fibroblasts and endothelial cells
		Stimulates chemotaxis
IL-1	Interleukin	Stimulates fibroblast production of proteoglycans, collagen, and proteases (MMP-1, MMP-3, and others)
TNF-α	TNF	Stimulates macrophage production of proteases
		Increases vascular permeability
		Inhibits collagen synthesis
Endothelin		Stimulates contraction of smooth muscle cells and myofibroblasts
Scatter factor (HGF)		Stimulates motility and proliferation of epithelial and endothelial cells

[a] These cytokines have all been found in injured tissues and are thought to participate in wound healing on the basis of *in vitro* models and effects on cultured cells. Common acronyms are: PDGF, platelet-derived growth factor; VEGF, vascular endothelial growth factor (also known as VPF or vascular permeability factor) TGF, transforming growth factor; EGF, epidermal growth factor; HB-EGF, heparin-binding EGF-like growth factor; FGF, fibroblast growth factor; KGF, keratinocyte growth factor; IGF, insulin-like growth factor; IL-1, interleukin-1; TNF, tumour necrosis factor; HGF, hepatocyte growth factor. (Reproduced from Gailit, J. and Clark, R.A.F. (1994), table 2, p. 719, © 1994, with permission from Elsevier Science.)

crosslinks is increased, the amount of mature tri-functional cross-links is low, and collagen is more readily extracted from the wound tissue. The collagen content increases through the next few weeks, with the gradual alignment of the collagen fibres with the long axis of the tendon/ligament. There is a slow transformation from loose fibrillar areas of types I and III collagen and pericellular type IV and V collagen to a dense network of parallel type I collagen fibre bundles (Watkins *et al.* 1985). Collagen maturation proceeds slowly but may not approach the normal composition, structure, and material properties even after many months (Banes *et al.* 1984).

In the rabbit MCL injury model, collagen turnover was greatest 3–6 weeks after injury, with increased synthesis of type III collagen compared to type I collagen, and the rate returned toward the normal after 40 weeks (Patterson-Kane *et al.* 1997; Amie *et al.* 1987). The collagen fibrils were initially a homogeneous population of small average diameter, and after 40 weeks there was a progressive increase in the proportion of slightly larger fibrils, but even

at 2 years approximately 90 per cent of the fibrils were small (Frank *et al.* 1997). Although the collagen concentration reached normal by 14 weeks, the mechanical strength of the ligament scar was 30 per cent of control values after 40 weeks, and there was a positive correlation with the HP cross-link density (Frank *et al.* 1995). In gene expression studies, injured human ligaments (ACL) were shown to express much higher quantities of mRNA for types I and III collagen, biglycan, lumican, and TIMP-1 and lower levels of versican, and there was no change in decorin and fibromodulin mRNA compared to that of normal ligaments (Boykiw *et al.* 1998; Lo *et al.* 1998). Types I and III collagen, biglycan, and TIMP-1 mRNA levels were raised even 1 year after injury (Lo *et al.* 1998). Thus, although the injured ACL demonstrates the ability to produce 'scar-like' molecules, healing is slow and there is a prolonged remodelling phase resulting in a low quality repair. Attempts to improve the repair of tendon and ligament must influence the cellular activity so as to promote the resolution of this extended remodelling phase and the restoration (as far as possible) of the normal matrix composition and organization.

Proteases in tendon and ligament injury

Proteolytic activity is an essential component of tissue repair, required to remove damaged matrix and remodel the resulting scar tissue so that it more closely resembles the normal tissue structure. Since most matrix proteolysis is thought to occur in the extracellular compartment, most importance is generally attributed to the MMP family described above. However, other proteinases such as the cathepsins may be implicated to some degree, and some matrix turnover may take place within the cell after phagocytosis, although there is relatively little research of these processes in tendon and ligament.

MMP-1 (interstitial collagenase) is stimulated by inflammatory mediators such as IL-1 during the inflammatory and proliferative phases of wound healing, declining in the later remodelling stages (Ågren et al. 1992). In slowly remodelling wounds, such as in the cornea, elevated levels of MMP-1 are found up to 9 months after injury (Girard et al. 1993). Acute wounds contain MMP-2 (72 kDa gelatinase) and MMP-9 (92 kDa gelatinase), but levels are higher and remain elevated in chronic wounds such as leg ulcers (Salo et al. 1994; Wysocki et al. 1993). The factors that stimulate MMP expression and activity are not well characterized, although, in addition to inflammatory mediators and cytokines, proteolytic fragments of matrix molecules such as fibronectin and tenascin may directly stimulate proteolysis (Grinnel et al. 1992).

Few studies have been conducted on protease expression in human tendon ruptures. A study of ruptured supraspinatus tendons showed co-localization of IL-1 and MMP-1 at the wound margin (Gotoh et al. 1997). An analysis of MMPs extracted from ruptured supraspinatus has confirmed that there was an increase in the amount of *active* MMP-1 in the tendon (not just levels of MMP-1 protein) (Fig. 1.1.9) (Riley et al. 2002). There was also a decrease in MMP-2 and MMP-3 activities compared to those of control tendons. The increase in MMP-1 was associated with increased turnover of the matrix collagen as measured by pentosidine cross-link analysis and racemization of aspartate (Bank et al. 1999; Riley et al. 2002). The change in MMP activity may not represent an acute response, however, since ruptures of the supraspinatus are usually a consequence of a long-standing degenerative process. Thus it is not known if the change in matrix remodelling activity precedes or follows supraspinatus tendon rupture. In contrast to the supraspinatus tendon, ruptured ACL showed an absence of MMP-1 and MMP-2 activity in the tissue remnant even 1 year after injury (Spindler et al. 1996). The lack of a matrix remodelling response could explain, at least in part, why the ACL (unlike the MCL) often fails to heal (Andriacchi et al. 1988).

Effects of exercise and mobilization on tendon and ligament repair

The use of controlled motion and exercise in the management of tendon and ligament injuries is now generally accepted. However, there is still considerable variation in the rehabilitation programme following tendon repair, despite objective evidence showing the benefits of early mobilization using techniques such as functional casting (for example) compared to rigid plaster casts (Stehno-Bittel et al. 1998). Animal models have shown how non-repaired tendons rapidly lose a substantial proportion of their matrix, demonstrating

the importance of early repair (Wiig et al. 1997). Prolonged immobilization after surgery has deleterious effects on the quality of repair, preventing the return to near-normal strength of transected rat Achilles tendon after 15 days immobilization (Murrell, G.A.C. 1994). There are a variety of other complications of an extended immobilization period following injury, including muscle atrophy, joint stiffness, cartilage deterioration, adhesions, and thrombosis (Stehno-Bittel et al. 1998). Tension, applied cyclically or as a constant load, has a positive influence on the intrinsic fibroblast response and the strength of repair. It promotes cell proliferation and migration, facilitating the alignment of fibroblasts and the amount of synthesized collagen (Graham et al. 1984; Slack et al. 1984; Mass et al. 1983; Tanaka et al. 1995; Iwuagwu and McGrouther 1998). Early passive mobilization of repaired tendons, using rubber bands or other devices to control or limit extension or flexion, results in better gliding function (reduced adhesions) and increased mechanical strength compared to immobilized tendons (Woo et al. 1981; Gelberman et al. 1982). Other data show the benefits of early active mobilization compared to passive mobilization, particularly in zone 2 flexor tendon repair, although care must be taken not to provoke re-rupture (Baktir et al. 1996; Bainbridge et al. 1994). Applied load has been shown to affect the orientation of fibroblasts, which become aligned with the direction of load (Eastwood et al. 1998). It also has profound effects on the synthesis of matrix, with differences in the quantity, composition, and orientation of matrix depending on the direction (tension or compression) of the applied load as discussed above. There are also thought to be positive benefits as a result of improved nutrient provision, particularly for repair within the tendon sheath (Gelberman et al. 1988). However more experimental work with controlled studies is required to define the optimum postoperative mobilization regime, designed to promote reorganization and remodelling of the repaired tendon/ligament so that higher strength and better function can be achieved.

Effects of exogenous agents on tendon/ligament repair
Growth factors

The application of exogenous, recombinant growth factors to damaged and healing ligaments and tendons has been attempted in a number of studies with variable levels of success. Bone morphogenetic protein 13 (BMP13, otherwise known as cartilage-derived morphogenetic protein 2 (CDMP-2) or growth differentiation factor 6 (GDF-6)), a member of the TGFβ superfamily of growth factors, improved the mechanical strength of repairing rat tendons by 39 per cent compared to controls, 8 days after injury (Forslund and Aspenberg 2001). GDF-5 (CDMP-1) also resulted in increased repair strength at 2 weeks, similarly to GDF-6 (Aspenberg and Forslund 1999). BMP-2 has been used to enhance the healing of tendon to bone in the canine (Rodeo et al. 1999). PDGF-BB increased the load to failure and stiffness of the healing MCL compared to untreated controls (Batten et al. 1996; Hildebrand et al. 1998). Application of PDGF within 24 hours after injury was more effective compared to application after 48 hours (Batten et al. 1996). The effect was dependent on dose, although structural properties never approached that of uninjured controls. Combinations of PDGF with a single additional growth factor (TGFβ, FGF, or IGF-1) did not result in significant improvement above PDGF alone (Hildebrand et al. 1998; Letson and Dahners 1994). bFGF promoted neovascularization and the organization of collagen fibre bundles in defects of canine ACL between 6 and 24 weeks post-injury (Kobayashi *et al.* 1997). PDGF-AB and TGFβ2, applied separately, had no significant effect on the healing of rabbit MCL at 3 to 12 weeks after injury (Woo *et al.* 1999).

Nonsteroidal anti-inflammatory drugs (NSAIDs)

NSAIDs are commonly used in the treatment of ligament and tendon injuries (Almekinders 1990; Almekinders and Almekinders 1994; Almekinders and Temple 1998). Their pharmacological target is cyclo-oxygenase (prostaglandin synthase), a key enzyme in the formation of prostaglandins that mediate the sensation of pain and inflammation in the tissues (Vane 1971). Studies of their effects on tendon healing have been inconclusive, with some studies showing deleterious effects on the repair quality and others showing no effect or even an increase in mechanical strength (Carlstedt 1987; Kulick *et al.* 1986; Thomas *et al.* 1991). *In vivo* studies on both normal and healing tendons have shown an increase in the proportion of insoluble collagen, thought to be evidence of a decrease in collagen breakdown and an increase in cross-linked collagen (Vogel 1977; Carlstedt *et al.* 1986). *In vitro* studies have shown that some NSAIDs (indomethacin, naproxen) may inhibit cell proliferation and matrix proteoglycan synthesis, while others (diclofenac, aceclofenac) have no effect and may even stimulate cell activity (Riley *et al.* 2001). The significance of these findings to the *in vivo* situation is not known. Studies using a topical NSAID (ketoprofen) showed that levels of NSAID accumulate in the peritendinous tissues and reach levels many times higher than circulating plasma concentrations (Rolf *et al.* 1997). The rationale behind NSAID use in chronic tendon pain is uncertain, since inflammation is generally not a feature of these conditions and prostaglandin levels are not increased in the fluid surrounding painful tendons (Almekinders and Temple 1998; Alfredson *et al.* 1999; Alfredson *et al.* 2000; Alfredson *et al.* 2001). There is also doubt about the effectiveness of NSAID treatment for ligament injuries (Almekinders 1990; Vane 1971).

Corticosteroids

There are many case reports describing rupture, often bilateral, of Achilles and other tendons after long-term oral corticosteroid therapy (Haines 1983; Potasman and Bassan 1984; Newnham *et al.* 1991; Kotnis *et al.* 1999). These ruptures are associated with a reduced collagen content and decreased mechanical strength as a result of decreased collagen synthesis over a long period of time. Local injections of steroid, sometimes given only once, have also been associated with tendon rupture, particularly in the Achilles (Clark *et al.* 1995; Smith *et al.* 1999). However, a review of the literature has shown that there are very few well controlled studies of the effects (and effectiveness) of corticosteroid injections on tendinopathy, particularly in the Achilles (Shrier *et al.* 1996). If there is a decrease in tendon strength it is in the first few weeks after injection, although there is no effect if the paratenon is injected rather than the tendon itself (Shrier *et al.* 1996). Other studies have suggested that it is the mode of delivery that is important (Martin *et al.* 1999).

The results of animal studies are somewhat paradoxical and often contradictory. Short-term treatment with prednisolone, either orally or injected locally, has been shown to increase the strength of normal tendons, increasing both the total amount of collagen and the proportion of insoluble collagen (Oxlund 1984). Long-term treatment reduced the tendon dry weight but increased the stiffness, although the ultimate mechanical strength of the tissue was unchanged. These effects are similar to those of NSAIDs such as indomethacin, with inhibition of both collagen synthesis and collagen degradation, although the effects of corticosteroids are more rapid and dramatic (Vogel 1977). Two different effects of corticosteroids are suggested to act on the tissue: (1) in the early period, a relatively fast increase in the stability of collagen; (2) over the long-term, a progressive reduction in collagen content caused by an inhibition of collagen synthesis.

In a rat model of Achilles tendon injury, multiple injections of hydrocortisone around the tendon were shown to have no deleterious effect on the repair quality up to 9 weeks post-injury (McWhorter *et al.* 1991). In contrast, repeated injections of triamcinolone into the subacromial space of the rat shoulder resulted in focal inflammation, necrosis, and collagen fragmentation of the rotator cuff (Tillander *et al.* 1999). A single injection of dexa-methasone had no effect on the healing of rat (Campbell *et al.* 1996). However, single injections of triamcinolone or betamethasone in rabbit MCL injury reduced the quality of repair (Wiggins *et al.* 1994; Wiggins *et al.* 1995). Thus the effects on tendons vary according to the species, timing, dosage, and type of corticosteroid preparation.

Anabolic androgenic steroids

The use and abuse of anabolic androgenic steroids (AAS) has been associated with tendon rupture. However, the literature is mostly case reports and far from conclusive (Laseter and Russell 1991; Visuri and Lindholm 1994). There is also a documented case of ligament rupture associated with the use of AAS, but this appears to be exceptional (Visuri and Lindholm 1994). Some microscopic studies have shown ultrastructural changes in the tendon collagen (Michna 1986; Miles *et al.* 1992), while clinical studies of ruptured tendon showed no significant changes (Evans *et al.* 1998). Supraphysiological doses of AAS have been shown to stimulate the synthesis of collagen types I and III and decrease collagen degradation in athletes (Parssinen *et al.* 2000). AAS are generally thought to promote muscle hypertrophy when combined with an exercise programme (Laseter and Russell 1991) and may also have some effect on immobilized and non-exercised muscle (Taylor *et al.* 1999). Although some studies have reported transitory inhibitory effects on collagen synthesis at very high doses (Karpakka *et al.* 1992), the main reported effects on tendon are an increase in stiffness so that the tendon absorbs less energy (Miles *et al.* 1992; Inhofe *et al.* 1995). The altered mechanical properties are related to changes in the crimp morphology of the collagen fascicles (Wood *et al.* 1988). There are reported to be no changes in fibril diameter, collagen type, or ultimate strength, and the change in mechanical properties is reversible (Inhofe *et al.* 1995). The combination of increased muscle hypertrophy and a stiffer, less elastic tendon is thought to account for the incidence of rupture. The stimulation of collagen synthesis by AAS (such as norethandrolone) may result in an improved repair response post-injury. However, there is a lack of hard evidence, and even the effects of AAS on athletic performance are largely anecdotal (Mottram and George 2000).

Miscellaneous factors and their effects on tendon and ligament repair

A variety of other factors and interventions are used in the treatment of tendon and ligament injuries, although few have shown clinical benefit in controlled trials. *In vitro* studies have shown benefit from the addition of vitamins (A, C, and E) (Greenwald *et al.* 1991) and exogenous electric currents (Cleary *et al.* 1988;

Fujita *et al.* 1992). The sulfated GAG heparin, an anticoagulant and stimulator of neovascularization, improved the collagen fibre organization of injured rabbit Achilles tendons (Williams *et al.* 1986). Related compounds such as the synthetic polymer GAG polysulfate (GAGPS) have shown promise in the treatment of chronic tendinopathies, perhaps as a consequence of their inhibitory effects on proteolytic activities (Akermark *et al.* 1995). The addition of hyaluronan has been suggested to promote healing as well as inhibit adhesion formation, although the effect on tendon repair has been questioned (Wiig *et al.* 1986; Wiig *et al.* 1997). Protease inhibitors such as aprotinin and chemical agents such as 5-fluorouracil have also been used to inhibit tendon adhesions (Komurcu *et al.* 1997; Akali *et al.* 1999). Low-energy laser photostimulation stimulated the synthesis of collagen by 26 per cent in healing rabbit Achilles tendons, perhaps as a consequence of an effect on growth factor synthesis by the resident fibroblasts (Reddy *et al.* 1998). However, when combined with mechanical loading, there were no significant improvements in the tissue biomechanics (Reddy *et al.* 1998)and there were only moderate improvements when combined with both ultrasound and mechanical loading (Gum *et al.* 1997). Therapeutic ultrasound resulted in increased tensile strength and elasticity of healing chicken tendons, if applied during the early stages of healing (Enwemeka 1989; Stevenson *et al.* 1986). However no therapeutic effect of ultrasound was reported in a similar study of repaired cockerel tendon (Turner *et al.* 1989). Extracorporeal shock wave therapy (ESWT) has recently been used in the treatment of tendon injuries and pathology such as rotator cuff tendinitis, plantar fasciitis, and calcific tendinitis (Fritze 1998; Speed and Hazleman 1999; Haake *et al.* 2001). Studies in animals have shown some benefit in the treatment of tendon injury, although the data presented were of a preliminary nature (Orhan *et al.* 2001). Some studies have shown negative effects such as necrosis, fibrosis, and inflammation if high-energy flux densities are used (Rompe *et al.* 1998). Systematic reviews of the literature have revealed the lack of controlled trials for ESWT and many of the commonly used modalities (Fritze 1998; Huang *et al.* 2000).

Chronic tendon pathology

Terminology

The terminology of chronic tendon pathology is both confused and confusing (Maffulli *et al.* 1998). A variety of different classifications is present in the literature, and there is no consensus as to the best or most appropriate term to describe specific conditions. This confusion is due to the incomplete understanding of the pathological nature of the condition, primarily because diagnosis is imprecise and not based on an objective assessment. Terms such as tendinitis imply that there is inflammation, although there is little evidence of any inflammatory process in histological studies. Conditions are consequently best considered as either acute or chronic, whether caused by trauma, repeated microtrauma ('overuse'), or the result of an insidious process of clinically silent (pain-free) degeneration. Unless the presence of inflammation or degeneration has been unequivocally demonstrated, most tendon pain and dysfunction is best described as a 'tendinopathy'. A variety of chronic tendinopathies have been described, although basic entities commonly encountered are 'spontaneous' tendon rupture, painful tendinopathy, and calcific tendinitis. The histopathology and biochemistry of these conditions is considered below, preceded by an overview of their aetiology.

Table 1.1.7 Factors implicated in the development of chronic tendinopathy

Intrinsic factors	Extrinsic factors
Age	Occupation
Vascular perfusion	Sport
Nutrition	Physical load
	Excessive force
Anatomical variants	Repetitive loading
Leg-length discrepancy	Abnormal/unusual movement
Malalignments (e.g. genu valgum)	
Bony impingement (e.g. acromiom)	Training errors
	Poor technique
Joint laxity	Fast progression
	High intensity
Muscle weakness/imbalance	Fatigue
Gender (?)	Shoes and equipment
Body weight	Environmental conditions Temperature
Systemic disease	Running surface

Aetiology of tendinopathy

The aetiology of most chronic tendinopathy is linked to multiple factors, both intrinsic and extrinsic (Table 1.1.7). These factors have been extensively reviewed elsewhere (Uhthoff and Sano 1997; Huang *et al.* 2000; Kannus 1997; Józsa and Kannus 1997; Józsa and Kannus 1997; Waterston *et al.* 1997; Teitz *et al.* 1997). Salient points are discussed here and throughout this volume where appropriate. Many tendon lesions, whether spontaneous ruptures or painful tendinopathies, are commonly associated with a reduction in vascular perfusion, particularly at specific sites in the supraspinatus and the Achilles (Waterston *et al.* 1997; Rathbun and MacNab 1970). However, this association and the importance of vascular perfusion has been questioned in other studies (Brooks *et al.* 1992; Ahmed *et al.* 1998; Astrom and Westlin 1994). Since most tendon ruptures occur in the fifth decade, age-related changes are usually implicated, although ruptures of the Achilles are most common in a younger, physically active population with a mean age in the mid-thirties (Astrom and Westlin 1994). In most tendon ruptures there tends to be a preponderance of males to females, although it is uncertain whether this is directly associated with gender (Józsa and Kannus 1997). There is a strong association with particular sports and activities that result in high levels of stress being applied to specific sites. Genetic factors have been implicated, since a proportion of individuals tend to suffer from multiple types of soft tissue pathology such as Dupuytren's contracture, frozen shoulder, and various tendinopathies (Nirschl and Pettrone 1973). However, no genetic abnormality that is specifically implicated in tendinopathy has yet been identified. Leg-length discrepancies and other anatomical variants, such as the shape and slope of the acromion in the shoulder, are implicated in some individuals. Lifestyle factors are also likely to be important, and the combination of a more sedentary existence with increased leisure time, recreational sports, and a propensity to obesity may account for the greater incidence in the developed world.

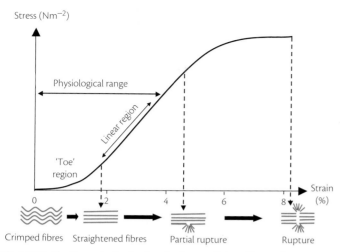

Fig. 1.1.13 The theoretical basis of tendon 'overuse' injury. The tendon stress–strain curve is used to illustrate the theoretical basis of tendon overuse injury. Strains of up to 4 per cent result in the stretching out of the crimped collagen fibres and do not damage the tendon. Strains above this level cause microscopic failure of fibrils within the tissue. If damage exceeds the ability of the tissue to repair, the tendon will rupture. (Reproduced from Stanish *et al.* (2000), © 2000 with permission from Oxford University Press.)

'Overuse' pathology—a mechanical model of tendon injury

Most chronic tendinopathy is not associated with a single traumatic event, but is thought to be the consequence of repeated exposure to low-magnitude forces. Thus an overuse injury has been defined as a long-standing or recurring problem in the musculoskeletal system that arises during or soon after exertion due to repetitive micro-trauma (Butler *et al.* 1978; Kannus 1997; Józsa and Kannus 1997). This concept now appears to be almost universally accepted and is usually explained with reference to the tendon stress-strain curve (Fig. 1.1.13).

Low levels of strain, up to a 2 per cent increase in the original length, are accommodated in normal tendon by the stretching out of the crimped collagen fibrils. This represents the 'toe' region of the stress–strain curve. Strains of up to 4 per cent are generally thought to represent the normal physiological range. Strains beyond this level result in fibril damage. Repeated stretching of the tendon results in accumulated damage that weakens the tendon. If the amount of damage exceeds the ability of the tendon cells to repair the matrix, the tendon will fail and rupture. The cellular response to mechanical strain is consequently a key factor in overuse pathology, and a failure of the cells to adapt to mechanical demands may precipitate the pathology (Leadbetter 1992). The concept of tendon fatigue has been further developed by *in vitro* models that demonstrate that repeated loading at low levels of strain will result in tendon rupture. Different tendons vary in their 'time-to rupture' and this correlates with the stresses experienced by the tendons *in vivo*. Thus specific tendons are thought to be 'engineered' to a minimum quality required for their normal function.

The ability of the tendon cell population to adapt, or to respond to tendon damage, is consequently thought to be a key factor in overuse tendinopathy (Leadbetter 1992). Some researchers have questioned whether mature tendons are capable of adaptation, suggesting that exercise can only lead to deleterious effects on the adult (equine) tendon matrix (Smith *et al.* 1999). In addition, exercise-induced hyperthermia, which can lead to an increase in

temperature of several degrees in the core of the tendon, may be damaging to both tenocytes and matrix (Wilson and Goodship 1994). These factors depend on the levels and type of exercise, and may not be relevant to common clinical conditions, even in endurance athletes. Ageing, systemic diseases, nutritional factors, hormones, and drugs are all potentially able to have an impact on the tenocyte activities (see above). Reduced vascular perfusion, as a result of age or trauma, may also have a deleterious effect on the tenocytes. Thus the two major theories about the pathogenesis of tendinopathy, a mechanical theory and a vascular theory, are often linked and probably implicated to some degree in most tendinopathy. For example, damage to the vasculature as a result of microtrauma may increase intratendinous or intrasynovial pressure, obliterating vessels and beginning a vicious cycle of decreased blood flow, tissue hypoxia, and fibre degeneration (Leadbetter 1992). The cell and blood vessel proliferation seen in painful tendinopathy and, less commonly, in spontaneous tendon rupture is assumed to represent a reparative response that is secondary to the initial lesion.

What is the cause of chronic tendon pain?

The model of overuse pathology presented above does not account for the onset of tendon pain. Damage to the vasculature and the cellular response to disrupted matrix has been suggested to precipitate an inflammatory response, resulting in oedema and pain. However, in the absence of any evidence of inflammation (see below), other causes of pain must be considered. The deterioration in material properties may result in the stimulation of stretch receptors in the tendon. Alternatively, receptors may be triggered by swelling in the tendon as a result of oedema, fibrosis, or (in some cases) calcific deposits. Very few studies have addressed the role of innervation in the perception of tendon pain, and it is not known whether the distribution of nociceptors is altered in tendinopathy. Some recent studies have identified nerve endings and neuropeptides (substance P and calcitonin gene-related peptide (CGRP)) at the site of the lesion in tendinopathies, although it was unclear whether this distribution was different from normal (Sanchis-Alfonso *et al.* 2001). It is interesting to note that, in a degenerative intervertebral disc, the in-growth of nerve endings accompanies the in-growth of blood vessels and is associated with the disc pathology (see Chapter 1.4).

Studies of fluids around painful tendons have led to new insights into the potential cause of pain in chronic tendinopathy. Using a microdialysis technique, Alfredson and co-workers found no difference in the amount of prostaglandin E_2 (PGE_2) around the patellar tendon in 'jumper's knee' compared to normal (Alfredson *et al.* 2001). A similar result was found in Achilles tendinopathy and around the extensor carpi radialis brevis tendon in patients with tennis elbow, confirming the absence of 'classic' inflammation (Alfredson *et al.* 1999; Alfredson *et al.* 2000). However, the levels of the neurotransmitter glutamate were significantly increased in all three tendinopathies relative to controls (Alfredson *et al.* 1999; Alfredson *et al.* 2000; Alfredson *et al.* 2001). Glutamate and glutamate *N*-methyl-D-aspartate receptor 1 (NMDAR1) have also been detected within Achilles tendons, located to nerve fibres, both in tendinopathy specimens and in controls (Alfredson . *et al.* 2000). Since glutamate is a potent mediator of pain in the central nervous system (CNS), it was suggested that glutamate NMDAR1 antagonists may be useful in the treatment of tendon pain. It has also been reported that substance P, another neuropeptide associated with the sensation of pain, is increased in the subacromial bursa in patients with rotator cuff tendinopathy (Gotoh *et al.* 1998). The amount of substance P was shown to correlate with the degree of motion pain as assessed by a visual analogue scale. Whether this was due to an increase in the release of substance P or an increase in the number of nerve fibres was not clear, although immunohistochemistry showed more nerve fibres in bursal tissues of patients with a perforated rotator cuff (Gotoh *et al.* 1998). Apart from the modulation of pain, substance P and other neuropeptides may have additional effects, regulating the local circulation and perhaps mediating neurogenic inflammation in and around the tendon.

Neurogenic inflammation and chronic tendinopathy

The pro-inflammatory role of neuropeptides such as substance P has been described with respect to the induction and progression of joint inflammation in other arthritides (O'Byrne *et al.* 1990; Garrett *et al.* 1992). More recently it has been proposed that the release of substance P and CGRP may be implicated in tendon (and ligament) pathology (Hart *et al.* 1999; Hart *et al.* 1999). Hart *et al.* have proposed that regulatory units composed of nerve endings and mast cells reside in and around the tendon (Fig. 1.1.14). The release of neurotransmitters stimulates mast cell degranulation, releasing a variety of mediators (including growth factors) that influence oedema, angiogenesis, fibroblast proliferation, and many other aspects of cell activity. Biomechanical stimulation of these units may comprise part of the normal regulatory system, maintaining the tissue and also contributing to the adaptive response to increased load (Fig. 1.1.15). Excessive stimulation of these neural-mast cell 'units' may contribute to overuse pathology. Since the extent of innervation and vascularization probably varies between different tendons (and ligaments), the potential for the development of neurogenic dysfunction also varies. This theory potentially links mechanical stimulation of the paratenon, which is more richly innervated, and tissue changes in the tendon mid-substance. The association with tissue remodelling has not been conclusively proved, although substance P and CGRP can directly modulate (reduce) the expression of MMP-1 and MMP-3, at least *in vitro* (Hart *et al.* 1999; Hart and Reno 1998). Thus innervation, and the stimulation of neuropeptide release by strain or friction at the tendon surface, are thought to be important for both normal tendon function and pathology.

Histopathology of tendinopathy

'Spontaneous' tendon rupture

The sudden rupture of tendons during low or moderate levels of activity, occurring without any preceding clinical symptoms such as pain or swelling, is often described as a spontaneous tendon rupture. However, the majority of ruptures are not truly spontaneous, since only rarely are they caused by excessive load acting on normal tendon. In most histopathological studies there is an absence of inflammatory cells and degeneration of the tendon matrix. Consequently this condition is attributed to 'tendinosis' (Khan *et al.* 1999; Chard *et al.* 1994). Very rarely, ruptures are associated with chronic systemic diseases such as rheumatoid arthritis, systemic lupus erythmatosus (SLE), uraemia (haemodialysis), and diabetes, but these represented only 3 per cent of cases in one large study (Nirschl and Pettrone 1973). Other diseases directly affecting the tendon such as xanthoma and tendon tumours are very rare causes of rupture. Most ruptures of normal tendons as a result of

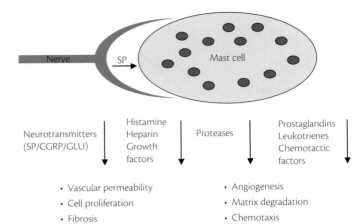

Fig. 1.1.14 Neurogenic inflammation. Schematic diagram illustrating the theoretical basis of neurogenic inflammation in tendon and ligament. Nerve endings in close proximity to mast cells release neuropeptides such as substance P (SP), calcitonin gene-related peptide (CGRP), and glutamate (GLU). Neuropeptides may have direct effects on the local cell population, but also stimulate mast cell degranulation, modulating a variety of different processes. (Modified and reproduced from Hart *et al.* (1995), © 1995, with permission from the American Association of Orthopaedic Surgeons.)

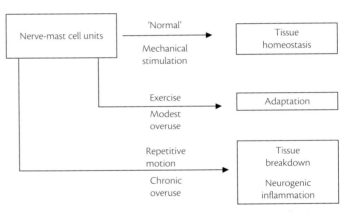

Fig. 1.1.15 Neurogenic control of tissue homeostasis. Nerve-mast cell units may function to modulate tissue homeostasis and the adaptive response to exercise. Excessive stimulation may result in negative effects on the tissue architecture. (Modified and reproduced from Hart *et al.* (1995), © 1995, with permission from the American Association of Orthopaedic Surgeons.)

excessive force tend to be avulsion injuries at the bone insertion, but these are also relatively rare.

The incidence of spontaneous tendon rupture has increased in recent years, and is more common in developed countries. Some tendons are more commonly affected than others, with the Achilles representing 45 per cent of all ruptures in one large study, followed by long head of biceps brachii (30 per cent), patellar (6 per cent), extensor pollicus longus (5 per cent), and quadriceps (4 per cent) (Nirschl and Pettrone 1973). Rotator cuff pathology, usually affecting the supraspinatus, was not included in this particular study, although complete ruptures and partial thickness tears are also very common at this site.

Ruptures tend to be more commonly found at particular sites within tendons. In the supraspinatus, a site at or near the bone insertion is usually affected (Codman 1934; Sano *et al.* 1998).

In the patellar and quadriceps tendons, ruptures are also usually close to the bone insertion (Nirschl and Pettrone 1973; King *et al.* 2000). In the Achilles, 83 per cent of ruptures occur in the tendon mid-substance, 3–6 cm from the calcaneus. In 12 per cent of cases, ruptures are found at the myotendinous junction and 5 per cent occur at the bone insertion (Nirschl and Pettrone 1973).

A number of features of matrix degeneration (tendinosis) have been described. In a heterogeneous group of 891 spontaneously ruptured human tendons, degenerative changes were found in the majority (97 per cent) (Nirschl and Pettrone 1973). The most frequent observation was hypoxic cell changes (44 per cent), followed by 'mucoid degeneration' (GAG accumulation), often accompanied by cell rounding (21 per cent). 'Tendolipomatosis' (lipid accumulation) was seen in 73 tendons (8 per cent), with lipid deposits interspersed between the collagen fibres. Calcifying tendi-

nopathy, with deposits of calcium on or between collagen fibres, was seen in 43 tendons. Similar degenerative changes were observed in non-ruptured cadaver tendons, but significantly less frequently, affecting 35 per cent of the sample. Other studies have shown an absence of degeneration in cadaver tendons from sites such as the biceps brachii (radius insertion) and Achilles (mid-substance), demonstrating that degeneration is not an inevitable consequence of ageing (Chard *et al.* 1994; Maffulli *et al.* 2000).

Chard *et al.* investigated degenerative changes in cadaver supraspinatus tendons and found that a significant proportion showed degenerative changes, the most common of which was GAG accumulation between the collagen fibrils (18 per cent), followed by a rounding up of the tendon cells to form regions with the appearance of fibrocartilage (8.5 per cent) (Fig. 1.1.16) (Chard *et al.* 1989; Chard *et al.* 1994). Other observations included

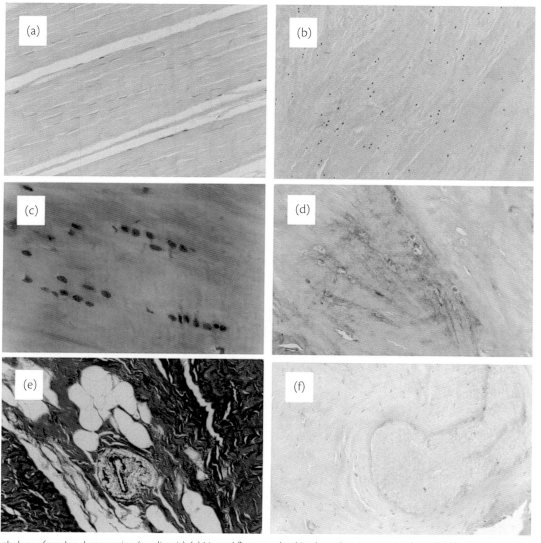

Fig. 1.1.16 Histopathology of tendon degeneration (tendinosis). (a) Normal flexor tendon histology, showing organized, parallel fibre bundles and long thin tenocytes dispersed throughout the matrix (H&E). (b) Ruptured supraspinatus tendon, showing hyaline (glassy) appearance, loss of matrix organization and rounded, shrunken nuclei (H&E). (c) Fibrocartilaginous change in supraspinatus tendon, showing rounded tenocytes in 'Indian file' (H&E). (d) Glycosaminoglycan (GAG) accumulation ('mucoid degeneration') in supraspinatus tendon, showing GAG (blue) surrounding rounded cells in the matrix (alcian blue/H&E). (e) Intimal hyperplasia of blood vessel and lipid droplets in the matrix (Elastin Ponceau S). (f) Calcium deposit in degenerate tendon, showing intense (blue) staining for GAG (Alcian Blue/H&E). (Reproduced from Chard *et al.* (1994), © 1994, with permission from BMJ publishing group.)

a reduction in cellularity, lipid deposits, calcification, and intimal hyperplasia of blood vessels. The severity of degeneration tended to increase with age, with the majority showing moderate to severe degeneration above the age of 60 (Riley *et al.* 2001). However, it was rare to find a normal supraspinatus tendon even in individuals under the age of 40, and less than 10 per cent of tendons in those over the age of 80 were considered normal. All specimens of ruptured supraspinatus tendons showed more severe degeneration, with the major change being a loss of cell number and disorganization of the matrix (Riley *et al.* 2001).

Other studies have described a variety of features that can be interpreted as indicators of tendon matrix degeneration, including a reduction in the size of fascicles, microtears of fascicles, the presence of granulation tissue, disruption of the 'tide mark', dystrophic calcification, and bony spurs (Uhthoff and Sano 1997; Sano *et al.* 1998; Sano *et al.* 1997). Degeneration was more prominent toward the articular side than the bursal side of the rotator cuff, and more severe degeneration was found in ruptured tendons (Sano *et al.* 1997). Weakness of the tendon was correlated with the severity of degeneration at the insertion, not at the tendon mid-substance or 'critical zone'. However, similar degenerative changes were found in all three rotator cuff tendons, demonstrating that additional factors must be involved in the pathogenesis of supraspinatus tendon pathology (Sano *et al.* 1999).

Studies have differed over whether there is any evidence of repair (granulation tissue) in ruptured tendons. There have been observations of hypervascular areas with fibroblast proliferation in close proximity to avascular regions of limited cellularity. Cell and vessel proliferation, sometimes described as an angiofibroblastic response (Nirschl and Pettrone 1973), is thought to represent a repair process, although there was no evidence of repair activity at the proximal tendon stumps (Fukuda *et al.* 1990). The cause of dysfunction in the supraspinatus has been linked to a combination of mechanical weakening and pain secondary to impingement caused by a swollen tendon (Uhthoff and Sano 1997).

Painful tendinopathy

Similar histopathological features of degeneration have been identified in the mid-substance of tendons affected by chronic pain such as the Achilles, patellar, posterior tibialis, and common extensor tendons at the lateral epicondyle (tennis elbow) (Fig. 1.1.17) (Chard *et al.* 1994; King *et al.* 2000; Puddu *et al.* 1976; Mosier *et al.*

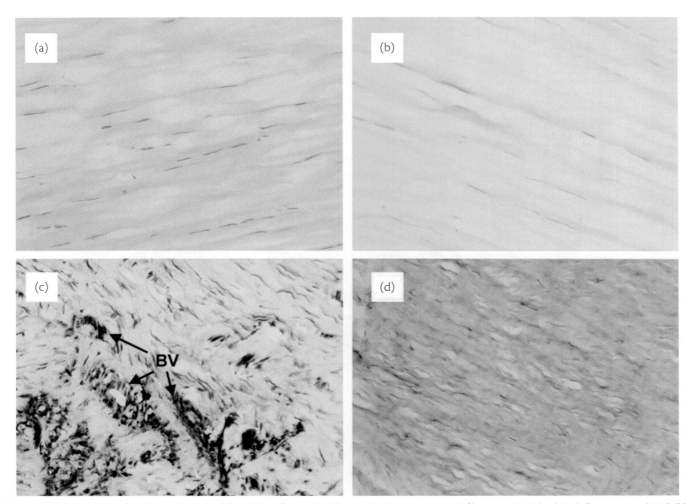

Fig. 1.1.17 Histopathology of painful tendinopathy. (a) Histology of normal Achilles tendon, showing organized, fibrous matrix with relatively few tenocytes (H&E). (b) Relative absence of glycosaminoglycan (GAG) in normal Achilles (toluidine blue). (c) 'Angiofibroblastic' activity in painful Achilles tendinopathy, showing increase in cell number and blood vessels (BV). (d) Increased GAG (blue) in painful tendinopathy, showing distribution throughout matrix (toluidine blue).

1999; Tallon *et al.* 2001). Very few (if any) specimens show evidence of inflammation such as chronic inflammatory cells (macrophages). Typical observations in Achilles tendinopathy include abnormal fibre structure and arrangement, focal variations in cellularity (both increased and decreased), rounded nuclei, and an increased non-collagenous matrix (Tallon *et al.* 2001; Movin *et al.* 1997). Increased vascularity was found in 65 per cent of pathological specimens and in 28 per cent of controls (Movin *et al.* 1997). The amount of proteoglycan was increased, found interspersed between the fibrils, sometimes as vacuolated 'lakes' (Movin *et al.* 1997).

In the Achilles, pain may be located at the insertion or in the tendon mid-substance (Puddu *et al.* 1976; Myerson and McGarvey 1998). At the insertion, degenerative features include longitudinal fissures and transverse tears in the fibrocartilage, bony spurs, and granulation tissue (Myerson and McGarvey 1998; Rufai *et al.* 1995). There is an association of calcification with mucoid degeneration (GAG infiltration), and the bony spurs form by a process of endochondral ossification following vascular invasion of the fibrocartilage (Rufai *et al.* 1995; Benjamin *et al.* 2000). In non-insertional Achilles tendon pain, the underlying tendinosis may or may not be associated with inflammation of the paratenon (paratenonitis) (Puddu *et al.* 1976). Other studies have shown that inflammation of the paratenon is only rarely found in Achilles tendinopathy (Astrom and Rausing 1995).

Calcific tendinitis

Relatively few detailed histopathological studies of calcific tendinitis have been published. Two theories have dominated the literature regarding the possible pathogenesis of the condition. Some authors believe that mineralization results from necrotic, degenerative changes in the tendon (Urist *et al.* 1964; Codman 1934). Indeed, calcific deposits are a common feature of degenerative tendinopathy, and found in many different tendons (Jarvinen *et al.* 1997; Riley *et al.* 1996). In contrast, others have postulated that calcification is the result of an endochondral transition, with mineral deposition occurring in a cartilaginous rudiment following chondrogenic metaplasia of the tenocytes (Uhthoff 1975; Uhthoff *et al.* 1976). Studies of calcific tendinitis in supraspinatus tendons have not supported this hypothesis, showing an absence of type II collagen and alkaline phosphatase, both of which should be associated with chondrogenesis (Archer *et al.* 1993). Uhthoff *et al.* recognized that there are two separate conditions associated with calcification of soft tissues (Uhthoff and Sarkar 1991). One is degenerative and the other a cell-mediated process that is self-limiting and will eventually resolve. The nature and size of the deposit varies markedly, and a distinction must be made between mineralization and ossification (the formation of bone) (Rooney 1994). The formation of bone in tendon is normal in some tendons, particularly in the avian, and can also develop spontaneously in pathological conditions such as myositis ossificans, ankylosing spondylitis, and diffuse idiopathic skeletal hyperostosis (DISH) (Rooney 1994). Bone also develops following mid-point tenotomy of rodent Achilles tendons, with the formation of a cartilaginous intermediate in the regenerating granulation tissue (Rooney *et al.* 1992; Rooney *et al.* 1993). Osteogenic precursor cells were thought to derive from the tendon cells themselves, and not from circulating progenitors (Rooney 1994; Rooney *et al.* 1993). We have recently demonstrated endochondral ossification in some Achilles and

patellar tendinopathy specimens, resulting in discrete mineralized bony deposits (Fenwick *et al.* 2002). These deposits showed a cartilaginous tissue consisting of type II collagen and the presence of both osteoblasts and osteoclasts within the bony nodule (Fig. 1.1.18). Tendons and ligaments appear to have an in-built capability to undergo cartilaginous and osteogenic transformation in certain pathological conditions and potentially as a result of trauma (Rooney 1994).

Biochemistry and molecular pathology of chronic tendinopathy

There have been relatively few biochemical studies of chronic tendinopathy, and most have been of material collected at the end-stage of the condition after tendon rupture. Studies of ruptured supraspinatus tendons have found a small but significant decrease in total collagen content, and an increased proportion of type III collagen relative to type I collagen (Riley *et al.* 1994). There was an increase in matrix proteoglycans and glycoproteins such as tenascin-C (Riley *et al.* 1996). These changes in composition are generally consistent with wound repair as described above. This analysis supports the contention that accumulated micro-injuries result in a gradual deterioration in the quality of the tendon matrix. There is a transformation from a tendon consisting of predominantly organized type I collagen fibrils, to a tissue consisting of randomly organized, small-diameter fibrils of types I and III collagen. Similar changes are found in animal tendons, after both acute tendon injuries and in chronic tendinopathies, and these changes have been shown to persist, resulting in permanently altered mechanical properties of the tissue (Williams *et al.* 1980; Watkins *et al.* 1985; Silver *et al.* 1983).

Although some of the changes found in ruptured tendons are likely to be the result of the tendon rupture and not the cause, there are other reasons to suspect that a change in collagen turnover precedes and predisposes to tendon rupture. A study of the molecular age of the collagen network by an analysis of pentosidine content demonstrated that up to 50 per cent of the collagen in control (cadaver) supraspinatus tendons had been replaced over the lifetime of the individual (Fig. 1.1.8) (Bank *et al.* 1999). An even greater proportion of collagen, up to 90 per cent of the total, was replaced in ruptured supraspinatus tendons (Bank *et al.* 1999). These data have since been supported by an analysis of the racemization of the amino acid aspartate, another indicator of the molecular age of the protein network (Riley *et al.* 2002). Since there were undetectable levels of immature collagen cross-links in these specimens, the data were consistent with increased remodelling of the collagen over a long time period—long enough to allow the maturation of the tri-functional HP cross-links.

Increased collagen turnover in supraspinatus tendons has been associated with several members of the MMP family. In control supraspinatus tendons, levels of MMP-1, MMP-2, and MMP-3 activity were significantly higher compared to those in normal biceps brachii tendons, which showed little or no collagen turnover (Fig. 1.1.9) (Riley *et al.* 2002). In ruptured supraspinatus tendons, there were increased levels of MMP-1 activity, reduced levels of MMP-2 and MMP-3, and increased collagen denaturation and turnover (Riley *et al.* 2002). MMP-3 (stromelysin 1) is thought to be a key regulatory enzyme in the control of matrix turnover, and a decline in this enzyme activity may represent a failure in the control of the normal remodelling process. Thus tendinopathy may

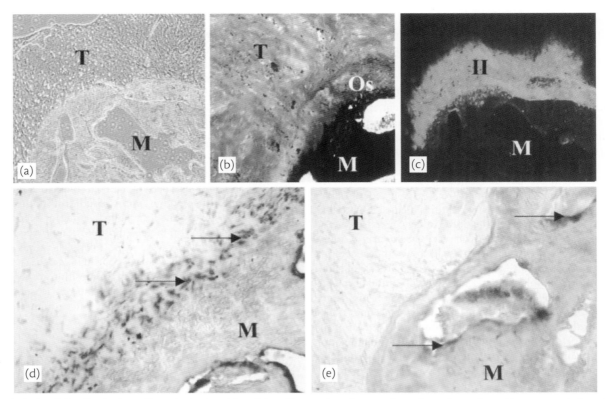

Fig. 1.1.18 Endochondral ossification in tendinopathy. A mineral deposit found in a specimen from patella tendinopathy was formed by a process similar or identical to endochondral ossification. Type II collagen was prominent in the matrix adjacent to the deposit, and markers of osteoblasts and osteoclasts were found in cells at the edge and within the deposit. (a) Phase contrast microscopy of mineral deposit. (b) Von Kossa staining of the calcific material (black), (c) Immunofluorescence staining of type II collagen (green). (d) Alkaline phosphatase activity, a marker of osteoblasts (red). (e) Tartrate-resistant acid phosphatase activity, a marker of osteoclasts (red). T, Tendon; M, Mineral deposit.

result from a failure to repair or maintain the tendon matrix in response to mechanical strain or microtrauma.

The key role of MMPs in chronic tendinopathy is further supported by the effect of a broad-spectrum inhibitor of metalloproteinases (Marimistat), which induces tendinopathy by an as yet unknown mechanism (Millar *et al.* 1998). Detailed studies are required to determine which metalloproteinase activities are implicated, whether an MMP, ADAM, or ADAM-TS enzyme. Interestingly, other compounds such as fluoroquinolone antibiotics, which can induce tendinopathy in some patients, have recently been shown to modulate MMP activity *in vitro*. Studies on canine tenocytes showed a stimulation of a caseinase activity (possibly MMP-3) by canine tenocytes treated with ciprofloxacin (Williams *et al.* 2000). We have shown no effect of ciprofloxacin on MMP-3 expression by human tenocytes, although pre-treatment with ciprofloxacin had a differential effect on the stimulation of MMPs by IL-1, increasing MMP-3 (protein) synthesis but not that of MMP-1 (Corps *et al.* 2002).

The importance of matrix remodelling activity in tendon was further emphasized in recent molecular studies of tendinopathy. Multiple changes in gene expression were detected in Achilles tendinopathy using cDNA arrays (Ireland *et al.* 2001). Of 265 genes that were analysed, 17 genes were upregulated and 23 were downregulated in degenerate tissue samples (Fig. 1.1.19). The absence of inflammation within the tendon was confirmed, and there were large increases in the expression of matrix genes such as collagen

types I and III that were consistent with an attempt at repair. Proteoglycan mRNAs, such as versican, biglycan, and a cell-surface-associated heparan sulfate proteoglycan (HSPG2), were increased although there was no change in decorin mRNA. Matrix glycoproteins such as laminin, SPARC (secreted protein, acidic and rich in cysteine), and tenascin-C were also increased. In addition to matrix genes, there were also changes in MMP expression. The greatest difference between normal and pathological specimens was in the level of MMP-3 (stromelysin), which was present in normal Achilles and absent in tendinopathy specimens. This change was shown to be reflected in the level of MMP-3 protein and was similar to that reported in degenerate supraspinatus tendons (above). The data support the hypothesis that MMP-3 activity is required for normal tendon maintenance, at least in highly stressed tendons such as the supraspinatus and the Achilles.

Despite many elegant hypotheses, the factors that regulate matrix synthesis and degradation in chronic tendinopathy have not been characterized. Matrix interactions, insoluble deposits, mechanical strain, and neuropeptides (to name but a few factors) may have a direct effect on the cellular expression of matrix and enzyme activities. Very few studies have attempted to address the role of specific growth factors and cytokines in tendinopathy.

A study of TGFβ expression in the Achilles showed that one isoform (TGFβ2) was predominant in the fibrillar matrix of both normal and pathological tendons (Fenwick *et al.* 2001). Although TGFβ2 was slightly increased in Achilles tendinopathy, an absence

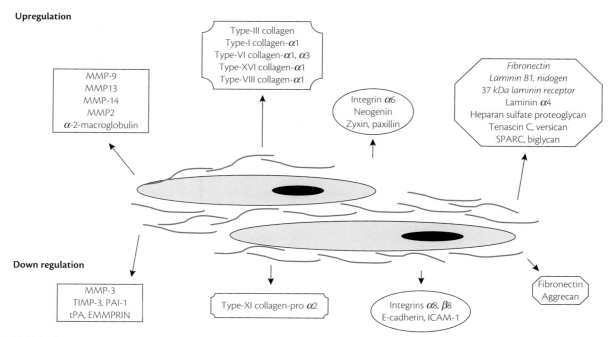

Upregulation

MMP-9
MMP13
MMP-14
MMP2
α-2-macroglobulin

Type-III collagen
Type-I collagen-α1
Type-VI collagen-α1, α3
Type-XVI collagen-α1
Type-VIII collagen-α1

Integrin α6
Neogenin
Zyxin, paxillin

Fibronectin
Laminin B1, nidogen
37 kDa laminin receptor
Laminin α4
Heparan sulfate proteoglycan
Tenascin C, versican
SPARC, biglycan

Down regulation

MMP-3
TIMP-3, PAI-1
tPA, EMMPRIN

Type-XI collagen-pro α2

Integrins α8, β8
E-cadherin, ICAM-1

Fibronectin
Aggrecan

Fig. 1.1.19 Multiple changes in gene expression in chronic tendinopathy. Differential expression of genes for ECM and cell-adhesion molecules in degenerate Achilles tendon compared to normal, as identified by ATLAS™ cDNA arrays (Clontech, USA). Major changes, such as the increased expression of collagen type I and type III, and decreased expression of MMP-3 and TIMP-3, were confirmed by real-time reverse transcription polymerase chain reaction. (Reproduced (modified) from Corps *et al.* (2002), © 2001, with permission from Elsevier Science.)

of one of the TGFβ signalling receptors (TGFβ-R1) suggested that TGFβ signalling was not actually taking place in the tendon. Consequently, a failure to control matrix degradation may result from a failure to upregulate TIMPs in response to TGF/3. This observation leads to the tentative hypothesis that the addition of growth factors such as TGFβ to facilitate tendon repair may be ineffective in chronic tendinopathy. It is also consistent with the hypothesis that the chronic nature of tendinopathy represents a failure to appropriately regulate the cell activities during tendon repair and remodelling. Currently there are no therapies for tendinopathy that specifically address this problem.

Future directions

More work needs to be done to characterize the heterogeneous cell populations that populate tendons and ligaments and to determine how these cells respond to injury. We need to understand how ageing affects cell activities in different soft connective tissues, and how alterations in matrix structure and composition modulate the cell response to injury and stress. The mechanical environment plays a fundamental role in the regulation of cell activity, and future studies will increase our understanding of the signal transduction pathways involved in the response to different stresses and strains.

Presently much of our knowledge of soft tissue injury and repair is derived from studies of acute injuries in immature animals. There is a relative dearth of information about chronic pathology due to the absence of animal models that recreate the conditions seen in patients. These models may be developed once the pathology is better described in humans, allowing us to test new treatments.

Little is known about early stages of the disease since most tissue samples reaching the laboratory come from the late or end-stage of the condition. Needle biopsies guided by ultrasound have recently been used to take small pieces of tendon from patients with chronic Achilles tendon pain, with no apparent ill effect (Movin *et al.* 1997). The application of ultrasensitive techniques of molecular analysis to these biopsy specimens may allow us to identify changes in gene and protein expression at earlier stages, potentially identifying new targets for future research.

Diagnosis of soft tissue pathology is currently difficult due to the lack of biopsy material, and the absence of objective methods and criteria to assess the pathological process. Advances in imaging technologies such as magnetic resonance imaging (MRI) and ultrasound have already led to significant improvements in the diagnosis of soft tissue pathology, and these techniques are going to become more sensitive, more affordable, and more widely used in the objective assessment of individual conditions. In the future, early changes in protein structure and composition may be monitored by non-invasive techniques such as nuclear magnetic resonance (NMR) spectroscopic analysis. Already the biochemical analysis of protein degradation products released into the bloodstream or synovial fluid is leading to their identification as potential markers for early tendon damage in horses, and a similar approach may be applied in human tendinopathies.

Based on the premise that much tendon and ligament pathology represents a failure by the resident cell population to adequately repair or maintain tissue after 'injury' (however caused), future treatment strategies may be targeted at improving the cellular activity in these tissues. Direct applications of recombinant growth factors such as TGFβ, PDGF, and IGF have been shown to have some possible benefit in animal models. However, application of these growth factors as proteins, given the proteolytic environment of many chronic wounds, may have little therapeutic use, particularly in the long term. There are problems of delivering these proteins and maintaining their concentration at the site of injury. An alternative strategy now being developed in animal models of tendon and ligament injury involves gene therapy. This can take a variety of forms, with one approach being to insert a gene encoding a particular growth factor into target cells at the wound site, increasing levels of expression and thus enhancing repair. Another approach is to apply small sequences of 'antisense' DNA, which bind to a specific gene and inhibit its expression, thus modulating some aspect of the wound healing response such as the formation of collagen fibrils. It is early days for these technologies, although the first clinical trials involving gene therapy on patients are now in progress.

Tissue repair requires a viable cell population that is able to respond to tissue injury and produce matrix of the correct composition and structure. All soft connective tissues are of mesenchymal origin, and contain a mixed population of cells. Some cells are less differentiated and specialized than others, and participate more actively in the repair response. Some of these cells may be derived from precursors known as 'stem cells', and enter tissues after injury or remain dormant in tissues as vascular 'pericytes'. Currently there is major research interest in developing ways to isolate and culture mesenchymal stem cells that may be used to repopulate sites of tendon injury and maintain the structure and composition of the tissue (Young *et al.* 1998).

Where tissues are extensively damaged, after cruciate ligament rupture, for example, there is currently no better option than to reconstruct the ligament, frequently using the central portion of the patient's own patellar tendon or hamstring. Alternative approaches with artificial materials such as carbon fibre have been disappointing. In the future, tissue engineering is likely to have a major impact on the reconstruction of soft tissues (Woo *et al.* 1999). Techniques are being developed so as to create whole tissues in culture that replicate the structure and composition of the original tissue. Cartilage, skin, ligaments, and tendons have all been constructed from stem cells and supporting three-dimensional matrices, and it is surely only a matter of time before artificially grown ligaments and tendons are surgically transplanted into patients.

Summary

Ligaments and tendons are more complex and heterogeneous than commonly thought. They are metabolically active and responsive to changes in their mechanical and chemical environment. Injury results in substantial and often permanent changes in the quantity and quality of the ECM. There are regional differences in the response to injury that are related to the tissue cellularity, vascularity, composition, and organization. The repair tissue can be affected and modulated by physical and chemical factors, although the precise conditions required to optimize repair have not been defined scientifically. In tendon, most pathology is degenerative, resulting either in a 'spontaneous' tendon rupture or chronic (painful) tendinopathy, sometimes associated with calcification. Degeneration has been shown to be an active, cell-mediated process involving increased levels of matrix remodelling, with the increased synthesis and degradation of matrix components mediated by a variety of enzymes. The source of pain in chronic tendinopathy is uncertain, since inflammatory mediators may not be present in the tendon, although mediators of pain and inflammation may be increased in the surrounding peri-tendinous tissues or fluids. Current forms of treatment are based largely on empirical observations and their effectiveness is questionable. More clinical and experimental work remains to be done to develop a scientific approach to therapy.

Acknowledgements

The author gratefully acknowledges past and present members of the Rheumatology Research Unit who have all contributed in some part to the work presented in this chapter. Funding for the various research projects conducted at the Rheumatology Research Unit was provided by the Arthritis Research Campaign, The Isaac Newton Trust, REMEDI, The Wishbone Trust, The Sybil Eastwood Trust, and the Cambridge Arthritis Research Endeavour (CARE).

References

Abbaszade, I., Liu, R.Q., Yang, F., Rosenfeld, S.A., Ross, O.H., Link, J.R., *et al.* (1999). Cloning and characterization of ADAMTS11, and an aggrecanase from the ADAMTS family. *J. Biol. Chem.* **274**, 23443–23450.

Adams, C.W.M. and Bayliss, O.B. (1973). Acid mucosubstances underlying lipid deposits in ageing tendons and atherosclerotic arteries. *Atherosclerosis* **18**, 191–195.

Ågren, M.S., Taplin, C.J., Woessner, J.F. Jr., Eaglstein, W.H., and Mertz, P.M. (1992). Collagenase in wound healing: Effect of wound age and type. *J. Invest. Dermatol.* **99**, 709–714.

Ahmed, I.M., Lagopoulos, M., McConnell, P., Soames, R.W., and Sefton, G.K. (1998). Blood supply of the Achilles tendon. *J. Orthop. Res.* **16**, 591–596.

Akali, A., Khan, U., Khaw, P.T., and McGrouther, A.D. (1999). Decrease in adhesion formation by a single application of 5-fluorouracil after flexor tendon injury. *Plast. Reconstr. Surg.* **103**, 151–158.

Akermark, C., Crone, H., Elsasser, U., and Forsskahl, B. (1995). Glycosaminoglycan polysulfate injections in lateral humeral epicondylalgia: a placebo-controlled double-blind trial. *Int. J. Sports Med.* **16**, 196–200.

Akeson, W.H., Amiel, D., and La Violette, D. (1967). The connective tissue response to immobility: a study of the chondroitin 4 sulphate and 6-sulphate and dermatan sulphate changes in periarticular connective tissues of control and immobilized knees of dogs. *Clin. Orthop. Rel. Res.* **51**, 183–197.

Alfredson, H., Thorsen, K., and Lorentzon, R. (1999). *In situ* microdialysis in tendon tissue: high levels of glutamate, but not prostaglandin E2 in chronic Achilles tendon pain. *Knee Surg. Sports Traumatol. Arthrosc.* **7**, 378–381.

Alfredson, H., Ljung, B.O., Thorsen, K., and Lorentzon, R. (2000). *In vivo* investigation of ECRB tendons with microdialysis technique—no signs of inflammation but high amounts of glutamate in tennis elbow. *Acta Orthop. Scand.* **71**, 475–479.

Alfredson, H., Forsgren, S., Thorsen, K., and Lorentzon, R. (2001). *In vivo* microdialysis and immunohistochemical analyses of tendon tissue demonstrated high amounts of free glutamate and glutamate NMDAR1 receptors, but no signs of inflammation, in jumper's knee. *J. Orthop. Res.* **19**, 881–886.

Alfredson, H., Forsgren, S., Thorsen, K., Fahlstrom, M., Johansson, H., and Lorentzon, R. (2001). Glutamate NMDAR1 receptors localised to nerves in human Achilles tendons. Implications for treatment? *Knee Surg. Sports Traumatol. Arthrosc.* **9**, 123–126.

Almekinders L.C. (1990). The efficacy of nonsteroidal anti-inflammatory drugs in the treatment of ligament injuries. *Sports Med.* **9**, 137–142.

Almekinders, L.C. and Almekinders, S.V. (1994). Outcome in the treatment of chronic overuse sports injuries: a retrospective study. *J. Orthop. Sports Phys. Ther.* **19**, 157–161.

Almekinders, L.C. and Temple, J.D. (1998). Etiology, diagnosis, and treatment of tendonitis: an analysis of the literature. *Med. Sci. Sports Exerc.* **30**, 1183–1190.

Amadio, P.C., Berglund, L.J., and An, K.-N. (1992). Biochemically discrete zones of canine flexor tendon: evaluation of properties with a new photographic method. *J. Orthop. Res.* **10**, 198–204.

Amiel, D., Frank, C., Harwood, F., Fronek, J., and Akeson, W.H. (1984). Tendons and ligaments: a morphological and biochemical comparison. *J. Orthop. Res.* **1**, 257–265.

Amiel, D., Foulk, R.A., Harwood, F.L., and Akeson, W.H. (1989). Quantitative assessment by competitive ELISA of fibronectin in tendons and ligaments. *Matrix* **9**, 421–427.

Amiel, D., Frank, C.B., Harwood, F.L., Akeson, W.H., and Kleiner, J.B. (1987). Collagen alteration in medial collateral ligament healing in a rabbit model. *Connect. Tiss. Res.* **16**, 357–366.

Andriacchi, T., Sabiston, P., DeHaven, K., Dahners, L., Woo, S.L.-Y., Frank, C., *et al.* (1988). Ligament: injury and repair. In *Injury and repair of the muskuloskeletal soft tissues* (ed. S.L.-Y. Woo and J.A. Buckwalter), pp. 103–128. American Academy of Orthopaedic Surgeons, Park Ridge, Illinois.

Archer, R.S., Bayley, J.I.L., Archer, C.W., and Ali, S.Y. (1993). Cell and matrix changes associated with pathological calcification of the human rotator cuff tendons. *J. Anat.* **182**, 1–12.

Aspenberg, P. and Forslund, C. (1999). Enhanced tendon healing with GDF 5 and 6. *Acta Orthop. Scand.* **70**, 51–54.

Astrom, M. and Westlin, N. (1994). Blood-flow in chronic Achilles tendinopathy. *Clin. Orthop. Rel. Res.* **308**, 166–172.

Astrom, M. and Rausing, A. (1995). Chronic Achilles tendinopathy. A survey of surgical and histopathologic findings. *Clin. Orthop.* **316**, 151–164.

Athanasou, N.A., West, L., Sallie, B., and Puddle, B. (1995). Localized amyloid deposition in cartilage is glycosaminoglycans-associated. *Histopathology* **26**, 267–272.

Aumailley, M. and Gayraud, B. (1998). Structure and biological activity of the extracellular matrix. *J. Mol. Med.* **76**, 253–265.

Bailey, A.J., Paul, R.G., and Knott, L. (1998). Mechanisms of maturation and ageing of collagen. *Mech. Ageing Dev.* **106**, 1–56.

Bailey, A.J., Robins, S.P., and Balian, G. (1974). Biological significance of the intermolecular crosslinks of collagen. *Nature* **251**, 105–109.

Bailey, A.J., Sims, T.J., Avery, N.C., and Miles, C.A. (1993). Chemistry of collagen cross-links: glucose-mediated covalent cross-linking of type-IV collagen in lens capsules. *Biochem. J.* **296**, 489–96.

Bainbridge, L.C., Robertson, C., Gillies, D., and Elliot, D. (1994). A comparison of post-operative mobilization of flexor tendon repairs with 'passive flexion-active extension' and 'controlled active motion' techniques. *J. Hand Surg. (Br.)* **19B**, 517–521.

Baktir, A., Türk, C.Y., Kabak, S., Sahin, V., and Kardas, Y. (1996). Flexor tendon repair in zone 2 followed by early active mobilization. *J. Hand Surg. (Br.)* **21B**, 624–628.

Banes, A.J., Link, G.W., Bevin, A.G., Peterson, H.D., Gillespie, Y., Bynum, D., *et al.* (1988). Tendon synovial cells secrete fibronectin *in vivo* and *in vitro*. *J. Orthop. Res.* **6**, 73–82.

Banes, A.J., Donlon, K., Link, G.W., Gillespie, Y., Bevin, A.G., Peterson, H.D. *et al.* (1988). Cell populations of tendon: a simplified method for isolation of synovial cells and internal fibroblasts. Confirmation of origin and biologic properties. *J. Orthop. Res.* **6**, 83–94.

Banes, A.J., Tsuzaki, M., Hu, P., Brigman, B., Brown, T., Almekinders, L., *et al.* (1995). PDGF-BB, and IGF-I and mechanical load stimulate DNA synthesis in avian tendon fibroblasts in vitro. *J. Biomech.* **28**, 1505–1513.

Bank, R.A., TeKoppele, J.M., Oostingh, G., Hazleman, B.L., and Riley, G.P. (1999). Lysylhydroxylation and non-reducible cross-linking of human supraspinatus tendon collagen: changes with age and in chronic rotator cuff tendinitis. *Ann. Rheum. Dis.* **58**, 35–41.

Batten, M.L., Hansen, J.C., and Dahners, L.E. (1996). Influence of dosage and timing of application of platelet-derived growth factor on early healing of the rat medial collateral ligament. *J. Orthop. Res.* **14**, 736–741.

Benjamin, M., Qin, S., and Ralphs, J.R. (1995). Fibrocartilage associated with human tendons and their pulleys. *J. Anat.* **187**, 625–633.

Benjamin, M. and Ralphs, J.R. (1998). Fibrocartilage in tendons and ligaments—an adaptation to compressive load. *J. Anat.* **193**, 481–494.

Benjamin, M., Rufai, A., and Ralphs, J.R. (2000). The mechanism of formation of bony spurs (enthesophytes) in the achilles tendon. *Arthritis Rheum.* **43**, 576–583.

Berenson, M.C., Blevins, F.T., Plaas, A.H.K., and Vogel, K.G. (1996). Proteoglycans of human rotator cuff tendons. *J. Orthop. Res.* **14**, 518–525.

Birch, H.L., Rutter, G.A., and Goodship, A.E. (1997). Oxidative energy metabolism in equine tendon cells. *Res. Vet. Sci.* **62**, 93–97.

Birk, D.E. and Mayne, R. (1997). Localization of collagen types I, III and V during tendon development. Changes in collagen types I and III are correlated with changes in fibril diameter. *Eur. J. Cell Biol.* **72**, 352–361.

Bornstein, P. (1992). Thrombospondins: structure and regulation of expression. *FASEB J.* **6**, 3290–3299.

Boykiw, R., Sciore, P., Reno, C., Marchuk, L., Frank, C.B., and Hart, D.A. (1998). Altered levels of extracellular matrix molecule mRNA in healing rabbit ligaments. *Matrix Biol.* **17**, 371–378.

Bray, D.F., Bray, R.C., and Frank, C.B. (1993). Ultrastructural immunolocalization of type-VI collagen and chondroitin sulphate in ligament. *J. Orthop. Res.* **11**, 677–685.

Briggs, M.D., Hoffman, S.M., King, L.M., Olsen, A.S., Mohrenweiser, H., Leroy, J.G., *et al.* (1995). Pseudoachondroplasia and multiple epiphyseal dysplasia due to mutations in the cartilage oligomeric matrix protein gene. *Nat. Genet.* **10**, 330–336.

Brooks, C.H., Revell, W.J., and Heatley, F.W. (1992). A quantitative histological study of the vascularity of the rotator cuff tendon. *J. Bone Joint Surg. (Br.)* **74B**, 151–153.

Butler, D.L., Grood, E.S., Noyes, F.R., and Zernicke, R.F. (1978). Biomechanics of ligaments and tendons. *Exer. Sport Sci. Rev.* **6**, 125–181.

Campbell, M.A., Tester, A.M., Handley, C.J., Checkley, G.J., Chow, G.L., Cant, A.E., *et al.* (1996). Characterization of a large chondroitin sulfate proteoglycan present in bovine collateral ligament. *Arch. Biochem. Biophys.* **329**, 181–190.

Campbell, M.A., Winter, A.D., Ilic, M.Z., and Handley, C.J. (1996). Catabolism and loss of proteoglycans from cultures of bovine collateral ligament. *Arch. Biochem. Biophys.* **328**, 64–72.

Campbell, R.B., Wiggins, M.E., Cannistra, L.M., Fadale, P.D., and Akelman, E. (1996). Influence of steroid injection on ligament healing in the rat. *Clin. Orthop.* 242–253.

Carlstedt, C.A. (1987). Mechanical and chemical factors in tendon healing. *Acta Orthop. Scand.* 58 (suppl. **224**), 7–75.

Carlstedt, C.A., Madsen, K., and Wredmark, T. (1986). The influence of indomethacin on collagen synthesis during tendon healing in the rabbit. *Prostaglandins* **32**, 353–358.

Cawston, T.E. (1998). Matrix metallo proteinases and TIMPs: properties and implications for the rheumatic diseases. *Mol. Med. Today* **4**(3), 130–137.

Cawston, T.E., Curry, V.A., Summers, C.A., Clark, I.M., Riley, G.P., Life, P.F., *et al.* (1998). The role of oncostatin M in animal and human connective tissue collagen turnover and its localization within the rheumatoid joint. *Arthritis Rheum.* **41**, 1760–1771.

Cawston, T.E. (1995). Proteinases and inhibitors. *Br. Med. Bull.* **51**, 385–401.

Cawston, T.E. and Billington, C. (1996). Metalloproteinases in the rheumatic diseases. *J. Pathol.* **180**, 115–117.

Chang, J., Most, D., Stelnicki, E., Longaker, M., Silberstein, F.C., Lineaweaver, C., *et al.* (1998). Gene expression of transforming growth factor -1 in rabbit zone II flexor tendon wound healing: evidence for dual mechanisms of repair. *Plast. Reconstr. Surg.* **100**, 937–44.

Chang, J., Most, D., Thunder, R., Mehrara, B., Longaker, M.T., and Lineaweaver, W.C. (1998). Molecular studies in flexor tendon wound healing: the role of basic fibroblast growth factor gene expression. *J. Hand Surg. (Am.)* **23A**, 1052–1058.

Chard, M.D., Wright, J.K., and Hazleman, B.L. (1987). Isolation and growth characteristics of adult human tendon fibroblasts. *Ann. Rheum. Dis.* **46**, 385–390.

Chard, M.D., Gresham, A., and Hazleman, B.L. (1989). Age related changes in the rotator cuff. *Br. J. Rheumàtal.* **28**, 19.

Chard, M.D., Cawston, T.E., Riley, G.P., Gresham, A., and Hazleman, B.L. (1994). Rotator cuff degeneration and lateral epicondylitis: a comparative histological study. *Ann. Rheum. Dis.* **53**, 30–34.

Chesney, J. and Bucala, R. (1997). Peripheral blood fibrocytes: novel fibroblast-like cells that present antigen and mediate tissue repair. *Biochem. Soc. Trans.* **25**, 520–524.

Chevalier, X., Groult, N., Larget-Piet, B., Zardi, L., and Hornebeck, W. (1994). Tenascin distribution in articular cartilage from normal subjects and from patients with osteoarthritis and rheumatoid arthritis. *Arthritis Rheum.* **37**, 1013–1022.

Chiquet, M. and Fambrough, D.M. (1984). Chick myotendinous antigen. II. A novel extracellular glycoprotein complex consisting of large disulfide-linked subunits. *J. Cell Biol.* **98**, 1937–1946.

Clark, J.M. and Harryman, D.T. II (1992). Tendons, ligaments, and capsule of the rotator cuff. Gross and microscopic anatomy. *J. Bone Joint Surg. (Am.)* **74A**, 713–725.

Clark, S.C., Jones, M.W., Choudhury, R.R., and Smith, E. (1995). Bilateral patellar tendon rupture secondary to repeated local steroid injections. *J. Accid. Emerg. Med.* **12**, 300–301.

Cleary, S.F., Li-Ming, L., Graham, R., and Diegelman, R.F. (1988). Modulation of tendon fibroplasia by exogenous currents. *Bioelectromagnetics* **9**, 183–194.

Codman, E.A. (1934). *The shoulder.* Todd Co., Boston, Massachusetts.

Cole, A.S., Cordiner-Lawrie, S., Carr, A.J., and Athanasou, N.A. (2001). Localised deposition of amyloid in tears of the rotator cuff. *J. Bone Joint Surg. (Br.)* **83B**, 561–564.

Cooper, R.R. and Misol, S. (1970). Tendon and ligament insertion: a light and electron microscopic study. *J. Bone Joint Surg. (Am.)* **52A**, 1–20.

Corps, A.N., Harrall, R.L., Curry, V., Hazleman, B.L., and Riley, G.P. (2002). Ciprofloxacin enhances the stimulation of matrix metalloproteinase-3 expression by interleukin-1 in human tendon derived cells. *Arthritis Rheum.* **46**(11), 3034–3040.

Creemers, L.B., Jansen, I.D.C., Docherty, A.J.P., Reynolds, J.J., Beertsen, W., and Everts, V. (1998). Gelatinase A (MMP-2) and cysteine proteinases are essential for the degradation of collagen in soft connective tissue. *Matrix Biol.* **17**, 35–46.

Dalton, S.E., Cawston, T.E., Riley, G.P., Bayley, I.J.L., and Hazleman, B.L. (1995). Human tendon biopsy samples in organ culture produce procollagenase and tissue inhibitor of metalloproteinases. *Ann. Rheum. Dis.* **54**, 571–577.

Dexter, T.M. and White, H. (1990). Growth factors: growth without inflation. *Nature* **344**, 380–381.

DiCesare, P., Hauser, N., Lehman, D., Pasumarti, S., and Paulsson, M. (1994). Cartilage oligomeric matrix protein (COMP) is an abundant component of tendon. *FEBS Lett.* **354**, 237–240.

Duance, V.C., Restall, D.J., Beard, H., Bourne, F.J., and Bailey, A.J. (1977). The location of three collagen types in skeletal muscle. *FEBS Lett.* **79**, 248–252.

Duffy, F.J., Seiler, J.G., Gelberman, R.H., and Hergrueter, C.A. (1995). Growth factors and canine flexor tendon healing: initial studies in uninjured and repair models. *J. Hand Surg.* **20A**, 645–649.

Dyer, R.F. and Enna, C.D. (1976). Ultrastructural features of adult human tendon. *Cell Tissue Res.* **168**, 247–259.

Eastwood, M., Mudera, V.C., McGrouther, D.A., and Brown, R.A. (1998). Effect of precise mechanical loading on fibroblast populated collagen lattices: morphological changes. *Cell Motil. Cytoskeleton* **40**, 13–21.

Elliott, D.H. (1965). Structure and function of mammalian tendon. *Biol. Rev.* **40**, 392–421.

Ellis, E.H., Spadaro, J.A., and Becker, R.O. (1969). Trace elements in tendon collagen. *Clin. Orthop. Rel. Res.* **65**, 195–198.

Enwemeka, C.S. (1989). The effects of therapeutic ultrasound on tendon healing. A biomechanical study. *Am. J. Phys. Med. Rehabil.* **68**, 283–287.

Evans, N.A., Bowrey, D.J., and Newman, G.R. (1998). Ultrastructural analysis of ruptured tendon from anabolic steroid users. *Injury* **29**, 769–773.

Everts, V., Van der Zee, E., Creemers, L., and Beertsen, W. (1996). Phagocytosis and intracellular digestion of collagen, and its role in turnover and remodelling. *Histochem. J.* **28**, 229–245.

Eyre, D.R., Paz, M.A., and Gallop, P.M. (1984). Cross-linking in collagen and elastin. *Ann. Rev. Biochem.* **53**, 717–748.

Fan, L., Sarkar, K., Franks, D.J., and Uhthoff, H.K. (1997). Estimation of total collagen and types I and III collagen in canine rotator cuff tendons. *Calcif. Tissue Int.* **61**, 223–229.

Faryniarz, D.A., Chaponnier, C., Gabbiani, G., Yannas, I.V., and Spector, M. (1996). Myofibroblasts in the healing lapine medial collateral ligament: possible mechanisms of contraction. *J. Orthop. Res.* **14**, 228–237.

Fenwick, S.A., Curry, V., Harrall, R.L., Hazleman, B.L., and Riley, G.P. (2002). Endochondral ossification in Achilles and patella tendinopathy. *Rheumatology,* in press.

Fenwick, S.A., Curry, V., Harrall, R.L., Hazleman, B.L., Hackney, R., and Riley, G.P. (2001). Expression of transforming growth factor-beta isoforms and their receptors in chronic tendinosis. *J. Anat.* **199**, 231–240.

Flint, M.H., Craig, A.S., Reilly, H.C., Gillard, G.C., and Parry, D.A.D. (1984). Collagen fibril diameters and glycosaminoglycan content of skins—indices of tissue maturity and function. *Connect. Tiss. Res.* **13**, 69–81.

Floridi, A., Ippolito, E., and Postacchini, F. (1981). Age-related changes in the metabolism of tendon cells. *Connect. Tissue Res.* **9**, 95–97.

Forslund, C. and Aspenberg, P. (2001). Tendon healing stimulated by injected CDMP-2. *Med. Sci. Sports Exerc.* **33**, 685–687.

Frank, C., McDonald, D., and Shrive, N. (1997). Collagen fibril diameters in the rabbit medial collateral ligament scar: A longer term assessment. *Connect. Tissue Res.* **36**, 261–269.

Frank, C., McDonald, D., Wilson, J., Eyre, D., and Shrive, N. (1995). Rabbit medial collateral ligament scar weakness is associated with decreased collagen pyridinoline crosslink density. *J. Orthop. Res.* **13**, 157–165.

Freeman, B.J. and Rooker, G.D. (1995). Spontaneous rupture of the anterior cruciate ligament after anabolic steroids. *Br. J. Sports Med.* **29**, 274–275.

Fritze, J. (1998). [Extracorporeal shockwave therapy (ESWT) in orthopedic indications: a selective review.] *Versicherungsmedizin* **50**, 180–185.

Fujioka, H., Wang, G.J., Mizuno, K., Balian, G., and Hurwitz, S.R. (1997). Changes in the expression of type-X collagen in the fibrocartilage of rat Achilles tendon attachment during development. *J. Orthop. Res.* **15**, 675–681.

Fujita, M., Hukuda, S., and Doida, Y. (1992). The effect of constant direct electrical current on intrinsic healing in the flexor tendon in vitro. An ultrastructural study of differing attitudes in epitenon cells and tenocytes. *J. Hand Surg. (Br.)* **17B**, 94–98.

Fukuda, H., Hamada, K., and Yamanaka, K. (1990). Pathology and pathogenesis of bursal-side rotator cuff tears viewed from *en bloc* histologic sections. *Clin. Orthop.* **254**, 75–80.

Fukuta, S., Oyama, M., Kavalkovich, K., Fu, F.H., and Niyibizi, C. (1998). Identification of types II, IX and X collagens at the insertion site of the bovine Achilles tendon. *Matrix Biol.* **17**, 65–73.

Gailit, J. and Clark, R.A.F. (1994). Wound repair in the context of extracellular matrix. *Curr. Opin. Cell Biol.* **6**, 717–725.

Garner, W.L., McDonald, J.A., Koo, M., Kuhn, C., and Weeks, P.M. (1989). Identification of the collagen producing cells in healing flexor tendons. *Plast. Reconstr. Surg.* **83**(5), 875–878.

Garrett, N.E., Mapp, P.I., Cruwys, S.C., Kidd, B.L., and Blake, D.R. (1992). Role of substance P in inflammatory arthritis. *Ann. Rheum. Dis.* **51**, 1014–1018.

Gelberman, R.H., Goldberg, V., An, K.-N., and Banes, A. (1988). Tendon. In *Injury and repair of the musculoskeletal soft tissues* (ed. S.L.-Y. Woo and J.A. Buckwalter), pp. 1–40. American Academy of Orthopaedic Surgeons, Park Ridge, Illinois.

Gelberman, R.H., Steinberg, D., Amiel, D., and Akeson, W.H. (1991). Fibroblast chemotaxis after wound repair. *J. Hand Surg. (Am.)* **16A**, 686–693.

Gelberman, R.H., Manske, P.R., Vande Berg, J.S., Lesker, P.A., and Akeson, W.H. (1984). Flexor tendon repair *in vitro*: a comparative histologic study of the rabbit, chicken, dog, and and monkey. *J. Orthop. Res.* **2**, 39–48.

Gelberman, R.H., Woo, S.L., Lothringer, K., Akeson, W.H., and Amiel, D. (1982). Effects of early intermittent passive mobilization on healing canine flexor tendons. *J. Hand Surg. (Am.)* **7A**, 170–175.

Gillard, G.C., Reilly, H.C., Bell-Booth, P.G., and Flint, M.H. (1979). The influence of mechanical forces on the glycosaminoglycan content of the rabbit flexor digitorum profundus tendon. *Connect. Tissue Res.* **7**, 37–46.

Gillis, C., Pool, R.R., Meagher, D.M., Stover, S.M., Reiser, K., and Willits, N. (1997). Effect of maturation and aging on the histomorphometric and biochemical characteristics of equine superficial digital flexor tendon. *Am. J. Vet. Res.* **58**, 425–430.

Girard, M.T., Matsubara, M., Kublin, C., Tessier, M.J., Cintron, C., and Fini, M.E. (1993). Stromal fibroblasts synthesize collagenase and stromelysin during long-term tissue remodelling. *J. Cell Sci.* **104**, 1001–1011.

Goldin, B., Block, W.D., and Pearson, J.R. (1980). Wound healing of tendon—i. physical, and mechanical and metabolic changes. *J. Biomech.* **13**, 241–256.

Gotoh, M., Hamada, K., Yamakawa, H., Tomonaga, A., Inoue, A., and Fukuda, H.O. (1997). Significance of granulation tissue in torn supraspinatus insertions: an immunohistochemical study with antibodies against interleukin-1, cathepsin, D., and matrix metalloprotease-1. *J. Orthop. Res.* **15**, 33–39.

Gotoh, M., Hamada, K., Yamakawa, H., Inoue, A., and Fukuda, H. (1998). Increased substance P in subacromial bursa and shoulder pain in rotator cuff diseases. *J. Orthop. Res.* **16**, 618–621.

Graham, M.F., Becker, H., Cohen, I.K., Merritt, W., and Diegelmann, R.F. (1984). Intrinsic tendon fibroplasia: documentation by *in vitro* studies. *J. Orthop. Res.* **1**, 251–256.

Greenlee, T.K. and Ross, R. (1967). The development of the rat flexor digital tendon, a fine structure study. *J. Ultrastruct. Res.* **18**, 353–376.

Greenwald, D., Mass, D., Gottlieb, L., and Tuel, R. (1991). Biomechanical analysis of intrinsic tendon healing *in vitro* and the effects of vitamins A and E. *Plast. Reconstr. Surg.* **87**, 925–930.

Grinnell, F., Ho, C.H., and Wysocki, A. (1992). Degradation of fibronectin and vitronectin in chronic wound fluid: analysis by cell blotting, immunoblotting, and cell adhesion assays. *J. Invest. Dermatol.* **98**, 410–416.

Gulcher, J.R., Nies, D.E., Alexakos, M.J., Ravikant, N.A., Sturgill, M.E., Marton, L.S., *et al.* (1991). Structure of the human hexabrachion (tenascin) gene. *Proc. Natl Acad. Sci., USA* **88**, 9438–9442.

Gum, S.L., Reddy, G.K., Stehno-Bittel, L., and Enwemeka, C.S. (1997). Combined ultrasound, electrical stimulation, and laser promote collagen synthesis with moderate changes in tendon biomechanics. *Am. J. Phys. Med. Rehabil.* **76**, 288–296.

Haake, M., Sattler, A., Gross, M.W., Schmitt, J., Hildebrandt, R., and Muller, H.H. (2001). [Comparison of extracorporeal shockwave therapy (ESWT) with roentgen irradiation in supraspinatus tendon syndrome—a prospective randomized single-blind parallel group comparison.] *Z. Orthop. Ihre Grenzgeb.* **139**, 397–402.

Haines, J.F. (1983). Bilateral rupture of the Achilles tendon in patients on steroid therapy. *Ann. Rheum. Dis.* **42**, 652–654.

Haralson, M.A. (1993). Extracellular matrix and growth factors: an integrated interplay controlling tissue repair and progression to disease. *Lab. Invest.* **69**, 369–372.

Hardingham, T.E. and Fosang, A.J. (1992). Proteoglycans: many forms and many functions. *FASEB J.* **6**, 861–870.

Hardingham, T.E. and Fosang, A.J. (1995). The structure of aggrecan and its turnover in cartilage. *J. Rheumatol.* 22 (Suppl. **43**), 86–90.

Harper, J., Amiel, D., and Harper, E. (1988). Collagenase production by rabbit ligaments and tendon. *Connect. Tissue Res.* **17**, 253–259.

Harper, J., Amiel, D., and Harper E. (1992). Inhibitors of collagenase in ligaments and tendons of rabbits immobilized for 4 weeks. *Connect. Tissue Res.* **28**, 257–261.

Hart, D.A., Frank, C.B., and Bray, R.C. (1995). Inflammatory processes in repetitive motion and overuse syndromes: potential role of neurogenic mechanisms in tendons and ligaments. In *Repetitive motion disorders of the upper extremity* (ed. S.L. Gordon, S.J. Blair, and L.J. Fine), pp. 247–262. American Association of Orthopaedic Surgeons, Rosemount, Illinois.

Hart, D.A., Kydd, A., and Reno, C. (1999). Gender and pregnancy affect neuropeptide responses of the rabbit Achilles tendon. *Clin. Orthop.* **365**, 237–246.

Hart, D.A., Archambault, J.M., Kydd, A., Reno, C., Frank, C.B., and Herzog, W. (1998). Gender and neurogenic variables in tendon biology and repetitive motion disorders. *Clin. Orthop.* **351**, 44–56.

Hart, D.A. and Reno, C. (1998). Pregnancy alters the *in vitro* responsiveness of the rabbit medial collateral ligament to neuropeptides: effect on mRNA levels for growth factors, cytokines, iNOS, COX-2, metalloproteinases and TIMPs. *Biochim. Biophys. Acta Mol. Basis Dis.* **1408**, 35–43.

Haut, R.C., Lancaster, R.L., and DeCamp, C.E. (1992). Mechanical properties of the canine patellar tendon: Some correlations with age and the content of collagen. *J. Biomech.* **25**, 163–173.

Hedbom, E. and Heinegård, D. (1993). Binding of fibromodulin and decorin to separate sites on fibrillar collagens. *J. Biol. Chem.* **268**, 27307–27312.

Heinegård, D., Hedbom, E., Antonsson, P., and Oldberg, A. (1990). Structural variability of large and small chondroitin sulphate/dermatan sulphate proteoglycans. *Biochem. Soc. Trans.* **18**, 209–212.

Hey, N.J., Handley, C.J., Ng, C.K., and Oakes, B.W. (1990). Characterisation and synthesis of macromolecules by adult collateral ligament. *Biochim. Biophys. Acta* **1034**, 73–80.

Hildebrand, A., Romarís, M., Rasmussen, L.M., Heinegård, D., Twardzik, D.R., Border, W.A., *et al.* (1994). Interaction of the small interstitial proteoglycans biglycan, and decorin and fibromodulin with transforming growth factor β. *Biochem. J.* **302**, 527–534.

Hildebrand, K.A., Woo, S.L., Smith, D.W., Allen, C.R., Deie, M., Taylor, B.J., *et al.* (1998). The effects of platelet-derived growth factor-BB on healing of the rabbit medial collateral ligament. An in vivo study. *Am. J. Sports Med.* **26**, 549–554.

Holz, U. (1980). [Achilles tendon rupture and achillodynia. The importance of tissue regeneration.] *Fortschr. Med.* **98**, 1517–1520.

Huang, H.H., Qureshi, A.A., and Biundo, J.J., Jr. (2000). Sports and other soft tissue injuries, tendinitis, bursitis, and occupation-related syndromes. *Curr. Opin. Rheumatol.* **12**, 150–154.

Inhofe, P.D., Grana, W.A., Egle, D., Min, K.W., and Tomasek, J. (1995). The effects of anabolic steroids on rat tendon. An ultrastructural, biomechanical, and biochemical analysis. *Am. J. Sports Med.* **23**, 227–232.

Iozzo, R.V. (1998). Matrix proteoglycans: from molecular design to cellular function. *Annu. Rev. Biochem.* **67**, 609–652.

Ippolito, E., Postacchini, F., and Ricciardi-Pollini, P.T. (1975). Biochemical variations in the matrix of human tendons in relation to age and pathological conoditions. *Ital. J. Orthop. Traum.* **1**, 133–139.

Ippolito, E., Natali, P.G., Postacchini, F., Accini, L., and de Martino, C. (1980). Morphological, immunological and biochemical study of rabbit achilles tendon at various ages. *J. Bone Joint Surg. (Am.)* **62A**, 583–598.

Ireland, D., Harrall, R.L., Holloway, G., Hackney, R., Hazleman, B., and Riley, G. (2001). Multiple changes in gene expression in chronic human Achilles tendinopathy. *Matrix Biol.* **20**, 159–169.

Iwuagwu, F.C. and McGrouther, D.A. (1998). Early cellular response in tendon injury: the effect of loading. *Plast. Reconstr. Surg.* **102**, 2064–2071.

Jarvinen, M., Józsa, L., Kannus, P., Jarvinen, T.L.N., Kvist, M., and Leadbetter, W. (1997). Histopathological findings in chronic tendon disorders. *Scand. J. Med. Sci. Sports* **7**, 86–95.

Johnston, R.B., Seiler, J.G., Miller, E.J., and Drvaric, D.M. (1995). The intrinsic and extrinsic ligaments of the wrist. A correlation of collagen typing and histologic appearance. *J. Hand Surg. (Br.)* **20B**, 750–754.

Jones, A.J. and Bee, J.A. (1990). Age and position related heterogeneity of equine tendon extracellullar matrix composition. *Res. Vet. Sci.* **48**, 357–364.

Józsa, L. and Kannus, P. (1997). Structure and metabolism of normal tendons. In *Human tendons. Anatomy physiology and pathology* (ed. L. Józsa and P. Kannus), pp. 46–95. Human Kinetics, Champaign, Illinois.

Józsa, L. and Kannus, P. (1997). Overuse injuries of tendons. *Human tendons: anatomy, physiology and pathology* (ed. L. Józsa and P. Kannus), pp. 164–253. Human Kinetics, Champaign, Illinois.

Józsa, L. and Kannus, P. (1997). Spontaneous rupture of tendons. In *Human tendons: anatomy, physiology and pathology* (ed. L. Józsa and P. Kannus), pp. 254–325. Human Kinetics, Champaign, Illinois.

Józsa, L., Kannus, P., Balint, J.B., and Reffy, A. (1991). Three-dimensional ultrastructure of human tendons. *Acta Anat. (Basel)* **142**, 306–312.

Józsa, L., Lehto, M., Kannus, P., Kvist, M., Reffy, A., Vieno, T., *et al.* (1989). Fibronectin and laminin in Achilles tendon. *Acta Orthop. Scand.* **60**, 469–471.

Józsa, L., Reffy, A., and Balint, B.J. (1984). The pathogenesis of tendolipomatosis—an electron microscope study. *Int Orthop SICOT* **7**, 251–255.

Józsa, L., Balint, B.J., and Reffy, A. (1980). Calcifying tendinopathy. *Arch. Orthop. Trauma Surg.* **97**, 305–307.

Kannus, P., Józsa, L., Jarvinen, T.A., Jarvinen, T.L., Kvist, M., Natri, A., *et al.* (1998). Location and distribution of non-collagenous matrix proteins in musculoskeletal tissues of rat. *Histochem. J.* **30**, 799–810.

Kannus, P. (1997). Etiology and pathophysiology of chronic tendon disorders in sports. *Scand. J. Med. Sci. Sports* **7**, 78–85.

Kannus, P. and Józsa, L. (1991). Histopathological changes preceding spontaneous rupture of a tendon. *J. Bone Joint Surg. (Am.)* **73A**, 1507–1525.

Karpakka, J.A., Pesola, M.K., and Takala, T.E. (1992). The effects of anabolic steroids on collagen synthesis in rat skeletal muscle and tendon. A preliminary report. *Am. J. Sports Med.* **20**, 262–266.

Kastelic, J., Galeski, A., and Baer, E. (1978). The multicomposite structure of tendon. *Connect. Tissue Res.* **6**, 11–23.

Kaushal, G.P. and Shah, S.V. (2000). The new kids on the block: ADAMTSs, and potentially multifunctional metalloproteinases of the ADAM family. *J. Clin. Invest.* **105**, 1335–1337.

Ker, R.F., Wang, X.T., and Pike, A.V.L. (2000). Fatigue quality of mammalian tendons. *J. Exp. Biol.* **203**, 1317–1327.

Khan, K.M., Cook, J.L., Bonar, F., Harcourt, P., and Astrom, M. (1999). Histopathology of common tendinopathies—Update and implications for clinical management. *Sports Med.* **27**, 393–408.

King, J.B., Cook, J.L., Khan, K.M., and Maffulli, N. (2000). Patellar tendinopathy. *Sports Med. Arthrosc. Rev.* **8**, 86–95.

Kobayashi, D., Kurosaka, M., Yoshiya, S., and Mizuno, K. (1997). Effect of basic fibroblast growth factor on the healing of defects in the canine anterior cruciate ligament. *Knee Surg. Sports Traumatol. Arthrosc.* **5**, 189–194.

Komurcu, M., Akkus, O., Basbozkurt, M., Gur, E., and Akkas, N. (1997). Reduction of restrictive adhesions by local aprotinin application and primary sheath repair in surgically traumatized flexor tendons of the rabbit. *J. Hand Surg. (Am.)* **22A**, 826–832.

Koob, T.J. and Vogel, K.G. (1987). Site related variations in glycosaminoglycan content and swelling properties of bovine flexor tendon. *J. Orthop. Res.* **5**, 414–424.

Koob, T.J., Clark, P.E., Hernandez, D.J., Thurmond, F.A., and Vogel, K.G. (1992). Compression loading *in vitro* regulates proteoglycan synthesis by tendon fibrocartilage. *Arch. Biochem. Biophys.* **298**, 303–312.

Kotnis, R.A., Halstead, J.C., and Hormbrey, P.J. (1999). Atraumatic bilateral Achilles tendon rupture: An association of systemic steroid treatment. *J. Accid. Emerg. Med.* **16**, 378–379.

Kulick, M.I., Smith, S., and Hadler, K. (1986). Oral ibuprofen: evaluation of its effect on peritendinous adhesions and the breaking strength of a tenorrhaphy. *J. Hand Surg. (Am.)* **11A**, 110–120.

Kumagai, J., Sarkar, K., and Uhthoff, H.K. (1994). The collagen types in the attachment zone of rotator cuff tendons in the elderly: an immunohistochemical study. *J. Rheumatol.* **21**, 2096–2100.

Kumagai, J., Sarkar, K., Uhthoff, H.K., Okawara, Y., and Ooshima, A. (1994). Immunohistochemical distribution of type I, II and III collagens in the rabbit supraspinatus tendon insertion. *J. Anat.* **185**, 279–284.

Kuno, K., Okada, Y., Kawashima, H., Nakamura, H., Miyasaka, M., Ohno, H., *et al.* (2000). ADAMTS-1 cleaves a cartilage proteoglycan, and aggrecan. *FEBS Lett.* **478**, 241–245.

Labat-Robert, J., Bihari-Varga, M., and Robert, L. (1990). Extracellular matrix. *FEBS Lett.* **268**, 386–393.

Lapiere, Ch.M., Nusgens, B., and Pierard, G.E. (1977). Interaction between collagen type I and type III in conditioning bundles organization. *Connect. Tissue Res.* **5**, 21–29.

Laseter, J.T. and Russell, J.A. (1991). Anabolic steroid-induced tendon pathology: a review of the literature. *Med. Sci. Sports Exerc.* **23**, 1–3.

Leadbetter, W.B. (1992). Cell-matrix response in tendon injury. *Clin. Sports Med.* **11**, 533–578.

Lee, J., Harwood, F.L., Akeson, W.H., and Amiel, D. (1998). Growth factor expression in healing rabbit medial collateral and anterior cruciate ligaments. *Iowa Orthop. J.* **18**, 19–25.

Lehto, M., Józsa, L., Kvist, M., Jarvinen, M., Balint, B.J., and Reffy, A. (1990). Fibronectin in the ruptured human Achilles tendon and its paratenon. An immunoperoxidase study. *Ann. Chir. Gynaecol.* **79**, 72–77.

Letson, A.K. and Dahners L.E. (1994). The effect of combinations of growth factors on ligament healing. *Clin. Orthop.* **308**, 207–212.

Lo, I.K.Y., Marchuk, L.L., Hart, D.A., and Frank, C.B. (1998). Comparison of mRNA levels for matrix molecules in normal and disrupted human anterior cruciate ligaments using reverse transcription polymerase chain reaction. *J. Orthop. Res.* **16**, 421–428.

Lundborg, G. and Rank, F. (1978). Experimental intrinsic healing of flexor tendons based upon synovial fluid nutrition. *J. Hand Surg.* **3**(1), 21–31.

Lundborg, G., Hansson, H.-A., Rank, F., and Rydevik, B. (1980). Superficial repair of severed flexor tendons in synovial environment. *J. Hand Surg.* **5**, 451–461.

Mackie, E.J., Halfter, W., and Liverani, D. (1988). Induction of tenascin in healing wounds. *J. Cell Biol.* **107**, 2757–2767.

Mackie, E.J. (1994). Tenascin in connective tissue development and pathogenesis. *Perspect. Dev. Neurobiol.* **2**, 125–132.

MacNab, I. (1973). Rotator cuff tendinitis. *Ann. R. Coll. Surg. Engl.* **52**, 271–287.

Maffulli, N., Ewen S.W.B., Waterston, S.W., Reaper, J., and Barrass, V. (2000). Tenocytes from ruptured and tendinopathic Achilles tendons produce greater quantities of type III collagen than tenocytes from normal Achilles tendons—An *in vitro* model of human tendon heating. *Am. J. Sports Med.* **28**, 499–505.

Maffulli, N., Khan, K.M., and Puddu, G. (1998). Overuse tendon conditions: time to change a confusing terminology. *Arthroscopy* **14**, 840–843.

Maffulli, N., Barrass, V., and Ewen, S.W. (2000). Light microscopic histology of Achilles tendon ruptures. A comparison with unruptured tendons. *Am. J. Sports Med.* **28**, 857–863.

Manske, P.R. and Lesker, P.A. (1984). Histologic evidence of intrinsic flexor tendon repair in various experimental animals. *Clin. Orthop. Rel. Res.* **182**, 297–304.

Margolis, R.U. and Margolis, R.K. (1994). Aggrecan-versican-neurocan family of proteoglycans. *Methods Enzymol.* **245**, 105–128.

Martin, D.F., Carlson, C.S., Berry, J., Reboussin, B.A., Gordon, E.S., and Smith, B.P. (1999). Effect of injected versus iontophoretic corticosteroid on the rabbit tendon. *South. Med. J.* **92**, 600–608.

Mass, D.P., Tuel, R.J., Labarbera, M., and Greenwald, D.P. (1993). Effects of constant mechanical tension on the healing of rabbit flexor tendons. *Clin. Orthop.* **296**, 301–6.

Matrisian, L.M. (1990). Metalloproteinases and their inhibitors in matrix remodelling. *Trends Genet.* **6**, 121–125.

Matrisian, L.M. (1992). The matrix degrading metalloproteinases. *BioEssays* **14**, 455–463.

McNeilly, C.M., Banes, A.J., Benjamin, M., and Ralphs, J.R. (1996). Tendon cells *in vivo* form a three dimensional network of cell processes linked by gap junctions. *J. Anat.* **189**, 593–600.

McWhorter, J.W., Francis, R.S., and Heckmann, R.A. (1991). Influence of local steroid injections on traumatized tendon properties. A biomechanical and histological study. *Am. J. Sports Med.* **19**, 435–439.

Mehr, D., Pardubsky, P.D., Martin, J.A., and Buckwalter, J.A. (2000). Tenascin-C in tendon regions subjected to compression. *J. Orthop. Res.* **18**, 537–545.

Merrilees, M.J., Tiang, K.M., and Scott, L. (1987). Changes in collagen fibril diameters across artery walls including a correlation with glycosaminoglycan content. *Connect. Tissue Res.* **16**, 237–257.

Merrilees, M.J. and Flint, M.H. (1980). Ultrastructural study of tension and pressure zones in a rabbit flexor tendon. *Am. J. Anat.* **157**, 87–106.

Michna, H. (1986). Organisation of collagen fibrils in tendon: changes induced by an anabolic steroid. I. Functional and ultrastructural studies. *Virchows Arch. B Cell Pathol. Incl. Mol. Pathol.* **52**, 75–86.

Miles, J.W., Grana, W.A., Egle, D., Min, K.-W., and Chitwood, J. (1992). The effect of anabolic steroids on the biomechanical and histological properties of rat tendon. *J. Bone Joint Surg. (Am.)* **74A**, 411–422.

Millar, A.W., Brown, P.D., Moore, J., Galloway, W.A., Cornish, A.G., Lenehan, T.J., *et al.* (1998). Results of single and repeat dose studies of the oral matrix metalloproteinase inhibitor marimastat in healthy male volunteers. *Br. J. Clin. Pharmacol.* **45**, 21–26.

Miller, R.R. and McDevitt, C.A. (1991). Thrombospondin in ligament, and meniscus and intervertebral disc. *Biochim. Biophys. Acta Gen. Subj.* **1115**, 85–88.

Moore, M.J. and De Beaux, A. (1987). A quantitative ultrastructural study of rat tendon from birth to maturity. *J. Anat.* **153**, 163–169.

Mosier, S.M., Pomeroy, G., and Manoli, A. (1999). Pathoanatomy and etiology of posterior tibial tendon dysfunction. *Clin. Orthop. Rel. Res.* **365**, 12–22.

Mottram, D.R. and George, A.J. (2000). Anabolic steroids. *Baillièr's Best. Pract. Res. Clin. Endocrinol. Metab.* **14**, 55–69.

Movin, T., Gad, A., Reinholt, P., and Rolf, C. (1997). Tendon pathology in long-standing achillodynia—biopsy findings in 40 patients. *Acta Orthop. Scand.* **68**, 170–175.

Movin, T., Guntner, P., Gad, A., and Rolf, C. (1997). Ultrasonography-guided percutaneous core biopsy in Achilles tendon disorder. *Scand. J. Med. Sci. Sports* **7**, 244–248.

Murphy, G., Willenbrock, F., Crabbe, T., O'Shea, M., Ward, R., Atkinson, S., *et al.* (1994). Regulation of matrix metalloproteinase activity. *Ann. NY Acad. Sci.* **732**, 31–41.

Murphy, G. and Willenbrock, F. (1995). Tissue inhibitors of matrix met-alloendopeptidases. *Methods Enzymol.* **248**, 496–510.

Murrell, G.A.C. (1994). Effects of immobilization on Achilles tendon healing in a rat model. *J. Orthop. Res.* **12**, 582–591.

Myerson, M.S. and McGarvey, W. (1998). Disorders of the insertion of the Achilles tendon and Achilles tendinitis. *J. Bone Joint Surg. (Am.)* **80A**, 1814–1824.

Nagase, H. (1994). Matrix metalloproteinases. A mini-review. *Contrib. Nephrol.* **107**, 85–93.

Nakamura, H., Fujii, Y., Inoki, I., Sugimoto, K., Tanzawa, K., Matsuki, H., *et al.* (2000). Brevican is degraded by matrix metalloproteinases and aggrecanase-1 (ADAMTS4) at different sites. *J. Biol. Chem.* **275**, 38885–38890.

Natsu-ume, T., Nakamura, N., Shino, K., Toritsuka, Y., Horibe, S., Ochi T. (1997). Temporal and spatial expression of transforming growth factor-β in the healing patellar ligament of the rat. *J. Orthop. Res.* **15**, 837–843.

Nessler, J.P., Amadio, P.C., Berglund, L.J., and An, K.-N. (1992). Healing of canine tendon in zones subjected to different mechanical forces. *J. Hand Surg. (Br.)* **17B**, 561–568.

Neuberger, A., Perrone, J.C., and Slack, H.G.B. (1951). The relative metabolic inertia of tendon collagen in the rat. *Biochem. J.* **49**, 199–204.

Newnham, D.M., Douglas, J.G., Legge, J.S., and Friend, J.A. (1991). Achilles tendon rupture: an underrated complication of corticosteroid treatment. *Thorax* **46**, 853–854.

Nielsen, H.M., Skalicky, M., and Viidik, A. (1998). Influence of physical exercise on aging rats. III. Life-long exercise modifies the aging changes of the mechanical properties of limb muscle tendons. *Mech. Ageing Dev.* **100**, 243–260.

Nirschl, R.P. and Pettrone, F.A. (1973). Tennis elbow. *J. Bone Joint Surg. (Am.)* **61A**, 832–839.

Niyibizi, C., Visconti, C.S., Kavalkovich, K., and Woo, S.L.-Y. (1994). Collagens in an adult bovine medial collateral ligament: immunofluorescence localization by confocal microscopy reveals that type XIV collagen predominates at the ligament-bone junction. *Matrix Biol.* **14**, 743–751.

Okuda, Y., Gorski, J.P., An, K.-N., and Amadio, P.C. (1987). Biochemical histological and biomechanical analyses of canine tendon. *J. Orthop. Res.* **5**, 60–68.

Oldberg, A., Antonsson, P., Lindblom, K., and Heinegård, D. (1992). COMP (cartilage oligomeric matrix protein) is structurally related to the thrombospondins. *J. Biol. Chem.* **267**, 22346–22350.

Oldberg, A., Antonnsson, P., Hedbom, E., and Heinegård, D. (1991). Structure and function of extracellular matrix proteoglycans. *Biochem. Soc. Trans.* **18**, 789–792.

Orhan, Z., Alper, M., Akman, Y., Yavuz, O., and Yalciner, A. (2001). An experimental study on the application of extracorporeal shock waves in the treatment of tendon injuries: preliminary report. *J. Orthop. Sci.* **6**, 566–570.

Oxlund, H. (1984). Changes in connective tisssues during corticotrophin and corticosteroid treatment. *Dan. Med. Bull.* **31**, 187–206.

O'Brien, M. (1992). Functional anatomy and physiology of tendons. *Clin. Sports Med.* **11**, 505–520.

O'Byrne, E.M., Blancuzzi, V., Wilson, D.E., Wong, M., and Jeng, A.Y. (1990). Elevated substance P and accelerated cartilage degradation in rabbit knees injected with interleukin-1 and tumor necrosis factor. *Arthritis Rheum.* **33**, 1023–1028.

Panossian, V., Liu, S.H., Lane, J.M., and Finerman, G.A.M. (1997). Fibroblast growth factor and epidermal growth factor receptors in ligament healing. *Clin. Orthop.* **342**, 173–180.

Parry, D.A., Barnes, G.R., and Craig, A.S. (1978). A comparison of the size distribution of collagen fibrils in connective tissues as a function of age and a possible relation between fibril size distribution and mechanical properties. *Proc. R. Soc. Lond B Biol. Sci.* **203**, 305–321.

Parssinen, M., Karila, T., Kovanen, V., and Seppala, T. (2000). The effect of supraphysiological doses of anabolic androgenic steroids on collagen metabolism. *Int. J. Sports Med.* **21**, 406–411.

Patterson-Kane, J.C., Parry, D.A., Birch, H.L., Goodship, A.E., and Firth, E.C. (1997). An age-related study of morphology and cross-link composition of collagen fibrils in the digital flexor tendons of young thoroughbred horses. *Connect. Tissue* Res. **36**, 253–26.

Patterson-Kane, J.C., Wilson, A.M., Firth, E.C., Parry, D.A.D., and Goodship, A.E. (1997). Comparison of collagen fibril populations in the superficial digital flexor tendons of exercised and nonexercised thoroughbreds. *Equine Vet. J.* **29**, 121–125.

Patterson-Kane, J.C., Wilson, A.M., Firth, E.C., Parry, D.A.D., and Goodship, A.E. (1998). Exercise-related alterations in crimp morphology in the central regions of superficial digital flexor tendons from young Thoroughbreds: a controlled study. *Equine Vet. J.* **30**, 61–64.

Peacock, E. (1957). The vascular basis for tendon repair. *Surg. Forum* **8**, 65–86.

Perez-Castro, A.V. and Vogel, K.G. (1999). *In situ* expression of collagen and proteoglycan genes during development of fibrocartilage in bovine deep flexor tendon. *J. Orthop. Res.* **17**, 139–148.

Perez-Tamayo, R. (1982). Degradation of collagen: pathology. In *Collagen in health and disease* (ed. J.B. Weiss and M.I.V. Jayson), pp. 135–159. Churchill Livingstone, Edinburgh.

Piening, C. and Riederer-Henderson, M.A. (1989). Neutral metalloproteinase from tendons. *J. Orthop. Res* **7**, 228–234.

Postacchini, F., Accinni, L., Natali, P.G., Ippolito, E., and de Martino, C. (1978). Regeneration of rabbit calcaneal tendon. *Cell Tissue Res.* **195**, 81–97.

Postacchini, F. and de Martino, C. (1980). Regeneration of rabbit calcaneal tendon maturation of collagen and elastic fibers following partial tenotomy. *Connect. Tissue Res.* **8**, 41–47.

Potasman, I. and Bassan, H.M. (1984). Multiple tendon rupture in systemic lupus erythematosus: Case report and review of the literature. *Ann. Rheum. Dis.* **43**, 347–349.

Potenza, A.D. (1963). Critical evaluation of flexor-tendon healing and adhesion formation within artificial digital sheaths. *J. Bone Joint Surg. (Am.)* **45A**, 1217–1233.

Prockop, D.J. and Kivirikko, K.I. (1995). Collagens: molecular biology, diseases, and potentials for therapy. *Annu. Rev. Biochem.* **64**, 403–34.

Puddu, G., Ippolito, E., and Postacchini, F. (1976). A classification of Achilles tendon disease. *Am. J. Sports Med.* **4**, 145–150.

Ralphs, J.R., Benjamin, M., and Thornett, A. (1991). Cell and matrix biology of the suprapatella in the rat: a structural and immunocytochemical study of fibrocartilage in a tendon subject to compression. *Anat. Rec.* **231**, 167–177.

Rathbun, J.B. and MacNab, I. (1970). The microvascular pattern of rotator cuff. *J. Bone Joint Surg. (Am.)* **52A**, 540–553.

Reddy, G.K., Stehno-Bittel, L., and Enwemeka, C.S. (1998). Laser photostimulation of collagen production in healing rabbit Achilles tendons. *Lasers Surg. Med.* **22**, 281–287.

Reddy, G.K., Gum, S., Stehno-Bittel, L., and Enwemeka, C.S. (1998). Biochemistry and biomechanics of healing tendon: Part II. Effects of combined laser therapy and electrical stimulation. *Med. Sci. Sports Exerc.* **30**, 794–800.

Rees, S.G., Flannery, C.R., Little, C.B., Hughes, C.E., Caterson, B., and Dent, C.M. (2000). Catabolism of aggrecan, and decorin and biglycan in tendon. *Biochem. J.* **350**(1), 181–188.

Reiser, K.M., Amigable, M., and Last, J.A. (1992). Nonenzymatic glycation of type I collagen. The effects of aging on preferential glycation sites. *J. Biol. Chem.* **267**, 24207–24216.

Riederer-Henderson, M.A., Gauger, A., Olson, L., Robertson, C., and Greenlee, T.K. Jr. (1983). Attachment and extracellular matrix differences between tendon and synovial fibroblastic cells. *IN VITRO* **19**, 127–133.

Riley, G.P., Harrall, R.L., Constant, C.R., Chard, M.D., Cawston, T.E., and Hazleman, B.L. (1994). Tendon degeneration and chronic shoulder pain: changes in the collagen composition of the human rotator cuff tendons in rotator cuff tendinitis. *Ann. Rheum. Dis.* **53**, 359–366.

Riley, G.P., Harrall, R.L., Constant, C.R., Chard, M.D., Cawston, T.E., and Hazleman, B.L. (1994). Glycosaminoglycans of human rotator cuff tendons: changes with age and in chronic rotator cuff tendinitis. *Ann. Rheum. Dis.* **53**, 367–376.

Riley, G.P., Harrall, R.L., Cawston, T.E., Hazleman, B.L., and Mackie, E.J. (1996). Tenascin-C and human tendon degeneration. *Am. J. Pathol.* **149**, 933–943.

Riley, G.P., Harrall, R.L., Constant, C.R., Cawston, T.E., and Hazleman, B.L. (1996). Prevalence and possible pathological significance of calcium phosphate salt accumulation in tendon matrix degeneration. *Ann. Rheum. Dis.* **55**, 109–115.

Riley, G.P., Curry, V., DeGroot, J., van El, B., Verzijl, N., TeKoppele, J.M., Hazleman, B.L., and Bank, R.A. (2002). Matrix metalloproteinase activities and their relationship with collagen remodelling in tendon pathology. *Matrix Biol.* **21**, 185–195.

Riley, G.P., Goddard, M.J., and Hazleman BL. (2001). Histopathological assessment and pathological significance of matrix degeneration in supraspinatus tendons. *Rheumatology* **40**, 229–230.

Riley, G.P., Cox, M., Harrall, R.L., Clements, S., and Hazleman, B.L. (2001). Inhibition of tendon cell proliferation and matrix glycosamino-glycan synthesis by non-steroidal anti-inflammatory drugs *in vitro*. *J. Hand Surg. (Br.)* **26B**, 224–228.

Rodeo, S.A., Suzuki, K., Deng, X.H., Wozney, J., and Warren RF. (1999). Use of recombinant human bone morphogenetic protein-2 to enhance tendon healing in a bone tunnel. *Am. J. Sports Med.* **27**, 476–488.

Rolf, C., Movin, T., Engstrom, B., Jacobs, L.D., Beauchard, C., and Le Liboux, A. (1997). An open, randomized study of ketoprofen in patients in surgery for Achilles or patellar tendinopathy. *J. Rheumatol.* **24**, 1595–1598.

Rompe, J.D., Kirkpatrick, C.J., Kullmer, K., Schwitalle, M., and Krischek, O. (1998). Dose-related effects of shock waves on rabbit tendo Achillis. A sonographic and histological study. *J. Bone Joint Surg. (Br.)* **80B**, 546–552.

Rooney, P. (1994). Intratendinous ossification. In *Mechanisms of development and growth* (ed. B.K. Hall), pp. 47–84. CRC Press, Boca Raton, Florida.

Rooney, P., Grant, M.E., and McClure, J. (1992). Endochondral ossification and *de novo* collagen synthesis during repair of the rat achilles tendon. *Matrix* **12**, 274–281.

Rooney, P., Walker, D., Grant, M.E., and McClure, J. (1993). Cartilage and bone formation in repairing Achilles tendons within diffusion chambers: evidence for tendon-cartilage and cartilage-bone conversion *in vivo*. *J. Pathol.* **169**, 375–381.

Rufai, A., Ralphs, J.R., and Benjamin, M. (1995). Structure and histopathology of the insertional region of the human achilles tendon. *J. Orthop. Res.* **13**, 585–593.

Sage, E.H. and Bornstein, P. (1991). Extracellular proteins that modulate cell-matrix interactions. SPARC, tenascin, and thrombospondin. *J. Biol. Chem.* **266**, 14831–14834.

Salo, T., Mäkelä, M., Kylmäniemi, M., Autio-Harmainen, H., and Larjava, H. (1994). Expression of matrix metalloproteinase-2 and -9 during early human wound healing. *Lab. Invest.* **70**, 176–182.

Sanchis-Alfonso, V., Rosello-Sastre, E., and Subias-Lopez, A. (2001). Neuroanatomic basis for pain in patellar tendinosis ('jumper's knee'): a neuroimmunohistochemical study. *Am. J. Knee Surg.* **14**, 174–177.

Sano, H., Uhthoff, H.K., Backman, D.S., Brunet, J.A., Trudel, G., Pham, B., *et al.* (1998). Structural disorders at the insertion of the supraspinatus tendon. Relation to tensile strength. *J. Bone Joint Surg. (Br.)* **80B**, 720–725.

Sano, H., Ishii, H., Yeadon, A., Backman, D.S., Brunet, J.A., and Uhthoff, H.K. (1997). Degeneration at the insertion weakens the tensile strength of the supraspinatus tendon: a comparative mechanical and histologic study of the bone-tendon complex. *J. Orthop. Res.* **15**, 719–726.

Sano, H., Ishii, H., Trudel, G., and Uhthoff, H.K. (1999). Histologic evidence of degeneration at the insertion of 3 rotator cuff tendons: a comparative study with human cadaveric shoulders. *J. Shoulder Elbow Surg.* **8**, 574–579.

Schechtman, H. and Bader, D.L. (1997). *In vitro* fatigue of human tendons. *J. Biomech.* **30**, 829–835.

Schlondorff, J. and Blobel, C.P. (1999). Metalloprotease-disintegrins: modular proteins capable of promoting cell–cell interactions and triggering signals by protein–ectodomain shedding. *J. Cell Sci.* **112**, 3603–3617.

Schmidt, C.C., Georgescu, H.I., Kwoh, C.K., Blomstrom, G.L., Engle, C.P., Larkin, L.A., *et al.* (1995). Effect of growth factors on the proliferation of fibroblasts from the medial collateral and anterior cruciate ligaments. *J. Orthop. Res.* **13**, 184–190.

Sciore, P., Boykiw, R., and Hart, D.A. (1998). Semiquantitative reverse transcription-polymerase chain reaction analysis of mRNA for growth factors and growth factor receptors from normal and healing rabbit medial collateral ligament tissue. *J. Orthop. Res.* **16**, 429–437.

Scott, J.E. (1990). Proteoglycan-collagen interactions and sub-fibrillar structure in collagen fibrils: implications in the development and remodelling of connective tissues. *Biochem. Soc. Trans.* **18**, 489–490.

Sell, D.R. and Monnier V.M. (1989). Isolation, purification, and partial characterization of novel fluorophores from aging human insoluble collagen-rich tissue. *Connect. Tissue Res.* **19**, 77–92.

Sell, D.R. and Monnier, V.M. (1989). Structural elucidation of a senescence cross-link from human extra-cellular matrix. Implication of pentoses in the aging process. *J. Biol. Chem.* **264**, 21594–21602.

Shaw, L.M. and Olsen, B.R. (1991). FACIT collagens: diverse molecular bridges in extracellular matrices. *TIBS* **16**, 191–194.

Shrier, I., Matheson, G.O., and Kohl, H.W., III. (1996). Achilles tendonitis: are corticosteroid injections useful or harmful? *Clin. J. Sport Med.* **6**, 245–250.

Silver, I.A., Brown, P.N., Goodship, A.E., Lanyon, L.E., McCullagh, K.G., Perry, G.C., *et al.* (1983). A clinical and experimental study of tendon injury, healing and treatment in the horse. *Equine Vet. J.* (Suppl. **1**), 1–24.

Siri, A., Knäuper, V., Veirana, N., Caocci, F., Murphy, G., and Zardi, L. (1995). Different susceptibility of small and large human tenascin-C isoforms to degradation by matrix metalloproteinases. *J. Biol. Chem.* **270**, 8650–8654.

Slack, C., Flint, M.H., and Thompson, B.M. (1984). The effect of tensional load on isolated embryonic chick tendon cells in organ culture. *Connect. Tissue Res.* **12**, 229–247.

Smith, R.K.W., Zunino, L., Webbon, P.M., and Heinegård, D. (1997). The distribution of cartilage oligomeric matrix protein (COMP) in tendon and its variation with tendon site, and age and load. *Matrix Biol.* **16**, 255–271.

Smith, R.K., Birch, H., Patterson-Kane, J., Firth, E.C., Williams, L., Cherdchutham, W., *et al.* (1999). Should equine athletes commence training during skeletal development? Changes in tendon matrix associated with development, ageing, and function and exercise. *Equine Vet. J. Suppl.* **30**, 201–209.

Smith, A.G., Kosygan, K., Williams, H., and Newman, R.J. (1999). Common extensor tendon rupture following corticosteroid injection for lateral tendinosis of the elbow. *Br. J. Sports Med.* **33**, 423–424.

Speed, C.A. and Hazleman, B.L. (1999). Calcific tendinitis of the shoulder. *New Engl. J. Med.* **340**, 1582–1584.

Spindler, K.P., Nanney, L.B., and Davidson, J.M. (1995). Proliferative responses to platelet-derived growth factor in young and old rat patellar tendon. *Connect. Tissue Res.* **31**, 171–177.

Spindler, K.P., Clark, S.W., Nanney, L.B., and Davidson, J.M. (1996). Expression of collagen and matrix metalloproteinases in ruptured human anterior cruciate ligament: an *in situ* hybridization study. *J. Orthop. Res.* **14**, 857–861.

Squier, C.A. and Magnes, C. (1983). Spatial relationships between fibroblasts during the growth of rat-tail tendon. *Cell Tissue Res.* **234**, 17–29.

Stanish, W.O., Curwin, S., and Mandel, S. (2000). *Tendinitisi its etiology and treatment*. Oxford University Press, New York.

Stehno-Bittel, L., Reddy, G.K., Gum, S., and Enwemeka, C.S. (1998). Biochemistry and biomechanics of healing tendon: Part I. Effects of rigid plaster casts and functional casts. *Med. Sci. Sports Exer.* **30**, 788–793.

Stetler-Stevenson, W.G. (1996). Dynamics of matrix turnover during pathologic remodelling of the extracellular matrix. *Am. J. Pathol.* **148**, 1345–1350.

Stevenson, J.H., Pang, C.Y., Lindsay, W.K., and Zuker, R.M. (1986). Functional, mechanical, and biochemical assessment of ultrasound therapy on tendon healing in the chicken toe. *Plast. Reconstr. Surg.* **77**, 965–972.

Tallon, C., Maffulli, N., and Ewen, S.W. (2001). Ruptured Achilles tendons are significantly more degenerated than tendinopathic tendons. *Med. Sci. Sports Exerc.* **33**, 1983–1990.

Tanaka, H., Manske, P.R., Pruitt, D.L., and Larson, B.J. (1995). Effect of cyclic tension on lacerated flexor tendons *in vitro*. *J. Hand Surg. (Am.)* **20A**, 467–473.

Taylor, D.C., Brooks, D.E., and Ryan, J.B. (1999). Anabolic-androgenic steroid administration causes hypertrophy of immobilized and nonimmobilized skeletal muscle in a sedentary rabbit model. *Am. J. Sports Med.* **27**, 718–727.

Teitz, C.C., Garrett, W.E., Miniaci, A., Lee, M.H., and Mann, R.A. (1997). Tendon problems in athletic individuals. *J. Bone Joint Surg. (Am.)* **79A**, 138–152.

Thomas, J.T., Taylor, D., Crowell, R., and Assor, D. (1991). The effect of indomethacin on Achilles tendon healing in rabbits. *Clin. Orthop. Rel. Res.* **272**, 308–311.

Tillander, B., Franzen, L.E., Karlsson, M.H., and Norlin, R. (1999). Effect of steroid injections on the rotator cuff: an experimental study in rats. *J. Shoulder. Elbow. Surg.* **8**, 271–274.

Tipton, C.M., Matthes, R.D., Maynard, J.A., and Carey, R.A. (1975). The influence of physical activity on ligaments and tendons. *Med. Sci. Sports* **7**, 165–175.

Tortorella, M.D., Burn, T.C., Pratta, M.A., Abbaszade, I., Hollis, J.M., Liu, R., *et al.* (1999). Purification and cloning of aggrecanase-1: a member of the ADAMTS family of proteins. *Science* **284**, 1664–1666.

Tremble, P., Chiquet-Ehrismann, R., and Werb, Z. (1994). The extracellular matrix ligands fibronectin and tenascin collaborate in regulating collagenase gene expression in fibroblasts. *Mol. Biol. Cell* **5**, 439–453.

Turner, S.M., Powell, E.S., and Ng, C.S. (1989). The effect of ultrasound on the healing of repaired cockerel tendon: is collagen cross-linkage a factor? *J. Hand Surg. (Br.)* **14B**, 428–433.

Uhthoff, H.K. and Sano, H. (1997). Pathology of failure of the rotator cuff tendon. *Orthop. Clin. N. Am.* **28**, 31–41.

Uhthoff, H.K. and Loehr, J.W. (1997). Calcific tendinopathy of the rotator cuff: pathogenesis, diagnosis, and management. *J. Am. Acad. Orthop. Surg.* **5**, 183–191.

Uhthoff, H.K. (1975). Calcifying tendinitis, an active cell-mediated calcification. *Virchows Arch. A* **366**, 51–58.

Uhthoff, H.K., Sarkar, K., and Maynard, J.A. (1976). Calcifying tendinitis. *Clin. Orthop. Rel. Res.* **118**, 164–168.

Uhthoff, H.K. and Sarkar, K. (1991). Classification and definition of tendinopathies. *Clin. Sports Med.* **10**, 707–720.

Uitto, J. (1979). Biochemistry of the elastic fibers in normal connective tissues and its alterations in diseases. *J. Invest Dermatol.* **72**, 1–10.

Urist, M.R., Moss, M.J., and Adams, J.M. (1964). Calcification of tendon. *Arch. Pathol.* **77**, 594–608.

Vailas, A.C., Tipton, C.M., Laughlin, H.L., Tcheng, T.K., and Matthes, R.D. (1978). Physical activity and hypophysectomy on the aerobic capacity of ligaments and tendons. *J. Appl. Physiol.* **44**, 542–546.

Vailas, A.C., Pedrini, V.A., Pedrini-Mille, A., and Holloszy, J.O. (1985). Patellar tendon matrix changes associated with aging and voluntary exercise. *J. Appl. Physiol.* **58**, 1572–6.

Van der Rest, M. and Garrone, R. (1990). Collagens as multidomain proteins. *Biochimie* **72**, 473–484.

Vandor, E., Józsa, L., and Balint, B.J. (1982). The lactate dehydrogenase activity and isoenzyme pattern of normal and hypokinetic human tendons. *Eur. J. Appl. Physiol. Occup. Physiol.* **49**, 63–68.

Vane, J.R. (1971). Inhibition of prostaglandin synthesis as a mechanism of action for aspirin-like drugs. *Nature* **231**, 232–235.

Visconti, C.S., Kavalkovich, K., Wu, J.J., and Niyibizi, C. (1996). Biochemical analysis of collagens at the ligament-bone interface reveals presence of cartilage-specific collagens. *Arch. Biochem. Biophys.* **328**, 135–142.

Visuri, T. and Lindholm, H. (1994). Bilateral distal biceps tendon avulsions with use of anabolic steroids. *Med. Sci. Sports Exerc.* **26**, 941–944.

Vogel, K.G. and Koob, T.J. (1989). Structural specialisation in tendons under compression. *Int. Rev. Cytol.* **115**, 267–293.

Vogel, K.G. and Heinegard, D. (1985). Characterisation of proteoglycans from adult bovine tendon. *J. Biol. Chem.* **260**, 9298–9306.

Vogel, K.G., Sandy, J.D., Pogány, G., and Robbins, J.R. (1994). Aggrecan in bovine tendon. *Matrix* **14**, 171–179.

Vogel, K.G., Ördög, A., Pogány, G., and Oláh, J. (1993). Proteoglycans in the compressed region of human tibialis posterior tendon and in ligaments. *J. Orthop. Res.* **11**, 68–77.

Vogel, H.G. (1983). Age dependence of mechanical properties of rat tail tendons (hysteresis experiments). *Akt. Gerontol.* **13**, 22–27.

Vogel, H.G. (1977). Mechanical and chemical properties of various connective tissue organs in rats as influenced by non-steroidal antirheumatic drugs. *Connect. Tissue Res.* **5**, 91–95.

von der Mark, K. (1981). Localization of collagen types in tissues. *Int. Rev. Connect. Tissue Res.* **9**, 265–324.

Waggett, A.D., Ralphs, J.R., Kwan, A.P.L., Woodnutt, D., and Benjamin, M. (1998). Characterization of collagens and proteoglycans at the insertion of the human Achilles tendon. *Matrix Biol.* **16**, 457–470.

Waterston, S.W., Maffulli, N., and Ewen, S.W.B. (1997). Subcutaneous rupture of the Achilles tendon: basic science and some aspects of clinical practice. *Br. J. Sports Med.* **31**, 285–298.

Watkins, J.P., Auer, J.A., Gay, S., and Morgan, S.J. (1985). Healing of surgically created defects in the equine superficial digital flexor tendon: collagen-type transformation and tissue morphologic reorganization. *Am. J. Vet. Res.* **46**, 2091–2096.

Webster, D.F. and Burry, H.C. (1982). The effects of hypoxia on human skin, and lung and tendon cells *in vitro. Br. J. Exp. Pathol.* **63**, 50–55.

Whitby, D.J. and Ferguson, M.W.J. (1991). The extracellular matrix of lip wounds in fetal, and neonatal and adult mice. *Development* **112**, 651–668.

Wiggins, M.E., Fadale, P.D., Barrach, H., Ehrlich, M.G., and Walsh, W.R. (1994). Healing characteristics of a type I collagenous structure treated with corticosteroids. *Am. J. Sports Med.* **22**, 279–288.

Wiggins, M.E., Fadale, P.D., Ehrlich, M.G., and Walsh, W.R. (1995). Effects of local injection of corticosteroids on the healing of ligaments. A follow-up report. *J. Bone Joint Surg. (Am.)* **77A**, 1682–1691.

Wiig, M., Hanff, G., Abrahamsson, S.-O., and Lohmander, L.S. (1997). Division of flexor tendons causes progressive degradation of tendon matrix in rabbits. *Acta Orthop. Scand.* **67**, 491–497.

Wiig, M., Abrahamsson, S.O., and Lundborg, G. (1996). Effects of hyaluronan on cell proliferation and collagen synthesis: a study of rabbit flexor tendons *in vitro. J. Hand Surg. (Am.)* **21A**, 599–604.

Wiig, M., Abrahamsson, S.O., and Lundborg, G. (1997). Tendon repair—cellular activities in rabbit deep flexor tendons and surrounding synovial sheaths and the effects of hyaluronan: an experimental study *in vivo* and *in vitro. J. Hand Surg. (Am.)* **22A**, 818–825.

Williams, I.F., McCullagh, K.G., and Silver, I.A. (1984). The distribution of types I and III collagen and fibronectin in the healing equine tendon. *Connect. Tissue Res.* **12**, 211–222.

Williams, I.F., Heaton, A., and McCullagh, K.G. (1980). Cell morphology and collagen types in equine tendon scar. *Res. Vet. Sci.* **28**, 302–310.

Williams, I.F., Nicholls, J.S., Goodship, A.E., and Silver, I.A. (1986). Experimental treatment of tendon injury with heparin. *Br. J. Plast. Surg.* **39**, 367–372.

Williams, R.J., III, Attia, E., Wickiewicz, T.L., and Hannafin, J.A. (2000). The effect of ciprofloxacin on tendon, paratenon, and capsular fibroblast metabolism. *Am. J Sports Med.* **28**, 364–369.

Wilmink, J., Wilson, A.M., and Goodship, A.E. (1992). Functional significance of the morphology and micromechanics of collagen fibres in relation to partial rupture of the superficial digital flexor tendon in racehorses. *Res. Vet. Sci.* **53**, 354–359.

Wilson, A.M. and Goodship, A.E. (1994). Exercise-induced hyperthermia as a possible mechanism for tendon degeneration. *J. Biomech.* **27**, 899–905.

Woo, S.L.-Y, Maynard, J., Butler, D., *et al.* (1988). Ligament, tendon and joint capsule insertions to bone. In *Injury and repair of the musculoskeletal soft tissues* (ed. S.L.-Y. Woo and J.A. Buckwalter), p. 156. American Academy of Orthopaedic Surgeons, Park Ridge, Illinois.

Woo, S.L.-Y., Gomez, M.A., Amiel, D., Ritter, M.A., Gelberman, R.H., and Akeson, W.H. (1981). The effects of exercise on the biomechanical and biochemical properties of swine digital flexor tendons. *J. Biomech. Eng.* **103**, 51–56.

Woo, S.L., Gomez, M.A., Woo, Y.K., and Akeson, W.H. (1982). Mechanical properties of tendons and ligaments. II. The relationships of immobilization and exercise on tissue remodelling. *Biorheology* **19**, 397–408.

Woo, S.L., Gomez, M.A., Sites, T.J., Newton, P.O., Orlando, C.A., and Akeson, W.H. (1987). The biomechanical and morphological changes in the medial collateral ligament of the rabbit after immobilization and remobilization. *J. Bone Joint Surg. (Am.)* **69A**, 1200–1211.

Woo, S.L., Gelberman, R.H., Cobb, N.G., Amiel, D., Lothringer, K., and Akeson W.H. (1981). The importance of controlled passive mobilization on flexor tendon healing. A biomechanical study. *Acta Orthop. Scand.* **52**, 615–622.

Woo, S.L., Hildebrand, K., Watanabe, N., Fenwick, J.A., Papageorgiou, C.D., and Wang, J.H. (1999). Tissue engineering of ligament and tendon healing. *Clin. Orthop.* S312–S323.

Wood, T.O., Cooke, P.H., and Goodship, A.E. (1988). The effect of exercise and anabolic steroids on the mechanical properties and crimp morphology of the rat tendon. *Am. J. Sports Med.* **16**, 153–158.

Wysocki, A.B., Staiano-Coico, L., and Grinnell, E (1993). Wound fluid from chronic leg ulcers contains elevated levels of metalloproteinases MMP-2 and MMP-9. *J. Invest. Dermatol.* **101**, 64–68.

Young, R.G., Butler, D.L., Weber, W., Caplan, A.I., Gordon, S.L., and Fink, D.J. (1998). Use of mesenchymal stem cells in a collagen matrix for Achilles tendon repair. *J. Orthop. Res.* **16**, 406–413.

1.2

Muscle

Michael Kjaer and Abigail Mackey

Introduction

Skeletal muscle is not only essential for human movement and performance, but is unfortunately also a common site for acute injuries related to physical activity and sports. The influence of exercise on skeletal muscle represents a wide range all the way from (i) physiological adaptation with regard to metabolism, morphology, and contractile properties, through (ii) physiological development of muscle hypertrophy, to (iii) pathological/physiological responses to heavy unaccustomed exercise with associated delayed onset of muscle soreness, and ending with (iv) muscle injury caused by either strain or contusion (and seldom laceration) trauma. In the present chapter we will focus on the muscle responses to acute stimuli that cause muscle injury of minor or larger magnitude, and the ensuing recovery.

Although treated clinically, muscle injury is one of the areas where much research is in its infancy. Whereas minor injury in the muscle can easily be provoked by intense eccentric activity of untrained muscle and studied thereafter, more severe acute muscle ruptures are more difficult to study in a systematic way, as they are very heterogeneous with regard to severity, occur in different muscles, and, in humans, do not allow for systematic tissue sampling in the recovery phase.

Types of skeletal muscle injury and mechanisms behind them (Table 1.2.1)

Strain injury

This type of injury is normally considered the 'classical muscle rupture', often occurring in hamstring (e.g. sprinters) or calf (e.g. tennis) muscle after explosive movements, and often affecting two-joint muscles. The term 'muscle rupture' is in fact somewhat inaccurate in that this type of injury is confined to the interphase between the muscle fibre and connective tissue, often in the myotendinous junction or the muscle–fascicle interphase. There is rarely a rupture of muscle fibres, but rather a disruption of the point of attachment of the individual muscle fibre to the matrix. Often the injury is located deep below the skin, so a clinically visible haematoma is rare.

Contusion injury

This injury, together with strain injury, represents over 90% of all acute muscle injuries, and often occurs in conjunction with direct contact with equipment or another athlete, typically as a result of a tackle (e.g. football), where a larger muscle like the quadriceps receives a contusion, which is followed by a tissue injury in which blood vessels are often damaged and a sizeable haematoma occurs. There is a varying degree of muscle fibre damage, and often these injuries recover relatively quickly depending on the clearance of the haematoma. Most of these injuries are minor and allow return to sports activity soon afterwards.

Complications with contusion injury

One of the rare complications of muscle injury is myositis ossificans, a bone–cartilage formation at the site of the injury. Although rare, myositis ossificans delays the return to activity, reduces joint motion, and is associated with pain during activity. No optimal treatment is currently documented. However, no non-surgical or surgical treatment has been shown to have any beneficial effect, and both local corticosteroid injection and surgical excision are used on an undocumented basis.

Laceration injury

This occurs infrequently in human exercise, but has been mentioned a lot because it is often used as an animal model to induce injury

Table 1.2.1 Types of muscle injury

Muscle strain injury
('Classical muscle rupture', often hamstring or calf muscle, explosive movements)
Obligatory position in the muscle fibre—connective tissue interphase, disruption of fibre—tendon–aponeurosis connection
Healing time depends on matrix tissue healing (8–12 weeks)
Muscle contusion injury
('Wooden leg', often quadriceps, contact/tackle with opponent)
Often marked intramuscular bleeding (between fibres), varying degree of muscle fibre damage
Healing time depends on extent of injury: minimal fibre damage, 1–2 weeks; larger fibre damage, 6–10 weeks
Muscle pain and soreness
('Delayed-onset muscle soreness', often day/days after unaccustomed heavy eccentric exercise)
Primarily a diffuse damage to the intramuscular connective tissue, only seldom muscle fibre rupture
Natural healing after 2–14 days; no need for treatment.

and study subsequent recovery. Clearly, laceration trauma will cause damage to muscle fibres, connective tissue, and vasculature.

Acute unaccustomed exercise and experimental exercise-induced injury

Unaccustomed exercise can result in muscle damage, especially when the muscle is subjected to lengthening (eccentric) contractions, such as that experienced by the quadriceps when running downhill or during the downward phase of a squat exercise. This type of muscle damage affects only some fibres, it is segmental in nature (i.e. affecting only certain areas along the length of a fibre), and complete regeneration occurs in healthy individuals. A common characteristic is the development of muscle soreness, which does not usually peak until 2–3 days after the exercise, hence the term delayed-onset muscle soreness (DOMS). This soreness can be severe, affecting the ability to walk downstairs, for example, if it is the quadriceps that is affected. In association with DOMS, a reduced range of motion of the joint and smaller relaxed joint angle is observed. Functionally, the affected muscle(s) usually suffers a dramatic drop (60% is not uncommon) in force-producing capacity, from which it can take up to 3–4 weeks to recover fully. What is perhaps surprising is that the muscle soreness, which one could imagine serves to prevent the person using the muscles too much while they are under repair, subsides long before the force-producing capacity has recovered. This has implications for individuals who return to repeat the same task (e.g. lifting the same weight) when in fact they are subjecting their muscles to loads that they are not really capable of lifting. Therefore susceptibility to further injury is possible during this period. It should be noted that activities involving only isometric or concentric muscle contractions may also induce DOMS, albeit to a lesser extent, in very untrained individuals.

Increased permeability of the sarcolemma is reflected by elevated circulating levels of creatine kinase (CK), which begin to increase after the damaging exercise, often to very high levels (~20 000 IU/l) where large muscle groups are involved, and can take up to 2 weeks to return to normal levels in extreme cases. Because of a delay in transport from the muscle to the circulation via the lymphatic system, circulating levels of CK may not peak until 4–8 days after the exercise, although exercise involving hundreds of repeated contractions, such as running, will accelerate transport to the circulation so that levels may peak as early as 24 hours after the exercise. Plasma concentrations of lactate dehydrogenase and myoglobin usually follow the same pattern, also reflecting increased membrane permeability of myofibres. Despite large inter-individual variation in these markers, they are useful for monitoring intra-individual day-to-day changes.

Indirect markers such as DOMS and CK are useful as non-invasive tools to assess the presence of exercise-induced injury. Examination of a muscle biopsy from the affected muscle can provide further evidence, but the merit of this is doubtful when muscle disease is not suspected. The most dramatic findings are from studies in animals where forced-lengthening contractions have resulted in histological signs of muscle damage in the form of inflammatory cell infiltration, fibres lacking desmin and dystrophin staining, and myofibre necrosis. This has also been demonstrated in humans, but is not always observed, perhaps because of the voluntary nature of human experiments. In support of this, if human muscle is stimulated using neuromuscular electrical stimulation, it is possible to reproduce many of the findings reported in animal studies (Crameri et al. 2007). Furthermore, it appears that performance of more physiological exercise induces more damage to the connective tissue component of skeletal muscle than to the contractile element, as long as the exercise is unaccustomed (Crameri et al. 2004). This is not surprising given that forces are transmitted, and therefore sensed by, skeletal muscle connective tissue. Adaptation of the force-bearing connective tissue and focal adhesion complexes results in a stronger structure for transmitting high forces, rendering the muscle more resistant to damage during subsequent bouts of the same exercise.

While the exact sequence of events remains to be uncovered, the general consensus regarding the cause of muscle damage at a cellular level is that increased activity of calcium-activated proteases, reactive oxygen species (ROS), and phospholipases results in structural degradation of the myofibre contractile components and sarcolemma (Ebbeling and Clarkson 1989; Allen et al. 2005). The role of calcium in muscle damage has been demonstrated in humans by administration of a calcium-channel blocker, which was associated with reduced desmin disruption and z-band streaming following forced lengthening (eccentric) contractions (Beaton et al. 2002). However, there is some debate about the order of events leading to altered calcium concentration in the myofibre. One relatively recent theory suggests that instability of sarcomeres on the descending limb of the length–tension relationship during eccentric contractions results in sarcomere disruption (Morgan 1990). Similarly, the mechanisms involved in the development of DOMS are not fully understood, but it is generally attributed to sensitization of nociceptors in the connective tissue. The mismatch of timing of events following unaccustomed exercise-induced damage has resulted in slow progress in research on this topic, especially when it is considered that the phenomenon of muscle soreness associated with unaccustomed exercise was documented more than a century ago (Hough 1902).

Diagnosis

Two important points determine the likelihood of a muscle injury: (i) the recognition by the patient of an acute event where either an unusual strain or contusion occurred, and sudden pain was felt; (ii) a sudden decrease in muscle function. In addition to this anamnestic information, the objective examination will reveal an area in relation to the relevant muscle that is swollen and painful upon palpation. Later, visible haematoma can appear, and often the contusion injuries are associated with larger haematoma than occur with strain injuries, as the latter are often deep intramuscular injuries. Confirmation of a muscle injury should be made using ultrasonography imaging (Aspelin et al. 1992; Thorsson et al. 1993), where a skilled examiner and good ultrasonography (US) equipment can visualize most injuries. Only in cases where discrepancy between symptoms, objective findings, and US exists, such as some myotendinous junction strain injuries, can it be justified to use MRI as an additional imaging technique (De Smet and Best 2000).

Development of the injury into repair and full recovery

Development of marked muscle injury

After the initial trauma it has been shown that three phases occur, and that these are fairly similar and independent of the type of severe muscle injury: (i) destruction phase, (ii) repair phase, and (iii) remodelling phase. In the destruction phase the damaged myofibres display necrosis, inflammatory cells are present, and a haematoma is formed. Necrosis develops after the sarcoplasmic damage to the fibres, and cytoskeletal material accumulates and acts as a barrier between the trauma and healthy tissue. The damage to blood vessels results in haematoma as well as an influx of inflammatory cells into the tissue. Macrophages and fibroblasts are activated and release growth factors and cytokines (TNF-α, FGF, TGF-β, HGF, IL-1β, IL-6), which then activate regeneration of the injured muscle cells (Chargé and Rudnicki 2004). Monocytes are transformed into macrophages which participate in proteolysis and phagocytosis of necrotic material.

In the repair phase regeneration of myofibres takes place as well as formation of connective scar tissue (Hurme *et al.* 1991). Following muscle cell damage satellite cells are activated, and proliferate and differentiate into myoblasts and form myotubes. These tubes fuse with surviving myofibres. Satellite cells are an important source of myonuclei in muscle repair, but progenitor cells from bone marrow and various mesenchymal tissues can also differentiate into a myogenic lineage.

Development of the unaccustomed exercise injury into repair and full recovery

With regard to experimental exercise-induced damage, the repair processes are primarily focused on the activity of a population of myogenic precursor cells, known as satellite cells (see Figure 1.2.1). An important feature of satellite cells, unlike post-mitotic myonuclei, is that they have the potential to re-enter the cell cycle and divide. The fate of these daughter cells usually falls into one of the following categories: (i) *de novo* synthesis of muscle tissue pre- and post-natally, (ii) donating myonuclei to facilitate muscle hypertrophy, (iii) forming new myofibre material to repair damaged segments, and (iv) replenishing the satellite cell pool. Many factors are known to activate satellite cells, and one of the best-known specific interactions is the action of Hepatocyte Growth Factor on the c-met receptor, located on quiescent satellite cells (Cornelison and Wold 1997). It is also known that quiescent murine satellite cells express VCAM-1, whose co-receptor is located on infiltrating leukocytes (Jesse *et al.* 1998), supporting a role for inflammation in the activation of satellite cells and subsequent regeneration. It is well established, that once activated, satellite cells proliferate, fuse together and fuse with existing myofibres to restore muscle function. Numerous human studies have shown that both long term (3–4 months) resistance training and a single bout of intense unaccustomed exercise result in enhanced numbers of satellite cells, fitting well with their roles in hypertrophy and regeneration, respectively (Kadi *et al.* 2005). While satellite cells do not display all of the traits of a stem cell, their regenerative potential has generated great interest in the context of muscle atrophy and muscle disease.

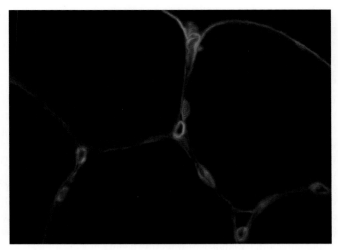

Fig. 1.2.1 A single satellite cell (outlined in red) located inside the laminin-rich border (green) of a muscle fibre cross-section of healthy human skeletal muscle. The satellite cell is identified by double-labelling immunofluorescent staining using an anti-CD56 antibody (347740, Becton Dickinson) and anti-laminin antibody (Z0097, Dako); nuclei are stained with 4′,6-diamidino-2-phenylindole (DAPI). Magnification 60×.

Treatments

Acute intervention: RICE

The classical first aid for muscle injury—Rest (R), Ice (I), Compression (C), and Elevation (E)—is widely used in attempts to limit further injury, reduce pain, and minimize bleeding and swelling. The scientific evidence for the effectiveness of these four steps of intervention on muscle injury remains undocumented, but some of the components have been shown to influence parameters of relevance for injury development and healing. It has been documented that rest will reduce the injury haematoma as well as the amount of connective tissue scarring (Järvinen and Lehto 1993), and compression has been shown to reduce injury zone blood flow, but it is not clear whether this will influence healing time after injury (Thorsson *et al.* 1987, 1997). Some recent studies have indicated that indirect compression on contusion muscle injuries in the quadriceps muscle by maximal knee flexion limited the haematoma and shortened the injury period (Engebretsen 2003). Substantial elevation (>30 cm) of the extremity above heart level is required to reduce flow, but it has never been documented to influence injury magnitude or healing time. Finally, application of cold/ice can reduce the intramuscular temperature superficially by several degrees and some studies have indicated that treatment of superficial injuries with ice results in limited haematoma and less inflammation (Hurme *et al.* 1993; Deal *et al.* 2002), but whether cold application will have any effect on the healing of deep muscle injuries remains unproven.

Recovery training

Early stimulation of the injured tissue promotes healing, but exactly how much should be performed and how early it should be started is not documented. It is known that leaving connective tissue unstimulated after injury will cause lack of alignment and alter the original morphology. Furthermore, early mobilization of muscle injury has been shown to cause better and faster capillary ingrowth into the damaged tissue, provide better regeneration of muscle fibres, and result in better alignment (Järvinen et al. 2005, 2007). Injury is associated with pain, but there is no proof that pain is directly associated with tissue damage; however, it is currently the best clinical sign of the borderline between successful and defective repair. For that reason, movement within the range of pain is encouraged in order to stimulate the tissue maximally without causing further damage to the tissue. It is shown in animal models that immediate remobilization after injury will result in re-ruptures and formation of larger scars (Järvinen and Sorvari 1975). The tissue can tolerate some loading after 24–48 hours and can at this time be subjected to stretching without pain, and the addition of heating may decrease muscle viscosity and increase muscle movement (Magnusson et al. 1995). The ideal duration of stretching is undocumented, and likewise the optimal amount of training in the following days has not been investigated scientifically. According to the loading pattern of different exercise types, isometric and dynamic exercise is preferable to eccentric exercise in order to avoid re-injury. There are two important points in rehabilitation after muscle injury. The first is to remember that muscle strain injuries are injuries to the connective tissue rather than to the muscle cell itself, and thus the time frame is often longer than expected. The second point is that although protein synthesis in intramuscular connective tissue adapts more slowly than the contractile protein of the muscle fibre, it has recently been shown that whereas muscle fibre protein responses depend strongly on the intensity of exercise (only high intensities will result in muscle hypertrophy), the adaptation of intramuscular connective tissue is independent of exercise intensity (Holm et al. 2008). This implies that although skeletal muscle cannot initially tolerate very high loads after injury, low exercise loads will be able to stimulate the connective tissue associated with the muscle and thus can optimize recovery in the very early stages after injury. It is important to note that even with optimal recovery training, there are signs of connective tissue ingrowth into the skeletal muscle (Nikolaou et al. 1987), which probably is an attempt to increase the resistance to future injuries, but potentially could mean a slight reduction in the future performance of the muscle–tendon unit.

Medical treatment

Treatment of pain and inflammation after muscle injury with glucocorticoids or non-steroidal anti-inflammatory drugs (NSAIDs) has been tried. Some studies have indicated a beneficial effect on early healing with use of NSAIDs, whereas others have shown no effect or even a detrimental effect on late healing outcome (Mishra et al. 1995; O'Grady et al. 2000). The use of glucocorticoids has been shown to delay elimination of haematoma and necrotic tissue and to prolong muscle regeneration and reduce the tensile strength of the tissue (Beiner et al. 1999).

Taking advantage of the analgesic properties of NSAIDs in order to continue training, not only when faced with injury, but also to alleviate DOMS, is common practice among keen sports participants. However, there is increasing evidence in the literature for negative effects of NSAIDs on skeletal muscle metabolism and growth (Mackey 2007). There is little doubt that NSAIDs are an invaluable tool in the treatment of injuries, but studies of whether NSAIDs can alleviate DOMS have shown that they have little or no effect. Evidence for a negative action of NSAIDs is based on the cyclo-oxygenase (COX) pathway, the target of NSAID action. Cell culture and animal models show quite clearly that COX activity, and its downstream prostaglandins, are important for skeletal muscle myogenesis at the key stages of proliferation, differentiation, and fusion. Convincing data from a recent study indicate that inhibition of COX activity by ingestion of ibuprofen can attenuate overload-induced hypertrophy in rats (Soltow et al. 2006). In this study, it was observed that the mass of the plantaris muscles of rats in the control group increased by 60% after 14 days of overload compared with only 30% in the group that consumed ibuprofen. As yet, there are few studies of the effects of NSAIDs in humans, but the available results indicate a negative influence on muscle protein synthesis and specifically on satellite cells. For example, 24 hours after a series of 100 eccentric contractions of the quadriceps, the fractional synthesis rate of mixed muscle protein was approximately halved by the ingestion of NSAIDs (Trappe et al. 2002), a good indicator that COX activity is necessary for the anabolic response of muscle to resistance exercise. With regard to satellite cells, ingestion of NSAIDs resulted in no change in satellite cell number following a 36 km run, in contrast with an increase of 27% in the placebo group (Mackey et al. 2007). Given the critical roles of satellite cells in muscle maintenance, growth, and regeneration, any block or delay in these processes could have consequences for the extent of muscle regeneration. Although the precise mechanisms by which NSAIDs exert this action remain to be fully uncovered, current knowledge certainly urges caution against the casual use of NSAIDs, especially in the treatment of DOMS.

Operation

Very little scientific data support a major role for surgical treatment of muscle rupture. As a general rule, skeletal muscle injury should be treated conservatively, and operative treatment has been shown to be beneficial only in special cases. Very large intramuscular haematoma and full or near-full ruptures of major muscles that are lacking sufficient agonist support can be operated on by removing haematoma or by suturing muscle to fascia (Almekinders 1991; Menetrey et al. 1999; Järvinen et al. 2005). Furthermore, it has been claimed that long-term extension pain (>6 months) can be helped with operative release of scar adhesions, but the scientific support is sparse.

Management of complications

It has been suggested that myositis ossificans can be treated by surgical removal of the bone–cartilage formation at the site of the injury. Although rare, myositis ossificans delays return to activity, reduces joint motion, and is associated with pain during activity. No optimal treatment is currently documented. No non-surgical or surgical treatment has been shown to have any beneficial effect, and both local corticosteroid injection and surgical excision are used on an undocumented basis. Some muscle injuries result in excessive scar formation that will lead to some symptoms in relation to exercise many months after the injury. Such complications are best dealt with by strength training to cause muscle hypertrophy and strengthening of the matrix tissue.

References

Allen, D.G., Whitehead, N.P., and Yeung, E.W. (2005). Mechanisms of stretch-induced muscle damage in normal and dystrophic muscle: role of ionic changes. *Journal of Physiology*, **567**, 723–35.

Almekinders, L.C. (1991). Results of surgical repair versus splinting of experimentally transected muscle. *Journal of Orthopaedics and Trauma*, **5**, 173–6.

Aspelin, P., Ekberg, O., Thorsson, O., Wilhelmsson, M., and Westlin, N. (1992). Ultrasound examination of soft tissue injury of the lower limb in athletes. *American Journal of Sports Medicine*, **20**, 601–3.

Beaton, L.J., Tarnopolsky, M.A., and Phillips, S.M. (2002). Contraction-induced muscle damage in humans following calcium channel blocker administration. *Journal of Physiology*, **544**, 849–59.

Beiner, J.M., Jokl, P., Cholewicki, J., and Panjabi, M.M. (1999). The effect of anabolic steroids and corticosteroids on healing of muscle contusion injury. *American Journal of Sports Medicine*, **27**, 2–9.

Chargé, S.B.P. and Rudnicki, M.A. (2004). Cellular and molecular regulation of muscle regeneration. *Physiological Reviews*, **84**, 209.

Cornelison, D.D. and Wold, B.J. (1997). Single-cell analysis of regulatory gene expression in quiescent and activated mouse skeletal muscle satellite cells. *Developmental Biology*, **191**, 270–83.

Crameri, R.M., Langberg, H., Magnusson, P., *et al.* (2004). Changes in satellite cells in human skeletal muscle after a single bout of high intensity exercise. *Journal of Physiology*, **558**, 333–40.

Crameri, R.M., Aagaard, P., Qvortrup, K., Langberg, H., Olesen, J., and Kjaer, M. (2007). Myofibre damage in human skeletal muscle: effects of electrical stimulation vs voluntary contraction. *Journal of Physiology*, **583**, 365–80.

Deal, D.N., Tipton, J., Rosencrance, E., Curl, W.W., and Smith, T.L. (2002). Ice reduces edema. A study of microvascular permeability in rats. *Journal of Bone and Joint Surgery, American Volume*, **84A**, 1573–8.

De Smet, A.A. and Best, T.M. (2000). MR imaging of the distribution and location of acute hamstring injuries in athletes. *AJR American Journal of Roentgenology*, **174**, 393–9.

Ebbeling, C.B. and Clarkson, P.M. (1989). Exercise-induced muscle damage and adaptation. *Sports Medicine*, **7**, 207–34.

Engebretsen, L. (2003). Akutte lårskader. In: R. Bahr and S. Mæhlum (eds), *Idretts-skader* (2nd edn), pp. 283–8. Gazette as, Oslo.

Holm, L., Reitelseder, S., Pedersen, T.G., *et al.* (2008). Changes in muscle size and MHC composition in response to resistance exercise with heavy and light loading intensity. *Journal of Applied Physiology*, **105**, 1454–61.

Hough (1902)

Hurme, T., Kalimo, H., Lehto, M., and Järvinen, M. (1991). Healing of skeletal muscle injury: an ultrastructural and immunohistochemical study. *Medicine and Science in Sports and Exercise*, **23**, 801–10.

Hurme, T., Rantanen, J., and Kaliomo, H. (1993). Effects of early cryotherapy in experimental skeletal muscle injury. *Scandinavian Journal of Medicine and Science in Sports*, **3**, 46–51.

Järvinen, M.J. and Lehto, M.U. (1993). The effects of early mobilisation and immobilisation on the healing process following muscle injuries. *Sports Medicine*, **15**, 78–89.

Järvinen, M. and Sorvari, T. (1975). Healing of a crush injury in rat striated muscle. 1. Description and testing of a new method of inducing a standard injury to the calf muscles. *Acta Pathologica Microbiologica Scandinavica A*, **83**, 259–65.

Järvinen TA, Järvinen TL, Kääriäinen M, Kalimo H, and Järvinen M. (2005). Muscle injuries: biology and treatment. *American Journal of Sports Medicine*, **33**, 745–64.

Järvinen TA, Järvinen TL, Kääriäinen M, *et al.* (2007). Muscle injuries: optimising recovery. *Best Practice & Research. Clinical Rheumatology*, **21**, 317–31.

Jesse, T.L., LaChance, R., Iademarco, M.F., and Dean, D.C. (1998). Interferon regulatory factor-2 is a transcriptional activator in muscle where it regulates expression of vascular cell adhesion molecule-1. *Journal of Cell Biology*, **140**, 1265–76.

Kadi, F., Charifi, N., Denis, C., *et al.* (2005). The behaviour of satellite cells in response to exercise: what have we learned from human studies? *Pflugers Archiv*, **451**, 319–27.

Mackey, A.L. (2007). Use of anti-inflammatory medication in healthy athletes—no pain, no gain? *Scandinavian Journal of Medicine and Science in Sports*, **17**, 613–14.

Mackey, A.L., Kjaer, M., Dandanell, S., *et al.* (2007). The influence of anti-inflammatory medication on exercise-induced myogenic precursor cell responses in humans. *Journal of Applied Physiology*, **103**, 425–31.

Magnusson, S.P., Simonsen, E.B., Aagaard, P., Gleim, G.W., McHugh, M.P., and Kjaer, M. (1995). Viscoelastic response to repeated static stretching in the human hamstring muscle. *Scandinavian Journal of Medicine and Science in Sports*, **5**, 342–7.

Menetrey, J., Kasemkijwattana, C., Fu, F.H., Moreland, M.S., and Huard, J. (1999). Suturing versus immobilisation of a muscle laceration. A morphological and functional study in a mouse model. *American Journal of Sports Medicine*, **27**, 222–9.

Mishra, D.K., Friden, J., Schmitz, M.C., and Lieber, R.L. (1995). Anti-inflammatory medication after muscle injury. A treatment resulting in short-term improvement but subsequent loss of muscle function. *Journal of Bone and Joint Surgery, American Volume*, **77**, 1510.

Morgan (1990)

Nikolaou, P.K., Macdonald, B.L., Glisson, R.R., Seaber, A.V., and Garrett, W.E., Jr (1987). Biomechanical and histological evaluation of muscle after controlled strain injury. *American Journal of Sports Medicine*, **15**, 9–14.

O'Grady, M., Hackney, A.C., Schneider, K., *et al.* (2000). Diclofenac sodium (Voltaren) reduced exercise-induced injury in human skeletal muscle. *Medicine and Science in Sports and Exercise*, **32**, 1191–6.

Soltow, Q.A., Betters, J.L., Sellman, J.E., Lira, V.A., Long, J.H., and Criswell, D.S. (2006). Ibuprofen inhibits skeletal muscle hypertrophy in rats. *Medicine and Science in Sports and Exercise*, **38**, 840–6.

Thorsson, O., Hemdal, B., Lilja, B., and Westlin, N. (1987). The effect of external pressure on intramuscular blood flow at rest and after running. *Medicine and Science in Sports and Exercise*, **19**, 469–73.

Thorsson, O., Leander, P., Lilja, B., Nilsson, P., Obrant, K.J., and Westlin, N. (1993). Comparing ultrasonography, magnetic resonance imaging and scintigraphy in evaluating an experimentally induced muscular hematoma. *Scandinavian Journal of Medicine and Science in Sports*, **3**, 110–16.

Thorsson, O., Lilja, B., Nilsson, P., and Westlin, N. (1997). Immediate external compression in the management of an acute muscle injury. *Scandinavian Journal of Medicine and Science in Sports*, **7**, 182–90.

Trappe, T.A., White, F., Lambert, C.P., Cesar, D., Hellerstein, M., and Evans, W.J. (2002). Effect of ibuprofen and acetaminophen on postexercise muscle protein synthesis. *American Journal of Physiology. Endocrinology and Metabolism*, **282**, E551–556.

1.3

Meniscus

Emma Blain and Victor Duance

Introduction

Menisci are present in several locations, e.g. the acromioclavicular joint (Tischer *et al.* 2009), the temporomandibular joint (Tanaka *et al.* 2008), and the tibiofemoral joint. All are susceptible to sports injuries, but the most prevalent are to the knee. Therefore only the meniscus of this joint will be considered in detail in this chapter.

The incongruence of the femoral and tibial articular surfaces of the knee joint is 'corrected' by the presence of two wedge-shaped 'semi-lunar' fibrocartilaginous structures, namely the medial and lateral menisci. The menisci perform highly specialized functions including load-bearing, shock absorption, joint lubrication, and stabilization, all critical roles for maintaining normal joint articulation (Brown 2004). In 1887, the meniscus was described as 'the functionless remains of a leg muscle' (Bland-Sutton 1887), but it was not until 1948 that the concept that 'meniscectomy is not wholly innocuous,' was reported (Fairbanks 1948), highlighting that the menisci were not redundant entities. Since these early observations, research into understanding the role of the meniscus has continued and has provided insights into the necessity of these 'semi-lunar' structures for normal knee joint function. The menisci provide important biomechanical functions to the knee, facilitating load transmission across the joint. This primary biomechanical function is fulfilled by the composition of the extracellular matrix (ECM), of which collagen is the principal component. The fibrils are arranged parallel to the periphery of the meniscus to provide the tissue with mechanical integrity. Interspersed within and/or bound to the collagen network are the non-collagenous components (proteoglycans and other glycoproteins), and embedded within this matrix is the predominant cell type—the fibrochondrocyte. The function, pathology, and strategies for repair of the meniscus have been key areas of research over the last decade, partly because of the magnitude of meniscal injuries within the population.

The structure, physiology, and function of the meniscus will be discussed in this chapter and compared with the pathological condition. Further, the strategies that are currently implemented and emerging techniques to repair the damaged meniscus will also be considered.

Anatomy and structure of the meniscus

The menisci are fibrous tissues comprising two separate wedge-shaped semi-lunar sections (medial and lateral) which are located in the space between the femoral condyles and the tibial plateau of the knee joint (Fig. 1.3.1(a)). These periarticular tissues are shaped to maximize their function as distributors of load within the joint. On gross inspection, the meniscus is a white, glossy, and smooth tissue. The proximal surface, which is in contact with the femoral condyle, is concave, whilst the distal surface, which is in contact with the tibial plateau, is flat or slightly convex.

Strong ligamentous horns attach the meniscus to the tibial plateau, and they are further tethered through attachments to the

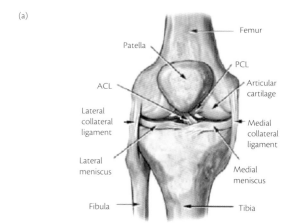

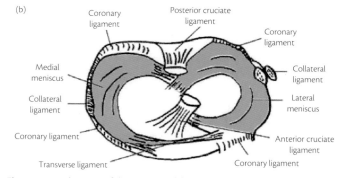

Fig. 1.3.1 A schematic of the meniscus. (a) Anterior view of the human knee joint: ACL, anterior cruciate ligament; PCL, posterior cruciate ligament. (b) Proximal view of a tibial plateau. The lateral and medial menisci (coloured) and associated capsular ligaments are shown.

capsular components of the joint, e.g. the collateral ligaments (Fig. 1.3.1(b)). The medial meniscus is semicircular and is smaller than the almost circular lateral meniscus. The peripheral region of the meniscus is covered by the synovial membrane and comprises vascularized tissue, whereas the inner region comprises an avascular, aneural, and alymphatic tissue. Histological and biochemical analyses demonstrate that the outer two-thirds of the meniscus is organized like fibrocartilage, whereas in some species the inner third is not dissimilar to hyaline cartilage. This disparity in organization reflects the tissue's ability to resist circumferential tensile loads occurring at the periphery of the meniscus, and resist compressive forces to which the inner region of the tissue is subjected.

Meniscal cell morphology

Embedded within the ECM of the meniscus is a sparse population of cells, referred to as 'fibrochondrocytes'—the term was designated to reflect their chondrocyte-like morphology and their synthesis of a fibrocartilaginous matrix. Historically, fibrochondrocytes were classified into two distinct populations: fusiform cells and fibrochondrocytes. The fusiform cells are present in the superficial margin of the meniscus (closest to the articular surface) and have been compared to the flatterned chondrocytes observed in the superficial zone of articular cartilage (Ghadially *et al.* 1978). The rounded fibrochondrocytes, lying interior to the superficial zone and constituting the majority of the meniscal tissue, are similar to chondrocytes distributed in the deep zone of articular cartilage (Ghadially *et al.* 1978).

In 2001, cells of the meniscus were further categorized and reclassified into four distinct cell populations based on extensive morphological differences, including cytoskeletal element localization and architecture, within these regions (Hellio Le Graverand *et al.* 2001a). These were reclassified as follows (Hellio Le Graverand *et al.* 2001a).

(i-ii) Two classes of cell present in the fibrocartilage region, in which the cells are highly elongated and exhibited long processes that extended from the body of the cell. These two cell types differ only in the number of cellular processes, with the cells closest to the inner hyaline-like region having very few.

(iii) A third cell type, rounded in morphology and devoid of projections, was detected in the inner hyaline-like region of the meniscus.

(iv) A fourth cell type with a fusiform or polygonal shape devoid of cytoplasmic projections is located within the superficial regions of the meniscus.

These diverse cell populations are rich in endoplasmic reticulum and Golgi apparatus, but minimal numbers of mitochondria are observed (McDevitt and Webber 1990), indicating that their function is to synthesize and maintain the meniscus ECM. As with articular cartilage, the major pathway for energy production in the meniscal fibrochondrocytes is via anaerobic glycolysis.

The distinct morphological characteristics of these cell populations reflect their divergence of function in the meniscus. Fibrochondrocytes located in the superficial margin, where load may first be experienced (i.e. during flexion and extension of the knee), may be adapted to respond to a mechanical stimulus. As a consequence, these cells may 'signal' to the cells of the inner region to synthesize components essential for withstanding this stimulus. Therefore the resultant matrix produced by these cell populations reflects their biomechanical environment and functional requirements.

Extracellular matrix composition of the meniscus

The meniscus is a dense connective tissue in which an extensive ECM is sparsely interspersed with fibrochondrocytes. As such, the matrix is an amalgamation of insoluble fibrils and soluble polymers that has evolved to withstand movement-derived loads. The meniscus ECM can be separated into four categories: water (comprising 70% of the tissue), collagens, proteoglycans, and non-collagenous proteins (e.g. elastin). Collectively, these macromolecules contribute to the biomechanical integrity of the meniscus, providing it with strength and resilience to load application. The ability to distribute load evenly across the joint surface depends on the arrangement of these macromolecules within the meniscus, highlighting the importance of correct ECM organization and composition. The components of the meniscus are presented in Table 1.3.1; however, the expression and/or relative abundance changes with age, species, pathology, and location within the tissue.

Collagens

Collagen constitutes approximately 60–70% of the dry weight of the meniscus (McDevitt and Webber 1990); the predominant form

Table 1.3.1 Extracellular matrix composition of the meniscus.

Extracellular matrix component	Macromolecule	Reference
Collagens (60–70% dry weight of meniscus)	Type I (95%[a]/40%[b])	Eyre and Muir 1975
	Type II (< 1%[a]/60%[b])	Cheung 1987
	Types III (~ 1%) and V (~ 1%)	Eyre and Wu 1983
	Type IV	Melrose et al. 2005\
	Type VI (2%)	Wu et al. 1987
Proteoglycans (2%[a]–8%[b] dry weight of meniscus)	Chondroitin SO_4^{2-}	Nakano et al. 1997
	Aggrecan (~ 55%[a]/ 80%[b])	Valiyaveettil et al., 2005
	Perlecan	Melrose et al. 2005
	Dermatan SO_4^{2-}	Scott et al. 1997
	Decorin and biglycan	
	Hyaluronan (10%[a]/5%[b])	Scott et al. 1997
Non-collagenous matrix proteins	Fibronectin (ED-A and ED-B isoforms)	Salter et al. 1995
	Thrombospondin	Miller and McDevitt 1991
	COMP	Muller et al. 1998
	Tenascin C	Salter et al. 1995
Other	Elastin (~ 0.6%)	Sweigart and Athanasiou 2001

[a]Outer region of the meniscus.
[b]Inner region of the meniscus.

is type I collagen which accounts for> 90% of the collagen in the tissue (dry weight) (Eyre and Muir 1975). In bovine meniscus, the outer two-thirds of the tissue is predominantly type I collagen, whereas the inner third comprises 40% type I collagen with the remaining 60% being type II collagen (Cheung 1987). Because of the presence of type II collagen in the inner region of the meniscus (Cheung 1987; Melrose *et al.* 2005), it is said to resemble articular cartilage, whereas the outer region is more fibrous in character.

Trace amounts of other collagen types, including types III, V, and VI, have been detected in the bovine meniscus (Eyre and Wu 1983). Polymerization of type I collagen with type III or V collagen to form heterotypic I–III and I–V fibres maximizes the ability of the meniscus to distribute load (Dudhia *et al.* 2004). The presence of types III and V collagen regulate type I collagen fibril diameter, resulting in a more compliant tissue. Type VI collagen constitutes approximately 2% of the dry weight of the bovine meniscus (Wu *et al.* 1987). The exact function of type VI collagen in the meniscus is still unknown. However, it is thought to participate in cell adhesion due to its ability to bind to integrins because of the presence of RGD sequence motifs in the short triple helix of type VI collagen (Marcelino and McDevitt 1995) as well as in other collagens,

matrix glycoproteins, and proteoglycans. The RGD sequence motif is recognized by many of the integrins, which are the cell surface receptors for ECM ligands. Therefore type VI collagen many be involved in cell signalling mechanisms. More recently, expression of type IV collagen has been detected in the ovine meniscus, mainly associated with blood vessels (Melrose *et al.* 2005) (Fig. 1.3.2), where it is localized in a dendritic pattern in the outer vascular zone, and also, but to a lesser extent, in the human inner meniscus (Marsano *et al.* 2007).

The orientation of collagen fibres across the meniscus is unique and three different layers have been identified (Petersen and Tillmann 1998): (1) a meshwork of small (~ 30nm diameter) collagen fibrils in the femoral and tibial surface regions; (2) a laminar superficial network (~150–200 µm deep) of radially or randomly orientated fibres; (3) circumferentially oriented collagen fibres with a small amount of radially oriented fibres, referred to as tie fibres (Petersen and Tillmann 1998, Kambic and McDevitt 2005). The presence of collagen fibres in a radial orientation at the periphery of the meniscus confers resistance to lateral spread and longitudinal splitting of the tissue. Therefore the unique organization of the collagen fibres in the meniscus reflects the mechanical properties of the

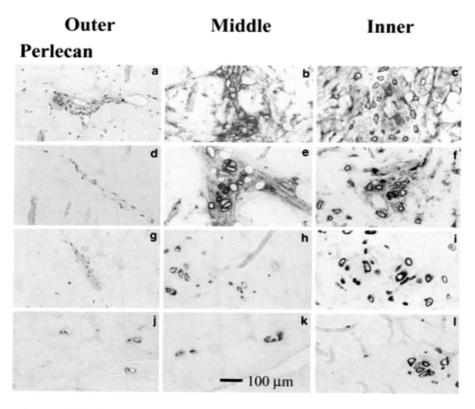

Type IV Collagen

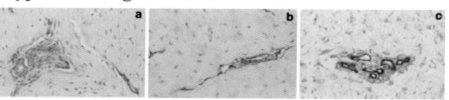

Fig. 1.3.2 Medium power views depicting spatial and temporal immunolocalizations of perlecan using MAb A76 to perlecan domain-1 in the outer (a, d, g, j), middle (b, e, h, k), and inner (c, f, i, l) zones of vertical coronal sections of lateral ovine menisci aged 7 months (a–c), 19 months (d–f), 7–8 years (g–i), and 10 years (j–l). Type IV collagen was also immunolocalized in 7-day-old meniscal sections for comparison (NovaRED chromogen). Scale bar 100µm. Perlecan is a prominent pericellular proteoglycan in small nests of oval to rounded cells of a chondrocytic morphology; these are prominent in the middle and inner meniscal zones up to 19 months of age and still evident but in lesser numbers in the inner zones of the 7- to 10-year-old meniscal sections (i, l). Reproduced with permission from Melrose, J. *et al.* (2005) *Histochemistry and Cell Biology*, **124**, 225–35, Springer.

tissue (discussed in the section below on biomechanical properties of the meniscus).

Proteoglycans

The functionality of the meniscus is not attributed exclusively to the presence of collagen fibres, but, as is evident with articular cartilage, is reliant on the presence of proteoglycans which impart the properties of hydration and ability to resist compression to the tissue (Nakano *et al.* 1997). Tissue hydration depends on the presence of large negatively charged proteoglycans in the ECM which causes imbibing of water and swelling pressure which is resisted by the collagenous network. Proteoglycan expression is more abundant in the inner two-thirds of the meniscus than in the outer third, as well as in the lateral relative to the medial side of the joint. Proteoglycans containing chondroitin sulphate glycosaminoglycans are the most abundant in both the inner and outer zones of the porcine meniscus, accounting for~ 80% and 50–56%, respectively (Nakano *et al.* 1997, Valiyaveettil *et al.* 2005). These large chondroitin-sulphate proteoglycans were identified as aggrecan (Adams *et al.* 1983). More recently, perlecan was identified in the inner hyaline part of the ovine meniscus; it is generally cell associated and diminishes significantly with age (Melrose *et al.* 2005) (Fig. 1.3.2). Perlecan is a heparan sulphate and/or chondroitin sulphate containing proteoglycan and is known to bind several growth factors, in particular members of the FGF family, which may be important in eliciting initial repair responses.

The second most abundant proteoglycans are those rich in dermatan sulphate glycosaminoglycans (Nakano *et al.* 1997). Interestingly, the distribution of these small dermatan sulphate proteoglycans is differentially expressed, with more concentrated levels of decorin in the outer region of the porcine meniscus and conversely more biglycan in the inner two-thirds of the tissue (Scott *et al.* 1997). Fibromodulin has also been detected in the inner region of the porcine meniscus (Scott *et al.* 1997). The function of biglycan in the inner region of the meniscus has been related to the greater compressive forces experienced. The prominence of decorin in the outer region, which is rich in type I collagen fibres, is associated with its function as a modulator of collagen fibrillogenesis.

Hyaluronan accounts for 4–5% of total glycosaminoglycan in the inner region and as much as 10% in the outer region of porcine meniscus (Nakano *et al.* 1997), fulfilling functions in regulating proteoglycan synthesis and, perhaps more unique to the meniscus, its involvement in meniscal tissue remodelling (Sonoda *et al.* 1997).

Non-collagenous matrix proteins

In addition to collagen and proteoglycans, the ECM of the meniscus also contains a cohort of non-collagenous matrix proteins. To date, elastin (McDevitt and Webber 1990), the ED-A and ED-B isoforms of fibronectin and tenascin-C (Salter *et al.* 1995), thrombospondin (Miller and McDevitt 1991), and COMP (cartilage oligomeric matrix protein) (Muller *et al.* 1998) have been identified. Their functions in the meniscus have not yet been identified, but all are involved in matrix assembly and/or regulating tissue homeostasis. Along with collagen, elastin is the other major fibrillar component of the meniscus. A combination of both mature and immature elastin fibres has been found within the inter-territorial region of adult meniscus; however, elastin only constitutes a small proportion of the meniscus (~ 0.6% dry weight) (McDevitt and Webber 1990). Although there have been no specific reports on elastin function in the meniscus, in other tissues elastin is involved in withstanding high tensile strains. Thus it is likely that the presence of elastin in the meniscus allows the tissue to revert to its original contour after cessation of a deforming load.

Biomechanical properties of the meniscus

The menisci serve several important biomechanical functions in the knee, including the dissipation of stresses across the articular cartilage, the ability to absorb shocks during dynamic loading, and assisting in joint lubrication. The menisci also fulfil a secondary biomechanical function by providing stability to the knee joint, in particular to a damaged knee where primary stabilizers may be deficient (e.g. the cruciate ligaments) (Dudhia *et al.* 2004). The importance of the menisci in dissipating mechanical loads has been highlighted in a recent survey showing that damaged menisci no longer give adequate protection to the underlying articular cartilage and generally result in early-onset osteoarthritis (OA) within 10–20 years (Lohmander *et al.* 2007).

Approximately 40–60% of the load acting on the knee is distributed by the menisci (Shrive *et al.* 1978). When a load is applied to the knee joint, the menisci are compressed/displaced (the lateral meniscus is displaced more than the medial meniscus during compression), but because of their semi-lunar architecture they transmit load away from the centre of the femoral condyles resulting in tensile stress towards the tibial plateau instead (Sweigart and Athanasiou 2001). The amount of force being transmitted through the knee joint also has some influence on how the joint components respond. When there is no force acting on the knee, the meniscus absorbs most of the load (Walker and Erkman 1975). However, when the force of body weight is applied, the lateral meniscus absorbs the majority of the load with the remainder divided between the medial meniscus and the articular cartilage (Walker and Erkman 1975). Overall, the lateral meniscus transmits 65–70% of the load, and the medial side transmits 40–50% (Dudhia *et al.* 2004); hence it is not surprising that damage to either or both menisci affects the biomechanical function of the tissue, disturbing normal joint articulation.

As previously discussed, the ability of the meniscus to withstand the biomechanical forces acting on the joint is a direct reflection of its intrinsic material properties in addition to its gross anatomical structure. The material properties of the meniscus are derived from the organization and interactions of the key ECM components, namely water, collagen, and proteoglycans. Interactions between these primary constituents result in the meniscus being a porous permeable composite material similar to articular cartilage (Dudhia *et al.* 2004). Application of load to the knee is effectively distributed by the menisci because of the orientation of the collagen fibres which confer tensile stiffness and strength to the tissue. Alignment of the collagen fibres in the direction of the applied load offers most resistance to stress; therefore the parallel arrangement of collagen fibres at the periphery of the tissue (i.e. circumferential) maximizes the ability of the meniscus to absorb and dissipate loads (Aspden *et al.* 1985). The presence of radially orientated collagen fibres influences the tensile properties of the meniscus, conferring stiffness on the tissue (Aspden *et al.* 1985).

Analysis of the tensile, compressive, and shear properties of meniscal tissue has been performed, but there has been great variability in outcomes, reflecting differences in species, specimen harvest, location, and size (reviewed by Sweigart and Athanasiou 2001).

Meniscal injuries

Contact sport is one of the primary causes of meniscal injuries which often arise in combination with ligament injuries, particularly when the medial meniscus is involved. The incidence of damage to the medial meniscus is approximately five times greater than damage to the lateral meniscus (Peterson and Renstrom 2001). Meniscal injuries are frequently caused by a twisting impact to the knee, and sports such as football, rugby, and squash, to name but a few, are principal contributors. Sports with the highest prevalence of meniscal injuries are football, basketball, and baseball—sports in which the knee is subjected to rotational and 'cutting' motions (Peterson and Renstrom 2001). Meniscal injuries can also be caused by hyperextension and hyperflexion of the knee, and again this can occur during particular sports activities. However, hyperextension or hyperflexion can also occur during normal body movement in elderly people, through actions such as deep knee bends, and meniscal degeneration is probably attributable to the decreased strength of the surrounding muscle/ligament supports.

Meniscal degeneration

As a consequence of their central anatomical and functional position in the knee joint, the menisci are prone to damage as a result of mechanical trauma, inflammation, altered metabolism, and/or degeneration of synovial joint components (e.g. articular cartilage degradation).

Age-related changes in the meniscus

Changes in ECM structure and composition in connective tissues with ageing and disease have been extensively studied; however, there is still a lack of basic understanding of the characteristics of the meniscus under these conditions. Early studies demonstrated that there were age-related increases in total collagen content in the developing human menisci, which remained static thereafter (Ingman et al. 1974). In a follow-up study, collagen content was found to increase from birth to 30 years and then remain constant until 80 years of age, after which a decline was observed (Ghosh and Taylor 1987). However, our own work indicated a steady loss of total collagen from 75% dry weight in 5-year-old human menisci to 65% in 80-year-old samples (Duance et al. 1999). We also found a decrease in type I collagen and an increase in type III collagen with age which probably changes the biomechanical properties of the tissue. Similarly, hexosamine, as an indicator of proteoglycan/hyaluronan content, decreased from birth to maturity, but increased slightly after 70 years of age (Ingman et al. 1974). Maturation and ageing of the human menisci are associated with an increased ratio of chondroitin-6-sulphate to chondroitin-4-sulphate, and an increase in keratan sulphate proteoglycans (McNicol and Roughley 1980). More recently, it has been shown that unlike aggrecan, which is constitutively expressed throughout life, perlecan expression declines markedly with the onset of age in ovine menisci (Melrose et al. 2005). Clearly, more research is required in this area to advance our knowledge of changes that occur in the meniscus with ageing, to understand the functional consequences of these changes, and to be able to discriminate between the effects of ageing and pathological events.

Pathology of the meniscus

The most common pathological condition of the tissue is meniscal tears (Mesiha et al. 2007); less common is separation from the tibial attachment or degeneration of the meniscus itself. Meniscal tearing can present in several forms, including longitudinal, radial, and complex tears (Brown 2004). The age distribution of those diagnosed with an isolated symptomatic meniscus lesion is very broad, with a mean age of 30 years for trauma-induced meniscal tears and a mean age of >40 years for those diagnosed with degenerative tears, which probably coincide with pre-existing joint cartilage damage (Lohmander et al. 2007).

The ability of the meniscus to repair itself naturally in vivo depends on the type of tear; a tear in the outer region can repair because of its vascularized nature, but the inner region, which is inherently avascular, appears to be incapable of adequate repair. Likewise, if a meniscal tear is longitudinal there is an increased chance of repair and restoration of the tissue's original function, whereas if the tear is in a radial orientation it is unable to repair because of disruption of the collagen structure (Sweigart and Athanasiou 2001).

Meniscal tears can heal via one of two processes: (1) the intrinsic ability of the meniscal cells to migrate, proliferate, and synthesize a matrix given the correct biological cue(s), or (2) extrinsic stimulation through neovascularization (Dudhia et al. 2004). The extrinsic pathway can only be activated in the outer region of the meniscus where vasculature is present. Mesenchymal stem cells and a supply of nutrients are attracted to a fibrin clot which acts as a natural scaffold for the proliferating cells (Dudhia et al. 2004). The formation of this fibrovascular tissue seals the defect and encourages new matrix synthesis and neovascularization. A more recent observation using an in vitro meniscal explant model suggests that the extrinsic pathway of repair is not unique to the outer region; explants from the avascular inner region exhibit similar healing potential and repair strength (Hennerbichler et al. 2007). It is possible that the regional differences in in vivo meniscal repair are a consequence of the additional vasculature of the outer region rather than inherent differences between the ECM and the cells residing in these tissue regions.

Based on a previous report that the annual incidence of meniscal injuries in the Danish population was 70 per 100 000, it has since been calculated that the cumulative risk of a meniscus injury leading to surgery, in a population aged 10–64 years, may be at least 15% (Lohmander et al. 2007); however, this number does not include meniscal injuries that are not diagnosed or treated by surgery. Although an estimate, it illustrates the potential magnitude of the clinical problem in which several reports indicate that, 10–20 years after a meniscal injury, every second patient develops OA (Lohmander et al. 2007), leading to significant pain, functional limitations, and a diminished quality of life.

Structure and function of osteoarthritic menisci

OA is a common, arguably age-related, connective tissue disorder that is characterized by focal areas of loss of articular cartilage in synovial joints accompanied by varying degrees of osteophyte formation, subchondral bone changes, and synovitis. In more advanced stages of OA, structural changes include joint space narrowing, subchondral sclerosis, and bone cyst formation. The development of magnetic resonance imaging (MRI) has increased our knowledge of the disease phenotype and, along with capsule thickening, there is evidence of maceration and extrusion of the menisci (Lohmander *et al.* 2007). MRI modelling of the medial and lateral tibiofemoral joints of symptomatic OA patients demonstrated that the positioning and degeneration of the menisci contributed to prediction of joint-space narrowing used as an outcome measure for OA progression (Hunter *et al.* 2006).

Even allowing for the wealth of evidence which shows an involvement of meniscal degeneration with OA progression, there is still limited knowledge on the biochemistry of OA menisci, as most interest has concentrated on the reverse, i.e. how removal of the menisci (meniscectomy) or joint instability predisposes the cartilage to development of OA. Although there is extensive information on the structural and biochemical changes in OA cartilage, we have yet to resolve what changes may be occurring in the meniscus.

Analyses of OA knees established a loss of collagen in degenerated menisci coincident with elevated levels of proteoglycans and non-collagenous proteins relative to age-matched control tissue (Ghosh *et al.* 1975). The loss of total collagen is primarily due to a loss of type I collagen; there is a slight increase in the type III collagen content of OA menisci. Type II collagen is present at a very low level in normal human menisci but increases dramatically in OA tissue. In addition, the level of hydroxylysyl pyridinoline, the mature collagen cross-link, decreases in OA menisci (Duance *et al.* 1999). These changes to the collagenous matrix suggest that the normal mechanical function of the meniscus in protecting the underlying articular cartilage is severely compromised and thus probably contributes to the degradation of the articular cartilage in OA. Increased fragmentation of decorin in degenerated human menisci has also been observed, although the proteolytic enzymes responsible for this cleavage have yet to be identified (Melrose *et al.* 2008). However, in these human studies it was unclear whether damage of the articular cartilage preceded meniscal degeneration or vice versa. To a certain extent, progress in answering this conundrum has been addressed by the use of animal models of joint instability. Adams *et al.* (1983) were the first to describe severe gross morphological changes in the menisci of a dog anterior cruciate ligament (ACL) transection model, where fibrillations and meniscal tears were observed. Menisci were shown to undergo extensive degeneration within as little as 3–8 weeks of joint destabilization induced by transection of the rabbit ACL (Hellio Le Graverand *et al.* 2001b). In this study, meniscal degeneration was most prominent in the medial compartment, where distinct morphological changes were observed across the tissue. The inner zone of the medial meniscus was characterized by fissures, depletion of cells, and the absence of proteoglycans, whereas the outer region exhibited increased cell number, abnormal organization of the collagen, and increased proteoglycan content (Hellio Le Graverand *et al.* 2001b). The gross morphological changes observed in the menisci, in particular the medial compartment, suggest that early alterations in the material properties of the meniscal tissue may lead to abnormal biomechanical function. The fact that, in this ACL transection model, structural and biochemical changes, resulting in significant degeneration of the medial meniscus, occurred prior to cartilage damage suggests that damage to the medial meniscus may initiate OA cartilage pathology in a mechanically compromised joint (e.g. with ACL damage).

Strategies for meniscal repair

Over the decades, many interventions have been designed and implemented to treat damaged meniscal tissue, including the infamous 'meniscectomy' procedure. However, most meniscal surgical options are fraught with difficulties, including persistent degeneration of the underlying cartilage and OA development. The field of tissue engineering has expanded and with it the opportunity to construct meniscal tissue, utilizing such materials as collagenous tissue, meniscal fibrochondrocytes, chondrocytes, synthetic scaffolds, and gene therapy as discussed below.

Meniscectomy

The first major type of repair technique developed for meniscal defects was 'meniscectomy', which involved complete removal of the meniscus. However, the complete removal of the meniscus inevitably led to cartilage erosion and the development of OA. Directly after the removal of the meniscus, the mechanical function of the knee joint is weakened, leading to greater application of stress to the articular cartilage which then compromises the integrity of this tissue. This is not surprising because after total meniscectomy increased forces of 235% would have to be dissipated across the tibiofemoral compartment in the absence of the menisci (Brown 2004). Partial meniscectomy, which is removal of a small portion of the meniscus, has been shown to cause less degenerative change in the articular cartilage than a complete meniscectomy, due in part to a more conservative increase in load (70%) across the tibiofemoral compartment (Brown 2004).

After the realization that total removal of the meniscus resulted in articular cartilage degeneration, preserving as much meniscal tissue as possible has led to a resurgence in repair of the meniscal tear. Several different modes of repair have been implemented, including suture, fibrin sealant, abrasion therapy, and induced vascularization (Lohmander *et al.* 2007). There is continuing research into the potential use of meniscal replacement by allograft, tendon autograft, or prostheses (Khetia and McKeon 2007; Schoenfeld *et al.* 2007; Verdonk *et al.* 2007; Stapleton *et al.* 2008). Transplantation of the menisci has had some success, although immunogenicity of meniscal allografts has made this procedure less attractive as a strategy for repair. Replacement of menisci with allograft tissue has met with success, particularly when patellar tendon has been used to replace the damaged menisci.

Cell-based approaches

In the last 10–15 years attempts at repairing damaged menisci have focused on the replacement of the tissue with either natural meniscal tissue or a synthetic replacement. Many *in vitro* and *in vivo* studies have been performed to engineer functional tissues such as cartilage and bone, but development of procedures for meniscal tissue engineering is still some way behind. Cells from a variety of different sources have been used. *In vitro* studies compared the potential repair capacity of cells derived from different regions of the meniscus (Mauck *et al.* 2007). Cells from the outer region of the meniscus of 3–6-month-old bovine calves showed greater plasticity in differentiation to chondrogenic, adipogenic, and osteogenic phenotypes. Although caution is required in extrapolating to mature human menisci, it is suggested that this greater plasticity would be beneficial in developing cell-based strategies for meniscal repair. Cells from alternative sources within the joint have been investigated (Marsano *et al.* 2006). Cells from articular cartilage, inner meniscus, fat pad, and synovial membrane were seeded on a hyaluronan non-woven mesh. When a hydrodynamic fluid flow system was used, only the articular cartilage cells generated a bizonal special organization with an inner and outer zone

similar in composition and biomechanical properties to the meniscus. A range of growth factors have been studied in investigations of enhancement of the matrix-forming capacity of meniscal cells. A combination of FGF2 and hypoxia (5% oxygen tension) has been shown to enhance significantly the chondrogenic potential of meniscal cells in culture and maybe a useful strategy during the cell expansion stage of any cell-based therapy (Adesida *et al.* 2006).

Several studies have investigated the use of stem cells to generate strategies for meniscal repair. Hoben *et al.* (2009) used human

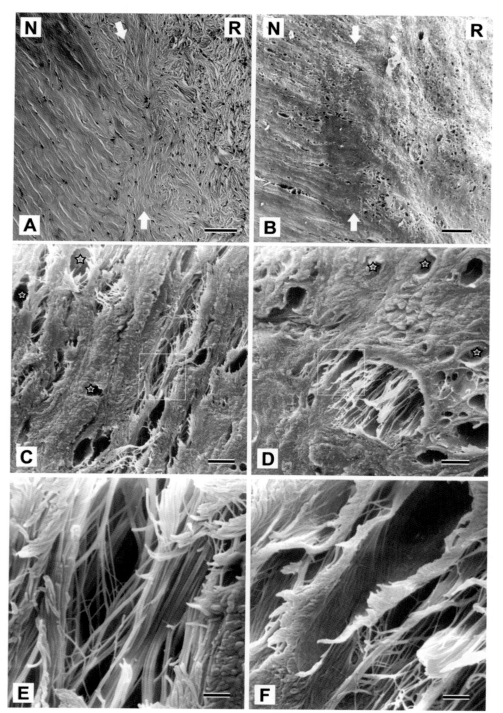

Fig. 1.3.3 (a) Toluidine blue histology and (b) scanning electron microscopy of a representative integration zone of repair tissue (R) with normal meniscus (N). The meniscal defect was filled with a cell-scaffold composite for 12 weeks. The arrows mark the integration zone. Magnification bars, 100µm. Normal meniscus (c, e) and repair tissue (d, f) at higher magnification. Asterisks indicate cell cavities; squares in (c, d) mark the region of collagen fibrils seen in (e, f). Magnification bars, 10 µm (c, d) and 2 µm (e, f). Reproduced from Angele, P. *et al.* (2008) *Journal of Biomedical Materials Research Part A*, **85**, 445–55. Reprinted with permission from John Wiley & Sons, Inc.

embryonic stem cells (hESCs) with a combination of growth factors to induce a fibrochondrogenic phenotype. Cells with BMP4 and TGF-β gave the best outcome with respect to type II collagen and GAG production. The co-culture of hESCs with fibrochondrocytes enhanced the fibrocartilage phenotype. It was found that CD44 expression was enhanced by the BMP4 and TGF-β treatment, enabling specific cell populations to be separated by flow cytometry for use in treatment strategies. Rabbit mesenchymal stem cells (MSCs) have been seeded onto a hyaluronan–gelatin construct for 14 days prior to implanting in a meniscal defect (Angele *et al.* 2008). These pre-cultured implants greatly enhanced the repair outcome in this animal model, demonstrating good integration of the tissue-engineered construct with the host tissue and identifying MSCs as an excellent source of cells for cell-based meniscal repair strategies (Fig. 1.3.3). Hyaluronan has also been used as a delivery vehicle for MSCs in a meniscectomy model of OA in the goat (Murphy *et al.* 2003). Interestingly, in addition to the reduced progression of the OA, there was clear evidence of regeneration of the removed meniscus, indicating the potential of these cells for tissue repair. A recent study attempted to enhance this potential by genetically modifying both meniscal cells and MSCs to express higher levels of TGF-β1 (Steinert *et al.* 2007). Genetically modified cells were seeded in a collagen–GAG matrix and used in an *in vitro* model of bovine meniscal repair. After 3 weeks there was enhanced repair with increased expression of meniscal genes. The use of virally transduced cells has a number of problems to be addressed but offers the possibility of overcoming some of the intrinsic lack of repair of the inner portion of the meniscus. However, a recent study using MSCs on a collagen scaffold found that the use of TGF-β1 to enhance stem cell differentiation inhibited construct integration (Pabbruwe *et al.* 2010). The use of a collagen based scaffold was found to be effective in repairing tears of the inner portion of the meniscus.

Concluding remarks

With our increasingly ageing and active population the incidence of meniscal injury will be greater in the future, leading to a higher incidence of osteoarthritis. Clearly, a better understanding of the biology of the meniscus and the links to degenerative joint disease are a priority in order to develop strategies to limit the incidence of meniscal damage. Significant advances in meniscal tissue repair/regeneration have been made recently. However, despite these advances more work needs to be done, including incorporating concepts from tissue engineering of other connective tissues, to potentiate the possibility of a tissue-engineered meniscus that resembles native tissue in terms of both biochemical and biomechanical characteristics. In particular, the histological, morphological, and biomechanical properties of tissue-engineered meniscal constructs must be better understood to facilitate this goal and improve the quality of life of our ageing society.

Acknowledgements

The authors would like to thank the Arthritis Research Campaign, UK, for financial support (EJB).

References

Adams, M.E., Billingham, M.E., and Muir, H. (1983). The glycosaminoglycans in menisci in experimental and natural osteoarthritis. *Arthritis and Rheumatism*, **26**, 69–76.

Adesida, A.B., Grady, L.M., Khan, W.S., and Hardingham, T.E. (2006). The matrix-forming phenotype of cultured human meniscus cells is enhanced after culture with fibroblast growth factor 2 and is further stimulated by hypoxia. *Arthritis Research and Therapy*, **8**, R61.

Angele, P., Johnstone, B., Kujat, R., *et al.* (2008). Stem cell based tissue engineering for meniscus repair. *Journal of Biomedical Materials Research A*, **85**, 445–55.

Aspden, R.M., Yarker, Y.E., and Hukins, D.W. (1985). Collagen orientations in the meniscus of the knee joint. *Journal of Anatomy*, **140** (Pt 3), 371–80.

Bland-Sutton, J. (1887). *Ligaments: Their Nature and Morphology*. H.K. Lewis, London.

Brown, J. (2004). Soft tissue injuries of the knee. *Surgery (Oxford)*, **22**, 40–4.

Cheung, H.S. (1987). Distribution of type I, II, III and V in the pepsin solubilized collagens in bovine menisci. *Connective Tissue Research*, **16**, 343–56.

Duance, V.C., Vaughan-Thomas, A., Wardale, R.J., and Wotton, S.F. (1999). The collagens of articular and meniscal cartilages. In: C.W. Archer, B. Caterson, M. Benjamin, and J.R. Ralphs (eds), *Biology of the Synovial Joint*. Harwood Academic, Amsterdam.

Dudhia, J., McAlinden, A., Muir, P., and Bayliss, M. (2004). The meniscus—structure, composition, and pathology. In: B. Hazleman, G. Riley, and C. Speed (eds), *Soft Tissue Rheumatology*. Oxford University Press.

Eyre, D.R. and Muir, H. (1975). Characterisation of the major CNBr-derived peptides of porcine type II collagen. *Connective Tissue Research*, **3**, 165–70.

Eyre, D.R. and Wu, J.J. (1983). Collagen of fibrocartilage: a distinctive molecular phenotype in bovine meniscus. *FEBS Letters*, **158**, 265–70.

Fairbanks, T.J. (1948). Knee joint changes after meniscectomy. *Journal of Bone and Joint Surgery, British Volume*, **30**, 664–70.

Ghadially, F.N., Thomas, I., Yong, N., and Lalonde, J.M. (1978). Ultrastructure of rabbit semilunar cartilages. *Journal of Anatomy*, **125**, 499–517.

Ghosh, P. and Taylor, T.K. (1987). The knee joint meniscus. A fibrocartilage of some distinction. *Clinical Orthopaedics and Related Research*, **224**, 52–63.

Ghosh, P., Ingman, A.M., and Taylor, T.K. (1975). Variations in collagen, non-collagenous proteins, and hexosamine in menisci derived from osteoarthritic and rheumatoid arthritic knee joints. *Journal of Rheumatology*, **2**, 100–7.

Hellio Le Graverand, M.P., Ou, Y., Schield-Yee, T., *et al.* (2001a). The cells of the rabbit meniscus: their arrangement, interrelationship, morphological variations and cytoarchitecture. *Journal of Anatomy*, **198**, 525–35.

Hellio Le Graverand, M.P., Vignon, E., Otterness, I.G., and Hart, D.A. (2001b). Early changes in lapine menisci during osteoarthritis development. Part I: cellular and matrix alterations. *Osteoarthritis and Cartilage*, **9**, 56–64.

Hennerbichler, A., Moutos, F.T., Hennerbichler, D., Weinberg, J.B., and Guilak, F. (2007). Repair response of the inner and outer regions of the porcine meniscus *in vitro*. *American Journal of Sports Medicine*, **35**, 754–62.

Hoben, G.M., Willard, V.P., and Athanasiou, K.A. (2009). Fibrochondrogenesis of hESCs: growth factor combinations and co-cultures. *Stem Cells and Development*, **18**, 283–92.

Hunter, D.J., Zhang, Y.Q., Tu, X., *et al.* (2006). Change in joint space width: hyaline articular cartilage loss or alteration in meniscus? *Arthritis and Rheumatism*, **54**, 2488–95.

Ingman, A.M., Ghosh, P., and Taylor, T.K. (1974). Variation of collagenous and non-collagenous proteins of human knee joint menisci with age and degeneration. *Gerontologia*, **20**, 212–23.

Kambic, H.E. and McDevitt, C.A. (2005). Spatial organization of types I and II collagen in the canine meniscus. *Journal of Orthopaedic Research*, **23**, 142–9.

Khetia, E.A. and McKeon, B.P. (2007). Meniscal allografts: biomechanics and techniques. *Sports Medicine and Arthroscopy Review*, **15**, 114–20.

Lohmander, L.S., Englund, P.M., Dahl, L.L., and Roos, E.M. (2007). The long-term consequence of anterior cruciate ligament and meniscus injuries: osteoarthritis. *American Journal of Sports Medicine*, **35**, 1756–69.

McDevitt, C.A. and Webber, R.J. (1990). The ultrastructure and biochemistry of meniscal cartilage. *Clinical Orthopaedics and Related Research*, **252**, 8–18.

McNicol, D. and Roughley, P.J. (1980). Extraction and characterization of proteoglycan from human meniscus. *Biochemical Journal*, **185**, 705–13.

Marcelino, J. and McDevitt, C.A. (1995). Attachment of articular cartilage chondrocytes to the tissue form of type VI collagen. *Biochimica Biophysica Acta*, **1249**, 180–8.

Marsano, A., Vunjak-Novakovic, G., and Martin, I. (2006). Towards tissue engineering of meniscus substitutes: selection of cell source and culture environment. *Conference Proceedings. IEEE Engineering in Medicine and Biology Society*, **1**, 3656–8.

Marsano, A., Millward-Sadler, S.J., Salter, D.M., *et al.* (2007). Differential cartilaginous tissue formation by human synovial membrane, fat pad, meniscus cells and articular chondrocytes. *Osteoarthritis and Cartilage*, **15**, 48–58.

Mauck, R.L., Martinez-Diaz, G.J., Yuan, X., and Tuan, R.S. (2007). Regional multilineage differentiation potential of meniscal fibrochondrocytes: implications for meniscus repair. *Anatomical Record*, **290**, 48–58.

Melrose, J., Smith, S., Cake, M., Read, R., and Whitelock, J. (2005). Comparative spatial and temporal localisation of perlecan, aggrecan and type I, II and IV collagen in the ovine meniscus: an ageing study. *Histochemistry and Cell Biology*, **124**, 225–35.

Melrose, J., Fuller, E.S., Roughley, P.J., *et al.* (2008). Fragmentation of decorin, biglycan, lumican and keratocan is elevated in degenerate human meniscus, knee and hip articular cartilages compared with age-matched macroscopically normal and control tissues. *Arthritis Research and Therapy*, **10**, R79.

Mesiha, M., Zurakowski, D., Soriano, J., Nielson, J.H., Zarins, B., and Murray, M.M. (2007). Pathologic characteristics of the torn human meniscus. *American Journal of Sports Medicine*, **35**, 103–12.

Miller, R.R. and McDevitt, C.A. (1991). Thrombospondin in ligament, meniscus and intervertebral disc. *Biochimica Biophysica Acta*, **1115**, 85–88.

Muller, G., Michel, A., and Altenburg, E. (1998). COMP (cartilage oligomeric matrix protein) is synthesized in ligament, tendon, meniscus, and articular cartilage. *Connective Tissue Research*, **39**, 233–44.

Murphy, J.M., Fink, D.J., Hunziker, E.B., and Barry, F.P. (2003). Stem cell therapy in a caprine model of osteoarthritis. *Arthritis and Rheumatism*, **48**, 3464–74.

Nakano, T., Dodd, C.M., and Scott, P.G. (1997). Glycosaminoglycans and proteoglycans from different zones of the porcine knee meniscus. *Journal of Orthopaedic Research*, **15**, 213–20.

Pabbruwe, M.B., Kaflenah, W., Tarlton, J.F., Mistry, S., Fox, D.J., and Hollander, A.P. (2010). Repair of meniscal cartilage white zone tears using a stem cell/collagen–scaffold implant. *Biomaterials*, **31**, 2583–91.

Petersen, W. and Tillmann, B. (1998). Collagenous fibril texture of the human knee joint menisci. *Anatomy and Embryology*, **197**, 317–24.

Peterson, L. and Renstrom, P. (2001). Meniscus injuries. In: *Sports Injuries: Their Prevention and Treatment* (3rd edn). Martin Dunitz, London.

Salter, D.M., Godolphin, J.L., and Gourlay, M.S. (1995). Chondrocyte heterogeneity: immunohistologically defined variation of integrin expression at different sites in human fetal knees. *Journal of Histochemistry and Cytochemistry*, **43**, 447–57.

Schoenfeld, A.J., Landis, W.J., and Kay, D.B. (2007). Tissue-engineered meniscal constructs. *American Journal of Orthopedics*, **36**, 614–20.

Scott, P.G., Nakano, T., and Dodd, C.M. (1997). Isolation and characterization of small proteoglycans from different zones of the porcine knee meniscus. *Biochimica Biophysica Acta*, **1336**, 254–62.

Shrive, N.G., O'Connor, J.J., and Goodfellow J,W. (1978). Load-bearing in the knee joint. *Clinical Orthopaedics and Related Research*, **131**, 279–87.

Sonoda, M., Harwood, F.L., Wada, Y., Moriya, H., and Amiel, D. (1997). The effects of hyaluronan on the meniscus and on the articular cartilage after partial meniscectomy. *American Journal of Sports Medicine*, **25**, 755–62.

Stapleton, T.W., Ingram, J., Katta, J., *et al.* (2008). Development and characterization of an acellular porcine medial meniscus for use in tissue engineering. *Tissue Engineering Part A*, **14**, 505–18.

Steinert, A.F., Palmer, G.D., Capito, R., *et al.* (2007). Genetically enhanced engineering of meniscus tissue using *ex vivo* delivery of transforming growth factor-beta 1 complementary deoxyribonucleic acid. *Tissue Engineering*, **13**, 2227–37.

Sweigart, M.A. and Athanasiou, K.A. (2001). Toward tissue engineering of the knee meniscus. *Tissue Engineering*, **7**, 111–29.

Tanaka, E., Detamore, M.S., and Mercuri, L.G. (2008). Degenerative disorders of the temporomandibular joint: etiology, diagnosis, and treatment. *Journal of Dental Research*, **87**, 296–307.

Tischer, T., Salzmann, G.M., El-Azab, H., Vogt, S., and Imhoff, A.B. (2009). Incidence of associated injuries with acute acromioclavicular joint dislocations types III through V. *American Journal of Sports Medicine*, **37**, 136–9.

Valiyaveettil, M., Mort, J.S., and McDevitt, C.A. (2005). The concentration, gene expression, and spatial distribution of aggrecan in canine articular cartilage, meniscus, and anterior and posterior cruciate ligaments: a new molecular distinction between hyaline cartilage and fibrocartilage in the knee joint. *Connective Tissue Research*, **46**, 83–91.

Verdonk, R., Almqvist, K.F., Huysse, W., and Verdonk, P.C. (2007). Meniscal allografts: indications and outcomes. *Sports Medicine and Arthroscopy Review*, **15**, 121–5.

Walker, P.S. and Erkman, M.J. (1975). The role of the menisci in force transmission across the knee. *Clinical Orthopaedics and Related Research*, **109**, 184–92.

Wu, J.J., Eyre, D.R., and Slayter, H.S. (1987). Type VI collagen of the intervertebral disc. Biochemical and electron-microscopic characterization of the native protein. *Biochemical Journal*, **248**, 373–81.

1.4

The intervertebral disc and the spine

Sally Roberts, Jai Trivedi, and Victor Duance

Introduction

Back problems are common in the general population, affecting approximately 80% of individuals at some time in their lives. It used to be thought that loading, activity levels, or certain types of activities (e.g. driving tractors or heavy goods vehicles) greatly influenced the incidence of back pain (Pope and Hansson 1992). However, the over-riding 'risk factor' for back pain in the general population is now known to be genetic (Sambrook *et al.* 1999; Battié *et al.* 2004). That withstanding, there are some clinical problems that are associated with certain sports. Examples include gymnasts, javelin throwers, divers, and trampolinists with hyperextension and hyperflexion injuries, rugby players and horse riders with burst fractures and spinal cord injuries, and wrestlers and weight trainers with stress fractures and spondylolysis. Some of these clinical problems are dealt with in Chapter 3.7. The objective of this chapter is to provide the basic understanding of how the tissues within the vertebral column function, what their normal anatomy and composition are, and what pathologies may predispose to particular sporting injuries.

Structure of the spine

The spine is composed of the vertebral column, which surrounds and protects the spinal cord. It consists of a series of vertebrae interspersed with cartilaginous intervertebral discs; each bone and adjacent discs is termed a 'motion segment' (Fig. 1.4.1). There is a system of ligaments binding the motion segments together: the anterior and posterior ligaments run the whole length of the spine, with smaller ligaments around the joints and between the vertebrae (ligamentum flavum, supra- and interspinous ligaments). Together these provide passive stability in combination with a series of muscles (which will not be addressed in this chapter) providing active stabilization.

The normal degree of flexibility and mobility of each motion segment varies considerably with location within the spine. The cervical region is the most mobile, the lumbar region is fairly mobile, and the thoracic is the least mobile due to the attachment of the ribs. It is the more mobile regions of the spine that generally give rise to problems, with the fused immobile sacrum and coccyx generally being injury free in sport.

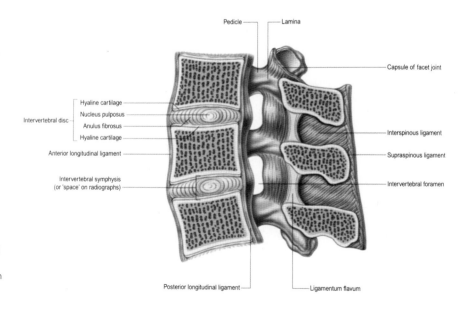

Fig. 1.4.1 Motion segments of the lumbar vertebrae showing the intervertebral disc, and the associated ligaments. Reproduced from *Gray's Anatomy* (Standring), with permission from Elsevier.

The vertebrae

Each vertebra (of which there are 24, plus the fused vertebrae within the sacrum and the coccyx) is a complex structure. One of the main functions must be to protect the spinal cord whilst permitting the off-shooting nerves to pass bilaterally to the parts of the body they control and feed back information to and from the central nervous system (CNS). There is a simpler, anterior portion of the vertebral body, interspaced and joined to each other by the cartilaginous intervertebral disc.

Each vertebra can be divided into three sections: the main vertebral body, the pedicle and the posterior processes. The main vertebral body has flat superior and inferior surfaces. It consists of a relatively thin outer shell of cortical bone and internally of trabeculae composed of cancellous bone. There are vertical and horizontal trabeculae that resist compressive and tensional forces respectively. Oblique trabeculae run from the vertebral body through the pedicle to the posterior processes and resist bending and shear forces. The ability of the vertebrae to resist these forces is often compromised in the elderly. There is a significant loss of trabeculae in osteoporosis, which can cause collapse of the vertebral body and serious disability.

Bone is a composite material comprising an organic extracellular matrix with the mineral calcium hydroxyapatite interspersed within and between the matrix (Schenk et al. 2002). The matrix is composed primarily of type I collagen but with minor amounts of types III and V collagen and, increasingly with ageing, the alpha 1 chain of type XI collagen. Type I collagen fibrils provide the principal mechanical strength of the tissue. The precise functions of the other collagen types are unknown, but they are thought to regulate fibril formation and fibril size, thus influencing the properties of the matrix. The extracellular matrix also contains a number of proteoglycans (PGs), in particular members of the small leucine rich family of PGs (SLRPs) including decorin, biglycan, and mimecan (osteoglycin) (Young 2003; Lamoureux et al. 2007). These proteoglycans modulate collagen fibril formation but are also known to bind growth factors important in regulating bone turnover and repair processes. A number of matrix glycoproteins, such as osteopontin and osteonectin, have also been isolated from the bone matrix (Schenk et al. 2002; Sodek et al. 2002; Young 2003). Osteopontin contains the RGD amino acid sequence motif recognized as a binding site for integrins, indicating that osteopontin is cell surface associated. Recent studies reveal that osteopontin is not bone specific but is expressed quite widely, and it has been implicated in cell migration and tumour cell metastasis (El-Tanani 2008). Osteonectin is an acidic glycoprotein that binds calcium hydroxyapatite and functions in bone to inhibit/regulate mineralization through its interaction with the collagenous component of the matrix. It is widely expressed in other tissues and has a variety of additional functions, including the regulation of growth factor activity, and is anti-adhesive for cell–matrix interactions. The mineral component of bone is primarily calcium hydroxyapatite. The initial deposition occurs in the gap zone of the collagen fibrils, which is mediated and regulated by the specific interactions of the proteoglycans and matrix glycoproteins with the collagen fibrils. Further mineral is deposited between the collagen fibrils, resulting in a fibrillar network embedded in the calcium hydroxyapatite crystals. The mineral does not contribute to the mechanical strength but provides rigidity to the bone structure.

The flat surfaces of the vertebral body provide a stable structure by resisting the longitudinal forces. To provide flexibility of the spine each vertebra is interposed with the intervertebral disc. This structure, although stable in the longitudinal axis, lacks any horizontal stability. The posterior processes of each vertebra allow flexibility but prevent excessive slippage or bending of each motion segment. The inferior articular process of one vertebra articulates with the superior articular process of the adjacent vertebra to form the zygapophyseal (facet) joint. These synovial joints function to prevent forward displacement and rotational dislocation of the intervertebral disc within the motion segment (Bogduk and Twomey 1996; Boszczyk et al. 1999). These joints are typical synovial joints with articular cartilage covering the bony processes enclosed within a joint capsule and synovial membrane lining. The limited biochemical studies undertaken have shown that the articular cartilage of these joints has a very similar composition to the articular cartilage of joints of the long bones such as the knee. It is primarily composed of type II collagen with lesser amounts of other collagen types such as types IX and XI as well as the major aggregating proteoglycan aggrecan (Duance et al. 1999; Eyre et al. 2006). The joint capsule is a fibrous structure composed primarily of type I collagen which encloses the joint. The anterior part of the capsule is replaced by the ligamentum flavum (see next section). The joint capsule also folds into the joint space to form a meniscoid structure which acts like a true meniscus by adding stability to the joint (Bogduk and Twomey 1996).

Ligaments

The spinal column is stabilized by a number of different ligaments: the anterior longitudinal ligament (ALL), the posterior longitudinal ligament (PLL), the interspinous and supraspinous ligaments, and the ligamentum flavum (Fig. 1.4.1).

The ALL and PLL are attached to the anterior and posterior aspects of the vertebral body of each vertebra. Deep-lying fibres attach to adjacent vertebrae whereas more superficial fibres span two, three, four, or five vertebrae. The short fibres of the ALL attach to the ring apophysis and are considered by some to be part of the annulus fibrosus. The ALL and PLL act to resist separation of the vertebral bodies during bending and extension of the spine, with the longer fibres acting over several motion segments (Bogduk and Twomey 1996).

The ligamentum flavum is composed of short thick fibres joining the medial and lateral laminae of adjacent vertebrae. Unlike the other ligaments of the spine, which are mostly composed of collagen, this ligament is 80% elastin and approximately 20% collagen, reflecting its highly elastic nature. It has a role in restoring the flexed lumbar spine to its normal extended position. The ligament maintains the intervertebral discs under a degree of prestressed tension. The elastic nature of this ligament also prevents it from buckling when not under tension and encroaching into the vertebral canal and potentially damaging the spinal cord.

The interspinous and supraspinous ligaments connect posterior processes of adjacent vertebrae. The interspinous ligament resists separation of the posterior processes and therefore limits the forward bending movements of the spine. The supraspinous ligament is not present along the whole spine being absent in the lower lumbar region. For the most part, the supraspinous ligament is not a true ligament but is largely composed of tendinous fibres from the back muscles (Bogduk and Twomey 1996).

The structure of ligaments is essentially similar to that of tendons (Benjamin 2004), being predominantly collagen with relatively large fibres composed principally of type I collagen. There are small amounts of other collagen types, namely types III, IV, V, VI XII, and XIV (Riley 2004). At the site of insertion into the bone most ligaments and tendons have a fibrocartilaginous appearance and composition with the presence of type II collagen and increased levels of proteoglycans such as aggrecan. As mentioned above, all ligaments contain some elastin, which distinguishes them from tendons. The amount of elastin varies considerably, generally from a few per cent up to the 80% quoted for the ligamentum flavum.

With increasing age, there is generally decreased mobility which relates to biochemical changes in the ligaments and intervertebral disc. The lumbar supraspinous and interspinous ligaments show a negative correlation in tensile strength with ageing and a decreased elastic modulus (Lida *et al.* 2002). This is similar to other ligaments in the body where these changes have been linked to decreases in hydration, glycosaminoglycan content and changes in collagen solubility/cross-linking. These changes reflect the lower cellular activity resulting in a failure to maintain and repair the matrix (Riley 2004). The intraspinous ligaments are the weakest of the posterior elements in resisting flexion, and are frequently found to have some degree of degeneration with age. Over-rotation of the spine tends to result in injury to the zygopophyseal joints, causing compaction (Barros *et al.* 2002; Nihei *et al.* 2003).

Intervertebral disc

The anterior vertebral body of each vertebra is interspersed by an intervertebral disc (IVD). Each intervertebral disc is morphologically composed of three distinct regions: the outer annulus fibrosus (AF), an inner core, the nucleus pulposus (NP) and the cartilaginous

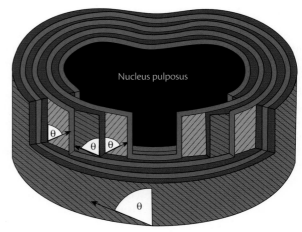

Fig. 1.4.3 Diagram showing the lamellar structure of collagen fibres in the annulus fibrosus. The lamellae are inclined to the long axis of the vertebral column by the angle θ. The inclination alternates to the left and right of the long axis in adjacent lamellae. (Adapted from Bogduk and Tworney (1996) by A. Hayes (2000)).

endplates on the superior and inferior surfaces. The IVD attaches to each vertebra via the cartilage endplate and the outer portion of the AF/ALL/PLL (Fig. 1.4.2).

The AF is composed of 10–20 lamellae of parallel bundles of collagen fibres oriented at 65° to the spinal axis with adjacent lamellae alternating their inclination to the right and left of the axis (Fig. 1.4.3). The fibres of the outer annulus and short fibres of the ALL and PLL merge with the ring apophysis of the adjacent vertebra (Sharpey's fibres), whereas the fibres of the inner annulus intercalate with the cartilaginous endplate. The outer AF is fibrous in nature and functions to resist tensional forces; it is populated with fibroblast-like elongated cells with long cellular processes. The inner AF is more fibrocartilaginous, with more rounded cells and functions to resist compression.

In young humans the NP is a gel-like structure rich in proteoglycans and with relatively sparse collagen fibrils. Embryologically the NP is derived from notochordal cells, but these disappear and are rarely found in the mature human IVD. Instead, the NP becomes populated with chondrocytic cells. The NP acts to resist compression dissipating the forces to the AF.

The cartilaginous endplates are located on the superior and inferior parts of the IVD. They are composed of hyaline cartilage and, along with the IVD itself, act as shock absorbers to protect the vertebrae from axial forces. They are also important for nutrition of the disc as it is avascular and the major route for nutrition is from the vasculature of the vertebral body (Fig. 1.4.4).

The composition of the IVD has been extensively studied over the past 20 years. Like other connective tissues, it is composed of collagens, proteoglycans, matrix glycoproteins, and water. The constituents vary considerably depending on the location within the disc. Collagen is the major constituent comprising around 50% of the dry weight in the AF and endplate, but only 15–20% in the NP. The major fibre-forming collagens, (types I and II) are the major constituents, with type I being predominant in the outer annulus and type II being the major component of the NP and cartilage endplate. The inner annulus is a mixture of types I and II, with an increasing proportion of type II towards the central NP.

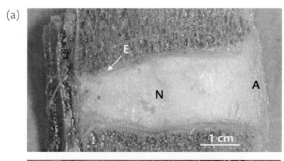

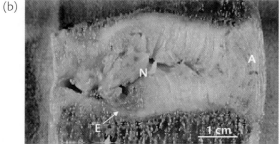

Fig. 1.4.2 Intervertebral discs from the lumbar region of (a) a 17-year-old male and (b) an 82-year-old female cut in the sagittal plane to demonstrate the central nucleus pulposus (N) and outer annulus fibrosus (A) with the thin cartilage endplates (E) at the interface of the disc and vertebral body. Bar = 1 cm.

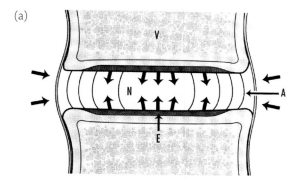

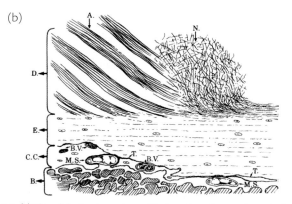

Fig. 1.4.4 (a) The adult disc depends on diffusion of nutrients and metabolites through the vasculature of either the anterior or posterior ligaments outside the annulus (A) or the vertebral body (V) and through the cartilage endplate (E). N, nucleus pulposus. (b) The marrow spaces (MS) and blood vessels (BV) in the calcified cartilage (CC) and bone (B) abutting the cartilage endplate (E) are important in supplying the nutrients to, and carrying the metabolites from, the cells of the disc (D), particularly those of the nucleus (N). A, annulus fibrosus; T, tidemark. (a): adapted from Holm *et al* 1981; b): adapted from Roberts *et al* 1989).

As with most connective tissues, there are smaller amounts of other collagen types and at least eight others, apart from types I and II, are known to be present in the IVD including types III, V, VI, IX, X, XI, XII, and XIV (reviewed by Duance and Roberts 2004). The proteoglycans account for approximately 10% of the dry weight of the AF, 15% of the endplate, and as much as 50% of the NP. Both large aggregating PGs and SLRPs are present. The large aggregating PGs are mainly aggrecan and versican, and the SLRPs include decorin, biglycan, fibromodulin, and lumican. Aggrecan and versican aggregate along with link protein on the glycosaminoglycan hyaluronan. In contrast to articular cartilage, a considerable proportion of the aggrecan and versican appears not to be aggregated with the hyaluronan. The combination of collagen and the proteoglycans reflects the functional and mechanical properties of the different regions of the disc, with the outer AF resisting predominantly tensional forces, while the endplate and NP, with a much higher proteoglycan content, resist compressive forces. The proteoglycans of the AF are important for the plasticity of this region. Additionally, elastin is found throughout the IVD, aligned with the collagen bundles in the outer AF but more randomly as large aggregates in the NP. In addition, it forms an elaborate network located particularly between lamellae, with cross-bridges connecting them (Yu *et al.* 2002, 2005). A number of matrix glycoproteins, including laminin, fibrillin and fibronectin, have also

been found, although their precise function in the IVD is largely assumed from studies of other tissues.

Significant changes occur to the IVD with age which probably render them more prone to injury and often ultimately result in disc degeneration (Fig. 1.4.2(b)). With age there is an increasing level of denatured type II collagen and a switch to type I collagen expression in the inner annulus and NP and type II expression in the inner and outer annulus (Hollander *et al.* 1996). This results in the distinction between the AF and the NP disappearing with age as they take on a similar fibrous appearance. In addition, changes have been observed in some of the minor collagenous components, but the functional significance of these changes is unclear. Age changes have also been identified in the collagen cross-link profile. There are reported decreases in the mature cross-link hydroxylysyl-pyridinoline which would result in a weakened tissue. However, on the other hand there is an increase in the amount of advanced glycation end products such as pentosidine (Duance *et al.* 1998). Increases in pentosidine and other similar cross-links are thought to increase the stiffness but decrease the elasticity of the tissue, making them less able to withstand mechanical loads. There is also a loss of proteoglycan resulting in a less hydrated tissue such that it is less resilient to compressive loading. There is an increase in the non-aggregating forms of the proteoglycan aggrecan, believed to be due to proteolytic degradation. The loss of these partially degraded PGs is the probable cause of the decreased tissue hydration. Clearly these age-related changes all act to compromise the correct mechanical functioning of the IVD.

Neural structures

The spinal cord is an extension of the brain, 45cm long, and runs within the vertebral canal to between the first and second lumbar vertebrae where it terminates in humans. There are 31 spinal nerves that connect to the spinal cord and emerge from the spinal column through the intervertebral foramina (Fig. 1.4.5). The intervertebral foramina are oval ellipsoid spaces that are bound by the pedicles inferiorly, the intervertebral disc and vertebral body anteriorly, and the zygapophysial joint posteriorly. The spinal nerve occupies up to 50% of the space, along with blood vessels, lymphatic vessels, and adipose tissue. The foramen may become smaller in cases of degenerative diseases affecting the IVD and osteoarthritis of the zygapophyseal joint. The spinal nerves are short with an anterior and a posterior part that connect to the spinal cord via the dorsal and ventral nerve roots. The dorsal roots carry only sensory fibres to the spinal cord, whereas the ventral roots carry mainly motor but some sensory nerves. Spinal nerves carry both somatic and visceral nerve fibres. The somatic efferent fibres innervate the skeletal muscles, whilst the afferent fibres carry impulses to the spinal cord from the skin, muscle, ligaments, and joints (Oliver and Middleditch 1991).

The spinal cord is protected by three layers of connective tissue known as the meninges. The outermost is the dura mater, the innermost is the pia mater, and the middle sheath is the arachnoid. The dura mater is attached to the bony skeleton of the vertebra such that movement results in forces being absorbed by the meninges. The dura mater also envelopes the emerging spinal nerves as they pass through the intervertebral foramina and then becomes the perineurium of these nerves. The spinal nerves are in general not attached to the intervertebral foramina and move freely on flexion of the spine. The dura mater is a fibrous tissue composed of

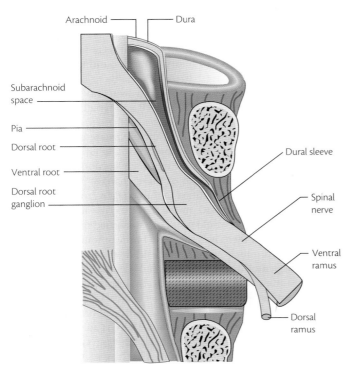

Arachnoid — — Dura

Subarachnoid space —

Pia —

Dorsal root —

Ventral root —

Dorsal root ganglion —

— Dural sleeve

— Spinal nerve

— Ventral ramus

— Dorsal ramus

Fig. 1.4. 5   A lumbar spinal nerve and its roots and meningeal coverings. Reproduced from *Gray's Anatomy* (Standring), with permission from Elsevier

longitudinal collagen fibres with a fine network of elastin fibres. The arachnoid is a thin sheath of loose connective tissue of collagen and elastin fibres in a lattice arrangement, allowing changes in length on movement of the spine. The innermost pia mater adheres closely to the nerve fibres of the spinal cord. It also forms the sheath of the dorsal and ventral roots of the spinal nerve. As with most connective tissue structures, there are age-related changes that reduce their plasticity and flexibility. Therefore the meninges are less able to accommodate the tensional stresses in the elderly as well as in young people, hence, affecting mobility (Oliver and Middleditch 1991). This lack of plasticity also renders these protective sheaths more prone to injury in the elderly.

Biomechanics of spinal structures

The motion segment

The motion segment is essentially a passive structure, responding to forces applied to it. *In vivo* the musculature is also involved in this response, providing an 'active' response. The intervertebral discs in the spine provide flexibility in addition to load-bearing. The primary function of the outer AF is to contain the hydrostatic pressure of the internal NP. Therefore the structure of the AF is exposed primarily to tensile stresses, whereas the NP is exposed to compression. The nucleus is able to withstand compression because of the high swelling pressure, which arises by virtue of the biochemical composition of the matrix. The high cationic charge of the glycosaminoglycan molecules within aggrecan attracts counteracting anions, which results in a high ionic charge and hence osmotic or swelling pressure of the disc matrix. This is resisted by

the tension arising in the collagen fibres, which are embedded in the aggrecan gel. Compressive stress measurements across a healthy adult disc show that the compressive stress is maintained throughout and across all the NP and inner AF before dropping off sharply at the outer AF. However, in more degenerate discs there are considerable peak stresses throughout the AF and reduced values in the NP, with the degree of change being greatest in the most degenerate discs (Adams *et al.* 1996).

There is a gradient of tensile properties across the disc with the outer AF being stiffer in tension than the inner AF. Much of the tensile strength of the AF is due not only to the collagen fibres within the disc matrix, but also to the interaction between collagen and other matrix components. However, compressive loading appears less important than bending of the spine as a cause of disc herniation or prolapse (Adams 1994). During bending the AF becomes stretched vertically, perpendicular to the endplates; the tensile strength is greater in the posterior outer AF (3.7 MN/m^2) than in the anterior (1.7 MN/m^2). In contrast, the PLL is not as strong as the ALL (Adams 1994).

The degree of elasticity of ligaments is important as well as their strength. The ligamentum flavum, for example, is strong (approximately three times as strong as the PLL) but has the highest amount of elastin of any ligament in the body, probably accounting for its high extensibility and ability to recover from strains of up to 80%. The function of the ligamentum flavum is to provide a smooth posterior lining to the spinal canal and resistance to bending of the motion segment. The ligaments of the facet joint capsule are believed to be even stronger and also resist bending within the motion segment, as do the interspinous and supraspinous ligaments (although the latter is weaker and absent in the lower lumbar region).

Most of the compressive strength of the healthy vertebral body appears to come from the trabecular bone with the vertebral cortices contributing 10–40% of the strength. However, this may increase to 75% in osteoporotic spines. The strength of the neural arch (fracture of which can result in spondylolysis) is estimated at 600–2800 N with 1–2 mm displacement.

Spinal cord

By necessity, movement of the spine must change the length and shape of the spinal cord and its surrounding tissues (the meninges; pia, arachnoid, and dura maters) since it is effectively 'tethered' at either end (by the dura to the foramen magnum cranially and the filum terminale caudally) and also down its length via the denticulate ligaments. This is in addition to the elasticity of the spinal cord and dura. When the spine is flexed the spinal cord elongates by up to 20% of its length; when this happens, the distance between the nerve fibres decreases, whereas in extension the space between them expands again. In extension, folds can also form in the meninges, particularly in the cervical region. Transient stretching of nerves alters their functioning, for example by reducing conduction as well as reducing the intraneural circulation, at least temporarily, but it does not damage axonal continuity. In pathological stretching, failure occurs in the short myelinated sections where the normally varying diameter of the nerve fibre is small.

The different regions of the spine are affected to varying degrees, with most change occurring in the cervical and lumbar regions. In both of these regions the spinal canal can elongate by approximately 3 cm, whereas in the thoracic region only 0.3 cm elongation occurs (Shacklock *et al.* 1994). Movement within the spine results not only in change in the length and shape of the spinal cord but also movement at its interface with the adjacent tissues (e.g. the cranium, spinal canal, or intervertebral discs). Similarly, spinal movement will result in altered loading or positioning of the nerve roots, which can vary depending on location within the spine. For example, on flexion of the spine the nerve roots above L3 angle more horizontally, whereas those below angle more vertically (because the dural theca converges towards the L4–5 segment).

Some sites within the spine are particularly susceptible to neural compromise, for example, the lower cervical region with its greater mobility than elsewhere or the L4–5 level, another region of high mobility, which is close to where the neural elements are strongly tethered by the dural ligaments. Other sites of compromise arise partly due to the anatomy of the interfacing tissue, for example, if the surrounding non-neural tissue (such as an osteophyte or bulging intervertebral disc) permits too little space for the nerve.

The nervous system is relatively mobile so that the neural structures can slide within the spinal canal. This can be used to help in diagnosing whether the source of symptoms is neural or non-neural. For example, if lumbar pain is altered by movement of the head, the pain is likely to be neurogenic, as non-neural structures in the lumbar region are not moved.

Pathologies and syndromes

Spondylolysis

Spondylolysis refers to a break in the pars interarticularis and is one of the most common disorders of the spine. It may or may not result in forward 'slippage' of one vertebra over another (spondylolisthesis). Spondylolysis in teenagers is usually sports related. It is particularly common in divers, dancers, and gymnasts who perform a high level of bending and twisting (Rothman and Wiltse 2004). Its incidence in female gymnasts is four times that of the general population. It is not thought to result from a single traumatic event, but occurs after repeated loading and has a genetic predisposition. The resulting fracture may remain un-united, or it can heal, with some sclerosis of the pars interarticularis (often slightly deformed in the shape of a hockey stick). Ossification of the ligamentum flavum and zygapophyseal joint may also occur, further stabilizing the structure.

If spondylosis does lead to a spondylolisthesis, this often renders high-level sport impossible because of the instability that ensues.

Low back pain

Back pain (as opposed to radicular pain) implies a somatic origin of the pain with many tissues capable of contributing to it including ligaments, zygophopyseal or facet joints, muscles, vertebrae, sacroiliac joints, thoracolumbar fascia, dura mater, and the intervertebral disc. In addition, the intervertebral disc is a major contributor to nerve root pain. The incidence of back pain is not restricted to a particular sport but is prevalent in several (Table 1.4.1).

The problems and limitations of diagnosis in sports patients with back pain and/or nerve root pain are the same as in the general population; accurate assessment of patients is hampered by the lack of reliable objective methods. Questionnaires such as the Oswestry Disability Index (ODI), which assess the impact on lifestyle, are often used to grade disability initially and monitor recovery. However, some symptoms in athletes may differ from those in

Table 1.4.1 Back pain in specific sports

Sport	Effect
Canoeists	22.5% suffered from 'lumbago'
Cross country skiers	64% suffered form back pain
Cyclists	30–73.2% suffer from back pain
Golfers	29–63% had back pain at some lifetime point
Gymnasts	86% of rhythmic gymnasts reported low back pain and 63% of Olympic female gymnasts have MRI abnormalities
Rowers	Mechanical back pain is the most common injury
Squash players	51.8% of competitive players reported back injury
Swimmers	37% suffer back pain especially with breaststroke and butterfly
Triathletes	32% suffer from low back pain
Windsurfers	Low back pain is the most common ailment
Yachtsmen and women	Lumbosacral sprain is the most common injury (29%)

Source: Thompson (2002).

the general population; for example, symptoms of disc prolapse may be subtle, in the form of tightness of the hamstrings and altered running pattern. Other individuals may be predisposed to other confounding problems; for instance, amenorrhoeic athletes will be at greater risk of osteoporotic vertebral collapse than the normal population. Careful questioning and knowledge of the sport can be useful in examining sports people with back pain; a useful enquiry is whether a specific incident led to the injury or the patient experienced similar symptoms previously. A detailed clinical history, with particular reference to training and to the characteristics of the sport, is often more important than many other investigations such as X-rays or MRI. Nonetheless, it is just as important to eliminate serious spinal pathology via checking for 'red flag' symptoms in these patients as in any others.

Scheuermann's disease

Juvenile thoracic kyphosis or Scheuermann's disease (defined as three or more vertebrae being wedged by more than 5°) is a hereditary condition that predisposes to progressive rounding of the back. It is normally pain free, but may lead to some discomfort associated with strenuous loading of the back; it is rarely found in athletes. However, young athletes can present with 'atypical' lumbar Scheuermann's disease with wedging commonly in the lower thoracic to mid-lumbar region of the spine. It is most commonly seen in young sports people (15–17 years old) such as rowers or gymnasts where repetitive flexion and extension of the spine might be common. These can result in multiple growth plate fractures, secondary bony deformation of the vertebrae, and subsequent changes in the disc space.

Inflammation

Inflammatory spondyloarthropathies are a group of related chronic inflammatory rheumatic diseases including ankylosing spondylitis. They involve inflammation of the axial skeleton entheses and have a strong association with the histocompatibility human leucocyte antigen (HLA-B27). The presence of HLA-B27, which varies widely with geographical location (occurring in 50% of some Native American tribes but in only 8% of Japanese (Balagué and Dudler 2004)), is believed to indicate an immunogenetic predisposition to an environmental trigger (most commonly a micro-organism) leading to occurrence of these diseases. The age of onset is usually at the end of the growth period (Goupille and Borenstein 2004). There is an initial inflammatory phase (osteolitis) of the entheses leading to limited erosion of the bone followed by a reactive phase with bone proliferation and periosteal opposition forming enthesophytes and possibly bone fusion and enthesopathy. In the general population the active phase might typically last for 6 months, followed by perhaps a 2-year latent phase before the cycle repeats itself (Goupille and Borenstein 2004).

The exact links between the presence of HLA-B27 and the clinical manifestation is unknown. At least 23 subtypes of HLA-B27 are now recognized, some of which have no association with, for example, ankylosing spondylitis. The population in which some of the 'risky' subtypes occur also appears to influence its presentation; for example, HLA-B2705 may predispose in some populations but is not a risk factor in West Africans (Balagué and Dudler 2004). Suggestions for how HLA-B27 could facilitate the disease include that the molecule may increase the intracellular survival rate of bacteria, enhance the pro-inflammatory response to some bacteria, or possibly via a tendency to misfold may lead to abnormal intracellular signalling. Furthermore, whilst HLA-B27 on chromosome 6 is undoubtedly associated with ankylosing spondylitis, it only accounts for 16–50% of the total risk, indicating that it is a polygenetic disease, possibly involving four other genes (suspects are on chromosomes 2,10, 16, and 19).

The axial skeleton, particularly the sacroiliac joint, is almost always affected at some time in ankylosing spondylitis, being the first manifestation in 75% of patients. Typically, patients present with morning stiffness and sometimes pain which can be relieved by exercise (less so in younger patients); it occurs predominantly in males (males-to-female ratio 10:1) and is often associated with other disorders (e.g. in males, chronic bacterial urethritis (Reiter's syndrome) (75%), ulcerative colitis (20%), or psoriasis (5%)). Affected athletes can be treated with anti-inflammatory drugs or biologics (e.g. TNF-α antagonists) during an acute phase. Sporting activities can be continued in the early stages of the disease or during symptom-free periods, although they may have to be limited at other times (Peterson and Renstrom 2001).

Spinal cord injuries

Ten to fifteen per cent of all spinal cord injuries occur in sports people. Some factors are particularly relevant to this and perhaps contribute to the occurrence of these injuries in sports people. One such 'risk factor' is youth! This is in part due to the greater elasticity of the young spinal cord, the cervical region of which can stretch by up to 3 cm in length. This may lead to SCIWORA (spinal cord injuries without obvious radiological abnormalities). In this syndrome a child has a spinal cord injury, frequently complete, with no radiographic evidence of a dislocation or fracture; it constitutes approximately 15–20% of spinal cord injuries in children (Chambers and Akbarnia 1994) but is much less common in adults. Fractures or displacement of the epiphyseal endplates in joints may contribute to SCIWORA, with the cartilage possibly injuring the spinal cord or nerve roots. Similarly, the relatively large head and vertical facet joints can make dislocation more likely in a younger individual.

Therefore training regimes in sports proper should restrict loading to less than body weight until after skeletal maturity. In high-risk sports, such as football and gymnastics, spine boards should be readily available. In the older sports person, spinal stenosis has been found in a large percentage with neck injuries that have resulted in permanent neurological deficit, quadriplegia, or even death (Boden and Jarvis 2008).

Ligamentous hyperlaxity

This can lead to hypermobility, which may be seen as advantageous in gymnastics and can even be increased with training. It is not likely to cause problems with normal levels of activity, but it can be accentuated with extreme levels of training, concentrating extension forces that may result in stress fractures of the pars interarticularis. The hyperlaxity may be characterized by (i) genu recurvatum, (ii) hyperextension at the elbows, or (iii) flat-footedness. The hyperlaxity may influence radiological imaging, falsely giving the impression of ligament injury when there may be none (e.g. pseudo-subluxation in the cervical spine).

However, it should always be borne in mind that the unexpected can happen, even in sports people. For example, the spine can have both primary (benign and malignant) and metastatic tumours in the vertebral body, thus replacing the marrow and cancerous bone, rendering it liable to premature fracture.

Summary

Ten to twenty per cent of all sports-related injuries involve the spine, so it is an important part of the musculoskeletal system in sport. With an ageing population and an emphasis on healthier living and more involvement in sporting activity the prevalence of these injuries is likely to increase. Greater knowledge of the age-related changes that occur in the connective tissue structures of the spine will help in our understanding of these injuries and enable better management of the repair and rehabilitation processes necessary to resume an active lifestyle.

Acknowledgments

We are grateful for funding from the European Community's Framework 7 Programme (FP7, 2007–2013) under grant agreement no. HEALTH-F2–2008–201626 (Genodisc) to support this work (SR).

References

Adams, M.A. (1994). Biomechanics of the lumbar motion segment. In: J.D.Boyling and N. Palastanga (eds), *Grieve's Modern Manual Therapy: The Vertebral Column*, pp. 109–30. Churchill Livingstone, New York.

Adams, M.A., McNally, D.S., and Dolan, P. (1996). 'Stress' distributions inside intervertebral discs: the effects of age and degeneration. *Journal of Bone and Joint Surgery*, **78B**, 965–72.

Balagué, F. and Dudler, J. (2004). Ankylosing spondylitis. In: H. Herkowitz, J. Dvorak, G. Bel, and D. Grob (eds), *The Lumbar Spine*, pp. 712–26. Lippincott–Williams & Wilkins, Philadelphia, PA.

Barros, E.M., Rodrigues, C.J., Rodrigues, N.R., Oliveira, R.P., Barros, T.E., and Rodrigues, A.J., Jr. (2002). Aging of the elastic and collagen fibres in the human cervical interspinous ligaments. *Spine Journal*, **2**, 57–62.

Battié, M.C., Videman, T., and Parent, E. (2004). Lumbar degeneration: epidemiology and genetic influences. *Spine*, **29**, 2679–90.

Benjamin, M. (2004). The structure and function of tendons. In: B. Hazleman, G. Riley and C. Speed (eds), *Soft Tissue Rheumatology*, pp. 9–19. Oxford University Press.

Boden, B.P. and Jarvis, C.G. (2008). Spinal injuries in sports. *Neurologic Clinics*, **26**, 63–78.

Bogduk, N. and Twomey, L. (1996). *Clinical Anatomy of the Lumbar Spine*. Churchill Livingstone, New York.

Boszczyk, B.M., Boszczyk, A.A., Putz, R., Buttner, A., Benjamin, M., and Milz, S. (1999). An immunohistochemical study of the dorsal capsule of the lumbar and thoracic facet joints. *Spine*, **26**, E338–43.

Chambers, H.G. and Akbarnia, B.A. (1994). Thoracic, lumbar and sacral spine fractures and dislocation. In: S.L. Weinstein (ed.), *The Pediatric Spine*. Raven Press, New York.

Duance, V. and Roberts, S. (2004). The intervertebral disc—structure, composition and pathology. In: B. Hazleman, G. Riley, and C. Speed (eds), *Soft Tissue Rheumatology*, pp. 54–79. Oxford University Press.

Duance, V.C., Crean, J., Sims, T., *et al.* (1998). Changes in collagen cross-linking in degenerative disc disease and scoliosis. *Spine*, **1**, 2545–51.

Duance, V.C., Vaughan-Thomas, A., Wardale, R.J., and Wotton, S.F. (1999). Collagens of articular, growth plate and meniscal cartilages. In: B. Caterson, C.W. Archer, M. Benjamin, and J. Ralphs (eds), *Biology of the Synovial Joint*, pp. 135–63. Harwood Academic, Amsterdam.

El-Tanani, M.K. (2008). Role of osteopontin in cellular signaling and metastatic phenotype. *Frontiers in Bioscience*, **13**, 4276–84.

Eyre, D.R., Weis, M.A., and Wu, J.J. (2006). Articular cartilage collagen: an irreplaceable framework? *European Cells and Materials*, **12**, 57–63.

Goupille, P. and Borenstein, D. (2004). Inflammatory spondyloarthropathies. In: H. Herkowitz, J. Dvorak, G. Bell, and D. Grob (eds), The Lumbar Spine, pp. 690–700. Lippincott–Williams & Wilkins, Philadelphia, PA.

Hayes, A.J. (2000). The development of the annulus fibrosus of the intervertebral disc. PhD thesis, University of Wales, Cardiff.

Hollander, A.P., Heathfield, T.F., Liu, J.J., *et al.* (1996). Enhanced denaturation of the alpha (II) chains of type-II collagen in normal adult human intervertebral discs compared with femoral articular cartilage. *Journal of Orthopaedic Research*, **14**, 61–6.

Holm, S., Maroudas, A., Urban, J.P., Selstam, G., and Nachemson, A. (1981). Nutrition of the intervertebral disc: solute transport and metabolism. *Connective Tissue Research*, **8**(2), 101–19.

Lamoureux, F., Baud'huin, M., Duplomb, L., Heymann, D., and Redini, F. (2007). Proteoglycans: key partners in bone cell biology. *BioEssays*, **29**, 758–71.

Lida, T., Abumi, K., Kotani, Y., and Kaneda, K. (2002). Effects of aging and spinal degeneration on mechanical properties of lumbar supraspinous and interspinous ligaments. *Spine J.* Mar-Apr;2(2): 95–100.

Nihei, A., Hagiwara, K., Kikuchi, M., Yashiro, T., and Hoshino, Y. (2003). Histological investigation of rabbit ligamentum flavum with special reference to differences in spinal levels. *Anatomical Science International*, **78**, 162–7.

Oliver, J. and Middleditch, A. (1991). *Functional Anatomy of the Spine*. Butterworth Heinemann, Oxford.

Peterson, L. and Renstrom, P. (2001). Back. In: *Sports Injuries:Their Prevention and Treatment*, pp. 207–30. Martin Dunitz, London.

Pope, M.H. and Hansson, T. (1990). Vibration of the spine and low back pain. *Clinical Orthopaedics and Related Research*, **279**, 49–59.

Riley, G. (2004). Tendon and ligament biochemistry and pathology. In: B. Hazleman, G. Riley, and C. Speed (eds), *Soft Tissue Rheumatology*, pp. 20–53. Oxford University Press.

Roberts, S., Menage, L., and Urban, J.P.G. (1989). Biochemical and structural properties of the cartilage end-plate and its relation to the intervertebral disc. *Spine*, **14**, 166–74.

Rothman, S.L.G. and Wiltse, L. (2004). Imaging in the evaluation of lumbar and lumbosacral spondylolysis and spondylolisthesis. In: H. Herkowitz, J. Dvorak, G. Bell, and D. Grob (eds), *The Lumbar Spine*, pp. 565–78. Lippincott–Williams & Wilkins, Philadelphia, PA.

Sambrook, P.N., MacGregor, A.J., and Spector, T.D. (1999). Genetic influences on cervical and lumbar disc degeneration: a magnetic resonance imaging study in twins. *Arthritis and Rheumatism*, **42**, 366–72.

Shacklock, M.O., Butler, D.S., and Slater, H. (1994). The dynamic central nervous system: structure and clinical neurobiomechanics. In: J.D. Boyling and N. Palastanga (eds), *Grieve's Modern Manual Therapy: The Vertebral Column*, pp. 21–38. Churchill Livingstone, New York.

Schenk, R.K., Hofstetter, W., and Felix, R. (2002). Morphology and chemical composition of connective tissue: Bone. In: P.M. Royce and B. Steinmann B (eds), *Connective Tissue and Its Heritable Disorders*, pp. 67–120. Wiley-Liss, New York.

Sodek, J., Zhu, B., Huynh, M.H., Brown, T.J, and Ringuette, M. (2002). Novel functions of the matricellular proteins osteopontin and osteonectin/SPARC. *Connective Tissue Research*, **43**, 308–19.

Thompson, B. (2002). How should athletes with chronic low back pain be managed in primary care?. In: D. MacAuley and T. Best (eds), *Evidence-Based Sports Medicine*, pp. 216–38. BMJ Books, London.

Young, M.F. (2003). Bone matrix proteins: their function, regulation and relationship to osteoporosis. *Osteoporosis International*, **14**, S35–42.

Yu, J., Winlove, C.P., Roberts, S., and Urban, J.P.G. (2002). Elastic fibre organisation in the bovine intervertebral disc. *Journal of Anatomy*, **201**, 465–75.

Yu, J., Fairbank, J.C.T., Roberts, S., and Urban, J.P.G. (2005). The elastic fibres network of the anulus fibrosus of the normal and scoliotic human intervertebral disc. *Spine*, **16**, 1815–20.

1.5

Articular cartilage

Simon Roberts

Introduction

Synovial joints allow the efficient and controlled movement necessary for sport with a biological shock-absorbing bearing of hyaline cartilage. This is an extremely low friction surface, with a coefficient of one-sixth of that of ice on ice, lower than most man-made bearing materials. It has viscoelastic properties allowing dynamic congruity and minimization of transmitted pressure and impact.

Hyaline cartilage is a highly specialized tissue consisting of a pre-stressed extracellular collagen and proteoglycan matrix, unusually containing absolutely no nerve supply, blood supply, or lymphatic drainage. Chondrocytes are highly differentiated and are the only type of mature cell which exists within normal articular cartilage, making up less than 5% of the total volume of the tissue. This means that each chondrocyte has a relatively large domain of influence. In keeping with the exclusively diffusional nutrition, chondrocytes have a slow metabolic rate and oxygen usage, approximately one-fiftieth of that of hepatocytes. Normal turnover times for the extracellular matrix in adults is measured in years, although chondrocytes can be stimulated both chemically and mechanically to accelerate this (Buckwalter and Mow 2003; Einhorn *et al.* 2007; Roberts 2007).

Biological properties

Cells

There are distinct populations of chondrocytes through the thickness of the articular cartilage (Fig. 1.5.1). Superficially, the cells are tangentially orientated and elliptically shaped and approximately three times as densely packed as in the deeper zones, possibly reflecting the greater availability of nutrition as well as the greater demand for matrix turnover as a result of increased exposure to injury on the surface. In the mid zone, the cells appear to be more rounded and randomly distributed, whereas in the deepest zone, again, round cells are here found arranged in a more columnar fashion, orientated perpendicular to the tide mark. Cell density also changes with age being much greater in skeletally immature individuals, but remaining fairly constant throughout adulthood. In the absence of injury, there is little if any cell division, but a mitotic response to injury does occur and, importantly, harvested chondrocytes can be induced to proliferate extensively in-vitro. Deeper zone cells are found to proliferate much more readily than those from the superficial zones and are preferred for therapeutic use in autologous chondrocytes transplantation although progenitor cells have been identified in superficial layers (Dowthwaite *et al.*

2004; Hiraoka *et al.* 2006). The cells have intracytoplasmic filaments which are attached to the cell membrane by integrins allowing the cell to respond to mechanical stimuli. This is not a simple process and one which remains to be fully elucidated.

Extracellular matrix

The extracellular matrix consists of approximately 80% water by weight. The structural macromolecules include collagens, proteoglycans, and non-collagenous proteins. All these are synthesized by the chondrocytes.

Collagen

Collagen is the most common protein in the body and comprises a family of at least 19 members, all of which have a superhelix of twisted triple helical alpha chains. They contribute approximately 60–80% of the dry weight of hyaline cartilage, of which approximately 90% is type II collagen. This is a fibrillar collagen consisting of a repeating tripeptide pattern of glycine, proline, and hydroxyproline. The amino acid chains coil round each other with glycine at the centre of the helix, forming a collagen molecule, with many collagen molecules aligning into parallel sheets. A number of

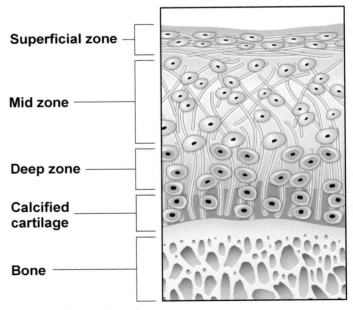

Fig. 1.5.1 Adult articular cartilage.

different types of cross-links are formed between the fibrils, some of which can be reduced or broken, perhaps allowing for physiological modification, but also giving us a means of measuring collagen turnover. At least 30 genes are involved in the synthesis of collagens, but type II is derived from a single gene, with the alpha chains transcribed from mRNA and hydroxylated and glycosylated in the endoplasmic reticulum before being secreted as a large precursor procollagen. The C and N terminals are subsequently enzymatically cleaved, allowing telopeptide measurement as a clinical indicator of collagen synthesis. Type II collagen is thought to be primarily responsible for resisting the swelling pressure within the matrix created by the proteoglycans.

As with the cells, there is a variation in the distribution and morphology of the extracellular matrix constituents with respect to depth. Type I collagen, also found widely in skin and bone, is distributed predominantly in the superficial zone where it may be able to resist mechanical abrasion. The superficial zone consists of collagen fibres lying predominantly parallel to the articular surface descending through the mid zone to the deep zone where they become orientated perpendicular to the underlying bone (Fig. 1.5.1). Types IX and XI collagen bind covalently to type II and may serve to stabilize the fibrils. The contribution of the other types of collagen (mostly types VI and X) to the function of articular cartilage is less clear.

Proteoglycans

Proteoglycans are the second-largest component of the dry weight of articular cartilage. As opposed to the collagens, they can be considered to give articular cartilage its resistance to compression. The highest concentration is in the deepest zone. Proteoglycans consist of a central protein core to which many glycosaminoglycan chains (long unbranched chains of disaccharides containing an amino acid, including keratan sulphate, chondroitin sulphate, and dermatan sulphate) are attached. Each disaccharide has a sulphate or carboxylate group which is negatively charged, leading to a high density of negatively charged ions repelling each other electrostatically, holding the chains out straight, and inflating the matrix. They also attract cations, which in turn lead to an increase in osmolality and thereby pressure (Donnan effect). In this way, the articular cartilage is 'prestressed' to resist compression. In the absence of restraining collagen, it is estimated the proteoglycans would expand to five times their volume in cartilage. A reduction in resistance to this swelling, with a commensurate decrease in concentration of proteoglycan and stiffness to compression, is an early sign of degenerative change in articular cartilage.

Articular cartilage consists of several kinds of proteoglycan. The most important and most common is aggrecan, a large aggregating proteoglycan with a molecular weight of 1.5–2.5 kDa. These large molecules (aggregates) form via one of three globular zones in the central protein core of the individual proteoglycan monomer attaching to a spine of hyaluronan (hyaluronic acid) (Fig. 1.5.2). This linkage is stabilized via a link protein which is coded by an independent gene. The hyaluronan molecule is synthesized at the cell membrane, enforcing extracellular assembly of the macromolecule.

Other minor components include lipids and non-collagenous proteins and glycoproteins such as fibronectin, fibromodulin and cartilage oligomeric protein whose roles are not well understood.

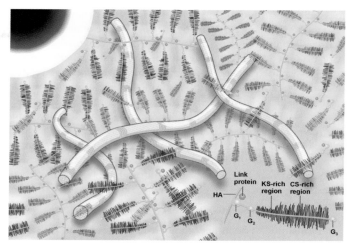

Fig. 1.5.2 Aggregating proteoglycan.

Mechanical properties

Articular cartilage needs to bear and distribute applied load and to lubricate movement. Although articular cartilage is stiff in tension as described above, compared with the underlying bone, it is 1000 times less stiff in compression (especially the superficial zone), but whereas bone will fail at a strain of 1%, cartilage can undergo strains of 50% or more without macroscopic failure. The thickness depends on the pressure which needs to be borne and varies inversely with joint congruity, with much thicker cartilage cover in the knee compared with the highly congruous ankle. Thinner cartilage also tends to be stiffer (Shepherd and Seedhom 1999). Its mechanical properties are both time and direction dependent. There is a rapid elastic deformation response to an applied stress, but the viscoelastic properties are a result of the biphasic nature of the material which allows fluid flow through the matrix. A constant load will lead to progressive deformity (creep) until equilibrium is reached, whereas a constant deformation will require a progressive decrease in stress (stress relaxation). Because of this deformability, joint congruity can be increased dynamically, which correspondingly decreases the contact pressure. The anisotropic orientation of the extracellular macromolecules is responsible for the material's ability to respond to forces in physiological directions.

Under compression during joint loading, interstitial fluid flows toward the leading and trailing edges. Secondly, increased interstitial pressure leads to ultrafiltration and the formation of a viscous surface gel.

Injury

Chondrocytes in articular cartilage have a limited capacity to remodel the extracellular matrix by varying the rates of synthesis and degradation of matrix components. Articular cartilage has recently been shown to contain a population of stem cells which may be able to repopulate an area of injury, contrary to what has traditionally been believed (Hiraoka *et al.* 2006). There is evidence of mechanotransduction, very likely mediated by the intracytoplasmic filaments, but some chondrocytes have a cilium which may also contribute to this. This allows mature chondrocytes to respond to mechanical stimuli by varying the rate of production of matrix. Cyclical physiological levels of change in hydrostatic pressure lead to increased proteoglycan synthesis, whereas static compression or reduced loading lead to a decrease. Age-related degradation of matrix constituents leads to a softening of articular cartilage with a relatively increased water content before structural failure occurs with surface fibrillation and subsequent fissuring and macroscopic loss of hyaline cartilage.

In the absence of a blood supply the response to articular cartilage injury is not inflammatory, and of course pain cannot be felt in the absence of any innervation. Injuries have been classified as follows:

(1) occult disruption of matrix macromolecules;

(2) mechanical disruption of the articular surface;

(3) mechanical disruption of both articular cartilage and subchondral bone.

Only the last of these can lead to exposure of the articular cartilage to the subchondral bone's blood supply and hence formation of granulation tissue and an inflammatory response. The response to partial thickness injury is poorly understood, but changes have been demonstrated in various growth factors including platelet-derived (PDGF), basic fibroblast (bFGF), insulin-like (IGF-I and IGF-II), and transforming (TGF-β) growth factors, some of which have mitogenic roles while others upregulate synthetic processes and protective cytokines.

There is some evidence that repetitive blunt trauma may lead to stiffening of the articular surface by thickening of the deeper zones and the tide mark. The interaction between the articular surface and the subchondral bone is clearly demonstrated on magnetic resonance scanning where injury can leave an intact articular surface, but with dramatic subchondral changes and increased fluid, often described as a 'bone bruise'.

Clinical features

Articular cartilage damage

Hunter in 1743 is widely quoted as saying that 'from Hippocrates down to the present time, we shall find, that an ulcerated cartilage is universally allowed to be a very troublesome disease; that it admits of a cure with more difficulty than a carious bone; and that when destroyed it is never recovered'(Hunter 1995). In 1851 Paget agreed saying that 'there are, I believe, no instances in which a lost portion of cartilage has been restored'. The healing response to partial-thickness lacerations differs from that in full-thickness injuries, which again differs from the healing with an osteochondral injury. Joints are designed to prevent adhesions and superficial lacerations have very little, if any, capacity for spontaneous healing. A more significant primarily reparative, as opposed to regenerative, healing response occurs in full-thickness defects where access to blood and pluripotential mesenchymal cells allows an inflammatory response. There is some metaplasia of fibroblasts in the early granulation tissue to chondrocytes, with cartilage-specific matrix proteins being produced some weeks after injury. There is also a flow of matrix from the uninjured to the injured area. There appears to be little improvement in the quality of the tissue beyond 3 months post-injury. It does appear that there are biological differences between different animals, different ages, different joints, and even different parts of the same joint, as well as between individuals with different demands. Whilst it may be difficult to understand teleologically why some tissues, notably the central nervous system and the articular surface of joints, have such a limited capacity for regeneration, there are still a number of therapeutic options that are particularly applicable to athletes.

Osteoarthritis

Osteoarthritis is a condition affecting not just the articular cartilage, but all the tissues within the joint, particularly thickening and stiffening of the synovium and capsule. It should be considered a different condition from that of an isolated chondral defect in the joint of an athlete, although it may of course follow this. The aetiology is still the subject of debate and is probably multifactorial, with familial, biological, and mechanical elements. Macroscopically, the early changes are of softening of the cartilage and fibrillation with cleft formation. Microscopically, there is decreased glycosaminoglycan and proteoglycan staining, and ultrastructurally there is increasing disorganization of the collagen fibrils. The articular cartilage is thinner and softer than normal with an increased water content and new bone is laid down, leading to both subchondral sclerosis and marginal osteophytes.

Normal healthy articular cartilage is in equilibrium—with the same rate of production as breakdown. Biochemically, in the early stages of osteoarthritis, there is little quantitative change in the collagen, but there is loss of both quality and quantity of proteoglycans, specifically aggrecan. There is an increase in catabolic enzymes, notably the matrix metalloproteinase family, combined with a decrease in their regulatory tissue inhibitors (TIMPs). A number of cytokines, including interleukins and other growth factors, have altered levels and ratios in the osteoarthritic joint.

The role of exercise in the prevention or acceleration of osteoarthritis in either previously normal or injured joints is controversial. There is some evidence that 'excessive' use, particularly impact loading, may increase the risk of subsequent osteoarthritis, but more evidence that overuse of a *previously injured* joint (especially an unstable or incongruent joint) leads to a high risk of premature degenerative change (Saxon *et al.* 1999; Buckwalter and Martin 2004).

Treatment options for articular cartilage injuries

Therapeutic interventions can be divided into specific interventions aimed at re-creating a normal or near-normal articular surface and those aimed at maximizing the function in the absence of healing. The latter applies particularly to the management of osteoarthritis where there is a generalized loss of articular cartilage in association with changes to the subchondral bone and biological changes in the other soft tissues. Here, measures include simple analgesia, but advice on weight loss, the prescription of moderate aerobic exercise including local muscle strengthening, and maintenance of mobility are important. The role of 'neutraceuticals' such as glucosamine and chondroitin remains to be clarified. There does appear to be some evidence of significant symptom relief.

Similarly, more invasive interventions of injection therapy with either steroid or hyaluronan derivatives have some scientific support in the literature. A review of this is available in the Cochrane database (Bellamy *et al.* 2006). The role of arthroscopic lavage and debridement has recently been the source of considerable debate following the study by Moseley *et al.* (2002) who found no benefit for arthroscopic surgery versus sham surgery in a randomized controlled trial. Simple washout has a very limited therapeutic effect in the absence of any mechanical symptoms for which there may be a specific surgical treatment.

A number of surgical procedures have been promoted for the treatment of isolated chondral defects as opposed to osteoarthritis, particularly in young adults who wish to maintain a high level of activity. In this case the most important aspect is to address the cause of the chondral defect wherever possible. This may involve joint stabilization; in the knee this may involve reconstruction of the patellofemoral joint or ligament so as to optimize the biomechanics. There is little point in attempting to re-create an articular surface if it is immediately going to be overloaded or damaged in the same way as the native surface. An absolute contraindication to any attempt at articular cartilage reconstruction is either static or dynamic malalignment.

Although there may be a history of acute injury, an athlete who has a chondral defect will typically present with chronic symptoms of post-exertional swelling and poorly localized discomfort, often with mechanical symptoms. Any catching or locking may well be helped by an arthroscopic procedure to excise unstable chondral flaps which may improve the congruity of the articular surface and may reduce the inflammatory pain with which this is associated. However, this would do nothing to either unload or resurface the defect and cover the subchondral bone.

There are three groups of surgical procedures which attempt to re-create the articular surface of a sportsman's joint.

1. **Marrow stimulation** This was first described by Pridie (1959), modified as 'abrasion chondroplasty', and popularized more recently and modified as microfracture by Steadman (Steadman *et al.* 2001, 2003, 2001). This is a procedure to penetrate the subchondral bone, allowing pluripotential mesenchymal cells to populate the chondral defect via an inflammatory granulation tissue which remodels with an element of chondral metaplasia. The vascularized tissue initially produced will be predominantly type I collagen and fibrocartilage, effectively a reparative scar rather than regenerative articular cartilage. The surgery is an outpatient arthroscopic procedure which involves thorough debridement of all unstable chondral material leaving a stable full-thickness-contained chondral defect with a perpendicular margin of healthy cartilage. The base of the lesion is curetted before being penetrated with one of a set of variously angled arthroscopic awls perpendicular to the subchondral bone surface. Multiple penetrations are made far enough apart to prevent the punctures coalescing so as to maintain the integrity of the bone plate. The procedure is not a major intervention, but is associated with a prolonged period (about 2 months) of reduced joint loading post-operatively. During this period movement is encouraged (often helped by a continuous passive motion machine) progressively to encourage congruity of the regenerate articular surface. The expected time to return to sport is 4 months.

2. **Osteochondral transfer** Macroscopic osteochondral grafts can be used to re-create the articular surface instantly. These grafts may be either be autologous, taken from a supposedly less important area of the same joint's articular surface, or use allografts. The latter procedure has the obvious advantage of not harvesting exactly the same area of articular surface in the patient as it re-creates. The procedure is most commonly described as mosaicplasty, whereby multiple cylindrical osteochondral plugs of around 1 cm in diameter are taken with a core reamer and gently tapped into correspondingly sized recipient drill holes in the defect to progressively produce a congruous filling of the articular surface defect. The cylindrical plugs fit together to form a mosaic-like surface (Hangody *et al.* 2001). Multiple small plugs fill a higher proportion of the defect with smaller triangular gaps, but there are difficulties seating each of the grafts to exactly the same level with stability so that no plug is either standing proud and subject to increased stress or recessed and non-load bearing. Problems with the procedure, apart from donor site morbidity, are lateral integration of the articular surface, and the difficulty in matching both thickness and shape of the donor and recipient sites. This is especially difficult in the tibial plateau and the ankle, where the typical defect lies at the shoulder of the talus, and the surface defect is of both the superior and side (medial or lateral) surface. For these reasons, artificial composite plugs which can be sized to fit are now commercially available, but few results have yet been reported. The procedure can be done on an outpatient basis, and often arthroscopically, but weight-bearing is still restricted until bony union of the grafts is expected.

3. **Autologous chondrocyte transplantation (ACT)** There are a number of variants of this tissue engineering procedure first popularized by Brittberg and colleagues in 1987 (Brittberg *et al.* 1994). The classical Gothenburg technique is a two-stage procedure in which small amounts of normal articular cartilage are harvested full-thickness arthroscopically with a gouge or curette, usually from either the lateral or intercondylar margin of the femoral condyle. The deepest cells in the biopsy are the most important, and a bleeding subchondral surface is desirable for the donor site's repair. In the laboratory, the chondrocytes are released from the matrix enzymatically using a collagenase, washed, and cultured in the patient's own serum. This continues over a period of approximately 3 weeks before a second surgical procedure, this time with formal arthrotomy, is undertaken to debride the chondral defect (rather less aggressively than in the microfracture technique so as to maintain the avascularity of the bone surface). After carefully measuring the size and shape of the defect, a matching patch of periosteum is taken, usually from the subcutaneous tibia, and sutured to the normal surrounding articular cartilage keeping the deep (cambial) layer on the subchondral bone side using fine absorbable sutures (Fig. 1.5.3). An attempt is made to achieve a waterproof seal, sometimes with the help of fibrin glue, before filling the 'blister' cavity with a suspension of the cultured chondrocytes (Fig. 1.5.4). There are now a number of variants of this procedure including the use of various matrices, either semi-synthetic membranes or three-dimensional structures, to provide a scaffold allowing some degree of primary stability of the articular surface. A number of synthetic substances have been used for this including synthesized collagen membranes and hyaluronan composites. Techniques are now available to do this

Overview of ACI Surgical Procedure

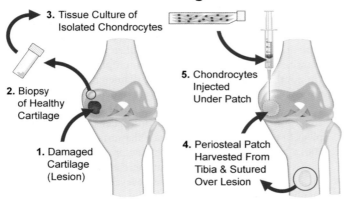

3. Tissue Culture of Isolated Chondrocytes

2. Biopsy of Healthy Cartilage

1. Damaged Cartilage (Lesion)

5. Chondrocytes Injected Under Patch

4. Periosteal Patch Harvested From Tibia & Sutured Over Lesion

Fig. 1.5.3 Overview of autologous chondrocyte transplantation.

minimally invasively and attempts are being made to optimize the biology of the procedure with other biologically active compounds. Rehabilitation following this procedure is even slower than for the preceding two, but runs along similar lines, with or without a short period of static splintage; partial weight-bearing is necessary for several weeks (Bailey *et al.* 2003). Follow-up histology suggests that the regenerate articular surface takes well over a year to mature.

There are a number of hybrid techniques which attempt to contain the 'super-clot' produced by microfracture underneath a membrane similar to that used for ACT. 'Paste grafting' has been recommended primarily to fill an osteochondral defect with a more homogenous osteochondral paste (Stone *et al.* 2006).

Results in athletes

It is always important to look for the cause of the articular problem—whether it was due to a one-off injury, or whether there is a

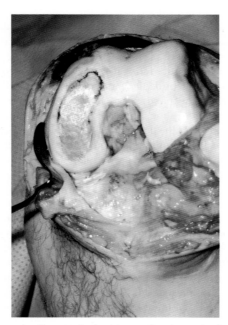

Fig. 1.5.4 Operative photograph of autologous chondrocyte implantation.

treatable contributory cause such as malalignment, instability, or a problem in training or technique. It is a waste of time to send 'good cartilage after bad' and any predisposing cause must be addressed. There is conflicting evidence in the literature about the relative efficacy of the three treatment procedures and considerable difference in expert opinion, whether in high-demand athletes or the general population. Over the last 10 years osteochondral grafting has fallen out of favour, but it has recently been popularized with the introduction of synthetic composite cylindrical plugs which remove the disadvantage of donor site morbidity. No good studies are available as yet. Microfracture remains popular as a relatively minor surgical intervention with low risk, although it does carry with it a substantial investment for the athlete in both time and effort for recovery. A minimum of 4 months out of full training is usually required to allow the regenerated articular surface to mature. It has also been suggested that, by penetrating the subchondral bone, there may be bone sclerosis and the complex architecture and interrelation of the constituents of the articular surface may be damaged, and that this may interfere with any subsequent attempt to re-create a normal type II collagen hyaline-like articular surface using a cultured chondrocyte technique.

As Moseley has noted, there is a large placebo effect associated with arthroscopy (Moseley *et al.* 2002). Many patients have very significant relief from simple debridement of unstable chondral flaps, at least in the medium term, but probably not as good as from reparative procedures (Dozin *et al.* 2005; Fu *et al.* 2005; Hubbard 1987).

The results of the microfracture in high-demand athletes have been reported to be good and excellent in two-thirds to three-quarters of cases in the medium term (Mithofer *et al.* 2005; Steadman *et al.* 2003). It seems to be maximally effective at 2 years especially in young (under 35 years) athletes with small lesions (less than 400 mm^2). Seventy-six per cent of American National Football League players and 77% of high-demand athletes returned to play following the procedure (Steadman *et al.* 2006). In another study, two-thirds of athletes rated their outcome as good or excellent follow-up after more than 2 years, but subsequent deterioration was noted in nearly half (Mithöfer *et al.* 2006).

Mosaicplasty has also been studied in sportsmen. Hangody and Szerb (2006) reported results from 96 professional athletes across various sports and various joints, most of whom had other corrective procedures such as ligament reconstruction or realignment. It is difficult to draw any firm conclusions from this about its role in sport.

A multicentre case series of ACT in 45 soccer players at a mean of 41 months reported 72% good and excellent results, rather worse than published series in the general population. Eighty-three per cent of competitive players returned to sport, of whom 80% returned to the same or higher level. It may be that the longer-term results will be better in ACT since this is more likely to produce hyaline cartilage, and perhaps this approach should be preferred in the adolescent (Mithofer *et al.* 2005; Micheli *et al.* 2006).

Comparisons have been made between mosaicplasty and ACT (Bentley *et al.* 2003), with significantly better results with ACT in a short-term randomized trial. No difference was found in another study, with a tendency to the opposite conclusion (Dozin *et al.* 2005).

Knutsen *et al.* (2007)found no significant difference between microfracture and ACT in a careful randomized trial of 80 patients at 5-year follow-up.

Comparative studies do not always compare like with like, since ACT, unlike mosaicplasty, has limited capacity to address a bony as opposed to a cartilage defect. Younger and lighter patients with a short duration of pre-operative symptoms have a better outcome, as do non-smokers, but their demands are higher. It is postulated that since ACT aims to increase the amount of hyaline cartilage, the long-term results may be better than those of procedures which aim for a fibrocartilaginous repair. Therefore a surrogate endpoint may be the normality of the surface in the short to medium term, whether this is mechanical (stiffness, edge integration) or biological (biopsy assessment of histology and histochemistry). This would tend to favour ACT (Saris *et al.* 2008).

There is no consensus on the optimal surgical management of either traumatic or atraumatic chondral lesions. After correcting predisposing causes as far as possible, especially malalignment, range of motion, and instability, it would seem reasonable to reserve mosaicplasty (whether autologous or synthetic) for symptomatic osteochondral lesions deeper than 1 cm, typically following osteochondritis dissecans. In the younger patient, or the patient whose main desire is for a good long-term result in the presence of a large lesion even with a prolonged rehabilitation, ACT may be preferred. The author's practice is to tend toward microfracture, at least in the first instance, as a reasonable compromise between the extent of surgery and damage to the subchondral bone, and a high proportion of good and excellent results are obtained within a reasonable period of post-operative rehabilitation. However, attention to surgical detail and post-operative rehabilitation is considered to be vital.

The future

Improvements in the biology of cartilage regeneration may come from growth factors such as TGF-β, IGF, bFGF, and the bone morphogenetic proteins or from gene therapy. In reality, they may be more likely to come from the use of stem cells which, given the right environment, may be able to synthesize the appropriate cocktail of growth factors with respect to time throughout the healing process. Technical advances will tend to reduce the invasiveness of the surgical procedure and to minimize the period of recovery by providing a temporary three-dimensional scaffold to load-share with the regenerate articular cartilage through an accelerated rehabilitation period.

For further information the reader is referred to a reviews of arthroscopic treatment for osteoarthritis (Steadman *et al.* 2007), microfracture (Williams and Harnly 2007), and ACT (Jones and Peterson 2006; Wasiak *et al.* 2006), and an overview by Marcacci *et al.* (2007).

Glenoid and acetabular labra

The concavity of both shoulder and hip articular surfaces is usually described as being deepened by a fibrocartilaginous lip which forms a transition between capsular soft tissues and the articular cartilage and subchondral bone. Histologically, however, the tissue is fibrous rather than fibrocartilaginous (Moseley and Overgaard 1962), with a few elastin fibres, and it is variable in size, morphology, and attachment. The extent to which the glenoid socket is deepened (and therefore its contribution to glenohumeral stability) is variable, but may be up to 50% (Howell and Galinat 1989), and there is often an overhanging intra-articular 'meniscoid' flap

of labrum which may appear as a cleft. This can be mistaken for a tear both on imaging and at arthroscopy.

Injuries to the labrum may lead to either mechanical symptoms or pain exactly similar to the symptoms of meniscal pathology in the knee. The glenoid labrum is most commonly injured antero-inferiorly where the anterior band of the inferior glenohumeral ligaments sweeps up along the anterior glenoid margin and almost parallel to it. As well as attaching to the glenoid neck, it blends with the labrum to insert over relatively long transition zones of ligament, fibrocartilage, and mineralized fibrocartilage and onto bone, attaching at an acute angle. Typically, this complex is avulsed from the glenoid margin during anterior dislocation, forming Bankart's 'essential' lesion which de-tensions the ligament complex, allowing a pocket of lax capsule into which recurrent dislocations can occur as well as decreasing the socket depth. The long head of the biceps brachii is inserted partly via the superior labrum into the superior glenoid and supraglenoid tubercle, and this attachment is often injured in throwing athletes leading to a SLAP (superior labrum anterior to posterior) tear. The injury may occur either by the humeral head 'pushing' the posterosuperior labrum in external rotation or 'pulling' during the follow-through phase of throwing.

Pathology in the hip is rather different in that there are no capsular or tendon attachments. The labrum does deepen the socket and may have a restraining role, altering the marginal flow of synovial fluid and affecting the joint's lubrication. Labral tears are associated with dysplasia leading to overload (Haene *et al.* 2007) and with femoroacetabular impingement (Philippon *et al.* 2007).

References

Bailey, A., Goodstone, N., Roberts, S., *et al.* (2003). Rehabilitation after Oswestry autologous chondrocyte implantation: the Oscell protocol. *Journal of Sports Rehabilitation*, **12**, 104–18.

Bellamy, N., Campbell, J., Robinson, V., Gee, T., Bourne, R., and Wells, G. (2006). Viscosupplementation for the treatment of osteoarthritis of the knee. *Cochrane Database of Systematic Reviews*, Vol **2**. CD005321, no. 2.

Bentley, G., Biant, L.C., Carrington, R.W., *et al.* (2003). A prospective, randomised comparison of autologous chondrocyte implantation versus mosaicplasty for osteochondral defects in the knee. *Journal of Bone and Joint Surgery, British Volume* **85**, 223–30.

Brittberg, M., Lindahl, A., Nilsson, A., Ohlsson, C., Isaksson, O., and Peterson, L. (1994). Treatment of deep cartilage defects in the knee with autologous chondrocyte transplantation. *New England Journal of Medicine*, **331**, 889–95.

Buckwalter, J.A. and Martin, J.A. (2004). Sports and osteoarthritis. *Current Opinion in Rheumatology*, **16**, 634–9.

Buckwalter, J.A. and Mow, V.C. (2003). Basic science and injury of articular cartilage, menisci and bone. In: DeLee, J.C. and Drez, D (eds), *Orthopaedic Sports Medicine* (2nd edn), pp. 67–120. W.B. Saunders, Philadelphia, PA.

Dowthwaite, G.P., Bishop, J.C., Redman, S.N., *et al.* (2004). The surface of articular cartilage contains a progenitor cell population. *Journal of Cell Science*, **117**, 889–97.

Dozin, B., Malpeli, M., Cancedda, R., *et al.* (2005). Comparative evaluation of autologous chondrocyte implantation and mosaicplasty: a multicentered randomized clinical trial. *Clinical Journal of Sport Medicine*, **15**, 220–6.

Einhorn, T.A., O'Keefe, R.J, and Buckwalter, J.A. (2007). *Orthopaedic Basic Science: Foundations of Clinical Practice* (3rd edn). Rosemont, IL, American Academy of Orthopaedic Surgeons.

Fu, F.H., Zurakowski, D., Browne, J.E., *et al.* (2005). Autologous chondrocyte implantation versus debridement for treatment of full-thickness chondral defects of the knee: an observational cohort study with 3-year follow-up. *American Journal of Sports Medicine*, **33**, 1658–66.

Haene, R.A., Bradley, M., and Villar, R.N. (2007). Hip dysplasia and the torn acetabular labrum: an inexact relationship. *Journal of Bone and Joint Surgery, British Volume*, **89**, 1289–92.

Hangody, L. and Szerb, I. (2006). Mosaicplasty in chondral defects of high demand athletes. In: Zanasi S., Brittberg M., and Marcacci, M. (eds), *Basic Science, Clinical Repair and Reconstruction of Articular Cartilage Defects: Current Status and Prospects*, pp. 627–30. Timeo Editore, Bologna.

Hangody, L., Feczko, P., Bartha, L., Bodo, G., and Kish, G. (2001). Mosaicplasty for the treatment of articular defects of the knee and ankle. *Clinical Orthopaedics and Related Research*, **391** (Suppl), 328–36.

Hiraoka, K., Grogan, S., Olee, T., and Lotz, M. (2006). Mesenchymal progenitor cells in adult human articular cartilage. *Biorheology*, **43**, 447–54.

Howell, S.M. and Galinat, B.J. (1989). The glenoid–labral socket. A constrained articular surface, *Clinical Orthopaedics and Related Research*, **243**, 122–5.

Hubbard, M.J. (1987). Arthroscopic surgery for chondral flaps in the knee. *Journal of Bone and Joint Surgery, British Volume*, **69**, 794–6.

Hunter, W. (1995). Of the structure and disease of articulating cartilages. 1743. *Clinical Orthopaedics and Related Research*, **317**, 3–6.

Jones, D.G. and Peterson, L. (2006). Autologous chondrocyte implantation. *Journal of Bone and Joint Surgery, American Volume*, **88**, 2502–20.

Knutsen, G., Drogset, J.O., Engebretsen, L., *et al.* (2007). A randomized trial comparing autologous chondrocyte implantation with microfracture. Findings at five years. *Journal of Bone and Joint Surgery, American Volume*, **89**, 2105–12.

Marcacci, M., Kon, E., Zaffagnini, S., *et al.* (2007). Arthroscopic second generation autologous chondrocyte implantation. *Knee Surgery, Sports Traumatology, Arthroscopy*, **15**, 610–19.

Micheli, L., Curtis, C., and Shervin, N. (2006). Articular cartilage repair in the adolescent athlete. Is autologous chondrocyte implantation the answer? *Clinical Journal of Sport Medicine*, **16**, 465–70.

Mithöfer, K., Peterson, L., Mandelbaum, B.R., and Minas, T. (2005). Articular cartilage repair in soccer players with autologous chondrocyte transplantation: functional outcome and return to competition. *American Journal of Sports Medicine*, **33**, 1639–46.

Mithöfer, K., Williams, R.J., Warren, R.F., Wickiewicz, T.L., and Marx, R.G. (2006). High-impact athletics after knee articular cartilage repair: a prospective evaluation of the microfracture technique. *American Journal of Sports Medicine*, **34**, 1413–18.

Moseley, H.F. and Overgaard, B. (1962). The anterior capsular mechanism in recurrent anterior dislocation of the shoulder. *Journal of Bone and Joint Surgery, British Volume*, **44B**, 913–27.

Moseley, J.B., O'Malley, K., Petersen, N.J., *et al.* (2002). A controlled trial of arthroscopic surgery for osteoarthritis of the knee. *New England Journal of Medicine*, **347**, 81–8.

Philippon, M., Schenker, M., Briggs, K., and Kuppersmith, D. (2007). Femoroacetabular impingement in 45 professional athletes: associated pathologies and return to sport following arthroscopic decompression. *Knee Surgery, Sports Traumatology, Arthroscopy*, **15**, 908–14.

Pridie, K.H. (1959). A method of resurfacing osteoarthritic knee joints. *Journal of Bone and Joint Surgery, British Volume*, **41B**, 618–619.

Roberts, S. (2007). Articular cartilage. In: V. Cassar-Pullicino and J. B. Richardson (eds), *Basic Science for the FRCS (Trauma and Orthopaedics)*, pp. 15–22. Institute of Orthopaedics, Oswestry.

Saris, D.B., Vanlauwe, J., Victor, J., *et al.* (2008). Characterized chondrocyte implantation results in better structural repair when treating symptomatic cartilage defects of the knee in a randomized controlled trial versus microfracture. *American Journal of Sports Medicine*, **36**, 235–46.

Saxon, L., Finch, C., and Bass, S. (1999). Sports participation, sports injuries and osteoarthritis: implications for prevention. *Sports Medicine*, **28**, 123–35.

Shepherd, D.E. and Seedhom, B.B. (1999). Thickness of human articular cartilage in joints of the lower limb. *Annals of the Rheumatic Diseases*, **58**, 27–34.

Steadman, J.R., Rodkey, W.G., and Rodrigo, J.J. (2001). Microfracture: surgical technique and rehabilitation to treat chondral defects. *Clinical Orthopaedics and Related Research*, **391** (Suppl), 362–9.

Steadman, J.R., Miller, B.S., Karas, S.G., Schlegel, T.F., Briggs, K.K., and Hawkins, R.J. (2003). The microfracture technique in the treatment of full-thickness chondral lesions of the knee in National Football League players. *Journal of Knee Surgery*, **16**, 83–6.

Steadman, J.R., Rodkey, W.G., and Briggs, K.K. (2006). The microfracture technique in the treatment of articular cartilage injuries in the athlete. In: Zanasi S., Brittberg M., and Marcacci, M. (eds), *Basic Science, Clinical Repair and Reconstruction of Articular Cartilage Defects: Current Status and Prospects*, pp. 623–26. Timeo Editore, Bologna.

Steadman, J.R., Ramappa, A.J., Maxwell, R.B., and Briggs, K.K. (2007). An arthroscopic treatment regimen for osteoarthritis of the knee. *Arthroscopy*, **23**, 948–55.

Stone, K.R., Walgenbach, A.W., Freyer, A., Turek, T.J., and Speer, D.P. (2006). Articular cartilage paste grafting to full-thickness articular cartilage knee joint lesions: a 2- to 12-year follow-up. *Arthroscopy*, **22**, 291–9.

Wasiak, J., Clar, C., and Villanueva, E. (2006). Autologous cartilage implantation for full thickness articular cartilage defects of the knee. *Cochrane Database of Systematic Reviews*, Vol. 3, CD003323.

Williams, R.J. and Harnly, H.W. (2007). Microfracture: indications, technique, and results. *Instructional Course Lectures*, **56**, 419–28.

1.6

Bone

Leanne Saxon

Introduction

Sports participation has numerous positive health benefits; however, it is also associated with an increased risk of injury. While bone injuries in sport are less frequent than ligament tears, contusions, or surface wounds, they can be debilitating for an athlete because of the time needed for recovery. In this chapter I describe the incidence and cost of bone injuries in sport, fundamentals of bone biology and repair, risk factors associated with fractures, stress fractures, and periostitis, and review both current and possible future recommendations for the treatment of bone-related injuries.

Incidence of bone-related injuries in sport

Bone fractures account for 18–20% of all sport-related injuries treated in hospital emergency departments (Finch *et al.* 1998; Burt and Overpeck 2001; MMWR 2002; Schneider *et al.* 2006). This contrasts with dislocations, torn ligaments, and surface or open wounds that make up the majority (Finch *et al.* 1998; Burt and Overpeck 2001; MMWR 2002; Schneider *et al.* 2006). Conversely, if one considers all the sport-related injuries recorded (including those not seen by a doctor), fractures only account for 5–6%, with the most common being contusions; stress fractures represent 3% and the most frequent bone-related injury is shin splints at 12% (Watson 1993). The bones of the arms and legs are most likely to break, and the spine or skull are rarely involved. Bones of the legs and feet are most susceptible to stress fractures, which are most common in ballet dancers, long-distance runners, and a subset of male athletes with thin bones (Crossley *et al.* 1999).

Approximately 15% of all fractures in children involve the growth plate (physis). Competitive sports (e.g. hockey, soccer, and baseball) account for 34% of growth-plate injuries, and recreational activities (e.g. cycling, skateboarding, and skiing) account for 22% (Peterson *et al.* 1994; Caine *et al.* 2006). American football is the sport most often connected with acute physeal fractures; however, most other sports are also represented (Lombardo and Harvey 1977; Goldberg and Aadalen 1978; Benton 1982; Peterson *et al.* 1994; Caine *et al.* 2006). Growth-plate injuries may produce irreversible damage, such as reducing or completely inhibiting growth (Caine *et al.* 2006). Overuse injuries, which include stress fractures of the long bones, account for approximately 50% of injuries in children (Micheli 1986; Dalton 1992). These injuries may be devastating to the athlete, but when recognized early and diagnosed accurately they respond well to conservative treatment and rest.

Basic concepts of bone biology

The human skeleton is comprised of 206 bones that function together to provide a rigid weight-bearing structure, attachment sites for muscles, tendons, and ligaments, protection of vital organs, calcium and phosphate homeostasis, immune function, and haemopoiesis (blood cell formation).

Bone first appeared more than 500 million years ago in primitive fish. The internal skeleton of these fish was comprised of cartilage. In the evolutionary branch that led to humans, most of the cartilage was replaced by bone (Martini 2001). Bone matrix makes up more than 90% of bone volume (Buckwalter *et al.* 1995a). It is a composite material consisting of water (10%), an organic component (20%), and an inorganic component (65%). The organic component is mostly made up of collagen fibres and the inorganic component is a mixture of calcium salts (calcium phosphate, calcium carbonate) (Buckwalter *et al.* 1995a). The calcium salts are organized around the collagen fibres and account for 80–90% of the variance in bone strength (Buckwalter *et al.* 1995a). The collagen fibres provide flexibility that allows bone to respond to forces by bending rather than breaking (Buckwalter *et al.* 1995a). Therefore the composition of bone results in a strong yet flexible structure that provides some resistance to breaking.

Bone tissue on a macroscopic level is non-homogeneous, porous, and anisotropic. Although porosity can vary from 5% to 95%, most bone tissues either have very low or very high porosity. As a result we usually distinguish between two types of bone (Fig. 1.6.1). The first type is **trabecular** or **cancellous** bone with 50–95% porosity, which is usually found in cuboidal bones, flat bones, and at the end of long bones, and comprises ~20% of the total skeleton (Buckwalter *et al.* 1995b). The pores are interconnected and filled with marrow (a tissue composed of blood vessels, nerves, and various types of cells, whose main function is to produce blood cells), while the matrix has the form of plates and struts called trabeculae, with a thickness of about 200 μm (Martin *et al.* 1998). Trabeculae are typically orientated in the direction that strains are applied, but also have extensive cross-branching. Given the high surface area to volume ratio, cancellous bone has a relatively high rate of bone turnover or remodelling. Therefore cancellous bone is sensitive to physical activity and bone loss with ageing (Buckwalter *et al.* 1995b).

The second type is **cortical** or **compact** bone, which is a densely compacted tissue found on the outer surface of bone. It provides a strong protective layer and comprises ~80% of the total skeleton. In long bones, cortical bone forms the diaphysis and there is little

Compact Bone & Spongy (Cancellous Bone)

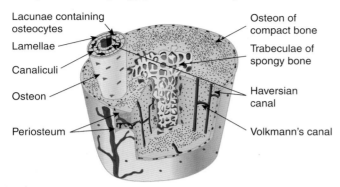

Fig. 1.6.1 Cross-section showing trabecular and cortical bone anatomy.

or no cancellous bone in this region. Cortical bone has 5–10% porosity and is made up of different types of pores. Vascular porosity is the largest (50 μm in diameter) formed by the Haversian canals (aligned with the long axis of bones) and Volkmanns's canals (transverse canals connecting Haversian canals with capillaries and nerves). Other porosities are associated with lacunae (cavities that are interconnected by microscopic canals called canaliculi) and the space between collagen and hydroxyapatite (around 10 μm). Cortical bone is made up of functional units called osteons which consist of layers of bone matrix, or lamellae, that surround the central Haversian canals.

Throughout life, both types of bone can be produced by two different tissues—woven and lamellar bone. The skeletal embryo consists of woven bone, which is later replaced by lamellar bone. Normally there is no woven bone in the skeleton after 4–5 years of age, but it reappears during fracture repair. Woven bone is formed quickly, consists of poorly organized collagen fibres with randomly distributed osteocytes (osteoblasts that have become embedded in mineralized collagen), and is shorter lived than lamellar bone (Baron 1999). Lamellar bone is formed slowly, is highly organized, and has parallel fibres that make it stronger than woven bone.

Bone is a living material and can adapt to changes in its local environment. Physical activity causes bones to become strong, while inactivity weakens them. High-impact activities, such as gymnastics, cause thickening and strengthening of the weight-bearing bones, whereas non-weight-bearing activities, such as swimming and cycling, provide minimal benefit to bone strength (Courteix *et al.* 1998). Bones are also able to react to other stimuli, such as fractures; the cells within the bone are able to remove the dead bone at the fracture and replace it with healthy new bone. Bones respond to the changes in their environment through processes called modelling or remodelling.

During childhood and adolescence, bone growth, shape, size, and strength mostly result from bone modelling. This means that bone formation and resorption can occur simultaneously on different surfaces (Buckwalter *et al.* 1995b). Therefore bone shape is modified, resulting in a larger outer bone diameter (periosteal apposition), a larger medullary cavity (due to endocortical bone resorption), or a smaller medullary cavity (due to endocortical bone formation) (Ruff and Hayes 1982). Modelling allows not only the development of normal bone architecture during growth, but also the modulation of this architecture and mass when loading (or

exercise) conditions change. When bone strain exceeds a modelling threshold (i.e. during high impact exercise), bone formation increases to augment bone mass and strength, and lower the strains within bone. When strains are below the modelling threshold (i.e. everyday activities), bone formation remains inactive. Because the forces on bone increase by a factor of 20 between birth and maturity, bone modelling ensures that bones are strong enough to withstand these strains and to prevent microdamage (Frost 1997).

In childhood, and primarily during adulthood, bone resorption and formation occur sequentially, at the same location, via osteoclasts (bone-resorbing cells) and osteoblasts (bone-forming cells). As a result, an equal amount of bone is resorbed and replaced so that the bone mineral content (BMC) neither increases nor decreases, and bone shape remains the same. This process is called bone remodelling and is vital for maintaining a skeleton that is biomechanically and metabolically competent. It also serves to remove microdamage, replace dead and hypermineralized bone, and adapt the bone's architecture to local stresses (Mundy 1999). Bone-remodelling sites can occupy 4–10% of a bone's surface and result in approximately one-fifth of the skeleton being replaced in a year (Recker 1993). In old age, the rate of remodelling increases, and because bone resorption is faster than bone formation, bone loss occurs (Buckwalter *et al.* 1995b) which leads to cortical thinning and increased porosity, trabecular thinning, complete loss of trabecular plates, and loss of connectivity (Seeman 1997).

Cartilage or endochondral ossification

Cartilage is a type of dense connective tissue composed of cells called chondrocytes that produce a large amount of extracellular matrix that is comprised of collagen fibres and is rich in proteoglycan and elastin fibres. Cartilage is classified as elastic, hyaline, or fibrocartilage, which differ in the relative amounts of the three main components, and is found on the articular surface of bones, rib cage, ear, nose, bronchial tubes, and intervertebral discs. Cartilage has limited repair capabilities; because the chondrocytes are bound in lacunae, they cannot migrate to damaged areas. Also, because hyaline cartilage does not have a blood supply, the deposition of new matrix is slow. Damaged hyaline cartilage is usually replaced by fibrocartilage scar tissue (Buckwalter *et al.* 1995a).

Early in fetal development, most of the skeleton is cartilaginous. This temporary cartilage is gradually replaced by bone (endochondral ossification), a process that ends at puberty and is only observed again during fracture repair. In contrast, the cartilage in the joints remains unossified throughout life and is therefore permanent. Adult hyaline articular cartilage is progressively mineralized at the junction between cartilage and bone. It is then termed articular calcified cartilage. Adult articular calcified cartilage is penetrated by vascular buds, and new bone is produced in the vascular space via a process similar to endochondral ossification (see section below on biology of fracture healing) (Buckwalter *et al.* 1995a).

The role of cortical bone and its microarchitecture in bone strength

Much of our understanding of the relationship between bone strength and the risk of fracture has been gained from research into osteoporosis. Osteoporosis is a disease characterized by a low bone density and deterioration of its structural quality, leading to weakness and fragility, and increased risk of fracture. This disease mostly affects older men and post-menopausal women but the research findings in this field can also be applied to athletes.

Bone mineral density (BMD, g/cm²) serves as a surrogate measure of the mechanical competence of bones and is used as an indirect measure of an individual's fracture risk. However, there is considerable overlap in BMD between people with and without fractures (Schuit et al. 2004). Thus, the strength and rigidity of bone is determined not only by the amount of material but also by the arrangement of the material in space. Geometric measures such as bone diameter, cortical thickness and porosity, and trabecular thickness and number can explain up to 40% of the variation in bone strength amongst individuals (Bousson et al. 2006). Biomechanical studies have evaluated the relative contributions of the different parameters relating to bone strength and found, for instance, that the best predictors of fracture load at the distal radius are measures of cortical bone mass, cortical area, and cortical width (Augat et al. 1996b). Similarly, male athletes who have a history of tibial stress fracture have a smaller cortical bone diameter but no difference in BMD compared with those who have never sustained a stress fracture (Crossley et al. 1999).

The material properties of bone (mineral, protein, and water) also play a critical role in determining a bone's resistance to fracture. The mineral constituent of bone can resist compression forces effectively, but it has relatively poor ability to withstand tensile strains (stretching) (Augat and Schorlemmer 2006). (Tensile strength is mostly determined by the quality and quantity of the collagen fibres within bone.) Unfortunately for athletes, with each step taken tensile stresses are applied to one side of the bone and this can increase the risk of stress fractures. Stiffness of cortical bone is predominantly associated with BMC, whereas its toughness is associated with collagen quality (Zioupos and Currey 1998). However, there is a trade-off: with increasing mineralization, bone becomes brittle and requires less energy to fracture, and if collagen denatures, cortical bone toughness is reduced (Zioupos et al. 1999). Other components that determine bone strength include mineral crystal size and bone porosity.

Bone is also anisotropic, i.e. it demonstrates different strength or mechanical integrity depending on the direction of the load. Thus, in an accidental fall, the direction in which the athlete falls also determines whether the bone will fracture. Cortical bone has very low porosity and its anisotropy is mainly controlled by lamellar and osteonal orientation (Fig. 1.6.1). Reilly and Burstein (1975) demonstrated that, as a result of its anisotropy, the strength of a cortical human bone was 104 MPa in a longitudinal compression test and 131 MPa in a transverse compression test. In contrast, trabecular bone has a higher porosity and its anisotropy is determined by trabecular orientation. Homminga et al. (2002) found that individuals with osteoporotic fractures of the hip do not have weaker bone tissue; rather, they display greater trabecular anisotropy, with over-adapted strength in the primary loading plane and under-adapted bone in the non-primary loading plane. Thus, although cortical bone is stronger in the transverse non-primary loading direction, which is a direction athletes may fall when playing sport (i.e. on their side), trabecular bone is not.

Rapid bone growth during puberty also increases a young athlete's risk of fracture (Bonjour et al. 1994). During this phase bone mineral accrual is delayed in relation to linear growth, rendering the bone temporarily more porous and more subject to injury.

Large epidemiological studies have found that 27–40% of girls and 42–51% of boys sustain at least one fracture during growth (Jones et al. 2002; Cooper et al. 2004). The peak incidence of fractures in girls occurs between 11 and 12 years of age and in boys between 13 and 14 years of age; corresponding to the age of peak height velocity, and precedes peak BMC velocity by nearly a year in both sexes (Bailey et al. 1989). This phase is also accompanied by structural changes that result in a thicker and more fragile growth plate. The growth spurt may also increase muscle–tendon tightness about the joints and decrease flexibility, thus further increasing the young athlete's risk of a growth-plate injury (Caine et al. 2006).

These findings highlight the need for clinicians to be aware of a young athlete's susceptibility to injury during puberty and to measure not only BMD but also the structural properties of bone when assessing an athlete's risk of fracture. The assessment of bone geometry is becoming readily accessible with the use of magnetic resonance imaging (MRI), peripheral quantitative computed tomography (pQCT), and ultrasound. However, the inclusion of material properties is difficult, given that bone biopsies are the only option and are not necessarily informative of cortical bone properties. Rather, they provide information about trabecular bone (because of the location of extraction).

Fractures

A fracture appears when an accidental load exceeds the physiological range, thus inducing stresses over and above the maximum strength that bone has achieved during growth and through exercise. There are two main causes of fracture: direct trauma (e.g. an impact on the leg) or indirect trauma (e.g. when the foot is trapped, causing the athlete to fall awkwardly and break a leg). Fractures are potentially serious injuries, damaging not only bone but also soft tissue surrounding the area (tendons, ligaments, muscles, nerves, blood vessels, and skin).

When the fractured ends of a bone pierce the skin, the injury is an **open** or **compound** fracture; when the skin remains undamaged, it is a **closed** or **simple** fracture. There is a great risk of infection to the bone with compound fractures; they require antibiotic treatment and usually surgical treatment (debridement). Fractures can be either simple or multi-fragmentary (formally comminuted). Simple fractures occur along one line, splitting the bone into two pieces, while multi-fragmentary fractures involve the bone splitting into multiple pieces (Fig. 1.6.2). A simple closed fracture is much easier to treat and has a better prognosis than an open contaminated fracture. Various types of fracture are defined in

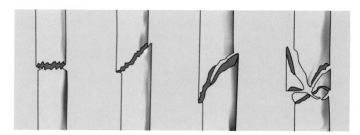

Fig. 1.6.2 Different types of fracture (from left): transverse fracture, oblique fracture, spiral fracture, and comminuted fracture. Reproduced with kind permission from Dunitz Publishing.

Table 1.6.1 Skeletal fracture classification

Type	Description
Compression	Collapse of the bone
Transverse	Fracture at a right angle to the bone's long axis
Oblique	Fracture diagonal to the bone's long axis
Spiral	Fracture where at least one part of the bone has been twisted
Comminuted	Fracture results in several fragments
Compacted	Fracture caused when bone fragments are driven into each other
Linear	Fracture that is parallel to the bone's long axis
Complete	Fracture in which bone fragments separate completely
Incomplete	Fracture in which the bone fragments are still partially joined
Articular	Fracture that involves an adjacent articular joint surface
Avulsion	Fracture where the bone has been torn away from the muscle and ligament

Table 1.6.1, and symptoms associated with a fracture and the recommended response are described in Table 1.6.2.

The doctor's role is to correct any displacement (fracture gap) and/or angulation, control bleeding, reduce pain, and improve blood supply. The fractured ends are realigned as precisely as possible by manipulation with or without surgery. In the latter case, internal fixation of the fracture is achieved by the use of steel wires, plates, screws, rods, pins, or nails. Internal fixation usually requires the application of a cast or a brace; some cases allow early immobilization without a cast. External fixation may be used for open fractures. These injuries take longer to heal than injuries without displacement or angulation (Peterson and Renstrom 2004).

If the fracture has not been displaced, the injured limb is immobilized and supported by the application of a cast, boot, or brace. After a cast is applied, the athlete must be aware of any increased pain, swelling, or tingling sensation distal to the cast. This may indicate poor circulation or deep vein thrombosis (blood clots).

Table 1.6.2 Symptoms associated with a fracture and what the athlete or trainer should do in response to a suspected fracture

Features suggesting that a fracture has occurred:
- Swelling and progressive bruising in the injured area.
- Tenderness and pain around the site of injury caused by both movement and loading of the limb.
- Deformity and abnormal mobility of the fractured limb.
- Sometimes fractures may cause few or none of these symptoms. This can be the case for fractures of the femoral neck or the humerus when fractured ends are driven into each other, becoming firmly impacted and giving the fracture stability.

When a fracture is suspected, the athlete or trainer should:
- Cover an open injury with a sterile compress, a clean bandage, or cloth.
- Immobilize the limb by splinting or bracing.
- Elevate the injured limb.
- Arrange for transport to hospital for treatment and X-ray examination as soon as possible.

If this occurs, the athlete must seek medical advice immediately (Peterson and Renstrom 2004). The length of time in a cast or brace depends on the location, severity of the fracture, and the rate of healing. A fracture to the wrist may be immobilized for 4–6 weeks, whereas a fracture of the lower leg is likely to be in a cast or brace for 12 weeks, and an equal period of time is needed to undergo rehabilitation after removal of the cast (Peterson and Renstrom 2004).

Biology of fracture healing

Bone healing is unique, given that after a fracture the injured site regenerates back to its original structural and biomechanical integrity. The repair process falls into two types depending on the mechanical stability of the fracture site.

1. Primary (direct, osteonal) fracture healing occurs under conditions of rigid stabilization. In this process the fracture gap ossifies via intramembranous bone formation without the formation of a callus.

2. Secondary (indirect, spontaneous) fracture healing occurs when the site is less stable and involves the formation of a callus to form a biological splint to stabilize the fracture.

During primary fracture healing, the fractured cortices repair 'directly' by osteonal remodelling across the cortex. Osteoclasts begin the process by forming a cutting cone across the fracture site. Osteoblasts then lay down lamellar bone behind the osteoclasts, creating a new secondary osteon; eventually the damaged area is healed by the formation of numerous secondary osteons. During this process, there is little or no bone formation by the endosteum or periosteum (inner and outer bone surfaces, respectively) (Goodship and Cunningham 2001). It takes months or years to complete and is less common than secondary fracture healing given that the fracture must be extremely stable for direct healing to occur. Clinically, this process occurs when fractures are stabilized by rigid fixation such as compression plating.

There are two types of primary healing: (i) contact healing, when there is direct contact between the fracture ends allowing lamellar bone to form immediately, and (ii) gap healing, where the gap is< 200–500 µm and is primarily filled with woven bone that is subsequently remodelled into lamellar bone. Larger gaps are repaired by indirect bone healing (partially filled with fibrous tissue that undergoes secondary ossification) (Doblare and Garcia 2003).

Secondary or indirect fracture healing consists of three phases: (i) reactive, (ii) reparative, and (iii) remodelling. Understanding the molecular mechanisms that regulate the phases of bone healing and regeneration are of immense importance for the athlete, the coach, and the clinician. The increasing use of pharmacological modifiers of the healing process make elucidation of these mechanisms essential for determining the safety of specific drugs for the athlete.

The inflammatory phase begins the day the bone is fractured and lasts for about 2–3 weeks. During this phase, the periosteum of the bone lifts and a haematoma due to rupture of blood vessels forms between the bone ends. Macrophages and other cells associated with the immune response remove damaged and necrotic (dead) tissue and generate a loose aggregate of cells, interspersed with blood vessels known as granulation tissue (Doblare and Garcia 2003).

The haematoma releases a large number of signalling molecules that activate mesenchymal cells which are critical for initiating the correct repair response and populating the wound site. These molecules include inflammatory cytokines, such as interleukins (IL-1, IL-6, IL-11), prostaglandins (PGs), tumour necrosis factor (TNF-α and TNF-β), macrophage-colony stimulating factor (M-CSF), receptor activator for nuclear factor κ B ligand (RANKL), osteoprotegrin (OPG), and transforming growth factor (TGF-β) (Bolander 1992). Bone also releases several growth factors at the site of fracture including bone morphogenic proteins (BMPs), TGF-β, platelet-derived growth factor (PDGF), insulin-like growth factors (IGF-I, IGF-II), and basic and acidic fibroblast growth factors (FGFs) (Augat *et al.* 2005). The release of FGFs is likely to play an important role in the initial phase of healing since they have shown angiogenic properties (blood vessel formation) and mitogenic activity (encourage cell division) on the osteoblast lineage (Claes *et al.* 2002).

The secondary reparative healing phase begins about 2–3 weeks after the injury and usually lasts 4–8 weeks. During this phase the pain and swelling decrease, and an external (periosteal) callus and an internal (intramedullary) callus are formed. The external hard callus is made up of rapidly formed woven bone and is located beneath the damaged periosteum. This intramembranous bone formation is initiated by mesenchymal or precursor cells which differentiate directly into bone-forming osteoblasts (without a preceding cartilage step). At the same time an internal soft callus is formed by chondrogenesis (cartilage formation). This endochondral bone formation is produced by mesenchymal cells which directly differentiate into chondrocytes (cartilage cells), unlike intramembranous ossification (Goodship and Cunningham 2001).

These two new tissues grow in size until they unite, eventually bridging the fracture gap, restoring some of the bone's original strength and forming the fracture callus. The chondrocytes hypertrophy and calcify, and blood vessels from the external callus penetrate deep into the internal callus, resulting in woven bone being synthesized on calcified cartilage cores of the callus. This continues until all the cartilage is converted to woven bone. The next stage involves remodelling the woven bone to lamellar bone (either cortical or cancellous depending on the site of fracture) and resorbing the external callus that is no longer needed since the fracture ends have been bridged and stabilized (Shapiro 2008).

The final bone remodelling phase begins 8–12 weeks after the injury and results in the restoration of the bone's original shape, with little or no evidence of scar tissue as would be seen following injury in other musculoskeletal tissue (Fig. 1.6.3). It will also correct any deformities that may remain as a result of the injury and remove any unnecessary callus. This has the advantage that no residual stress concentration remains and the strength and stiffness of the bone returns to pre-fracture values.

Although bone has the ability to self-repair and treatment methods have improved over the past few decades, 5–10% of fractures still show delayed healing. Many of these injuries persist for more than 9 months and are thus termed non-unions. Many athletes would benefit from the methods available for treating these delayed unions and non-unions (Einhorn 1995). Below are a number of factors to consider in order to improve the athlete's chance of recovering full mechanical function.

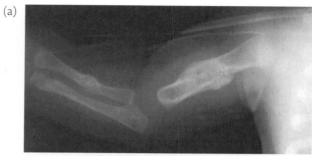

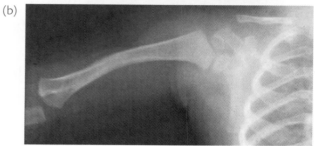

Fig. 1.6.3 (a) Radiograph of a displaced mid-diaphyseal humeral fracture illustrates endochondral bone repair with callus at 3 weeks post-injury in a patient with osteogenesis imperfecta. Note the more advanced healing of previous radius and distal ulna fractures. (b) Radiograph of the same humerus at 1 year post-injury showing complete repair with excellent remodelling. Shapiro, F. (2008). Bone development and its relation to fracture repair. The role of mesenchymal osteoblasts and surface oseteoblasts. European Cells and Materials, 15, 53–76. With kind permission of reproducing from ecmjournal.org

Factors influencing bone repair/bone formation

Mechanical loading

Bone modifies its architecture to adapt to its mechanical environment. Therefore it is critical for athletes to begin physical rehabilitation within days of fracture or surgery (Duncan and Turner 1995). Animal studies have shown that rates of healing, tissue ossification, and stiffness are enhanced by cyclic mechanical loading (Goodship and Kenwright 1985; Gardner *et al.* 1998) (Fig. 1.6.4). However, the benefits of loading depend on how the loads/activities are applied. For instance, cyclic tensile (stretching) strains provide no additional benefit to bone healing compared with regular weight-bearing activities (Augat *et al.* 2001). Furthermore, shear (twisting) movement may delay healing time and reduce the number of bridged fractures compared with compressive (squeezing) axial (vertical) loads (60% vs. 100%) (Augat *et al.* 2003). However, the findings reported in the literature are not consistent. A rehabilitation programme incorporating shear movements was associated with successful healing in humans (Sarmiento *et al.* 1996). Also, shear movement resulted in superior or similar healing results when compared with axial movements in animals (Park *et al.* 1998; Bishop *et al.* 2006). Thus the benefits of shear compared with axial motion may depend on the timing, strain magnitude, and/or fracture gap size.

Strain magnitude, or the amount of applied force, is perhaps the most important variable to consider during the rehabilitation process. Animal studies have shown that relatively low loads promote callus formation and increase bone strength (Kenwright and

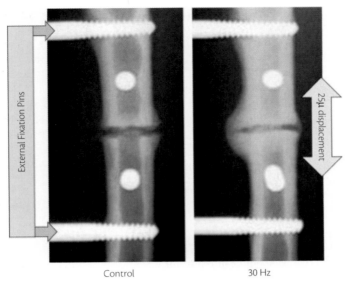

External Fixation Pins

25μ displacement

Control   30 Hz

Fig. 1.6.4 These radiographs show the marked difference in the size and maturity of the callus 10 weeks postopearatively in a control (left) and an experimental (right) animal. The experimental animal was exposed to short daily periods (17 minutes) of low-magnitude high-frequency cyclical interfragmentary motion, 5 days per week. While there is some endochondral bone formation evident in both radiographs at 10 weeks, the extent and maturity of the periosteal callus is much greater on the experimental animal, contributing to the increased functional stiffness of the fracture gap. Reproduced with permission from Goodship, A.E., Lawes, T.J., and Rubin, C.T. (2009). Low-magnitude, high-frequency (30 Hz), mechanical signals accelerate and augment endochondral bone repair: preliminary evidence of efficacy. *Journal of Orthopaedic Research*, **27**, 922–30.

Goodship 1989; Claes *et al.* 1998; Hannouche *et al.* 2001; Yamaji *et al.* 2001; Zhang *et al.* 2007), whereas high loads or no loads at all may have a deleterious effect (Hannouche *et al.* 2001). Zhang *et al* (2007) found that application of low loads (0.5N) at 5 Hz (5 cycles/second) distal to the site of fracture during the reparative and remodelling phase accelerates bone healing in mice compared with sham-loaded controls (Zhang *et al.* 2007). One of the few prospective randomized studies published on humans showed that the application of a controlled axial displacement of 1.0 mm at 0.5 Hz for 30 min/day, starting within a week of surgery, reduced fracture healing time (22 weeks vs. 29 weeks) and was associated with a lower rate of secondary surgery compared with patients with limited movement (Kenwright *et al.* 1991). Similar findings were reported earlier by this group (Kenwright *et al.* 1986; Kenwright 1989). Temporary distraction followed by compression (where the two ends of the bone are separated and then closed together) may also accelerate fracture healing; however, this is only possible in patients who have external fixation (where rods or pins drilled into the bone pierce the skin to provide a rigid support) (Claes *et al.* 2008).

It has also been proposed that the magnitude of stress determines the fate of mesenchymal stem cells; low strains and low hydrostatic pressure favour bone formation by intramembraneous ossification, high compressive strains favour cartilage formation, and high strains and high hydrostatic pressure lead to connective tissue (Claes and Heigele 1999). Cell proliferation and TGF-β production are also increased in the presence of low strains but are decreased during larger strains (Claes *et al.* 1998). Therefore, based on these findings, the magnitude of load should vary depending on the athlete's phase of recovery.

Strain rate, or the time to peak load, is another variable to consider when designing activities to enhance bone healing. Fractures stimulated at a moderate strain rate (40 mm/s) showed faster gains in BMC and stiffness than those stimulated at slow (2 mm/s) and fast (400 mm/s) rates (Goodship *et al.* 1993, 1998). High-frequency loads that are low in magnitude (20–30 Hz) may enhance fracture healing (Fig. 1.6.4) or show no additional benefit than regular weight-bearing activity (Goodshipe *et al.* 2009; Wolf *et al.* 2001). On the other hand, periods of rest in between loading cycles appear to enhance healing time. Mice with tibia fractures exposed to 100 cycles, with rest periods of 9 seconds in between each cycle, showed greater rates of fracture healing than mice undergoing no loading or continuous loading (Gardner *et al.* 2008).

It is important to note that many loading modalities are often ineffective when fractures are immobilized by a cast. Thus a loading modality that does not require direct contact with the fracture site and induces small mechanical strain is well suited for accelerating fracture healing. The timing at which the loads are applied is also critical. Delaying mechanical stimulation until after the reparative phase eliminates the beneficial effects of cyclic loads (Goodship *et al.* 1998). However, full weight-bearing activity should be introduced slowly and not too early. Steadily increasing weight-bearing will enhance mechanical stiffness of the callus tissue and bone formation at the healing front (Augat *et al.* 1996a).

Low-intensity ultrasound (LIUS)

Low-intensity ultrasound (LIUS) is a form of mechanical energy that is transmitted through and into living tissue as acoustic pressure waves. Ultrasound is absorbed at a rate proportional to the density of the tissues through which it passes. It has been proposed that the mechanical strains produced by these pressure waves in biological tissue stimulate the biochemical events that enhance fracture healing (Claes and Willie 2007).

Animal studies have shown that LIUS accelerates the fracture healing process by a factor of 1.5 (Pilla *et al.* 1990). Similarly, in humans LIUS applied for 20 min/day within a week of fracture is associated with a significant reduction (38%) in healing time (Heckman *et al.* 1994). Similar results were reported by Kristiansen *et al* (1997) in a prospective double-blind study of 61 patients with Colles' fractures treated with a cast (Kristiansen *et al.* 1997). No adverse reactions or complications were observed. Several groups have also demonstrated that LIUS may influence the inflammatory and soft callus formation phases of fracture healing but has little to no effect during the remodelling phase (Claes and Willie 2007). Based on these studies, the US Food and Drug Administration (FDA) has approved the use of LIUS for healing fresh fractures. Similar promising results have been reported in the treatment of delayed unions or non-unions (Duarte 1983, Warden *et al.* 2000).

Electromagnetic fields

Several investigators have proposed applying an electrical field at the site of fracture to mimic the positive effects of fluid flow through the bone. Electromagnetic (EM) fields can be delivered by direct current stimulation using implanted electrodes (invasive), or by capacitive coupling (non-invasive). In capacitive coupling two external electrodes are placed on either side of the injured limb and are attached to an appropriate voltage source. The voltage applied to the external electrodes produces an internal electric field.

In clinical settings, EM fields have been used in the treatment of delayed unions and non-unions for 30 years in several departments (Sedel *et al.* 1981), and various devices have been approved by the FDA. In a long-term prospective study performed on 35 non-unions treated by stimulation with capacitive coupling, positive results were found in 14 (Sedel *et al.* 1981). Only one randomized double-blind study of the use of EM fields in the treatment of non-unions has been performed. Twenty-three patients with non-unions 28 months after the injury were treated with capacitative-coupling EM stimulation for 21 weeks, and 11 patients were treated with a placebo unit. Healing was achieved in 60% of the patients treated with EM, whilst none of the fractures in the control group healed. Although these are promising results, they need to be confirmed in a larger cohort.

How does mechanical loading enhance fracture healing?

Although it is well understood that fracture repair is influenced by mechanical loading, the mechanism by which this occurs is still being elucidated. It is proposed that when bone is subjected to mechanical stress, strain gradients are created, resulting in pressure gradients in the interstitial fluid. These drive fluid flow through the small cavities in bone (canaliculi) from regions of high to low pressure, exposing bone cells (osteocytes) to fluid shear stress as well as electric potentials. As a result, these cells stimulate the secretion of growth factors and new bone formation. This notion is supported by a number of fracture healing studies that have shown an increase in various bone formation markers in response to mechanical strain (extracellular matrix proteins, bone-specific alkaline phosphatase marker, TGF-β_1, FGF-β, BMPs) (Mikuni-Takagaki 1999; Nomura and Takano-Yamamoto 2000).

EM treatment has also been associated with an increase in the secretion of growth factors and may indirectly enhance fracture healing by raising the temperature (Hannouche *et al.* 2001). Ultrasound appears to enhance fracture healing by having a direct effect on cell physiology. It increases the incorporation of calcium ions in cultures of cartilage and bone cells and stimulates the expression of numerous genes involved in the healing process including aggreca, IGF, and TGF-β (Hannouche *et al.* 2001).

Physical rehabilitation

Physical rehabilitation is critical for the athlete and may allow an early return to training and competition. After the first 48 hours, an active rehabilitation programme may commence. This approach has developed because prolonged rest is neither necessary nor desirable and fails to utilize the athlete's motivation for a speedy recovery. Immobilization can lead to muscle hypotrophy, decline in biomechanical properties of ligaments and bone, and changes in articular cartilage biochemistry. Exercises, within the athlete's pain limits, will enhance local circulation, help absorb any haematomas, restore muscular and ligament strength and flexibility, promote new bone formation, and maintain cardiovascular fitness. Exercise regimes need to be properly supervised by a physiotherapist and progressed accordingly. Muscles inside a plaster cast can be exercised isometrically (i.e. the joint and muscle are worked against an immovable force), or if movement is possible dynamic exercises can be incorporated (Peterson and Renstrom 2004). Activities often include joint and muscle stretching, pool therapy, and weight training. To accelerate healing, within a week of fracture therapists may introduce ultrasound at 20 min/day of 1 MHz sine waves repeating at 1 kHz, average intensity 30 mW/cm^2, and pulse width 200 μs (Claes and Willie 2007). If fracture healing is delayed, EM stimulation is also recommended. Over time, physical therapy will not only aid in the recovery of the injury but also restore the athlete's physical capabilities to their pre-injury state.

Fracture geometry

Fracture geometry is defined by the fracture type and gap size. It is perhaps the most fundamental determinant of fracture healing time. In comminuted fractures and fractures with large butterfly fragments, angulation and displacement of the fragments may result in delayed healing (Pankovich *et al.* 1981). Transverse fractures that have not been repositioned correctly and lack adequate fixation frequently result in delayed union or non-union (Koch *et al.* 2002). However, if stable fixation is achieved, transverse fractures can heal faster than oblique fractures (Aro *et al.* 1991).

A fracture also heals faster with a smaller interfragmentary gap, but never heals if the gap is too large (e.g. critical gap) (Augat *et al.* 1998). The size of the gap also determines how effective interfragmentary movement is on healing; the same amount of micromovement applied to a smaller gap increases bone formation, but may diminish new bone formation and delay healing in larger gaps (Yamaji *et al.* 2001). This may be because small fracture gaps will produce higher values of strain for a similar amount of axial movement.

Biological regulators of bone healing

A number of regulators play an important role during the fracture healing process. There are too many to discuss in detail, but one of the best examples is cyclo-oxygenase-2 (COX-2). This enzyme is released at inflammation sites and produces pro-inflammatory prostaglandins. When animals are treated with a COX-2-selective non-steroidal anti-inflammatory drug (NSAID), prostaglandin production is inhibited and fracture healing fails (Simon *et al.* 2002). Normal fracture healing also fails in mice homozygous for a null mutation in the COX-2 gene. This confirms that COX-2 activity is necessary for normal fracture healing and that the negative effects of NSAIDs on fracture healing are caused by the inhibition of COX-2 activity and not by a drug side effect (Simon *et al.* 2002). As a result of these findings and others, prostaglandin receptor agonists are being developed to promote bone healing (Paralkar *et al.* 2003), and the use of NSAIDs should be viewed cautiously.

It is generally accepted that once cells enter the wound, their proliferation and differentiation are determined by the type and level of growth factors present at the site of fracture. BMPs (members of the TGF-β superfamily) are the only factors known to stimulate bone formation by inducing mesenchymal stem cells to differentiate into osteoblasts. Therefore it is proposed that increasing the concentration of these growth factors in depleted areas will accelerate fracture repair. As a result, a number of investigators have supplemented biomaterials with growth factors and found that they promote bone healing in large defects in rabbits, sheep, dogs, and rats (Sciadini *et al.* 1997; Cook *et al.* 1998; Arnaud *et al.*

1999) and in models of spinal fusion in dogs and monkeys (Sandhu *et al.* 1997; Zdeblick *et al.* 1998). Clinical studies using hBMPs (extracted from human bone) or recombinant BMPs (produced by genetic engineering) have been successful in healing non-union fractures in humans (Riedel and Valentin-Opran 1999; Johnson and Urist 2000).

Although promising, these findings need to be evaluated in a larger number of patients before they are approved and commonly prescribed. The dose of BMP implanted in each trial was significantly higher than that found in bone and may trigger unwanted side effects. Thus studies focusing on how to deliver a slow release of BMPs and reduce the dose implanted have been performed. Several investigators have used poly-hydroxyester foams (Okada and Toguchi 1995; Schrier and DeLuca 1999; Zhu *et al.* 2000), whilst others are considering gene delivery systems by transducing bone marrow cells with a gene encoding for a growth factor and implanting these into the site of fracture (Vukicevic *et al.* 1995). Thus, the optimum delivery system for growth factors is still a matter of debate (Niyibizi and Kim 2000).

Medication

Other potential drug therapies to accelerate fracture healing include bisphosphonates. Early evidence suggests they may produce earlier healing, but they also hinder strengthening of the fracture (Li *et al.* 2001). Recent evidence suggests that intermittent injections of parathyroid hormone (PTH) can accelerate fracture healing, especially when the callus is becoming mineralized (Skripitz and Aspenberg 2001; Seebach *et al.* 2004). Further clinical trials are needed before these forms of medication are generally prescribed for fracture healing. Until then, the decision to prescribe these drugs and others (reviewed by Aspenberg 2005) will have to be taken on an individual basis and judged on a risk–benefit basis (Fleisch 2001).

Angiogenesis

Fracture healing, like any tissue repair process, results in increased blood flow to the surrounding tissues. Thus it is speculated that interactions between the blood vessels and the periosteum facilitate intramembraneous bone formation. The mesenchymal stem cells located in the blood vessel walls are likely to contribute to this (Bouletreau *et al.* 2002). The importance of vascularization during fracture repair has been demonstrated in several studies, suggesting that treatment with broad-spectrum angiogenic (blood vessel formation) inhibitors prevents fracture healing and the formation of callus and woven bone (Street *et al.* 2002). In contrast, treatment with vascular endothelial growth factor (VEGF) improves fracture healing (Geiger *et al.* 2007).

VEGF promotes new blood vessel formation through the stimulation of endothelial cell division and is associated with more rapid regaining of mechanical strength, and with increased mineralization of the callus and cartilage formation (Peng *et al.* 2002; Street *et al.* 2002). VEGF expression has been found in conjunction with Ang 1 and Ang 2 (Carvalho *et al.* 2004; Lehmann *et al.* 2005). These regulators of angiogenesis, in particular new vessel formation, are expressed throughout the chondrogenic phase of healing and reach maximum levels of expression during the late phases of endochondral bone remodelling and formation (Gerstenfeld and Einhorn 2006). Thus VEGF appears to be essential for normal angiogenesis, callus formation, and mineralization. In time VEGF (in conjuction

with BMPs) may prove to be a beneficial treatment for athletes with specific types of defects, especially those with non-union fractures.

Mesenchymal stem cell regulators

Adult mesenchymal stem cells (MSCs) have the ability to divide and create a clone or a more differentiated cell type. These cells play an important role during fracture repair and reside in a number of tissues, such as the periosteum, bone marrow, trabecular bone, blood vessels, and synovial fluid (Bielby *et al.* 2007). During direct fracture healing MSCs located in perivascular sites provide a source of osteoprogenitors, whereas during indirect fracture healing MSCs located in the periosteum provide a source of progenitors for osteoblasts to form without a preceding cartilage step during intramembraneous bone formation. Conversely, during endochondral bone formation MSCs in the periosteum and marrow stroma provide the progenitors for chondrogenesis (Bielby *et al.* 2007). A number of factors are involved in the overall recruitment, differentiation, and proliferation of different MSC populations: the TGF-β superfamily of proteins, BMPs, growth and development factors (GDFs), Wnts (proteins that activate the Wnt signalling pathway involved in growth and normal physiological processes in adults), and the FGF and IGF families (Gerstenfeld and Einhorn 2006).

A recent animal study showed that MSCs can be recruited from the circulation and/or remote sites and used for fracture healing (Shirley *et al.* 2005). Labelled MSCs injected intravenously into a rabbit vein were identified at the fracture site 3 weeks post-osteotomy. More surprisingly, cells implanted into a remote non-injured marrow cavity 48 hours after osteotomy were more prevalent at the fracture site than those injected intravenously or directly implanted into the fracture gap. Also, MSCs injected into a remote marrow site 4 weeks prior to fracture were detected in the callus 4 weeks after injury. A limitation of these data is that it is unclear whether these cells were MSCs before and after *in vitro* (in culture) manipulation. Phase I and II trials are currently underway to determine the potential use of MSCs for treating bone defects in humans (Sinden 2001).

Bone marrow stromal fibroblasts (BMSFs) are also candidates for accelerating fracture healing. These cells, unlike MSCs, do not have the capacity for self-renewal but can differentiate into bone cells (Maniatopoulos *et al.* 1988). For these reasons, researchers are currently finding ways to attach BMSFs to scaffolds that can form a template for bone formation and bridge large defects in bone. Animal studies are already demonstrating that this approach can increase bone formation (Bruder *et al.* 1998). Once again these results are promising, but further studies are needed before moving to clinical trials.

Stress fractures

Stress fractures (also called fatigue or insufficiency fractures) are generally the result of repeated loading of the skeleton over a period of time and are probably preceded by periostitis (inflammation of the periosteum). If the accumulation of microdamage is faster than repair by remodelling, microcracks can multiply to produce macrocracks and a complete fracture. Stress fractures normally occur in athletes who engage in repetitive activities, such as ballet and

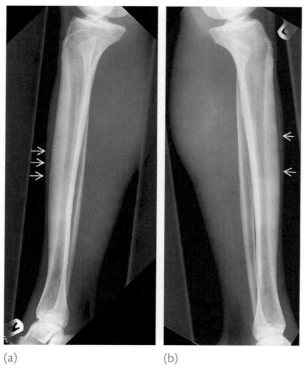

(a)   (b)

Fig. 1.6.5 X-ray of the right (a) and left (b) tibia showing multiple wedge-shaped stress fractures of the anterior cortex in a 26-year-old male professional ballet dancer. The so-called 'dreaded black lines' indicate regions of high tension stress and correspond to areas of pain experienced during jumping exercises for 8 weeks. Reproduced from Berger, F.H., De Jonge, M.C., and Maas, M. (2007). Stress fractures in the lower extremity. The importance of increasing awareness amongst radiologists. *European Journal of Radiology*, **62,** 16–26. Copyright © 2007 with permission from Elsevier.

long-distance running. Stress fractures account for 0.7–20% of all sports medicine clinic injuries (Fredericson *et al.* 2006). The symptoms of stress fracture include pain with activity, swelling, and bruising.

Plain radiographs can be used to diagnose stress fractures; however, only 40–50% of X-rays will show changes initially (Fig. 1.6.5). X-rays are generally better for showing indicators of bone healing, such as new periosteal bone formation, areas of sclerosis (hard bone), and callus, 2–3 weeks after the injury. Given the potential for misdiagnosis initially, it is important to repeat X-rays if the first is negative but symptoms persist. A triple bone scan is 100% sensitive. In some cases a computed tomography (CT) scan can be helpful in evaluating a stress fracture, and MRI performed 3 weeks after the onset of symptoms can separate stress fractures from a suspected bone tumour or infection (Peterson and Renstrom 2004).

Animal experiments show that the incidence and size of the microcracks varies depending on whether the region is exposed to tensile or compressive strains. Microcracks accumulate more rapidly in regions exposed to tensile strains but their growth is limited. Conversely, cracks are started less easily in compressive cortices but their growth is not constrained (Burr *et al.* 1998). Microcracks tend to cut across osteons in compression, but are stopped by osteonal cement lines (or boundary of an osteon) in tension (Carter and Hayes 1977; Griffin *et al.* 1997). Thus the cement line interfaces

keep damage to a minimum and prevent the formation of a fatal crack (Norman and Wang 1997). Furthermore, interruption of crack propagation allows time for bone remodelling to occur, replacing the damaged tissue with new tissue.

Incidence

Stress fractures occur in healthy individuals at all ages from 7 years upwards. The inadequately trained are more likely to suffer stress fractures, which should be suspected in any athlete who complains of bone pain, particularly in the legs, during exercise. Stress fractures occur in the tibia in 46% of cases, in the fibula in 12%, in the metatarsal bones in 15%, and in the femur in 6–8% (Bennell *et al.* 1996b; Peterson and Renstrom 2004). The calcaneus, navicular bone, humerus, pelvis, and vertebrae are also affected, but less frequently. A potentially serious location is the femoral neck; such stress fractures often need surgical treatment to ensure healing and to prevent dislocation and vascular necrosis of the head of femur. Stress fractures are bilateral in 25% of cases and multiple in 8–12%. They do not occur twice at the same site. Runners typically sustain stress fractures in the lower third of the fibula, usually 5–7 cm (2–3 inches) above the lateral malleolus. High jumpers usually sustain stress fractures in the upper third of the fibula (Peterson and Renstrom 2004).

Risk factors

There are two theories of the origin of stress fractures (Peterson and Renstrom 2004). The **fatigue theory** states that during long periods of repetitive effort, such as running, the muscles pass their peak of endurance and are no longer able to support the skeleton when the foot strikes the ground. Therefore the load is transferred directly to the skeleton, its tolerance is eventually exceeded, and a fracture occurs. Modelling experiments show that if the quadriceps muscle is paralysed, ground reaction forces at heel strike increase (Jefferson *et al.* 1990). Moreover, with muscle fatigue, knee flexion occurs earlier in the gait cycle (Nyland *et al.* 1994), reducing stride rate (Clarke *et al.* 1985) and increasing the impact during heel strike (Voloshin *et al.* 1998). Gait changes caused by fatigue increase the peak vertical ground reaction force from 2.4 to 3.0 times body weight (by about 25%) (Nyland *et al.* 1994).

The second theory explaining the origin of stress fractures is the **overload theory** which is based on the fact that certain muscle groups contract in such a way that they cause the bones to which they are attached to bend. For example, the contraction of the calf muscles causes the tibia to bend forwards like a drawn bow. After repeated contractions the innate strength of the tibia is exceeded and it breaks (Peterson and Renstrom 2004).

Anatomical factors are also likely to increase the athlete's risk of stress fracture. For instance, athletes who have a smaller bone width and/or increased hip rotation show a greater incidence. Athletes with leg-length discrepancy, or excessively high or low foot arches, also have increased incidence of stress fractures (Peterson and Renstrom 2004). Middle- and long-distance running or playing basketball are also associated with increased risk of stress fracture (Bennell *et al.* 1996b), and these injuries are more common in young people and women (Nattiv 2000) (Fig. 1.6.6). There is a trend for a greater incidence in women with menstrual disturbances and eating disorders (Bennell *et al.* 1996a), and a reduced risk in women taking oral contraceptives (Cobb *et al.* 2007).

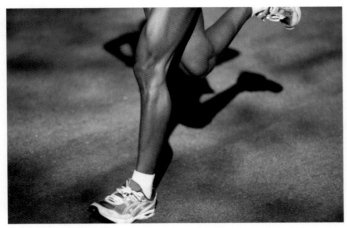

Fig. 1.6.6 Increased running volume, a hard running surface, and the use of worn or inadequate shoes is associated with an increased risk of periostitis or shin splints. Other contributing factors include structural or functional abnormalities of the foot or ankle. Copyright © Mark Atkins-Fotolia.com

Table 1.6.3 Summary of the symptoms associated with stress fractures and the recommended treatment

Symptoms associated with stress fractures
- The pain is activity related. In the first week of symptoms pain is felt during activity but not at rest. When training is intense, the pain increases and a dull ache may persist after exercise. Pain can be detected at night.
- Local swelling and tenderness can be felt over the fracture area.
- Symptoms appear gradually in 50% of cases and acutely without apparent injury in the other 50%.

Treatment of stress fractures
- The most important treatment for a stress fracture is rest.
- Apply ice packs over the injury for 20–30 minutes, every 3–4 hours, for 2–3 days or until the pain goes away.
- Runners should only run if there is no pain, or change activities, such as from running to swimming.
- Take anti-inflammatory medicine.
- Wear a plaster cast or walking boot for 2–6 weeks if the pain is severe or if the fracture is located in the tibia or the foot.
- Surgery in some cases. This may involve pinning the fracture and rehabilitation may take up to a year.

What types of activities induce microdamage?

Important questions for athletes are: What type of load produces microdamage? Is it the magnitude of the load, the strain rate, or the number of impacts, or all of the above? Animal experiments show that repetitive normal strains initiate microdamage. Forced jumping produced cracks in rabbit tibia after 10 days. With continued jumping, some of these cracks accumulated into fractures (Li *et al.* 1985). These findings were confirmed in another rabbit model where repetitive non-traumatic loads induced stress fractures in most animals within 6 weeks (Burr *et al.* 1990) and damage to the bone appeared as early as 4 days after loading (Burr *et al.* 1990). These data support the epidemiological data that show a high incidence of stress fractures in long-distance runners (Fredericson *et al.* 2006).

Although normal loads at a high frequency may initiate microdamage, heavy loads at a normal frequency (e.g. running 100 m carrying a second person) or at a high frequency (e.g. intensive weight training) also increase the risk of stress fracture. Significant microdamage was produced in dog forelimbs subjected to three-point bending at 1500 or 2500 microstrains ($\mu\varepsilon$) for 10 000 cycles, but not when subjected to lower strains or fewer cycles (Burr *et al.* 1985). Frost, an expert in bone biomechanics, supports this theory. Based on fatigue, clinical, and pathological studies, he suggests that there is a strain threshold of 2000 $\mu\varepsilon$ above which microdamage occurs (Frost 1989).

In addition to continuous and large-magnitude strains, a high strain rate or time to peak (e.g. jumping) will also damage bone (Fyhrie *et al.* 1998). Cortical bone specimens showed greater fatigue, as measured by a loss in stiffness, when cyclically loaded in uniaxial tension for a million cycles at a high strain rate than at a low strain rate (Schaffler *et al.* 1989). This fatigue corresponded to increased microcracks in bone. Thus, prolonged normal strains, high strain rates and large-magnitude loads, characteristic of vigorous activities, are more damaging to bone than lower physiological strain rates and lower-magnitude loads.

It is important to note that microcracks exist to some extent in normal healthy bone; thus they may play a role in the normal turnover process as well as in the adaptive response to mechanical stimuli or exercise. In fact, some researchers believe that the accumulation of microdamage is a stimulus for bone remodelling (Martin and Burr 1982; Prendergast and Taylor 1994; Doblare and Garcia 2003). However, it is when there is a loss of mechanical properties that bone damage occurs and microcracks accumulate, leading to macrocracks and potentially complete fracture. Table 1.6.3 lists the symptoms that athletes need to be aware of when they suspect a stress fracture and the recommended treatment.

When can an athlete return to normal activities?

Everyone recovers from an injury at a different rate. An athlete can return to training when their stress fracture has healed, but it cannot be predicted exactly how many days or weeks it will be after their injury. In general, the longer the symptoms existed before treatment started, the longer it will take to recover. The goal of rehabilitation is to return to normal training as soon as it is safely possible. If the athlete returns too soon, it may worsen their injury.

How can athletes prevent stress fractures?

Stress fractures are caused by overuse. The best way to avoid stress fractures is for the athlete to listen to their body and not force themselves to peform activities when in pain. Athletes should also assess their training methods with their coach and pay attention to footwear and equipment (replace shoes every 500–1100 km (300–700 miles)). It is important to consider the degree of progression in training volume and ensure that it is no more than 10% per week. Other risk factors for stress fractures include the 'female triad' of menstrual disturbances, low bone density, and dietary problems (Cobb *et al.* 2003, 2007). Bone geometry and biomechanical abnormalities should also be analysed. Ensure that muscle strength in the legs is adequate, as this will stop them from becoming fatigued too quickly.

Medial tibial stress syndrome (periostitis, shin splints)

Medial tibial stress syndrome (periostitis or shin splints) is the result of chronic inflammation of the muscular attachment and bony changes (outer bone layer) along the posteromedial border of the tibia in the middle to distal region. This condition is likely to be a preliminary stage in the stress fracture of the tibia (Peterson and Renstrom 2004). An athlete with shin splints will experience tenderness along the posteromedial border of the tibia in the middle to distal third regions (tenderness is usually more localized with stress fractures). Radiographs are usually normal with shin splints; however, bone scans (i.e. radio-isotope scanning) will show shin splints as linear streaking over the tibia (in stress fractures the uptake is localized). The incidence of shin splints is the highest of all bone-related sports injuries—12% vs. only 5% for fractures (Watson 1993).

What causes shin splints in athletes?

Factors contributing to shin splints include excessive forefoot pronation, angular displacement during running due to structural or functional differences in foot and ankle, increased external rotation of the femur with the hip extended, varus hindfoot deformity, and increased double heel strikes during dancing for ballet dancers (Thacker *et al.* 2002). Also, unskilled runners will often over-stride and land heavily with each foot strike. As a result, they forcefully plantar flex the foot (the forefoot rapidly slaps the ground), and stretch (eccentric contraction) the muscles of the anterior shin (tibialis anterior, extensor digitorum longus, and hallucis longis). External factors also associated with shin splints include low calcium intake among female athletes, increased training volume, hard running surface, and the use of worn or inadequate shoes (Thacker *et al.* 2002) (Fig. 1.6.6). Table 1.6.4 summarizes the approach that athletes should adopt for recovery from shin splints.

How can athletes prevent shin splints?

Only a few randomized controlled trials have addressed this question. Three out of four found no improvement with shock-absorbing insoles, and only one study showed a significant reduction in the incidence of shin splints compared with controls (Thacker *et al.* 2002). To date, the best advice is based primarily on expert opinion

Table 1.6.4 Recommended treatment for shin splints.

- Rest is the key to treating shin splints.
- Ice and drugs such as NSAIDs to reduce pain and inflammation in the early stages.
- Stretch the muscles of the lower leg, in particular the tibialis posterior.
- During weight-bearing activity, wear shock-absorbing insoles to reduce impact on the lower leg.
- Maintain fitness with other non-weight-bearing exercises such as swimming, cycling, or running in water.
- After the initial acute stage, and particularly before training, apply heat and/or use a heat retainer or shin and calf support. These supports will apply compression to the lower leg and help reduce muscle strain and increase blood flow to the area.
- For some athletes, symptoms can be relieved by fasciotomy, but surgery is not always successful and pain is often relieved without surgery.

and clinical experience, and includes screening for anatomical risks, adequate overall physical conditioning, appropriate diet, warm-up exercises, good running shoes, avoidance of over striding and heavy heel strike, balanced muscle development, minimizing running on hills and hard surfaces, and rehabilitation of limbs previously injured (Thacker *et al.* 2002).

Conclusion

Fracture repair is a complex and multifactorial process, but with the right biological and mechanical environment bone can restore itself to its previous structural and biomechanical integrity. For athletes whose healing is compromised there are promising signs for future use of alternative techniques to enhance fracture healing or for the treatment of non-unions. Although participating in sport increases an athlete's risk of bone-related injuries, it may also provide long-term skeletal benefits when they have retired. The increased BMD that athletes often accrue because of their intense training and weight-bearing activity will help to decrease their risk of fragility fractures later in life. The measures athletes can take to reduce their risk of injury or to accelerate recovery time so that they can return to training/competition as soon as possible are highlighted in this chapter.

References

Arnaud, E., De Pollak, C., Meunier, A., Sedel, L., Damien, C., and Petite, H. (1999). Osteogenesis with coral is increased by BMP and BMC in a rat cranioplasty. *Biomaterials*, **20**, 1909–18.

Aro, H.T., Wahner, H.T., and Chao, E.Y. (1991). Healing patterns of transverse and oblique osteotomies in the canine tibia under external fixation. *Journal of Orthopaedic Trauma*, **5**, 351–64.

Aspenberg, P. (2005). Drugs and fracture repair. *Acta Orthopaedica*, **76**, 741–8.

Augat, P. and Schorlemmer, S. (2006). The role of cortical bone and its microstructure in bone strength. *Age and Ageing*, **35** (Suppl 2), ii27–31.

Augat, P., Merk, J., Ignatius, A., *et al.* (1996a). Early, full weightbearing with flexible fixation delays fracture healing. *Clinical Orthopaedics and Related Research*, **328**, 194–202.

Augat, P., Reeb, H., and Claes, L.E. (1996b). Prediction of fracture load at different skeletal sites by geometric properties of the cortical shell. *Journal of Bone and Mineral Research*, **11**, 1356–63.

Augat, P., Margevicius, K., Simon, J., Wolf, S., Suger, G., and Claes, L. (1998). Local tissue properties in bone healing: influence of size and stability of the osteotomy gap. *Journal of Orthopaedic Research*, **16**, 475–81.

Augat, P., Merk, J., Wolf, S., and Claes, L. (2001). Mechanical stimulation by external application of cyclic tensile strains does not effectively enhance bone healing. *Journal of Orthopaedic Trauma*, **15**, 54–60.

Augat, P., Burger, J., Schorlemmer, S., Henke, T., Peraus, M., and Claes, L. (2003). Shear movement at the fracture site delays healing in a diaphyseal fracture model. *Journal of Orthopaedic Research*, **21**, 1011–17.

Augat, P., Simon, U., Liedert, A., and Claes, L. (2005). Mechanics and mechano-biology of fracture healing in normal and osteoporotic bone. *Osteoporosis International*, **16** (Suppl 2), S36–43.

Bailey, D.A., Wedge, J.H., McCulloch, R.G., Martin, A.D., and Bernhardson, S.C. (1989). Epidemiology of fractures of the distal end of the radius in children as associated with growth. *Journal of Bone and Joint Surgery*, **71A**, 1225–31.

Baron, R. (1999). *Anatomy and Ultrastructure of Bone*. Lippincott–Williams & Wilkins, Philadelphia, PA.

Bennell, K.L., Malcolm, S.A., Thomas, S.A., *et al.* (1996a). Risk factors for stress fractures in track and field athletes. *American Journal of Sports Medicine*, **24**, 810–7.

Bennell, K.L., Malcolm, S.A., Thomas, S.A., Wark, J.D., and Brukner, P.D. (1996b). The incidence and distribution of stress fractures in competitive track and field athletes. A twelve-month prospective study. *American Journal of Sports Medicine*, **24**, 211–17.

Benton, J.W. (1982). Epiphyseal fractures in sports. *Physician and Sportsmedicine*, **10**, 63–71.

Bielby, R., Jones, E., and McGonagle, D. (2007). The role of mesenchymal stem cells in maintenance and repair of bone. *Injury*, **38** (Suppl 1), S26–32.

Bishop, N.E., Van Rhijn, M., Tami, I., Corveleijn, R., Schneider, E., and Ito, K. (2006). Shear does not necessarily inhibit bone healing. *Clinical Orthopaedics and Related Research*, **443**, 307–14.

Bolander, M.E. (1992). Regulation of fracture repair by growth factors. *Proceedings of the Society for Experimental Biology and Medicine*, **200**, 165–70.

Bonjour, J.P., Theintz, G., Law, F., Slosman, D., and Rizzoli, R. (1994). Peak bone mass. *Osteoporosis International*, **4** (Suppl 1), 7–13.

Bouletreau, P.J., Warren, S.M., Spector, J.A., *et al.* (2002). Hypoxia and VEGF up-regulate BMP-2 mRNA and protein expression in microvascular endothelial cells: implications for fracture healing. *Plastic and Reconstrive Surgery*, 109, 2384–97.

Bousson, V., Le Bras, A., Roqueplan, F., *et al.* (2006). Volumetric quantitative computed tomography of the proximal femur: relationships linking geometric and densitometric variables to bone strength. Role for compact bone. *Osteoporosis International*, **17**, 855–64.

Bruder, S.P., Kraus, K.H., Goldberg, V.M., and Kadiyala, S. (1998). The effect of implants loaded with autologous mesenchymal stem cells on the healing of canine segmental bone defects. *Journal of Bone and Joint Surgery. American Volume*, **80**, 985–96.

Buckwalter, J.A., Glimcher, M.J., Cooper, R.R., and Recker, R. (1995a). Bone biology. Part I: Structure, blood supply, cells, matrix and mineralization. *Journal of Bone and Joint Surgery*, **77A**, 1256–75.

Buckwalter, J.A., Glimcher, M.H., Cooper, R.R., and Recker, R. (1995b). Bone biology. Part II: Formation, form, modeling, remodeling, and regulation of cell function. *Journal of Bone and Joint Surgery*, **77A**, 1276–89.

Burr, D.B., Martin, R.B., Schaffler, M.B., and Radin, E.L. (1985). Bone remodeling in response to *in vivo* fatigue microdamage. *Journal of Biomechanics*, **18**, 189–200.

Burr, D.B., Milgrom, C., Boyd, R.D., Higgins, W.L., Robin, G. and Radin, E.L. (1990). Experimental stress fractures of the tibia. Biological and mechanical aetiology in rabbits. *Journal of Bone and Joint Surgery. British Volume*, **72**, 370–5.

Burr, D.B., Turner, C.H., Naick, P., *et al.* (1998). Does microdamage accumulation affect the mechanical properties of bone? *Journal of Biomechanics*, **31**, 337–45.

Burt, C.W. and Overpeck, M.D. (2001). Emergency visits for sports-related injuries. *Annals of Emergency Medicine*, **37**, 301–8.

Caine, D., Difiori, J., and Maffulli, N. (2006). Physeal injuries in children's and youth sports: reasons for concern? *British Journal of Sports Medicine*, **40**, 749–60.

Carter, D.R. and Hayes, W.C. (1977). Compact bone fatigue damage: a microscopic examination. *Clinical Orthopaedics and Related Research*, **127**, 265–74.

Carvalho, R.S., Einhorn, T.A., Lehmann, W., *et al.* (2004). The role of angiogenesis in a murine tibial model of distraction osteogenesis. *Bone*, **34**, 849–61.

Claes, L.E. and Heigele, C.A. (1999). Magnitudes of local stress and strain along bony surfaces predict the course and type of fracture healing. *Journal of Biomechanics*, **32**, 255–66.

Claes, L. and Willie, B. (2007). The enhancement of bone regeneration by ultrasound. *Progress in Biophysics and Molecular Biology*, 93, 384–98.

Claes, L.E., Heigele, C.A., Neidlinger-Wilke, C. *et al.* (1998). Effects of mechanical factors on the fracture healing process. *Clinical Orthopaedics and Related Research*, **355** (Suppl), S132–47.

Claes, L., Eckert-Hubner, K., and Augat, P. (2002). The effect of mechanical stability on local vascularization and tissue differentiation in callus healing. *Journal of Orthopaedic Research*, **20**, 1099–1105.

Claes, L., Augat, P., Schorlemmer, S., Konrads, C., Ignatius, A., and Ehrnthaller, C. (2008). Temporary distraction and compression of a diaphyseal osteotomy accelerates bone healing. *Journal of Orthopaedic Research*, **26**, 772–7.

Clarke, T.E., Cooper, L.B., Hamill, C.L., and Clark, D.E. (1985). The effect of varied stride rate upon shank deceleration in running. *Journal of Sports Science*, **3**, 41–9.

Cobb, K.L., Bachrach, L.K., Greendale, G., *et al.* (2003). Disordered eating, menstrual irregularity, and bone mineral density in female runners. *Medicine and Science in Sports and Exercise*, **35**, 711–19.

Cobb, K.L., Bachrach, L.K., Sowers, M., *et al.* (2007). The effect of oral contraceptives on bone mass and stress fractures in female runners. *Medicine and Science in Sports and Exercise*, **39**, 1464–73.

Cook, S.D., Salkeld, S.L., Brinker, M.R., Wolfe, M.W., and Rueger, D.C. (1998). Use of an osteoinductive biomaterial (rhOP-1) in healing large segmental bone defects. *Journal of Orthaedic Trauma*, **12**, 407–12.

Cooper, C., Dennison, E.M., Leufkens, H.G., Bishop, N., and Van Staa, T.P. (2004). Epidemiology of childhood fractures in Britain: a study using the general practice research database. *Journal of Bone and Mineral Research*, **19**, 1976–81.

Courteix, D., Lespessailles, E., Peres, S.L., Obert, P., Germain, P., and Benhamou, C.L. (1998). Effect of physical training on bone mineral density in prepubertal girls: a comparative study between impact-loading and non-impact-loading sports. *Osteoporosis International*, **8**, 152–8.

Crossley, K., Bennell, K.L., Wrigley, T. and Oakes, B.W. (1999). Ground reaction forces, bone characteristics, and tibial stress fracture in male runners. *Medicine and Science in Sports and Exercise*, **31**, 1088–93.

Dalton, S.E. (1992). Overuse injuries in adolescent athletes. *Sports Medicine*, **13**, 58–70.

Doblare, M. and Garcia, J.M. (2003). On the modelling bone tissue fracture and healing of the bone tissue. *Acta Científica Venezolana*, **54**, 58–75.

Duarte, L.R. (1983). The stimulation of bone growth by ultrasound. *Archives of Orthopaedic and Trauma Surgery*, **101**, 153–9.

Duncan, R.L. and Turner, C.H. (1995). Mechanotransduction and the functional response of bone to mechanical strain. *Calcified Tissue International*, **57**, 344–58.

Einhorn, T.A. (1995). Enhancement of fracture-healing. *Journal of Bone and Joint Surgery. American Volume*, **77**, 940–56.

Finch, C., Valuri, G., and Ozanne-Smith, J. (1998). Sport and active recreation injuries in Australia: evidence from emergency department presentations. *British Journal of Sports Medicine*, **32**, 220–5.

Fleisch, H. (2001). Can bisphosphonates be given to patients with fractures? *Journal of Bone and Mineral Research*, **16**, 437–40.

Fredericson, M., Jennings, F., Beaulieu, C., and Matheson, G.O. (2006). Stress fractures in athletes. *Topics in Magnetic Resonance Imaging*, **17**, 309–25.

Frost, H.M. (1989). Transient-steady state phenomena in microdamage physiology: a proposed algorithm for lamellar bone. *Calcified Tissue International*, **44**, 367–81.

Frost, H.M. (1997). On our age-related bone loss: insights from a new paradigm. *Journal of Bone and Mineral Research*, **12**, 1539–46.

Fyhrie, D.P., Milgrom, C., Hoshaw, S.J., *et al.* (1998). Effect of fatiguing exercise on longitudinal bone strain as related to stress fracture in humans. *Annals of Biomedical Engineering*, **26**, 660–5.

Gardner, M.J., Ricciardi, B.F., Wright, T.M., Bostrom, M.P., and Van Der Meulen, M.C. (2008). Pause insertions during cyclic *in vivo* loading affect bone healing. *Clinical Orthopaedics and Related Research*, **466**, 1232–8.

Gardner, T.N., Evans, M., and Simpson, H. (1998). Temporal variation of applied inter fragmentary displacement at a bone fracture in harmony with maturation of the fracture callus. *Medical Engineering and Physics*, **20**, 480–4.

Geiger, F., Lorenz, H., Xu, W., *et al.* (2007). VEGF producing bone marrow stromal cells (BMSC) enhance vascularization and resorption of a natural coral bone substitute. *Bone*, **41**, 516–22.

Gerstenfeld, L.C. and Einhorn, T.A. (2006). Fracture healing: the biology of bone repair and regeneration. In: J. Lian and S. Goldring (eds), *Primer on the Metabolic Bone Diseases and Disorders of Mineral Metabolism* (6th edn). ASBMR, Washington, DC.

Goldberg, V.M. and Aadalen, R. (1978). Distal tibial epiphyseal injuries: the role of athletics in 53 cases. *American Journal ofSports Medicine*, **6**, 263–8.

Goodship, A.E. and Cunningham, J.L. (2001). Pathophysiology of functional adaptation of bone in remodeling and repair *in vivo*. In: S.C. Cowin (ed.), *Bone Mechanics Handbook* (2nd edn). CRC Press, Boca Raton, FL.

Goodship, A.E. and Kenwright, J. (1985). The influence of induced micromovement upon the healing of experimental tibial fractures. *Journal of Bone and Joint Surgery. British Volume*, **67**, 650–5.

Goodship, A.E., Watkins, P.E., Rigby, H.S., and Kenwright, J. (1993). The role of fixator frame stiffness in the control of fracture healing. An experimental study. *Journal of Biomechanics*, **26**, 1027–35.

Goodship, A.E., Cunningham, J.L., and Kenwright, J. (1998). Strain rate and timing of stimulation in mechanical modulation of fracture healing. *Clinical Orthopaedics and Related Research*, **355** (Suppl), S105–15.

Griffin, L.V., Gibeling, J.C., Martin, R.B., Gibson, V.A., and Stover, S.M. (1997). Model of flexural fatigue damage accumulation for cortical bone. *Journal of Orthopaedic Research*, **15**, 607–14.

Hannouche, D., Petite, H., and Sedel, L. (2001). Current trends in the enhancement of fracture healing. *Journal of Bone and Joint Surgery. British Volume*, **83**, 157–64.

Heckman, J.D., Ryaby, J.P., McCabe, J., Frey, J.J., and Kilcoyne, R.F. (1994). Acceleration of tibial fracture-healing by non-invasive, low-intensity pulsed ultrasound. *Journal of Bone and Joint Surgery. American Volume*, **76**, 26–34.

Homminga, J., McCreadie, B.R., Ciarelli, T.E., Weinans, H., Goldstein, S.A., and Huiskes, R. (2002). Cancellous bone mechanical properties from normals and patients with hip fractures differ on the structure level, not on the bone hard tissue level. *Bone*, **30**, 759–64.

Jefferson, R.J., Collins, J.J., Whittle, M.W., Radin, E.L. and O'Connor, J.J. (1990). The role of the quadriceps in controlling impulsive forces around heel strike. *Proceedings of the Institute of Mechanical Engineers Part H*, **204**, 21–8.

Johnson, E.E. and Urist, M.R. (2000). Human bone morphogenetic protein allografting for reconstruction of femoral nonunion. *Clinical Orthopaedics and Related Research*, **371**, 61–74.

Jones, I.E., Williams, S.M., Dow, N., and Goulding, A. (2002). How many children remain fracture-free during growth? A longitudinal study of children and adolescents participating in the Dunedin Multidisciplinary Health and Development Study. *Osteoporosis International*, **13**, 990–5.

Kenwright, J. (1989). The influence of cyclical loading upon fracture healing. *Journal of the Royal College of Surgeons of Edinburgh*, **34**, 160.

Kenwright, J. and Goodship, A.E. (1989). Controlled mechanical stimulation in the treatment of tibial fractures. *Clinical Orthopaedics and Related Research*, **241**, 36–47.

Kenwright, J., Richardson, J.B., Goodship, A.E., *et al.* (1986). Effect of controlled axial micromovement on healing of tibial fractures. *Lancet*, **ii**, 1185–7.

Kenwright, J., Richardson, J.B., Cunningham, J.L., *et al.* (1991). Axial movement and tibial fractures. A controlled randomised trial of treatment. *Journal of Bone and Joint Surgery. British Volume*, **73**, 654–9.

Koch, P.P., Gross, D.F., and Gerber, C. (2002). The results of functional (Sarmiento) bracing of humeral shaft fractures. *Journal of Shoulder and Elbow Surgery*, **11**, 143–50.

Kristiansen, T.K., Ryaby, J.P., McCabe, J., Frey, J.J., and Roe, L.R. (1997). Accelerated healing of distal radial fractures with the use of specific, low-intensity ultrasound. A multicenter, prospective, randomized, double-blind, placebo-controlled study. *Journal of Bone and Joint Surgery. American Volume*, **79**, 961–73.

Lehmann, W., Edgar, C.M., Wang, K., *et al.* (2005). Tumor necrosis factor alpha (TNF-alpha) coordinately regulates the expression of specific matrix metalloproteinases (MMPS) and angiogenic factors during fracture healing. *Bone*, **36**, 300–10.

Li, C., Mori, S., Li, J., *et al.* (2001). Long-term effect of incadronate disodium (YM-175) on fracture healing of femoral shaft in growing rats. *Journal of Bone and Mineral Research*, **16**, 429–36.

Li, G.P., Zhang, S.D., Chen, G., Chen, H., and Wang, A.M. (1985). Radiographic and histologic analyses of stress fracture in rabbit tibias. *American Journal of Sports Medicine*, **13**, 285–94.

Lombardo, S.J. and Harvey, J.P., Jr (1977). Fractures of the distal femoral epiphyses. Factors influencing prognosis: a review of thirty-four cases. *Journal of Bone and Joint Surgery. American Volume*, **59**, 742–51.

Maniatopoulos, C., Sodek, J., and Melcher, A.H. (1988). Bone formation *in vitro* by stromal cells obtained from bone marrow of young adult rats. *Cell and Tissue Research*, **254**, 317–30.

Martin, R.B. and Burr, D.B. (1982). A hypothetical mechanism for the stimulation of osteonal remodelling by fatigue damage. *Journal of Biomechanics*, **15**, 137–9.

Martin, R., Burr, D., and Sharkey, N. (1998). *Skeletal Tissue Mechanics*. Springer-Verlag, new York.

Martini, F. (2001). *Fundamentals of Anatomy and Physiology*. Prentice Hall, Upper Saddle River, NJ.

Micheli, L.J. (1986). Pediatric and adolescent sports injuries: recent trends. *Exercise and Sport Sciences Reviews*, **14**, 359–74.

Mikuni-Takagaki, Y. (1999). Mechanical responses and signal transduction pathways in stretched osteocytes. *Journal of Bone and Mineral Metabolism*, **17**, 57–60.

MMWR (2002). Nonfatal sports and recreational related injuries treated in emergency departments—United States, July 2000–June 2001. *Morbidity and Mortality Weekly Report*, **51**, 736–40.

Mundy, F. (1999). *Bone Remodelling*. Lippincott–Williams & Wilkins, Philadelphia, PA.

Nattiv, A. (2000). Stress fractures and bone health in track and field athletes. *Journal of Science and Medicine in Sport*, **3**, 268–79.

Niyibizi, C. and Kim, M. (2000). Novel approaches to fracture healing. *Expert Opinion on Investigational Drugs*, **9**, 1573–80.

Nomura, S. and Takano-Yamamoto, T. (2000). Molecular events caused by mechanical stress in bone. *Matrix Biology*, **19**, 91–6.

Norman, T.L. and Wang, Z. (1997). Microdamage of human cortical bone: incidence and morphology in long bones. *Bone*, **20**, 375–9.

Nyland, J.A., Shapiro, R., Stine, R.L., Horn, T.S., and Ireland, M.L. (1994). Relationship of fatigued run and rapid stop to ground reaction forces, lower extremity kinematics, and muscle activation. *Journal of Orthopaedic and Sports Physical Therapy*, **20**, 132–7.

Okada, H. and Toguchi, H. (1995). Biodegradable microspheres in drug delivery. *Critical Reviews in Therapeutic Drug Carrier Systems*, 12, 1–99.

Pankovich, A.M., Tarabishy, I.E., and Yelda, S. (1981). Flexible intramedullary nailing of tibial-shaft fractures. *Clinical Orthopaedics and Related Research*, **160**, 185–95.

Paralkar, V.M., Borovecki, F., Ke, H.Z., *et al.* (2003). An EP2 receptor-selective prostaglandin E2 agonist induces bone healing. *Proceedings of the National Academy of Sciences of the USA*, **100**, 6736–40.

Park, S.H., O'Connor, K., McKellop, H., and Sarmiento, A. (1998). The influence of active shear or compressive motion on fracture-healing. *Journal of Bone and Joint Surgery. American Volume*, **80**, 868–78.

Peng, H., Wright, V., Usas, A.,*et al.* (2002). Synergistic enhancement of bone formation and healing by stem cell-expressed VEGF and bone morphogenetic protein-4. *Journal of Clinical Investigation*, **110**, 751–9.

Peterson, H.A., Madhok, R., Benson, J.T., Ilstrup, D.M., and Melton, L.J, 3rd (1994). Physeal fractures. Part 1: Epidemiology in Olmsted County, Minnesota, 1979–1988. *Journal of Pediatric Orthopedics*, **14**, 423–30.

Peterson, L. and Renstrom, P. (2004). *Sports Injuries. Their Prevention and Treatment*. Informa Healthcare, London.

Pilla, A.A., Mont, M.A., Nasser, P.R., *et al.* (1990). Non-invasive low-intensity pulsed ultrasound accelerates bone healing in the rabbit. *Journal of Orthopaedic Trauma*, **4**, 246–53.

Prendergast, P.J. and Taylor, D. (1994). Prediction of bone adaptation using damage accumulation. *Journal of Biomechanics*, **27**, 1067–76.

Recker, R.R. (1993). *Bone Histomorphometry. Techniques and Interpretation*. CRC Press, Boca Raton, FL.

Reilly, D.T. and Burstein, A.H. (1975). The elastic and ultimate properties of compact bone tissue. *Journal of Biomechanics*, **8**, 393–405.

Riedel, G.E. and Valentin-Opran, A. (1999). Clinical evaluation of rhBMP-2/ACS in orthopedic trauma: a progress report. *Orthopedics*, **22**, 663–5.

Ruff, C. and Hayes, W. (1982). Subperiosteal expansion and cortical remodeling of the human femur and tibia with aging. *Science*, **217**, 945–7.

Sandhu, H.S., Kamin, L.E., and Toth, J.M. (1997). Experimental spinal fusion with recombinant human bone morphogenetic protein-2 without decortication of osseous elements. *Spine*, **22**, 1171–80.

Sarmiento, A., McKellop, H.A., Llinas, A., *et al.* (1996). Effect of loading and fracture motions on diaphyseal tibial fractures. *Journal of Orthopaedic Research*, **14**, 80–4.

Schaffler, M.B., Radin, E.L. and Burr, D.B. (1989). Mechanical and morphological effects of strain rate on fatigue of compact bone. *Bone*, **10**, 207–14.

Schneider, S., Seither, B., Tonges, S., and Schmitt, H. (2006). Sports injuries: population based representative data on incidence, diagnosis, sequelae, and high risk groups. *British Journal of Sports Medicine*, **40**, 334–9.

Schrier, J.A. and Deluca, P.P. (1999). Recombinant human bone morphogenetic protein-2 binding and incorporation in PLGA microsphere delivery systems. *Pharmaceutical Development and Technology*, **4**, 611–21.

Schuit, S.C., Van Der Klift, M., Weel, A.E., *et al.* (2004). Fracture incidence and association with bone mineral density in elderly men and women: the Rotterdam Study. *Bone*, **34**, 195–202.

Sciadini, M.F., Dawson, J.M., and Johnson, K.D. (1997). Bovine-derived bone protein as a bone graft substitute in a canine segmental defect model. *Journal of Orthopaedic Trauma*, **11**, 496–508.

Sedel, L., Christel, P., Duriez, J., *et al.* (1981). [Acceleration of repair of non-unions by electromagnetic fields]. *Revue de Chirurgie Orthopédique et Réparatrice de l'Appareil Moteur*, **67**, 11–23.

Seebach, C., Skripitz, R., Andreassen, T.T., and Aspenberg, P. (2004). Intermittent parathyroid hormone (1–34) enhances mechanical strength and density of new bone after distraction osteogenesis in rats. *Journal of Orthopaedic Research*, **22**, 472–8.

Seeman, E. (1997). From density to structure: growing up and growing old on the surfaces of bone. *Journal of Bone and Mineral Research*, **12**, 1–13.

Shapiro, F. (2008). Bone development and its relation to fracture repair. The role of mesenchymal osteoblasts and surface osteoblasts. *European Cells and Materials*, **15**, 53–76.

Shirley, D., Marsh, D., Jordan, G., McQuaid, S., and Li, G. (2005). Systemic recruitment of osteoblastic cells in fracture healing. *Journal of Orthopaedic Research*, **23**, 1013–21.

Simon, A.M., Manigrasso, M.B., and O'Connor, J.P. (2002). Cyclo-oxygenase 2 function is essential for bone fracture healing. *Journal of Bone and Mineral Research*, **17**, 963–76.

Sinden, J. (2001). What therapeutic products could arise from stem cell research? In: *Stem Cells: Therapies of the Future*. Available online at: http://ec.europa.eu/research/quality-of-life/stemcells/proceedings.html

Skripitz, R. and Aspenberg, P. (2001). Implant fixation enhanced by intermittent treatment with parathyroid hormone. *Journal of Bone and Joint Surgery. British Volume*, **83**, 437–40.

Street, J., Bao, M., Deguzman, L., *et al.* (2002). Vascular endothelial growth factor stimulates bone repair by promoting angiogenesis and bone turnover. *Proceedings of the National Academy of Sciences of the USA*, **99**, 9656–61.

Thacker, S.B., Gilchrist, J., Stroup, D.F., and Kimsey, C.D. (2002). The prevention of shin splints in sports: a systematic review of literature. *Medicine and Science in Sports and Exercise*, **34**, 32–40.

Voloshin, A.S., Mizrahi, J., Verbitsky, O., and Isakov, E. (1998). Dynamic loading on the human musculoskeletal system—effect of fatigue. *Clinical Biomechanics*, **13**, 515–20.

Vukicevic, S., Stavljenic, A., and Pecina, M. (1995). Discovery and clinical applications of bone morphogenetic proteins. *European Journal of Clinical Chemistry and Clinical Biochemistry*, **33**, 661–71.

Warden, S.J., Bennell, K.L., McMeeken, J.M., and Wark, J.D. (2000). Acceleration of fresh fracture repair using the sonic accelerated fracture healing system (SAFHS): a review. *Calcified Tissue International*, **66**, 157–63.

Watson, A.W. (1993). Incidence and nature of sports injuries in Ireland. Analysis of four types of sport. *American Journal of Sports Medicine*, **21**, 137–43.

Wolf, S., Augat, P., Eckert-Hubner, K., Laule, A., Krischak, G.D., and Claes, L.E. (2001). Effects of high-frequency, low-magnitude mechanical stimulus on bone healing. *Clinical Orthopaedics and Related Research*, **385**, 192–8.

Yamaji, T., Ando, K., Wolf, S., Augat, P., and Claes, L. (2001). The effect of micromovement on callus formation. *Journal of Orthopaedic Science*, **6**, 571–5.

Zdeblick, T.A., Ghanayem, A.J., Rapoff, A.J., *et al.* (1998). Cervical interbody fusion cages. An animal model with and without bone morphogenetic protein. *Spine*, **23**, 758–66.

Zhang, P., Sun, Q., Turner, C.H., and Yokota, H. (2007). Knee loading accelerates bone healing in mice. *Journal of Bone and Mineral Research*, **22**, 1979–87.

Zhu, G., Mallery, S.R., and Schwendeman, S.P. (2000). Stabilization of proteins encapsulated in injectable poly (lactide-co-glycolide). *Nature Biotechnology*, **18**, 52–7.

Zioupos, P. and Currey, J.D. (1998). Changes in the stiffness, strength, and toughness of human cortical bone with age. *Bone*, **22**, 57–66.

Zioupos, P., Currey, J.D., and Hamer, A.J. (1999). The role of collagen in the declining mechanical properties of aging human cortical bone. *Journal of Biomedical Materials Research*, **45**, 108–16.

Training, recovery and adaptation

Ken van Someren and Glyn Howatson

Introduction

Organized physical training in the pursuit of sporting excellence is not a recent phenomenon. Reports of structured athletic training programmes date back to the ancient Greeks, when they were used for both military and Olympic preparation. Despite an extensive history, it was not until the mid to late twentieth century that what is now considered a scientific approach to training theory developed. The description of the General Adaptation Syndrome by Dr Hans Selye in 1956, which examined the relationship between training stress and adaptation, and the work of Metveyev, Harre, and others in the 1970s and 1980s developed the foundation of training theory and its application to athletic training programmes.

The recent momentum in the sport and exercise sciences, with disciplines including sports medicine, exercise physiology, biochemistry, and genetics, has elucidated many of the acute and chronic responses to athletic training that are outlined in this chapter. Such advances have been due both to the increased professionalism of modern sport and the financial rewards that can accompany sporting success, and to technological developments in the human sciences. Despite the quantity and quality of scientific research in this field, sport and exercise science has in many ways been one step behind sports coaching. A primary focus of much of the research over the last few decades has been to investigate and describe the acute and chronic responses to training practices currently employed by sports coaches. Sceptics might argue that whilst this has successfully satisfied the scientific enquiry of sport and exercise scientists, it has had limited impact on informing the training methods adopted by many coaches. As understanding of this field develops, and with an increasing number of applied sport doctors and scientists working in elite sport, so the extent to which science and medicine leads the coaching and training processes has increased. Many coaches now utilize the knowledge and evidence base presented by the sport and exercise sciences in their everyday work; indeed, many work alongside multidisciplinary teams of sport doctors and scientists who share responsibility for the preparation and performance of the athlete.

This chapter describes the principles of training that underpin successful athletic training programmes and examines the physiological adaptation to different types of physical training. It also outlines the effects of training on the musculoskeletal system, with a focus on exercise-induced muscle damage, and provides a critical review of some of the recovery strategies adopted by many athletes in an attempt to enhance the adaptive response to training.

Principles of training

Successful training programmes are built upon sound principles that have underpinned training for many decades and have been evaluated and supported through scientific enquiry. Whilst these principles provide a framework in which the coach and scientist can develop the physical training, they do not provide a complete training programme. It is the skill, knowledge, and understanding of the sport, the event, and the individual athlete on the part of the coach that allows the principles to be used to prescribe an effective training programme. This is often referred to as the 'art of coaching' and there are many examples of world-class coaches whose training strategies have been developed through trial and error rather than a scientifically driven evidence base. For those doctors and scientists working in this field, the integration of the science and art of training is one of the most interesting challenges they face.

Progressive overload

The overload principle states that the repetitive stressing or overloading of a physiological system will induce a response and adaptation. In the context of physical training, a training session that stresses the athlete will result in the structural and functional adaptation of physiological systems to effect an improvement in performance. The principle of progressive overload dictates that the overload must be increased as the athlete adapts to the training so as to achieve ongoing reorganization of physiological systems and performance enhancement. For decades, research in sport science and medicine has examined the chronic responses (adaptations) to physical training; however, it is only recently that some of the acute molecular responses to a training stimulus have been identified.

Training load, and therefore the scale of the overload, can be described and measured in three dimensions: volume, intensity, and frequency. Volume simply refers to the amount of work performed within the training bout(s) and is described in units of time or distance. Intensity refers to the effort of the training load and can be described in either absolute terms (e.g. speed, power output) or relative terms (e.g. rating of perceived exertion, percentage of maximum oxygen consumption, percentage of maximum heart rate). More sophisticated methods to quantify training intensity include the classification of training intensity according to exercise domains that are categorized by metabolic thresholds (e.g. anaerobic threshold or lactate threshold, respiratory compensation or lactate turn-point). Frequency refers to how often the training load is performed and may be considered on a daily, weekly, monthly, or even a longer-term basis.

It is the interplay of the training volume, intensity, and frequency that determines the training load and therefore the consequent adaptation to the training. The quantification of training load so as to accurately record what an athlete undertakes, and therefore better understand the responses to a specific training stimulus, is a considerable challenge for the coach and scientist. Whilst constant load training bouts (e.g. cycling at 200 W or running at 14 km/h for a specified period) can be quantified using a number of methods, as described above, this is more problematic for stochastic training involving periods of variable intensity (e.g. interval training or team sports). In addition, in many team sports, match play is a very significant part of the total training load—the discontinuous stochastic nature of match play make quantification of the load difficult. Current techniques include the use and analysis of heart rate and time–motion data, including GPS (global positioning systems), and accelerometry, to quantify this imposed training load.

Recovery and reversibility

Recovery is often the most overlooked component of any training programme, with coaches and athletes sometimes reluctant to reduce training load for fear of compromising performance gains. Recovery between training bouts within a programme is essential not only to allow recovery from the previous bout and therefore enable the athlete to undertake the next, but also to permit the physiological adaptation to the training load. Given that the fundamental goal of any training programme is to elicit such adaptation and the consequent improvement in performance, the principle of recovery is of paramount importance to the training process.

Insufficient recovery will limit the athlete's ability to undertake subsequent training bouts, resulting in the inability to achieve the required intensity and therefore the intended adaptations. Periods of inadequate recovery within a training programme may be intentionally prescribed by coaches to induce a temporary state of overreaching, which may induce specific adaptations and increase an athlete's capacity for training load. However, longer periods of inadequate recovery have been associated with overtraining or the unexplained underperformance syndrome (Budgett et al. 2000), with consequences including maladaptation to training, a performance decrement, and long-term health implications for the athlete.

The principle of reversibility relates to detraining or the loss of training-induced adaptations, which also results in a decrement in performance. Whilst the human body demonstrates a remarkable ability to undergo structural and functional adaptation to training-induced stress, this is only a transient response. In the same way that the training overload must be progressive to ensure ongoing adaptation, if the overload is excessively reduced or terminated then adaptations will be reversed. However, training load may be reduced for a relatively short period to maintain a component of fitness and is typically reduced during the taper phase of a training programme so as to achieve peak performance at competition (Mujika et al. 2004).

Training specificity

The principle of specificity states that training-induced adaptations are specific to the type of training performed; this applies with respect to the mode of exercise performed and the intensity of the training load. Whilst there may be some transfer across limbs, muscle contraction types and training intensities, adaptations are typically realized in the specific movement patterns and the physiological capacities stressed through the training load. Of course, this raises the question as to why many athletes engage in cross-training (i.e. undertaking a mode of exercise other than one's primary sport) and what benefits may be conferred. In addition to providing an alternative mode of exercise during rehabilitation from injury, cross-training may provide central adaptation to the cardiorespiratory system, allowing the development of aerobic power. Cross-training is often prescribed in the general preparatory phase of a training plan; it is sometimes considered to provide a base upon which sport-specific fitness can be developed.

Different training types all induce differing physiological stresses, to which the rate of recovery, adaptation, and detraining is also quite varied. Therefore it is impossible to provide definitive guidelines on how the principles of progressive overload and recovery and reversibility should be applied to the prescription of training programmes to optimize adaptation and performance.

Individuality

The principle of individuality states that no two individuals will respond to a given training load in the same manner; consequently, individualization of the training programme is required to optimize the physiological adaptation and performance improvement for the athlete. It is well established that genetic factors play a significant role in athletic ability, with genotype accounting for as much as 80% of the variability between individuals in their response and adaptation to training (Bouchard et al. 1992). It is therefore imperative that individual characteristics are taken into account when considering all of the above training principles. The physiological assessment of an athlete provides an objective evaluation of both their current phenotype and their response to training and can therefore be used to inform and evaluate the efficacy of the training programme on an individual basis.

Types of training

The enhancement of athletic performance requires specific training, targeted to elicit the required physiological adaptations. Types of training and their consequent adaptations are discussed here within the following classifications: endurance; high intensity; strength and power.

Endurance training

Endurance training involves both cardiorespiratory and muscular endurance and is typically characterized by long-duration, low-intensity bouts of cyclical exercise (e.g. running, swimming, rowing). Such training may be performed as continuous exercise or as interval training, which comprises the repetition of exercise bouts to develop aerobic endurance capacity. Interval training was brought to popular attention in the 1930s by Rudolf Harbig, a German 800 m world record holder; the repetition of intervals allows the athlete to complete a greater volume of training at the appropriate intensity in any one training session. The principal aim of endurance training is to improve cardiorespiratory fitness and metabolic efficiency of the exercising muscle. The specific physiological adaptations to this type of training are discussed in the next section.

The volume of endurance training may be quantified and prescribed according to the duration of the continuous exercise bout or of the intervals performed within the training session. The intensity of the training load may be considered in absolute terms (e.g. running speed, power output); however, given the principle of individualization, the load may also be prescribed in relation to the individual's physiological capacity. Maximum oxygen consumption (VO_2max), fractional utilization, and lactate parameters are correlated with endurance performance in many sports and are commonly used to prescribe training intensity on an individual basis.

High-intensity training

High-intensity training is performed at perimaximal and supramaximal intensities (i.e. $\geq VO_2$max) and results in considerable metabolic fatigue (e.g. substrate depletion; accumulation of metabolites). High-intensity training therefore comprises repetitive short bouts of exercise interspersed with recovery periods. The principal aim of high-intensity training is to elicit adaptations in anaerobic capacity; however, recent evidence indicates that such training is also effective in developing VO_2max (Billat *et al.* 2000). High-intensity training is generally quantified and prescribed in absolute terms – e.g. speed; power output. The use of relative measures becomes redundant for high-intensity training due to the lag time in the response of heart rate and oxygen consumption when the athlete is performing at perimaximal or supramaximal intensities for short durations.

The importance of high-intensity training for middle-distance running was illustrated in the 1980s by the training methods employed by Sebastian Coe (the 1984 Olympic medallist in 800 m and 1,500 m). Coe's training adopted a greater volume of high-intensity training than had previously been considered appropriate for middle-distance running. Coe's success turned coaching and scientific attention to the role of high-intensity training and the importance of anaerobic capacity for middle-distance events.

Strength and power training

Muscular strength and power is an important component of fitness for many sports; whilst the relative importance of these attributes is a function of the physiological demands of the sport, strength and power training is often a significant part of training programmes for many sports. Strength is defined as the ability to produce muscular force to overcome a resistance; power is the rate at which work is performed. Strength is often typified by slow movements overcoming high resistances, whilst power is typified by dynamic movements; however, there is considerable overlap between the physiological bases of these components.

Strength and power may be effectively developed through resistance training; although this is typically gym-based, it may also be performed by adding resistance to specific sport activities (e.g. running against a resistance; the use of resistance around the hulls of rowing boats and kayaks). Whilst this approach ensures the principle of specificity, it is often difficult to elicit the same level of resistance and force production as that possible in the gym environment; for this reason maximum strength and power development often necessitate gym-based resistance training.

Power training is sometimes synonymous with speed training, in which the principal aim is to develop sport-specific speed.

Whilst all sports require an element of speed, it is the short-duration, high-intensity events (e.g. 100 m running; 50 m swimming) that make the greatest demands on this component of fitness. Such training comprises very short-duration repetitions, typically performed at a higher intensity than that achieved during the sport event, with long recovery periods to allow restoration of cellular homeostasis.

Adaptation to training

The energetic demands and the physiological profiles of elite performers have been widely reported in a number of sports and provide the context in which the principles of training may be applied. An understanding of the physiological factors that determine performance aids the sport scientist and coach in the prescription of appropriate physical training regimens that target specific physiological adaptations.

Training overload results in a series of inter-related molecular responses, stimulating protein synthesis that in turn manifests structural and functional adaptations (Coffey and Hawley 2007). It is these responses that underpin developments in physiological capacity and performance. The response to training is described by the supercompensation cycle, which has been developed from Selye's model of the General Adaptation Syndrome (Selye 1956). The cycle comprises four components: training load, fatigue, recovery and adaptation (Fig. 1.7.1). The initial component is the exercise bout, which causes an acute and temporary performance decrement resulting from energy substrate depletion, metabolic by-product accumulation and other causes of central and peripheral fatigue. Following exercise, a condition of fatigue and reduced performance capacity persists until homeostasis is restored. The final component of the cycle is that of adaptation or supercompensation, in which the structural and functional cellular adaptations are achieved. These adaptations elicit a higher level of homeostasis and therefore physiological capacity, resulting in a gain in athletic performance.

The duration of each component of the cycle depends upon the type and load of training performed. For instance, the repletion of intramuscular glycogen is a slower process than the restoration of intracellular high energy phosphates and therefore requires a

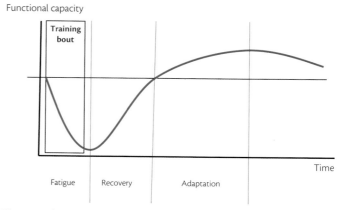

Fig. 1.7.1 The supercompensation cycle, illustrating the phases of fatigue, recovery, and adaptation subsequent to a training load.

greater period of recovery. Similarly, high-intensity exercise, including unaccustomed eccentric contractions, results in damage of the myofibrillar structure, which can take days to weeks to be repaired. This temporary disruption to skeletal muscle is termed exercise-induced muscle damage and is discussed in detail later in this chapter.

The principle of individualization dictates that the temporal pattern of the supercompensation cycle will differ between athletes; it is only through the objective monitoring of the individual response to training that this detail can be described.

The supercompensation cycle suggests that subsequent training bouts should be performed at the peak of the training-induced adaptation in order to optimize adaptation. Unfortunately, it is seldom practical or possible to identify this point; further, the fact that many athletes are required to develop more than one component of fitness or physiology in their training makes this approach inappropriate. Therefore coaches and scientists must alternate the types of training and heavy, moderate, and light loads to ensure adaptation in all aspects of the training. In an effort to expedite the supercompensation cycle and maximize training-induced adaptations, many athletes adopt recovery strategies as part of their training. Popular strategies include massage, cryotherapy, and nutritional interventions, and these are discussed later in this chapter.

Adaptation to endurance training

Endurance training may take the form of long-duration continuous training or interval training, and may be performed at intensities of up to approximately 100% $VO_{2\,max}$. In accordance with the principle of specificity, the physiological adaptations to endurance training are intensity dependent; they have recently been reviewed by Midgley et al. (2006, 2007). Investigations of endurance events have identified the physiological capacities that determine endurance performance (Bassett and Howley 2000; Ingham et al. 2002). These physiological determinants of endurance performance are routinely used as a basis for the evaluation of performance progression and adaptation to training. The relationships between these determinants and performance are presented in Fig. 1.7.2.

Maximum oxygen uptake (VO$_{2\,max}$)

Maximum oxygen uptake is defined as the highest rate at which oxygen is utilized to resynthesize adenosine triphosphate (ATP) for aerobic energy metabolism. It is a function of both oxygen delivery to the exercising muscle and oxygen consumption within the muscle cell. For more than 30 years maximum oxygen uptake has been shown to correlate with endurance exercise performance

(Costill et al. 1973), with elite endurance athletes typically exhibiting superior measures. Many of the studies reporting strong relationships between $VO_{2\,max}$ and performance have done so in heterogeneous groups of athletes; when homogeneous groups are investigated this relationship is not as strong (Basset and Howley 1997).

The identification of the limiting factor to maximum oxygen uptake has long been debated, with much focus on the central versus the peripheral argument. Central factors include pulmonary function, cardiac morphology (particularly left ventricular volume and mass), and haematological parameters (including blood volume and erythrocyte mass). Peripheral factors include intramuscular aerobic enzyme concentration and activity, intramuscular muscle capillary density, mitochondrial density, myoglobin content, and muscle fibre phenotype.

Oxygen delivery, and therefore central factors, are likely to determine the upper limit for maximum oxygen consumption in whole-body exercise (Bassett and Howley 2000); however, peripheral factors (i.e. the ability of the muscle cell to consume oxygen) may be the limitation when exercise is not whole body and utilizes only a small muscle mass.

Fractional utilization and lactate parameters

Fractional utilization is the percentage of VO_{2max} that can be maintained during competition without premature fatigue and is determined by factors including economy and a range of lactate parameters that are highly correlated with endurance performance (Nicholson and Sleivert 2001). There are numerous techniques to identify relevant lactate parameters (Bishop et al. 1998), though the lactate threshold and lactate turn-point are perhaps the most commonly used and are highly correlated with endurance performance.

The lactate threshold identifies the exercise intensity at which blood lactate accumulates and is reported to demarcate the transition from predominant fat metabolism to predominant carbohydrate metabolism. It is most closely correlated with performance in events in which competition pace is similar to the exercise intensity associated with the lactate threshold (e.g. marathon running). The lactate turn-point identifies the exercise intensity at which there is a further and rapid accumulation of blood lactate; it is reported to represent the exercise intensity beyond which a significant anaerobic energy contribution is required, thus resulting in metabolic fatigue. The exercise intensity associated with the lactate turn-point can typically be sustained for approximately 45 minutes in well-trained athletes.

Economy

Economy is defined as the oxygen cost of a given absolute exercise intensity and is an important determinant of endurance capacity. Endurance athletes specializing in longer-duration events tend to exhibit superior levels of economy than their shorter-distance counterparts; in addition, economy is more closely associated with endurance performance than is $VO_{2\,max}$ in elite athletes (Conley and Krahenbuhl 1980). An improvement in economy confers a lower rate of energy expenditure at a given pace; this prolongs endurance performance through glycogen sparing, reduced heat production, and delayed metabolic acidosis. Economy is a function of the integration of physiological and biomechanical factors, including metabolic efficiency, elasticity of the muscle–tendon unit, and mechanical efficiency; however, the effects of endurance training on economy are unclear (Saunders et al. 2004a).

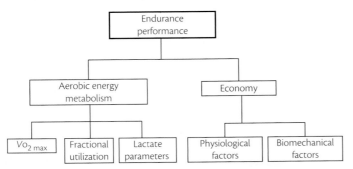

Fig. 1.7.2 Determinants of endurance performance.

Adaptation to high-intensity training

Unlike the adaptations to endurance training that occur at both central and peripheral sites, adaptations to high-intensity training are peripheral, occurring predominantly within the muscle cell. The primary adaptations that result from high-intensity training are increased capacities of the adenosine triphosphate–creatine phosphate (ATP–CP) energy system and the anaerobic glycolytic system (van Someren 2006). An increased capacity of the ATP–CP energy system is manifested through an increase in intramuscular ATP and CP stores, intramuscular free creatine stores, and the concentration and activity of specific enzymes (creatine kinase, myokinase). An increased capacity of the glycolytic system is achieved by increases in glycolytic enzymes (e.g. phosphofructokinase (PFK), phosphorylase) and intracellular and extracellular buffering capacities.

Differences in fibre composition between trained and untrained individuals, and indeed between trained and untrained muscles within individuals, are evidence that long-term training and not heredity alone determine muscle fibre characteristics. Contrasting muscle fibre compositions in athletes of different sports (Gollnick *et al.* 1972) and an increase in the percentage of slow-twitch fibres of up to 36% in response to endurance training (Gollnick *et al.* 1973) have been reported; however, the transition towards a predominance of fast-twitch fibres as a result of high-intensity training is less well documented. Selective muscle fibre hypertrophy is also evident with training. Clarkson *et al.* (1982) identified that although there was no difference in the percentage fibre composition of the biceps brachii and vastus lateralis in sprint kayakers, the fast-twitch fibres in the biceps brachii exhibited hypertrophy and an increase in the percentage of total muscle area (as opposed to number) compared with the vastus lateralis. Therefore both muscle fibre composition and selective fibre hypertrophy are a consequence of specific physical training. Contemporary understanding of skeletal muscle indicates that the categorization of fibres into three discrete types is probably overly simplistic; rather, there is a continuum of fibre types based on a number of biochemical characteristics, all of which exhibit adaptation to exercise training.

High-intensity training has also recently been demonstrated to be a potent stimulus for adaptation in $VO_{2\,max}$ (Billat *et al.* 2000). This is probably due to the perimaximal work intensity and the high rates of oxygen consumption achieved during such training. Therefore it is probable that training designed to develop anaerobic capacity will have some effect on $VO_{2\,max}$, a fact that may be particularly important for athletes participating in middle-distance events in which there is a large anaerobic and aerobic energy contribution, and in which performance has been correlated with both aerobic and anaerobic capacities.

Adaptation to strength and power training

Adaptation to strength and power training can be categorized as myogenic and neurological. The principal myogenic adaptation is hypertrophy, whereby muscle fibres enlarge due to an accretion of contractile and non-contractile muscle tissue. Indeed, a number of studies have shown that maximal force-generating capacity is related to the cross-sectional area of muscle. Evidence suggests that although all muscle fibres undergo hypertrophy in response to strength and power training, it is the type II fibres that demonstrate the more profound response to such a stimulus. There has been much scientific debate as to whether hyperplasia (an increase in the number of muscle fibres) is an adaptation to training in human muscle. Although satellite cell proliferation and myotube formation has been observed *in vitro*, this is generally considered to be part of the tissue repair process specific to the repair of damaged or necrotic fibres rather than evidence of an increase in the number of muscle fibres.

Neurological adaptations are related to the recruitment of motor units. An increase in the number and synchronicity of motor unit recruitment during maximal voluntary contractions is seen in response to training. This provides a greater level of force production, which may be further enhanced by a reduction in the activation of the antagonist muscle.

There is growing evidence that mechanical damage to the muscle cell may be a potent stimulus for hypertrophy. This exercise-induced muscle damage is commonly caused by eccentric exercise in which mechanical disruption to the cell is produced. Indeed, eccentric resistance training has consistently been shown to yield greater levels of hypertrophy than concentric resistance training (e.g. Hortobágyi *et al.* 1996).

For many athletes, particularly those competing in middle-distance events, the need for concurrent development of strength and power together with endurance poses a challenge. For over 25 years it has been known that concurrent training significantly impedes the development of strength and power, yet it does not reduce the adaptation to endurance training (Hickson 1980). Recent work has elucidated the interaction of the molecular responses to resistance and endurance training, thus providing explanation of this phenomenon. The activation of AMPK (AMP-activated protein kinase) in response to endurance training appears to reduce muscle hypertrophy through the inhibition of mTOR (mammalian target of rapamycin), which is activated in response to resistance training (Nader 2006). Current research is examining how nutritional interventions and the timing and periodization of such training can be manipulated so as to maximize adaptation to both resistance and endurance training.

Skeletal adaptation

In addition to the profound effects of physical training on the muscular system, the skeletal system also undergoes adaptation to a training load. Bone tissue demonstrates plasticity to compression, tension, and shear stresses that are routinely experienced during exercise. Increases in bone mineral density (BMD) are promoted particularly by weight-bearing exercise, with athletes typically demonstrating a higher bone density than the non-athletic population.

Despite the positive effects associated with regular exercise for bone health, some highly trained female athletes experience menstrual cycle disturbance that can have negative effects on BMD. Menstrual cycle irregularity is caused by a disruption of hypothalamic function, which is probably precipitated by a negative energy balance (Zanker and Hind 2007). Hypothalamic dysfunction results in reduced secretion of gonadotrophin-releasing hormone (GnRH); this in turn suppresses anterior pituitary secretion of follicle-stimulating hormone (FSH) and luteinizing hormone (LH), which downregulates ovarian function and oestrogen secretion. Given the association with negative energy balance, there is a higher prevalence of menstrual disruption in endurance athletes or those competing in weight-categorized sports and sports where extreme leanness is considered an aesthetic benefit.

Compromised BMD is seen in female athletes with menstrual disruption and is probably a result of both increased bone turnover loss exacerbated by oestrogen suppression and reduced bone formation as a consequence of hypothalamic dysfunction. Consequently, bone fractures are more common in amenorrhoeic athletes, with slower fracture healing rates, than in athletes with normal menstrual function (Carbon *et al.* 2006). Although low BMD can be reversed with the resumption of normal menstrual cycle, it is likely that athletes experiencing amenorrhea during adolescence will never attain optimal BMD since this is the time that peak mineral accretion rates are normally experienced (Nichols *et al.* 2007).

Exercise-induced muscle damage

High-intensity exercise, particularly when incorporating unaccustomed eccentric contractions, can result in temporary muscle damage. This is termed exercise-induced muscle damage (EIMD) and is a short-term training-induced injury that is experienced by many athletes. The adaptive response to such injury demonstrates the high degree of plasticity of skeletal muscle following an imposed training stress.

Eccentric contractions occur when the external force is greater than that being exerted by the muscle and hence lead to the muscle lengthening whilst tension is generated (Armstrong *et al.* 1991), which occurs as a natural consequence of human movement. In addition, the forces that can be generated by eccentric contractions may far exceed the force generated during concentric (shortening) or isometric (stationary) contractions (Woledge *et al.* 1985). For these reasons, athletes often engage in high-intensity exercise that incorporates a large eccentric component in order to overload the neuromuscular system in an attempt to maximize the benefits of training. The EIMD that results from eccentric exercise typically manifests itself as a temporary decrease in force production, joint position sense and reaction time, a rise in passive muscle tension, increased muscular soreness and swelling of the involved muscle group, and an increase of intramuscular proteins such as creatine kinase (CK) found in blood (Fig. 1.7.3).

The magnitude of damage is generally greater in the upper limb than in the lower limb. This is probably due to the lower limb being regularly exposed to prior bouts of eccentric exercise for daily locomotion, such as descending stairs. Conversely, the upper limb is non-weight-bearing and most individuals are unaccustomed to high intensity eccentric loading using this limb.

Mechanisms of exercise-induced muscle damage

Despite substantial research investigating EIMD and the associated soreness, the mechanisms responsible for damage, repair, and adaptation from eccentric muscle actions are not clear. The cause of EIMD and soreness has been previously attributed to metabolic ischaemia or hypoxia, which may occur during prolonged endurance exercise such as marathon running. Although soreness is evident following this type of exercise, earlier work failed to acknowledge the substantial eccentric component involved during running. As a consequence it seems that any ischaemia occurring during running will probably only further exacerbate damage incurred from the eccentric contractions. Metabolic stress and lactic acidosis are unlikely causes of EIMD given the lower metabolic cost and lactate response of eccentric exercise. In addition, lactic acidosis in the muscle and blood lactate return to a state of homeostasis within a relatively short period of time and cannot explain the observed negative effects of reduced force production and soreness for several days following the damaging bout of exercise.

It is likely that EIMD is caused by two inter-related mechanisms: (i) the mechanical strain induced during eccentric contractions results in primary damage to the myofibril; (ii) further cellular disruption associated with the inflammatory response (McHugh 2003). Evidence has demonstrated that eccentric contractions generate more force than other contraction types, but in addition the lengthening of the sarcomeres is non-uniform under eccentric conditions, which results in some myofilaments being stretched and no longer able to overlap within the sarcomere (Proske and Allen 2005). Consequently, when the myofilaments are stretched beyond the overlap, the passive structures assume more tension and undergo what is termed 'popping' (Morgan and Proske 2004), resulting in a visible deformation of the myofibres which is evident immediately after exercise, as shown in Fig. 1.7.4. Muscle soreness does not become apparent until several hours after the bout of exercise and tends to peak around 48 hours later, suggesting that the soreness component is linked with secondary damage and not the initial events of the exercise bout.

The processes that follow the primary phase of damage are initiated by a disruption of the intracellular Ca^{2+} homeostasis. Eccentric exercise leads to a loss of sarcoplasmic reticulum membrane integrity and a disruption in Ca^{2+} homeostasis. The influx of the Ca^{2+} into the cytosol initiates a cascade of events that cause further

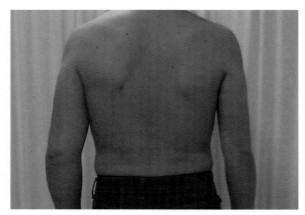

Fig. 1.7.3 Swelling of the left upper arm following damaging exercise.

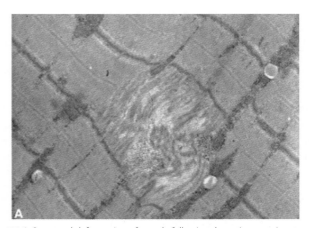

Fig. 1.7.4 Structural deformation of muscle following damaging exercise. Reproduced from Jones *et al* (2004), with permission from Elsevier.

damage to cellular structures (Gissel and Clausen 2001). The Ca^{2+} disruption results in the activation of proteolytic and lipolytic pathways that lead to cell membrane degradation, inflammatory cell infiltration and the subsequent production and activation of reactive oxygen species, fibre necrosis (in extreme cases), and ultimately regeneration of the fibres some days later.

A number of factors may contribute to the magnitude and susceptibility of an individual response to damaging exercise. Evidence shows that fast-twitch fibres are more, though not exclusively, susceptible to damage from eccentric exercise. Faster eccentric contractions may also result in greater damage than slower contractions, which may be the result of reduced cross-bridge formation during higher speeds. Although the damage response can occur from submaximal loads, more damage tends to occur when the exercise is maximal and is carried out at longer muscle lengths or on the descending limb of the length–tension curve as this places greater strain on the passive structure within the sarcomere. Although these factors are important in the magnitude of the damage response, current evidence suggests that eccentric contractions, regardless of the speed, muscle length, or intensity, cause the most damage when the exercise bout is novel or unaccustomed. Furthermore, it has recently been proposed that there is a genetic component that influences the magnitude of the damage response from eccentric exercise (Clarkson *et al.* 2005).

Prevention and treatment of EIMD

Despite the benefits of high-intensity training incorporating eccentric contractions, the resultant EIMD can compromise subsequent training sessions because of residual muscle pain, restriction of movement and reduced capacity to exercise at the required intensity. There are many preventative and therapeutic recovery strategies used to attenuate the negative effects of EIMD, thereby accelerating recovery from training and in theory enabling the athlete to complete the next bout of training sooner and therefore achieve a greater training stimulus. Whilst EIMD is a consequence of a specific and extreme training overload, it serves as an effective model with which to examine the efficacy of strategies employed to reduce training stress and/or promote recovery.

Antioxidant supplementation

The initial events caused by unaccustomed eccentric exercise that result in EIMD elicit an inflammatory response in which phagocytosis and neutrophil respiratory burst result in the production of reactive oxygen species (ROS), thereby imposing an oxidative stress upon the tissue. ROS have been implicated in the secondary damage that follows the initial mechanical disruption, although the exact nature of the relationship between EIMD, muscle soreness, and ROS production is unclear. It has been proposed that dietary antioxidants such as vitamins C and E reduce ROS production and oxidative stress imposed by EIMD.

There is evidence that vitamin C supplementation attenuates symptoms of EIMD and soreness when the supplementation period is for 1–2 weeks prior to the damaging bout of exercise; however, short duration supplementation before or after exercise has little or no protective effect (Howatson and van Someren, 2008). There is less compelling evidence of the protective effects of vitamin E supplementation; in addition, the co-ingestion of vitamins C and E has no benefit over and above that of vitamin C

supplementation alone. Unfortunately, differences in dose, supplementation period, and exercise interventions adopted in previous studies make it difficult to draw definitive conclusions on the efficacy of vitamin C and E supplementation. Tart Montmorency cherry juice is another dietary antioxidant, containing melatonin and anthocyanins that have anti-inflammatory properties. In contrast to vitamins C and E, supplementation for 4 days prior to and 4 days following damaging exercise reduces muscle soreness and attenuates loss of muscle force on subsequent days (Connolly *et al.* 2006). In addition, supplementation for 5 days prior to and for 2 days following a Marathon reduces interlenkin-6 and C-reactive protein (both inflammatory markers) and oxidative stress, and accelerates recovery of muscle function (Howatson *et al.* 2010).

Carbohydrate and protein

Muscle glycogen resynthesis can be impaired following high-intensity eccentric exercise. When eccentric contractions are performed following glycogen-depleting exercise, not only is muscle glycogen diminished following the exercise, but resynthesis is also significantly reduced in the following 48 hours. The lower carbohydrate uptake in the eccentrically exercised muscle may be due to inflammatory cells competing with muscle cells for blood glucose; however, a carbohydrate-rich diet in the days following eccentric exercise can help to increase intramuscular carbohydrate storage (Costill *et al.* 1990). Although a high carbohydrate diet in the days following damaging eccentric contractions may be of benefit in restoring muscle glycogen stores, there is no scientific evidence to suggest that there is any benefit from carbohydrate alone in reducing the negative effects of EIMD.

There has been only limited research examining the role of protein supplementation in preventing or alleviating symptoms of EIMD. Nosaka *et al.* (2006) showed that amino acid supplementation taken before and immediately after damaging exercise does not reduce signs and symptoms of EIMD; however, when extended for several days after the bout, some benefits are seen in reducing soreness, but not in muscle function. Branch chain amino acids have also been examined; however, the efficacy of supplementation in reducing symptoms of EIMD is unclear and further research is required to elucidate the role of protein supplementation in the prevention and treatment of EIMD.

The co-ingestion of protein and carbohydrate, compared with carbohydrate alone, may provide synergistic effects in attenuating muscle damage when ingested during and immediately after repeated exhaustive endurance cycling (Saunders *et al.* 2004b). A carbohydrate and protein cocktail can increase the time to exhaustion and reduce muscle damage from prolonged endurance exercise. Although cycling is not an eccentric-biased activity, there may be applications for athletes engaged in strenuous high-intensity eccentric exercise.

β-Hydroxy-β-methylbutyrate (HMB)

HMB is a downstream metabolite of the branched-chain amino acid leucine and its ketoacid α-ketoisocaproate. HMB has recently gained popularity as a dietary supplement in humans, particularly among strength athletes who may carry out significant volumes of high-intensity eccentric contractions. It has been suggested that it has a prophylactic effect in attenuating muscle protein degradation and reducing EIMD following intense physical training. Although no direct evidence exists as to the exact mechanisms for these effects, HMB has been hypothesized to act as a precursor for cholesterol synthesis via its metabolism, and thus provide a carbon source for cholesterol synthesis, or perhaps to serve as a structural component within the cell membrane. An increase in intracellular cholesterol could enhance cell membrane integrity, particularly the sarcolemma and sarcoplasmic reticulum, which may help to maintain Ca^{2+} homeostasis and reduce the efflux of intramuscular proteins following unaccustomed or intense exercise.

HMB supplementation taken during short training periods of 3–8 weeks reduces muscle protein degradation and increases muscle mass and strength in recreational exercisers; however, the effects may be less profound in well-trained athletes. To date, only limited data are available examining the effects of HMB supplementation on muscle damage resulting from a single bout of eccentric resistance exercise. Short-term supplementation prior to damaging exercise is of limited value, but longer-duration supplementation (~ 14 days) reduces the decrement in muscle force production (van Someren et al. 2005). However, these findings are limited to relatively untrained individuals and it is unknown what response may occur in highly trained athletes.

Non-steroidal anti-inflammatory drugs (NSAIDs)

NSAIDs (e.g. ibuprofen, aspirin, naproxen, diclofenac, flurbiprofen, and ketoprofen) are perhaps the most widely known therapy in the treatment of inflammatory related pathologies which include EIMD and muscle soreness. NSAIDs inhibit the synthesis of prostaglandin, a mediator of the inflammation process and pain during acute inflammation, by inhibiting the metabolism of arachidonic acid via the cyclo-oxygenase (COX-1 and COX-2) pathway. The administration of NSAIDs as a preventative and/or therapeutic intervention has been extensively reviewed (Baldwin-Lanier 2003). Prophylactic administration of over-the-counter doses of NSAIDs has been shown on a number of occasions to significantly reduce soreness and, in some cases, to reduce the appearance of CK in blood and enhance the recovery of muscle function following maximal eccentric exercise.

The performance benefits of NSAID administration are less clear. Tokmakidis et al. (2003) administered 400 mg of ibuprofen every 8 hours for 48 hours following eccentric exercise; although there was less muscle soreness and CK on the day after the exercise bout, there was no effect on maximum strength, vertical jump performance, or range of motion. Donnelly et al. (1990) reported that doses of 1200 mg ibuprofen administered prior to downhill running for 45 minutes, together with a further 600 mg every 6 hours for 72 hours post-exercise, had no effect on muscle soreness or strength. Peterson et al. (2003) used over-the-counter maximum doses of ibuprofen (1200 mg/day) and acetaminophen (4000 mg/day) following damaging exercise with no effect on the inflammatory response 24 hours post-exercise.

Evidence is currently equivocal for the use of NSAIDs in the prevention and/or reduction of the signs and symptoms associated with EIMD. The use of higher doses of NSAIDs in future research has been advocated by some (Sayers et al. 2001), although caution should be exercised as the habitual or chronic use of NSAIDs may produce adverse effects causing further medical complications. Furthermore, inflammation is the body's natural response to EIMD, and the use of pharmacological agents may inhibit protein synthesis, thus attenuating the damage–repair–adaptation cycle of skeletal muscle following eccentric exercise. Tissue protein synthesis following high-intensity eccentric exercise is inhibited by the administration of over-the-counter doses of ibuprofen and acetaminophen (Trappe et al. 2002). Indeed, inhibited muscle regeneration and hypertrophy following NSAID administration has been demonstrated in animal models (Soltow et al. 2006). Given that the effects of NSAIDs on EIMD are equivocal, the lack of performance benefits, and the potential negative long-term consequences of administration, their use as an effective strategy to prevent or treat symptoms of EIMD is not recommended.

Stretching

Stretching is proposed to decrease the passive and/or active stiffness of skeletal muscle, making it more compliant to eccentric contractions and thereby reducing the amount of primary mechanical damage. Pre-exercise stretching may provide a possible intervention to attenuate the magnitude of muscle damage, though a brief meta-analysis of five studies (Herbert and Gabriel 2002) found that stretching reduced soreness in the days following exercise by approximately 2% and suggested that this effect was too small to be worthwhile. However, other work has shown that passive stretching performed prior to damaging eccentric contractions reduces the inflammatory response, presumably because of a reduced primary damage to the myofibril (Pizza et al. 2002).

In contrast, static stretching performed prior to eccentric exercise seems less beneficial and has little or no effect on muscle soreness, maximal force, or the CK response; however, these observations are restricted to female patients. Therefore it is possible that gender may account for these findings as oestrogen may provide protection against damage in skeletal muscle, and consequently females might respond to damaging exercise in a different manner to males, depending upon menstrual cycle phase (Kendall and Eston 2002).

Current literature reporting the efficacy of stretching to prevent or reduce EIMD suggests only minimal effects in reducing muscle soreness and no meaningful effect on performance. However, other stretching protocols, such as proprioceptive neuromuscular facilitation (PNF) and ballistic or dynamic stretching techniques may be of benefit, and present a direction for future research.

Massage

Massage is a widely used therapy in the treatment of athletic muscle soreness and micro-injury and many athletes are convinced by its potential to alleviate muscle soreness. The exact mechanisms by which massage might be effective are not clear; however, there is some support for its use in the treatment of exercise-induced muscle soreness. Massage techniques such as petrissage, effleurage, and tapotement delivered in the hours following damaging eccentric exercise reduce muscle soreness and the appearance of CK in blood, probably because of reduced neutrophil accumulation, prostaglandin production, and consequent pain. However, the effects of massage on muscle function are less convincing, with very little evidence of attenuated decrements in muscle strength or accelerated recovery from damaging exercise. This may be due in part to a number of methodological limitations in the literature (e.g. inadequate therapist training, different massage techniques used, insufficient duration of treatment, and inconsistent treatment between subjects) that have been highlighted in a previous review of sports massage (Moraska 2005).

Electrotherapeutic modalities

Electrical modalities are commonly used in the treatment of injury and the rehabilitation of a range of musculoskeletal problems;

however, the use of electrical therapies to reduce symptoms associated with muscle damage has not been extensively examined.

Transcutaneous electrical nerve stimulation (TENS) has been used for the management of muscle soreness and inflammation. Any effects of TENS are proposed to be attributed to the 'pain gate control theory' (Melzack and Wall 1965), which suggests that presynaptic pain fibres are inhibited by stimulation of large sensory fibres in the muscle. Indeed, muscle soreness is reduced by the application of TENS when administered in the days following the damaging bout of exercise; however, there is no evidence that the force-generating capacity of muscle recovers faster with the use of TENS.

Microcurrent electrical neuromuscular stimulation, which has a similar hypothetical basis to TENS, appears to have no effect on muscle function, soreness, or muscle stiffness when applied at any time in the first 72 hours following a damaging bout of exercise. In contrast, electromembrane microcurrent therapy significantly attenuates the increase in CK and the decrease in muscle stiffness and muscle strength at 24 hours, although, perhaps surprisingly, it has no effect on muscle soreness. The mechanisms for these observations are not fully understood, although it is hypothesized that the disturbances in Ca^{2+} homeostasis that are a consequence of damaging eccentric exercise may be reduced by such treatments (Lambert et al. 2002).

Another electrotherapeutic modality that may assist in treating EIMD is high-voltage pulsed current (HVPC), which is applied via a short-duration pulse monophasic waveform directly through electrodes applied to the skin surface. Although HVPC has been demonstrated to alleviate muscle soreness in animal models, probably because of a reduction in oedema formation, there is not yet evidence that it is of benefit to humans in reducing soreness or returning muscle function at an accelerated rate.

Ultrasound converts electrical energy into sound waves that penetrate the skin surface. It is a commonly used therapeutic modality and is proposed to increase circulation, accelerate metabolism, and control the sensation of pain. Muscle soreness is reduced when ultrasound treatment is applied for 20 minutes 24 hours following damaging exercise. When ultrasound therapy is delivered in conjunction with a topically administered anti-inflammatory cream there may be greater benefits in reducing soreness when compared with ultrasound alone (Ciccone et al. 1991). It is proposed that the combined treatment allowed for an increase in blood flow to the damaged tissue whilst simultaneously reducing the inflammatory response, oedema, and hence secondary damage. Despite ultrasound being routinely used in clinical environments, many of the benefits are based on anecdote and the empirical evidence to support its effects and the mechanisms by which it may benefit are scarce.

Electrical therapies show some promise in the treatment of EIMD, particularly for the management of pain; however, there are a number of potential issues when using these instruments. Electrical media often require specialist training to administer and the equipment itself can be expensive. There are currently no evidence-based guidelines on the dose and frequency of application concerning electrical therapies, making it somewhat difficult to determine the appropriate treatment strategy. It has been suggested that the prescription of ultrasound treatment strategies is based on guesswork (Robertson 2002); at present, this also applies to other electrical modalities. Therefore there is a need to elucidate the efficacy of electrical therapies using standardized guidelines based on documented evidence. However, given that these therapies target

isolated muscles, the application of such findings may be of limited value in an athletic environment in which individuals rarely experience such isolated muscle damage and soreness.

Cryotherapy

Cryotherapy is the application of cold for therapeutic purposes. It is usually applied during the acute stage of trauma and is proposed to diminish the undesirable effects of soft tissue injury by reducing the inflammatory response, swelling, oedema, haematoma, and pain. The therapeutic effects are proposed to be a consequence of analgesia of the injured tissue, hypometabolism of the tissue (thereby reducing the negative effects of any inflammatory induced tissue hypoxia), and a vascular response whereby blood flow and haematoma formation is retarded. The most commonly used methods of cryotherapy include ice application, ice massage, and cold water immersions.

Single treatments of ice massage have only limited effect in the treatment of muscle damage and soreness, regardless of when in the first 72 hours post-exercise they are administered. There is generally an immediate reduction in soreness which is probably due to the analgesic effects of the cold; however, this is transient and lasts only for a short period following the treatment. More importantly, this reduced soreness is mirrored by a reduction in the force-generating capacity of muscle; hence single treatments of ice massage may be contraindicated in the management of EIMD. Repeated applications of ice massage following eccentric exercise has been shown to be equivocal, with evidence of attenuated CK efflux at 72 hours post-exercise but with effect on muscle soreness or function (Howatson and van Someren 2003; Howatson et al. 2005).

Cold water immersion is another form of cryotherapy that has become popular among athletes, although the evidence to support its use is relatively weak. Paddon-Jones and Quigley (1997) found no effects on signs and symptoms of EIMD using a protocol of 20 minutes of cold water immersions ($5 \pm 1°C$), separated by 60 minutes and repeated five times following eccentric exercise. However, it is possible that such an aggressive approach may have elicited the Hunting reaction, which is brought about when tissue temperature falls below ~18°C and there is periodic vasodilation and rewarming of the tissue, which may eliminate any potential benefits of cryotherapy. A less aggressive treatment regimen involving immersion in water at 15°C for 15 minutes every 12 hours for 3 days following eccentric exercise resulted in significantly less muscle stiffness and lower CK levels in blood, but with no effects on muscle soreness or strength (Eston and Peters 1999). A recent study has examined the practice of intermittent ice-water immersion, which is perhaps an extreme form of cold water immersion (Sellwood et al. 2007). Immersion in ice-water (5°C), repeated three times and interspersed with 1 minute periods out of the water, resulted in no changes in CK, muscle function, or swelling, but increased muscle soreness. Similarly no effect was found when cold water immersions repeated every 24 hours were used for a longer duration (12 minutes with more temperate water (12°C) following damaging plyometric exercise (Howatson et al. 2009). However, cold water immersion has had some success in facilitating recovery during repeated days of fatiguing cycling (Vaile et al. 2008).

Cryotherapy appears an attractive strategy to combat the signs and symptoms of EIMD because it offers a quick, simple, and, if required, whole-body intervention. Experimental support for cryotherapy suffers the same limitations as electrotherapies in that there are no evidence-based guidelines for the appropriate frequency, duration, and temperature of these interventions. Indeed, there are many anecdotal reports of the widespread use of part- or whole-body cold water immersion following competition and training by athletes in an attempt to enhance recovery. In contrast, however, the empirical evidence regarding the physiological benefits of cryotherapy on muscle function and soreness are equivocal.

Exercise

Many physical therapists prescribe light exercise in the presence of muscle soreness; however the appropriate mode, intensity, and duration are not known. Exercise may be one of the most effective strategies to temporarily alleviate muscle soreness, although the analgesic effect is only temporary and pain tends to resume soon after the exercise has stopped. Exercise is purported to increased blood flow, removed noxious waste products, and increase endorphin release, thereby causing an analgesic effect. However, the research-based evidence pertaining to the efficacy of exercise as a treatment in attenuating symptoms of EIMD remains equivocal.

Most athletes precede training or competition with a period of exercise performed as a warm-up to prepare for the demands of the bout and possibly to reduce the risk of injury. However, in the case of exercise-induced muscle damage, there is little evidence to support this practice to reduce the incidence and symptoms of EIMD. A comparative examination of active warm-up (i.e. exercise) and passive warm-up (i.e. using pulsed short-wave diathermy) showed that neither method has any beneficial effect on creatine kinase activity, swelling, muscle function, or soreness (Evans *et al.* 2002). Exercise is sometimes prescribed therapeutically following damaging exercise. Although there is some evidence that this reduces soreness, this is by no means unequivocal.

Repeated bout effect

The signs and symptoms of EIMD following eccentric exercise can be greatly attenuated following a second bout of a similar magnitude. This protection or adaptation is commonly referred to as the repeated bout effect (RBE) and has been demonstrated using the lower and upper limbs. The RBE not only provides protection that occurs within a few days, but the benefits may last for several months following the initial bout.

Several theories have been mooted as potential mechanisms for the RBE; these include mechanical, cellular, neural, and enhanced excitation–contraction (E–C) coupling as well as a growing body of evidence of an altered inflammatory response and/or change in reactive oxidative species during and after the repeated bout. It is likely that all these theories identify mechanisms for the RBE and have been reviewed in detail previously (McHugh 2003).

Early investigations have clearly demonstrated the RBE by showing an attenuation of indirect damage indices such as muscle soreness, blood CK, and muscle function following the repeated bout using upper and lower limb models. In addition, direct evidence for the RBE has also been demonstrated (Hortobágyi *et al.* 1998); biopsy revealed reduced focal damage to the myofibrils in two-thirds of subjects on the second day following the repeated bout and all subjects showed minimal soreness, CK elevation, and decrement in muscle function. More recent investigations support earlier work concerning the RBE and demonstrate compelling and conclusive evidence of an attenuation of the signs and symptoms of EIMD following a repeated bout of eccentric exercise.

When eccentrically biased exercise is performed before the signs and symptoms of EIMD resulting from a prior bout of exercise have subsided, the extent of muscle damage is not exacerbated further (Nosaka *et al.* 2002a). However, this does not indicate a RBE being manifested immediately post-exercise; rather it suggests that the focal damage to the stress-susceptible fibres during the initial bout reduces the potential for further damage to these fibres during the repeated bouts. In addition, the ability to generate force during subsequent bouts is greatly inhibited, almost certainly as a result of the damage inflicted from the initial bout, and therefore the force generated during subsequent bouts may be insufficient to precipitate further damage.

In the context of athletic training, if the skeletal muscle has residual damage from eccentric contractions, further insults of exercise are unlikely to incur further detriments in performance or inhibit the recovery process. However, if the purpose of further exercise bouts (prior to full recovery) is to elicit training-induced adaptations, the exercise stimulus from the repeated bout might be insufficient to achieve this. In addition, the capacity for the muscle to generate force is greatly reduced and may put unnecessary strain on other passive structures which could potentially lead to injury.

Interestingly, the RBE may be manifested by an initial bout that causes only minimal damage and soreness, with a low volume bout of eccentric exercise providing protection against damage in a subsequent high-volume bout of eccentric exercise (Howatson *et al.* 2007). However, the magnitude of the RBE following a low-volume initial bout is less profound than that elicited by a high-volume initial bout (Howatson *et al.* 2007), suggesting that the level of protection conferred is at least in part proportional to the initial training load imposed and the resultant damage.

Exercise intensity is another factor that determines the RBE. It is well established that lower levels of muscle damage result from submaximal bouts of eccentric exercise when compared with maximal eccentric exercise and the implications of this on the RBE has been examined. Eight weeks of submaximal (50% voluntary isometric maximum) concentric or eccentric training has been shown to provide no protection against muscle damage during subsequent maximal eccentric exercise carried out at the end of the training period (Nosaka and Newton 2002b). Therefore, although the initial bout of exercise need only cause modest muscle damage to induce the RBE, this exercise must be of maximal intensity to confer protection for subsequent maximal exercise. This finding is another practical illustration of the training principle of specificity.

The length of muscle during the initial bout of exercise may also affect the RBE. Eccentric muscle actions carried out at shorter muscle lengths (i.e. on the ascending limb of the length–tension curve) provide little or no protection against a subsequent bout at longer muscle lengths. This is probably attributable to little or no damage occurring from the initial bout carried out at shorter muscle lengths, because of a substantial overlap within the sarcomeres, and hence active tension can be generated by contractile elements within the myofilaments. As a consequence there is less mechanical stress and therefore a reduced stimulus for adaptation imposed on the structures responsible for passive tension, which is required to maintain myofibrillar integrity at longer muscle lengths. Therefore it is important for athletes to conduct muscle contractions over the entire anatomical range to maximize the full potential of the RBE from the initial bout. The adaptation to damaging exercise has been reported to last several months (Nosaka *et al.* 2005) although, anecdotally, many strength and conditioning coaches and clinicians engaged in rehabilitation and preventative interventions report that athletes tend to suffer from muscular soreness and reduced function after far shorter lay-off periods between bouts.

The adaptive RBE response to a single bout of eccentric exercise is probably the only intervention that has consistently shown a positive prophylactic effect in attenuating EIMD. A number of factors should be considered when conducting potentially damaging exercise, particularly when the exerciser is expected to complete further bouts of eccentric-biased exercise. If the exercise bout is unaccustomed, it is prudent to commence with a low-volume high-intensity bout so as to both reduce the initial damaging effects and therefore reduce the impact on subsequent training bouts, and to confer a RBE against subsequent high-volume bouts performed in future training sessions.

Recovery from training

It should be recognized that exercise-induced muscle damage is an extreme response to physical training, and whilst athletes may experience signs and symptoms associated with muscle damage when they commence high-intensity training or modify their training programme, this is probably not a regular occurrence. In contrast, the fatigue and decrement in performance capacity that results from any training bout is frequently experienced by athletes. Many of the recovery strategies discussed above are also used on an ongoing basis in an attempt to promote recovery from all types of training. Whilst the use of some of these strategies is based on sound evidence, many are based only on anecdotal reports.

Among the most popular strategies employed by athletes on a regular basis are contrast bathing and the wearing of compression garments. Contrast bathing involves the repeated and alternate immersion in hot and cold water and is proposed to reduce inflammation and accelerate the removal of metabolic by-products. The use of compression garments has become very popular, particularly in team sport players, with garments being worn during and/or following exercise. Compression garments are proposed to reduce oedema and increase the clearance of metabolic by-products; however, there has been limited research to support of refute this. These and other recovery strategies used to promote recovery from training have recently been reviewed (Barnett 2006).

Recovery strategies and training adaptation

A mechanism by which many of the popular recovery strategies are proposed to be effective is the reduction of inflammation following a severe bout of training. Whilst it is widely believed that the management of this inflammatory response following exercise is beneficial, the important biological functions of inflammatory cells must not be ignored. Neutrophils have been implicated in the exacerbation of muscle damage, in part through the oxidative stress caused by phagocytosis; however, they play an essential role in the function of macrophages and the repair and regeneration of injured tissue (Butterfield *et al.* 2006).

The management of training-induced fatigue and injury so as to promote both recovery and adaptation is as yet an inexact science. There is recent but limited evidence that the use of recovery strategies may in fact interfere with the supercompensation cycle and attenuate adaptation to a training stimulus. Yamane *et al.* (2006)

demonstrated that when cold water immersion was adopted following endurance or resistance training sessions during a 4–6-week programme the adaptation to the training stimulus was blunted. In contrast, Howatson *et al.* (2009) reported the repeated bout effect to be unaffected by a cold water immersion recovery strategy following plyometric exercise, demonstrating that cold water immersion does not attenuate the rapid and profound adaptation to a single bout of damaging exercise. The work of Yamane and colleagues does however question the use of such a strategy to promote recovery from normal physical training, though more extensive research is required to elucidate both the acute and chronic effects of recovery strategies.

Summary

Athletic training programmes are based on well-established principles that have been developed and validated by empirical evidence and scientific enquiry. An understanding of the physiological determinants of performance in sports events informs the prescription and planning of training to achieve specific adaptations. Gains in performance are underpinned by structural and functional adaptation of physiological systems, which in turn are manifested by molecular responses to a given training load. The stress–response relationship of training stimulus and adaptation is specific to the type and load of the training performed and to the individual. One of the most profound examples of the stress–response relationship can be seen in exercise-induced muscle damage and the RBE, which demonstrate both the sometimes negative acute effects of unaccustomed high-intensity exercise and the adaptability of skeletal muscle to a training stimulus. The use of strategies to promote recovery and adaptation to training is widespread; however, the evidence base to support the use of many such strategies is limited at present.

References

Armstrong, R.B., Warren, G.L. and Warren, J.A. (1991). Mechanisms of exercise-induced muscle fibre injury. *Sports Medicine*, **12**, 184–207.

Baldwin-Lanier, A. (2003). Use of anti-inflammatory drugs following exercise-induced muscle injury. *Sports Medicine*, **33**, 177–85.

Barnett, A. (2006). Using recovery modalities between training sessions in elite athletes: does it help? *Sports Medicine*, **36**, 781–96.

Bassett, D.R. and Howley, E.T. (1997). Maximum oxygen uptake: 'classical' versus 'contemporary' viewpoints. *Medicine and Science in Sports and Exercise*, **29**, 591–603.

Bassett, D.R. and Howley, E.T. (2000). Limiting factors for maximum oxygen uptake and determinants of endurance performance. *Medicine and Science in Sports and Exercise*, **32**, 70–84.

Billat, V.L., Slawinski, J., Bocquet, V., *et al.* (2000). Intermittent runs at the velocity associated with maximal oxygen uptake enables subjects to remain at maximal oxygen uptake for a longer time than intense but submaximal runs. *European Journal of Applied Physiology*, **81**, 188–96.

Bishop, D., Jenkins, D.G., and MacKinnon, L.T. (1998). The relationship between plasma lactate parameters, Wpeak and 1-h cycling performance in women. *Medicine and Science in Sports and Exercise*, **30**, 1270–5.

Bouchard, C., Dionne, F.T., Simoneau, J.A., and Boulay, M.R. (1992). Genetics of aerobic and anaerobic performances. *Exercise and Sport Science Reviews*, **20**, 27–58.

Budgett, R., Newsholme, E., Lehmann, M., *et al.* (2000). Redefining the overtraining syndrome as the unexplained underperformance syndrome. *British Journal of Sports Medicine*, **34**, 67–8.

Butterfield, T.A., Best, T.M., and Merrick, M.A. (2006). The dual roles of neutrophils and macrophages in inflammation: a critical balance between tissue damage and repair. *Journal of Athletic Training*, **41**, 457–65.

Carbon, R.J., Whyte, G., Budgett. R., and McConnell, A.L. (2006). Medical conditions and training. In: G. Whyte (ed.), *The Physiology of Training*, pp. 191–228. Churchill Livingstone, Edinburgh.

Ciccone, C.D., Leggin, B.G., and Callamaro, J.J. (1991). Effects of ultrasound and trolamine salicylate phonophoresis on delayed-onset muscle soreness. *Physical Therapy*, **71**, 666–75.

Clarkson, P.M., Kroll, W., and Melchionda, A.M. (1982). Isokinetic strength, endurance, and fiber type composition in elite American paddlers. *European Journal of Applied Physiology*, **48**, 67–76.

Clarkson, P.M., Hoffman, E.P., Zambraski, E., *et al.* (2005). ACTN3 and MLCK genotype associations with exertional muscle damage. *Journal of Applied Physiology*, **99**, 564–9.

Coffey, V.G. and Hawley, J.A. (2007). The molecular bases of training adaptation. *Sports Medicine*, **37**, 737–63.

Conley, D.L. and Krahenbuhl, G. (1980). Running economy and distance running performance of highly trained athletes. *Medicine and Science in Sports and Exercise*, **12**, 357–60.

Connolly, D.A.J., McHugh, M.P., and Padilla-Zakour, O.I. (2006). Efficacy of a tart cherry juice blend in preventing the symptoms of muscle damage. *British Journal of Sports Medicine*, **40**, 679–83.

Costill, D.L., Thomason, H., and Roberts, E. (1973). Fractional utilization of the aerobic capacity during distance running. *Medicine and Science in Sports and Exercise*, **5**, 248–52.

Costill, D.L., Pascoe, D.D., Fink, J.W., Robergs, R.A., Barr, S.I. and Pearson, D. (1990). Impaired muscle glycogen after eccentric exercise. *Journal of Applied Physiology*, **69**, 46–50.

Donnelly, A.W., Maughan, R.J., and Whiting, P.H. (1990). Effects of ibuprofen on exercise-induced muscle soreness and indices of muscle damage. *British Journal of Sports Medicine*, **24**, 191–5.

Eston, R. and Peters, D. (1999). Effects of cold water immersion on the symptoms of exercise-induced muscle injury. *Journal of Sports Sciences*, **17**, 231–8.

Evans, R.K., Knight, K.L., Draper, D.O., and Parcell, A.C. (2002). Effects of warm-up before eccentric exercise on indirect markers of muscle damage. *Medicine and Science in Sports and Exercise*, **34**, 1892–9.

Gissel, H. and Clausen, T. (2001). Excitation-induced Ca^{2+} influx and skeletal muscle cell damage. *Acta Physiologica Scandinavica*, **171**, 327–34.

Gollnick, P.D., Armstrong, R.B., Saubert, C.W., Piehl, K., and Saltin, B. (1972). Enzyme activity and fiber composition in skeletal muscle of untrained and trained men. *Journal of Applied Physiology*, **33**, 312–19.

Gollnick, P.D., Armstrong, R.B., Saltin, B., Saubert, C.W., Sembrowich, W.L., and Shepherd, R.E. (1973). Effect of training on enzyme activity and fiber composition of human skeletal muscle. *Journal of Applied Physiology*, **34**, 107–11.

Herbert, R. and Gabriel, M. (2002). Effects of stretching before and after exercising on muscle soreness and risk of injury: systematic review. *British Journal of Sports Medicine*, **325**, 1–5.

Hickson, R.C. (1980). Interference of strength development by simultaneously training for strength and endurance. *European Journal of Applied Physiology and Occupational Physiology*, **45**, 255–63.

Hortobágyi, T., Hill, J.P., Houmard, J.A., Fraser, D.D., Lambert, N.J., and Israel, R.G. (1996). Adaptive responses to muscle lengthening and shortening in humans. *Journal of Applied Physiology*, **80**, 765–72.

Hortobágyi, T., Houmard, J., Fraser, D., Dudek, R., Lambert, J., and Tracy, J. (1998). Normal forces and myofibrillar disruption after repeated eccentric exercise. *Journal of Applied Physiology*, **84**, 492–8.

Howatson, G. and van Someren, K.A. (2003). Ice massage: effects on exercise-induced muscle damage. *Journal of Sports Medicine and Physical Fitness*, **43**, 500–5.

Howatson, G. and van Someren, K.A., (2008). The prevention and treatment of exercise-induced muscle damage. *Sport Medicine*, **38**, 1–21.

Howatson, G., Gaze, D., and van Someren, K.A. (2005). The efficacy of ice massage in the treatment of exercise-induced muscle damage. *Scandinavian Journal of Medicine and Science in Sports*, **15**, 416–22.

Howatson, G., Goodall, S., and van Someren, K.A. (2009). The influence of cold water immersions on adaptation following a single bout of damaging exercise. *European Journal of Applied Physiology*, **105**, 615–211.

Howatson, G., McHugh, M.P., Hill, J., Brouner, J., Jewell, A., van Someren, K.A., and Shave, R. Howatson, S.A. (2010). The effects of a tart cherry juice supplement on muscle damage, inflammation, oxidative stress and recovery following Marathon running. *Scandinavian Journal of Medicine and Science in Sports*, DOI: 10.1111/j. 1600-0838.2009.01005.x).

Howatson, G., van Someren, K.A., and Hortobágyi, T. (2007). The repeated bout effect after maximal eccentric exercise. *International Journal of Sports Medicine*, **28**, 557–63.

Ingham, S.A., Whyte, G.P., Jones, K., and Nevill, A.M. (2002). Determinants of 2,000 m rowing ergometer performance in elite rowers. *European Journal of Applied Physiology*, **88**, 243–6.

Jones, D.A., Round, J., and dettaan, A., (2004). **Skeletal Muscle-From Molecules to Movement. ATextbook of Muscle Physiology for Sport, Exercise and Physiotherapy and medicine.** Churchill Livingstone: London, UK.

Kendall, B. and Eston, R. (2002). Exercise-induced muscle damage and the protective role of estrogen. *Sports Medicine*, **32**, 103–23.

Lambert, M.I., Marcus, P., Burgess, T., and Noakes, T.D. (2002). Electro-membrane microcurrent therapy reduces signs and symptoms of muscle damage. *Medicine and Science in Sports and Exercise*, **34**, 602–7.

McHugh, M. P. (2003). Recent advances in the understanding of the repeated bout effect against muscle damage from a single bout of eccentric exercise. *Scandinavian Journal of Medicine and Science in Sports*, **13**, 88–97.

Melzack, R. and Wall, P.D. (1965). Pain mechanisms: a new theory. *Science*, **19**, 971–9.

Midgley, A.W., McNaughton, L.R., and Wilkinson, M. (2006). Is there an optimal training intensity for enhancing the maximal oxygen uptake of distance runners? Empirical research findings, current opinions, physiological rationale and practical recommendations. *Sports Medicine*, **36**, 117–32.

Midgley, A.W., McNaughton, L.R., and Jones, A.M. (2007). Training to enhance the physiological determinants of long-distance running performance. Can valid recommendations be given to runners and coaches based on current scientific knowledge? *Sports Medicine*, **37**, 857–80.

Moraska, A. (2005). Sports massage. A comprehensive review. *Journal of Sports Medicine and Physical Fitness*, **45**, 370–80.

Morgan, D.L. and Proske, U. (2004). Popping sacromere hypothesis explains stretch-induced muscle damage. *Clinical and Experimental Pharmacology and Physiology*, **31**, 541–5.

Mujika, I., Padilla, S., Pyne, D., and Busso, T. (2004). Physiological changes associated with the pre-event taper in athletes. *Sports Medicine*, **34**, 891–927.

Nader, G.A. (2006). Concurrent strength and endurance training: from molecules to man. *Medicine and Science in Sports and Exercise*, **38**, 1965–70.

Nichols, D.L., Sanborn, C.F., and Essery, E.V. (2007). Bone density and young athletic women. An update. *Sports Medicine*, **37**, 1001–14.

Nicholson, R.M. and Sleivert, G.G. (2001). Indices of lactate threshold and their relationship with 10-km running performance. *Medicine and Science in Sports and Exercise*, **33**, 339–42.

Nosaka, K. and Newton, M. (2002a). Repeated eccentric exercise bouts do not exacerbate muscle damage and repair. *Journal of Strength and Conditioning Research*, **16**, 117–22.

Nosaka, K. and Newton, M. (2002b). Concentric or eccentric training effect on eccentric exercise-induced muscle damage. *Medicine and Science in Sports and Exercise*, **34**, 63–9.

Nosaka, K., Newton, M.J. and Sacco, P. (2005). Attenuation of protective effect against eccentric exercise-induced muscle damage. *Canadian Journal of Applied Physiology*, **30**, 529–42.

Nosaka, K., Sacco, P., and Mawatari, K. (2006). Effects of amino acid supplementation on muscle soreness and damage. *International Journal of Sport Nutrition and Exercise Metabolism*, **16**, 620–35.

Paddon-Jones, D.J. and Quigley, B.M. (1997). Effects of cryotherapy on muscle soreness and strength following eccentric exercise. *International Journal of Sports Medicine*, **18**, 588–93.

Peterson, J.M., Trappe, T.A., Mylona, E., *et al.* (2003). Ibuprofen and acetaminophen: effects on muscle inflammation after eccentric exercise. *Medicine and Science in Sports and Exercise*, **35**, 892–6.

Pizza, F.X., Koh, T.J., McGregor, S.J., and Brooks, S.V. (2002). Muscle inflammatory cells after passive stretches, isometric contractions, and lengthening contractions. *Journal of Applied Physiology*, **92**, 1873–8.

Proske, U. and Allen, T.J. (2005). Damage to skeletal muscle from eccentric exercise. *Exercise and Sport Sciences Reviews*, **33**, 98–104.

Robertson, V.J. (2002). Dosage and treatment response in randomized clinical trials of therapeutic ultrasound. *Physical Therapy in Sport*, **3**, 124–33.

Saunders, M.J., Kane, M.D., and Todd, K. (2004a). Effects of a carbohydrate–protein beverage on cycling endurance and muscle damage. *Medicine and Science in Sports and Exercise*, **36**, 1233–8.

Saunders, P.U., Pyne, D.B., Telford, R.D., and Hawley, J.A. (2004). Factors affecting running economy in trained distance runners. *Sports Medicine*, **34**, 465–85.

Sayers, S.P., Knight, C.A., Clarkson, P.M., van Wegan, E.H., and Kamen, G. (2001). Effect of ketoprofen on muscle function and sEMG activity after eccentric exercise. *Medicine and Science in Sports and Exercise*, **33**, 702–10.

Sellwood, K.L., Brukner, P., Williams, D., Nichol, A., and Hinman, R. (2007). Ice-water immersion and delayed-onset muscle soreness: a randomised controlled trial. *British Journal of Sports Medicine*, **41**, 392–7.

Selye, H. (1956). *The Stress of Life*. McGraw-Hill, New York

Soltow, Q.A., Betters, J.L., Sellman, J.E., Lira, V.A, Long, J.H., and Criswell, D.S. (2006). Ibuprofen inhibits skeletal muscle hypertrophy in rats. *Medicine and Science in Sports and Exercise*, **38**, 840–6.

Tokmakidis, S.P., Kokkinidis, E.A., Smilios, I., and Douda, H. (2003). The effects of ibuprofen on delayed muscle soreness and muscular performance after eccentric exercise. *Journal of Strength and Conditioning Research*, **17**, 53–9.

Trappe, T.A., White, F., Lambert, C.P., Cesar, D., Hellerstein, M., and Evans, W.J. (2002). Effect of ibuprofen and acetaminophen on postexercise muscle protein synthesis. *American Journal of Physiology, Endocrinology and Metabolism*, **282**, E551–6.

Vaile, J., Halson, S., Gill, N., and Dawson, B. (2008). Effect of Hydrotherapy on Recovery from Fatigue. *International Journal of Sports Medicine*, **29**, 539–44.

van Someren, K.A. (2006). The physiology of anaerobic endurance training. In: G. Whyte (ed.), *The Physiology of Training*, pp. 85–115. Churchill Livingstone, Edinburgh.

van Someren, K.A., Edwards, A.J., and Howatson, G. (2005). Supplementation with β-hydroxy-β-methylbutyrate (HMB) and α-ketoisocaproic acid (KIC) reduces signs and symptoms of exercise-induced muscle damage in man. *International Journal of Sport Nutrition and Exercise Metabolism*, **15**, 413–24.

Woledge, R.C., Cutin, N.A., and Homsher, E. (1985). Energetic aspects of muscle contraction. *Monographs of the Physiological Society*, **41**, 1–357.

Yamane, M., Teruya, H., Nakano, M., Ogai, R., Ohnishi, N., and Kosaka, M. (2006). Post-exercise leg and forearm flexor muscle cooling in humans attenuates endurance and resistance training effects on muscle performance and on circulatory adaptation. *European Journal of Applied Physiology*, **96**, 572–80.

Zanker, C. and Hind, K. (2007). The effect of energy balance on endocrine function and bone health in youth. *Medicine and Sport Science*, **51**, 81–101.

Principles of biomechanics and their use in the analysis of injuries and technique

Sharon Dixon

Introduction

Biomechanics, defined literally, is the mechanics of living systems. Human biomechanics involves the study of mechanical aspects of human movement. It is the science studying the internal and external forces experienced by the human and the effects of such forces. Nigg and Herzog (2007) highlight that forces may result in movement of body segments, deformation of biological materials, or biological changes in the tissue(s) on which they act. Thus biomechanics can involve the study of human movement and factors that affect this movement, deformation of biological structures and factors that influence this, and the biological effects of locally acting forces on living tissue (e.g. effects on growth development or injuries).

This chapter introduces the concepts of biomechanics and describes the tools used in biomechanics to measure aspects such as force and movement. Basic biomechanics of common activities are included, with a specific focus on running. Finally, a case study of a runner is used to highlight the possible application of biomechanical methods in a clinical setting. Since methods for measuring deformation of biological structures and for studying the effects of forces acting on living tissue are generally limited to research, this chapter will focus on methods for monitoring human movement and the factors influencing this movement.

Biomechanical principles

The study of biomechanics is traditionally approached by the quantification of movement (kinematics) and force (kinetics). In general, human movement involves both linear and angular motion. As an athlete runs, their centre of gravity experiences linear motion, with displacement in the vertical, forward (anterior), and medial-lateral directions. This linear motion is achieved by the angular rotation of body segments—the arms and legs. For the study of human movement, it is generally convenient to analyse the linear and angular aspects of motion separately. Thus, the areas of kinematics and kinetics are usually subdivided into linear and angular aspects: linear kinematics and angular kinematics; linear kinetics and angular kinetics.

Linear kinematics

Linear kinematics involves measurement of the motion characteristics of position, velocity, and acceleration. For the runner illustrated in Fig 1.8.1, it may be of interest to monitor the linear motion of a marker placed on the hip. To achieve this, a reference frame is required. This is illustrated in two dimensions as the y and z axes. Thus the location of the hip marker at any point in time is represented by the coordinates (y,z). If medial-lateral motion is of interest, a third axis can be added to provide medial-lateral position. For the two-dimensional situation illustrated in Fig. 1.8.1(A), the y coordinate quantifies the location of the hip relative to the z axis. Thus, as the runner travels forward, this value will increase. The z coordinate quantifies the height of the marker. Thus, if vertical oscillation of the hip is of interest, this coordinate can be monitored. Therefore the quantification of position or displacement of a

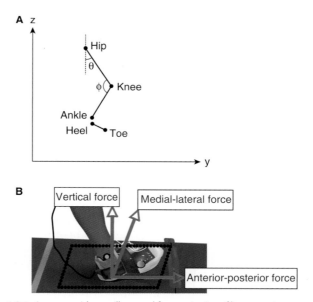

Fig. 1.8.1 A runner with axes illustrated for monitoring of linear motion.

single point in this way can provide useful information on human movement.

For the runner illustrated in Fig. 1.8.1(B), the coach or practitioner may be more interested in velocity than position. The velocity in the horizontal and vertical directions can be determined as separate velocity components, or can be combined to provide a resultant velocity. Velocity is defined as the change in position per unit time, calculated using the equation

$$\text{velocity} = (\text{position}_{final} - \text{position}_{initial})/(\text{time}_{final} - \text{time}_{initial})$$

$$= (\text{change in position})/(\text{change in time}) \quad (1)$$

Thus, if one is concerned with average horizontal velocity over a period of time, this can be calculated by subtracting the y coordinate at the end of the time period from the y coordinate at the start, and dividing this by the time taken to move between the two points. An example of where horizontal velocity of the hip marker may be useful is in gait analysis when one wants to ensure that the walking or running performances being analysed all have similar velocities. The average velocity can be monitored and runs outside the required velocity range can be discarded.

Assessment of linear acceleration can also be useful in the analysis of human movement. For example, an athletics coach monitoring sprint starts may be interested in the rate at which maximum velocity is achieved. A sprinter may perform repeated sprint starts and get feedback on the acceleration achieved. Acceleration is defined as the rate of change of velocity with respect to time, calculated using the equation

$$\text{accleration} = (\text{velocity}_{final} - \text{velocity}_{initial})/(\text{time}_{final} - \text{time}_{initial})$$

$$= (\text{change in velocity})/(\text{change in time}) \quad (2)$$

If a coach is interested in the acceleration of an athlete during the first 10 metres of a race, they can determine the velocity at 10 metres, subtract the velocity at the start (zero), and then divide by the time taken to reach the 10 metre point of the race. Smaller time periods can be selected to monitor the changes in acceleration within the 10 metres, or even within each step.

Angular kinematics

Angular kinematics is the analysis of angular motion. Angular motion occurs about an axis of rotation that is perpendicular to the plane in which the motion takes place. Virtually all human movement involves the rotation of body segments, where the segments rotate about joint centres. Figure 1.8.1 illustrates some example joint angles for a runner. These joint angles are calculated using the position information (coordinates) for the relevant joint centres. For example, with information on the coordinates of the hip, knee, and ankle, it is possible to calculate the knee angle using basic trigonometry.

The measurement of joint angles can be very useful for analysis of performance and injury. Figure 1.8.2 illustrates the time histories for the right and left sides of the knee joint angle during running for a runner with patellofemoral pain on the left side. The graph clearly illustrates a greater amount of knee flexion on the left side, which may be linked with this pain. This information can be combined with kinematic data for other relevant joints, the patient history, and a podiatry and/or physiotherapy assessment to help in identifying the cause of injury, selecting an appropriate

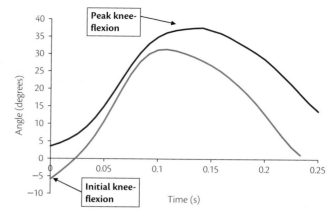

Fig. 1.8.2 Knee angle time history during running for right (red) and left (blue) sides.

intervention, and monitoring rehabilitation. Thus monitoring joint angles can be useful in a clinical setting.

Angular velocity, defined as the angular displacement per unit of time, can also be useful in the analysis of human movement. For example, the average knee flexion velocity for the left knee illustrated in Fig. 1.8.2 can be determined by subtracting the knee angle at initial ground contact (2.1°) from the peak knee flexion angle (38.5°) and dividing this by the time period from initial ground contact to peak angle. Knee flexion velocity may vary, for example in response to pain (Anderson and Herrington 2003) or shoe–surface compliance (Hardin *et al.* 2004).

Angular acceleration is defined as the rate of change in angular velocity with respect to time. If joint rotations are being used to develop a high velocity, such as during a sprint start or in throwing and kicking, it is beneficial to accelerate optimally. For example, during a ball throw the elbow joint is flexed and then extended. At the start of the extension phase, the joint angular velocity is zero instantaneously as the joint moves from flexing to extending. The extension phase then involves achieving as high a velocity as possible in the range of motion available before release of the ball. Therefore the thrower aims to increase the velocity as quickly as possible; this rate of change of velocity is acceleration. The greater the angular acceleration, the greater is the velocity at the point of release. Therefore an ability to optimize angular accelerations at relevant joints is vital to those in sports where release velocity determines the performance.

Linear kinetics

Kinetics is concerned with the causes of motion—the forces that act on a system. Fundamental to the study of kinetics are the laws of motion, described by Sir Isaac Newton. According to Newton's principles, objects move when a force is applied that is greater than the resistance of the object to movement. Forces may be described as non-contact or contact forces, where the non-contact force of most relevance to human motion is gravity. Contact forces are those acting as a result of contact between two objects. Contact forces can be internal or external to the body. Examples of internal forces include joint and muscle forces. In general, it is not possible to measure internal forces unless within a research project (and this is still relatively rare due to ethical considerations).

External forces of relevance to the analysis of human movement include ground reaction forces and friction.

Ground reaction force is the reaction from the ground during contact. The runner in Fig 1.8.1 pushes against the ground with a force and the ground pushes back with an equal force in the opposite direction. The ground reaction force can be measured using a force platform, usually sited flush with the running surface. In Fig. 1.8.1(B) a force plate is positioned below the running surface, as indicated by the rectangular contact area marked (Fig. 1.8.1(B)). The force is typically broken down into three orthogonal components: F_x (medial-lateral), F_y (anterior-posterior), and F_z (vertical).

Ground reaction force data have been used to study many types of human movement. During ground contact, the force changes continually, resulting in a force–time profile such as that illustrated in Fig. 1.8.3 for running. Figure 1.8.3 illustrates the vertical force F_z, which during running has by far the highest magnitude of the three components. The profile provided in Fig. 1.8.3 is for a heel–toe runner. The initial peak is termed the passive or impact peak and occurs during the initial impact. The later peak is called the active peak, and occurs as a result of the active muscle forces applied to propel the runner off the ground. Force–time profiles can also be presented for the two horizontal components F_x and F_y. These may be of more relevance for stopping and turning movements, where substantially larger horizontal forces occur compared with those seen for running.

Friction is the force acting parallel to the interface of two interacting surfaces. It is a force that opposes motion, or impending motion. It exists whenever one body moves, or tends to move, across the surface of another. Without friction humans could not move. An understanding of factors influencing friction can help a coach, player, or clinician in the choice of equipment and allow them to assess the techniques used when moving on a specific surface. An understanding of design factors influencing friction is also useful for the development of optimal features in equipment such as sports shoes and playing surfaces. For surface interactions where parts of an object indent another, such as football studs in turf or running spikes in a track surface, the resistance to motion is commonly referred to as traction.

The force of friction is proportional to the normal force between the two surfaces. Consider a tennis player changing direction on a court surface. As the foot contacts the surface, a horizontal force is applied. Sliding friction is the force that opposes any sliding motion between the surface of the shoe sole and the surface of the court.

As the applied force increases, the friction force increases. When sliding does not occur, the value of the friction force is equal to the magnitude of the applied force. If sliding does occur, this indicates that the applied force has exceeded a specific limit. This limit depends on the properties of the court surface and the surface of the shoe sole. It also depends on the normal (vertical) force applied.

The friction value that occurs just before sliding commences is known as limiting friction. For two dry surfaces, the limiting friction F is equal to the normal reaction force R multiplied by a constant. The value of this constant depends only on the nature of the surfaces. The symbol used to represent the friction constant, known as the coefficient of friction, is μ. The relationship between the frictional force, the normal force, and the coefficient of friction is given

$$F = \mu R \qquad (3)$$

The greater the coefficient of friction, the greater is the interaction of the surface molecules. For the tennis player turning on a court surface, a greater coefficient of friction results in a greater horizontal force being required to induce sliding; thus sliding is less likely. It is important to acknowledge that the coefficient of friction, and thus the likelihood of sliding, is influenced by the properties of both the shoe and the surface.

Angular kinetics

To determine the influence that an external force has on movement, an understanding of moment of force, or torque, is required. The influence that a force has on the rotation of a body will be influenced by both its magnitude and its location on the body. For example, for someone in the propulsive phase of running, the force applied by the calf muscles will influence the motion, but so will the line of action of the muscle relative to the point of rotation (the ankle). The perpendicular distance d from the centre of rotation to the line of action of the force is the moment arm, or lever arm. The product of the force magnitude and the moment arm is termed the moment of force (moment = force × d). The relationship between force, moment arm and moment is illustrated in Fig. 1.8.4.

The muscle moment causing (or tending to cause) motion can be increased by an increase in muscle force and/or an increase in moment arm length. The moment arm length is influenced by both the anatomy of the individual (the origin and insertion of the muscle) and the joint angle. For the running example illustrated, as the ankle joint flexes, the moment arm length will change, influencing the muscle force required to apply a defined moment.

Whilst it is rarely possible or practical to directly measure the muscle force or the line of action of the muscle for a defined individual, it is possible to use biomechanical techniques to estimate

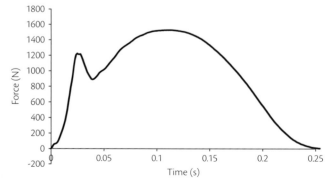

Fig. 1.8.3 Typical vertical ground reaction force–time profile for running.

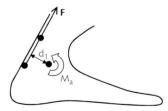

Fig. 1.8.4 Relationship between Achilles tendon force, moment arm, and ankle moment for the foot segment.

muscle moments. This can be demonstrated for the ankle moment during running. The collection of synchronized force and kinematic data, combined with anatomical information such as segment mass and centre of gravity, allows estimation of ankle joint moment. The methodology used to estimate joint moments in this manner is termed inverse dynamics. A detailed explanation of this technique is beyond the scope of this chapter, but it be found in numerous textbooks (Zatsiorsky 2002; Nigg and Herzog 2007). The inverse dynamics approach is used in biomechanics research to investigate relationships between factors such as joint moment and injury or treatment intervention (Milner *et al.* 2007; MacLean *et al.* 2006), but is also increasingly used in a clinical environment to detect deficiencies in muscle function (Lohmann Siegel *et al.* 2006). The concept of support moment has been used to describe the combined action of the ankle, knee, and hip moments to prevent collapse of the lower limb during ground contact in walking and running (Winter 1980). If one of the joints is dysfunctional, perhaps due to disease or injury, the other joints compensate for this to avoid collapse. Therefore monitoring of joint moments in a clinical environment can detect joint moments (and thus muscle function) that are not contributing effectively, and consider interventions to aid in treatment or rehabilitation.

Measurement and analysis tools

Collection of kinematic data

Using the example of human running, the concepts of position, velocity, and acceleration have been introduced. Video-based or automated optoelectronic systems are typically used to obtain kinematic data. A standard commercial camcorder can provide adequate recording of human movement for the biomechanical assessment of most human movements for use in a coaching or clinical environment. Standard video cameras operating with the PAL system, as utilized in the UK, collect data at 25 frames per second (25 Hz), which can be divided into 50 fields per second (50 Hz) with appropriate software. In the US NTC system, video is recorded at 30 frames or 60 fields per second. Unless analysing motion that involves high accelerations, such as impacts, these sampling rates are generally sufficient. If higher sampling rates are required, high-speed video or cinefilm cameras can be utilized.

The main limitation of video-based systems for biomechanical analysis of human movement is the time taken to obtain some of the data. For the video recording itself, the camera must be placed in an optimal location to view the field of interest. The camera should also be positioned normal to the plane of movement to minimize errors introduced by movements out of the recorded plane. The recording of the video only takes as long as the activity itself, and so is not time consuming. The time taken to obtain data from the video recording depends on the specific data required. It is possible to obtain some indication of position, velocity, and acceleration simply by playing the video back on a standard television or computer monitor, placing an acetate sheet on the screen and marking the points of interest. Calculations to obtain measurements of position, velocity, and acceleration can be achieved using these markings and suitably placed axes. This is acceptable for occasional measurements, but would not be ideal for collecting large quantities of data.

Increasingly, commercially available computer software is a realistic option for taking measurements from video, both financially

and in terms of the required technical understanding. Software such as SiliconCoach (www.siliconcoach.com) and Dartfish (www.dartfish.com) allow the determination of both linear and angular kinematic measures directly from the screen. For example, video clips are replayed within the software and the user can click with the computer mouse on selected body landmarks. Selection of the hip, knee, and ankle will allow instantaneous calculation of the knee angle for an observed video frame. This form of software can be beneficial for quick feedback in a coaching environment and for clinical analysis of relevant joint angles.

Automated motion analysis systems are also increasingly available. These imaging systems monitor the movement of specific markers directly, without the requirement for the user to identify the location of the marker on a screen. With most automated systems the markers are passive, typically spherical markers covered with reflective tape or paint. Such systems include VICON (Oxford, UK) and ProReflex (Qualisys, Gothenburg, Sweden). In general, the software cannot differentiate between different passive markers. Thus the user must identify them for at least one frame of the motion. This is not necessary with active marker systems such as Codamotion (Charnwood Dynamics, Leicestershire, UK), which uses small infrared light-emitting diodes (LEDs) to allow the software to recognize individual markers and avoid the requirement for marker identification by the user.

Automated systems can be extremely useful for providing data quickly, or even in real time. This can be beneficial in a clinical environment, where immediate feedback to the practitioner and the patient/client can greatly enhance the service provided. Immediate feedback on technique can also be provided to the performer and coach for performance enhancement. Whilst use of such systems in the outdoor field environment has been limited by the lack of control over lighting conditions, improvements in these systems are increasing their applicability to coaching.

Automated motion analysis systems can also be synchronized with force platforms, allowing the determination of joint moments, particularly useful in the analysis of human gait in a clinical setting.

Collection of kinetic data

Traditionally, tools for the collection of kinetic data have not been utilized by coaches or clinicians as extensively as motion analysis systems. This has probably been influenced by both the cost of force-measuring devices and the limited application of force platforms. Since, outside a research environment, a force plate provides data on the resultant force, rather than on the force acting on parts of the body, the relevance of force-plate data is not always clear. Details of the location of the resultant force relative to the centre of gravity of the performer can be useful for skills such as somersaults in gymnastics (Hay 1993). Similarly, in some clinical settings, details regarding the location of the point of application of the resultant force relative to the centre of gravity can be beneficial when considering balance problems (Gefen *et al.* 2002). However, in general, force platforms have limited application in a clinical or coaching setting.

The application of force-measuring technology in sports medicine has increased with the development of pressure-measuring systems. These systems provide detail on the distribution of force across the contacting surface. Pressure-measuring devices are available in the form of discrete sensors, pressure plates, or pressure insoles. Discrete sensors can be useful if localized loads at defined locations are important. For example, for a diabetic patient with leg ulcers, pressure sensors can be placed over ulcer sites and the influence of footwear interventions on loads can be investigated. Pressure plates are generally used for the collection of barefoot data during walking or running. Commercial systems are now frequently utilized in a clinical environment for the identification of characteristic pressure patterns (e.g. Giacomozzi and Martelli 2006). For example, the relative contact area in the midfoot during gait can be used to classify someone as having a high, 'normal', or low arch. These dynamic data can complement clinical information such as static anatomical measures and patient history. The pressure data can be collected for walking or running, depending on the activity associated with injury/disease. Some examples of pressure patterns for running are provided in Fig. 1.8.5 (see Chapter 1.9 for details of the application of pressure systems for the analysis of walking gait in a clinical environment). Pressure insoles are placed within footwear to measure the influence of footwear interventions (Dixon and Stiles 2003) or to quantify foot function in a more realistic environment than obtained when using barefoot data collection (Cavanagh *et al.* 1998).

Basic mechanics of running and clinical applications

Running is a skill that is integral to the majority of sports, and as a result it has undergone extensive research compared with other sports skills. Whilst there are still aspects of running that we do not understand, the general characteristics of running biomechanics have been described in detail. The reader is directed to Cavanagh (1990) for detailed information on distance running, and the textbook by Bosch and Klomp (2005) for details of both distance and sprint running. This section provides a brief description of the biomechanics of heel–toe running, which is characteristic of most distance runners, and includes examples of the application of the dynamic biomechanical analysis of runners in a clinical environment to aid in the management of injury.

The description of kinematics provided earlier in this chapter focused on two-dimensional sagittal plane analysis of motion, which is often sufficient for movements that are predominantly in one plane. Whilst running does occur mainly in the sagittal plane, the relatively small movements out of this plane are frequently associated with injury. For example, excessive pronation (eversion), occurring in the frontal plane, and tibial internal rotation, occurring in the transverse plane, have been linked to injuries such as medial knee pain and Achilles tendon pathology. With appropriate cameras and software it is possible to collect kinematic data in three dimensions, allowing monitoring of these movements. This section describes typical movements of key joints in all three planes during relaxed heel–toe running.

Ankle dorsi/plantarflexion

The amount of motion of the ankle joint may influence the occurrence of injury. This motion can be measured by taking standing values as zero. At initial ground strike, the foot will typically be

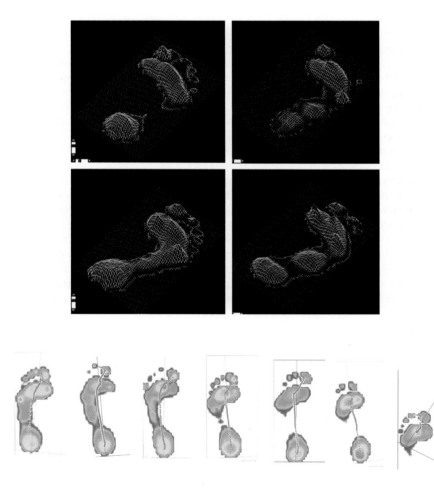

Fig. 1.8.5 Examples of typical pressure patterns for running.

pointing slightly upwards, resulting in a heel strike with the ground. The lower leg is inclined backwards at this time. Therefore at ground strike the ankle is usually in a neutral or slightly dorsiflexed position. Immediately after ground strike, the foot quickly rotates forward as the forefoot makes ground contact. Therefore a small amount of ankle plantarflexion usually occurs. Once the foot is flat on the ground, the forward rotation of the lower leg results in ankle dorsiflexion occurring as the leg bends to absorb the impact with the ground. Following maximum ankle dorsiflexion, occurring around the middle of the ground contact phase, plantarflexion of the ankle joint occurs to help in the propulsion phase of the running step.

The maximum amount of ankle dorsiflexion provides an indication of the contribution of the ankle joint to the cushioning phase of running. This value can be measured for an athlete and compared with the range of 15°–25° documented in the literature (Milliron and Cavanagh 1990).

Knee flexion/extension

Knee flexion/extension is also usually monitored using the standing values as zero. During running, the knee typically strikes the ground with a small amount of flexion. The knee then flexes (bends), reaching a peak flexion of around 40° during midstance (Milliron and Cavanagh 1990). From here, extension of the knee occurs as the body is propelled forwards. The amount of knee flexion exhibited at ground strike and the maximum knee flexion can be monitored to highlight any differences from the patterns typically seen during running.

Pronation and supination

Figure 1.8.6 illustrates the rearfoot angle, used to indicate pronation (eversion) and supination (inversion). Supination and pronation are natural phases of running gait. Typically the foot is supinated at ground strike, resulting in the outside of the foot striking the ground first. The foot then rolls onto the inside, indicating pronation. Pronation is a necessary part of running gait, contributing to the absorption of impact forces and allowing adjustment to uneven surfaces. However, the maximum pronation angle is of interest because 'excessive' pronation has been associated with the occurrence of overuse injuries.

Since running shoes are typically directed at different running styles, this information can inform the selection of appropriate footwear. Runners exhibiting around 8°–12° of pronation have

been classified as 'normal' pronators (Clarke *et al.* 1984; Edington *et al.* 1990). Therefore a neutral shoe is most likely to suit these runners. Those with 12°–18° of pronation may benefit from the additional supportive features of a stability shoe. Runners with more than 18° of pronation have been classed as 'excessive' pronators, and may require a motion control shoe. Those exhibiting less than 8° of pronation may benefit from a cushioned shoe because of the reduced natural cushioning they experience owing to reduced pronation. Whilst the amount of pronation is only one factor that can be used to help in the identification of an appropriate type of footwear, these measurements add significantly to the information available when making this selection.

Internal tibial rotation

The amount of internal rotation of the lower leg during ground contact is likely to be influenced by the amount of pronation. As the foot rolls inwards, the tibia (lower leg) experiences internal rotation and subsequently rotation of the knee occurs internally. The average runner experiences in the region of 8°–12° of internal rotation in the period immediately following ground contact. In gait analysis of running performed in the EXBiRT Laboratory at the School of Sport and Health Sciences, University of Exeter, we have found internal tibial rotation data particularly useful. It is often possible to identify whether someone is pronating (everting) excessively through a combination of static analysis and visual observation. Similarly, ankle and knee flexion–extension may be relatively easy to detect. However, the internal rotation of the tibia in the sagittal plane requires a three-dimensional analysis to detect this movement confidently.

Clinical example

A case study of a runner is provided to illustrate the possible clinical application of dynamic gait analysis data. The runner is a 30-year-old female averaging 30 miles per week and competing in distances from 5 km to the half-marathon. At the time of the examination she was experiencing left medial knee pain. During the examination she underwent a combined podiatry and dynamic gait analysis assessment.

The podiatry analysis revealed 6° of rearfoot varus (inversion) for both sides when in the subtalar neutral position (see Chapter 2.7 for more details of the definition and collection of podiatry measures). The calcaneus was vertical when in relaxed standing. The subtalar joint range of motion was 12° inversion to 8° eversion for the left side, and 18° inversion to 10° eversion for the right. Additional observations included an ankle equinus, where the forefoot is dropped in relation to the rearfoot. On the left side, restricted ankle dorsiflexion was observed. In addition, the wear pattern on the sole of the running shoes revealed wear on the central heel for the left shoe, rather than the lateral wear more typically associated with heel–toe running.

The collection of dynamic gait data revealed similar patterns of ankle dorsiflexion for left and right sides at the start of ground contact, with both sides contacting the ground in a slightly dorsiflexed orientation. However, the peak ankle dorsiflexion was only 15.6° for the left side compared with 23.8° for the right. Similar patterns of knee flexion were exhibited for both sides, with around 5° of flexion at ground strike and a maximum knee flexion in the region of 35°. The rearfoot movement data showed similar values of peak pronation (eversion) for both sides of around 11°. However, the

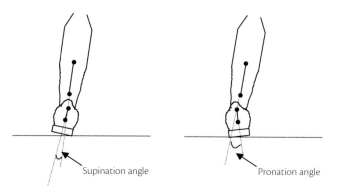

Fig. 1.8.6 Illustration of rearfoot inversion–eversion movement (right leg).

Supination angle

Pronation angle

initial supination (inversion) angle at heel strike was close to zero (neutral) for the left side compared with 4.2° for the right side. The internal tibial rotation data indicated greater internal rotation for the left side (10.3°) than for the right side (5.4°). The collection of barefoot pressure data for the runner indicated no midfoot ground contact during running.

In summary, the runner demonstrated lower static range of motion of the subtalar joint for the left side, no initial inversion during running for the left side, ankle equinus for both sides, low ankle dorsiflexion for the left side (static and dynamic), and high internal rotation for the tibia for the left side. The following characteristics were highlighted from the combined podiatry and dynamic biomechanical data:

◆ an ankle equinus for both sides, compensated for by rearfoot pronation (relatively high for both sides);

◆ restricted static joint motion at the ankle and subtalar joints for the left side, resulting in low initial inversion and low peak ankle dorsiflexion during running;

◆ high internal rotation of the tibia for the left side probably as compensation for restricted ankle flexion, providing the necessary cushioning during impact.

It was suggested that the high internal rotation of the tibia resulted in high or unaccustomed knee loading and thus was linked to the left medial knee pain. The runner was prescribed heel lifts for both sides to reduce the requirement for compensatory pronation due to the ankle equinus. Calf stretches were recommended as initial treatment for the restricted ankle joint motion.

This case study has been used to illustrate the possibility of supplementing the traditional podiatry assessment of athletes with a dynamic gait analysis. Combination of the skills and experience of a podiatrist with those of a sports biomechanist has provided the athlete with a more comprehensive assessment. In particular, knowledge of the influence of restricted static motion on ankle dorsiflexion and tibial rotation during running provided additional evidence to inform the resultant prescription.

A key problem with the use of gait analysis in this way is the fact that most athletes only seek a gait assessment when they are injured. Thus, if unusual characteristics of gait are identified, it is not possible to know whether these are a result of the recent injury or a contributing factor to the injury. Therefore it is suggested that, ideally, athletes, particularly those at the elite level, should have gait data collected when injury free and that this information should be kept for future comparison if they become injured.

Conclusion

This chapter has introduced basic biomechanical principles, using the example of running to illustrate most of the key concepts. In particular, linear and angular kinematics and kinetics have been described. The tools available to a practitioner or coach for collecting kinematic and kinetic data have also been described, highlighting some of the strengths and limitations of the equipment. The skill of heel–toe running has been described in some detail, with a case study provided to illustrate how these data can be applied in a clinical setting.

The application of biomechanics in sports medicine is in its infancy, with much scope for greater and improved use. For example, despite the use of automated motion analysis systems to provide joint kinematics and joint moments for clinical populations, particularly those with cerebral palsy and the application of pressure systems for diabetic populations, the use of these systems to address sports injury issues, such as those illustrated in the case study, is relatively rare. The increased use of this combined approach will increase our understanding of injury mechanisms and methods of treatment and rehabilitation. It will also increase our confidence in using such an approach.

References

Anderson, G. and Herrington, L. (2003). A comparison of eccentric isokinetic torque production and velocity of knee flexion angle during step down in patellofemoral syndrome patients and unaffected subjects. *Clinical Biomechanics*, **18**, 500–4.

Bosch, F. and Klomp, R. (2005). *Running: Biomechanics and Exercise Physiology Applied in Practice*. Elsevier, Amsterdam.

Cavanagh, P.R. (ed.) (1990). *Biomechanics of Distance Running*. Human Kinetics, Champaign, IL.

Cavanagh, P.R., Perry, J.E., Ulbrecht, J.S., *et al.* (1998). Neuropathic diabetic patients do not have reduced variability of plantar loading during gait. *Gait Posture*, **7**, 191–9.

Clarke, T.E., Frederick, E.C., and Hamill, J. (1984). The study of rearfoot movement in running. In: E.C. Frederick (ed.), *Sports Shoes and Playing Surfaces*, pp. 166–189. Human Kinetics, Champaign, IL.

Dixon, S.J. and Stiles, V.H. (2003). Shoe–surface interaction in tennis. *Sports Engineering*, **6**, 1–10.

Edington, C.J., Frederick, E.C., and Cavanagh, P.R. (1990). Rearfoot motion in distance running. In: P.R. Cavanagh (ed.), *Biomechanics of Distance Running*, pp. 135–64. Human Kinetics, Champaign, IL.

Gefen, A., Megido-Ravid, M., Itzchak, Y., and Arcan, M. (2002). Analysis of muscular fatigue and foot stability during high-heeled gait. *Gait Posture*, **15**, 56–63.

Giacomozzi, C. and Martelli, F. (2006). Peak pressure curve: an effective parameter for early detection of foot dysfunctional impairments in diabetic patients. *Gait Posture*, **23**, 464–70.

Hardin, E.C., van den Bogert, A., and Hamill, J. (2004). Kinematic adaptations during running: effects of footwear, surface and duration. *Medicine and Science in Sports and Exercise*, **36**, 838–44.

Hay, J.G. (1993). *The Biomechanics of Sports Techniques* (4th edn). Prentice-Hall, Englewood Cliffs, NJ.

Lohmann Siegel, K., Kepple, T.M., and Stanhope, S.J. (2006). Using induced accelerations to understand knee stability during gait of individuals with muscle weakness. *Gait Posture*, **23**, 435–40.

MacLean, C., McClay Davis, I., and Hamill, J. (2006). Influence of a custom orthotic intervention on lower extremity dynamics in healthy runners. *Clinical Biomechanics*, **21**, 623–30.

Milliron, M.J. and Cavanagh, P.R. (1990). Sagittal plane kinematics of the lower extremity during distance running. In: P.R. Cavanagh (ed.), *Biomechanics of Distance Running*, pp. 65–106. Human Kinetics, Champaign, IL.

Milner, C., Hamill, J., and Davis, I. (2007). Are knee mechanics during early stance related to tibial stress fracture in runners? *Clinical Biomechanics*, **22**, 697–703.

Nigg, B.M. and Herzog, W. (2007). *Biomechanics of the Musculo-skeletal System*. John Wiley, Chichester.

Winter, D.A. (1980). Overall principle of lower limb support during stance phase of gait. *Journal of Biomechanics*, **13**, 923–7.

Zatsiorsky, V.M. (2002). *Kinetics of Human Motion*. Human Kinetics, Champaign, IL.

1.9

Gait analysis

Sophie Roberts and Sharon Dixon

Introduction

Gait analysis describes the process of systematically quantifying mechanical aspects of walking or running to aid in the examination of a patient/client. In the publication *Gait Analysis: An Introduction*, Whittle (2002) identifies the eye as being the first tool in this assessment, with technology being available to supplement this visual analysis. Technological analysis tools include two-dimensional (2D) video, three-dimensional (3D) motion analysis, pressure plates, and pressure insoles. The application of technology has increased our understanding of human gait substantially. This chapter introduces the basic tools of gait analysis and highlights specific considerations when selecting appropriate tools for the assessment of walking gait. Details of running gait are provided in Chapter 1.8.

Typical walking gait

Variability is present in the gait of healthy individuals, with variables such as joint range of motion, muscle activation, and ground reaction forces differing between subjects. However, there exists a generally accepted 'normal' pattern of gait and an expected range for the variables measured in gait analysis. Deviation from this range constitutes unusual or 'abnormal' gait. The use of gait analysis allows the identification of abnormal characteristics of gait and the investigation of interventions aimed at correcting gait patterns. Measurements of gait for healthy individuals provide the benchmark against which pathological gait can be assessed, and thus it is important to have gait measurements from healthy subjects.

Walking gait is typically assessed using the gait cycle—the time interval between two successive occurrences of a specific event in the walking gait pattern; this event is most frequently initial ground contact. Major events in the gait cycle are:

(1) initial contact

(2) opposite toe-off

(3) heel rise

(4) opposite initial contact

(5) toe-off

(6) feet adjacent

(7) tibia vertical.

The stance or support phase lasts from initial contact to toe-off, and the swing phase from toe-off to initial contact. The stance phase itself can be further divided into four phases: loading response, mid-stance, terminal stance, and pre-swing. Similarly, the swing phase can be divided into the phases of initial swing, mid-swing, and terminal swing. These phases are illustrated in Fig. 1.9.1.

Measurements of the timings of key events in the gait cycle can provide an initial indication of typical gait patterns for healthy subjects. In each gait cycle there are two periods of double support where both feet are in contact with the ground. At this stage, the leading leg has just landed on the ground and is in the phase of weight acceptance. The trailing leg is just about to leave the ground and is in the pre-swing phase. The trailing leg leaves the ground and undergoes the swing phase, while the other leg experiences single support. Initial contact then occurs for the swing phase leg, initiating a second double-support phase. Whilst varying with the speed of walking, the stance phase typically constitutes 60% of the cycle and the swing phase 40%.

Assessment of foot placement can also be valuable in gait analysis (Fig. 1.9.2). The distance between two successive placements of the same foot is termed stride length, and consists of one step from each foot. The left and right step lengths for healthy individuals are usually of similar length, but frequently these differ for those with pathological gait patterns. The side-to-side distance between the mid-heel of each foot, or base of support, is frequently assessed. In addition, the amount of toe-out or toe-in, the angle between the line of progression and the longitudinal axis of the foot, can provide a useful measure in the characterization of gait.

Cadence, the number of steps taken per minute, also provides a useful measure. The average healthy adult has a natural cadence of around 96–138 steps per minute, with this figure tending to be higher for children and lower for older adults (Whittle 2002). Cadence combines with step length to determine the walking speed, with an increase in either variable increasing the speed of walking.

The basic characteristics of gait described above can be used to assess walking gait objectively without the requirement for advanced technology. More detailed analysis of gait, such as measurement of joint angles and underfoot pressures, can be performed using the equipment described in the following sections.

Eyeball gait assessment

It is not essential to use complicated computer technology to observe the way in which a person walks, especially in a clinical setting. However, it is difficult to see intricate movements of joints without looking at slow-motion video playback or more complex gait analysis methods. Gross movement patterns can be observed

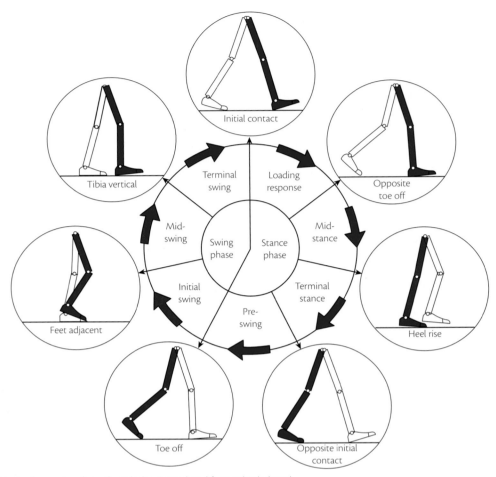

Fig. 1.9.1 Positions of the leg for a gait cycle by the right leg. Reproduced from Whittle (2001).

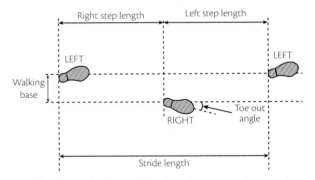

Fig. 1.9.2 Terminology for characterizing foot placement on the ground.

easily by eye and can provide valuable information on the way a person walks, which can easily be included in a patient's examination and can help in diagnosis and aetiology of the clinical problem. Eyeball assessment of gait can be carried out in any environment, including a corridor or a clinic room, and is not confined to a biomechanics laboratory or specified walkway.

During gait, the majority of movement occurs in the sagittal plane, and therefore it is easy to assess movement patterns in this plane compared with the frontal or transverse planes, where smaller movements occur. An example of a movement pattern which

is easy to assess by eye in the sagittal plane is the range of ankle dorsiflexion and plantarflexion a person is demonstrating during walking. By assessing the timing of the heel lift and angle of plantarflexion at propulsion, it is possible to identify the functional range of the ankle joint during dynamic gait.

Frontal and transverse movements are harder to see with the naked eye. However, they can provide information on the efficiency of the patient's gait. An example of a movement pattern which is easy to assess by eye in the frontal plane is head movement. When standing behind a person and watching them walk away from you, you can observe the side-to-side movement of the head to see if it moves more to one side than the other or whether the person holds their head at a constant angle whist walking. An example of a transverse plane movement which is easy to see with the naked eye is the abduction angle of the foot, indicating whether the person rotates their foot into excessive abduction or adduction during gait. Table 1.9.1 illustrates movement patterns which occur in all three planes during gait and are possible to see by eye.

Eyeball assessment of gait can be carried out by all healthcare professionals treating the patient with a musculoskeletal complaint and provides an overview of gait efficiency and gait compensation in closed kinetic chain walking. Gross movement patterns can be monitored and compared and can be conjugated with a physical examination to provide a clearer picture of the patient biomechanical structure and function. However, important movement

Table 1.9.1 Movement patterns during walking viewed by the naked eye

What movement pattern	What to look for	Which aspect to look from
First MTP joint movement	Dorsiflexion of hallux at push-off and whether propulsion occurs straight, medially, or laterally. Is there an abductory twist?	Side view and anterior view
Ankle movement	Speed of heel lift, dorsiflexion angle through mid-stance, plantar flexion angle at propulsion	Side view and posterior view
Knee movement	Does knee reach full extension at push-off at propulsion? Does the knee excessively internally rotate?	Side view and anterior view
Hip movement	Do the hips drop on one side excessively or on both? Is there excessive lateral sway? Is there reduced hip extension?	Side view, posterior and anterior view
Swing phase leg movements	Is there circumflexion (swing out) of the leg? Does the ankle dorsiflex?	Anterior and posterior view
Arm swing	Is it symmetrical? Is it abducted? Does it cross the mid-line of the body?	Anterior view
Shoulder and head position	Are the shoulders symmetrical? Is the head straight?	Anterior view

MTP, metatarsophalangeal.

patterns can be missed if they are occurring too fast for the naked eye to see, are occurring in a plane that is difficult to view, or are looked at by an untrained eye.

Two-dimensional video analysis

The next step from eyeball assessment of gait is 2D video analysis which permits slow motion playback of the footage recorded of the patient's gait. Again, this is a cheap and relatively easy method of gait analysis to perform in a clinical situation and permits a more detailed analysis of biomechanical function because of the frame-by-frame playback ability (Fig. 1.9.3). The main problem with 2D video is the misleading effect that different camera angles can create. If the camera is not at right angles to the plane of movement of the subject or the joint of interest, true representation of the movement pattern can be distorted. Analysis of the patient whilst walking on a treadmill helps to reduce the effect of misleading camera angles; however, there is then the question of whether this is a true

representation of the patient's gait, especially if the patient is not familiar with walking on a treadmill. There is recent evidence that treadmill and overground walking gait are essentially the same (Riley *et al.* 2007), but this may not be true for clinical populations. If walkway analysis is used instead of treadmill analysis, sagittal (side view) analysis becomes very difficult as it is only possible to analyse the time period when the movement of interest is at direct right angles to the camera.

The equipment used for 2D video analysis should be considered carefully. A wide-angle lens can be useful for capturing the movements of both the upper and lower body. Additionally, the sampling rate of the video camera should be high enough to capture the speed of gait assessed. The sampling rate of a commercially available video camera (25–30 Hz) is generally sufficient for walking gait. A higher sampling rate is required for some aspects of running gait. If the sampling rate of the video analysis equipment is too low, intricate movements will be missed. A tripod should be used to hold the camera steady during filming. Table 1.9.1 provides examples of movement patterns which can be assessed by eye; however, these movement patterns can be assessed in more detail using 2D video gait analysis

Three-dimensional motion analysis

Many of the limitations identified for 2D video analysis can be overcome by using a three-dimensional (3D) motion analysis system. Markers are placed at defined locations on the body, allowing the development of joint coordinate systems to monitor 3D motion. These systems generally utilize four or more cameras positioned around the area that the patient will walk/run through, requiring that all markers on the body can be viewed by at least two cameras. Segment orientation and joint motions can then be monitored in three dimensions. For example, the 3D orientation of the foot at ground contact can be quantified in terms of its sagittal plane inclination to the ground, the level of ab-adduction and the inversion–eversion heel angle. Similarly, knee joint flexion–extension, ab-adduction, and internal–external rotation can be monitored throughout the gait cycle.

These systems are relatively expensive and take some time to set up and to become familiar with. However, they do provide valuable

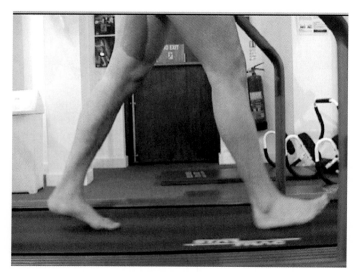

Fig. 1.9.3 A frame taken from 2D video assessment.

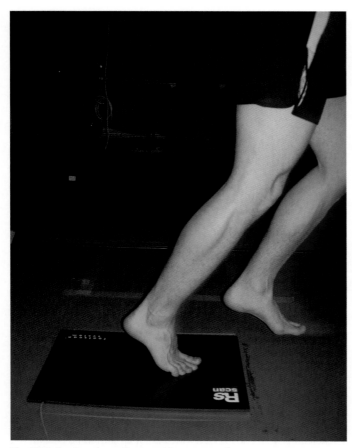

Fig. 1.9.4 Barefoot data collection with a pressure plate.

information, particularly if movements out of the sagittal plane are of interest. For example, internal rotation of the tibia is difficult to detect using the naked eye or 2D video techniques. Rearfoot eversion is frequently a variable of particular interest in gait analysis and can often be monitored satisfactorily with 2D analysis. However, the movement of more concern may be the internal rotation of the tibia. Three-dimensional motion analysis systems can measure this variable directly and highlight any unusual or excessive movement patterns (see Chapter 1.8).

Pressure platform analysis

A pressure platform measures the distribution of vertical force across the foot plantar surface. The main application of a pressure platform is to assess the interaction of the foot with the ground to obtain an indication of the actual function of the foot without any interfering variables such as footwear or orthotics (Fig 1.9.4). These systems are usually very user friendly and simple to use in clinical practice. Using a pressure platform, it is possible to look at pressure and force changes underneath the foot throughout the gait cycle, as well as tracking the gait cycle timings and comparing limb symmetry. It is also useful for assessing the centre of pressure to track the progression of the foot through the gait cycle. The centre of pressure is shown by the software calculating the central point of the pressure loading of the foot on the platform during each time frame. It is important to note that the centre of pressure does not

equate to the body centre of mass; they are different parameters in their own right.

In a clinical environment, pressure platform analysis can be useful for looking at sagittal function during gait, first metatarsophalangeal (MTP) joint loading characteristics, and heel/forefoot loading characteristics. It should be noted that transverse loads cannot be assessed using a pressure platform because frictional forces cannot be measured. Pressure platform equipment has been used extensively in the fields of diabetes and rheumatology to predict ulceration sites and quantify the peak pressures in these fragile areas (Giacomozzi and Martelli 2006; Schmiegel *et al.* 2008).

There are a number of pressure platforms on the market, all with slightly different technologies, which can be used in a clinical environment. These systems generally employ capacitive sensors (e.g. Novel emed, Munich) or conductor sensors (e.g. Tekscan F-scan, Boston, MA) to provide a uniform array of sensors across the plate surface. The majority of commercially available pressure plate systems operate at a sampling rate of 25–100 Hz, which is generally sufficient for the assessment of human walking. Higher sampling rates are increasingly available, and are particularly suitable for the assessment of running. The system software is able to determine between left and right footsteps and average a set of individual footsteps to provide a more overall picture of function. However, looking at an average footstep may not be representative of a typical step since this footstep never actually occurred.

When taking measurements with a pressure platform, ideally the platform is embedded into a walkway so that its surface is flush with the walking surface. This discourages the subject from purposely placing their foot onto the platform and allows a more representative footstep for normal gait. In clinical practice, two or three footsteps are usually recorded. However, if the first footstep analysed is classified as good data in terms of the whole foot striking within the platform and the subject felt that it was a normal footstep for them, this footstep is analysed. The number of footsteps before the foot strikes the platform may be important, although there is evidence of little difference in gait variables when single-step protocols are compared with multi-step (mid-gait) approaches (Harrison and Folland 1997). Other studies have reported changes in temporal and peak pressure values with different methods for initiation and termination of the walking trial (Wearing *et al.* 1999). Therefore a mid-gait trial appears preferable, if space permits, but acceptable data can also be obtained within a limited space. In this situation, a two-step protocol is recommended (Bus and de Lange 2005).

When interpreting barefoot plantar pressure measurements, prior biomechanical assessment information should ideally be obtained to aid interpretation and focus the pressure assessment. For example, if the patient presents with a hallux limitus, you can focus on the forefoot and the first MTP joint area. It is possible with the software to mask certain areas of the foot and analyse parameters specifically in these areas. This is done by dividing up specified areas of the foot pressure picture for local analysis in that area. For example, the heel area is marked and the loading duration of both feet in this mask is compared. The difficulty in masking the foot is the identification of anatomical landmarks in the data. For example, how can you identify exactly where the heel is? It is impossible to identify exactly where the calcaneus finishes by looking at a pressure picture. The Footpressure Interest Group have been able to identify a standard mask procedure which helps to

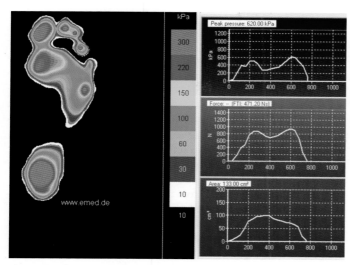

Fig. 1.9.5 Software screen for typical pressure data analysis.

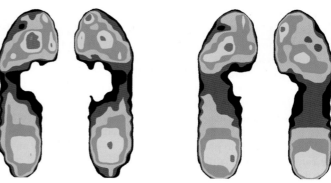

Fig. 1.9.6 Pressure images of before and after orthotic intervention.

obtain repeatability when using masks to analyse pressure data. Figure 1.9.5 shows an example of how a footstep can be divided up into estimated anatomical regions. Table 1.9.2 provides sample variables for typical pressure data analysis.

In-shoe pressure analysis

In-shoe pressure analysis is the measurement and analysis of plantar pressure from inside the shoe using a pressure measurement insole linked to a computer system. This can provide information on how the shoe is interacting with the foot. This is useful in clinical practice as it allows biomechanical analysis in the environment in which the patient is being injured, for example in the aggravating footwear or during the aggravating movement pattern. As the subject walks, readings are taken from the pressure measurement insoles at varying sampling rates depending on the type of measurement system. The data collected are transported via cable, Bluetooth, or a data-storage device to a computer where software permits biomechanical analysis. Systems using Bluetooth or data-storage devices allow wireless data collection which can be useful in sports medicine when the data need to be taken with the subject on the track, on grass, on the tennis court, or during skiing for example. Here, the term 'wireless' indicates that no wired connection directly from the subject to the computer is required. However, wires are still required to transmit the data to the storage device, which is usually carried by the subject on a belt. Thus, in some

situations, wires may interfere with natural movement. This is not usually a problem for analysis of walking and running gait.

There are a number of commercially available pressure insole systems which can be used in a clinical environment (e.g. RScan insole, RScan International, Belgium; Novel pedar, Munich; Tekscan F-scan, Boston). Data are usually collected over a number of footsteps to allow analysis of step-to-step variation, with 10 footsteps from each foot being a typical number to collect. If too much data is collected in the clinical setting, there will be too much data to analyse in one go and no benefit will be obtained. Readings can be taken in different types of footwear, before and after exercise programmes, and before and after movement pattern training in sport to identify differences in biomechanical function. It is also possible to analyse orthotic function by taking a baseline reading in the shoe without the orthotic and then placing the pressure measurement insole over the top of the orthotic in the shoe and repeating the data collection process. The two sets of data can then be compared to assess the effect of the orthotic device (Fig. 1.9.6). In situations where the primary concern is with the effect of an orthotic on loads on specific areas of the foot, such as with diabetic patients, in-shoe pressure analysis is clearly preferred to a pressure plate system.

Parameters assessed are similar to those of the pressure platform systems; however, it must be appreciated that the shoe distorts the data to some extent and this should be taken into consideration when analysing the data. For example, at propulsion the shoe is held onto the foot by the laces or the upper, and this will create pressure and forces on the plantar surface of the foot when the foot is not applying load. The system still provides data on the load experienced by the plantar surface of the foot, but both the function of the foot and the shoe are being quantified. Synchronization

Table 1.9.2 Sample variables for analysis of pressure data

Parameter	What can it show you?	Clinical implication
Force–time curve	The peak forces underneath the foot over time frames throughout each footstep	Provides an idea of gait efficiency, lower limb symmetry
Peak pressure loading	Shows areas of high loading and where the foot is loading throughout the gait cycle	Can show foot biomechanical dysfunction by comparing loading pattern with the normal events of the gait cycle
Centre of pressure	Where the pressure is progressing through the foot throughout the footstep	Can indicate excessive lateral and medial loading
Can indicate lower limb asymmetry
Pressure–time integral	Combines time and pressure parameters which provide information on how long the peak pressure is occurring	Can indicate for how long areas of peak pressure (e.g. under metatarsal heads) are being loaded

of the in-shoe pressure data with video footage is desirable as it makes it easier to identify the different phases of the gait cycle. Again, in-shoe pressure measurement systems do not measure frictional forces which are an important part of the propulsive phase of gait. There is also limited clinical research on the data analysis of some of the parameters examined in clinical practice.

One area which has been researched quite extensively is the use of in-shoe pressure analysis in diabetic medicine where areas of high and prolonged plantar loading can lead to tissue breakdown and ulceration due to poor tissue viability. In-shoe pressure analysis can be used to quantify these areas of high pressure and show the degree of off-loading or redistribution of pressure that an orthotic can create to protect the delicate areas of the foot.

The force data are very useful when analysing in-shoe gait to determine whether the shoe is providing sufficient shock absorption and also when analysing the different phases of gait, such as impact, mid-stance, and propulsion. The force–time curve is plotted on a graph for each footstep showing the changes in forces over time. The force–time curve can be analysed for step-to-step variation and lower limb symmetry, and can be used to track the forces through the contact, mid-stance, and propulsive phases. A force–time curve for good sagittal function is a double-peaked curve with clear differentiation between the different phases of gait. An example of a force–time curve is shown in Fig. 1.9.7.

Other parameters that can be assessed in clinical practice are changes in peak pressure during dynamic loading, the centre of pressure, contact time, and the mean pressure picture. Again, masks can be applied to the data to analyse certain areas of the foot; for example, the rearfoot section of the foot can be masked to look at heel loading patterns. When assessing the changes in peak pressure during dynamic loading, the loading pattern should be compared with what should be taking place during the events of the gait cycle described earlier in this chapter. For example, initial contact should take place on the lateral aspect of the heel; therefore loading should be seen in this area at this point in the gait cycle.

There are many more parameters that can be assessed, for example pressure–time integral, medial-lateral force indices, and time to peak pressure. However, analysis of many parameters can be time consuming and often confirms the findings previously described in

a clinical setting. The analysis software is often able to average all the footsteps and show a representation of an average of all of the footsteps; again, it is argued that looking at an average footstep does not necessarily represent a typical footstep since this step never actually occurred.

As with all the analysis tools described, there are limitations in using in-shoe pressure analysis, with the most important being that in-shoe pressure analysis is a 2D tool which is being used to analyse a 3D function. A huge number of variables affect the data, including step-to-step variation, movement of the foot in the shoe, wearing equipment which alters movement patterns, and variation in gait speed. An assessment of musculoskeletal structure and function should be carried out before in-shoe pressure data is analysed as the information is required to interpret the pressure data. The limited sampling rate of the data may also limit the application of in-shoe pressure analysis. Most commercially available systems sample at 50–100 Hz, which is generally adequate for walking but may not be sufficient if assessing running gait.

How can biomechanical dysfunction affect the gait cycle?

It is rare to find a person with a normal gait pattern and quantifying 'normal' has been shown to be difficult in the field of biomechanical research. Most people have some form of biomechanical dysfunction which can affect the way in which their musculoskeletal system functions, and it is important to consider that biomechanical dysfunction generally worsens with age so it is constantly changing and should be monitored over time. Gait analysis can identify and help quantify the way in which biomechanical dysfunction affects gait.

Decreased joint range of motion or inflexibility of muscles can alter normal movements in the gait cycle as well as joint hypermobility and muscle weakness. For example, if the ankle joint is restricted in motion, perhaps because of calf muscle inflexibility, compensation may occur through subtalar joint pronation (to achieve more dorsiflexion) or the knee may compensate by flexing more during the gait cycle. These gait compensations will be visible during gait. Similarly if a first MTP joint is reduced in dorsiflexion, propulsive mechanics will be affected and an abductory twist or excessive inversion or eversion of the foot may be noticed at push-off.

As previously emphasized, biomechanical assessment information is essential before analysing gait so that if gait compensations are observed, their causes may be predicted. For example, an excessively flexed knee position may be noticed at initial heel contact. This may be caused by inflexibility of the hamstring muscle group, weakness of the quadriceps to extend the knee fully, weakness of the hip flexors, or a combination of all these factors. Another example is the identification of a prolonged mid-stance phase of the foot with a delayed heel lift. This may be caused by weakness of the tibialis posterior muscle, weakness of the calf muscle, hypermobility of the subtalar joint, reduced ankle joint motion, or again a combination of all these factors.

Sometimes a large degree of step-to-step variation can be observed in gait, and this can be confusing when trying to determine gait features and potential gait dysfunctions or compensations. Step-to-step variation can be related to biomechanical

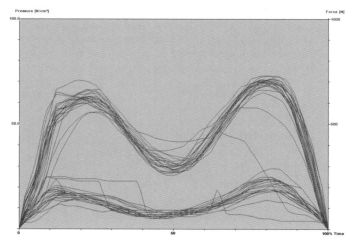

Fig. 1.9.7 A sample force–time curve.

dysfunction, for example poor core stability where recruitment of stability muscles is so weak or misfiring that the person is unable to create a controlled repetitive movement pattern. Gait features that are often observed together with a large degree of step-to-step variation are an abducted base of gait, excessive arm abduction, and excessive pelvic motion during gait. Proprioception should also be assessed together with biomechanical dysfunction.

Factors affecting gait

Numerous factors should be taken into consideration when assessing gait in a clinical setting. The speed of gait can affect the gait pattern markedly, so that if gait is assessed during very slow walking more instability features, such as step-step variation and a wide base of gait, may be noticed than for someone walking at a faster pace. The gait cycle relies on momentum and inertia, and therefore if not enough momentum is generated during gait, stability measures are taken by the central nervous system at the level of the brain. Therefore it is important to ask the patient to walk at their preferred speed during gait analysis so that compensations do not occur.

Another factor which can affect gait is the environment in which a patient is walking. For example, gait can often deteriorate if the patient is walking on an uneven path or walkway or when asked to walk on a treadmill with which they are unfamiliar. Open spaces or crowded pavements or corridors can also create changes in gait, as can different footwear which can either ease or impede gait depending on the type of footwear and what is optimum for the patient.

As already mentioned, biomechanical dysfunction can affect gait and compensation for this should be identified during gait analysis. Fatigue is another factor that can affect gait; for example, if a patient is asked to walk further than they can normally manage, gait can change. It can be useful to observe this clinically as it can provide information on the mechanism of injury. The final factor, which is perhaps the most important factor, is pain. If the patient is in pain when walking, gait compensations which mask the mechanism of injury may occur. For example, if the patellofemoral joint is being aggravated by poor knee stability due to weakness of the gluteus medius and quadriceps muscles, the patient may recruit other muscles to stabilize the knee and protect the joint. This may create a limp in the gait pattern and, as a consequence, instability around the knee may not be identified. Similarly, if excessive foot pronation has overloaded the plantar fascia and created plantar fasciitis pain, the patient may walk with a supinated gait to reduce the load on the plantar fascia and 'protect' the area. The pronatory cause of the plantar fasciitis will not be identified during gait analysis.

Conclusion

Writing in 2002, Whittle stated that gait analysis had 'come of age', being routinely used as a clinical tool for assessment of patients, particularly those with cerebral palsy. He expressed the desire that, following its success in this application, the use of gait analysis would spread to other patient groups. Certainly gait analysis is increasingly available for the assessment of walking gait for different patient groups, and the increased experience of practitioners in the interpretation and use of data obtained from gait analysis will further increase its application. Despite this availability, many practitioners are unable to make optimum use of gait reports because of either their limited experience with this type of data or, frequently, the unnecessary complexity of the gait report.

Sheldon (2005) questions whether gait analysis has come of age. This author highlights that gait analysis is not sufficiently exploited in clinical applications and that this is only likely to come about through the development of more user-friendly interfaces and clearer explanations of key data. With improved data collection and processing procedures, it is anticipated that gait analysis will become a routine feature of health checks in the future, particularly in specific clinical population groups and elite athletes.

References

Bus, S.A. and de Lange, A. (2005). A comparison of the 1-step, 2-step, and 3-step protocols for obtaining barefoot plantar pressure data in the diabetic neuropathic foot. *Clinical Biomechanics*, **20**, 892–9.

Giacomozzi, C. and Martelli, F. (2006). Peak pressure curve: an effective parameter for early detection of foot dysfunctional impairments in diabetic patients. *Gait and Posture*, **23**, 464–70.

Harrison, A.J. and Folland, J.P. (1997). Investigation of gait protocols for plantar pressure measurement of non-pathological subjects using a dynamic pedobarograph. *Gait and Posture*, **6**, 50–5.

Riley, P.O., Paolini, G., Croce, U.D., Paylo, K.W., and Kerrigan, D.C. (2007). A kinematic and kinetic comparison of overground and treadmill walking in healthy subjects. *Gait and Posture*, **26**, 17–24.

Schmiegel, A., Rosenbaum, D., Schorat, A., Hilker, A., and Gaubitz, M. (2008). Assessment of foot impairment in rheumatoid arthritis patients by dynamic pedobarography. *Gait and Posture*, **27**, 110–14.

Sheldon, S.R. (2005). Quantification of human motion: gait analysis—benefits and limitations to its application to clinical problems. *Journal of Biomechanics*, **37**, 1869–80.

Wearing, S.C., Urry, S., Smeathers, J.E., and Battistutta, D. (1999). A comparison of gait initiation and termination methods for obtaining plantar foot pressures. *Gait and Posture*, **10**, 255–63.

Whittle, M. (2002). *Gait Analysis: An Introduction*. Butterworth Heinemann, Oxford.

1.10

Epidemiology and injury surveillance in sports medicine

John Orchard, Hugh Seward, and Wayne Hoskins

Basis for injury surveillance in sport

Injury surveillance has for many years been considered fundamental to injury prevention in sport (van Mechelen *et al.* 1992; van Mechelen 1997; Finch 2006). The seminal paper by van Mechelen and colleagues in 1992 described a sequence for achieving injury prevention in sport, with injury surveillance typically being the fundamental first step behind the injury prevention process. Despite this observation, there has been little agreement about the best methodology for injury surveillance and few published examples in the literature of long-term multi-recorder reliable injury surveillance systems.

Advancements on the van Mechelen paradigm have been described, including the Translating Research into Injury Prevention Practice (TRIPP) paradigm (Table 1.10.1) (Finch 2006). This new paradigm correctly points out that it is not enough to have an understanding of reversible risk factors from scientific studies. The risk factors must also be reversible in the 'real world' and, even then, sports governing bodies must support the implementation of policies designed to reduce risk. These steps should not be trivialized when we consider the delay of decades between the knowledge that smoking was a major health hazard and belated government intervention to reduce its prevalence.

The largest hurdle with respect to the van Mechelen process is actually the first—achieving reliable long-term injury surveillance. It has only been in very recent years that individual researchers and research groups working in particular sports have banded together

to attempt to produce consensus statements (Orchard *et al.* 2005; Fuller *et al.* 2006, 2007) rather than persisting with differing, and often incompatible, definitions. Even now, these consensus statements have not yet been properly tested for reliability (Fuller 2007).

Nevertheless the basic van Mechelen formula should be robust enough to ensure eventual success in preventing sports injuries. There is no reason to believe that sports injuries will permanently defy prevention with a scientific approach (surveillance/risk factors/ interventions) similar to that successful in preventing conditions as diverse as traffic accidents and cardiovascular disease (Orchard 2008). The New Zealand government body entitled the Accident Compensation Corporation (ACC) (http://www.acc.co.nz/index.htm) is probably the world's most prominent example of successful implementation of such an approach, demonstrating substantial injury and cost savings from programmes applied to an entire country (Gianotti and Hume 2007).

Definition of an injury

It has been very difficult to achieve a universal definition of an injury in sport (Noyes *et al.* 1988). Many definitions require time to be lost from matches/competition or training for an injury to be considered significant (Meeuwisse and Love 1997). These definitions may exclude certain injuries such as minor concussions or lacerations. Injuries have also been defined by their presentation to medical care. These forms of definition make comparisons between studies and groups within studies difficult, as there is much variation in injury rates based on threshold of presentation (Orchard and Hoskins 2007).

A broad injury definition adopted as early as 1986 by the European Council of Football in Holland is 'any injury acquired during a game or practice, causing one or more of the following: reduction of activity, the need for treatment or medical advice and/ or negative social and economic consequences' (Schmidt-Olsen *et al.* 1991). This definition would potentially capture far more conditions than one based on activity reductions alone, but may lead to serious difficulties in compliance. Some experts have suggested that an injury should be based on anatomical 'proof' of tissue damage (Mitchell and Hayen 2005). Again, this is based on a sound theoretical argument but is difficult to comply with in practice. The three most common ways to define an injury are summarized in Table 1.10.2.

Table 1.10.1 TRIPP framework (developed from van Mechelen)

Stages of injury prevention (TRIPP)	van Mechelen stage
1. Injury surveillance	Stage 1
2. Establish aetiology and mechanisms of injury	Stage 2
3. Develop possible preventive measures	Stage 3
4. 'Ideal conditions' scientific evaluation of preventive programmes	Not included
5. Describe implementation of preventive programmes in 'real world'	Not included
6. Monitor success of intervention	Stage 4

Source: Finch 2006

Table 1.10.2 Comparison of injury definitions

Method of definition	Advantage	Disadvantage	Relative injury rate
Time loss from competition (and/or practice) only	Objective, reliable, can be independently verified (if game time only is used)	Excludes from definition some injuries which are considered significant (e.g. mild concussion, lacerations)	Lower than the 'true' injury rate but a reliable measure; can be used for comparative studies
Injuries which require medical treatment	Inclusive of the full spectrum of 'significant' injuries	Final rate is very user dependent (on the role that medical care has within a team and compliance with any study)	Higher rate which is closer to the 'real' injury rate but perhaps unreliable and subjective
Anatomical 'tissue' diagnosis	Most objective	Very costly and impractical for all injuries at this stage; may be used when studying one injury type only	Can be compared with other studies using the same imaging protocol in single-injury studies

Meeuwisse and Love (1997) stated what is an obvious but often overlooked point: 'Few, if any, [injury surveillance] systems will be capable of capturing all [defined] injuries. Recognising this, it is important to estimate the direction and extent of bias introduced by under-reporting'. The authors of one long-standing injury surveillance system, conducted on the professional Australia Football League (AFL) competition, assert that they achieve 100% compliance (Orchard and Seward 2002). They suggest that this is because the definition of injury equates (only) to conditions causing a match to be missed, with defined injury episodes recorded by reporters who are independent of the data collectors at each club. The AFL itself requires information on which players miss matches through injury for the purposes of checking compliance with the competition salary cap. Because of the independent checking of defined injuries, the authors claim that the annual survey does in fact capture 100% of defined injuries and is therefore reliable (Orchard and Hoskins 2007).

'Missed match only' injury definitions are used in other sports such as rugby league (Gissane *et al.* 2002; Hoskins *et al.* 2006), but have not generally not been used in football (soccer) because it is believed that such a definition does not capture important injuries (Hagglund *et al.* 2005; Brooks and Fuller 2006; Fuller *et al.* 2006). One study (McManus 2000) assessed intra- and inter-rater reliability of a data collection form in rugby union, but this study compared the data collection for defined events rather than which events passed the threshold for inclusion. There is one study in football (soccer) which compared a 'tissue damage' definition with 'training or match time loss' definition (Walden *et al.* 2005). This study, using the same recorders for two different definitions, found 765 injuries in total according to 'tissue damage' and 715 injuries in total according to the 'time loss' definition and concluded that there was 'no significant difference in the risk for injury between tissue injuries and time-loss injuries'. Our view is that this study clearly shows that either or most probably both of these injury definitions are *not* reliable, as quite obviously a definition based on 'tissue damage' *should* yield a *far greater* injury incidence than one based on 'time loss from training or matches', since in all codes of football it is very common for a player to suffer symptomatic tissue damage but continue to train and play. This study suggests to us that the ability of medical recorders to accurately capture injuries at the mild end of the spectrum is extremely limited.

A practical way to ask whether an injury definition is reliable is: 'If, say, the team doctor and team physiotherapist both had to

independently determine which conditions met the criteria for a survey injury, would they provide exactly the same list?' (Orchard and Hoskins 2007). Without even needing to test the hypothesis further, it is clear that definitions which rely on either radiological abnormalities or medical presentations are probably inherently biased (Hagglund *et al.* 2005). If the team doctor consulted players for 80 distinct injuries over the season, but the team physiotherapist consulted players for 180 injuries over the same season, the inter-recorder reliability between the two based on a medical presentation definition would be very poor. If football team A decides to use MRI routinely (i.e. for most injuries and for 'screening') whereas football team B only uses MRI when a clinical diagnosis is in doubt, it may appear as if team A has a higher injury incidence than team B. This does not mean that these injury definitions should never be used, just that they are not reliable tools for injury surveillance where the objective is to reliably compare injury rates between different teams and/or seasons. If an administrator or insurance company is budgeting for professional service utilization, it is perfectly sensible to use a definition based on medical presentation (Meeuwisse and Love 1997), just as a study looking at the development of a gradual-onset overuse injury detected by radiological screening may appropriately base the definition on tissue damage (Cook *et al.* 2000).

In the sport of rugby league, a large number of studies have been performed using a definition of an injury requiring a 'missed match' (Gissane *et al.* 2002; Hoskins *et al.* 2006) Eight separate studies using the 'missed match' definition have found injury incidence rates of 34.4, 38.7, 39.8, 40.3, 44.0, 44.9, 45.5, and 52.3 injuries per 1000 player hours, strongly suggesting that these studies are directly comparable and therefore that such an injury definition is reliable. However, studies using broader definitions uncover far greater numbers of injuries but have wildly varying injury incidence rates, for example 114.3, 160.6, 346.0, and 824.7 injuries per 1000 player hours (Hoskins *et al.* 2006). Although these studies had slight variations in their definition of an injury, all were 'tissue damage/any medical presentation' definitions and therefore might have been expected to yield similar injury incidence. In rugby league sevens, two studies from New Zealand and Australia using exactly the same 'medical presentation' definition found injury incidences of 497.6 and 283.5 injuries per 1000 player hours (King *et al.* 2006) which, given that the sports were played under the same rules, suggests that methodological limitations were responsible for the large discrepancy between studies.

However, there are some legitimate criticisms of an injury definition based on missed match time only (Orchard and Hoskins 2007).

1. It is not particularly useful for individual sports where competition only occurs rarely (e.g. track and field, gymnastics, swimming).

2. It subjects the threshold for reporting injuries to a bias when the time between matches deviates from a standard schedule (e.g. one game per week).

3. There is a strong bias against defined injuries occurring in the last match of a season, as there are no further matches available to be missed.

4. Players who use painkillers (including local anaesthetic injections) to play are not considered 'injured' if they never miss a match.

5. It may encourage data collectors, in the interests of efficiency, to only record injuries on a weekly basis (i.e. when it has been determined that a match has been missed) rather than on the day of injury occurrence. Theoretically, there may be some loss of accuracy for some components of data collection (e.g. injury mechanism) because of the delay of a few days if weekly rather than daily injury recording is made.

6. Some healthcare resources (e.g. treatment costs) must still be devoted to injuries which do not cause missed playing time, and indeed quality treatment may allow a player to continue participation with an injury which normally would have caused missed playing time.

7. Including the examples above, there are injuries of some importance which are not captured by such a definition, for example injuries that still allow a player to continue during a season, but require surgery and rehabilitation when the season is completed.

Despite the criticisms listed above, the most important injuries from a player's (and team's) perspective tend to be those which cause missed match time. From the perspective of injury surveillance where comparisons between teams (different recorders) are to be made, all injuries are important, but for the purposes of comparison, it is most important that the recording is reliable.

A broad definition, which eliminated some or all these described limitations, would be superior presuming it could be implemented with reliability (Hodgson *et al.* 2007). However, the broader alternatives may lack the demonstrated reliability to be useful as consensus or comparison definitions in team sports (Orchard and Hoskins 2007). Broad definitions are currently more suitable for individual sports, single-team studies not planning comparison with other studies, and studies which focus on a single injury category, particularly those injuries which do not necessarily cause missed playing time (e.g. facial lacerations, concussion). The debate about whether broad or narrow definitions are superior (Fig. 1.10.1) for team sports hinges on whether the ideal alternative (broad) is reliable in the real world (Orchard and Hoskins 2007; Hodgson *et al.* 2007).

Injury rates: incidence and exposure

Injury incidence is a measurement of the number of injuries presenting in a defined population over a certain time period.

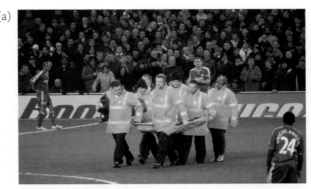

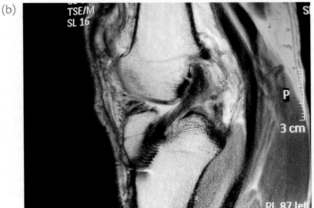

Fig. 1.10.1 Injury definitions can be based on either (a) loss of participation time and medical presentation or (b) actual tissue damage (irrespective of effect on competition).

The numerator in a calculation of injury incidence is the number of defined injuries occurring, relying on the definition of injury previously discussed. Unfortunately, there are also substantial methodological considerations when choosing the denominator for determining injury incidence. These involve selection of both the population exposure and the time exposure.

The simplest choice for cohort is the entire population. Knowing, for example, the number of anterior cruciate ligament (ACL) injuries which occur in a given country in a given year can allow the generation of a population ACL incidence rate. This would be expressed in the unit of number of ACL injuries per person per year. However, a disadvantage is that this does not take into account the relative exposure of individuals within the population. If the population incidence of ACL injuries changes over time, it is difficult to assess whether this is due to certain sports becoming more risky or simply more of the population being exposed to a particular sport.

If a cohort less than the entire population is desired for study, which is usual, decisions must be made as to who is part of the cohort and what the criteria are for joining or leaving it.

Time at risk also presents a dilemma, particularly for training. Match exposure is usually relatively straightforward, as matches last for a defined period of time. However, there are still issues, such as whether a player should be considered exposed to injury when not on the playing field but otherwise engaging in match duties (such as a baseball pitcher warming up in the 'bull pen'). Another consideration is whether exposure time should include 'added time' such as the time taken for stoppages or injuries.

With respect to training, a difficulty is that training is less structured than a match. A training 'session' may occur at a team's training venue over a period of, say, 3 hours, but certain individuals may be actually engaged in physical training for varying proportions of that time. Alternatively, athletes may complete individual training away from the group or team, making recording problematic. The most difficult dilemma is that regarding injuries which have an insidious onset, such as tendinopathies and stress fractures. Should they be considered to be match injuries, training injuries, or both, given that loading during both match time and training time has contributed to the development of the injury? These considerations can be debated and a universal decision made as part of a consensus statement for that sport (Orchard et al. 2005; Fuller et al. 2006, 2007).

With the options available, it is possible to report injury incidence alternatively as follows.

1. For specific activities, such as matches or training, in units of 'injuries occurring per x player hours' for those specific activities.

2. For all injuries, as an annual or seasonal injury incidence, once the cohort and length of season has been defined, in units of 'injuries occurring per team/squad (of x players) per season (of duration y)'.

Although injury incidence has generally been recorded using the former method (match or training injuries per player hour of exposure), future studies may shift towards an approach of preferring a seasonal incidence measurement. Bahr (2009) has written that many gradual-onset overuse injuries are not able to be adequately measured if authors insist on focussing on injuries with an acute onset. Orchard et al (2009) have found that the apparent onset of overuse injuries in cricket is three to four weeks after the aggravating event. If the injuries are assigned to the match or training session in which symptoms first appeared, the actual aggravating factors may be overlooked. Finally injury incidence must be defined as referring to new injuries only, recurrent injuries only, or new and recurrent injuries combined. It is usually a default for injury incidence to refer to new injuries only, if it is not specified. A 'recurrence rate' can be the proportion of the incidence of recurrent injuries to the incidence of new (or combined) injuries.

Injury rates: injury prevalence and severity

Incidence is the number of new occurrences of an injury (or disease) for a defined population over a defined time period. However, this rate does not take into account injury severity. Based on incidence, sprained ankles (for example) are far more common than knee ACL injuries in most sports, yet knee ACL injuries may extract a relatively greater toll on the individual athletes as their severity (per injury) is much greater.

Average injury severity (often defined as average time loss per individual injury) is a concept which is agreed to by most authors (Fuller 2007) and considered important to record.

The injury rate which is the product of incidence and severity is also considered important, but there is conjecture about the best term to use to describe this concept. Fuller prefers the term injury risk (therefore risk = incidence × severity)(Fuller 2007), whereas Orchard and others prefer the term injury prevalence (therefore prevalence = incidence × severity) (Lower 1995; Orchard and Seward 2002; Orchard et al. 2006).

A difficulty with the use of the term 'risk' is that it can be confused with concepts like risk ratios, which refer to incidence only. A difficulty with the use of the term 'prevalence' is that in epidemiology, prevalence sometimes refers to this concept ('point prevalence' or the percentage of the population with a condition at any given time) but sometimes does not ('period prevalence' or the rate at which the population will suffer from a condition over a time period, including a sum of the onset of new cases and pre-existing ongoing cases). We suggest that prevalence in sport is most easily expressed in percentage terms (the proportion of athletes in a cohort suffering from an injury at any given time). Therefore prevalence is therefore proportional to incidence and severity.

Unfortunately, even when expressed in these simple terms, prevalence is subject to the same considerations as can be applied to the definition of an injury. Should the prevalence of patellar tendinopathy in a basketball team be:

(1) the percentage of players who are unable to play basketball at any given time, due to patellar tendinopathy?

(2) the percentage of players who are limited in either a match or training situation by patellar tendinopathy at any given time?

(3) the percentage of players who are currently suffering from patellar tendon pain at any given time?

(4) the percentage of players who have an abnormal patellar tendon on imaging at any given time?

Obviously the debate about which of the suggestions for prevalence is the 'true' prevalence of patellar tendinopathy has analogous arguments to the debate about what actually defines an injury. In a similar outcome to the debate on definition of an injury, the best answer may depend on the context of the question. When studying a specific injury (like patellar tendinopathy) it may be most appropriate to use a symptomatic or tissue damage definition. When trying to compare overall injury prevalence between teams and between different competitions, it is probably more reliable to use a prevalence method based on inability to play matches. In professional athletes, the prevalence of any symptom of pain at any given time probably approaches 100% and therefore becomes relatively meaningless. It is far more relevant to compare a prevalence figure of, say, 15% of the squad being unavailable for selection through injury with other squads or years.

Prevalence is quite commonly reported in general medical studies but rarely in sporting injury papers (Lower 1995). This may be because of the difficulty in a sporting population of monitoring an entire cohort prospectively over a period of time, which must be done to measure average prevalence accurately.

A dilemma for those researchers reporting on prevalence is how to deal with an athlete who leaves a cohort (i.e. decides to stop playing a certain sport) if the reason for leaving is injury itself. An athlete with an enforced injury retirement, who is thereby eliminated from the cohort under study, is not considered by prevalence measures, which means that an extra measure may be required to fully understand the impact of injury.

Injury cost is usually proportional to prevalence, although it is not generally reported in scientific papers. It is most relevant to insurance companies who deal with sporting injuries, although these companies do not tend to report their balance sheets in the scientific literature.

Injury rates: permanent impairment and retirement from sport

'Rate of sporting retirement through injury' is another measure that has rarely been reported in the scientific literature, although it is known to be high in professional American football (Pitts and Popovich 1993). When comparing sporting injuries with medical illnesses this is an important measurement, which is analogous to mortality, whereas injury incidence and prevalence are analogous to morbidity. A related injury measure, which has more often been reported, is the incidence of long-term disability (e.g. major joint osteoarthritis) subsequent to retirement from sport (Deacon et al. 1997; Nicholas et al. 2007; Oztürk et al. 2008).

Injury classification

The gold standard for classification of medical conditions is the International Classification of Diseases (ICD). However, ICD codes have rarely been used in sports medicine for classification as they contain a huge amount of detail for diagnoses that are not needed but very little detail for the common diagnoses in sports medicine. The earliest comprehensive system published in the sports medicine field was the National Athletic Injury/Illness Reporting System (NAIRS) Medical Terminology Codebook (Levy 1988). This system has been used by many sports in North America but has not been extensively taken up worldwide, possibly for copyright reasons. The Orchard Sports Injury Classification System (OSICS) was specifically developed for the AFL injury survey (Orchard 1993, 1995). This attempted to provide codes that were simple and user-friendly (important in the early stages of the study when there was paper recording) but with enough detail to give specific independent medical diagnoses. A major influence on the development of codes within OSICS was the publication of two Australian general sports medicine textbooks (Brukner and Khan 1993; Bloomfield et al. 1995). It was felt that diagnoses which warranted a discrete paragraph in textbooks of this level should have their own discrete injury code. The codes were also designed so that they reflected the body part and the pathology type. Therefore they can be collated to give the injury rate by body part and injury type.

OSICS has been expanded since the original version; this has been done as systems have become partially or fully computerized and the need for diagnostic detail has taken precedence over the need for brevity on a printed sheet (Rae and Orchard 2007; Orchard et al. 2010). On returning to the realm of the printed page in a report, the value of being concise is very important. OSICS has many hundred individual codes and therefore reports should not attempt to produce a table with every OSICS code as a row heading. However, OSICS has become popular internationally, mainly because of its copyright-free status and availability for download on the Internet (http://www.injuryupdate.com.au/research/OSICS. htm).

A further sport-specific injury classification system known as the Sport Medicine Diagnostic Coding System (SMDCS) was developed in 1991 and has been used extensively in the North American setting (Meeuwisse and Wiley 2007). It has been mapped to the consensus categories proposed by the international definitions for football and rugby injuries, which will possibly lead to greater uptake worldwide.

Injury mechanism and risk factor assessment

Injury mechanism and risk factors are critical for understanding injury causation and therefore creating hypotheses for prevention (Bahr and Krosshaug 2005). However, injury mechanism is a further area which is difficult to define and classify. Bahr and Krosshaug have described how many factors combine to create the 'injury environment' including player factors, game/opponent factors, rules, biomechanics, etc. As can be seen from Table 1.10.3, a description of injury mechanics needs to be sports specific.

Consensus definitions and universal components of an injury surveillance system

In order to best be able to compare injury rates between different studies, it has been recommended that consensus definitions for various sports be developed (Orchard et al. 2005; Fuller et al. 2006, 2007). To date, four international consensus statements have been published on injury definitions in cricket (Orchard et al. 2005), football (soccer) (Fuller et al. 2006), rugby union (Fuller et al. 2007) and tennis (Pluim et al. 2009). In addition, recommendations for data collections have been made in rugby league (King et al. 2009) and Olympic sports (Junge et al. 2008). Consensus statements face many challenges, including determining standards for exposure time and choice of cohorts. However, the most difficult dilemma for consensus statements is the proposed injury definition for surveillance systems in team sports. Consensus statements should encourage assessment for reliability and functionality of the definitions. In order to be useful in a consensus statement any proposed injury definition should be highly reliable. If it is not, the original problem of inability to make a proper comparison between different teams, seasons, and studies has not been solved by the use of the consensus definition.

Cricket, one of the sports with published consensus definitions (Orchard et al. 2005), based this on slight modifications from a successful surveillance system with a narrow injury definition and apparent long-term reliability (based on low standard deviations in injury incidence between teams) (Orchard et al. 2006). The few published injury incidence rates of different studies using the consensus definitions show compatible results (Mansingh et al. 2006; Orchard et al. 2006). Football (soccer) and rugby have chosen to use broader definitions, which will capture more injury events but may lead to issues in reliability. Future publications can be assessed to help determine whether the goal of reliability has been achieved by these definitions.

Most of the useful components of an injury reporting system were described as early as 20 years ago (Lindenfeld et al. 1988) (Table 1.10.4). As discussed in this chapter, this plan is essentially correct, but its simplicity does not give an accurate picture of the difficulty in standardizing each stage of the process. Some of the problems which may be encountered have been described previously (Hunter and Levy 1988) and include:

◆ self-selection of players into certain groups may bias results (e.g. ankle-taping)

Table 1.10.3 Categories of injury mechanism descriptions with examples of elements and descriptions

Category	Elements	Examples of factors describing the injury mechanism			
		Non-contact ACL injury in basketball	ACL injury a mogul skiing jump landing	Knock-out in boxing	Lower leg stress fracture in football
Playing (sports) situation	Team action	Fast break	Course steepness	Uppercut, hook	Exposure to matches and training (total load)
	Skill performed before and at the point of injury	Zone defence	Jump elements (e.g. twist, helicopter)	Counter-attack	Midfielder with defensive and offensive tasks (i.e. many runs in matches and training)
	Court position	Charging	Jump height and length	Foot work	Hard-working team
	Player position	Cutting		Forced into the corner/to the ropes	Frequency of duels
	Ball handling	Setting up for a shot		Ring-side referee decision	
		Defensive rebound		Inter-boxer distance	
		Man-to-man defence			
Athlete/opponent behaviour	Player performance	Effort	Rhythm and balance before the jump	Awareness	Effort
	Opponent interaction	Disturbance by opponent	Concentration	Aggressiveness	Toe–heel runner
	Player attention	Intention	Balance	Punching power	Jumping technique
		Foot firmly fixed to the floor	Boot binding release	Punching speed	Duel technique
		Intention	Visual control	Balance	
		Technical foul	Jumping technique		
			Over-rotation		
			Falling technique		
Whole-body biomechanics	Coarse description, often static, of whole body kinematics and kinetics	Sideways translation	Linear and angular momentum	Centre-of-mass velocity	Stride length
		Rotation of the body around the fixed foot	Energy absorption	Punching force	Stride frequency
		Speed at impact	Centre of mass to the rear	Punching direction	Vertical excursion
		Foot in front of centre of mass		Weight distribution on the legs	Ground reaction forces
					Knee flexion angle
Joint/tissue biomechanics	Detailed description of joint/tissue kinematics and kinetics	Valgus moment	Shear forces	Energy transfer	Bending moment
		Pivot shift of the tibia relative to the femur	Anterior drawer	Head acceleration	Shear forces
		Notch impingement	Intercondylar lift-off, loading rate	Pressure distribution and localization	Surface/shoe dynamics

Reproduced wih permission from Bahr, R. and Krosshaug, T. (2005). *British Journal of Sports Medicine*, **39**, 324–9.

Table 1.10.4 Components of injury reporting systems

Component		Description
I	Population	Defining a cohort (e.g. player roster) is important to ascertain the denominator of the injury rates
II	Injury rate	Defining injuries and time-at risk is important to give an accurate rate
III	Injury conditions	Reporting of injury mechanism gives general information, but studying risk factors for all players (injured and non-injured) is needed to ascertain causation
IV	Injury	An injury classification system is needed to divide injuries into categories
V	Treatment	Tests, surgery, medications, etc. are all useful to survey
VI	Results	Results may be reported by (a) time loss, (b) tissue damage, or (c) permanent impairment

Summarized from Lindenfeld *et al.* (1988)

- observational bias can occur between different teams
- difficulty in controlling retrospective associations with injury
- compliance if information requested is tedious or too onerous
- difficulty with compliance if forms are not pretested
- bias introduced by players dropping out of study
- recall bias if information is not completed at the time of injury
- funding sources may diminish as results take a long time to produce.

A review of the major injury surveillance systems in use in North America (USA and Canada) found that they have evolved over the past two decades (Meeuwisse and Love 1997). The designs used have been case series (1970s onwards), cohort design with exposure estimation (1980s onwards), and cohort design with exposure measurement (1990s onwards). Future evolution will be into cohort design studies with exposure measurement using consensus definitions tested for reliability.

References

Bahr, R. (2009). No injuries, but plenty of pain? On the methodology for recording overuse symptoms in sports. *Br. J. Sports Med.*, **43**(13), 966–72.

Bahr, R. and Krosshaug, T. (2005). Understanding injury mechanisms: a key component of preventing injuries in sport. *British Journal of Sports Medicine*, **39**, 324–9.

Bloomfield, J., Fricker, P., and Fitch, K. (eds) (1995). *Textbook of Science and Medicine in Sport*, Blackwell, Melbourne.

Brooks, J. and Fuller, C. (2006). The influence of methodological issues on the results and conclusions from epidemiological studies of sports injuries: illustrative examples. *Sports Medicine*, **36**, 459–472.

Brukner, P. and Khan, K. (1993) *Clinical Sports Medicine*. McGraw-Hill, Sydney.

Cook, J.L., Khan, K.M., Kiss, Z.S., Purdam, C.R., and Griffiths, L. (2000) Prospective imaging study of asymptomatic patellar tendinopathy in elite junior basketball players. *Journal of Ultrasound Medicine*, **19**, 473–9.

Deacon, A., Bennell, K., Kiss, Z., Crossley, K., and Brukner, P. (1997). Osteoarthritis of the knee in retired, elite Australian Rules footballers. *Medical Journal of Australia*, **166**, 187–90.

Finch, C. (2006). A new framework for research leading to sports injury prevention. *Journal of Science and Medicine in Sport*, **9**, 3–9.

Fuller, C. (2007). Managing the risk of injury in sport. *Clinical Journal of Sport Medicine*, **17**, 182–7.

Fuller, C., Molloy, M., Bagate, C., *et al.* (2007). Consensus statement on injury definitions and data collection procedures for studies of injuries in rugby union. *Clinical Journal of Sport Medicine*, **17**, 177–181.

Fuller, C., Ekstrand, J., Junge, A., *et al.* (2006). Consensus statement on injury definitions and data collection procedures in studies of football (soccer) injuries. *British Journal of Sports Medicine*, **40**, 193–201.

Gianotti, S. and Hume, P. (2007). A cost–outcome approach to pre and post-implementation of national sports injury prevention programmes. *Journal of Science and Medicine in Sport*, **10**, 436–46.

Gissane, C., Jennings, D., Kerr, K., and White, J. (2002). A pooled data analysis of injury incidence in rugby league football. *Sports Medicine*, **32**, 211–16.

Hagglund, M., Walden, M., Bahr, R., and Ekstrand, J. (2005). Methods for epidemiological study of injuries to professional football players: developing the UEFA model. *British Journal of Sports Medicine*, **39**, 340–6.

Hodgson, L., Gissane, C., Gabbett, T., and King, D. (2007). For debate: Consensus injury definitions in team sports should focus on encompassing all injuries. *Clinical Journal of Sport Medicine*, **17**, 188–191.

Hoskins, W., Pollard, H., Hough, K., and Tully, C. (2006). Injury in rugby league: a review. *Journal of Science and Medicine in Sport*, **9**, 46–56.

Hunter, R. and Levy, I. (1988). Vignettes. *American Journal of Sports Medicine*, **16**, S25–37.

Junge, A., Engebretsen, L., Alonso, J.M. *et al.* (2008). Injury surveillance in multi-sport events: the international Olympic Committee approach. *Br. J. Sports Med.*, **42**(6), 413–21.

King, D., Gabbett, T., Dreyer, C., and Gerrard, D. (2006). Incidence of injuries in the New Zealand National Rugby League Sevens Tournament. *Journal of Science and Medicine in Sport*, **9**, 110–18.

King, D.A., Gabbett, T.J., Gissane, C., Hodgson, L. (2009). Epidemiological studies of injuries in rugby league: suggestions for definitions, data collection and reporting methods. *J. Sci. Med. Sport*, **12**(1), 12–19.

Levy, I. (1988). Formation and sense of the NAIRS athletic injury surveillance system. *American Journal of Sports Medicine*, **16**, S132–3, S201–21.

Lindenfeld, T., Noyes, F., and Marshall, M. (1988). Components of injury reporting systems. *American Journal of Sports Medicine*, **16**, S69–80.

Lower, T. (1995). Injury data collection in the rugby codes. *Australian Journal of Science and Medicine in Sport*, **27**, 43–7.

McManus, A. (2000). Validation of an instrument for injury data collection in rugby union. *British Journal of Sports Medicine*, **34**, 342–7.

Mansingh, A., Harper, L., Headley, S., King-Mowatt, J., and Mansingh, G. (2006). Injuries in West Indies Cricket 2003–2004. *British Journal of Sports Medicine*, **40**, 119–23.

Meeuwisse, W. and Love, E. (1997). Athletic injury reporting: development of universal systems. *Sports Medicine*, **24**, 184–204.

Meeuwisse, W. and Wiley, J. (2007). The Sport Medicine Diagnostic Coding System. *Clinical Journal of Sport Medicine*, **17**, 205–207.

Mitchell, R. and Hayen, A. (2005). Defining a cricket injury. *Journal of Science and Medicine in Sport*, **8**, 357–8.

Nicholas, S., Nicholas, J., Nicholas, C., Diecchio, J., and McHugh, M. (2007). The health status of retired American football players: Super Bowl III revisited. *American Journal of Sports Medicine*, **35**, 1674–9.

Noyes, F., Lindenfeld, T., and Marshall, M. (1988). What determines an athletic injury (definition)? Who determines an injury? (occurrence). *American Journal of Sports Medicine*, **16**, S65–8.

Orchard, J. (1993). Orchard Sports Injury Classification System (OSICS). *Sport Health*, **11**, 39–41.

Orchard, J. (1995). Orchard Sports Injury Classification System (OSICS). In: J. Bloomfield, P. Fricker, and K. Fitch (eds), *Science and Medicine in Sport*, pp. 674–681. Blackwell, Melbourne.

Orchard, J. (2008). Preventing sports injuries at the national level: time for other nations to follow New Zealand's remarkable success. *British Journal of Sports Medicine*, **42**, 392–3.

Orchard, J. and Hoskins, W. (2007). For debate: Consensus injury definitions in team sports should focus on missed playing time. *Clinical Journal of Sport Medicine*, **17**, 192–6.

Orchard, J. and Seward, H. (2002). Epidemiology of injuries in the Australian Football League, seasons 1997–2000. *British Journal of Sports Medicine*, **36**, 39–45.

Orchard, J., Newman, D., Stretch, R., Frost, W., Mansingh, A., and Leipus, A. (2005). Methods for injury surveillance in international cricket. *Journal of Science and Medicine in Sport*, **8**, 1–14.

Orchard, J., James, T., and Portus, M. (2006). Injuries to elite male cricketers in Australia over a 10-year period. *Journal of Science and Medicine in Sport*, **9**, 459–467.

Orchard, J., James, T., Portus, M., Kountouris, A. and Dennis, R. (2009). Fast bowlers in cricket demostrate up to 3- to 4-week delay between high workloads and increased risk of injury. *Am. J. Sports Med.*, **37**(6), 1186–92.

Orchard, J., Rae, K., Brooks, J. *et al.* (2010). Revision, uptake and coding issues related to the open access Orchard Sports Injury Classification System (OSICS) versions 8,9 and 10.1. *Open Access Journal of Sports Medicine*, **Volume 1**, in press.

Oztürk, A., Ozkan, Y., Ozdemir, R., *et al.* (2008). Radiographic changes in the lumbar spine in former professional football players: a comparative and matched controlled study. *European Spine Journal*, **17**, 136–41.

Pitts, B. and Popovich, M. (1993). Aftermath of an NFL career: injuries. In: *American College of Sports Medicine Annual Conference*. National Football League Players Association, Seattle.

Pluim, B.M., Fuller, C.W., Batt, M.E. *et al.* (2009). Consensus statement on epidemiological studies of medical conditions in tennis, April 2009. *Br. J. Sports Med.*, **43**(12), 893–7.

Rae, K. and Orchard, J. (2007). The Orchard Sports Injury Classification System (OSICS) Version 10. *Clinical Journal of Sport Medicine*, **17**, 201–4.

Schmidt-Olsen, S., Jorgensen, U., Kaalund, S., *et al.* (1991). Injuries among young soccer players. *American Journal of Sports Medicine*, **19**, 273–5.

van Mechelen, W. (1997). Sports injury surveillance systems: 'one size fits all'? *Sports Medicine*, **24**, 164–168.

van Mechelen, W., Hlobil, H., and Kemper, H. (1992). Incidence, severity, aetiology and prevention of sports injuries: a review of concepts. *Sports Medicine*, **14**, 82–99.

Walden, M., Hagglund, M., and Ekstrand, J. (2005). Injuries in Swedish elite football—a prospective study on injury definitions, risk for injury and injury pattern during 2001. *Scandinavian Journal of Medicine and Science in Sports*, **15**, 118–25.

SECTION 2

Clinical principles

Assessment and management

Mike Hutson

Assessment of injury

Individuals undertaking exercise include those engaged in aerobic activities as part of a healthy lifestyle, those engaged in an active fitness or rehabilitation programme relevant to acute or chronic conditions such as cardiovascular disease, respiratory problems, and musculoskeletal disorders, and the committed competitive athlete with high performance targets. Accordingly, those injured as a consequence of exercise or sport attend medical practitioners in diverse circumstances. Urgency of assessment of the full impact of injury clearly varies across the spectrum from the life-threatening situation on the field of play (or other sports/recreational exercise location, for instance poolside or roadside) to one in which a chronic condition can be evaluated in the relative comfort of the clinician's consulting room. Irrespective of the circumstances, the primary requirement is the establishment of an accurate diagnosis. The process of assessment is aided when relevant by an appropriate index of suspicion with respect to those injuries that are not often seen outside sporting and recreational activity (e.g. throwers' elbow and shin splints). Diagnosis of tissue injury is followed by a full assessment of its impact on the function of the surrounding structures, and subsequently assessment of impairment of sporting capacity in general. Evaluation is made of the aetiological factors associated with the development of injury, the behavioural responses, including motivation and health prioritization, and the individual's standard of performance (actual and potential). Clinical assessment (and reassessment) is a constant theme throughout the text.

Assessment
Diagnosis of tissue damage—aided by history and clinical examination
Impact on surrounding anatomical structures
Functional impairment
Sporting capacity

It is regrettable that, within the clinical curriculum of the medical student and junior doctor, a limited amount of time is devoted to musculoskeletal problems, represented within the medical disciplines by orthopaedics, rheumatology, musculoskeletal medicine, and sports and exercise medicine. A paradox exists in that, although soft tissue problems of all kinds constitute a high proportion of the workload of doctors in general practice and in hospital-based traumatology or emergency medicine practice, there is little opportunity

during training to hone the skills required for examination of the musculoskeletal system. Therefore clinical examination procedures are described in some detail in this book. Historically, basic examination procedures for musculoskeletal complaints were laid down by, amongst others, James Cyriax in his *Textbook of Orthopaedic Medicine* (Cyriax 1982). The examination protocol devised by Cyriax, augmented by additional sport-specific tests, continues to be used by many clinicians. Alternatively, expansion of the traditional orthopaedic surgical or rheumatological examination protocol of 'look, feel, move' by the addition of techniques, often described as 'special tests', such as ligament stress testing and joint loading tests makes it possible to build from basic principles in an orderly fashion, thus reducing the likelihood of diagnostic error because of inadequate musculoskeletal examination.

The established sports physician is expected to have achieved and retained a high level of clinical diagnostic competency, predicated on manual examination skills. The budding and as yet inexperienced sports physician (and indeed the general public) may be forgiven for thinking that in the twenty-first century clinical evaluation takes second place to, or is subjugated by, technological investigation, particularly in view of the well-publicized high-tech medical diagnostic advances of recent years. In high-profile circumstances, for instance professional sports under constant gaze, MRI appears to have become an essential first-line tool. However, judicious use of such investigative aids should take second place to clinical examination predicated on a sound understanding of basic anatomy and physiology. *MRI is not a substitute for a good history and physical examination*. In general, imaging should only be undertaken to provide additional information, which is then considered in conjunction with the clinical examination findings. Controversially, some contemporary pedagogical strategies rely heavily on problem-solving (otherwise referred to as problem-based learning (PBL)), apparently to the detriment of acquisition of a sound knowledge of anatomy and functional pathology, and of pathophysiology. The sports and exercise medicine (SEM) practitioner, particularly the clinician who focuses on the musculoskeletal injury component of SEM, should not forget the benefits of a sound knowledge of functional anatomy and good manual diagnostic skills in the detection of tissue dysfunction.

Predisposing factors to injury

Acute injuries demand urgent clinical assessment, augmented if necessary by radiological or other investigations. Loss of function of the affected tissue or anatomical region may be substantive.

With severe soft tissue or neural injuries, neuromuscular compromise may cause profound and relatively obvious disability. Under other circumstances, additional clinical or laboratory-based tests must be performed to identify more subtle functional impairment. Commonly, the need is to translate diagnosis and functional loss into the most appropriate management strategy. The situation with chronic or 'overuse' injuries is equally challenging; in addition to anatomy, a basic knowledge of the **technical aspects** and **biomechanical forces** involved in sporting activities is required. By way of illustration, track athletes run anticlockwise both in their events and during training, so that asymmetrical forces are continually being applied to their lower limbs in particular. Javelin throwers may have an overhead style, or tend to sling; the forces applied to their shoulders and elbows are different in the two styles. Tennis players may use a single- or a two-handed backhand, imposing different stresses on the trunk and upper limbs, and so on. Numerous examples of the physical forces applied to the body during exercise and sport are given throughout this book. Technical factors are particularly relevant when considering overuse injury. The reader is referred to Table 3.11.2 in Chapter 3.11 for an example of factors that need to be considered during the analysis of overuse injuries. It is helpful to categorize **predisposing factors** as 'intrinsic' and 'extrinsic', although many injuries are the consequence of the interaction of factors from both groups.

An example of an **intrinsic factor** is abnormal joint mobility some (anatomical) distance away from the site of injury. A squash player with a limited range of hip rotation as a result of early degenerative disease may develop low back pain when excessive rotational stress is transferred repeatedly to the lumbar spine. Weakness or tightness of one group of muscles acting about a joint may result in injury elsewhere. For instance, tight hamstrings may be responsible for low back problems or for injury to compensating muscle groups. Age and gender affect injury predisposition.

Extrinsic factors that contribute to injury are also explored in greater detail in the individual chapters which follow. Training schedules, playing surfaces, and the quality and appropriateness of protective devices (e.g. gum shields and visors) and equipment, including footwear, racquets, and bicycles, should be investigated and documented where relevant. Although 'holistic' medicine is enjoying much popularity in the twenty-first century, it has surely always been incumbent upon medical practitioners to develop a breadth of vision for every patient—a facet of their skills in which they are trained from the first weeks of the clinical curriculum in medical school. Sports injuries need no less perspicacity than other medical conditions that are recognizably 'stress' related. When injuries in children are considered, the relationship and interactions between the expectations and ambitions of the patient, parents, coaches, and teachers become even more important.

History

The history given by the patient should, of course, be revealing. However, patience is often required by the interviewer, particularly with chronic or recurrent problems, as relevant information often has to be requested and sometimes 'teased out' once the symptoms that are deemed to be associated with the complaint have been outlined by the patient. Clinicians often develop instinctive and sometimes distinctive styles of inquiry, but basic requirements are the identification of past medical history, concurrent health problems,

and factors that could affect the development of the symptoms and their cause, in addition to current complaints. Hand or foot dominance is recorded. The relationship or possible relationship to competition, training, use of equipment, type of footwear and clothing, and changes in routines is established. Menstrual irregularities and eating preferences are noted when relevant. Visceral pathology may present as a musculoskeletal problem, so that when interviewing a patient with shoulder pain, for instance, enquiries should be made about concurrent or previous symptoms which might suggest referred pain (usually from the neck) or raise the suspicion of gastrointestinal, respiratory, or cardiac disease. Systemic symptoms such as weight loss, fever and sweats indicate the possibility of a systemic inflammatory process, infection, or metastases.

An attempt should be made to identify the patient's primary complaint—pain, stiffness, 'giving way', weakness, clicking, etc.—and, if necessary, 'translate' the symptom described into a meaningful medical concept. For instance, patients often refer to 'stiffness' in situations in which 'ache' is implied and perception of loss of active movements or mobility is not intended, or 'toothache' to describe a nagging ache. As is the case with most musculoskeletal complaints, whether associated with sport or otherwise, pain is common. A past history of the complaint and any relevant investigations and treatment (including physiotherapy, injections, surgery, and medication) should be recorded. Indeed, a full past medical history and a sporting history should always be included. It is useful to enquire about the patient's understanding of the nature of the problem, for instance as provided by a previously attended clinician.

Onset

With **acute** injuries, the circumstances of the 'incident' and/or onset of symptoms should be established. Collisions with other persons involved in the sport or with inanimate objects are common, particularly in contact sports. The position of the affected limb or spine at the time of injury and an assessment of the mechanical forces applied to it should be established if possible. Immediate sensations such as a 'tearing feeling', a 'pop', or a 'crack' are suggestive of tissue disruption, including ligament tear, tendon tear, and fracture. A feeling of being struck on the back of the calf by a squash ball following a shot from an opponent is often the initial response of the player with a partial tear of the medial head of gastrocnemius. Associated symptoms such as loss of use of the affected limb, numbness, and inability to weight-bear or to continue with the relevant activity clearly indicate a significant injury. Information on the progress or lack of it from the time of the incident or onset of symptoms to the clinical assessment should be gained. A more gradual onset of symptoms is expected with **chronic** injuries.

Pain

The exact site of the pain, and its quality, associations, referral patterns, and severity, should be established. Pain on active movement of the injured area is to be expected. Additional information is required about whether the discomfort is related only to the sporting activity, or whether other situations evoke symptoms (such as lying on 'that side' at night, or during mundane day-to-day activities). Nocturnal pain may suggest serious pathology such as neoplasm or infection, but is also common in some soft tissue conditions, such as rotator cuff pathology at the shoulder. A visual analogue scale (VAS) can be used to register the severity of the pain, which is particularly useful in monitoring progress. Constant and unremitting pain suggests serious pathology. Constant burning pain is more likely to be neuropathic (which is more frequently seen in pain management clinics, when psychosocial factors often 'drive' the symptoms, than in sports injury clinics).

Stiffness

This common symptom may be used to indicate difficulty with movement associated with a feeling of tightness or a nagging ache, or both. Stiffness is a common complaint in the early stages following soft tissue injury. Early morning stiffness lasting for more than 15 minutes is a cardinal feature of ankylosing spondylitis and is also a feature of inflammatory joint disease. It is also common in decompensated spines that are degenerate or overused. Effused joints, pathological tendons, and contused or overused muscles feel 'stiff'.

'Giving way'

The expression 'giving way' is often used to describe instability associated with ligamentous incompetence at weight-bearing joints, particularly the knee. Further inquiry is necessary. For instance, elucidation of whether giving way at the knee is secondary to impingement (e.g. loose body, meniscus tear, or patellofemoral syndrome) is necessary. Patients usually use other descriptors for subjective instability at non-weight-bearing joints such as 'throwing out' or 'sliding out' at the shoulder. Instability at the shoulder often manifests as painful syndromes such as impingement. Subacromial dysfunction is often secondary to instability in the under-40 age group. On a cautionary note, 'abnormalities' on clinical examination may be very common and are not always symptomatic. They may be sport specific. For instance, laxity of the connective tissue restraints at the shoulder (e.g. in competitive swimmers and canoeists) and at the elbow (e.g. in throwers, particularly baseball pitchers) is to be expected, and the question of causation (with respect to a symptom complex) should be given due thought.

'Clicking, clunking, catching, and crunching'

Clicking is a common sensation, particularly when there is increased arousal or awareness by the patient 'focusing' on the injury site. It is not always significant, although it may be associated with joint hypermobility, tendon lesions, or degenerative changes (e.g. in the knee). Clunking may be used to describe abnormal intra-articular movement associated with pathology of the glenoid labrum at the shoulder or the acetabular labrum. A catching sensation is experienced when tissue is pinched, for instance in subacromial impingement. 'Crunching' is sometimes the preferred descriptor for any of the above conditions. 'Snapping' is usually applied by the clinician to a clinical syndrome, for instance snapping scapula and snapping hip. 'Locking' (and subsequent early unlocking) of a joint is characteristic of an intra-articular loose body.

'Weakness'

Neuromuscular dysfunction of all types gives rise to muscle weakness that is evident on clinical testing by manual resistance. However, weakness of a specific muscle or muscle group is not always obvious to the patient. Discomfort in the posterior thigh is often the primary complaint in the 'hamstring syndrome'—a good example of a 'disconnect' between the nerve supply at spinal level and the hamstring, which is found on examination to be weak. Nerve root entrapment causes sensory changes in many (but not all) patients in addition to radicular pain and a subjective feeling of 'weakness' or simply an inability to undertake accustomed tasks or sporting activities. Weakness secondary to musculotendinous lesions, such as acute rotator cuff tears or tears of the Achilles tendon, demands urgent musculoskeletal assessment; disconcertingly, weakness secondary to chronic degradation of these tendons may be less obvious to the patient and cause delay in referral or self-referral. Systemic neurological disease may present in sports enthusiasts, as in all population groups, and should not be forgotten when painless weakness, with or without altered sensation, is a presenting symptom. Apparent muscle weakness may be the consequence of pain inhibition.

'Swelling'

Joint swelling is usually accurately perceived by the patient, although the significance of immediate swelling, indicating haemarthrosis (which merits urgent evaluation), is less often appreciated. In undergraduate clinical training the contrasting characteristics of joint effusion and haemarthrosis are universally taught, but the implications less commonly so. Blood in a joint is an irritant and, as a general rule, should be aspirated whenever possible. Identification of the underlying cause should be explored vigorously. Soft tissue swelling is common to many soft tissue injuries, infections, and inflammatory disorders. The patient's attention may have been drawn to a 'lump' or swelling by regional discomfort, when the clinical finding is a normal tissue, such as the xiphisternum or a prominent rib in a slightly asymmetrical ribcage. Neoplasms may present as painless swellings.

Relieving and exacerbating factors

A record is kept of aggravating (or 'exacerbating') factors, such as use of the affected limb or trunk or the sleeping position. The relationship to day-to-day activities in addition to sporting activities is important. Factors that relieve are also recorded, for instance analgesics, rest, or possibly activity. Generally, pain from soft tissue injuries is expected to lessen with rest, including the adoption of the recumbent position. However, lying on an injured shoulder or trochanteric bursitis is painful. Nocturnal pain raises the suspicion of neurogenic, vascular, bony, infective, or neoplastic conditions. Early morning stiffness is characteristic of an inflammatory component of the injury or a frank inflammatory condition.

When injury is acute, particularly when extrinsic forces are involved, the direction of the externally applied forces should be established if possible. When injury is of a more chronic nature the history is quite different, as exemplified by the phases of discomfort experienced during the development of painful Achilles tendinosis:

(i)   discomfort (plus stiffness) after activity;

(ii) discomfort during the initiation of activity, subsequently improving ('run-off') during further activity and worsening afterwards;

(iii) discomfort worsening during activity, associated with functional impairment;

(iv) discomfort of sufficient severity to prevent activity.

Clinical examination

Once a historical perspective of the symptoms and relevant background information have been gained from the patient, augmented when necessary from bystanders, coach, parent, or paramedic, the establishment of a diagnosis requires the application to the musculoskeletal system of examination techniques which previously may not have been used extensively or perfected by many doctors. An appreciation must be gained of the importance of an examination routine that is founded upon sound neuromusculoskeletal principles, so that an **assessment of function** may be included. A recommended clinical appraisal comprises the following, preferably in the stated order:

(1) observation ('inspection')

(2) active movements

(3) passive movements, including stress tests

(4) resisted, ie isometric, muscle contraction (selective tissue tension)

(5) palpation

(6) neurological and vascular examination

(7) additional clinical tests of function ('special tests').

The importance of **observation** (or 'inspection') cannot be overstated. Visual scanning is second nature to experienced clinicians, but knowledge of the ranges of 'normality', for instance those associated with dominant-side muscle hypertrophy, minor congenital or developmental body asymmetries, posture, foot type, and leg length inequalities has to be acquired by trainees. This part of the examination necessitates inspection of the trunk and the limbs from all angles, looking for asymmetries and relatively conspicuous deformities. Local inspection may reveal swellings, including joint effusions, callosities, deformities, malalignments, discoloration, and muscle wasting, some of which may be subtle to the inexperienced eye. Gait, which is of particular importance to hip and lower limb injuries, is observed and categorized (e.g. antalgic, Trendelenburg, or waddling). For further information on abnormal gait patterns the reader is directed to Chapter 3.8. Guarding may be evident at this or later stages of the examination.

Active movements constitute a screening test for neuromuscular and joint function. Range of movements and abnormal movements (for instance 'hitching' at the shoulder) are recorded. The **passive movements** are compared with the active range of movement, and offer information on joint function and the integrity of the periarticular and intra-articular structures, including menisci, and may be further subdivided into:

- range of motion (around physiological axes)

- 'joint play' (movements not under voluntary control)

- provocative (stress) testing, e.g. for impingement, ligamentous competency, and joint integrity.

Muscle contraction against manual resistance should be undertaken methodically as it differentiates neural from muscle dysfunction. Note that **palpation** is usefully postponed until after assessment of movements and neuromuscular function, at which stage the clinician should have gained an insight into the nature and anatomical site of the injury. Gentle superficial palpation may be followed by palpation of the deeper structures; tenderness, swellings, muscle hypertonus, and gaps (such as tears of supraspinatus or Achilles tendon) are routinely searched for. A knee effusion may be ballotted. Warmth, with or without erythema over an olecranon or infrapatellar burstis, is indicative of infection. Bone percussion (for stress fracture) and soft tissue percussion or pressure over nerves (in the form of Tinel's test) is undertaken when indicated.

Special tests are described throughout the text. Footwear should be closely examined when indicated. The only compromise to a systematic examination of this type should be when, as a result of a history of acute trauma and the disposition of the patient or of the injured area, a fracture is suspected: gentle handling and palpation of the injured site may be followed by early X-ray, prior to more extensive examination procedures if appropriate (thereby conforming to the orthopaedic *surgical* system of 'look, feel, move').

Illustration of this schedule of examination, as an introduction at this stage to the clinical section of the textbook, may be made by reference to the shoulder, an anatomical region that is a frequent source of (diverse) complaints by the sportsperson.

- Observation identifies deformities of the bones (e.g. a fracture, old or new, of the clavicle) or of the joints of the shoulder girdle (e.g. a dislocation of the sternoclavicular, acromioclavicular, or glenohumeral joint), lesions of the soft tissues (e.g. rupture of the long head of biceps), wasting of muscles, hypertonicity of muscles (a 'hunched' shoulder), and other abnormalities such as winging of the scapula.

- Active abduction provides information in particular on the integrity of the rotator cuff and subacromial space.

- Passive movements are the best guide to capsular contracture.

- Resisted muscle contraction is a definitive clinical test for rotator cuff tear or tendinosis.

- Palpation confirms the anatomical site of lesions by identification of tenderness, swelling, or defect (e.g. a palpable gap in the supraspinatus tendon).

- Provocative (stress) testing is useful for a focused evaluation of the rotator cuff, impingement, instability, and intra-articular lesions (such as a tear of the glenoid labrum).

- Joint play (translatory) movements assist with assessment of acromioclavicular or glenohumeral joint instability.

Regrettably, but understandably, eponymous labelling is still prevalent (e.g. Neer's sign, Hawkins test, Yergason test, Speed's manoeuvre); more descriptive labelling is also commonplace (such as 'empty can', 'drop arm', 'sulcus sign', 'cross arm', 'clunk sign', 'load and shift'). For the junior clinician, there seems little alternative to studying and practising these clinical tests to perfection. Even then, the diagnostic accuracy (or discriminatory capacity) of many clinical tests is limited (Hegedus *et al.* 2008) or unknown. (As a footnote, clinicians have a duty in an era of evidence-based medicine to use diagnostic tests and treatment procedures that are of proven value. Regrettably, with respect to diagnosis of musculoskeletal conditions, not all manual tests appear to have been subjected to inter-observer reliability or validity studies.)

Further investigations, such as X-rays, arthrography, ultrasound scans, bone scans, CT scans, MRI scans, haematology, etc., should be considered where relevant. Full assessment relies on an understanding that, just as there is a wider range of normal parameters in

ECG tracings in an athlete than in the non-sporting population, so 'abnormal' findings on investigations for somatic complaints, such as are seen in X-rays of 'footballer's ankle' (marginal osteophytes and avulsion fragments) or on bone scans of long-distance runners (scattered increased uptake in the bones of the lower limbs), are simply a manifestation of recurrent physical stress. Therefore interpretation must be made with due care. **It is worth repeating that imaging must always be interpreted in the clinical context as correlation of clinical with imaging findings is often poor**. This is no less important in magnetic resonance imaging, often considered to be the 'ultimate' high-tech investigation, than in investigations that offer less image resolution. With a good understanding of patho-anatomy and pathophysiology, the MRI scan or other expensive investigation can be ordered appropriately (with discretion), thereby making best use of healthcare resources. Early imaging confirmation of a suspected clinical diagnosis, particularly one that could lead to serious sequelae, may be very helpful (Figs 2.1.1 and 2.1.2). Imaging may also be useful in circumstances in which the suspected condition (e.g. de Quervain's tenovaginitis (Fig. 2.1.3)) may be difficult to differentiate from other local pathology (e.g. osteoarthritis of the first metacarpophalangeal joint)

Functional assessment

Additional information about functional loss or impairment may be required as part of the initial assessment or subsequent review process following injury. Functional assessment is also made under other circumstances, for instance prior to participation in sport or as part of a pre-employment assessment. Weakness (and/or discomfort) may only be revealed by repetitive muscle contraction or joint movement, which is undertaken under close monitoring in the consulting room, in the laboratory, or at the training ground. An analogy in the broader field of sports medicine or cardiology is the ECG exercise test to detect ST segment inversion as an indicator of coronary artery insufficiency. Similarly, neuromuscular dysfunction may be detected during endurance exercise on an ergometer such as treadmill, bicycle, or rowing ergometer. For the purpose of a sophisticated functional assessment, repetitive sport-specific

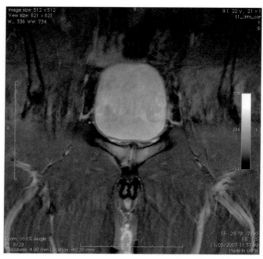

Fig. 2.1.2 MRI in 'symphysitis pubis'. Extensive marrow oedema of the pubic bones with fat saturation of the symphysis pubis is seen in this T2-weighted image.

activity may initially be undertaken as a screening procedure, followed when appropriate by more dedicated tests for function of individual nerves, muscles, and tendons, ligaments, or joints.

A basic functional assessment of the feet may be made by simple tests such as bilateral and unilateral tiptoeing, squatting, and heel-walking. The reader is recommended to become familiar with the more detailed assessment procedures described in relevant chapters of this book. Injury profiles in the lower limbs are often profoundly influenced by foot type and weight-bearing dynamics. Examination of footwear, for instance distortion and wear pattern, provides considerable additional information about the dynamics of running and weight-bearing movements associated with the patient's sport(s). When indicated, inspection of equipment may also be revealing.

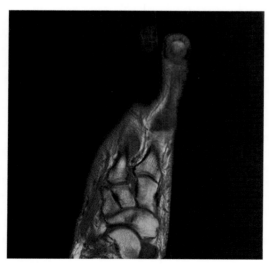

Fig. 2.1.1 MRI of left foot, demonstrating a stress fracture of the navicular.

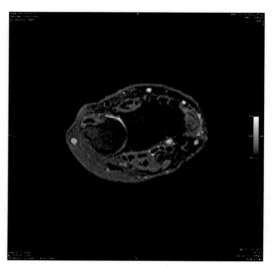

Fig. 2.1.3 MRI demonstrating thickening of the tendons of abductor pollicis longus and extensor pollicis brevis in de Quervain's tenovaginitis.

Investigations

Investigative procedures are well covered in the relevant chapters in this textbook. Suffice it to state at this juncture that hardly a year has gone by over the decade prior to the publication of this book in which advances in image resolution, availability, and expansion of target disorders in MRI, diagnostic ultrasound, or the equivalent in some other techniques have not been observed. Under these circumstances, the sports clinician has a most important responsibility to achieve and maintain a high level of clinical acumen and understanding of the relative (and possibly changing) merits of each technological investigation in order to apply appropriate evidence-based and cost-effective criteria to their use.

Diagnostic process

1. History (anamnesis)
2. Manual examination and functional assessment
3. Investigation when indicated
4. Reassessment following treatment

Reassessment

The diagnostic process should incorporate a review of progress whenever feasible and appropriate. The impact of the initial consultation, through the traditional holistic 'laying on of hands' role of a physician, irrespective of the prescription of drugs or interventional procedure, on symptoms from whatever cause should be assessed after a period of time that is relevant to the complaint. *Ex juvantibus* diagnosis (and associated management strategies) may be useful if the situation has been reached in which the diagnosis is not crystal clear following evaluation, and further action is considered desirable (Blomberg 2006). Under these circumstances, a 'trial' clinical intervention may be deemed to have diagnostic in addition to therapeutic value, and is not infrequently or unreasonably used throughout medical practice in general, for good ethical and empirical reasons. This is as useful in the era of evidence-based medicine, perhaps more appropriately described as evidence-informed practice (EIP), as in past decades. Clinical examination should be undertaken at each patient contact, unless there is convincing reason otherwise; how else can we relate the subjectivity of symptomatic progress, or conversely the failure to improve, to the perceived goal and benefits of objective evaluation?

Management

When underpinned by an appropriate level of knowledge of biomechanics in addition to functional anatomy and sports physiology, management of injury may incorporate a spectrum of treatment modalities prior to rehabilitation of the patient to a satisfactory level of sport-specific fitness.

Management of athletic injury requires substantially more than 'treatment' of an injured area. Patients need advice on a number of other aspects, including maintenance of overall fitness during recovery. Maintenance of a reasonable level of general fitness should be a priority, commencing within a day or two of the injury whenever possible and subsequently whilst specific treatment strategies are applied. Athletes (and other interested parties or stakeholders

such as managers) also require a prognosis. Of course this may need to be altered during the treatment and rehabilitation phase, but keeping the injured person and associated personnel, if applicable, 'in touch' with the current situation is important. If physical treatment is desirable, it is necessary to have a wide knowledge of the benefit of the spectrum of therapeutic modalities, and preferably a sound professional working relationship with the therapist of choice. It is erroneous to assume automatically that ice and ultrasound, for instance, cure all soft tissue lesions; more critical evaluation of the options is required before prescribing or recommending defined therapeutic regimes. A physical therapist needs, above all else, an accurate diagnosis. The therapist will probably have more experience in the usefulness of modalities such as effleurage, friction massage, laser therapy, etc. than the referring practitioner. However, it is incumbent upon the referring doctor to offer guidance, and thereby encourage suitable feedback of information on patients' progress. Multidisciplinary teamwork is necessary for many complex injuries; early collaboration is often critical to satisfactory progress.

Management

Treatment—aided by specific diagnosis

Rehabilitation

Prevention of further injury—aided by knowledge of aetiological factors

---

Depending on the type, severity, and duration of the injury, it is often necessary for the patient to progress from the therapy room to the rehabilitation arena, where functionally relevant progressive strengthening, proprioceptive, and flexibility exercises may be performed. (The derangement following injury of the proprioceptive reflex secondary to disturbance to or disruption of the articular mechanoreceptors found in joint capsules and ligaments was well described by Wyke (1972)). Isotonic, isometric, plyometric, and isokinetic exercises all have their place; they should be combined with suitable stretching schedules. **The emphasis is on coordination, proprioception, peripheral muscle strength and flexibility and core muscle control, allied to recovery of technical skills**. In view of the accessibility to most if not all athletes of gymnasia and health clubs, in which sophisticated equipment is commonly available for both training and rehabilitation, it is increasingly important for progress to be monitored by the practitioner or therapist and for prescriptive exercises to be relevant to both the injury and the sport. It is often forgotten that strengthening exercises which are performed primarily for muscle groups around the site of injury may impose stresses on other parts of the body—this is particularly relevant to the prevention of spinal injury during the rehabilitation of an injured limb.

Liaison with the coach or trainer should be considered to be an important aspect of both assessment and management. The coaches of athletes, particularly those in the younger age groups with considerable aptitude, may well be able to furnish useful information regarding the cause of injury which has not otherwise been disclosed; conversely, they need guidance on the reduction of potentially damaging physical stress during the subsequent resumption of training. Situations frequently arise when a telephone call to the coach of an up-and-coming tennis starlet, for instance, reveals the existence of abnormal biomechanical stress associated with faulty serving technique. Hyperextension of the spine on a tennis service or excessive forearm rotation on the forehand is not uncommon. Unless such information is presented to the physician, and a flawed technique identified and corrected, recurrence of injury is to be expected. The reader is referred particularly to Chapter 2.8 in which the principles of rehabilitation and prevention of injury are fully explored from the perspective of an experienced physiotherapist.

Overall, the patient needs reassurance, whenever possible, regarding the likelihood of a satisfactory outcome, as their worst fears are not always overtly expressed. The parents of an adolescent with Osgood–Schlatter syndrome (an example of a condition that is preferably not referred to as 'disease') often need a positive statement that the 'lump' is not a tumour, and likewise the patient with a thigh swelling from a rectus femoris tear. These and other considerations will be explored more fully in subsequent chapters. In this branch of medicine, in which the frustration of injury is often compounded by a psychological 'low' secondary to inactivity, sympathetic understanding is required. Too many patients inappropriately receive a bland prescription for absolute rest, or an unhelpful reaction such as, 'I am not surprised that you have leg pain if you run 70 miles a week'. Patients, quite rightly, expect advice for injuries that have occurred in an era when physical recreation and sport are encouraged, not least by the government-backed Sport for All and Exercise for Health campaigns in past decades. The abrogation by some members of the medical profession of their responsibility to provide a caring service on the grounds that sports injuries are 'self-induced' is unacceptable.

Internationally, sports medicine as a discipline has advanced steadily over recent years. In the UK, an Intercollegiate Academic Board of Sports and Exercise Medicine was created in 1998. This reflected the increasing desire and greater awareness of the need for sports medicine (as a component of SEM—sports and exercise medicine) to develop as a consultant-led speciality service within the National Health Service. Sports and exercise medicine was recognized as a stand-alone specialty in the UK in February 2005, and the Faculty of Sport and Exercise Medicine was officially launched at the Royal College of Physicians, London, in September 2006. At the time of going to press with this textbook, training programmes have commenced, and there is continuing discussion concerning the future role of specialist SEM physicians within the healthcare system in the UK. Irrespective of such employment issues, it is anticipated that a vast number of doctors of first contact (in general practice and in hospital accident and emergency departments) will continue to bear the brunt of an ever-increasing workload with respect to those injured in recreational exercise and sport.

Philosophy

An adequate history is important in musculoskeletal and sports medicine. James Cyriax, who devised orthopaedic medicine in the UK and stimulated the development of manual/musculoskeletal medicine globally, taught that many diagnoses should be strongly suspected from the history alone. To balance this view, it is not unusual for atypical presentations to occur—perspicacity is required. Furthermore, the subjective description of pain has little discriminative validity; behavioural responses may be perceived as a better guide to disability. (It should be noted that disability is

essentially a behavioural concept, whereas functional 'impairment' demands greater objectivity.) Frustratingly, in many overuse injuries there may be a paucity of physical signs; re-examination of the patient when the affected area is subjected to stress (e.g. measurement of compartment pressures in the lower leg immediately after exercise) may be required to establish the diagnosis. More refined investigations, such as CT or MRI scanning, may be necessary.

That there is an art to learning and to the practical application of knowledge is not an original concept. However, it is as applicable to assessment of sports injuries as it is in other medical disciplines. Just as the medical student attempting a final MB understands the need for a sound written and practical examination technique to provide the examiner with evidence of his or her clarity of thought, so the practising physician requires the logical application of functional anatomy and biomechanics (allied to sports techniques) for the purpose of correct diagnosis and management. All too often these basic principles are forgotten. When the physician is faced with a history of localized pain, there is a tendency for 'hands-on' palpatory techniques in the painful area to be employed too often and too rapidly without due attention either to history (the patient often supplies both diagnosis and aetiological factors if given the chance) or to clinical assessment of the function of the structure containing the lesion and of the musculoskeletal system adjacent to the lesion. Using by way of illustration the distribution of pain from the C5 nerve root or from tissues innervated by C5, this is felt in the upper arm, particularly in the region of the deltoid insertion, and often radiates to the radial border of the wrist. Deltoid lesions may be incorrectly diagnosed (they are extremely rare), and useless injections given to the site of the pain in the upper arm. However, functional assessment of the cervical spine and shoulder will reveal the real *site* of the lesion, which may be found, for instance, in the neck, causing nerve-root pressure, or in the shoulder joint, causing referred C5 dermatomal pain. Given the opportunity, the patient may recall the neck stiffness and pain which had temporarily been forgotten when the presentation was of persistent arm pain. The pathological lesion may then be treated appropriately.

Furthermore, problem-solving should relate to the likely sequelae if an injury is misdiagnosed or mistreated. The simple (stable) ankle sprain, involving the lateral collateral ligament of the ankle, may give rise to greater problems from an overcautious approach that incorporates immobilization, thus increasing proprioceptive deficit, than from early mobilization; a discriminating functional assessment is a prerequisite. Although functional stability, provided by external or internal splintage, is the desired outcome when acute bony or ligamentous instability is identified, early joint mobilization is still desirable (Noyes *et al.* 1974). Bone has an excellent blood supply and therefore may be expected to heal well. However, management of the less well-vascularized soft tissues, particularly ligaments and tendons, requires sensitive judgement. The capsule, articular cartilage, and surrounding muscles react adversely to immobilization, while ligament requires suitable apposition if ruptured. Ligament heals in a more physiological fashion, i.e. with parallel rather than haphazard collagen deposition, if the joint is allowed some degree of natural movement *during* healing, hence the use of cast-bracing techniques for the weight-bearing joints of the lower limbs. In this way, muscle tone and articular cartilage nutrition are also maintained.

Overall, whatever tissue has been damaged, the desired primary objective is restoration of normal joint function.

The responsibility of the sports physician in advising and assessing potential participants in different sporting and recreational activities receives special attention in subsequent chapters. The popularity of certain endurance activities practised for aerobic fitness, such as long-distance running, is directly proportional to the incidence of overuse injury. However, the injuries sustained are usually only temporarily disabling, and as far as is known do not appear to cause those degenerative joint conditions in the lower limb associated with years of participation in sports such as soccer which involve greater shearing forces and impact loading. Endurance events such as marathons and competitive squash racquets place substantial demands on competitors' cardiovascular and other physiological resources: pre-participation screening procedures, although considered contentious because of their time-consuming and often financially unrewarding nature, should be invoked whenever possible. Furthermore, sports physicians, in conjunction with sports associations, should be prepared to advise individuals, sports clubs, and communities in general on the inherent dangers relating to their particular sport. This responsibility extends to the provision of suitable first-aid facilities, and early management of injury advice to teachers, coaches, and trainers.

Profiling prior to sports participation and fitness testing following injury is considered in Chapter 2.8. Prevention of injury is a major topic, and is explored throughout the text.

References

Blomberg, S (2006). A pragmatic management strategy for low-back pain—an integrated multimodal programme based on antidysfunctional medicine. In: M. Hutson and R. Ellis (eds), *Textbook of Musculoskeletal Medicine*, p 516. Oxford University Press

Cyriax, J. (1982). *Textbook of Orthopaedic Medicine, Vol. I: Diagnosis of Soft Tissue Lesions* (8th edn). Baillière Tindall, London.

Hegedus EJ, Goode A, Campbell S, *et al.* (2008). Physical examination test of the shoulder: a systematic review with meta-analysis of individual tests. *British Journal of Sports Medicine*, **42**, 80–92.

Noyes, F.R., Torvik, P.J., Hyde, W.B., *et al.* (1974). Biomechanics of ligament failure II. An analysis of immobilisation, exercise and reconditioning effects in primates. *Journal of Bone and Joint Surgery*, **56A**, 1406–18.

Wyke, B. (1972). Articular neurology—a review. *Physiotherapy*, **58**, 94–9.

2.2

Radiology

Philip Bearcroft

Introduction

A number of radiological techniques are available for the evaluation of the injured athlete. In this chapter each technique will be considered in turn. The technique will be explained first in terms of technical aspects together with variations on the basic theme. Then the strengths and weaknesses of each technique will be described together with specific clinical uses. Understanding the strengths and weaknesses of these techniques will allow a rational approach to imaging of these patients, leading to a rapid accurate diagnosis and effective treatment process.

Plain radiographs

Technical aspects

A conventional plain radiograph is produced when film coated with photographic emulsion is exposed to ionizing radiation in the form of X-rays, which have been produced by a stationary X-ray tube. Energy values in the range 60–120 kV are typical for diagnostic radiology purposes. Different body parts cause varying degrees of X-ray attenuation, from high attenuation for bone and calcified structures, through intermediate attenuation from soft tissues, to low attenuation for fat and gas. The resulting contrast on the film produces an image which is determined by the different relative attenuations of the various anatomical structures imaged (Fig. 2.2.1(a)). Most radiographs are now taken using digital imaging techniques. This allows them to be viewed on computers via a picture archive and communication system (PACS) rather than on physical hard copy film. There are two main ways of achieving a digital image. In the first, **computed radiography**, the exposed plate must be processed by a computer before the image is composed. In the second, **direct radiography**, the exposed plate is wired to the computer directly and the images are read off instantaneously. The computer monitors are then used to display the images.

It is an axiom of good radiographic practice that radiographs of extremities should be taken in two orthogonal planes, particularly when there has been a history of injury. For all parts of the body, standard projections have been defined representing a minimum of a frontal and lateral projection, allowing a standardized technique to be followed (Swallow and Naylor 1996). The annotation of the frontal radiograph (e.g. anteroposterior, dorsiplanar, or dorsipalmar) corresponds to the direction of travel that the X-ray photons take through the anatomical structure. Alternative or additional views may be necessary when the anatomical region is complex or is orientated in a different plane. For example, an axial plane of the shoulder is often performed instead of the lateral view as it gives more information about the acromioclavicular joint and the acromion. Similarly, an oblique projection is required to evaluate fully the upper sacrum in the form of an anteroposterior radiograph with 15° cephalad angulation. A detailed catalogue of imaging projections is beyond the scope of this book and the interested reader is referred to a suitable book of radiographic positioning (Swallow and Naylor 1996).

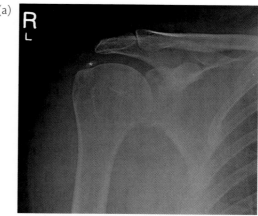

(a)

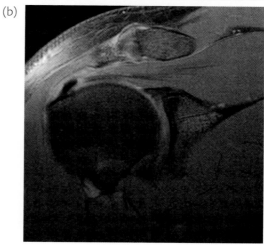

(b)

Fig. 2.2.1 (a) Calcific tendonitis. A small area of soft tissue calcification (asterisk) is seen projected over the supraspinatus tendon. It is seen as white because the calcification has blocked X-ray photons passing through the soft tissues. (b) Corresponding MRI picture. The area of calcification is dark on all sequences as there are no free water protons to return a signal.

Variations

In **tomography** the film and tube move in opposite directions during a prolonged X-ray exposure. The movement's geometry dictates that only a single plane within the imaging volume remains in focus during the exposure, and this imaged slice must necessarily be parallel to the film. The technique has now been largely replaced by other tomographic techniques (especially CT and MRI). In **fluoroscopy**, the radiographic film or plate is imaged by an image intensifier, which can be likened to a video camera sensitive to the X-ray photons. The resulting image is projected on a television screen in real time, and as the patient moves, the changes are reflected on the screen. This can be particularly useful in the dynamic assessment of an extremity, for example in the evaluation of dynamic instability of the wrist, but it is more commonly used in relation to sports injuries to guide intervention procedures such as steroid injections into joints or nerve root blocks.

Stress views may give indirect evidence of ligamentous injury. The joint is imaged while under active or passive force and ligamentous injury will allow widening of the joint space, which can be captured radiographically. For example, the clenched fist view can be useful for demonstrating static disruption of the scapholunate ligament.

In **angiography**, a thin catheter up to 1 m long is introduced into the arterial tree from the femoral or brachial artery and the technique allows visualization of the arterial tree. Although angiography techniques are used widely in medical practice, there are few indications for their use in the treatment of patients with sports injuries.

Strengths

Plain radiography has a historical heritage dating back over 100 years, and the raw materials are inexpensive and universally available. The resulting images are readily understood by clinicians. The spatial resolution is excellent, allowing detailed analysis of small structures. Plain films are particularly useful in the diagnosis of bone abnormalities or when soft tissue disorders involve calcification (Fig. 2.2.1(a)).

Weaknesses

In terms of the injuries commonly encountered in sports, the main weakness of plain radiographs is the recognized lack of soft tissue contrast resolution. This is because all structures of soft tissue density have essentially the same attenuation values, and therefore differences between soft tissue structures will not be conspicuous in the absence of mineralization or calcification. The other main disadvantage relates to the ionizing nature of X-ray radiation, and the potential resulting adverse side effects (Table 2.2.1).

Specific clinical uses

Radiographs in two projections perpendicular to each other are generally the first examination that is required for the evaluation of sports injuries, and in many cases are the only diagnostic images needed. This is because it is important to visualize the underlying bone when evaluating soft tissue complaints and to exclude underlying primary bone abnormalities presenting with secondary soft tissue symptoms. In addition, in the context of sports injury, evaluation of the adjacent bone is important to exclude either bony fracture or tendon–bone avulsion. Plain film provides an easy method of assessing joint abnormalities, particularly degenerative changes, and for monitoring changes longitudinally over time. For example, radiographs are useful to confirm the alignment after external or internal fixation, and to demonstrate reduction after manipulation of displaced fractures. The degree of fracture healing with callus formation can be monitored serially and complications of bony injury can be assessed. Soft tissue calcification after severe muscle trauma (e.g. myositis ossificans) can also be assessed radiographically.

In addition, plain radiographs can provide useful diagnostic information in the patient who presents with a soft tissue mass. For example, the mass may exhibit areas of calcification such as phleboliths, which are pathognomonic of a haemangioma or the typical soft tissue changes of myositis ossificans.

Summary

Plain radiographs are usually the first and may be the only radiographic investigation required in the context of sports injury. They are universally available and are low cost. They are accurate for diagnosing the majority of bone abnormalities related to sports injuries, but they are more limited when the abnormality arises within the soft tissues. They are also a useful adjunct to other imaging techniques in the evaluation of soft tissue injuries, but it is the remaining imaging modalities considered later that have contributed most to our understanding of the processes that underlie sport injuries and healing.

Table 2.2.1 Typical effective doses from diagnostic medical exposures

Procedure	Typical effective dose (mSv)	Equivalent number of chest radiographs	Approximate equivalent period of natural background radiation[a]
Extremity joint	<0.01	<0.5	<1.5 days
CXR	0.02	1	3 days
Hip	0.3	15	7 weeks
Pelvis	0.7	35	4 months
Lumbar spine	1.3	65	7 months
Bone scintigram (^{99m}Tc)	4	200	1.8 years
CT abdomen or pelvis	10	500	4.5 years

[a]UK average background radiation, 2.2 mSv per year; regional averages range from 1.5 to 7.5 mSv per year.
Source: RCR Working Party (1998). *Making the Best Use of a Department of Clinical Radiology* (4th edn), p.13. Royal College of Radiologists, London.

Arthrography

Technical aspects

The technique of arthrography was devised at a time when many of the other imaging techniques in this chapter were not available. A fundamental problem of plain radiography is its inability to visualize soft tissue structures directly. Arthrography involves the injection of a radio-opaque contrast agent into a joint to distend the joint space. As a result, additional information about the soft tissue structures related to the joint is available (Resnick 1995). The contrast agent used contains iodine bound to large macromolecules.

The contrast medium molecule increases the X-ray attenuation of photons passing through the area injected. The technique is performed with fluoroscopic guidance to ensure that the needle tip is appropriately sited and then plain radiographs are taken using a conventional technique to image the area under investigation. Details of each injection are outside the scope of this chapter, and the interested reader is referred elsewhere for further details (Resnick 1995).

The technique is interventional, in that it requires percutaneous injection, and therefore contraindications to arthrography include a blood dyscrasia that would make a haemarthrosis following the injection more likely, or infection in the cutaneous or subcutaneous tissues overlying the joint, which would increase the risk of septic arthritis.

Variations

The basic technique of arthrography was used with plain radiographs and has now generally been replaced wherever MRI and other techniques are available. However, the basic technique can be combined with MR and CT contrast agents, allowing MR arthrography and CT arthrography, respectively, and these techniques are practised widely. The arthrographic technique is also the basis of many injection techniques, for example steroid injections into joints where a small injection of contrast medium will be used to ensure that the needle tip is intra-articular. This is particularly the case for deeper joints such as the hip, sacroiliac, or subtalar joints which can be difficult to palpate clinically.

Strengths

Conventional arthrography is potentially universally available wherever fluoroscopic facilities are present, and it is inexpensive and reliable. It is easily learned and well tolerated by the patient. Indeed, many patients prefer arthrography to MRI, probably because of the personal contact between clinician and patient (Blanchard et al. 1997). Nevertheless, with the advent of MRI, the use of arthrography has become more limited to specific indications as discussed below, or if MRI is contraindicated.

Weaknesses

The main weakness is that the technique is invasive, requiring an intra-articular injection of contrast medium. In addition, the information that arthrography provides is by its very nature indirect—soft tissues themselves are not directly visualized, but information about them is deduced from the pattern of contrast medium distribution. The patient is also exposed to ionizing radiation during the initial fluoroscopy time and the subsequent series of plain radiographs. Therefore the technique may result in a radiation exposure 5–10 ten times greater than the corresponding plain radiograph technique.

Specific clinical uses

In the diagnosis of sports injuries, conventional arthrography plays very little role unless MRI is either unavailable or contraindicated. In these situations, conventional arthrography can be useful in the shoulder, where it can be used to diagnose full-thickness rotator cuff tears and partial tears that involve the articular surface. Radio-opaque contrast medium (10–15 ml) is injected into the joint, and the concept behind the technique relates to the anatomical fact that the roof of the joint is comprised of the tendons of the rotator cuff, especially supraspinatus and infraspinatus, covered by joint synovial lining. Therefore a full-thickness rotator cuff tear in one of these tendons would be associated with capsular damage, which will allow contrast medium to pass from the joint into the subacromial subdeltoid bursa. In a normal individual there is no communication between the bursa and the joint. The accuracy of shoulder arthrography for the detection of full-thickness tear is excellent (Ahovuo et al. 1984). A partial tear does not extend from the articular to the bursal surface (Fig. 2.2.2).

The main use for shoulder arthrography is in the diagnosis of capsulitis (frozen shoulder), for which it is the only diagnostic test that has been found useful. The condition results in a radiologically tight joint with reduced volume, and during the injection procedure it is manifest as a reduction in the amount of contrast medium that can be injected into the shoulder before the patient experiences pain, followed in some individuals by early lymphatic filling and a tight joint on visual inspection of resulting images with obliteration of the axillary recess and irregularity of the capsular insertion.

The distension of the shoulder by contrast medium during the procedure is associated in some with a reduction in the symptoms, and this led to the suggestion that capsulitis can be treated hydrostatically using this technique (Andrenn and Lundberg 1965). The joint is filled with water and local anaesthetic, allowing increased pain tolerance during the next few hours, during which intense physiotherapy is used to help loosen up the tight joint.

Diagnostically, the injection of local anaesthetic into a joint as part of an arthrographic procedure can be informative, as the failure of the pain to improve after local anaesthetic injection implies that it may not be arising from the suspect joint. For example, hip pain is common and may be non-specific, and it may coexist with a

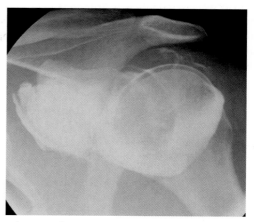

Fig. 2.2.2 Arthrogram of a partial-thickness supraspinatus tear. During the arthrogram, contrast medium passed into the supraspinatus tendon, but not into the bursa, indicating that there is a tear which is only partial thickness.

source of back pain. Injection of local anaesthetic into the hip can help resolve whether the pain is arising from the back or the hip.

Summary

Arthrography is a technique that involves ionizing radiation and percutaneous injection of intra-articular contrast medium, and has largely been replaced by other imaging techniques, particularly MRI. Where there are contraindications to the use of MRI, contrast arthrography retains a role. The technique also forms the basis of MR arthrography and CT arthrography, which are widely used techniques and are discussed elsewhere in this chapter.

Ultrasound

Technical aspects

In this technique, high-frequency pulses of sound are used to generate cross-sectional information. The sound frequency used (3–15 MHz) is inaudible to the human ear (range of hearing approximately 10 Hz–20 kHz). It was the advent of ultrasound probes capable of working at frequencies above 7.5 MHz that allowed the use of ultrasound in the musculoskeletal system generally, and in the study of patients with sports injuries in particular. The sound bounces off internal structures, and the echoes are received and recorded by the same transducer and converted into an image.

Reflections will be greatest at interfaces between tissues of differing acoustic impedance and, in general, areas of more detailed anatomical complexity will return a more heterogeneous image compared with the more uniform image corresponding to a homogeneous organ or region. The higher the frequency used, the higher will be the spatial resolution, but conversely the shallower will be the depth of the image.

Variations

Doppler ultrasound provides information about internal structures that are moving. In addition to recording the depth and intensity of echoes returned from these structures, the transducer also detects any alteration in frequency of the received sound which would result if the interface being imaged is moving with regard to the length of the transducer. For example, blood flow within a vessel can be recorded in a graphic format as a function of time, and this can be displayed on the screen alongside the image.

Colour Doppler and power Doppler techniques are extensions of the Doppler technique where, rather than a single Doppler gate, every pixel in part of the image is assessed for frequency change and its reflected sound, and a colour map is constructed to represent this directional information, where the colour of each pixel corresponds to the size of the frequency change. Colour Doppler imaging provides useful information in relation to tendinosis in the form of the degree of neovascularization (Fig. 2.2.3). The true relevance of this increased vascularity has yet to be determined, but many authors consider it to be related to clinical symptoms (Weinberg *et al.* 1998; Zanetti *et al.* 2003).

Unlike most of the other imaging techniques discussed in this chapter, ultrasound is a dynamic test, and the limb can be moved or stressed dynamically during the procedure. Therefore ultrasound is particularly good at, for example, guiding therapeutic intervention allowing real-time guidance of needles for steroid injections. In addition, conditions that relate to clicking or clunking

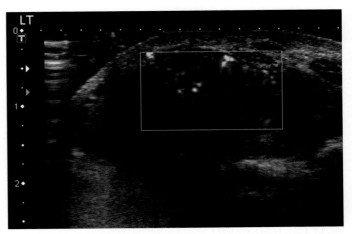

Fig. 2.2.3 Ultrasound image of neovascularization synovitis. Areas of blood flow are identified by the use of power Doppler and displayed as an overlay on the grey-scale image.

of joints or soft tissues are well assessed with ultrasound. This is commonly used, for example, in the snapping hip syndrome, where the iliopsoas tendon snaps over the iliopectineal eminence (Pelsser *et al.* 2001), and also in assessment of the snapping of the peroneal tendon (Raikin *et al.* 2008).

Portable ultrasound machines are finding a particular niche in the evaluation of patients with sports injuries, as they are portable and can be taken to the side of the pitch or track during the game. Much research and development has been focused on the design of the transducers, and while there remains potentially a large difference between the quality of images available from the top-end ultrasound machines available in hospital departments and those from smaller office-based niche ultrasound machines, the latter provide useful and detailed information, particularly at the time of the injury.

Strengths

Ultrasound enjoys certain unique properties that make it ideally suited to the evaluation of patients with sports injuries. It is non-invasive, does not involve ionizing radiation, is painless to the patient, has no known side effects, and exhibits excellent spatial resolution for evaluating soft tissue complaints. For example, ultrasound has 5–10 times better spatial resolution than MRI (Fig. 2.2.4).

Weaknesses

The major weakness of ultrasound is that the accuracy depends on the operator in a way that is not applicable to other imaging techniques. The hard-copy images that are available are often difficult to interpret accurately by another operator, unless a systematic approach to layout has been adopted, and therefore the clinician or therapist is reliant on the original reporter's interpretation of the images. Ultrasound requires a detailed knowledge of anatomy, and there is a long steep learning curve during which time the results of the apprentice sonographer may be less accurate than those quoted in the literature. The technique is not able to visualize intrinsic bone abnormalities, and therefore must be combined with plain film radiographs or other imaging techniques to ensure that bony abnormalities have not been missed.

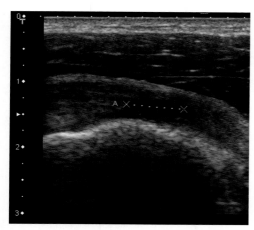

Fig. 2.2.4 A full-thickness tear of the supraspinatus tendon on ultrasound. Note the scale on the left. The entire image represents only 3 cm of soft tissue depth, and the tear is 6 mm deep. This represents high spatial resolution with respect to CT and MRI in particular.

Specific clinical uses

In the athlete, sonography has revolutionized the imaging of **shoulder** impingement and rotator cuff disease. The supraspinatus tendon is the most common tendon to undergo impingement changes (Kieft *et al.* 1988), and this tendon is well visualized sonographically. Complete tears of the supraspinatus tendon can be detected with high accuracy on ultrasound (Dinnes *et al.* 2003) (Fig. 2.2.4). However, ultrasound does not have a role in the evaluation of internal derangements of the joint, including instability (Table 2.2.2).

Injuries around the **elbow** are well suited to sonographic evaluation. Lesions at the common extensor origin (tennis elbow) and common flexor origin (golfer's elbow) are largely a clinical diagnosis, but ultrasound is useful in demonstrating the degree of tear or retraction. Loose bodies within the elbow are also detectable by ultrasound, particularly if there is an effusion. In young athletes, cartilaginous fracture or dislocation of the radial head can be diagnosed on ultrasound.

In the **wrist and hand**, ultrasound can be useful for the evaluation of tendon injuries and degenerative processes. Ultrasound is also good at assessing the degree of tenosynovitis that often accompanies tendon injuries (Fig. 2.2.3). Unexplained pain in an athlete

may be due to the presence of a ganglion, which is particularly well evaluated on ultrasound (Teefey *et al.* 2004).

In the **hip**, ultrasound is good at detecting excess fluid within the joint at all ages, and the dynamic nature of ultrasound makes it useful in detecting the underlying cause of painful clicks resultant from soft tissue structures (e.g. snapping iliopsoas tendon). Fluid within the iliopsoas bursa is another potential mimic of hip pathology, and such bursitis is easily demonstrated sonographically.

In the **knee**, ultrasound is generally not the first-line investigation in the evaluation of a sporting injury. Because of the inability of ultrasound to see into the joint, internal derangements of the knee, which are so common in this context, cannot be evaluated accurately. Fluid in the semimembranosus gastrocnemius bursa (Baker's cyst) is an exception, and its size and position can be documented using ultrasound. Patella tendonopathy is also well evaluated sonographically, and dynamic assessment of the interaction between the inferior pole of the patella and the patellar tendon can be useful in patients with deep infrapatellar tendinosis (Fredberg and Bolvig 1999).

In the **foot**, the superficial position of the various tendons that are related to the ankle mean that ultrasound is particularly useful in their evaluation. The posterior tibial tendon and the Achilles tendon are the most commonly injured tendons, and ultrasound can be useful to detect the presence of tendonopathy and quantify the degree of any damage. Neovascularization can be detected on power Doppler imaging, and its relevance needs to be determined (Alfredson and Ohberg 2005; Kristoffersen *et al.* 2005). Tendons of the foot and toes are occasionally ruptured, and the advent of high-frequency transducers has allowed even these tiny structures to be followed peripherally to detect disruption, and to identify the anatomical site of the torn ends prior to surgery.

Ultrasound has found widespread use in the evaluation of **muscle tears**, both at the time of injury and in the following weeks where it can be used to monitor healing. In grade I injuries, the abnormal area may be seen as an area of increased echogenicity (Takebayashi *et al.* 1995). More severe injuries involve hypo-echoic regions which indicate fluid adjacent to the myotendonous junction or the epimysium, depending on the site of the tear. The presence of haematoma is also well evaluated with ultrasound, and the changes of myositis ossificans will be seen on ultrasound before they are seen on plain film. Ultrasound is less well suited than MRI to monitoring the resolution of tears as they become less conspicuous

Table 2.2.2 Common uses of MRI and ultrasound

	Ultrasound	MRI
Shoulder	Rotator cuff damage including biceps	Rotator cuff damage (surgical patients), entrapment syndromes, labral abnormalities and instability
Elbow	Common flexor and common extensor tendinopathy Distal biceps rupture	Osteochondral lesions, loose bodies
Wrist/hand	Overuse injuries of the tendons, tenosynovitis, ganglion cyst	TFCC injury, AVN of scaphoid fracture
Hips/pelvis	Inguinal hernia. bursitis, snapping iliopsoas tendon, muscle injury	Labral abnormality, AVN, stress fracture, adductor tendonopathy, osteitis pubis, symphyseal cleft
Knee	Patella and quadriceps tendons, collateral ligaments, cysts	Cruciate ligaments, meniscal injury, osteochondral injuries, patella injuries, posterolateral corner
Foot/ankle	Achilles tendinosis and tear, ligamentous injuries, plantar fasciitis	Talar dome defects following injury, coalition

TFCC, triangular fibrocartilage complex; AVN, avascular necrosis.

compared with MRI over time. Complications such as scar formation or development of an intramuscular cyst are features that can be evaluated sonographically.

Summary

Ultrasound is a relatively inexpensive radiation-free form of imaging that is particularly suited to soft tissue abnormalities. Its application has exploded over the last 10 years because of the advent of high-frequency ultrasound probes, and it has found many uses in the evaluation of patients with sports injuries. In many institutions ultrasound is a first-line diagnostic technique for the majority of soft tissue injuries. It has no known adverse side effects in the range of power used for diagnostic imaging.

Computed tomography (CT)

Technical aspects

CT uses ionizing radiation in the form of X-rays to produce multiple parallel cross-sectional images. Most modern CT devices comprise a multiple array of X-ray detectors that move around the patient circumferentially, while the patient, who is lying on a table, passes longitudinally through the device. The images that are produced are intrinsically digital and, unlike the other images, the digital information is quantitative. The CT density of each pixel within the image is linearly proportional to the X-ray attenuation of the voxel, or volume element within the body, on a scale of attenuation values where the unit of measurement is called a Hounsfield unit (HU). Internal calibration of the CT scanning system defines water to have a value of 0 HU, and room air to have a value of -1000 HU. Thereafter all other CT values can be represented on a visual grey scale, and the displayed pixels produce the resulting image. Typical attenuation values are given in Table 2.2.3.

Several parameters are selectable by the CT scanning system operator, and some of these have a fundamental effect on the eventual image. The reconstructed slice thickness is an obvious example, but in addition the method of reconstruction can be altered to accentuate either soft tissues or bones. CT scanning can be performed in conjunction with the injection of intravenous contrast medium. This iodinated contrast medium passes intravenously into the extracellular fluid in proportion to a combination of blood flow and capillary permeability.

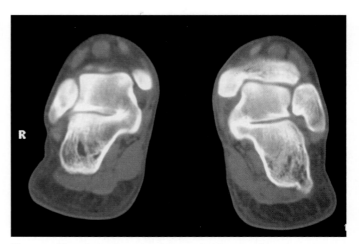

Fig. 2.2.5 Bilateral talocalcaneal coalition on CT. The coronal reconstruction shows the bony bar between the talus and calcaneus on each side.

Variations

The images are acquired axially, but can then be reconstructed into coronal, sagittal, or oblique orientations (Fig. 2.2.5). Surface-rendered three-dimensional (3D) reconstructions involve recreating a surface shaded virtual image from the original two-dimensional slices. To produce the 3D image, the computer picks out only those pixels from contiguous slices that have Hounsfield attenuation values that correspond to bone. The computer then paints the 3D image by deducing what a picture would look like if light was shone onto the virtual 3D reconstruction (Prokop 2003).

CT arthrography involves imaging a joint after the intra-articular injection of iodinated contrast medium that has often been diluted. This allows soft tissue structures that otherwise would not have been seen on CT to be outlined in contrast medium, in a way analogous to MR arthrography (Fig. 2.2.6). Its main use is in the area where anatomy is complex, where overlying structure may obscure detail, and it is also often the best way to determine whether or not a cartilaginous or calcified body within a joint is loose.

Table 2.2.3 Typical attenuation values for various body tissues and fluids

Tissue type	Standard value (HU)
Bone (compact)	>250
Bone (spongy)	130 ± 100
Muscle	45 ± 5
Liver	65 ± 5
Fat	−65 ± 10
Lung tissue	−750 ± 150
Blood (venous whole blood)	55 ± 5
Exudate (>30 g protein / l)	>18 ± 2
Transudate (<30 g protein / l)	<18 ± 2

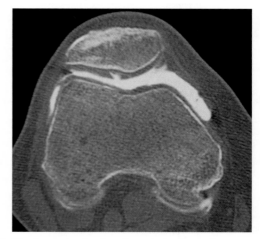

Fig. 2.2.6 CT arthrography showing a fissure in patellar cartilage.

Strengths

The strength of CT scanning arises from its cross-sectional nature: the problem with overlapping structures that affects plain radiography acutely is less of a problem with CT. Similarly, unlike plain radiographs where the patient may be required to assume an uncomfortable position during exposure, with CT scanning the patient is required only to lie supine and remain still during the acquisition of the slices, which takes only 5–10 seconds.

Weaknesses

Although CT is excellent for demonstration of complex fractures, the main weakness in relation to imaging patients with sports injuries is that soft tissue structures generally have attenuation values within a narrow range, and therefore are not well differentiated, even when abnormal. Therefore oedematous soft tissue and adjacent normal soft tissue cannot be differentiated. Thus, other than for issues relating to either bone or soft tissue calcification, CT has little role in the evaluation of sporting injuries.

The risks associated with CT imaging are related primarily to the patient's exposure to ionizing radiation, and a CT of the abdomen or pelvis is associated with a radiation dose many times that of a plain film (Table 2.2.1). The injection of intravenous contrast medium may be associated with complications such as minor allergic reactions, which can occur in up to 5% of injections with certain ionic contrast agents. More severe allergic reactions resulting in hospital admission can also occur (approximately 1:40 000 injections with older contrast agents).

Specific clinical uses

Because the Hounsfield units of bone are significantly higher than those of adjacent structures, bony detail or calcified abnormalities are particularly well differentiated with CT. For this reason, CT is the preferred technique for complex bony injuries. It is also useful in certain circumstances where calcification within a mass is suspected, for example myositis ossificans, which is best appreciated with CT (Fig. 2.2.7). In addition, CT can be used to guide injections, particularly in intervention related to the spine (nerve root blocks, facet joint injections, etc).

Summary

CT is a technique that uses ionizing radiation to create a series of radiological slices through the area of interest. These slices can be

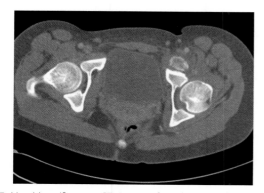

Fig. 2.2.7 Myositis ossificans on CT. An area of curvilinear calcification is seen in the adductors on the left 3 months after injury.

analysed in a number of different planes. Its main use in sports injury is in the assessment of complex fractures and the evaluation of soft tissue injuries that involve calcification such as myositis ossificans. The radiation dose to the patient is relatively high with this technique.

Magnetic resonance imaging (MRI)

Technical aspects

MRI is an imaging modality ideally suited to the investigation of sports injuries. It is a technique that does not use ionizing radiation, and it can generate cross-sectional images in any arbitrary plane. The image is produced by placing a patient in a strong homogeneous magnetic field (typically in the range 0.5–1.5 Tesla (T), where 1 T corresponds to approximately 10 000 times the strength of the Earth's magnetic field). As a result, the body's water protons are affected. A radiofrequency pass is then applied at exactly the correct frequency to promote some of these protons into a higher-energy state, and as they drop back into the lower-energy state, a faint electromagnetic pulse is transmitted back from the body. This pulse is detected by the coils within the MRI system and converted into an image.

In a **T1-weighted** image the intensity of each pixel is related to the rate at which protons release this energy to adjacent macromolecules; conversely, in a **T2-weighted** image the intensity of each pixel relates to the ability of the protons to release energy to surrounding protons. A **proton-density**-weighted image is a corresponding map of the number of protons that are available to absorb energy in this way, and this in turn is related to quantity of free water. Therefore the image generated by MRI is a representation of certain fundamental quantum physical characteristics of free water protons. Details of how the MR images are constructed lie outside the scope of this book, but common terms used in MRI are given in the glossary in Table 2.2.4. Much of the complexity of MRI relates to the profusion of sequences, and sequences still continue to be developed and improved. However, the acquisition of the image takes place over several minutes, during which time the patient must remain still or the resulting images will be ruined.

In general, T1-weighted sequences are useful for demonstrating and evaluating anatomical structures, but any pathological processes are generally not well visualized; an abnormal structure will frequently have a signal on T1-weighted images that is identical to that of adjacent normal soft tissue structures. Therefore it will remain inconspicuous. However, on T2-weighted sequences those parts of the image which contain a higher proportion of fluid (which is usually an indication of abnormality such as inflammation, infection, trauma, etc.) are generally brighter and therefore more conspicuous. A large number of techniques for maximizing the conspicuity of pathological processes are available. Central to this is the desire to render a signal from normal structures, such as fat, dark so that abnormal structures, which will be bright, will stand out. Therefore the majority of examinations include some form of **fat saturation**, and the combination of fat saturation with fast spin–echo sequences is particularly useful in the evaluation of the musculoskeletal system generally, and sports injuries in particular. When this is not available or suitable, an alternative is the 'short tau inversion recovery' (**STIR**) sequence, which is frequently encountered in the evaluation of sports injuries. Further complexity is created as in many cases there is inconsistency in the terminology

Table 2.2.4 Glossary of terms used in magnetic resonance imaging

Fat saturation	A technique to render the signal from fat dark. On *FSE* T2-weighted images (commonly used in musculoskeletal applications) fat is bright, as is the lesion being evaluated. By selectively darkening the normal adjacent fat, the lesion becomes more conspicuous. An alternative fat saturation technique is STIR.
FSE (fast spin echo)	A technique to increasing the speed of a *spin echo* sequence. Can be used with *T1-*, *T2-*, or *PD*-weighted images, and with or without *fat saturation*.
Gradient	Spatial variation of some physical quantity, such as magnetic field.
Gradient echo	One of the two fundamental MR imaging sequences. The term relates to the way that the *protons* are refocused after they have been excited by using a magnetic field *gradient*.
PD (proton density or spin density)	Density of free water protons in a given volume. Therefore it is one of the principal determinants of the strength of the MR signal.
Proton	A positively charged nucleon, i.e. a hydrogen nucleus. Although all protons are affected by the magnetic field, it is those hydrogen nuclei that are part of free water molecules that contribute most significantly to the radiological image.
Spin	A spin is another name for a *proton*.
Spin echo (SE)	One of the two fundamental imaging sequences. In SE imaging, the *protons* are refocused after they have been excited by applying a second radiofrequency pulse.
STIR (short tau inversion recovery)	A technique to suppress signal from tissues with a short T1 value. Fat has a particularly short (low) T1 value, so STIR is a technique to produce *fat saturation*.
T1 (pronounced 'T-one')	Spin–lattice or longitudinal relaxation time measured in milliseconds. It is a measure of the rate that excited protons release their energy to surrounding larger macromolecules ('the lattice').
T2 (pronounced 'T-two')	Spin–spin or transverse relaxation time measured in milliseconds. It is a measure of the rate that excited protons release their energy to other adjacent protons.

used by different competing manufacturers for what may fundamentally be the same sequence.

Variations

Contrast medium in MRI is frequently used to evaluate sports injuries. The agent used is **gadolinium-DTPA** which is a paramagnetic agent and increases the rate which energy can be transferred from protons by acting as a ready receptor for that extra energy. The molecule is usually injected intravenously, and the degree of enhancement is related to both the perfusion of the structure in question and the permeability of the capillaries. In the context of trauma or inflammation, perfusion and permeability are often both increased and therefore the abnormal structure will enhance. The effect of this enhancement is seen on T1-weighted images, and these sequences are often combined with fat saturation to make the enhancement even more conspicuous.

In **MR arthrography**, contrast medium is introduced into the joint and this provides additional information relating to the internal structures of the joint. This can be achieved in one of two ways. In **direct MR arthrography** dilute gadolinium (typically diluted 1:500 to 1:1000) is injected directly into the joint. The alternative approach, **indirect MR arthrography**, involves injecting the contrast medium intravenously and excising the joint in question. The result is that contrast medium passes from the capillaries in the synovium into the joint fluid, thereby enhancing the internal contents of the joint.

The conventional MR scanning system is comprised of an elongated doughnut-shaped construction containing the super cooled wire coil that produces the strong magnetic field. Such an arrangement was the easiest way to achieve the field strengths when the technique was in its infancy. The patient passes into the centre of the coil, and some patients find this uncomfortable or, if they are overtly claustrophobic, intolerable. Developments in coil design have taken several paths over the past 15 years, and other geometries have been devised such as the double-doughnut design, which allows an interventionist to access the patient between the doughnuts, and a horizontal design where the magnetic field is orientated perpendicular to the floor. These **open MR scanning systems** represent alternatives to the conventional doughnut design.

In addition, niche **low-field-strength magnets** have been devised and these have the potential to revolutionize the availability of MRI. They are self-contained MRI systems that can be wheeled into almost any room without any special preparation. They are cheaper and are particularly useful for the assessment of extremities (wrists, knees, etc). They work at lower field strength (typically 0.02T). Imaging time is typically longer, but their small foot print and manoeuvrability make them convenient to install near emergency departments or even in the community.

High-field-strength magnets (typically 3T or above) are also being more commonly deployed, particularly in the research environment. Their future benefits need to be determined. It appears that they offer the ability to detect changes in osteoarthritis earlier by providing more information relative to the articular cartilage (Eckstein *et al.* 2007), and there is potential for them to be useful in the investigation of soft tissue injuries.

More recently interest in **diffuser tensor imaging** (DTI) has raised the possibility of studying muscle architecture and structure (Deng *et al.* 2007). In future DTI may become a useful tool for following up subtle skeletal muscle changes, which may be a consequence of age, atrophy, or disease (Galban *et al.* 2004). In addition, important information about muscle biomechanics and joint function may be obtained with new MR contrasts such as T2 mapping, spectroscopy, blood oxygenation level dependent (BOLD) imaging and molecular imaging. These new techniques are currently in the research arena, but may allow more accurate determination of sporting injuries in the future (Gold 2003).

Strengths

Over the past 15 years, MRI has become crucial to the evaluation of sport injuries, and this success is due to many factors. As a proton imaging technique, MRI is sensitive in detecting areas of increased free water, and most sporting injuries involve either altered morphology of the affected structure or oedema (increased tissue free water). In addition, the ability to image in any orthogonal plane, or indeed in any random plane, means that the abnormality in question can be visualized longitudinally and in transverse, which aids diagnosis. Furthermore, sequences can be tailored by altering the various imaging parameters and this allows specific diagnoses to be made. Most diagnoses can be made without the use of intravenous contrast medium, but alteration in perfusion and permeability related to injury can also be evaluated by the use of contrast medium. Finally, the technique does not appear to be associated with any biological hazard to the individual patient and avoids the use of ionizing radiation.

Weaknesses

MRI relies on expensive hardware and specially designed buildings supported by complicated software and peripherals. This means that the start-up and running costs of MRI are higher than the other modalities, and this has slowed the rate at which MRI has been widely introduced. In many countries MRI remains a scarce resource. In addition, because of the elongated tunnel design of most MR systems, approximately 1–2% of individuals cannot tolerate the examination because of claustrophobia. There are also some situations in which MRI is contraindicated, as it would not be safe for the patient to enter the strong magnetic field. These include the presence of a pacemaker or previous surgical implants of certain metallic clips (e.g. some intracerebral surgery aneurysm clips). Metallic foreign bodies, particularly in the orbits, can also be a particular problem with MRI and would prohibit its use.

A major disadvantage of MRI is that, although it enjoys high sensitivity for detecting abnormalities, this is not always associated with a high degree of specificity. The areas of high signal on the fluid-sensitive sequence result from an increase in the amount of free water in the area being imaged, but MRI cannot differentiate the cause of this increase. For example, this increase may be due to trauma, but could also be due to infection or tumour.

Therefore it is important to review MRI examinations in conjunction with other information, particularly plain films and clinical findings. The clinical information must be conveyed to the radiologist in some detail as the examination can be tailored to the clinical question if that information is available. This results from the fact that there are many different ways of obtaining an examination; for example 'MR knee' can be performed in a multitude of ways depending on the specific question being asked.

Specific clinical uses

At the **shoulder**, MRI can differentiate between rotator cuff tendinosis and full-thickness rotator cuff tears, and has the advantage over ultrasound in that it also shows a degree of any degenerative change affecting the acromioclavicular joint and the shape of the acromion, both of which are important aetiological factors in the development of rotator cuff tears and in patient management. The majority of such tears affect the supraspinatus tendon and, in addition to the tear itself, secondary signs include fluid within the subacromial subdeltoid bursa, atrophy of the supraspinatus muscle, cranial migration of the humeral head, and impingement cysts affecting the greater tuberosity of the humerus. Calcific tendonitis is essentially a plain film diagnosis, but areas of calcification are well demonstrated on MRI as a signal void on all sequences (Fig. 2.2.1(b)). Capsulitis (frozen shoulder) is difficult to evaluate on MRI and is largely considered a clinical diagnosis. Conventional arthrography is the only imaging technique that can confirm the

diagnosis of capsulitis. Glenohumeral joint instability affects a younger age group than those affected by rotator cuff impingement, and MR arthrographic techniques (direct or indirect) are ideally suited to the evaluation of these patients. Similarly, pain arising in athletes involved with overhead arm activity is best evaluated by MR arthrographic techniques. These techniques allow accurate delineation of the glenoid in particular, and tears, which might be missed on conventional MR, are demonstrated by the presence of contrast medium which gets into the tear to make it more readily visible.

The complicated 3D anatomy at the **elbow** means that the imaging protocols must be tailored to the clinical question. Repetitive injuries such as osteochondritis dissecans, which commonly occur in young athletes, is an important indication for MRI of the elbow, and both the integrity of the cartilage and loose bodies can be demonstrated. Epicondylitis (tennis elbow, golfer's elbow) can also be detected on MRI, although generally these diagnoses remain clinical and ultrasound is most useful for confirmation of diagnosis. Biceps tendon rupture most commonly occurs proximally, and results in the typical 'popeye' appearance of the anterior musculature of the upper arm, but tendon injuries at the bicipital tuberosity of the radius are also well demonstrated on MRI.

MRI of the **wrist and hand** has been revolutionized in the past 10 years by the advent of small dedicated wrist coils, which comfortably accommodate the size of the wrist. This permits an increase in the spatial resolution, allowing accurate assessment of small structures such as the triangular fibrocartilage. Another common indication for MRI in the wrist relates to the assessment of fractures of the scaphoid; MRI is sensitive at demonstrating the presence of a fracture, and it can be useful in patients with anatomical snuff box tenderness in whom plain films are negative (Bretlau *et al.* 1999). MRI can also be used to provide prognostic information relating to the risk of avascular necrosis of the proximal fragment in cases of non-union (Sakuma *et al.* 1995). In these cases, the proximal pole of the scaphoid is of low sequence on both the T1- and T2-weighted sequences, and if gadolinium is given intravenously, the proximal pole will fail to enhance. Ganglions are the most common cause of wrist lumps in adults, and are a common cause of pain in athletes. MRI is the best imaging modality for assessing the presence and extent of a ganglion, as it allows the size of the lesion, and also the extent into any underlying joint, to be assessed in a way that is difficult to achieve with ultrasound or other imaging techniques.

Pain arising from the region of the **hip** may be due to one of a large number of causes, including cartilage and labral abnormalities of the hip itself, abnormalities arising from adjacent bursae, muscle injuries, avulsion injuries from greater tuberosity or ischium, iliopsoas snapping, osteitis pubis, or referral from the spine. Therefore MRI represents a good screening tool for the athlete with hip pain, and it is also useful for following up patients serially after injury. MR arthrography of the hip, which is usually performed as a direct procedure, gives exquisite information with regard to the labrum and is useful in patients with suspected femoroacetabular impingement. In addition, stress fractures are well demonstrated on MRI as a linear low-signal structure on all sequences, often surrounded by bone oedema when acute (Fig. 2.2.8). The distension and oedema associated with bursitis make MRI a suitable diagnostic tool for its detection, such as in the case of iliopsoas bursitis or trochanteric bursitis.

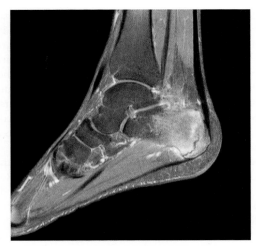

Fig. 2.2.8 Stress fracture of the calcaneus on MRI. The fracture line is well seen, and there is surrounding oedema. This condition can mimic other causes of hindfoot pain.

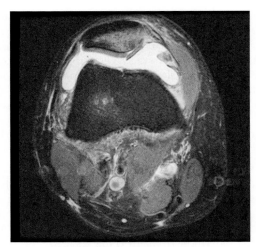

Fig. 2.2.10 Patellar cartilage fracture on MRI. The medial portion of the patellar cartilage is detached after an acute injury.

MRI of the **knee** was one of the earliest and most successful applications of MRI, and complemented the developing technique of knee arthroscopy. Meniscal and cruciate ligaments are demonstrated with high accuracy at all field strengths from 0.2 to 1.5 T (Cotten *et al.* 2000). The normal meniscus appears as a bow-tie-shaped structure, which is of low signal on all sequences. Disruption or tear of the architecture of the meniscus results in areas of increased signal on proton density or T2-weighted sequences, and can be seen extending to the articular surface (Fig. 2.2.9). Most tears are demonstrated in the sagittal plane. The cruciate ligaments are intracapsular but extra-synovial, and tears are a common cause of pain in the injured athlete. The accuracy of MRI exceeds 90% in demonstration of these lesions. Collateral ligaments are injured by excess valgus or varus force applied to the knee. The diagnosis is normally clinical, but such injuries can coexist with other injuries, and when present, MRI is accurate at detecting sprains and tears, and quantifying the grade of the injury. As in other sites, MRI is an accurate way of demonstrating fractures that are occult on plain films, particularly stress fractures, depending on the circumstance.

Anterior knee pain requires sequences in the axial plane to evaluate the patellar cartilage, and MRI is particularly suited to the demonstration of chondromalacia patellae and acute fractures of the cartilage (Fig. 2.2.10). The extent and degree can be quantified, as can underlying bony complications (Cotten *et al.* 2000). The height of the patella in relation to the tibia is also an important aetiological factor in knee pain. The height of the patella in the normal population is documented (Shabshin *et al.* 2004) and a high patella (patella alta) is associated with development of chondromalacia patellae and patellar dislocation.

Cysts and bursae around the knee are common, and can arise with a number of situations. They are well imaged by MRI. A ganglion cyst is represented by a well-defined, and often multiloculated, cystic structure, which may have the beaded appearance resulting from the adjacent development of multiple small component cysts, and the underlying joint is typically normal. However, a meniscal cyst develops as a result of fluid being forced through a meniscal tear into the adjacent soft tissues, and therefore a necessary prerequisite for its diagnosis is the presence of an adjacent meniscal tear. There are many named bursae in relation to the knee, the most common being the semimembranosus gastrocnemius bursa (Baker's cyst, popliteal cyst). Patellar tendonitis is well imaged in the sagittal plane by MRI, although ultrasound is usually considered a better way of assessing it.

At the **ankle**, the Achilles tendon is the largest and strongest tendon in the human body, and tendon abnormalities are well evaluated by MRI. The normal tendon can be differentiated from early tendinosis, cystic degeneration, partial-thickness tear, or full-thickness tear (Fig. 2.2.11). The presence of a complete tear is associated with extensive adjacent soft tissue abnormalities, in addition to haematoma formation and tendon fragmentation. However, patients with the possibility of an acute complete Achilles tendon rupture are best imaged with ultrasound because of its dynamic nature. The posterior tibial, long flexor, and peroneal tendons are also well seen on MRI (Fig. 2.2.12). Lateral ligament injuries can be well demonstrated on MRI, but medial ligament injuries are more difficult to evaluate fully. Generally, these are considered a clinical diagnosis. MRI is accurate acutely, but once the inflammation has subsided the ligament laxity that sometimes is associated with

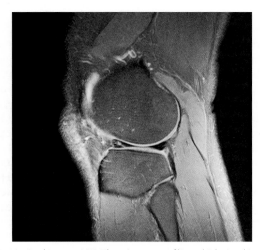

Fig. 2.2.9 Meniscal tear on MRI. There is an area of linear high signal in the anterior third of the lateral meniscus, extending to the inferior surface.

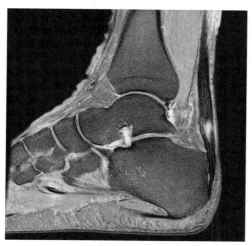

Fig. 2.2.11 Achilles partial-thickness tear on MRI. A focal area of high signal is seen within an expanded Achilles tendon, indicating the site of the partial tear.

healing is not an MRI diagnosis. Accessory muscles occur at many sites, but the most common site is the accessory soleus muscle where the soleus inserts separately into the calcaneus rather than joining the gastrocnemius muscles to form the Achilles tendon. Diagnosis is readily made on axial MRI.

MRI has a pivotal role in the evaluation of the **spine**, particularly in the context of low back pain, and is the most useful test for evaluating the presence of the prolapsed disc in the athlete. In addition, pars interarticularis defects, whether congenital or due to stress injury, which are commonly seen in the athlete are well evaluated on MRI (Campbell and Grainger 2000).

Muscle injuries are among the most common injuries that the athlete will suffer, and MRI is often considered the preferred method in the diagnosis of these injuries and in the follow-up of these patients to assess healing. Fat-saturated proton density and T2-weighted images are the most sensitive techniques for diagnosis of tears, and the time taken to return to sport can be predicted

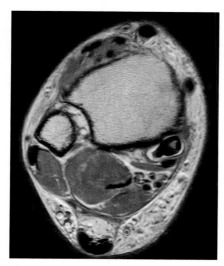

Fig. 2.2.12 Tibialis posterior tendinosis. The tendon is swollen and high signal is seen within it. There is fluid in the associated tendon sheath.

semiquantitatively based on changes seen on MRI (Slavotinek *et al.* 2002; Connell *et al.* 2004). The parameters that are relevant include an estimated volume of muscle injury, the percentage cross-sectional area of abnormal muscle, and the craniocaudal length of the muscle abnormality adjacent to the musculotendinous junction. The last of these probably has the strongest association with rehabilitation of patient time. During the repair or healing phase, there is a gradual resolution of the amount of fluid between the muscle fascicles and in relation to the epimysium, and therefore the increased T2 signal decreases over time.

Soft tissue masses in the athlete are usually trauma related, but it must be born in mind that masses such as sarcoma do occur in these patients and must be differentiated from causes related to injury. MRI has become the most useful technique for the assessment of the soft tissue mass, particularly if sarcoma is suspected. However, MRI fails to detect calcification, and if myositis ossificans is considered the most likely cause for an area of swelling, a CT might be preferred.

Summary

As previously emphasized, plain film in two orthogonal planes is the most commonly used imaging modality, but MRI has become the cornerstone of imaging of the athlete when other modalities have left uncertainty. This is because of its supreme sensitivity to increased free water which allows it to demonstrate the oedema associated with trauma, tumour, inflammation, or degeneration. The abnormality can be imaged in the plane which is the most suitable for its evaluation, and the technique avoids the biohazard associated with ionizing radiation. The equipment and the maintenance costs are expensive, and although costs are reducing every decade, they still remain significant.

Nuclear medicine scintigraphy

Technical aspects

The most commonly performed nuclear medicine examination in the context of sport injuries and stress fractures is the standard planar bone scintigram with technetium-99m (^{99m}Tc) labelled methylene diphosphonate (MDP). Common to all scintigraphic techniques, a radioactive substance which undergoes radioactive decay by emitting gamma rays, which can be considered identical to X-rays, is injected intravenously. These gamma rays are detected by a gamma camera. Many modern gamma cameras are able to resolve two points of separate foci when positioned as close as 5–8 mm apart. As soon as the tracer has been injected intravenously, the area of concern can be imaged in the arterial phase of the injection (the **radionuclide angiogram**) which represents blood distribution in the body. Approximately 3–5 minutes later the **blood pool image** is available, which represents the intra- and extravascular distribution of tracer. Finally, approximately 2–4 hours after the injection, the **bone scan image** is produced, which reflects osteoblastic uptake of the injected tracer. When all three sets of images are acquired, this is called a **three-phase bone scan**. Occasionally a fourth phase is performed after 24 hours when there is an improved ratio of bone to soft tissue uptake of tracer that can make a lesions more conspicuous, although as ^{99m}Tc has a radioactive half-life of 6 hours, imaging at or after 24 hours is associated with very much reduced overall activity.

Variations

Other specialized techniques, such as **leucocyte scintigraphy** where white blood cells are labelled and injected back into the body for imaging areas of inflammation, are used less commonly. **Single-photon emission computed tomography** (SPECT) involves acquiring images at various angles and reconstructing the images into tomograms, or slices, at various planes through the body part imaged. This allows improved spatial localization over planar scintigraphy. **Positron emission tomography** (PET) is not yet widely available. It has widespread uses in oncology but its application to the evaluation of sport-related injuries has still to be determined. More recently, PET has been combined with CT data, resulting in the **PET–CT** technique, but like PET, this does not yet have much applicability to sporting injuries.

Strengths

The main advantage of planar bone scintigraphy is that the entire skeleton and all the joints can be imaged at a single sitting, without any increase in the radiation dose compared with a scan to look at a few joints only. This is unlike radiography, where multiple additional examinations have an associated increased radiation burden. Bony abnormalities are detected with great sensitivity, and scintigraphy can identify sites of altered bone metabolism before detection by other imaging modalities is possible. In the evaluation of soft tissue disorders, a bone scintigram can help by excluding or confirming underlying bone or joint abnormalities. A negative scintigram has a high negative predictive value for excluding underlying bony involvement by a rheumatological process.

Weaknesses

Although highly sensitive, the abnormalities demonstrated are not specific for any particularly pathology, and may indeed reflect the secondary bone response to the underlying primary problem. The radiation dose of the injectate is high compared with plain film radiography (Table 2.2.1), and the spatial resolution of scintigraphy is one or more orders of magnitude less than that of other imaging modalities.

Specific clinical uses

Although [^{99m}Tc]MDP bone scintigrams have a limited role in the diagnosis of soft tissue disorders associated with sport, they can be very useful for excluding underlying bone or joint abnormality (such as arthritis, avascular necrosis, tumours, or fractures), and can help in the diagnosis of reflex sympathetic dystrophy syndrome (complex regional pain syndrome type 1). In the **spine**, scintigraphy (in particular SPECT) can be useful for assessing disease activity of facet joint arthropathy and spondylolysis. In the **pelvis**, sacroiliitis is commonly assessed by bone scintigraphy, and although the diagnosis is usually made by visual inspection of the images, quantative analysis can be helpful, particularly in disease monitoring. In the **lower limb**, stress fractures in the tibia and metatarsal (March fracture) and to a lesser extent the femur can be a cause of diffuse pain. The bone scintigram is particularly sensitive at detecting, staging, and monitoring stress fracture (Matin 1988).

Summary

Bone scintigraphy is the most commonly used nuclear medicine imaging technique in the evaluation of a sporting injury, particularly for consideration of a stress fracture. In established stress fracture, MRI is the preferred imaging technique but bone scintigraphy is very sensitive in detecting the early bone responses to excessive stress. The technique involves ionizing radiation, which is an order of magnitude greater than that involved in extremity plain radiography.

Imaging guidelines

A combination of the ionizing nature of X-rays and the imperfect accuracy of radiological tests has generally resulted in the international development of guidelines for the use of radiological examinations. Many European guidelines are based on the book by the UK Royal College of Radiologists (RCR) covering guidelines for all routine radiological examinations and aim to clarify the most appropriate use in such examinations (RCR Working Party 2007). The timeliness of this publication is illustrated by the rapidity with which the guidelines have been taken up internationally. Although, as has been stressed on several occasions in this chapter, plain films remain the mainstay for significant injuries in sport, soft tissue abnormalities most commonly involve imaging using either ultrasound or MRI. There is much variation between institutions as to preference for ultrasound or MRI in any particular circumstance, but well-established indications for ultrasound and MRI are listed in Table 2.2.2.

Conclusion

The differentiation of sports injuries can be difficult because of the multitude of underlying causes. It is important to understand the strengths and weaknesses of the different imaging techniques, so that the correct use of imaging modalities is promoted. This will lead to an earlier accurate diagnosis, which in many cases helps to prevent the development of chronic pain or complications.

The use of these imaging modalities in specific sporting injuries is considered in the remaining chapters of this book.

References

Ahovuo, J., Paavolainen, P., and Slatis, P. (1984). The diagnostic value of arthrography and plain radiography in rotator cuff tears. *Acta Orthopaedica Scandinavica*, **55**, 220–3.

Alfredson, H. and Ohberg, L. (2005). Neovascularisation in chronic painful patellar tendinosis—promising results after sclerosing neovessels outside the tendon challenge the need for surgery. *Knee Surgery, Sports Traumatology, Arthroscopy*, **13**, 74–80.

Andrenn, L. and Lundberg, B. (1965). Treatment of rigid shoulders by joint distension during arthrography. *Acta Orthopaedica Scandinavica*, **36**, 45–53.

Blanchard, T.K., Bearcroft, P.W., Dixon, A.K., *et al.* (1997). Magnetic resonance imaging or arthrography of the shoulder: which do patients prefer? *British Journal of Radiology*, **70**, 786–90.

Bretlau, T., Christensen, O.M., Edstrom, P., Thomsen, H.S., and Lausten, G.S. (1999). Diagnosis of scaphoid fracture and dedicated extremity MRI. *Acta Orthopaedica Scandinavica*, **70**, 504–8.

Campbell, R.S. and Grainger, A.J. (2000). Routine thin slice MRI effectively demonstrates the lumbar pars interarticularis. *Clinical Radiology*, **55**, 984.

Connell, D.A., Schneider-Kolsky, M.E., Hoving, J.L., *et al.* (2004). Longitudinal study comparing sonographic and MRI assessments of acute and healing hamstring injuries. *AJR American Journal of Roentgenology*, **183**, 975–84.

Cotten, A., Delfaut, E., Demondion, X., *et al.* (2000). MR imaging of the knee at 0.2 and 1.5 T: correlation with surgery. *AJR American Journal of Roentgenology*, **174**, 1093–7.

Deng, X., Farley, M., Nieminen, M.T., Gray, M., and Burstein, D. (2007). Diffusion tensor imaging of native and degenerated human articular cartilage. *Magnetic Resonance Imaging*, **25**, 168–71.

Dinnes, J., Loveman, E., McIntyre, L., and Waugh, N. (2003). The effectiveness of diagnostic tests for the assessment of shoulder pain due to soft tissue disorders: a systematic review. *Health Technology Assessment*, **7**, iii1-166.

Eckstein, F., Mosher, T., and Hunter, D. (2007). Imaging of knee osteoarthritis: data beyond the beauty. *Current Opinion in Rheumatology*, **19**, 435–43.

Fredberg, U. and Bolvig, L. (1999). Jumper's knee. Review of the literature. *Scandinavian Journal of Medicine and Science in Sports*, **9**, 66–73.

Galban, C.J., Maderwald, S., Uffmann, K., de Greiff, A., and Ladd, M.E. (2004). Diffusive sensitivity to muscle architecture: a magnetic resonance diffusion tensor imaging study of the human calf. *European Journal of Applied Physiology*, **93**, 253–62.

Gold, G.E. (2003). Dynamic and functional imaging of the musculoskeletal system. *Seminars in Musculoskeletal Radiology*, **7**, 245–8.

Kieft, G.J., Bloem, J.L., Rozing, P.M., and Obermann, W.R. (1988). Rotator cuff impingement syndrome: MR imaging. *Radiology*, **166**, 211–14.

Kristoffersen, M., Ohberg, L., Johnston, C., and Alfredson, H. (2005). Neovascularisation in chronic tendon injuries detected with colour Doppler ultrasound in horse and man: implications for research and treatment. *Knee Surgery, Sports Traumatology, Arthroscopy*, **13**, 505–8.

Matin, P. (1988). Basic principles of nuclear medicine techniques for detection and evaluation of trauma and sports medicine injuries. *Seminars in Nuclear Medicine*, **18**, 90–112.

Pelsser, V., Cardinal, E., Hobden, R., Aubin, B., and Lafortune, M. (2001). Extraarticular snapping hip: sonographic findings. *AJR American Journal of Roentgenology*, **176**, 67–73.

Prokop, M. (2003). General principles of MDCT. *European Journal of Radiology*, **45** (Suppl. 1), S4–10.

Raikin, S.M., Elias, I., and Nazarian, L.N. (2008). Intrasheath subluxation of the peroneal tendons. *Journal of Bone and Joint Surgery*, **90**, 992–99.

RCR (Royal College of Radiologists) Working Party (2007). *Making the Best Use of a Department of Radiology* (6th edn). Royal College of Radiologists, London.

Resnick, D. (1995). Arthrography, tenography and bursography. In: D. Resnick (ed.), *Diagnosis of Bone and Joint Disorders* (3rd edn), pp. 277–409. W.B. Saunders, Philadelphia, PA.

Sakuma, M., Nakamura, R., and Imaeda, T. (1995). Analysis of proximal fragment sclerosis and surgical outcome of scaphoid non-union by magnetic resonance imaging. *Journal of Hand Surgery (Edinburgh)*, **20**, 201–5.

Shabshin, N., Schweitzer, M.E., Morrison, W.B., and Parker, L. (2004). MRI criteria for patella alta and baja. *Skeletal Radiology*, **33**, 445–50.

Slavotinek, J.P., Verrall, G.M., and Fon, G.T. (2002). Hamstring injury in athletes: using MR imaging measurements to compare extent of muscle injury with amount of time lost from competition. *AJR American Journal of Roentgenology*, **179**, 1621–8.

Swallow, R.A. and Naylor, E. (eds) (1996). *Clarke's Positioning in Radiography* (11th edn). Heinemann Medical, Oxford.

Takebayashi, S., Takasawa, H., Banzai, Y., *et al.* (1995). Sonographic findings in muscle strain injury: clinical and MR imaging correlation. *Journal of Ultrasound in Medicine*, **14**, 899–905.

Teefey, S.A., Middleton, W.D., Patel, V., Hildebolt, C.F., and Boyer, M.I. (2004). The accuracy of high-resolution ultrasound for evaluating focal lesions of the hand and wrist. *Journal of Hand Surgery*, **29**, 393–9.

Weinberg, E.P., Adams, M.J., and Hollenberg, G.M. (1998). Color Doppler sonography of patellar tendinosis. *AJR American Journal of Roentgenology*, **171**, 743–4.

Zanetti, M., Metzdorf, A., Kundert, H.P., *et al.* (2003). Achilles tendons: clinical relevance of neovascularization diagnosed with power Doppler US. *Radiology*, **227**, 556–60.

Key references

Connell, D.A., Schneider-Kolsky, M.E., Hoving, J.L., *et al.* (2004). Longitudinal study comparing sonographic and MRI assessments of acute and healing hamstring injuries. *AJR American Journal of Roentgenology*, **183**, 975–84.

Kristoffersen, M., Ohberg, L., Johnston, C., and Alfredson, H. (2005). Neovascularisation in chronic tendon injuries detected with colour Doppler ultrasound in horse and man: implications for research and treatment. *Knee Surgery, Sports Traumatology, Arthroscopy*, **13**, 505–8.

Slavotinek, J.P., Verrall, G.M., and Fon, G.T. (2002). Hamstring injury in athletes: using MR imaging measurements to compare extent of muscle injury with amount of time lost from competition. *AJR American Journal of Roentgenology*, **179**, 1621–8.

Takebayashi, S., Takasawa, H., Banzai, Y., *et al.* (1995). Sonographic findings in muscle strain injury: clinical and MR imaging correlation. *Journal of Ultrasound in Medicine*, **14**, 899–905.

Zanetti, M., Metzdorf, A., Kundert, H.P., *et al.* (2003). Achilles tendons: clinical relevance of neovascularization diagnosed with power Doppler US. *Radiology*, **227**, 556–60.

Review articles and chapters

The following are review articles or book chapters:

Eckstein, F., Mosher, T., and Hunter, D. (2007). Imaging of knee osteoarthritis: data beyond the beauty. *Current Opinion in Rheumatology*, **19**, 435–43.

Fredberg, U. and Bolvig, L. (1999). Jumper's knee. Review of the literature. *Scandinavian Journal of Medicine and Science in Sports*, **9**, 66–73.

Gold, G.E. (2003). Dynamic and functional imaging of the musculoskeletal system. *Seminars in Musculoskeletal Radiology*, **7**, 245–8.

Matin, P. (1988). Basic principles of nuclear medicine techniques for detection and evaluation of trauma and sports medicine injuries. *Seminars in Nuclear Medicine*, **18**, 90–112.

Prokop, M. (2003). General principles of MDCT. *European Journal of Radiology*, **45** (Suppl. 1), S4–10.

RCR (Royal College of Radiologists) Working Party (2007). *Making the Best Use of a Department of Radiology* (6th edn). Royal College of Radiologists, London.

Resnick, D. (1995). Arthrography, tenography and bursography. In: D. Resnick (ed.), *Diagnosis of Bone and Joint Disorders* (3rd edn), pp. 277–409. W.B. Saunders, Philadelphia, PA.

Swallow, R.A. and Naylor, E. (eds) (1996). *Clarke's Positioning in Radiography* (11th edn). Heinemann Medical, Oxford.

2.3

Neurophysiological investigation of injuries sustained in sport

Gerard Mullins and Julian Ray

Introduction

The continued growth of recreational and competitive sports has been accompanied by an increased incidence of nerve injuries that have been traditionally associated with other types of occupational injury (Krivickas and Wilbourn 1998). Peripheral nerves are susceptible to injury in the athlete because of excessive physiological demands (Feinberg *et al.* 1997). The most common mechanisms of nerve injuries associated with physical activity include compression or entrapment (e.g. median and ulnar neuropathies), traction injuries (e.g. brachial plexopathies and 'stingers'), repetitive strain, direct trauma causing ischaemia to nerves or laceration of nerves (e.g. dislocation of shoulder with brachial plexopathies), and indirect trauma due to associated fractures or haematoma formation (radial nerve injury in patients with humeral shaft fractures) (Stewart 1999).

When assessing athletes with nerve injury, an understanding of the physiology of nerve injury and repair is necessary. Nerve fibres are composed of axons, over half of which are enclosed in a myelin sheath. Axons are responsible for propagating action potentials and the myelin sheath acts as an insulating layer to facilitate conduction. According to the widely used Seddon classification (Seddon *et al.* 1943), nerve injuries can be subdivided into three types (Table 2.3.1).

In reality nerve injuries encountered in athletes are frequently mixed. The aim of the neurophysiologist is to accurately diagnose and localize nerve injuries. In addition, it is possible to assess severity and to classify the type of nerve injury with detailed neurophysiological investigations. This is important as this information will enable the referring physician to plan treatment and to provide the athlete with an accurate prognosis and projected recovery time.

The electrodiagnostic techniques employed in assessing patients are nerve conduction studies (NCS) and needle electromyography (EMG). In daily clinical practice these should be considered as an extension of the clinical examination.

Nerve conduction studies

The principles of nerve conduction involve the extracellular recording of intracellular events in nerve fibres. NCS are usually recorded by stimulating the action potential of a nerve by applying an electrical impulse to the overlying skin with a stimulating electrode and recording from electrodes placed over a distal muscle or a cutaneous sensory nerve. Motor, sensory, and mixed nerve responses can be recorded from the median, ulnar, radial, and musculocutaneous nerves in the upper limb, and from the peroneal, tibial, and sural nerves in the lower limb.

Motor conduction studies

Motor conduction studies are obtained by stimulating a motor nerve at one or more sites along its course and recording the resultant motor response or compound motor action potential (CMAP) with electrodes placed over the muscle being studied. The CMAP

Table 2.3.1 Classification of nerve injury (Data from John D. Stewart 1999)

Neuropraxia (mild)
Focal demyelination after focal injury
◆ e.g. acute ulnar nerve compression in cyclists
◆ demyelination blocks velocity of nerve conduction ⇒weakness
Usual rapid recovery
◆ repair of small section of demyelination restores conduction
Axonotmesis (moderate)
Preservation of nerve sheath
Sufficient trauma to cause axonal loss (Wallerian degeneration)
May regrow 1–2mm/day
Neurotmesis (severe)
Disruption of nerve sheath + axonal loss
Cut, stretch or crush lesions
◆ traumatic stretch injury (e.g. brachial plexu
◆ intraoperative nerve injury (e.g. axillary nerve, femoral)
Will not recover as nerve sheath disrupted
◆ operative repair essential

represents the depolarization of muscle fibres innervated by a motor nerve, and responses are usually in the millivolt (mV) range (Preston and Shapiro 2005).

The active electrode is placed over the muscle belly with the reference electrode placed distally over the muscle tendon. It is useful if the patient activates the muscle voluntarily so that the muscle belly can be identified. The stimulating electrode is placed over the nerve with the cathode closest to the recording electrode and the nerve is stimulated orthodromically. The current is increased until the CMAP no longer increases in size; then stimulation is increased by a further 20% to ensure a supramaximal response.

The CMAP is analysed to determine distal motor latency (DML), amplitude, duration, and conduction velocity. DML is defined as the time from the stimulus to the initial CMAP deflection from the baseline. It is a function of transmission along the motor nerve and neuromuscular junction, and depolarization across the muscle. Amplitude reflects the number of muscle fibres depolarized. To calculate the conduction velocity, the nerve is stimulated at two or more sites (distal or close to the recording muscle and at a proximal site in the motor nerve) and is calculated by dividing the distance between these two points by the nerve conduction time (i.e. velocity = distance/time). If there is a loss of motor axons the CMAP amplitude will be reduced, but distal latency and conduction velocity should be preserved (unless there is a severe axonal loss). In demyelinating nerve injuries, the distal latency is prolonged if the area of demyelination is in the distal portion of the motor nerve (e.g. carpal tunnel syndrome), motor conduction velocity may be slowed, and the CMAP can have a prolonged duration and a dispersed morphology. If the area of demyelination lies between distal and proximal stimulating sites, this may result in a conduction block, which as defined as a reduction of more than 50% reduction in CMAP between distal and proximal stimulation sites.

In addition to orthodromic stimulation of the motor nerve resulting in the CMAP, impulses also propagate antidromically to the anterior horn cell which stimulates a portion of the anterior horn cells to send another impulse othodromically resulting in a smaller late motor response known as the F wave. Calculation of the F wave latency allows assessment of conduction in the proximal portion of the motor nerve and nerve roots (Preston and Shapiro 2005).

Sensory nerve conduction studies

Sensory nerve conduction studies represent the summation of all sensory nerve action potentials and are recorded as the sensory nerve action potential (SNAP). Sensory nerve fibres have a lower stimulation threshold than motor nerve fibres and so a lower current is usually required to achieve supra-maximal stimulation. SNAPs are much smaller in amplitude (microvolts (μV)) than motor responses (millivolts) and are more susceptible to environmental factors and electrical interference (Preston and Shapiro 2005).

The SNAP is recorded by placing a pair of recording electrodes over the nerve, with the active electrode placed closest to the stimulator and the reference electrode placed approximately 2–3 cm away. The sensory nerves can be stimulated orthodromically with a standard stimulating electrode or antidromically by using a ring electrodes on the fingers. Finger ring electrodes can also be used to record orthodromic stimulated sensory responses on the fingers.

The time between stimulation of the nerve and the first deflection from the baseline (onset latency) or to the peak of the SNAP (peak latency) is measured first. The SNAP amplitude is the summation of all depolarized sensory fibres. The sensory velocity represents the speed along the largest myelinated sensory fibres and is calculated by dividing the distance D between the stimulating (cathode) and recording active electrode by the onset latency (i.e. sensory velocity = D/onset latency). Axonal lesions cause a reduction in the SNAP amplitude, while onset latency and conduction velocity are usually preserved. Demyelinating lesions may cause delayed onset latency, slowing of sensory conduction velocity, increased duration of the SNAP wave form, and reduction in the SNAP amplitude (Seddon *et al.* 1943).

All sensory fibres are derived from the dorsal root ganglion which lies in the exit foramina of the vertebrae. Sensory nerve conduction can assess the integrity of the sensory nerve distal to the dorsal root ganglion, but does not allow assessment of sensory fibres proximal to this. This explains why patients with radiculopathies have entirely normal sensory nerve conduction despite significant sensory symptoms.

Needle electromyography

Needle EMG records the extracellular electrical activity from muscle fibres by insertion of a needle in the muscle belly. EMG is performed using a standard EMG machine, an EMG needle (usually concentric needles), an earth electrode, gloves, and a cooperative patient. Accurate identification of surface landmarks for each muscle is necessary to insert the needle and to determine how best to get the patient to correctly rest and activate the muscle. The electromyographer must sample sufficient muscle groups to answer the clinical question. Recordings are made from each muscle at rest, during slight voluntary contraction, and during maximal voluntary contraction (Preston and Shapiro 2005).

During rest insertion activity and spontaneous activity are assessed. A small degree of insertion electrical activity is normal as a result of potentials generated at the muscle endplate (endplate spikes and endplate noise) but these are short lived. Any spontaneous activity outside the endplate zone is abnormal. Sometimes spontaneous activity needs to be triggered by moving the EMG needle in the muscle, by muscle contraction, or by percussion over the muscle. Increased spontaneous activity is seen in denervated muscles and in a number of other conditions. The most common types of abnormal muscle activity seen are fibrillation potentials, positive sharp waves, fasciculation potentials and complex repetitive discharges.

Fibrillation potentials and positive sharp waves are due to spontaneous discharges from individual muscle fibres. On EMG fibrillation potentials sound like 'rain on a tin roof' whereas positive sharp waves have a dull 'pop' sound. Both are a marker of acute and active denervation, but can also be seen in myopathies.

Complex repetitive discharges are seen as a result of chronic denervation and are generated by spontaneous depolarization of a single denervated muscle fibre with direct spread to adjacent muscle fibres. These have a 'machine-like' sound on EMG.

Fasciculation potentials are spontaneous discharges that originate in the axon of the motor nerve. Fasciculations have an irregular firing rate. The morphology can either be that of a simple motor unit or be complex and larger. Fasciculations can often be seen clinically as brief twitches in the muscle belly. They are a feature of chronic denervation.

After assessment of the muscle at rest, the next goal is to evaluate the muscle motor unit action potentials (MUAPs) during minimal and maximal voluntary contraction. The MUAP is best assessed during minimal voluntary activity.

A normal motor action potential has three phases (Fig. 2.3.1). The duration of the MUAP varies from muscle to muscle but most are less than 15 ms. The amplitude also varies from muscle to muscle, with most MUAPs having amplitude 0.5 to 3 mV.

With chronic denervation, collateral sprouting to the denervated motor unit from adjacent motor units (i.e. re-innervation) occurs. This leads to MUAPs of larger amplitude, longer duration, and an increased number of phases (polyphasia). In acutely denervated muscles (before re-innervation has time to occur), the morphology of the MUAP is unchanged. If there is severe or complete denervation, with no nearby surviving axons, the only means by which re-innervation can occur is by regrowth of axons. This will lead to partial re-innervation of the original muscle fibres. The MUAPs in early re-innervation are termed nascent MUAPs and are of small amplitude and polyphasic.

Normally increased contraction of a muscle corresponds to an increase in the recruitment of MUAPs. As recruitment increases, MUAPs begin to overlap producing the interference pattern. The interference pattern is reduced in acute and chronic denervated muscles, consequently individual motor potentials can be discerned (Fig. 2.3.2).

The investigation of the upper limb injuries seen in athletes:

Brachial plexus

The brachial plexus is formed from the anterior primary rami of the lower cervical and upper thoracic nerve roots (C5 to T1) and carries motor, sensory, and autonomic fibres w supply the upper limb. The long thoracic nerve arises directly from the C6–C7 nerve roots and can be affected in isolation in some patients. Most nerves to the upper limb are derived from the cords (Ferrante 2004). There is an increasing body of literature describing brachial plexus injuries encountered in sports.

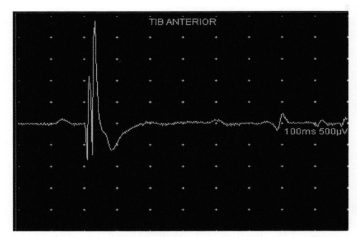

Fig. 2.3.2 A chronic denervated MUAP. This MUAP has an amplitude of 3.5 mV and a duration of 20 ms

'Stingers' or 'burners' are common in athletes who play contact sports (e.g. American football, rugby, and wrestling) (Feinberg 2000). They are due to traction (from a lateral flexion injury to the neck) or a direct blow to the upper trunk of the brachial plexus (Weinberg *et al.* 2003). Patients complain of a sudden onset of severe pain and burning in the shoulder on impact, which is followed variably by weakness in the affected limb (Weinberg *et al.* 2003). Many recover within minutes, but 5–10% are more serious, presenting with a neurological deficit lasting several hours or longer. There have been reports of isolated long thoracic nerve palsies in weightlifters, thought to be due to stretch injury of the long thoracic nerve. There have also been cases of brachial plexopathies in swimmers caused by compression of the lower trunk of the brachial plexus by a cervical rib or fibrous band. One case was due to compression of the lower trunk by a hypertrophied scalenus anticus muscle (Katirji and Hardy 1995). The brachial plexus is vulnerable to injury after shoulder dislocations, and can be seen in contact sports such as rugby, soccer, and wrestling.

Patients can present with a variety of symptoms and signs, depending on the part of the brachial plexus injured, so it is the role of electrophysiological investigations to confirm that a patient's symptoms are due to a brachial plexopathy, to localize the lesion accurately (trunks or cord), and to assess severity of the injury. In addition, it is necessary to exclude other possible causes for the patient's symptoms such as focal neuropathies that mimic a brachial plexus injury.

As sensory nerve fibres originate in the dorsal root ganglion, sensory responses are often abnormal in patients with brachial plexus injuries. Sensory responses are recorded from the median, ulnar, radial, medial cutaneous, and lateral cutaneous nerves of the forearm from symptomatic and unaffected sides. A 50% difference in amplitude of sensory responses is significant (Ferrante and Wilbourn 2002).

Motor studies from median and ulnar nerves are also recorded. As well as excluding multiple entrapment neuropathies, motor studies also provide other important information (Preston and Shapiro 2005). In severe axonal injuries, CMAPs can be reduced or even absent. Median and ulnar F latencies are prolonged in lower trunk brachial plexopathies. The brachial plexus can be stimulated

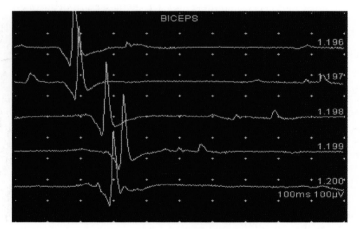

Fig. 2.3.1 Normal MUAPs. Each MUAP has three phases, and has an amplitude between 0.5 and 3 mV and a duration of 10 ms. The MUAPS here have an amplitude of 0.5 mV and a duration of 10 ms.

directly at Erb's point (2–3 cm above the clavicle) when investigating upper trunk brachial plexopthies.

Needle EMG will detect acute and chronic denervation changes in an affected limb. Needle EMG from muscles supplied by all trunks, cords, and branches of the brachial plexus is necessary to localize the level of brachial plexus injury accurately (Ferrante and Wilbourn 2002). For example, an upper trunk plexopathy will show denervation in muscles whose nerve supply originates in the upper trunk (i.e. deltoid, biceps, spinati, and brachioradialis) but will be essentially normal from muscles where the nerve supply originates from the lower trunk. However, a number of brachial plexopathies are patchy and involve more than one trunk.

Needle EMG in patients with severe axonal injury (axonotmesis, neurotmesis) exhibits florid spontaneous activity accompanied by absent voluntary effort in the muscles studied. This indicates a poor prognosis, and surgical exploration and nerve repair require consideration.

Axillary neuropathy

Axillary nerve injuries are common in athletes who play contact sports, especially rugby, American football, and ice hockey. The mechanism of injury is often a direct blow to the anteriorlateral deltoid muscle, simultaneous contralateral neck flexion and ipsilateral shoulder depression, and secondary to shoulder dislocations (Perlmutter and Apruzzese 1998).

There are no sensory nerve conduction studies of use in patients with axillary neuropathies. However, sensory nerves in the affected limb should be examined to exclude a brachial plexopathy. Motor studies can be obtained by stimulating the axillary nerve in the axilla and Erb's point and recording the CMAP with an electrode over the deltoid muscle.

Needle EMG will show denervation with or without re-innervation (depending on the time after the injury that the investigation is performed) in the deltoid and rhomboid muscles, but EMG of other muscles supplied by nerves originating in the upper trunk of the brachial plexus (supraspinatus, infraspinatus, biceps, and brachioradialis) will be normal (Preston and Shapiro 2005).

Ulnar neuropathy

The ulnar nerve is derived from the medial cord and descends in the upper arm where it passes through the medial head of the triceps muscle and then continues medially to pass through the olecranon groove at the elbow. The nerve gives off motor branches in the forearm to flexor carpi ulnaris (FCU) and flexor digitorum profundus (FDP) and then extends along the medial forearm. It enters the wrist through a fibrocartilaginous canal (Guyon's canal). In the canal it gives off a sensory branch to the palmar surface of digits 4 and 5, motor branches to the hypothenar muscles, and then continues as the deep palmar branch to supply the remaining intrinsic hand muscles (interossei and medial lumbricals). The nerve is vulnerable to compression at the elbow and less commonly at the wrist (Stewart 1999; Preston and Shapiro 2005).

Ulnar neuropathy at the elbow is a common disorder seen in the 'throwing athlete' (volleyball players, baseball players, and tennis players) (Chen et al. 2001; Cain et al. 2003; Ozbek et al. 2006). Ulnar neuropathy can also be caused by forceful poling in cross-country skiing, and appears to be the consequence of extension of the elbow with concomitant contraction of the flexor carpi ulnaris and triceps while driving the arm and shoulder downwards and

behind the body (Fulkerson 1980). There have also been cases of compressive ulnar neuropathy in high-performing cyclists.

Distal ulnar neuropathies are uncommonly seen in routine clinical practice, but have been identified in cyclists ('handlebar palsy') (Capitani and Beer 2002; Patterson et al. 2003) and golfers (White and Johnson 2003; Hsu et al. 2005). It is thought that prolonged grip pressures on handlebars or the forceful grasp of a golf club handle in the palm causes a focal entrapment neuropathy in Guyon's canal at the wrist.

The aim of nerve conduction studies is to confirm the ulnar neuropathy and localize the site of compression. Patients with ulnar neuropathy of the elbow can have a reduced ulnar SNAP compared with the unaffected side. Motor studies are recorded by stimulating the ulnar nerve at the wrist, 2 cm below the elbow, and 4–8 cm above the elbow and recording the CMAPS from electrodes placed on the abductor digiti minimi (ADM). In cases of ulnar entrapment, focal slowing of motor conduction is seen across the elbow (less than 50 m/s or a decrease in the velocity across the elbow of greater than 10 m/s compared with the motor velocity in the forearm). In addition, where there is focal demyelination at the site of compression, conduction block can sometimes be demonstrated as a drop in the CMAP potential of greater than 20% between stimulation below and above the elbow. In some cases the CMAP morphology is dispersed. In severe axonal injuries the CMAP potential can also be significantly reduced in the forearm. EMG of ulnar innervated muscle can determine the extent of axonal involvement, with prognosis proportional to the degree of denervation seen. All ulnar innervated hand and forearm muscles are examined, as well as other non-ulnar innervated C8–T1 muscles (e.g. abductor pollicis brevis) to exclude a lower trunk brachial plexopathy or a lower cervical radiculopathy (Preston and Shapiro 2005).

The electrodiagnostic findings in an ulnar neuropathy at the wrist depend on whether the nerve is compressed proximal or distal to the deep palmar branch. In all cases of ulnar neuropathy at the wrist it is necessary to perform motor studies recording from the ADM and the first dorsal interosseous muscle (FDIO). In distal ulnar neuropathies the DML to the FDIO and ADM may be prolonged, with a reduced CMAP compared with the responses from the contralateral side. In more distal lesions (i.e. compression distal to the motor supply to the ADM) the DML to the FDIO is prolonged compared with the DML to the ipsilateral FDIO. The normal DML to the FDIO is less than 4.5 ms, with a latency of less than 1.3 ms to he normal side being normal. EMG shows denervation in the intrinsic hand muscle with sparing of the FCU and FDP (as the motor branches to these muscles are given off in the forearm) (Preston and Shapiro 2005).

Median neuropathy

Carpal tunnel syndrome is caused by compression of the median nerve at the wrist and is the most common entrapment neuropathy, occurring in 8% of the population (Preston and Shapiro 2005). The pathophysiology of carpal tunnel syndrome is usually focal demyelination at the site of compression and can be associated with secondary axonal loss (Stewart 1999). It may be caused by repetitive work-related activity. Sports such as motor cycle racing, Formula One racing (Masmejean et al. 1999), rock climbing (Holtzhausen and Noakes 1996), wheelchair athletics (Boninger et al. 1996; Jackson et al. 1996), weightlifting, golf, and swimming have all been associated with an increased incidence of carpal tunnel syndrome.

Carpal tunnel syndrome can be diagnosed clinically, but neurophysiology remains the gold standard for confirming median nerve compression at the wrist as a range of other conditions can present with similar symptoms (e.g. C6–C7 radiculopathy). The aim of neurophysiology is to confirm slowing of median conduction across the carpal tunnel. Sensory nerve conduction studies are performed by stimulating sensory fibres with ring electrodes over digits 2 and 3 (median) and digit 5 (ulnar) and recording the SNAP with recording electrodes over the median and ulnar nerve at the wrist. Slowing of median compared with ulnar sensory conduction of 10 m/s or more is significant. In more severe cases the SNAP can have reduced amplitudes secondary to axonal loss. Motor studies reveal slowing of distal median motor conduction as a prolonged DML and a modest prolongation of F latency. In severe cases, the CMAP amplitudes may be reduced due to motor axon loss. There are a group of patients in whom all the routine tests discussed above are normal (up to 15%). In such patients more sensitive studies need to be performed. Two of the most frequently used include comparing the median and ulnar palm to wrist mixed nerve latency and to comparing DMLs with the second lumbrical (median) and second dorsal interosseous (ulnar) muscles (Preston and Shapiro 2005).

Nerve conduction studies can also be used to assess the severity of carpal tunnel syndrome. Mild carpal tunnel syndrome is associated with sensory slowing only. Moderate carpal tunnel syndrome is also associated with sensory slowing. In addition, sensory axons are lost (reduced SNAP amplitude) and motor slowing (prolonged DML but less than 6.5 μs) is seen. In severe carpal tunnel syndrome sensory axons are lost resulting in absent SNAPs; there is also more marked motor slowing (DML >6.5 μs) and motor axons may be lost (reduced CMAP amplitude). Patients with mild carpal tunnel syndrome may respond to conservative measures, but surgical intervention is usually required in cases of moderate and severe carpal tunnel syndrome.

Needle EMG of abductor pollicis brevis may show denervation and re-innervation in moderate and severe cases. It is also necessary to examine proximal median innervated muscle (flexor pollicis longus, flexor digitorum profundus, and pronator teres) to exclude a more proximal median neuropathy. In addition, at least one other non-median innervated C8–T1 muscle must be sampled (FDIO) to exclude a lower trunk brachial plexopathy and a non-median innervated C6–C7 muscle (e.g. triceps) should be sampled to exclude a radiculopathy.

Radial neuropathy

Most radial nerve injuries seen in athletes are associated with fractures of the humerus. Patients present variable weakness of extensor muscles in the arm, depending on the level of the lesion. Humeral fractures are seen in contact sports, but can also be due to muscular forces occurring in the act of throwing (Ogawa and Yashida 1998; Curtin et al. 2005). Examples reported include baseball, softball, and javelin throwing. Approximately 18% of humeral shaft fractures are associated with a radial nerve palsy, and it is most commonly seen with fractures that occur in the middle and distal thirds (Holstein–Lewis fracture). The radial nerve can be damaged by laceration (most common in fractures of the distal third of the humerus) or by entrapment at the fracture site by bone fragments or ruptured tendons (Stewart 1999).

Posterior interosseous nerve palsies are due to focal compression of the posterior interosseous nerve in the forearm in a tendinous canal known as the 'radial tunnel' or supinator tunnel. This is most commonly encountered in carpenters, but is also very rarely seen in athletes. Cases have been reported in patients who perform repetitive manual tasks involving pronation and supination of the arm (Dickerman et al. 2002) (weightlifters) and athletes involved in rackets sports (tennis) (Pfandl et al.1992).

The superficial radial nerve response is obtained by stimulating the nerve approximately 10 cm proximal to the radial head and recording the response over the nerve at the anatomical snuff box. The SNAP is usually normal in athletes with a posterior interosseous nerve palsy and in patients with radial neuropathies due to focal demyelination of the radial nerve secondary to entrapment. The SNAP is abnormal if there has been significant axonal injury (nerve laceration associated with humeral fractures), but can be normal in the acute setting (before Wallerian degeneration has occurred) (Preston and Shapiro 2005).

Radial motor studies are an important component of the assessment. The CMAP is obtained by placing recording electrodes over the extensor indices proprius muscle. The nerve is then stimulated in the forearm, at the elbow, above the elbow (proximal and distal to the spiral groove), and at the axilla. It is important to compare responses with the opposite side. Focal areas of entrapment can be identified as slowing of motor conduction, conduction block, and/or dispersion of the CMAP amplitudes at the site of demyelination/entrapment. For example, in patients with 'radial tunnel syndrome' (posterior interosseous nerve palsy due to compression in the forearm) it is sometimes possible to demonstrate focal demyelination in the forearm (Preston and Shapiro 2005).

Needle EMG helps to differentiate the level of the lesion. In patients with a pure posterior interosseous nerve palsy, denervation is seen only in the finger and wrist extensors supplied by this nerve (extensor indicis proprius, extensor digitorum communis, extensor carpi ulnaris, extensor pollicis brevis, and supinator muscles). The nerves to the extensor carpi radialis and brachioradialis leave the radial nerve proximal to the posterior interosseous nerve, so EMG of these muscles is normal. When the radial nerve is injured at the level of the spiral groove or in the distal forearm, these two muscles will also be weak and EMG will exhibit signs of denervation. A proximal radial nerve lesion is very uncommon, but when it occurs it will result in denervation in the triceps muscle. EMG of the deltoid (axillary nerve) is necessary to exclude a posterior cord brachial plexopathy and EMG of the C7 paraspinal muscles helps to exclude a radiculopathy (Preston and Shapiro 2005).

Investigation of the lower limb:

Exercise-related leg pain is a common problem in sports medicine. There are many common causes of such symptoms, including stress fractures and muscle compartment syndromes. There are also a number of less common but important conditions including nerve entrapment syndromes. We will now focus on the investigation of the most common nerve entrapments and nerve injuries seen in the lower limbs of athletes.

Peroneal neuropathy.

Peroneal neuropathy is the most common mononeuropathy in the lower extremity seen in the neurophysiological department. Patients present with footdrop and sensory symptoms over the dorsum of the foot and lateral calf muscle (Stewart 1999). The most common site of injury is at the fibular head following trauma, stretch injury during exercise or prolonged squatting, and compression (e.g. above knee plaster casts to immobilize a fracture). Several sports have been implicated in causing peroneal nerve injuries in this fashion (McCrory *et al.* 2002; MacDonald *et al.* 2002; Adam *et al.* 2005). Rarely, the superficial peroneal sensory nerve can be compressed by tight-fitting boots ('ski boot neuropathy') (Preston and Shapiro 2005).

Motor studies are performed by placing a recording electrode over the extensor digitorum brevis muscle in the foot. The nerve is stimulated at three sites: the ankle (between the malleoli on the dorsal aspect of the ankle), below the knee (just inferior to the fibular head), and above the knee. Focal slowing and conduction block can localize the lesion to the fibular head. Sensory responses from the superficial peroneal nerve are usually reduced and can be absent (Preston and Shapiro 2005).

Needle EMG is important to exclude an L5 radiculopathy and sciatic nerve injuries. In pure common peroneal neuropathies, denervation is limited to tibialis anterior, peroneus longus, and extensor hallucis longus. Denervation in the ipsilateral tibialis posterior (tibial nerve) indicates an L5 radiculopathy, and denervation in the short head of biceps femoris indicates a sciatic neuropathy (Preston and Shapiro 2005).

Tarsal tunnel syndrome

Tarsal tunnel syndrome results from compression of the distal tibial nerve under the flexor retinaculum at the ankle. It presents with malleolar pain, burning, and sensory loss over the heel. Symptoms are exacerbated by weight-bearing (Preston and Shapiro 2005). Numerous sports-related activities have been associated with triggering tarsal tunnel syndrome, in particular those that impose heavy burdens on the ankle joints such as sprinting, jumping, marathon running, and judo (Kinoshita *et al.* 2006).

Bilateral tibial and peroneal motor responses and F latencies, sural sensory responses, and medial and lateral plantar mixed nerve responses are performed. The medial plantar nerve is stimulated over the medial sole and the mixed nerve response is recorded over the medial ankle. The lateral mixed plantar nerve is stimulated over the lateral sole and again recorded over the medial ankle. In patients with tarsal tunnel syndrome the tibial distal motor latency is prolonged, and medial and lateral plantar mixed nerve responses are either reduced or absent on the symptomatic side. Needle EMG should also be performed to exclude an S1 radiculopathy (Preston and Shapiro 2005).

Lumbosacral radiculopathies

Spinal roots may be injured by direct and indirect trauma during contact sports. Bilateral sacral radiculopathy in a cyclist has also been reported (Pardal-Fernández *et al.* 2005). Most cases seem to be due to disc prolapse and/or degenerative disc disease.

Lower limb sensory nerve conduction studies are usually normal. This helps exclude other causes of the patient's symptoms such as lumbosacral plexopathies and peripheral neuropathies. The main reason for performing detailed nerve conduction studies is to exclude an entrapment neuropathy. Some subtle abnormalities can be seen in motor conduction studies with prolongation of F latencies, and if the pathophysiology involves axonal injury, motor CMAP amplitudes can be reduced.

EMG holds the key to making a neurophysiological diagnosis of a radiculopathy. In nerve root compression there are signs of chronic and partial denervation. The key is to sample at least two muscles innervated by the same myotome but different nerves, and to examine muscles from several myotomes to exclude multilevel radiculopathies. It is also helpful to examine the paraspinal muscles as these are supplied directly by the nerve roots (Preston and Shapiro 2005).

Meralgia paraesthetica

Several cases of meralgia paraesthetica have been reported in bodybuilders, footballers, and runners (Szewczyk *et al.* 1994; Ulkar *et al.* 2003). It is postulated that the lateral femoral cutaneous nerve is prone to compression by fibrous bands and hypertrophied muscles. It presents with burning sensory symptoms over the anterior lateral thigh, which tend to be exacerbated by physical activity and therefore can limit performance (Preston and Shapiro 2005). Surgical decompression is often necessary in order for the athlete to resume full activity.

Routine lower limb motor and sensory nerve conduction studies and needle EMG are normal. It is possible to stimulate the nerve directly. The lateral femoral cutaneous SNAP is either absent or significantly reduced on the symptomatic side compared with the asymptomatic side.

Conclusions

Nerve conduction studies and EMG are simple and safe investigations. When used as an adjunct to clinical assessment, a detailed neurophysiological investigation adds greatly to the clinical diagnosis, prognosis and therapeutic decisions in the ever growing number of patients seen with sports related nerve injuries. As more amateur athletes take to the gyms, sports fields, track and courts, it is likely we will see many more patients in the future with the injuries detailed in this text. Clear communication with neurophysiology services plays a major role in the management of these patients.

References

Adam, F., Roren, A., and Chauvin, M. (2005). Uncommon aetiology of peroneal compartment syndrome. *Annales Françaises d'Anesthésie et de Rèanimation*, **24**, 432–4.

Boninger, M.L., Robertson, R.N., Wolff, M., and Cooper, R.A. (1996). Upper limb nerve entrapments in elite wheelchair racers. *American Journal of Physical Medicine & Rehabilitation*, **75**, 170–6.

Cain, E.L., Jr Dugas, J.R., Wolf, R.S., and Andrews, J.R. (2003). Elbow injuries in throwing athletes: a current concepts review. *American Journal of Sports Medicine*, **31**, 621–35.

Capitani, D. and Beer, S. (2002). Handlebar palsy: a compression syndrome of the deep terminal (motor) branch of the ulnar nerve in biking. *Journal of Neurology*, **249**, 1441–5.

Chen, F.S., Rokito, A.S., and Jobe, F.W. (2001). Medial elbow problems in the overhead-throwing athlete. *Journal of the American Academy of Orthopaedic Surgeons*, **9**, 99–113.

Curtin, P., Taylor, C., and Rice, J. (2005). Thrower's fracture of the humerus with radial nerve palsy: an unfamiliar softball injury. *British Journal of Sports Medicine*, **39**, e40.

Dickerman, R.D., Stevens, Q.E., Cohen, A.J., and Jaikumar, S. (2002). Radial tunnel syndrome in an elite power athlete: a case of direct compressive neuropathy. *Journal of the Peripheral Nervous System*, **7**, 229–32.

Feinberg, J.H. (2000). Burners and stingers. *Physical Medicine and Rehabilitation Clinics of North America*, **11**, 771–84.

Feinberg, J.H., Nadler, S.F., and Krivickas, L.S. (1997). Peripheral nerve injuries in the athlete. *Sports Medicine*, **24**, 385–408.

Ferrante, M.A. (2004). Brachial plexopathies: classification, causes, and consequences. *Muscle & Nerve*, **30**, 547–68.

Ferrante, M.A. and Wilbourn, A.J. (2002). Electrodiagnostic approach to the patient with suspected brachial plexopathy. *Neurologic Clinics*, **20**, 423–50.

Fulkerson, J.P. (1980). Transient ulnar neuropathy from Nordic skiing. *Clinical Orthopaedics and Relat Research*, **153**, 230–1.

Holtzhausen, L.M. and Noakes, T.D. (1996). Elbow, forearm, wrist, and hand injuries among sport rock climbers. *Clinical Journal of Sport Medicine*, **6**, 196–203.

Hsu, W.C., Chen, W.H., and Oware, A. (2005). Distal ulnar neuropathy in a golf player. *Clinical Journal of Sport Medicine*, **15**, 189–90.

Jackson, D.L., Hynninen, B.C., Caborn, D.N., and McLean, J. (1996). Electrodiagnostic study of carpal tunnel syndrome in wheelchair basketball players. *Clinical Journal of Sport Medicine*, **6**, 27–31.

Katirji, B. and Hardy, R.W., Jr (1995). Classic neurogenic thoracic outlet syndrome in a competitive swimmer: a true scalenus anticus syndrome. *Muscle & Nerve*, **18**, 229–33.

Kinoshita, M., Okuda, R., Yasuda, T., and Abe M. (2006). Tarsal tunnel syndrome in athletes. *American Journal of Sports Medicine*, **34**, 1307–12.

Krivickas, L.S. and Wilbourn, A.J. (1998). Sports and peripheral nerve injuries: report of 190 injuries evaluated in a single electromyography laboratory. *Muscle & Nerve*, **21**, 1092–4.

McCrory, P., Bell, S., and Bradshaw, C. (2002). Nerve entrapments of the lower leg, ankle and foot in sport. *Sports Medicine*, **32**, 371–91.

MacDonald, P.B., Strange, G., Hodgkinson, R., and Dyck, M. (2002). Injuries to the peroneal nerve in professional hockey. *Clinical Journal of Sport Medicine*, **12**, 39–40.

Masmejean, E.H., Chavane, H., Chantegret, A., Issermann, J.J., and Alnot, J.Y. (1999). The wrist of the Formula 1 driver. *British Journal of Sports Medicine*, **33**, 270–3.

Ogawa, K. and Yoshida, A. (1998). Throwing fracture of the humeral shaft. An analysis of 90 patients. *American Journal of Sports Medicine*, **26**, 242–6.

Ozbek, A., Bamaç, B., Budak, F., Yenigün, N., and Colak, T. (2006). Nerve conduction study of ulnar nerve in volleyball players. *Scandinavian Journal of Medicine and Science in Sports*, **16**, 197–200.

Pardal-Fernández, J.M., Godes-Medrano, B., and Jerez-García, P. (2005). Bilateral sacral radiculopathy in a cyclist. *Electromyography and Clinical Neurophysiology*, **45**, 155–60.

Patterson, J.M., Jaggars, M.M., and Boyer, M.I. (2003). Ulnar and median nerve palsy in long-distance cyclists. A prospective study. *American Journal of Sports Medicine*, **31**, 585–9.

Perlmutter, G.S. and Apruzzese, W. (1998). Axillary nerve injuries in contact sports: recommendations for treatment and rehabilitation. *Sports Medicine*, **26**, 351–61.

Pfandl, S., Wetzel, R., Hackspacher, J., and Puhl, W. (1992). Supinator tunnel syndrome—a differential diagnosis of so-called tennis elbow. *Sportverletzung Sportschaden*, **6**, 71–6.

Preston, D.C. and Shapiro, B.E. (2005). *Electromyography and Neuromuscular Disorders: Clinical–Electrophysiologic Correlations* (2nd edn). Butterworth Heinemann, Oxford.

Seddon, H.J., Medawar, P.B., and Smith, H. (1943). Rate of regeneration of peripheral nerves in man. *Journal of Physiology*, **102**, 191–215.

Stewart, J.D. (1999). *Focal Peripheral Neuropathies*. Lippincott–Williams & Wilkins, Philadelphia, PA.

Szewczyk, J., Hoffmann, M., and Kabelis, J. (1994). Meralgia paraesthetica in a body-builder. *Sportverletzung Sportschaden*, **8**, 43–5.

Ulkar, B., Yildiz, Y., and Kunduracioğlu, B. (2003). Meralgia paresthetica: a long-standing performance-limiting cause of anterior thigh. *American Journal of Sports Medicine*, **31**, 787–9.

Weinberg, J., Rokito, S., Silber, J.S. (2003). Etiology, treatment, and prevention of athletic 'stingers'. *Clinics in Sports Medicine*, **22**, 493–500.

White, J.C. and Johnson, R.K. (2003). Unusual entrapment neuropathy in a golf player. *Neurology*, **60**, 885.

2.4

Therapeutic modalities

Cathy Speed

Introduction

Therapeutic modalities can be defined as thermal, mechanical, electrical, or electromagnetic energies used for the treatment of medical complaints. A range of such modalities is used in the treatment of sports injuries, particularly soft tissue injuries (Table 2.4.1). These include thermal agents, ultrasound, and electrical agents. The basis for the use of specific modalities and the existing evidence relating to their clinical effects are outlined in this chapter.

Thermal agents

Cryotherapy

Cryotherapy involves the application of cold in the temperature range 0–18°C to have therapeutic effects upon tissue to a depth of 5 cm (Table 2.4.2). Cryotherapy may be delivered in the form of ice packs, ice immersion, ice bags, or ice massage, with the aim of limiting the effects of the acute injury upon a tissue (Table 2.4.3). Standard treatments last for 15–20 minutes. During this time, cell metabolism is reduced by almost 20%, which is considered to be beneficial by reducing the hypoxic damage by the inflammatory process. Nevertheless inflammation is an important component of the healing process and excessive use of cold is inappropriate.

Table 2.4.1 Therapeutic modalities in sports injuries

Thermal agents	Cold
	Packs, immersion, bags, controlled therapy units
	Heat
	Superficial
	Heat packs/lamps
	Paraffin baths
	Immersion
	Deep
	Short-wave diathermy
	Ultrasound
	Laser
Ultrasound	'Standard' therapeutic ultrasound
	Low-intensity pulsed ultrasound
	Phonophoresis
Electrical agents	Neuromuscular electrical stimulation (NMES)
	Transcutaneous electrical stimulation (TENS)
	Interferential
	Iontophoresis
Others	Laser
	Extracorporeal shock wave therapy

Table 2.4.2 Local effects of thermal agents

Cold	Heat
Vasoconstriction	Vasodilatation
Reduced cellular metabolic rate	Increased cellular metabolic rate
Reduction in inflammation Reduced inflammatory mediators Reduced prostaglandin synthesis Reduced capillary permeability	Increase in inflammation Increased inflammatory mediators Increased capillary permeability
Decreased pain Reduced sensitivity of afferent neurons Reduced sensitivity of muscle spindles	Decreased pain Stimulates free nerve endings, blocking pain pathways
Decreased muscle spasm	Decreased muscle spasm

Treatment is usually applied every 2 hours, although controlled continuous treatment can be delivered using cold therapy units. Cryotherapy is continued during the acute phase of the injury, which may vary in duration between individuals.

Cryotherapy is generally safe, but frostbite with excessive or inappropriate use has been reported. The risk is increased by the use of reusable cold packs which contain antifreeze and are stored

Table 2.4.3 Indications/contraindications for the use of thermal agents in soft tissue injuries

Cold	Heat
Indications	Indications
Acute injury	Subacute/chronic injuries
Acute/chronic pain	Subacute/chronic pain
After initial rehabilitation sessions	Subacute/chronic muscle spasm
Muscle spasm	Soft tissue stiffness, joint contractures
	Resolution of haematomas
Contraindications	Contraindications
Open wounds	Acute injuries
Circulatory insufficiency	Open wounds
Sensory deficit	Circulatory insufficiency
Raynaud's phenomenon	Sensory deficit
	Neoplasms

below freezing, and by failure to place a moist towel between the ice pack and the skin.

Heat

Many of the effects of heat upon tissue are the opposite to those of cold. Heat therapy can be superficial, when the skin temperature is raised to 40–45°C and tissue at depths less than 2 cm is heated, or deep, penetrating to 5 cm. Heat is avoided in acute injuries on the basis that it will promote the inflammatory response and increase cell metabolism. With the initial application of heat, the skin temperature rises rapidly for the first 10–15 minutes until vasodilatation balances the heat being delivered and the patient may (falsely) believe that the modality has cooled. With continued application of heat at a stable temperature, rebound vasoconstriction may occur as a protective mechanism.

Superficial heat treatment in the form of packs, an infrared lamp, or a paraffin bath is usually applied for 15–20 minutes and can be repeated several times daily. Deep heat treatment can be delivered using short-wave diathermy or some of the other devices described below.

Short-wave diathermy

Short-wave diathermy delivers high-frequency electromagnetic energy that is absorbed by tissues, resulting in a heating effect. Treatment is delivered in either continuous or pulsed forms, with the former causing a greater heating effect. Fat and muscle, which have a high water content, are selectively heated at depths of up to 5 cm.

Short-wave diathermy is used in deep-seated injuries, including bursitis, muscle injuries, and some tendinopathies. Contra-indications include local ischaemia, circulatory disturbance, sensory deficit, pregnancy, bleeding disorders, malignancy, and sensitive areas.

Ultrasound*

With the exception of thermal agents, ultrasound is the most commonly used modality in the management of soft tissue injuries (Speed 2001).

Characteristics of therapeutic ultrasound

Ultrasound is a form of acoustic energy consisting of inaudible high-frequency mechanical vibrations that may produce thermal or non-thermal effects upon the tissue. Ultrasound waves are created when a generator produces electrical energy that is converted to acoustic energy through mechanical deformation of a piezoelectric crystal located within the transducer. Ultrasound causes molecular collision in a medium, which allows its transmission by propagation of the wave through vibration of molecules, and a progressive loss of the intensity of the energy (**attenuation**) occurs with passage through the tissue due to absorption and/or dispersion.

Therapeutic ultrasound has a frequency range of 0.75–3 MHz, with most ultrasound units set at a frequency of 1 or 3 MHz. Ultrasound at a frequency of 1 MHz is absorbed primarily by tissues at a depth of 3–5 cm. The lower the frequency of the waves, the greater is the depth of penetration and the lower the absorption. Thus 1 MHz ultrasound is recommended for deeper injuries, particularly in those patients with considerable subcutaneous fat, whereas a frequency of 3 MHz is suggested for more superficial lesions at depths of 1–2 cm.

---

* This section is partly taken from Speed, C.A. (2001). Therapeutic ultrasound in soft tissue lesions. *Rheumatology*, **40**, 1331–6.

Table 2.4.4 Definitions used in ultrasound therapy

Term	Definition
Power	Total amount of energy in an ultrasound beam (watts)
Acoustic impedance of a tissue	Product of the density of the tissue and the speed that ultrasound will travel through it.
Attenuation	Progressive loss of energy during passage through tissue
Beam non-uniformity ratio (BNR)	Variability of the beam intensity: the ratio of the maximum intensity of the transducer to the average intensity across the transducer face
Coupling medium	Substance that prevents the reflection of ultrasound at the soft tissue–air interface
Duty cycle	Percentage of time that ultrasound is delivered over one on–off cycle
Standing wave (hot spot)	Created when reflected ultrasound meets further waves being transmitted, with potential adverse effects on tissue.
Intensity (common examples)	
(1) Spatial averaged intensity (SA_I)	Intensity averaged over the area of the transducer; calculated by dividing the power output by the effective radiating area of the transducer head
(2) Spatial peak intensity (SP_I)	Maximum intensity over time
(3) Temporal peak intensity (or pulsed averaged intensity)	Peak intensity during the on period of pulsed ultrasound
(4) Temporal-averaged intensity (TA_I)	The average power during the on off periods of pulsed therapy
(5) Spatial averaged temporal peak intensity (SATP)	Maximum intensity occurring during a single pulse

Reproduced with permission from Speed, C.A. (2001). Therapeutic ultrasound in soft tissue lesions. *Rheumatology*, **40**, 1331–6.

The greater the density of the medium (tissue), the faster is the velocity of the ultrasound waves travelling through it. Low absorption (and therefore high penetration) of ultrasound waves is seen in tissues that are high in water content (e.g. fat), whereas absorption is higher in those tissue rich in protein (e.g. skeletal muscle). Tissue is characterized by its **acoustic impedance**, the product of its density and the speed that ultrasound will travel through it. When travelling through more than one tissue, some of the ultrasound will be transmitted to the next tissue and some will scatter at the boundaries that separate them—the larger the difference in acoustic impedance, the greater is the scattering. The percentage of energy reflected at the soft tissue–fat interface is 1% compared with 40% at the soft tissue–bone interface (McDiarmid and Burns 1987). When ultrasound energy reflected at tissue interfaces meets further waves being transmitted, a standing wave (hot spot) may be created, which has potential adverse effects upon tissue. This can be minimized by ensuring that the apparatus delivers a uniform wave, using pulsed waves (see below), and moving the transducer during treatment.

Since almost all energy is reflected away at the soft tissue–air interface, coupling media, in the form of water, oils, and most commonly gels, prevent reflection of the waves by excluding air from between the transducer and patient. Different media have different impedances. The criteria for any coupling medium are that its acoustic impedance should be similar to the impedance of the transducer, it absorbs little of the ultrasound passing through it, it remains free of air bubbles, and it allows easy movement of the transducer over the skin surface.

The larger the diameter of the effective radiating area of the face of the transducer, the more focused is the ultrasound beam produced. Energy is not evenly distributed within this beam, and the greatest non-uniformity occurs close to the transducer surface (near zone). The variability of the beam intensity is termed the beam non-uniformity ratio (BNR); the optimal value of the BNR is 1, but failing this it should be less than 8.

Therapeutic ultrasound can be pulsed or continuous. The former has on–off cycles and the amount of energy being delivered can be varied by adjusting the duration of either part of the cycle. Continuous ultrasound has a greater heating effect, but either form at low intensity will produce non-thermal effects.

Ultrasound 'dosage' can also be varied by altering its amplitude and intensity. There are various definitions of ultrasound intensity, and machines differ with respect to the definition chosen for their intensity setting.

Modified forms of ultrasound

Modified forms of ultrasound include *phonophoresis* and *Low Intensity Pulsed Ultrasound (LIPUS)*. Phonophoresis involves the use of ultrasound energy and its effects upon cell permeability for the transdermal delivery of low molecular weight drugs. LIPUS involves low energy, focussed ultrasound energy delivered and is discussed further below.

The physiological effects of ultrasound

Ultrasound may induce thermal and non-thermal physical effects in tissues (Table 2.4.6). When it is applied for thermal effects, non-thermal effects will also occur, but by alteration of the dose parameters non-thermal effects can be achieved in the absence of thermal effects. Reported thermal effects of ultrasound upon tissue include increased blood flow, reduction in muscle spasm, increased extensibility of collagen fibres, and a pro-inflammatory response. It is estimated that thermal effects occur with elevation of tissue temperature to 40–45°C for at least 5 minutes (Prentice 1994). Excessive thermal effects, seen in particular with higher ultrasound intensities, may damage the tissue. The use of ultrasound in subacute or chronic conditions aims to relieve pain and spasm, and to increase tissue extensibility in the 10 minutes after heating before the tissue cools. This may be of use in combination with stretching exercises to achieve optimal tissue length. Lengthening with thermal doses of ultrasound has been demonstrated in the ligament of normal knees (Ellis 1969) and in scar tissue (Noyes *et al.* 1974).

It has been suggested that the non-thermal effects of ultrasound are more important than thermal effects in the treatment of soft tissue lesions (Dyson and Suckling 1978). These non-thermal properties of ultrasound include **cavitation** and **acoustic microstreaming**. Cavitation takes the form of gas-filled bubbles that expand and compress due to ultrasonically induced pressure changes in tissue fluids (Wells 1977). As a result there is increased flow in the surrounding fluid. Stable (regular) cavitation is considered to be beneficial to injured tissue, whereas unstable (transient) cavitation is considered to cause tissue damage (Wells 1977). Acoustic microstreaming, the unidirectional movement of fluids along cell membranes, occurs due to the mechanical pressure changes within the ultrasound field. Microstreaming may alter cell membrane structure, function, and permeability (Dyson 1987),

Table 2.4.5 Variables that may affect the dosage of ultrasound delivered to target tissue

Frequency
Wavelength
Intensity
Amplitude
Effective radiating area of transducer head
BNR
Continuous/pulsed therapy
Coupling medium
Tissue composition
Movement of transducer

Table 2.4.6 Proposed effects of therapeutic ultrasound

Type of effect	Result
Thermal	Increase in tissue extensibility
	Increase in blood flow
	Modulation of pain
	Mild inflammatory response
	Reduction in joint stiffness
	Reduction of muscle spasm
Non-thermal	Cavitation
	Acoustic microstreaming
	In combination may result in stimulation of fibroblast activity, increase in protein synthesis, increased blood flow, tissue regeneration, bone healing

which has been suggested to stimulate tissue repair (Dyson and Suckling 1978). Effects of cavitation and microstreaming that have been demonstrated *in vitro* include stimulation of fibroblast repair and collagen synthesis, tissue regeneration, and bone healing (Dyson and Luke 1986; Pilla *et al.* 1990). Adverse effects of ultrasound have also been reported.

Most of our knowledge of the effects of ultrasound on living tissue has been gained from *in vitro* studies or animal models, and many have focused in particular on skin wounds and ulcers. It has been suggested that ultrasound interacts with one or more components of inflammation, and earlier resolution of inflammation (Young and Dyson 1990a), accelerated fibrinolysis (Harpaz *et al.* 1993), stimulation of macrophage-derived fibroblast mitogenic factors (Young and Dyson 1990b), heightened fibroblast recruitment (Young and Dyson 1990a), accelerated angiogenesis (Young and Dyson 1990c), increased matrix synthesis, denser collagen fibrils (Friedar 1998), and increased tissue tensile strength (Dyson and Luke 1986) have all been demonstrated *in vitro*. Such findings form the basis of the rationale for the use of ultrasound to promote and accelerate tissue healing and repair. However, as has been detailed in earlier chapters, the pathophysiology of many soft tissue lesions, in particular tendinopathies, and the mechanisms of healing of such lesions are poorly understood compared with those of skin. The effects of ultrasound upon these processes are not yet known.

Research on the use of ultrasound specifically in tendon healing is minimal and relates only to animals. Studies have used a range of regimes. Variable increases in tensile strength, increased mobility, improved alignment of collagen fibrils, and reduced inflammatory infiltrate and scar tissue in tenotomized rabbit and cockerel tendons (Enwemeka 1989) have been found in some studies but not in others (Roberts *et al.* 1982; Turner *et al.* 1989; Gan *et al.* 1995). These findings not only demonstrate the variety of therapeutic regimes (and definitions of treatment intensities), but also the conflicting evidence regarding the use of therapeutic ultrasound in tendon lesions, even in animal studies. Caution must be exercised in extrapolating these results to human tendon lesions, as differences exist between species in the types of collagen in tendon.

The evidence for clinical effect

Gam and Johanssen (1995) reviewed 293 papers published between 1953 and 1993 to evaluate the evidence of effect of ultrasound in the treatment of musculoskeletal pain. Twenty-two trials of a variety of soft tissue disorders comparing ultrasound treatment with sham ultrasound-treated, non-ultrasound-treated, and untreated groups were found. The studies were generally found to be methodologically lacking. Data from 13 studies were presented in a way that made pooling possible; no evidence was found for pain relief with ultrasound treatment. Further papers have been published on the subject of ultrasound treatment of soft tissue lesions, but few have added any support to its use (van der Heijden *et al.* 1997; Green *et al.* 2007).

It has been suggested that ultrasound may be particularly useful in the early stages after injury, whereas many studies have evaluated more chronic lesions (or are unspecified in duration). This has been addressed in part by the use of delayed-onset muscle soreness (DOMS) as a clinical model of acute inflammation. A reduction in pain and tenderness and increased muscle strength with pulsed ultrasound in DOMS in the quadriceps has been reported

Table 2.4.7 Possible reasons for the apparent lack of effect of therapeutic ultrasound in soft tissue lesions

Study design	Insufficient blinding
	Dissimilar groups at baseline, inadequate sample sizes
	Varied outcome measures, withdrawal from treatment
	Loss to follow-up
	Inadequate duration of follow-up
	Wide spectrum of pathologies within study group
Dosage of ultrasound	Varied between studies
	Varied between treatments
	Inappropriate dose
Inadequate calibration of machinery	Inappropriate dose
Inappropriate/ inadequate coupling medium	Inadequate delivery of ultrasound to injured site
True lack of effect	

(Hasson *et al.* 1990), but other studies have refuted this (Ciccone *et al.* 1991; Craig *et al.* 1999).

It is apparent that although ultrasound is used extensively in soft tissue injuries and there are rational theories for its use, sound evidence for its effectiveness in such conditions is lacking. While *in vitro* studies have demonstrated that many of the effects described earlier occur, these have failed to translate into *in vivo* success. The absence of evidence of benefit of ultrasound in soft tissue lesions may be due to a true lack of effect, but poor study design or technical factors may play a role (Table 2.4.7). Inadequate calibration of machines has also been noted (Pye and Milford 1992).

Low-intensity pulsed ultrasound (LIPUS)

Low-intensity pulsed ultrasound therapy (LIPUS) has been shown to be beneficial in accelerating fracture healing (Heckman *et al.* 1994; Kristiansen *et al.* 1997). It has been reported that 1.5 MHz ultrasound pulsed at 1 kHz, 20% duty cycle, 30 mW/cm^2 intensity accelerates the healing time in fresh tibia, radius, and scaphoid fractures by up to 40% (Pounder and Harrison 2008). Additionally, the same ultrasound signal has been shown to be effective in resolving all types of non-unions of all ages, following a wide range of

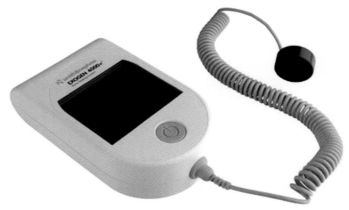

Fig. 2.4.1 A low-intensity pulsed ultrasound (LIPUS) unit. Courtesy of Smith & Nephew Inc.

fracture types and primary fracture management techniques. LIPUS has been demonstrated to accelerate *in vivo* all stages of the fracture repair process (inflammation, soft callus formation, and hard callus formation). In particular, accelerated mineralization has been demonstrated *in vitro* with increases in osteocalcin, alkaline phosphatase, vascular endothelial growth factor, and MMP-13 expression. Integrins, a family of mechanoreceptors present on a wide range of cells involved in the fracture healing process, have been shown to be activated by the ultrasound signal. Downstream of the integrin activation, focal adhesions occur on the surface of cells with the activation of multiple signalling pathways, which have been directly linked to the production of cyclo-oxygenase-2 (COX-2) and prostaglandin, which are key to the processes of mineralization and endochondral ossification in fracture healing. Hence, LIPUS is now commonly advocated in the treatment of fractures and stress injuries in the athlete (Pounder and Harrison 2008). Healing through osteogenesis at the tendon–bone junction has been demonstrated, and may help to speed postoperative healing after tendon repair (Rodeo 2007). However, although animal model work has suggested that LIPUS accelerates tendon healing (Takakura *et al.* 2002), human studies have not shown significant benefits in tendinopathies (Warden et al. 2008; D'Vaz *et al.* 2006). Notably, most studies involve those with chronic injuries; research in earlier cases is needed.

Extracorporeal shock wave therapy

Extracorporeal shock waves are focused single-pressure pulses of microsecond duration delivered using either an electromagnetic or an electrohydraulic generator. They represent one of the most effective approaches to the treatment of renal calculi. More recently, extracorporeal shock wave therapy (ESWT) has been used in the treatment of a number of musculoskeletal conditions, including non-union fractures, and soft tissue disorders such as calcifying tendonitis, plantar fasciitis, patellar tenidinopathy, and lateral epicondylitis, at doses of 10–20% of those used in lithotripsy of renal calculi (Delius 1994; Speed 2004). The rationale for such an approach is the stimulation in soft tissue lesions of promotion of healing, reduction of calcification, inhibition of pain receptors, or denervation to achieve pain relief, although the true effects have not been established. Hardware, doses, and treatment protocols vary, and there is a need for studies of different regimes in specific musculoskeletal conditions (Speed 2004).

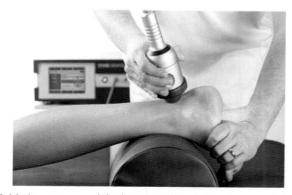

Fig. 2.4.2 An extracorporeal shock-wave machine dedicated to musculoskeletal conditions.

Electrical agents

Electrical agents have been used in the management of painful conditions since c.2500 BC. Stone carvings from this time have been found in Egyptian tombs, depicting the application of local fish to painful areas of the body. Such fish (e.g. *Malapterurus electricus*) contained organs which produced an electric charge. However, it was not until the mid-eighteenth century that electrical stimulation was delivered using a man-made device (Wesley 1759). The field received little attention until the publication of the gate control theory of pain in 1966, whereupon further interest in the use of electrical agents for pain control began to develop.

Several indications have been proposed for the use of electrical agents in the treatment of soft tissue injuries (Table 2.4.8). Electrical stimulation can be used for analgesic effects and to stimulate muscle contractions, limit disuse atrophy during the initial phase post-injury, reduce oedema, promote local muscle blood flow, and maintain range of motion. Soft tissue healing may be enhanced, but although evidence exists for benefit in superficial wounds, benefits in soft tissue musculoskeletal injuries are unproven.

A number of different forms of electrical stimulation are in common use in the management of soft tissue complaints. The dose of the electrical current being delivered varies according to the characteristics of the electrical generator, the frequency and amplitude of the current, the tissues through which it is passing, and whether the current is pulsed or continuous. Where the current is pulsed, dose is influenced by the pulse attributes (pulse frequency, period, duration, etc. as described for ultrasound). The size, position, number, and orientation of the electrodes, the space between them, and the degree of contact with the skin also influence the 'dose' of current being applied. Muscle is most effectively stimulated by application of the electrodes to motor points. Larger electrodes produce stronger but less selective contractions; the optimal interelectrode distance varies according to the site stimulated.

Neuromuscular electrical stimulation

Neuromuscular electrical stimulation (NMES), which involves high-amplitude pulses of longer duration, aims to stimulate and re-educate muscle, limit atrophy, maintain range of motion, and reduce muscle spasm. It is particularly useful in the early phases after injury/operation and is superior to no exercise at all. Improved local blood flow and reduced oedema are recorded. In the less acute patient it is not a substitute for active rehabilitation. Daily treatments can be given, but the response of the patient should be closely monitored. Contraindications include avulsions and musculotendinous

Table 2.4.8 Therapeutic uses of electrical currents in soft tissue injuries.

Pain control
Reduction of muscle spasm
Limitation of disuse atrophy
Re-education of muscle contraction
Promote local blood flow
Reduction of oedema
Promotion of tissue healing

lesions if it is considered that any increase in muscle tension may be detrimental.

Transcutaneous electrical nerve stimulation

In addition to neuromuscular stimulation, electrical stimulation may result in a reduction in pain in a format of lower-intensity high-frequency pulses. Transcutaneous electrical nerve stimulation (TENS) is a process that uses an electric current, transmitted through surface electrodes applied to the skin, to alter the perception of pain. The mechanism of pain reduction depends on the characteristics of the current and includes action on central mechanisms (release of endogenous opiates) and stimulation of the gate control mechanism. A variety of approaches to electrode placement have been described but direct placement over or around the painful site is common practice.

High-frequency (conventional) TENS involves pulses at high frequency and short duration and selectively stimulates A-delta fibres, closing the pain pathway gate to painful stimuli but opening it to sensory information. Onset of pain relief occurs within the initial 10 minutes of treatment and may persist for minutes to hours afterwards.

Low-frequency TENS, involving higher intensity but lower pulse frequency and shorter duration, results in pain relief, probably as a result of release of β-endorphins from the pituitary. Relief of pain may take longer to occur than with high TENS, but may be longer lasting; however, no overall difference in the degree of pain relief between the two types has been demonstrated. Since some degree of motor stimulation occurs, low TENS is best avoided in the acute phase of a musculotendinous injury.

Brief intense TENS involves stimulation at high intensity and high pulse frequency for long duration. Analgesia appears to be achieved through action at brainstem level, ultimately resulting in inhibition of release of substance P. Pain relief is generally of short duration.

The use of TENS units for pain control has several advantages. They are safe, non-addictive, easy to use, patient operated, and portable. Side effects are possible; they may cause skin irritation and, of course, may not be effective. They should not be used in a patient with a pacemaker or arrhythmia and must be used with caution in those with epilepsy. The patient should not operate a machine or drive during use. Although there is a theoretical risk of thermal burns, this is negligible.

When a TENS unit is given to a patient for pain control, specific instructions should be given with respect to application of electrodes, treatment time, intensity, pulse frequency, potential adverse reactions, and care of the machine.

Initial treatment should be less than 30 minutes and the response (including adverse reactions) should then be evaluated. Provided that the patient has tolerated the therapy, treatments can subsequently last up to an hour at a time, with a minimum of 30 minutes break at a time. The intensity produces strong tingling or buzzing under the electrodes, without discomfort. Recommendations for electrode placement include over or close to the painful area, over motor points, over a peripheral nerve supplying the cutaneous area over the site of pain, over the paraspinal region, or over peripheral nerves that supply the dermatome or myotome of the site of pain. Ultimately, the choice of electrode placement depends upon the condition involved and patient preference, and at times a degree of

trial and error (Walsh 1997). Unilateral or bilateral placement may be selected, and a minimum inter-electrode distance of the diameter of the electrode is recommended (Mannheimer and Lampe 1984). Some units require the use of gel for skin contact and tape to secure the electrodes. A diary of pain levels and machine use is often helpful in evaluating the response.

Interferential stimulation

Interferential therapy involves the generation of two alternating sine waves, one at constant high frequency and the other at variable frequency. This results in easy penetration of tissues, whereupon the interference between the two waves results in (proposed) biological effects upon tissues. It is suggested that these effects include analgesia, neuromuscular stimulation, and reduction of oedema, although, as is the case with so many modalities, evidence is lacking.

Iontophoresis

Iontophoresis involves the use of low-voltage electrical current to deliver medication into the skin or subcutaneous structures. Such medications include anaesthetics, analgesics, and NSAIDs. The transdermal route has obvious advantages over the systemic route, but there is no evidence for benefit from this approach.

Laser therapy

The use of lasers (**l**ight **a**mplification by **s**timulated **e**mission of **r**adiation) to cut and destroy tissue is well established. The same electromagnetic radiation, at much lower intensities, can elicit non-destructive physiological responses in tissues in the absence of significant heating ('cold laser' therapy). This phenomenon forms the basis for the use of 'laser therapy' in the management of a variety of soft tissue complaints.

An assortment of devices exists, including helium–neon, infra-red diodes, argon, and krypton lasers, with the first two types being the most commonly used. Treatment times are short (e.g. 30 seconds), with an output power in the range 1–75mW, and can be delivered as either pulsed or continuous, using a static or dynamic technique.

The proposed effects of laser therapy are analgesia and tissue healing, with the latter resembling the non-thermal effects proposed for therapeutic ultrasound. Laser energy commonly penetrates tissues at a depth of a few millimetres, although it is possible to stimulate tissues at a depth of up to 15 mm below the skin. Beneficial effects on tissue healing are proposed to occur through stimulation of the cellular and chemical aspects of the healing process, particularly in the early phases. Pain reduction may also take place through reduction of muscle spasm or altering nerve conduction velocity (Basford 1993). Nevertheless, the clinical utility of laser therapy remains unestablished.

Summary

A vast number of therapeutic modalities for the treatment of soft tissue complaints are in widespread use. Whilst there are numerous physiological rationales proposed for their use, further clinical research is needed to define their role(s) more clearly in the management of these conditions.

References

Basford, J.R. (1993). Laser therapy: scientific basis and clinical role. *Orthopedics*, **16**, 541–7.

Ciccone, C., Leggin, B., and Callamaro, J. (1991). Effects of ultrasound and trolamine salicylate on delayed-onset muscle soreness. *Physical Therapy*, **71**, 666.

Craig, J.A., Bradley, J., Walsh, D.M., Baxter, G.D., and Allen, J.M. (1999). Delayed onset muscle soreness: lack of effect of therapeutic ultrasound in humans. *Archives of Physical Medicine and Rehabilitation*, **80**, 318–23.

Delius, M. (1994). Medical applications and bioeffects of extracorporeal shock waves. *Shock Waves*, **4**, 55–72.

D'Vaz, A., Ostor, A., Speed, C., et al. (2006). Pulsed low-intensity ultrasound therapy for chronic lateral epicondylitis: a randomized controlled trial. *Rheumatology*, **45**, 566–70.

Dyson, M. (1987). Mechanisms involved in therapeutic ultrasound. *Physiotherapy*, **73**, 116–20.

Dyson, M. and Luke, D.A. (1986). Induction of mast cell degranulation in skin by ultrasound. *IEEE Transactions and Ultrasonics, Ferroelectrics and Frequency Control*, **UFFC-33**, 194.

Dyson, M. and Suckling, J. (1978). Stimulation of tissue repair by ultrasound: a survey of the mechanisms involved. *Physiotherapy*, **64**, 105–8.

Ellis, D.G. (1969). Cross-sectional area measurement for tendon specimens: a comparison of several methods. *Journal of Biomechanics*, **2**, 175–86.

Enwemeka, C.S. (1989). The effects of therapeutic ultrasound on tendon healing. A biomechanical study. *American Journal of Physical Medicine and Rehabilitation*, **68**, 283–7.

Friedar, S. (1988). A pilot study: the therapeutic effect of ultrasound following partial rupture of Achilles tendons in male rats. *Journal of Orthopaedic and Sports Physical Therapy*, **10**, 39.

Gam, A.N. and Johannsen, F. (1995). Ultrasound therapy in musculoskeletal disorders: a meta-analysis. *Pain*, **63**, 85–91.

Gan, B.S., Huys, S., Sherebrin, M.H., and Scilley, C.G. (1995). The effects of ultrasound treatment on flexor tendon healing in the chicken limb. *Journal of Hand Surgery (Edinburgh, Scotland)*, **20**, 809–14.

Green, S., Buchbinder, R., Glazier, R., and Forbes, A. (1998). Systematic review of randomised controlled trials of interventions for painful shoulder: selection criteria, outcome assessment and efficacy. *British Medical Journal*, **316**, 354–60.

Harpaz, D., Chen, X., Francis, C.W., et al. (1933). Ultrasound enhancement of thrombolysis and reperfusion *in vitro*. *Journal of the American College of Cardiology*, **2**, 1507–11.

Hasson, S, Mundorf, R, Barnes, W., Williams, J., and Fujii, M. (1990). Effect of pulsed ultrasound versus placebo on muscle soreness perception and muscular performance. *Scandinavian Journal of Rehabilitation Medicine*, **22**, 199–205.

Heckman, J.D., Ryaby, J.P., McCabe, J., Frey, J.J., and Kilcoyne, R.F. (1994). Acceleration of tibial fracture-healing by non-invasive, low-intensity pulsed ultrasound. *Journal of Bone and Joint Surgery*, **76A**, 26–34.

Kristiansen, T.K., Ryaby, J.P., McCabe, J., Frey, J.J., and Roe, L.R. (1997). Accelerated healing of distal radial fractures with the use of specific, low-intensity ultrasound. A multicentre, prospective, randomised, double-blind, placebo-controlled study. *Journal of Bone and Joint Surgery*, **79A**, 961–73.

McDiarmid, T. and Burns, P.N. (1987). Clinical applications of therapeutic ultrasound. *Physiotherapy*, **73**, 155.

Mannheimer, J.S. and Lampe, G.N. (1984). *Clinical Transcutaneous Nerve Stimulation*. F.A. Davis, Philadelphia, PA.

Noyes, F.R., Torvik, P.J., Hyde, W.B., and DeLucas, J.L. (1974). Biomechanics of ligamnt failure II. An analysis of immobilisation exercise and reconditioning effects in primates. *Journal of Bone and Joint Surgery. American Volume*, **56**, 1406–18.

Pilla, A. A., Figueiredo, M., Nasser, P., et al. (1990). Non-invasive low intensity pulsed ultrasound: a potent accelaerator of bone repair. In: *Proceedings of the 36th Annual Meeting*, Orthopaedics Research Society, New Orleans, LA.

Pounder, N.M. and Harrison, A.J. (2008). Low intensity pulsed ultrasound for fracture healing: a review of the clinical evidence and the associated biological mechanism of action. *Ultrasonics*, **48**, 330–8.

Prentice, W.E. (1994). Therapeutic Modalities in Sports Medicine (3rd edn). Mosby, St Louis, MO.

Pye, S.D. and Milford, C. (1994). The performance of ultrasound physiotherapy machines in Lothian Region, Scotland. *Ultrasound in Medicine and Biology*, **20**, 347–59.

Roberts, M., Rutherford, J.H., and Harris, D. (1982). The effect of ultrasound on flexor tendon repairs in the rabbit. *Hand*, **14**, 17–20.

Rodeo, SA. (2007). Biologic augmentation of rotator cuff tendon repair. *Journal of Shoulder and Elbow Surgery*, **16**(Suppl), S191–7.

Speed, C.A. (2001). Therapeutic ultrasound in soft tissue lesions. *Rheumatology*, **40**, 1331–6.

Speed, C.A. (2004). Extracorporeal shock wave therapy in the management of chronic soft tissue conditions: a critical review. *Journal of Bone and Joint Surgery. British Volume*, **86**, 165–71.

Takakura, Y., Matsui, N., Yoshiya, S., et al. (2002). Low-intensity pulsed ultrasound enhances early healing of medial collateral ligament injuries in rats. *Journal of Ultrasound in Medicine*, **21**, 283–8.

Turner, S.M., Powell, E.S., and Ng, C.S. (1989). The effect of ultrasound on the healing of repaired cockerel tendon. Is collagen cross-linkage a factor? *Journal of Hand Surgery (Edinburgh, Scotland)*, **14**, 428–33.

van der Heijden, G.J.M.G., van der Windt, D.A.W.M., and de Winter, A.F. (1997). Physiotherapy for patients with shoulder disorders: a systematic review of randomised controlled clinical trials. *British Medical Journal*, **315**, 25–30.

Walsh, D.M. (1997). The clinical application of TENS. In: D.M. Walsh (ed.), *TENS: Clinical Applications and Related Theory*, pp. 103–24. Churchill Livingstone, London.

Warden, S.J., Metcalf, B.R., Kiss, Z.S., et al. (2008). Low-intensity pulsed ultrasound for chronic patellar tendinopathy: a randomized, double-blind, placebo-controlled trial. *Rheumatology*, **47**, 467–71.

Wells, P.N.T. (1977). *Biomedical Ultrasonics*. Academic Press, London.

Wesley, J. (1759). *The Desideratum: Or Electricity Made Plain and Useful by a Lover of Mankind and of Common Sense*. Bailliere, Tindall and Cox, London.

Young, S. and Dyson, M. (1990a). The effects of therapeutic ultrasound on the healing of full thickness excised skin lesions. *Ultrasonics*, **28**, 175–80.

Young, S.R. and Dyson, M. (1990b). Macrophage responsiveness to therapeutic ultrasound. *Ultrasound in Medicine and Biology*, **16**, 809–16.

Young, S.R. and Dyson, M. (1990c). The effect of therapeutic ultrasound on angiogenesis. *Ultrasound in Medicine and Biology*, **16**, 261–9.

2.5

Pharmacological pain management in sports injuries

Cathy Speed

Introduction

The perception of pain is a biological mechanism which warns that damage has occurred and protects against further damage, allowing healing to occur. Acute pain often acts as an indicator of injury severity and progression or healing. The same may apply in some with chronic injuries, but in others pain may not correlate with tissue damage and/or may not be a sign that the tissue needs to be protected from mechanical stress. The management of most sports injuries involves early mobilization where possible, and pain management in the treatment of these injuries is important to allow rehabilitation to proceed and to ease distress. Modalities play an important role in this respect, and are discussed elsewhere (Chapter 2.4). Injection therapies are also discussed elsewhere (Chapter 2.6). Thorough counselling of the athlete is a priority to ensure that he/she understands what the pain represents, as this will be likely to affect compliance. For example, a degree of pain during eccentric exercise protocols in the rehabilitation of chronic tendinopathies would be anticipated, and would not contraindicate continuation of a set programme. In contrast, when an athlete is returning to sporting activities after injury, pain that is experienced during the activity would not be acceptable, and the athlete is also advised during this period that conclusions as to the tissue's reaction to activity should not be drawn until the day after the training session. Athletes should also be taught appropriate self-help strategies to manage their pain and when this involves medication, how and when to take it. Principles for the use of medications in pain management are given in Table 2.5.1.

Psychological influences on pain should not be underestimated. Athletes, like other individuals, vary in their psychophysiological responses to injury and pain. Many have a stress response, manifested physically and/or psychologically, which will exacerbate the situation. Introduction of simple self-help techniques that address the mind–body connection, such as relaxation and creative visualization or imagery, can be helpful. Athletes are strongly motivated, and tend to have high levels of body awareness, somatization, and anxiety. Support, reassurance, and honesty are key to their management, and thorough counselling and review in relation to their injury and management plan are a priority.

Table 2.5.1 Principles for the use of medications in pain management

- ◆ Counsel the athlete: purpose, prescription, potential adverse effects
- ◆ Never use to allow inappropriate activity
- ◆ Use short term; review regularly
- ◆ Use the lowest dose necessary for benefit
- ◆ Consider topical preparations
- ◆ Avoid misuse

Non-steroidal anti-inflammatory drugs (NSAIDs)

NSAIDs act both centrally and peripherally to relieve pain. The peripheral effects occur through inhibition of the cyclo-oxygenase (COX) pathway, inhibiting production of prostaglandin, and dampening the inflammatory process and associated pain (Fig. 2.5.1). Their mechanisms of action centrally are not well understood.

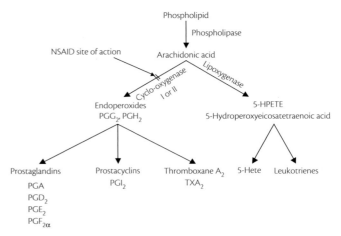

Fig. 2.5.1 Prostaglandin synthesis. Non-steroidal anti-inflammatory drugs impair prostaglandin synthesis by inhibiting the cyclo-oxygenase enzyme.

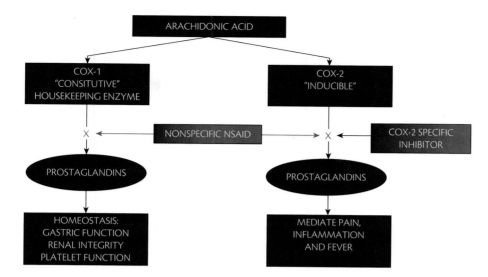

Fig. 2.5.2 Mechanism of pain: arachidonic acid cascade. Reproduced from Needleman, P. and Isakson, P.C. (1997) The discovery and function of COX-2. *Journal of Rheumatology*, **49** (Suppl), 6–8.

NSAIDs are divided into traditional non-selective NSAIDs and COX-2 selective inhibitors. The latter group was principally developed to limit adverse gastrointestinal effects. It has subsequently become clear that there are additional risks with both groups of NSAIDs that were previously underestimated, in particular cardiovascular effects (Figs 2.5.2 and 2.5.3).

NSAIDs and soft tissue healing

The limited evidence for benefit from the use of NSAIDs in the treatment of acute and chronic musculoskeletal injuries (Green *et al.* 2002; Kvien and Vitkil 2003) has not limited their use, and the accessibility of over-the-counter preparations makes self-medication very common. The principal rationale for their use in acute soft tissue injuries is to limit excessive inflammatory response and swelling, so that early mobilization and healing can occur. However, inflammation is an important component of the healing process, and inhibition of this phase could potentially delay full

recovery. In addition, whether they are superior to basic analgesics such as paracetamol (acetaminophen) in sports injuries is also doubtful (Green *et al.* 2002; Kvien and Vitkil 2003; Dalton and Schweinle 2006). For example, Dalton and Schweinle (2006) reported no difference between acetaminophen and ibuprofen in the treatment of grade I and II ankle sprains.

NSAIDs are taken by some athletes before and/or after a bout of exercise in an attempt to reduce delayed onset muscle soreness, and there is weak evidence for benefit in this respect although restoration of function is questionable (Tokmakidis *et al.* 2003). However, it appears that light physical activity is superior to an NSAID alone in relieving symptoms (Rahnana *et al.* 2005).

When the decision is taken to prescribe an NSAID, topical preparations should be used where possible. High levels of uptake into the Achilles tendon have been demonstrated with topical applications, with higher levels being achieved than those seen with oral preparations (Rolf *et al.* 1997).

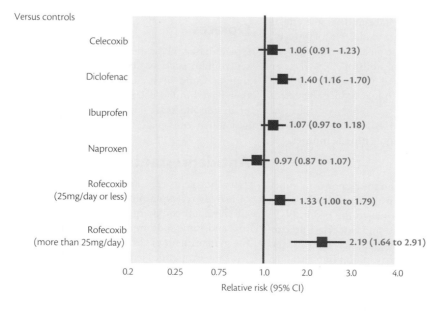

Fig. 2.5.3 Systematic review of observational studies to compare cardiovascular risks with NSAIDs and COX-2 inhibitors. Reproduced from McGettigan, P. and Henry, D.I. (2006). Cardiovascular risk and inhibition of cyclooxygenase: a systematic review of the observational studies of selective and nonselective inhibitors of cyclooxygenase 2. *Journal of the American Medical Association*, **296**, 1633–44.

Table 2.5.2 Side effects of non-steroidal anti-inflammatory drugs

Gastrointestinal
◆ Dyspepsia
◆ Ulceration
◆ Haemorrhage
◆ Perforation
Renal
◆ Acute renal failure (reversible or irreversible)
◆ Increased blood pressure
◆ Cardiac failure
Hepatic
◆ Variable (e.g. 'transaminitis')
◆ Hypersensitivity
◆ Rashes
◆ Bronchospasm
Haematological
◆ Haemolysis
◆ Thrombocytopenia
◆ Neutropenia
◆ Red cell aplasia
Drug interactions
◆ Reduced efficacy of diuretics (e.g. antihypertensive agents)
◆ Increased efficacy (e.g. anticonvulsants, digoxin, anticoagulants, lithium)

In **muscle injuries,** short-term use of different NSAIDs in the early phase of healing has been shown to lead to a decrease in the inflammatory cell reaction (Järvinen *et al.* 1992; Rahusen *et al.* 2001) with no adverse effects on the healing process, the tensile strength, or the ability of the injured muscle to contract (Järvinen *et al.* 1992; Dalton and Schweinle 2006). Furthermore, NSAIDs do not delay myofibre regeneration (Mishra *et al.* 1995). It has been proposed that their long-term use might have undesirable effects on the regenerating skeletal muscle (Mishra *et al.* 1995). However, detrimental effects were not reported in the most thorough experimental study (Thorsson *et al.* 1998). In addition, NSAIDs are sometimes used if there is a suspicion of impending myositis ossificans, in the hope that this approach might reduce the extent of heterotopic bone formation.

The principal issue remains that NSAIDs are not superior to analgesics in the management of most chronic muscle injuries.

NSAIDs and bone healing

Bone metabolism and repair is complex, and the response to injury involves an initial inflammatory response, with prostaglandins such as PGE_2 having a pivotal role in the response to the insult. PGE_2 acts to replicate and differentiate osteoblast and osteoclast precursors, which lead to increased bone resorption and new bone formation. It has been postulated that NSAIDs may inhibit bone healing, on the basis of inhibition of prostaglandin production. However, the evidence for this is limited, and some NSAIDs in some models have been shown to inhibit bone loss (Harder and An 2003).

There are conflicting results from studies of the effects of non-selective NSAIDs and COX-2 selective agents on bone healing in animal models, and furthermore there is little evidence from human studies of a negative impact on bone (Wheeler and Batt 2005). The conflicting results may be a function of the type of NSAID; proprionic NSAIDs (ibuprofen, naproxen, ketoprofen) may prevent bone loss in some circumstances, while acetic acid NSAIDs (indomethacin, diclofenac) may not. Reported effects of COX-2 selected inhibitors are also variable. Dose and duration of use may also be factors.

It has also been proposed that NSAIDs may cause a reduction in bone mass. There is no conclusive evidence of this. For example, in a study of over half a million patients on NSAIDs and 215 000 controls, no major effect of NSAIDs on risk of fracture was identified (Vestergaard and Moskelide 2003).

Although clinical data are lacking, it seems prudent to avoid the use of NSAIDs in the management of bone injuries and to replace them with other analgesics (Vuolteenaho *et al.* 2008).

NSAIDs: conclusions

In sports injuries, NSAIDs should only be prescribed for short-term use in situations where there is a true excessive inflammatory response, such as a bursitis or synovitis, and must be restricted in those with underlying cardiovascular or gastrointestinal disease. Concomitant prescription of a gastroprotective agent, usually a proton pump inhibitor, should be considered.

Acetaminophen (paracetamol)

The mechanism of action of acetaminophen remains uncertain. It does not have the ability to inhibit COX enzymes, although there has been a suggestion that it has some effect on COX-2 or even possibly a putative COX-3 isoenzyme (Hersh *et al.* 2005; Hinz *et al.* 2008). Other potential pathways include stimulation of descending inhibitory pathways or effects on *N*-methyl D-aspartate (NMDA) receptor activity. The precise mechanism of action remains elusive. Side effects are rare when acetaminophen is used in normal dose regimens.

Opiates

Opiate-based medications should be reserved for short-term use in severe pain such as that following fracture or major soft tissue trauma. Concerns about their abuse and adverse effects mean that they have limited use in the management of sports injuries. The main side effects are constipation and sedation. A synergistic interaction between opiates and NSAIDs is seen.

Antidepressants

Tricyclic agents (e.g. amitriptyline, doselupin) inhibit the uptake of 5-hydroxytryptamine (5-HT, serotonin), block H1 receptors and have anticholinergic effects, as well as blocking NMDA receptors and some sodium channels. These antidepressants are used in the management of chronic musculoskeletal pain, particularly that with a neuropathic element. Their antinociceptive effects are independent of their antidepressant actions, occurring at lower doses and after a shorter duration of treatment. The principal adverse effect of these agents is sedation (and for this reason they are

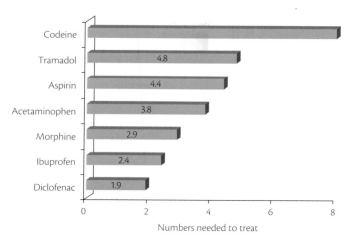

Fig. 2.5.4 Oxford League Table of common analgesics in acute pain. Reproduced from http://www.jr2.ox.ac.uk/bandolier/booth/painpag/Acutrev/Analgesics/Leagtab.html

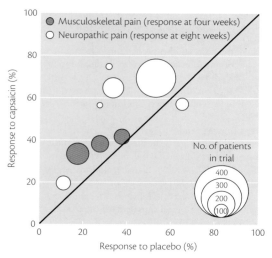

Fig. 2.5.5 Effects of capsaicin cream in chronic musculoskeletal conditions. L'Abbé plot showing response to capsaicin and placebo in individual randomised controlled trials. Reproduced from Mason, L *et al.* (2004) Systematic review of topical capsaicin for the treatment of chronic pain *BMJ*;328:991, with permission from BMJ Publishing Group Ltd.

usually prescribed to be taken at night), which may be unacceptable to the athlete. When used, it is recommended that very small doses are prescribed in the first instance (e.g. doselupin 25 mg nocte). It may take some weeks to see an effect on chronic pain.

Ion-channel blockade

Agents such as gabapentin and pregabalin block calcium channels and act as presynaptic inhibitors of the release of excitatory neurotransmitters. Their effectiveness in musculoskeletal pain has not been established, and they are rarely used in the context of sporting injuries. The principal side effect is sedation.

Approaches to bone healing and pain

Intravenous bisphosphonate therapy has been proposed as a useful approach in the treatment of stress fractures (Stewart *et al.* 2005). However, apart from a small uncontrolled study of five patients (Stewart *et al.* 2005), no other evidence to support its use is available, and the unknown long-term effects of this drug in a young population and potential adverse effects (such as, very rarely, osteonecrosis of the jaw) make it unlikely that this approach would be commonly indicated.

Parathyroid hormone (parathormone) therapy, which is increasingly used for osteoporosis, has been shown to accelerate fracture healing, and may have a role to play in the management of fractures in the athlete, particularly those with low bone mass, in the future (Barnes *et al.* 2008).

Calcitonin given subcutaneously or nasally is associated with pain relief in patients following acute osteoporotic vertebral fractures, but has not been assessed in sport-related bone injury.

Non-NSAID topical agents

Continuous topical glyceryl trinitrate treatment (e.g. 1.25 mg/24 h glyceryl trinitrate) has been advocated in the treatment of tendon pain and to promote healing (Hunte and Lloyd-Smith 2005; Paoloni *et al.* 2005). The mechanism of action is unknown but may be related to modulation of local nitric oxide levels. The main reported side effects are headaches (glyceryl trinitrate 53% vs.

placebo 45%) and rashes (glyceryl trinitrate 16% vs. placebo 12%) (Hunte and Lloyd-Smith 2005). The treatment can take several weeks to have an effect and therefore is reserved for those with recalcitrant soft tendinopathies.

Capsaicin is used for musculoskeletal pain disorders (e.g. ligamentous, local articular, back pain) or superficial neuropathic pain, which in the sportsperson may be due to local nerve trauma. It is extracted from chilli peppers and binds to nociceptors in the skin, causing an initial excitation of the neurons and a period of enhanced sensitivity to noxious stimuli, usually perceived as itching, pricking, or burning sensations. This is followed by a refractory period with reduced sensitivity and, after repeated applications, persistent desensitization. It is the ability of capsaicin to desensitize nociceptors that is exploited for therapeutic pain relief. It is available in strengths of 0.025% and 0.075%, and is applied three or four times daily. One-third of patients will report adverse effects, and in particular excessive burning sensation of the skin. Although not recommended for first-line treatment of soft tissue pain, it may prove a useful adjunct in chronic resistant cases (http://www.jr2.ox.ac.uk/bandolier/booth/painpag/topical/topcap.html).

References

Barnes, G.L, Kakar, S., Vora, S., Morgan, E.F., Gerstenfeld, L.C., and Einhorn, T.A. (2008). Stimulation of fracture-healing with systemic intermittent parathyroid hormone treatment. *Journal of Bone and Joint Surgery. American Volume*, **90** (Suppl 1), 120–7.

Dalton, J.D. Jr and Schweinle, J.E. (2006). Randomized controlled noninferiority trial to compare extended release acetaminophen and ibuprofen for the treatment of ankle sprains. *Annals of Emergency Medicine*, **48**, 615–23.

Green, S., Buchbinder, R., Barnsley, L., *et al.* (2002). Non-steroidal anti-inflammatory drugs (NSAIDs) for treating lateral elbow pain in adults. *Cochrane Database of Systematic Reviews* (2), CD003686.

Harder, A. and An, Y. (2003). The mechanisms of the inhibitory effects of nonsteroidal anti-inflammatory drugs on bone healing: a concise review. *Journal of Clinical Pharmacology*, **43**, 807–15.

Hersh, E.V., Lally, E.T., and Moore, P.A. (2005). Update on cyclooxygenase inhibitors: has a third COX isoform entered the fray? *Current Medical Research and Opinion*, **21**, 1217–26.

Hinz, B., Cheremina, O., and Brune, K. (2008). Acetaminophen (paracetamol) is a selective cyclooxygenase-2 inhibitor in man. *FASEB Journal*, **22**, 383–90.

Hunte, G. and Lloyd-Smith, R. (2005). Topical glyceryl trinitrate for chronic Achilles tendinopathy. *Clinical Journal of Sport Medicine*, **15**, 116–17.

Järvinen, M., Lehto, M., and Sorvari, T. (1992). Effect of some anti-inflammatory agents on the healing of ruptured muscle. An experimental study in rats. *Journal of Sports Traumatology*, **14**, 19–28.

Kvien, T.K., and Vitkil, K. (2003). Pharmacology for regional musculoskeletal pain. *Rheumatol.*, **17**, 137–50.

Mason, L., Moore, R.A., Derry, J., Edwards, J.E., and McQuey, H.J. (2004). Systematic review of topical capsaicin for the treatment of chronic pain. *Br Med. J.*, **328**(7446), 991.

Mishra, D.K., Fridén, J., Schmitz, M.C., and Lieber, R.L. (1995). Anti-inflammatory medication after muscle injury. A treatment resulting in short-term improvement but subsequent loss of muscle function. *Journal of Bone and Joint Surgery. American Volume*, **77**, 1510–19.

Paoloni, J.A., Appleyard, R.C., Nelson, J., and Murrell, G.A. (2005). Topical glyceryl trinitrate application in the treatment of chronic supraspinatus tendinopathy: a randomized, double-blinded, placebo-controlled clinical trial. *American Journal of Sports Medicine*, 2005 Jun; **33**(6): 806–13.

Rahnama, N., Rahmani-Nia, F., and Ebrahim, K. (2005). The isolated and combined effects of selected physical activity and ibuprofen on delayed-onset muscle soreness. *Journal of Sports Science*, **23**, 843–50.

Rahusen, F.T., Weinhold, P.S., and Almekinders, L.C. (2001). Nonsteroidal anti-inflammatory drugs and acetaminophen in the treatment of an acute muscle injury. *American Journal of Sports Medicine*, **32**, 1856–9.

Rolf, C., Movin, T., Engstrom, B., Jacobs, L.D., Beauchard, C., and Le Liboux, A. (1997). An open, randomized study of ketoprofen in patients in surgery for Achilles or patellar tendinopathy. *Journal of Rheumatology*, **24**, 1595–8.

Stewart, G.W., Brunet, M.E., Manning, M.R., and Davis, F.A. (2005). Treatment of stress fractures in athletes with intravenous pamidronate. *Clinical Journal of Sport Medicine*, **15**, 92–4.

Thorsson, O., Rantanen, J., Hurme, T., and Kalimo, H. (1998). Effects of nonsteroidal antiinflammatory medication on satellite cell proliferation during muscle contraction. *American Journal of Sports Medicine*, **26**, 172–6.

Tokmakidis, S.P., Kokkinidis, E.A., Smilios, I., and Douda, H. (2003). The effects of ibuprofen on delayed muscle soreness and muscular performance after eccentric exercise. *Journal of Strength and Conditioning Research*, **17**, 53–9.

Vestergaard, P. and Moskelide, L. (2003). Fracture risk associated with smoking: a meta-analysis. *Journal of Internal Medicine*, **254**, 572–83.

Vuolteenaho, K., Moilanen, T., and Moilanen, E. (2008). Non-steroidal anti-inflammatory drugs, cyclooxygenase-2 and the bone healing process. *Basic and Clinical Pharmacology and Toxicology*, **102**, 10–14.

Wheeler, P. and Batt, M.E. (2005). Do non-steroidal anti-inflammatory drugs adversely affect stress fracture healing? A short review. *British Journal of Sports Medicine*, **39**, 65–9.

2.6

Injection therapies in sports injuries

Cathy Speed

Introduction

Local injection therapies are utilized in the management of sports injuries in order to facilitate diagnosis (local anaesthetics), to manage pain and to aid in the process of healing. Routes and injectates for local injection therapies in the management of sports injuries are listed in Tables 2.6.1 and 2.6.2, respectively. Importantly, injections form only one component of a management strategy in sports injuries, which also includes correction of causative and provocative factors and appropriate rehabilitation.

Injection accuracy is also important, and injection under guidance, particularly using ultrasound, is becoming increasingly popular for this reason.

Local corticosteroid injections (LCSIs)

Local corticosteroid injections (LCSIs) are commonly used in musculoskeletal disorders in the general and sporting populations, and can be intra-articular or periarticular, with the latter delivered either around the lesion (e.g. peritendinous/tendon sheath infiltration) or into the lesion itself (e.g. intra-bursal injection). Steroid injections are also used for back pain in the context of epidural injections, and for diagnostic and therapeutic nerve blockades.

Intra-articular injections, most commonly used in joint disease, are also used in the treatment of capsulitis (e.g. adhesive capsulitis of the shoulder), with or without hydrodistension of the joint. As this is not a sporting-related injury it will not be discussed further here.

Table 2.6.1 Injection therapies in sports injuries: routes

- Intra-articular (degenerative joint pain, synoritis)
- Intra-sheath (tenosynovitis, adhesions)
- Intra-bursal (bursitis)
- Intra-tendinous (neovascularization, tendinosis)
- Intramuscular (muscle injuries)
- Local infiltration (carpal tunnel, trigger point, ligament, muscle)

Table 2.6.2 Injection therapies in sports injuries: injectates

- None (dry needling)
- Local anaesthetic (LA)
- Corticosteroids (± LA)
- Sclerosants
- Platelet Rich Plasma/Antologous conditioned plasma
- Botulinum toxins
- Heparin
- Actovegin
- Traumeel

Rationale for use and mechanisms of action

Corticosteroids have anti-inflammatory effects and are also likely to have many other effects upon alternative ('non-inflammatory') sources of pain that are poorly understood. Although inflammation is clearly evident in cases of bursitis and in early capsulitis, its role in tendinopathies is less clear. With the exception of some cases of tenosynovitis, most histological studies of a range of chronic tendon lesions have demonstrated alteration in cellular and extracellular components of the tendon and paratenon or sheath (Chard *et al.* 1994; Riley *et al.* 1994; Josza and Kannus 1997) and an absence of cellular evidence for inflammation (Chard *et al.* 1994; Riley *et al.* 1994). Hence the term 'tendinosis' is preferred to 'tendinitis', since the latter suggests inflammation. However, most histopathological studies of tendon have focused upon endstage non-healing lesions; it is not clear whether the degenerative features are primary or whether they are preceded by an inflammatory phase. Biochemical studies of inflammation in tendons are scant. Human tendon fibroblasts have been shown to produce prostaglandin E_2 (PGE_2) *in vitro* and *in vivo* in response to repetitive mechanical loading, and repetitive exposure of the tendon to PGE_2 can result in degenerative changes within tendons in animal models (Khan *et al.* 2005). However, normal levels of prostaglandin have been shown in painful Achilles tendon lesions in humans (Alfredson 1999).

Other mechanisms of tendon pain have been proposed, including triggering of nociceptive receptors by neurotransmitters such as substance P and biochemical irritants such as chondroitin sulphate extravasated by damaged tendon, and irritation of mechanoreceptors by vibration, traction, or shear forces. The influences of corticosteroid on such processes are undefined.

General indications for LCSIs in sports injuries

Peri-articular corticosteroid injections have little or no role to play in most acute sports injuries. They are also not indicated in the management of ligament and muscle injuries and do not appear to offer any advantage over dry needling in myofascial pain. Intra-articular injections are rarely indicated, as sports-related loading after such injections makes their effects short lived and can result in cartilage damage. The exceptions to this rule include the athlete with an underlying inflammatory arthritis or severe post-traumatic synovitis. Viscosupplement injections are preferred for masters' athletes with degenerative joint disease (see below). Ideally, local corticosteroid injections should be considered in soft tissue injuries in sportspeople when there is an excessive or chronic inflammatory response, chronic pain, and rehabilitation is inhibited.

Clinical evidence for the use of LCSIs in specific sports related injuries

Although there are a large number of publications relating to local corticosteroid injections which span the last five decades, the quality of these is limited and good evidence for benefit in many injuries is scant. Several methodological issues are relevant, including study design and accuracy of both diagnosis and injection. Many studies have been limited by small sample sizes and heterogeneity of study populations, unsuitable outcome measures, short-term follow-up, inadequate blinding, and lack of a true placebo. The increasing availability of imaging in the form of MRI and ultrasound should improve diagnostic reliability, and hence clinical studies in this field.

Injection accuracy is evidently of vital importance. A range of soft tissue and joint injections administered blindly, even by experienced operators, are inaccurate, and there is some evidence that accuracy correlates with efficacy [Jones *et al.* 1993; Eustace *et al.* 1997; Zingas *et al.* 1998; Henkus *et al.* 2006]. Hence, the use of ultrasound-guided injection is now increasingly advocated and with time may become standard practice.

Potential adverse effects of steroid injections

The specific incidence of side effects after LCSIs for soft tissue complaints, and the relevance of factors such as the steroid used, the tissue involved, the extent of the injury, the phase of healing at the time of injection, and post-injection events—particularly loading of the tissue—have not been established. Most unwanted effects of local LCSIs are minor, and include temporary pain after injection, a post-injection flare, facial flushing, local skin lesions, temporary menstrual irregularity, and post-menopausal haemorrhage (Speed 2001). Diabetics should be warned that a rise in blood glucose levels may occur and can last for approximately a week after injection. Many clinicians advise against the injection of corticosteroid near heavily loaded tissues, such as the Achilles and patellar tendons and the plantar ligament. Complete tendon rupture with loading after steroid injection is recognized, although the literature is limited to case reports. Sepsis is reported in 1/14 000–1/50 000 intra-articular/soft-tissue injections. Other commonly reported side effects include tissue atrophy and hypersensitivity reactions (Speed 2001). Potential adverse effects of LCSIs when administered in patients with plantar fasciitis include fascial rupture, infection, subcutaneous fat atrophy, skin pigmentation changes, peripheral nerve injury and muscle damage.

Resuscitation facilities should be available in the event of a rare severe reaction. Although corticosteroid arthropathy and osteonecrosis are rare (0.8%), they seem to affect mostly weight-bearing joints after intra-articular injections, highlighting the need to be particularly cautious in the athlete, who will undoubtedly load the joint more than most non-athletic patients.

Table 2.6.4 Potential unwanted effects of local corticosteroid injections

---

- Hypersensitivity—local or systemic
- Tissue atrophy
- Tendon rupture
- Infection—local or systemic
- Menstrual irregularities
- Post-injection 'flare' of symptoms
- Osteonecrosis/steroid arthropathy (intra-articular injections, weight-bearing joints)

Table 2.6.3 Indications and contraindications for the use of local corticosteroid injections in sports injuries.

Indications
- Reserve for chronic injuries after a failure of intensive use of other approaches
- Use when rehabilitation is inhibited by pain
- Ensure adequate attention has been given to correcting the cause

Contraindications
- Local or systemic infection
- Coagulopathy
- Tendon tear
- LCSIs are often unnecessary and should be avoided in the younger patient

Avoid intra-articular steroid injections wherever possible

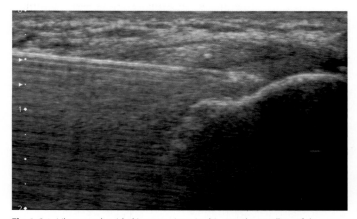

Fig. 2.6.1 Ultrasound-guided interventions, in this case dry needling of the Achilles tendon, are the preferred approach when needling or injection therapies are indicated.

Practical suggestions for use

Many of the recommendations for the use of LCSIs are based upon anecdote. There is no consensus with respect to environment (operating theatre, treatment room, or clinic), skin preparation, the use of LA, wearing gloves, the safe number of injections at one site, or the appropriate interval between injections. Agents differ with respect to their potency and solubility, with solubility inversely correlating with the duration of action (Table 2.6.5). There are few data on the absorption of corticosteroids from peritendinous injections, but methylprednisolone acetate remains in plasma for a mean of 16 days after periarticular injection. More soluble preparations that are short acting (e.g. hydrocortisone) or moderate acting (eg methylprednisolone) are recommended for soft tissue injections on the theoretical basis of likelihood of fewer side effects, and agents with low solubility should not be used for this purpose (Speed 2001).

LA mixed with the corticosteroid is commonly used to increase injection volume for wider dispersion and to lessen any pain with the injection (Speed 2001). This is common practice, although some manufacturers advise against mixing agents because it may cause clumping and precipitation of steroid crystals. There is no evidence of a difference in outcome between the addition of long-versus short-acting anaesthetic, nor is there evidence that injection of LA in advance of the corticosteroid is beneficial, with the exception of ensuring under ultrasound guidance that the needle is in place.

Local steroid injections in the vicinity of the Achilles or patellar tendon in the circumstances of a tear are frequently discouraged owing to the concerns about rupture of heavily loaded tendons and/or impairment of tissue repair where disruption is already present (Benazzo *et al.* 1996; Josza and Kannus 1997). In trigger-point therapy, there appears to be no benefit of infiltration of corticosteroid injection over LA or dry needling. Since the potential side effects are greater, they are reserved for use in the resistant trigger point.

Local anaesthetic injections and dry needling

Injections of LA alone are used for both diagnostic and therapeutic purposes in sports injuries. In sport-related pain syndromes, pain may be present only during specific dynamic situations, and identification of its source can be difficult. In other cases, multiple pathologies coexist and teasing out the specific source of pain can be a challenge. These situations can often be usefully addressed by guided injection into specific sites and dynamic stress testing to evaluate alteration in symptoms.

In some cases, the duration of analgesia obtained can exceed the duration of action of the LA, for reasons that are not fully understood.

Local injection of a trigger point with anaesthetic or saline in the patient with myofascial pain aims to mechanically disrupt the trigger point and, when LA is used, desensitize the area. Reduction of symptoms should facilitate a stretching and exercise programme to increase the range of motion and improve exercise tolerance.LA may have the advantage over dry needling in reducing post-injection soreness, but otherwise they seem to be equally effective. Where multiple muscle groups are involved, the use of dry needling or acupuncture is preferable. Trigger point and ligament injections can also be beneficial in the control of back pain, although, as with other injuries, they should be used to facilitate rehabilitation.

Side effects of LA injection are rare. Injection of large volumes into a highly vascular area may theoretically result in systemic effects. Adrenaline is not recommended in LAs for procedures involving the appendages because of the risk of ischaemic necrosis.

Dry needling is also used in chronic tendinopathies, as discussed below.

Platelet rich plasma, growth factors and bioactive proteins

The concept of using growth factors to accelerate the healing of injuries to muscle, tendon and ligament is a current focus of attention in the management of sports injuries. It is an exciting concept, since so many other forms of therapies are based on pain management rather than true healing of the condition. It is proposed that delivery of autologous bioactive growth factors derived from platelets (insulin-like growth factor-1, transforming growth factor-beta(1), basic fibroblast growth factor, platelet-derived growth factor (PDGF), epidermal growth factor, vascular endothelial growth factor (VEGF)) will promote healing, stimulating fibrocyte migration and inducing neovascular ingrowth (Molby *et al.* 2003). Although the overall evidence from animal model studies is encouraging (Wang *et al.* 2005), evidence of benefit in the human is limited to Level 4 evidence studies. Nevertheless, platelet rich

Table 2.6.5 Comparison of injectable corticosteroids

Preparation	Potency[a]	Concentration (mg/ml)	Solubility (% wt/vol)	Onset of action	Dose(mg)
Hydrocortisone acetate (Hydrocortistab)	1	25	0.002	Variable	5–25
Prednisolone acetate (Deltastab)	4	25	0.001	Variable	5–25
Methyprednisolone acetate (Depomedrone)	5	20, 40, 80	0.001	1–5 days	20–80
Tramcinolone acetonide (Adcortyl, Kenalog)	5	10, 40	0.004	Variable	5–40
Betamethasone sodium phosphate/acetate	25	6	NA	2–24 hours	0.25–2
Dexamethasone phosphate	25	4	0.01	2–24 hours	NA
Triamcinolone hexacetonide[b]	5	20	0.0002	Variable	NA[b]

[b]Insolubility makes it unsuitable for use in soft tissue injections.
[a]Hydrocortisone equivalents (per milligram).

plasma (PRP) therapies are now commonly used in articular, tendon, ligament, and muscle injuries. A helpful review by Foster and colleagues (2009) provides an insight into current practice in this field.

Normal platelet counts in blood are 150-350000/µL; PRP containing 1 000 000/µL in 5 ml of blood, is associated with the promotion of healing (Marx 2010). There are many PRP systems available, providing preparations that differ in their composition and in particular in their platelet concentrations. The basis process is that a sample of whole blood (e.g. 60–120 ml) is first anticoagulated then centrifuged once or twice to provide a harvest sample of PRP (e.g. 6–10 ml, 500 000–1000 000/µL) that is then clotted and the platelets activated to degranulate and release growth factors. There are also simpler systems that produce autologous conditioned plasma (ACP), lower in platelet concentrate (300 000–500 000/µL) and harvest sample (typically 2–5 ml from a 10 ml blood sample). The relative merits of different preparations, timing of treatment and appropriate schedules and best post-procedural protocols have yet to be established. However pathologies are likely to differ from each other in this respect.

Intra-tendinous sclerosant injections

Sclerosant injections, such as polidocinol, are also used in the treatment of chronic tendinopathies, targeting neovascularization, which is considered by many to be the prime source of pain in these lesions.

Alfredsson and coworkers have reported a number of studies in which they have targeted new vessels in chronic tendinopathies using intra-tendinous LA or sclerosant under ultrasound guidance, and have noted significant improvements in pain and function (Alfredson and Ohberg 2005a,b). One such study involved 20 consecutive patients (nine men and 11 women with a mean age of 50 years) with chronic painful mid-portion Achilles tendinopathy,

Table 2.6.6 Suggestions for practice in the use of local steroid injections in soft tissue lesions

---

- Informed consent should be obtained from the patient, who is warned of potential side effects and must be willing to follow post-injection guidelines
- The practitioner should have full knowledge of the local anatomy
- Select the finest needle that will reach the lesion
- The practitioner's hands and the patient's skin should be cleansed and a no-touch technique used
- Use short/medium-acting corticosteroid preparations in most cases, with LA
- Injection should be peritendinous; avoid injection into tendon substance
- The minimum interval between injections should be 6 weeks
- Use a maximum of three injections at one site
- Soluble preparations may be useful in those patients who have had hypersensitivity/local reaction to previous injection
- Details of the injection should be carefully recorded
- Do not repeat if two injections do not provide at least 4 weeks' relief
- Warn the patient of early post-injection local anaesthesia, to avoid initial overuse
- Advise a minimum post-injection rest of 2 weeks and avoid heavy loading for 6 weeks
- The patient should inform the doctor if there is any suggestion of infection or other significant adverse event

---

Reproduced from Speed, C.A. (2001). Fortnightly review: local corticosteroid injections in tendon lesions. *British Medical Journal*, **323**, 282–6.

who were randomized to injection treatment with either polidocanol (5 mg/ml) (group A) or lidocaine (5 mg/ml) + adrenaline (5 µg/ml) (group B) (Alfredson and Ohberg 2005a). Both substances have a local anaesthetic effect, but polidocanol also has a sclerosing effect. The patients and the treating physician were blinded to the substance injected. The short-term effects were evaluated after a maximum of two treatments 3–6 weeks apart. Before treatment, all patients had structural tendon changes and neovascularization demonstrated with ultrasonography (US) and colour Doppler. Under US and colour Doppler guidance, the injections targeted the area of neovascularization just outside the ventral part of the tendon. For evaluation, the patients recorded the severity of Achilles tendon pain during tendon loading activity, before and after treatment, on a visual analogue scale. Patients' satisfaction with treatment was also assessed. At follow-up (mean 3 months) after a maximum of two treatments, 5/10 patients in group A were satisfied with the treatment and had a significantly reduced level of tendon pain ($p < 0.005$). In group B, no patient was satisfied with treatment. In the pain-free tendons, but not in the painful tendons, neovascularization was absent after treatment. After completion of the study, treatment with polidocanol injections (cross-over in group B and additional treatments in group A) resulted in 10/10 and 9/10 satisfied patients in groups A and B, respectively.

The same workers reported similar improvements in painful patellar tendinosis in an uncontrolled study of sclerosant therapy to areas of neovascularization in 15 athletes (Alfredson and Ohberg 2005b).

Larger randomized controlled studies of this technique are needed. The procedure itself is lengthy, and the long-term consequences of this approach in isolation remain unclear.

Other sclerosant injections (prolotherapy)

Injection of various solutions, such as a mixture of dextrose 12.5%, glycerin 12.5%, phenol 1.25%, and lidocaine 0.25%, with the aim of producing a sclerosing effect to reduce pain and disability, has long been used to treat soft tissue and spinal pain. The evidence base is limited, treatment protocols are varied, and injection sites are often poorly defined but commonly involve ligamentous structures. Post-injection pain and stiffness are the most common side effects (Dagenais *et al.* 2005).

Botulinum toxins

Botulinum toxins (BTX) are purified proteins, produced by the anaerobic bacterium *Clostridium botulinum*, which block the presynaptic release of the neurotransmitter acetylcholine. There are as many as seven antigenically distinct botulinum neurotoxins, but only types A and B are in clinical use. They are used in the treatment of a number of painful conditions, and in the sporting context these include myofascial pain, muscular low back pain, and spasticity. However, they are rarely used, with the exception of paralympic athletes. Studies of BTX in myofascial disorders imply similar results to injection of saline or LA, and therefore BTX should be reserved for resistant cases.

Clinical effects are typically seen 3–10 days after injection. Pain relief is usually temporary, lasting weeks to months, and stretching and exercise therapy are important components of a successful outcome. When administered properly, the procedure is usually very safe, although reported side effects include injection site pain, muscle soreness, headache, fever, abdominal symptoms, a flu-like illness, rash, and antibody formation. The long-term side effects of regular injections are not known. The development of immunoresistance results in inefficacy of the treatment, but this can be limited by using the smallest possible effective dose and extending the interval between treatments as long as possible. Those who do develop resistance may benefit from the use of other botulinum toxin serotypes in the future. Muscle paralysis can occur with misplaced injections or excessive doses.

Other injections

Anti-TNF injections

Anti-TNF therapies are increasingly popular in the management of inflammatory joint disease. One small study has examined their potential in chronic tendinopathies [26].

Ultrasound-guided, peritendinous injections of adalimumab (tumor necrosis factor -alpha blocker) and anakinra (interleukin-1 receptor antagonist) were evaluated with regard to reducing pain, tendon thickness, and the blood flow in chronic Achilles tendinopathy. Peritendinous injections of adalimumab had a significant effect on pain sensation at rest in chronic Achilles tendinopathy but no effect on tendon thickness and contrary to all expectation, the tendon thickness in the anakinra-treated patients increased significantly after 12 weeks. Adalimumab showed a significant tendency to reduce the blood flow in the tendon over 12 weeks, whereas anakinra had no effect on the blood flow. The clinical application of these findings will undoubtedly be evaluated by future studies.

Hyaluronic acid injections

Viscosupplememt injections of hyaluronic acid are used in the management of osteoarthritis, and this is of particular relevance to masters athletes. Such injections are safe with a post-injection flare being the only significant frequently reported side effect. They have considerable advantage over corticosteroids in relation to potential adverse effects on soft tissue and cartilage and appear to have a longer duration of effect. They are also considered safe in younger adults. Most clinical research has focussed on osteoarthritis of the knee.

There are many products available, differing in their molecular weights, hyaluronic acid concentrations, numbers of injections recommended as an approved course of therapy, and source (some being extracted from avian proteins, some being artificially manufactured). Although higher molecular weight preparations have the advantage of requiring less frequent injections, they are associated with higher local side effects without necessarily a therapeutic advantage [27].

HA preparations have also been proposed as an approach in the management of soft tissue mediated pain. Enhanced tendon healing to bone has been demonstrated in rabbit models [28].

Others

Low dose heparin has been used in the management of Achilles tendinopathies, with the aim to limit the formation of adhesions. However, there is some evidence that there is no beneficial effect and it has been suggested that heparin may, in itself, cause a degenerative tendinopathy.

A calf-derived deproteinized haemodialysate, **Actovegin**, has been suggested to be useful in the management of Achilles paratenonitis, but a large, high-quality trial is needed.

Traumeel, a mixture of diluted extracts from minerals and medicinal plants including Arnica, is proposed to have anti-inflammatory properties. It is increasingly popular in the treatment of soft tissue injuries and in particular muscle strain injuries, but trials are lacking.

Peripheral somatosensory nerve blockade

Peripheral somatosensory nerve blocks are also used in the management of pain in a variety of musculoskeletal complaints, including those affecting the sportsperson. Common examples include carpal tunnel injection, suprascapular nerve block in the management of shoulder pain, and ilioinguinal nerve blocks. Some of these will be briefly mentioned here.

The *suprascapular nerve* supplies sensory nerves to the posterosuperior aspect of the shoulder, including major portions of the rotator cuff. There is some evidence to suggest that suprascapular nerve block using steroid/bupivacaine is temporarily effective in reducing pain in rotator cuff tendinitis and tears, improving movement range in tendinitis and is possible in an outpatient setting with little or no risk of complication. The benefit of using steroid and lignocaine over anaesthetic alone is questionable. Differing techniques for suprascapular nerve blockade have been described, including needle tip guided by superficial bony landmarks, and a near-nerve electromyographically guided technique.

Ilioinguinal nerve blockade can be useful in the sportsperson, usually male, with sportsman's abdominal wall syndrome. Typically, long acting local anesthetic and hydrocortisone are infiltrated under ultrasound guidance around the nerve, and the patient's pain assessed over the subsequent 4 hours. The injection is primarily used for diagnostic purposes.

Conclusions

A number of local injection therapies are available for the management of sports related injury and in particular soft tissue mediated pain. They should be reserved for the treatment of chronic soft-tissue lesions and as part of a programme that includes identification and correction of provocative factors. Although an increasing number of techniques and injectates are available, the current evidence for the use of many is scant. Accuracy of diagnosis and injection appears to be important for maximum benefit to be achieved.

References

Alfredson, H. (1999). *In situ* microdialysis in tendon tissue: high levels of glutamate, but not prostaglandin E_2 in chronic achilles tendon pain. *Knee Surgery, Sports Traumatology and Arthroscopy*, **7**, 378–81.

Alfredson, H. and Ohberg, L. (2005a). Neovascularisation in chronic painful patellar tendinosis–promising results after sclerosing neovessels outside the tendon challenge the need for surgery. *Knee Surgery, Sports Traumatology and Arthroscopy*, **13**, 74–80.

Alfredson, H. and Ohberg, L. (2005b). Sclerosing injections to areas of neo-vascularisation reduce pain in chronic Achilles tendinopathy: a double-blind randomised controlled trial. *Knee Surgery, Sports Traumatology and Arthroscopy*, **13**, 338–44.

Assendelft, W.J., Hay, E.M., Adshead, R., and Bouter, L.M. (1996). Local corticosteroid injections for lateral epicondylitis:a systematic overview. *British Journal of General Practice*, **46**, 209–16.

Chard, M.D., Cawston, T.D., Riley, G.P., *et al.* (1994). Rotator cuff degeneration and lateral epicondylitis: a comparative histological study. *Annals of the Rheumatic Diseases*, **53**, 30–4.

Crawford, F. (2002). Plantar heel pain (including plantar fasciitis). *Clinical Evidence*, **7**, 1091–1100.

Crawford, F., Atkins, D., Young, P., *et al.* (1999). Steroid injection for heel pain: evidence of short term effectiveness. A randomised controlled trial. *Rheumatology*, **38**, 974–7.

DaCruz, D.J., Geeson, M., Allen, M.J., and Phair, I. (1988). Achilles paratendonitis: an evaluation of steroid injection. *British Journal of Sports Medicine*, **22**, 64–5.

Dagenais, S., Haldeman, S., and Wooley, J.R. (2005). Intraligamentous injection of sclerosing solutions (prolotherapy) for spinal pain: a critical review of the literature. *Spine Journal*, **5**, 310–28.

Eustace, J.A., Brophy, D.P., Gibney, R.P., *et al.* (1997). Comparison of the accuracy of steroid placement with clinical outcome in patients with shoulder symptoms. *Annals of the Rheumatic Diseases*, **56**, 59–63.

Foster, T.E., Puskas, B.L., Mandelbaum, B.R., Gerhardt, M.B., and Rodeo, S.A. (2009). Platelet-Rich Plasma: from basic sciences to clinical applications. *Am. J. Sports Med.*, **37**, 2259–72.

Fredberg, U. and Ostgaard, R. (2008). Effect of ultrasound-guided, peritendinous injections of adalimumab and anakinra in chronic Achilles tendinopathy: a pilot study. *Scandinavian Journal of Medicine and Science in Sports*. Epub ahead of print.

Green, S., Buchbinder, R., Glazier, R., and Forbes, A. (2000). Interventions for shoulder pain. *Cochrane Database of Systematic Reviews*, **2**, CD001156.

Hay, E.M., Paterson, S.M., Lewis, M., *et al.* (1999). Pragmatic randomised controlled trial of local corticosteroid injection and naproxen for treatment of lateral epicondylitis of elbow in primary care. *British Medical Journal*, **319**, 964–8.

Hazleman, B., Riley, G., and Speed, C. (2004). *Soft Tissue Rheumatology*. Oxford University Press.

Henkus, H.E., Cobben, L.P., Coerkamp, E.G., Nelissen, R.G., and van Arkel, E.R. (2006). The accuracy of subacromial injections: a prospective randomized magnetic resonance imaging study. *Arthroscopy*, **22**, 277–82.

Jones, A., Regan, M., Ledingham, J., *et al.* (1993). Importance of placement of intra-articular steroid injections. *British Medical Journal*, **307**, 1329–30.

Josza, J. and Kannus, P. (1997). Overuse injuries of tendons. In: J. Josza and P. Kannus (eds), *Human Tendons*, pp. 164–253. Human Kinetics, New York.

Khan, M.H., Li, Z., and Wang, J.H. Repeated exposure of tendon to prostaglandin-E2 leads to localized tendon degeneration. *Clinical Journal of Sport Medicine*, **15**, 27–33.

Marx, R.E. (2001). Platelet-rich plasma (PRP): What is PRP and what is not PRP? *Implant Dent.*, **10**(4), 225–8.

Molloy, T., Wang, Y., and Murrell, G. (2003). The roles of growth factors in tendon and ligament healing. *Sport Medicine*, **33**, 381–94.

O'Connor, T. and Abram, S. (2003). *Atlas of Pain Injection Techniques*. Churchill Livingstone, London.

Reichenbach, S., Blank, S., Rutjes, A.W., *et al.* (2007). Hylan versus hyaluronic acid for osteoarthritis of the knee: a systematic review and meta-analysis. *Arthritis and Rheumatism*, **57**, 1410–18.

Riley, G.P., Harrall, R.L., Constant, C.R., *et al.* (1994). Tendon degeneration and chronic shoulder pain: changes in collagen composition of the human rotator cuff tendons in rotator cuff tendinitis. *Annals of the Rheumatic Diseases*, **53**, 359–66.

Speed, C.A. (2001). Fortnightly review: Local corticosteroid injections in tendon lesions. *British Medical Journal*, **323**, 382–6.

Speed, C.A. (2005). Shoulder pain. *Clinical Evidence*, **14**, 1543–60.

Waldman, S. (2000). *Atlas of Pain Management Techniques*. W.B. Saunders, Philadelphia, PA.

Wang, X.T, Liu, P.Y., and Tang, J.B. (2005). Tendon healing *in vitro*: modification of tenocytes with exogenous vascular endothelial growth factor gene increases expression of transforming growth factor beta but minimally affects expression of collagen genes. *Journal of Hand Surgery*, **30**, 222–9.

Yagishita, K., Sekiya, I., Sakaguchi, Y., Shinomiya, K., and Muneta, T. (2005). The effect of hyaluronan on tendon healing in rabbits. *Arthroscopy*, **21**, 1330–6.

Zingas, C., Failla, J.M., and van Holsbeeck, M. (1998). Injection accuracy and clinical relief of de Quervain's tendinitis. *Journal of Hand Surgery*, **23**, 89–96.

2.7

Orthotics

Sharon Dixon and Sophie Roberts

Introduction

An orthotic is a custom-made insole which fits inside a shoe with the purpose of changing the way in which the foot functions during both standing and dynamic gait. There are many theories regarding the influence of these devices on the foot and lower limb. It is widely accepted that the fundamental principle is that an orthotic encourages a change in the movement pattern of the foot, aiming to alleviate stress to musculoskeletal structures, and produce changes in muscle firing patterns. An example of how an orthotic works is when one is used to change the functioning position of the medial longitudinal arch of the foot by altering the orientation of the calcaneus and potentially reducing the demand on the tibialis posterior tendon.

There is evidence that orthotic devices are successful in alleviating lower limb injury, with reports that 70–80% of sports participants experiencing lower extremity injury, such as shin pain, knee pain, and plantar fasciitis, show a reduction in symptoms after wearing orthoses (James *et al.* 1978; D'Ambrosia and Douglas 1982; Donatelli *et al.* 1988; Nigg *et al.* 1999). In contrast, some studies have reported no change in injury incidence with orthotic use (Jenkins and Raedeke 2006). Whilst clinically it is generally accepted that orthotic devices produce positive outcomes, it remains unclear exactly how an orthotic influences lower extremity dynamics to produce these positive effects. Without a solid science base, it is difficult to determine exactly what an orthotic is trying to achieve. There are a number of theories which have directed clinicians in their clinical decision-making.

Theories of orthotic prescription and design

The theory of orthotic therapy was first introduced by Inman *et al.* (1981) and Root *et al.* (1971, 1977) in the 1970s and 1980s when they proposed a practical set of techniques for identifying biomechanical dysfunction and directing treatment approaches. Their work mainly focused on the functional importance of the subtalar joint as a reference position from which to identify foot types and control the foot position. Before this work was performed, orthotic therapy had been based on supporting the medial longitudinal arch in a static position.

Methods described by Root *et al.* (1971) for producing functional foot orthoses use subtalar joint neutral as a goal in orthotic prescription. This approach assumes that the foot functions most efficiently about a neutral position. A cast is made of the foot whilst in subtalar neutral and corrections are added if appropriate, with the aim being to encourage the foot to function about the subtalar neutral and to maintain a neutral forefoot orientation (Hunter *et al.* 1995). Corrections include intrinsic rearfoot posting (Darrigan and Ganley 1985), the inverted foot orthosis (Blake 1986), and the medial heel skive (Kirby 1992).

Several limitations of the initial approach to orthotic prescription described by Root *et al.* (1971) have been highlighted (Ball and Afheldt 2002). Root *et al.* (1971) provide two contradictory definitions of subtalar neutral, leading to varying interpretations of the approach. In addition, determination of non-weight-bearing subtalar neutral has been found to be unreliable (Evans *et al.* 2003), and the functional significance of subtalar neutral has been questioned (McPoil and Cornwall 1994). The subtalar neutral approach also relies primarily on static measures, which may not be appropriate when developing a device to influence dynamic locomotion. Despite these limitations, some of the Inman and Root ideas are retained in orthotic manufacture today, with many clinicians including at least some of the Root approaches in their prescription methods. To demonstrate this, Landorf *et al.* (2001) reported that 72% of podiatrists answering a questionnaire on orthotic prescription methods stated that they utilize functional foot orthoses most frequently, with the majority indicating that they prefer a modified Root style of orthosis.

The Root approach does not acknowledge the variation in subtalar joint axis orientation and the movement of this axis (Nester 1998). Thus alternative methods for prescription of orthotic devices which consider this variation have been developed. Kirby (1987, 2001) described subtalar joint axis theory, using subtalar axis palpation for determination of the orientation of the subtalar joint axis relative to the plantar surface of the foot. Kirby indicated how changes in the spatial location and orientation of the subtalar joint axis will influence the biomechanics of the foot during stance and thus should be determined to aid orthotic prescription. To highlight the implications of this approach, Kirby (2001) described how any variation in the location and orientation of the subtalar joint axis will influence the moment arm lengths of the muscle forces and the ground reaction force, affecting the pronation and supination moments. The balance of these moments will influence the resulting movement and the loads experienced by structures controlling pronation/supination. Thus, an understanding of the balance of these moments is argued to be critical in successful orthotic prescription. Examples of this approach include use of an inverted foot orthosis or a Kirby heel skive, both of which aim to provide a supinatory moment to reduce pronation movement. Both these interventions apply a force medial to the subtalar joint axis, where the amount of required force depends on the distance from the line of action of force to the subtalar joint axis. Thus the spatial location of the subtalar joint axis influences the effect of the force on joint motion.

The specific amount of intervention required in an orthotic has generally been based on trial and error (Payne *et al.* 2003). Payne and coworkers have described a supination resistance test to help determine the exact degree of intervention required (Noakes and Payne 2003; Payne *et al.* 2003). This procedure aims to quantify the resistance of the foot to a supinatory force, indicating the required moment for control of pronation. The methods described by Kirby and by Payne take a more functional approach than traditional Root techniques, with consideration of the forces and moments applied to the foot rather than focusing primarily on movement.

Dananberg (2000) has described an approach to orthotic prescription which considers the role of the forefoot in lower limb motion. This method focuses on the sagittal plane facilitation of the foot. It is suggested that, for efficient locomotion, the centre of gravity pivots over the first metatarsophalangeal joint during propulsion. For this sagittal plane motion to be achieved, adequate dorsiflexion of the metatarsophalangeal joint is required. If sufficient dorsiflexion does not occur (hallux limitus), the sagittal plane rotations of the lower limb are restricted and compensatory motions are required. For example, delayed heel lift and late midtarsal pronation during mid-stance may occur to allow forward motion. Suggested orthotic interventions to avoid the requirement for compensation are aimed at redirecting forces in the right direction at the right time. To achieve this optimally, measurements of pressure within the shoe are required (Payne *et al.* 2003). An alternative approach is to use a first ray cut-out, which is aimed at increasing plantar-flexion of the first ray, reducing the force required to dorsiflex the hallux. Such devices have been found to be successful in increasing dorsiflexion of the metatarsophalangeal joint in walking (Scherer *et al.* 2006).

In general, the approaches to orthotic prescription described so far have focused on the control of lower limb movement through a device with specific additions aimed at limiting undesirable movement or encouraging movement that is believed to be required. For example, the most common orthotic interventions aim to control the amount of pronation immediately following heel contact or during mid-stance. Nigg (2001) has suggested an alternative paradigm. Nigg highlighted that literature evidence has generally not supported the suggestion that interventions such as medial posting to control pronation do in fact limit this motion. Thus, the belief that orthotic devices act to align the skeleton was questioned. Instead, Nigg suggested that the body tries to maintain a preferred movement pattern regardless of the footwear and shoe insert/orthotic worn. Thus, if the footwear combination inhibits natural movement, increased muscle action is used in an attempt to maintain movement as close as possible to that preferred. This suggestion indicates that the most appropriate footwear/orthotic combination is one that allows the body to move naturally, minimizing the energy cost of muscle action to maintain natural movement. To test the suggestion that a footwear condition supporting natural joint motion will reduce muscle activation and that one counteracting natural motion will increase muscle activity, Mündermann *et al.* (2006) compared electromyography (EMG) for selected leg muscle groups for different types of orthoses. They reported a systematic change in EMG across subjects for specific orthotic interventions, with the lowest muscle activity associated with the control condition(no orthotic). Whilst this provides some support for the suggestion that there is a preferred movement pattern and that the introduction of an orthotic device which attempts to change this may increase muscle activity, the authors acknowledge the requirement for further work, particularly in the investigation of the long-term use of orthotic devices where subjects will be more familiar with the device.

From a practical standpoint, these different theories should be understood and applied where necessary according to the prescribing practitioner's clinical reasoning. It is generally not practical to obtain EMG data for different orthotic interventions, often limiting the practical application of the Nigg theory. More functional methods than the static approaches of Root and coworkers have been developed, and appear to provide logical tools to improve orthotic prescription. The degree of utilization of these newer techniques among practitioners is varied, and is dependent on their understanding of the proposed methodology and the appropriateness of the approach to the case in question.

Typical measures taken for orthotic prescription

Whatever the underlying philosophy of a particular podiatrist regarding orthotic prescription, a series of observations or measurements are generally taken to inform the prescription. It has been noted that this methodology can vary considerably between practitioners (Landorf *et al.* 2001).

Various biomechanical measurements are taken or estimated to aid the orthotic prescription process. These measurements are taken not only from the foot but from the whole lower limb to gain an understanding of the individual's biomechanical function. Information such as hamstring length, quadriceps length, gluteus medius strength, internal and external hip range of motion, and assessment of leg length equality are useful in formulating a prescription, as the feet can compensate for these biomechanical measures. For example, if a person demonstrates a very externally rotated hip position, controlling the foot with an orthotic with aggressive pronation control will potentially reduce the hip range of motion. Therefore in this case a reduced amount of subtalar joint pronation control will be used in the orthotic design.

Both a non-weight-bearing and weight-bearing assessment are generally made of the foot and ankle complex to aid quantification of structure and function. Some of the measures typically taken by one of the authors (SC) are described below. A non-weight-bearing assessment of the subtalar joint is used to assess in detail the range of motion and the position of the axis of the subtalar joint, which are both important factors in orthotic prescription. The range of motion of the subtalar joint is determined by placing the subject in either a prone or a supine position. The tibia is held steady with one hand and the other hand takes the subtalar joint through its range by gripping the lateral column of the foot, pushing the foot into inversion and eversion. The range of motion can either be assessed through estimation of the range or it can be measured using a goniometer (Fig. 2.7.1). If a goniometer is to be used to measure the subtalar range of motion, the subject should be placed in a prone position so that it is easy to place and read the goniometer. It should be noted that goniometric measurement of the subtalar joint has been shown to have poor reliability and repeatability,

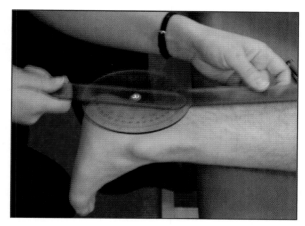

Fig. 2.7.1 Measurement of subtalar joint range of motion using a goniometer.

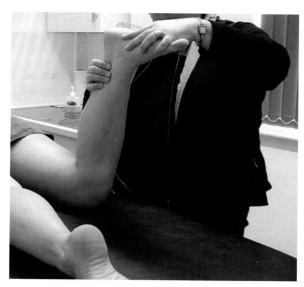

Fig. 2.7.2 Measurement of ankle dorsiflexion.

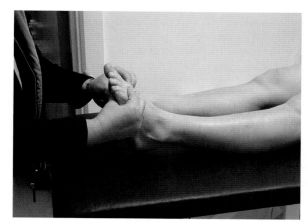

Fig. 2.7.3 Assessment of the metatarsals.

and therefore estimation of the range is often sufficient in the clinical field (Evans, Copper *et al.* 2003).

If excessive range of motion (approximately 20° of inversion and 10° of eversion) is found, the subtalar joint can be classed as hypermobile and therefore might indicate a requirement for more supportive features on the orthotic than for cases of normal subtalar range of motion. These features may include a deeper heel cup, a higher angle of varus wedging, a high arch height, and a medial heel skive (a raised section in the medial heel cup to buttress the medial calcaneus).

The position of the axis of the subtalar joint is also assessed to determine if it is a high or low axis or if it is medially deviated. Again, this affects the orthotic prescription. A foot with a low subtalar joint axis will show more inversion and eversion and therefore features in the orthotic design will focus on controlling the frontal plane movement of the calcaneus with perhaps a deeper heel cup. A foot with a high axis will have more abduction and adduction and therefore a deeper heel cup on the orthotic may cause irritation, particularly on the lateral side.

The position of the subtalar joint is determined by placing the subject in either a prone or a supine position and again taking the subtalar joint through its range of motion. If more abduction and adduction is noticed in relation to the amount of inversion and eversion, the axis is high, and if inversion and eversion is noticed more than abduction and adduction of the joint, the subtalar joint has a low axis. The assessment technique is based on observation and cannot be measured easily in a clinic without using three-dimensional motion analysis.

The ankle joint range of motion is also assessed to determine if foot pronation is a component of compensation for reduced ankle joint dorsiflexion (Fig. 2.7.2). The metatarsal parabola (the length of the metatarsals) is assessed (Figure 2.7.3) as well as the range of motion of the first metatarsophalangeal joint. These measures provide information on forefoot function during the propulsive phase of gait, informing decisions regarding the requirement of metatarsal head accommodations or metatarsal pads in the orthotic prescription.

In the weight-bearing assessment, the calcaneal angle and tibial angle are measured or estimated in a relaxed stance position and also in subtalar joint neutral position. The subtalar joint neutral position is obtained by inverting the joint so that both talar heads

are equally palpable both medially and laterally. The degree of rearfoot control added to an orthotic device is calculated by comparing the relaxed and neutral calcaneal position. The symmetry of the pelvis is also assessed in the standing position to check for leg length inequality so that appropriate leg length correction can be built into the orthotic if necessary.

The preceding paragraphs provide an overview of key measures used to develop an orthotic prescription. The reader is directed to orthotic textbooks for more detail on these and other clinical measurements used in the prescription process (Hunter *et al.* 1995).

Recent advances in the measurement of plantar pressure have provided an additional tool in the prescription of orthotic devices. Whilst it should be acknowledged that pressure data do not directly indicate patterns of movement, there is evidence that high pronators can be detected in shod running over a pressure plate (Dixon 2006), and that barefoot pressure data can provide valuable detail in the characterization of ground contact patterns (de Cock *et al.* 2006). In addition, the use of in-shoe pressure data, collected using pressure insoles placed at the plantar surface of the foot, to inform orthotic prescription has been advocated by Payne (2008). Systems such as the RSscan D3D software exploit the suggested relationship between plantar pressure and movement by utilizing barefoot pressure plate data to aid in the determination of an orthotic prescription. This software focuses on factors such as the balance of pressure between the medial and lateral sides of the foot to determine whether corrective devices are required (Dixon and McNally 2008).

Orthotic classification and indications for use

The spectrum of orthotic devices available for prescription by podiatrists and other health professionals is growing all the time, ranging from generic insoles to complex custom-made orthotics (Figure 2.7.4). Therefore it is important to classify the different types of orthotics and determine the indications for prescription for these types. It should be appreciated that onward referral to a specialist podiatrist or orthotist for the provision of custom-made orthotics is sometimes necessary as prefabricated insoles would not be an appropriate choice for the individual patient. Table 2.7.1 lists the range of insoles available for prescription:

Custom-made orthotics are usually manufactured in a laboratory or by a skilled clinician using information provided in a prescription together with an impression of the foot taken by plaster of Paris cast, a foam imprint, or more recently a three-dimensional electronic scan of the foot. There is much discussion as to whether the impression of the foot should be taken non-weight-bearing or weight-bearing; however, it is the author's opinion (SC) that as long as the prescription is modified accordingly, it does not matter.

The manufacturing process starts with a positive replica of the foot being created either from the cast/foam impression or on the computer from the three-dimensional scan. The replica of the foot is then modified according to the prescription. Without going into the complexity of the manufacturing process, modifications like arch height correction, heel expansion, heel skive resection, and forefoot correction are applied. If this process has been done by computer, the modified replica of the foot is machine milled from a block of medium density fibreboard (MDF).

The material used for the shell of the orthotic is then heat moulded around the replica of the foot. The choice of material for the shell of the orthotic device is selected by the prescribing practitioner. Materials range from carbon fibre to polypropylene to ethelyne vinyl acetate (EVA), depending on the rigidity required

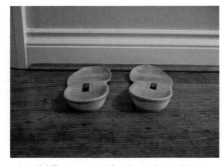

Fig. 2.7.4 Examples of different types of orthotic device: (a) a prescription device; (b) an off-the-shelf device.

for the orthotic device. The thickness of the shell material used also determines the rigidity of the device, and the degree of rigidity selected is usually based on patient weight and degree of pronation control required.

The shell is then trimmed and 'balanced' by applying rearfoot and forefoot control/wedging, again according to the prescription. The orthotic is then finished with external features such as topcovers, cushioning layers, metatarsal pads, and accommodations for metatarsal heads.

Provision of orthotics in sport

Orthotics play an important role in the management of the sports patient, with attention to detail required in the selection of the type of orthotic prescribed. Nigg *et al.* (1999) described several of the successes that have been gained with the use of soft orthotics, which are often preferred because of the impact forces created in most sports. The degree of pronation control or orthotic support must also be carefully considered in patients who participate in multidirectional sports, such as tennis, badminton, and football, where controlling the foot too much during lateral movement can predispose the individual to ankle inversion injuries or knee injuries.

The orthotic device must not be too bulky, or the patient may be pushed out of the sport-specific shoe with the consequence that support or protection is compromised. The mechanics of the foot during the sport should also be considered, and sometimes orthotics must be made specifically for the sport. Examples of this are cycling and skiing, where the foot performs different movements than during a gait cycle.

Several studies have focused on investigating the influence of othotic devices on lower limb biomechanics during running. Because of its suggested association with several lower limb injuries, the most frequently studied variable has been rearfoot eversion. However, these studies have provided equivocal evidence regarding the influence of orthotic devices on rearfoot control. There have been several reports of reductions in peak eversion and peak eversion velocity with orthotic use (Rodgers and Leveau 1982; Smith *et al.* 1986; Novick and Kelly 1990; McCulloch *et al.* 1993; Eng and Pierrynowski 1994; Mündermann *et al.* 2003; MacLean *et al.* 2006). This reduction in peak rearfoot eversion magnitude or velocity is an anticipated effect of devices aimed at controlling rearfoot eversion. However, there are also several studies that have reported no change in peak eversion or eversion velocity when wearing orthoses designed to control rearfoot movement (Blake and Ferguson 1992; Nawoczenski *et al.* 1995; Stacoff *et al.* 2000; Nigg *et al.* 2003). A less frequently documented effect of orthotic devices has been an increase in rearfoot inversion at initial ground strike (Eng and Pierrynowski 1994; Dixon and McNally 2008). This is consistent with the suggestion by Blake and Ferguson (1992) that encouraging a more inverted heel at ground strike is a function of orthotic devices, with the presence of an orthotic effectively acting to bring the ground up to meet the foot earlier in the movement phase. However, studies investigating the influence of orthotic devices have rarely investigated changes in initial inversion. The conflicting results regarding the influence of orthoses on rearfoot movement is likely to be contributed to substantially by construction of orthotic devices using different materials, different casting (moulding) methods, and different amounts of posting. Thus, for different orthotic prescriptions and construction

Table 2.7.1 An overview of orthotic types, features and indication for prescription

Types of orthotic	Who can prescribe it?	Features	Indication for prescription
Shop-sold prefabricated orthotics	Patients and all health professionals	Generally soft materials and mild support	Mild foot problems, patient independence
Health-professional-ordered prefabricated orthotics	All health professionals	Numerous types are available Standard prescription although degree of pronation control varies between types Material flexibility ranges Some have specific additional features	Mild to moderate foot or lower limb biomechanical dysfunction To test whether orthotic therapy is appropriate.
Custom simple insoles	All health professionals	Specific prescription Generally made with cork or EVA insole base with components added	To test whether orthotic therapy is appropriate Temporary treatment for acute problems Can be issued rapidly
Health-professional-modified prefabricated orthotics	Specialist health professionals	Modifications added to a standard prescription insole Material flexibility ranges	Mild to moderate foot or lower limb biomechanical dysfunction Lower cost for patient Can be issued rapidly
Custom-made orthotics	Specialist health professionals	Manufactured in laboratory or by skilled clinician according to a prescription 3D impression of foot is required for manufacture Numerous material options as well as additional features	Complex foot or lower limb biomechanical dysfunction

methods, it is important to independently assess the influence on lower extremity movement.

Recent biomechanical evidence points to influence of orthotic devices on ankle inversion moment (Mündermann *et al.* 2003; MacLean *et al.* 2006). As the heel strikes the ground and the foot moves into an everted orientation, an inversion moment acts to control this movement. It has been reported that medial wedging or posting reduces the inversion moment required to control this movement, thus reducing the load on medial structures controlling eversion (pronation). These findings support the use of functional approaches to orthotic prescription, such as those described by Kirby (2001) and Payne *et al.* (2003), which consider the moment acting about the subtalar joint when determining an orthotic prescription.

Summary and conclusions

Orthotic devices are popular among sporting populations as a treatment for lower limb injuries and, in general, these devices are successful in relieving symptoms. Whilst it has been assumed that this success is a result of changes in movement patterns, evidence to support this is limited. Several alternative explanations have been presented to suggest how a successful orthotic functions, including influencing joint moments and the encouragement of a preferred movement pattern. Each of these suggestions is based on sound scientific argument and is the subject of ongoing research.

The static measures originally described remain the foundation of orthotic prescription for many podiatrists, but these are supplemented by newer methods taking a more functional approach. These methods include the application of techniques such as determination of subtalar joint axis orientation and the supination resistance test. Increasingly, dynamic plantar pressure data are used to inform the orthotic prescription and forms of gait analysis are employed (see Chapter 1.9). It has been suggested that the

increased integration of gait analysis and podiatry measures will improve orthotic prescription because of the inclusion of dynamic gait data in the decision process (Dixon *et al.* 2008).

When looking at the efficacy of orthotics, it should be accepted that there is sometimes a limitation on what can be achieved. The lower limb mechanics of some patients are so pathological that an orthotic device can only provide a limited effect, for example in marked pes-planovalgus feet. Provision of the correct type of device for the patient and providing follow-up care are vitally important. One limitation of orthotic therapy is shoe fit. If an orthotic device is too wide for the shoe, it can completely alter the prescription it is providing. If a device is too narrow, the full affects of the prescription cannot be gained. Orthoses should be prescribed only after careful clinical reasoning and regular follow-up care should always be implemented.

References

Ball, K.A. and Afheldt, M.J. (2002). Evolution of foot orthotics. Part 1: Coherent theory or coherent practice. *Journal of Manipulative and Physiological Therapeutics*, **25**, 116–24.

Blake, R. (1986). Inverted functional orthosis. *Journal of the American Podiatric Medical Association*, **76**, 275–6.

Blake, R.L. and Ferguson, H. (1992). Extrinsic rearfoot posts. *Journal of the American Podiatric Medical Association*, **82**, 202–7.

D'Ambrosia, R. and Douglas, R. (1982). Orthotics. In: R. D'Ambrosia and D. Drez (eds), *Prevention and Treatment of Running Injuries*. Slack, Thorofare, NJ.

Dananberg, H.J. (2000). Sagittal plane biomechanics. American Diabetes Association. *Journal of the American Podiatric Medical Association*, **90**, 47–50.

Darrigan, R. and J. Ganley (1985). Functional orthoses with intrinsic rearfoot post. *Journal of the American Podiatric Medical Association*, **75**, 619–24.

de Cock, A., Willems, T., Witvrouw, E., Vanrenterghem, J., and de Clercq, D. (2006). A functional foot type classification with cluster analysis based on plantar pressure distribution during jogging. *Gait and Posture*, **23**, 339–47.

Dixon, S.J. (2006). Application of centre of pressure to indicate rearfoot inversion-eversion in shod running. *Journal of the American Podiatric Medical Association*, **96**, 305–11.

Dixon, S.J. and McNally, K. (2008). Influence of orthotic devices prescribed using pressure data on lower extremity kinematics and pressures beneath the shoe during running. *Clinical Biomechanics*, **23**, 593–600.

Dixon, S.J., McNally, K., *et al.* (2008). *Integration of podiatry assessment and gait analysis in the treatment of running injuries*. Presented at 13th Annual Congress of the European College of Sport Science, Estoril, Portugal.

Donatelli, R., Hurlburt, C., Conaway, D. and St Pierre, R. (1988). Biomechanical foot orthotics: a retrospective study. *Journal of Orthopaedic and Sports Physical Therapy*, **10**, 205–12.

Eng, J.J. and Pierrynowski, M.R. (1994). The effect of soft foot orthotics on three-dimensional lower limb kinematics during walking and running. *Physical Therapy*, **74**, 836–42.

Evans, A.M., Copper, A.W., Scharfbillig, R.W., Scutter, S.D., and Williams, M.T. (2003). Reliability of the foot posture index and traditional measures of foot position. *Journal of the American Podiatric Medical Association*, **93**, 203–13.

Hunter, S., Dolan, M.G., and Davies, J.M. (1995). *Foot Orthotics in Therapy and Sport*. Human Kinetics, Champaign, IL.

Inman, V., Ralston, H.J., and Todd, F. (1981). *Human Walking*. Williams & Wilkins, Baltimore, MD.

James, S., Bates, B., and Osternig, L.R. (1978). Injuries to runners. *American Journal of Sports Medicine*, **6**, 40–9.

Jenkins, W.L. and Raedeke, S.G. (2006). Lower-extremity overuse injury and use of foot orthotic devices in women's basketball. *Journal of the American Podiatric Medical Association*, **96**, 408–12.

Kirby, K.A. (1987). Methods for determination of the positional variations of the subtalar joint axis. *Journal of the American Podiatric Medical Association*, **77**, 228–34.

Kirby, K.A. (1992). The medial heel skive technique: improving pronation control in foot orthoses. *Journal of the American Podiatric Medical Association*, **82**, 177–88.

Kirby, K.A. (2001). Subtalar joint axis location and rotational equilibrium theory of foot function. *Journal of the American Podiatric Medical Association*, **91**, 465–87.

Landorf, K., Keenan, A., and Rushworth, R.L. (2001). Foot orthosis prescription habits of Australian and New Zealand podiatric physicians. *Journal of the American Podiatric Medical Association*, **91**, 174–83.

McCulloch, M.U., Brunt, D., and Vander Linden, D. (1993). The effect of foot orthotics and gait velocity on lower limb kinematics and temporal events of stance. *Journal of Orthopaedic and Sports Physical Therapy*, **17**, 2–10.

MacLean, C., Davis, I.M., Hamill, J. *et al.* (2006). Influence of a custom foot orthotic intervention on lower extremity dynamics in healthy runners. *Clinical Biomechanics*, **21**, 623–30.

McPoil, T. and Cornwall, M.W. (1994). Relationship between neutral subtalar joint position and pattern of rearfoot motion during walking. *Foot and Ankle International*, **15**, 141–5.

Mündermann, A., Nigg, B.M., Humble, R.N., and Stefanyshyn, D.J. (2003). Foot orthotics affect lower extremity kinematics and kinetics during running. *Clinical Biomechanics*, **18**, 254–62.

Mündermann, A., Wakeling, J.M., Nigg, B.M., Humble, R.N., and Stefanyshyn, D.J. (2006). Foot orthoses affect frequency components of muscle activity in the lower extremity. *Gait and Posture*, **23**, 295–302.

Nawoczenski, D.A., Cook, T.M., and Saltzman, C.L. (1995). The effect of foot orthotics on three-dimensional kinematics of the leg and rearfoot during running. *Journal of Orthopaedic and Sports Physical Therapy*, **21**, 317–327.

Nester, C.J. (1998). Review of literature on the axis of rotation of the foot. *Foot*, **8**, 111–18.

Nigg, B.M. (2001). The role of impact forces and foot pronation: a new paradigm. *Clinical Journal of Sport Medicine*, **11**, 2–9.

Nigg, B., Nurse, M.A., and Stefanyshyn, D.J. (1999). Shoe inserts and orthtoics for sport and physical activities. *Medicine and Science in Sports and Exercise*, **31** (Suppl), S421–28.

Nigg, B.M., Cole, G., Stefanyshyn, D., Mündermann, A., and Humble, N. (2003). Effect of shoe inserts on kinematics, center of pressure, and leg joint moments during running. *Medicine and Science in Sports and Exercise*, **35**, 314–19.

Noakes, H. and Payne, C. (2003). The reliability of the manual supination resistance test. *Journal of the American Podiatric Medical Association*, **93**, 185–9.

Novick, A. and Kelly, D. (1990). Position and movement changes of the foot with orthotic intervention during the loading response of gait. *Journal of Orthopaedic and Sports Physical Therapy*, **11**, 301–12.

Payne, C. (2008). Sagittal plane facilitation of the foot. Available online at: http://www.latrobe.edu.au/podiatry/sagittal.html (accessed 5 August 2008).

Payne, C., Munteanu, S., and Miller, K. (2003). Position of the subtalar joint axis and resistance of the rearfoot to supination. *Journal of the American Podiatric Medical Association*, **93**, 131–5.

Rodgers, M. and Leveau, B. (1982). Effectiveness of orthotic devices used to modify pronation in runners. *Journal of Orthopaedic and Sports Physical Therapy*, **4**, 86–90.

Root, M., Orien, W.P., and Weed, J.H. (1971). *Biomechanical Examination of the Foot*. Clinical Biomechanics, Los Angeles, CA.

Root, M., Orien, W.P., and Weed, J.H. (1977). *Normal and Abnormal Function of the Foot*. Clinical Biomechanics, Los Angeles, CA.

Scherer, P., Sanders, J., Eldredge, D.E., Duffy, S.J., and Lee, R.Y. (2006). Effect of functional foot orthoses on first metatarsophalangeal joint dorsiflexion in stance and gait. *Journal of the American Podiatric Medical Association*, **96**, 474–81.

Smith, L.S., Clarke, T.E., Hamill, C.L., and Santopietro, F. (1986). The effects of soft and semi-rigid orthoses upon rearfoot movement in running. *Journal of the American Podiatric Medical Association*, **76**, 227–32.

Stacoff, A., Reinschmidt, C., Nigg, B.M., *et al.* (2000). Effects of orthoses on skeletal motion during running. *Clinical Biomechanics*, **15**, 54–64.

2.8

Physiotherapy and rehabilitation

Lynn Booth

Introduction

In the broadest sense, there should be no difference in the way a physiotherapist treats a sprained ankle in an elderly patient, an active younger person, or an elite athlete—within reason the pathology and stages of healing remain the same. However proficient the physiotherapist, the process of inflammation and the stages of healing in an acute injury cannot be rushed. All the physiotherapist can do is provide the best environment for healing to occur.

However, it would be naive to suggest that there is no difference in treating injuries sustained during sport. One of the main differences between treating injuries which occur in sport, as opposed to those that occur in a more sedentary population, is the demand placed on the physiotherapist and other medical personnel by the athlete: 'When will I be fit?'; 'When can I start to train?'; 'Will I be ready by a specific date?'. Athletes frequently overestimate the seriousness of their injuries (Crossman and Jameson 1985). The ability to provide sound advice on all aspects of injury management without being swayed by any emotional considerations is particularly important for physiotherapists working within sport, especially if the physiotherapist is closely involved with the particular sport/team/athlete and appreciates the enormity, to either the individual or the team, of the injured athlete not being fully fit.

The role of physiotherapists in sport will depend on whether they work solely within a clinic environment or are involved at pitch/court/pool-side for training sessions and competition. Those physiotherapists involved at training/competition venues will see acute injuries as they occur and may be more involved with final stages of rehabilitation and with testing for fitness post-injury. Physiotherapists working within a sporting environment are more closely involved in providing an injury management service, which should include:

◆ profiling: musculoskeletal/movement analysis

◆ injury prevention

◆ injury assessment

◆ first aid/initial treatment

◆ treatment

◆ rehabilitation

◆ testing for fitness post-injury.

In the more elite sporting situation, the physiotherapist will have to work in an interdisciplinary environment, where collaboration between coaching, sports medicine, and sport science staff fosters an atmosphere designed not only to return athletes to full fitness as quickly as possible but also to assist in enhancing performance. In a multidisciplinary environment different disciplines may work alongside each other, but not necessarily in collaboration.

Profiling: musculoskeletal/movement analysis

Profiling has changed markedly over recent years. Unlike medical screening, it is not investigating for known pathological conditions; rather, it is trying to provide a picture of the athlete's physical make-up. The information gained is used to show an athlete's improvement, or otherwise. However, there are drawbacks: it is a 'snapshot' of the athlete's condition on that day and any comparison with previous or future tests should be viewed with caution—few musculoskeletal tests/examinations have been shown to have intertester, or even intratester, reliability.

Initially, profiling looked at more basic aspects such as joint, muscle, and neural mobility, basic core stability, and local muscle strength. This has now developed to a more functional approach, where the main bulk of the assessment is based on movement analysis. Inability of an athlete to perform an exercise effectively and efficiently leads the physiotherapist to undertake various other tests. The movements chosen progress from simple to more complex actions, and thus allow several areas of the body to be scrutinized at the same time. All the aspects tested should be relevant to the sporting actions to be performed. For example, a half-squat with a wooden pole raised above the head (Fig. 2.8.1) enables the assessors to view:

◆ foot posture

◆ spinal posture

◆ shoulder flexibility

◆ thoracoscapular stability and control

◆ lumbopelvic stability and control

◆ ankle dorsiflexion/calf flexibility

◆ quadriceps/gluteal dominance/control

◆ flexibility of latissimus dorsi.

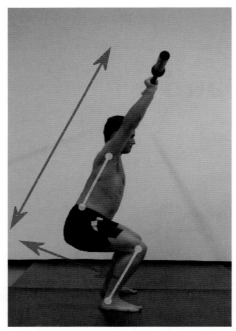

Fig. 2.8.1 Half-squat with wooden pole raised above the head. Photograph courtesy of England Golf.

Muscle imbalance between postural and phasic muscles will become evident during movement analysis. Reflex inhibition of shortened postural muscles will result in weakness of their phasic antagonists and synergists; the phasic muscle cannot be optimally strengthened because maximal activation and optimal training are prevented (Pieper and Schulte 1996).

In many sports the combined expertise of a physiotherapist and a strength and conditioning coach is used when undertaking movement analysis with an athlete. Their combined observational skills and anatomical and kinesiological knowledge are used to decide which aspects of the movement are the primary limiting factors and which are secondary compensations. For example, an athlete with poor gluteal control will try to become more quadriceps dominant by squatting with the knees further forwards over the toes, which may result in him/her appearing to have restricted ankle mobility or tight soleus if the heels rise during the squat. Factors outside the control of the athlete can combine to alter movement patterns; for example, a recent growth spurt in junior athletes may result in reduced muscle flexibility rather than a lack of commitment to an exercise programme.

Exercise programmes designed using the results from the profiling/movement analysis should have a two-pronged approach: they should not only improve performance but should also help to reduce the incidence of injury. Generally athletes, of any age, commit far better to an exercise programme that is designed to improve their sporting performance than one which is aimed at preventing injury.

Although there are some generic profiling and movement analysis tests that can be used for most sports, it is important to include assessments which make demands of the specific aspects of the sport, or even the position within a sport: a goalkeeper in football or field hockey will require different tests than an outfield player; in rugby, backs and forwards have different demands placed on

them during training and competition and will require different tests during the profiling/movement analysis.

Injury prevention

It would be unusual if, at some time in their sporting life, athletes did not sustain an injury which prevented them from training and playing. Obviously 'prevention is better than cure'. However, most athletes realise that they should have paid more attention to injury prevention after they have developed an injury! It is important that athletes are aware of the importance of injury prevention and that they take responsibility for this aspect of their training.

Sports physiotherapy should be a proactive service for athletes. Working at training and competition sites allows the physiotherapist to see the demands placed on the athlete and the opportunity for potential injury, which may be very different in training compared with competition. Some aspects of training may involve repetitive activities designed to hone a skill (technique) even though the sport itself is not repetitive in nature, giving a different type of injury in training to those usually sustained in competition. Clinic-based physiotherapists are usually more reactive to injuries/issues which appear in the clinic, and although advice and strategies to prevent recurrence will be provided, this is not as effective as preventing the initial problem from occurring.

Injuries can occur to anyone, but some athletes appear to be more at risk than others. This may be due to the demands of the sport, the type of training methods used, or undetected physical imbalances. Physiotherapists working within sport need to be vigilant; it is important not to 'switch off' during routine training sessions but to use the time to check for potential injuries (Table 2.8.1).

Proactive physiotherapy strategies should certainly reduce the incidence and severity of overuse injuries, but should also have an effect on the occurrence of acute injuries, particularly those that occur as a consequence of restricted mobility/strength/control in another area, for example acute hamstring strain due to restricted lumbopelvic mobility (Hoskins and Pollard 2005; Hunter and Speed 2007), or because of muscle imbalance between concentric quadriceps and eccentric hamstrings (Croisier *et al.* 2002).

Coaches and physiotherapists prescribe/teach/coach skill drills and exercises and modify techniques in an effort to prevent injury, a phase known as prehabilitation. However, many athletes view these exercises and drills as boring and often either ignore them or do not practise conscientiously. Discipline is required to continue with the proposed exercise regimes, and athletes should be encouraged to work at such (prehabilitation) regimes.

Injury assessment

Soft tissue injuries may involve muscle, ligament, tendon, capsular structures, and/or cartilaginous structures and can be categorized into three grades or degrees of severity of injury (Table 2.8.2).

Working in a clinic situation provides a clean and relatively unhurried environment in which to assess, diagnose and treat. Working 'pitch-side', even in relatively low-key competitions, places additional pressures on the physiotherapist: being observed by players, officials, and spectators; the pressure to make a decision quickly and allow the competition to continue; having to deflect 'helpful advice' from non-qualified onlookers; working in an unclean environment.

Table 2.8.1 Strategies in injury prevention

Possible problems	Comments
Physical imbalances	e.g. Muscle imbalance, adverse neural tension Should have been noted at musculoskeletal profiling/movement analysis
Inadequate preparation prior to training/competition	Exercises to improve mobility/flexibility should not be part of warm-up (see later)
Inadequate recovery after training/competition (cool-down)	Particularly if the next round of competition is in a short time
Unsuitable sports equipment and/or footwear for the task	New equipment/footwear, even though suitable, may also cause problems
Changes within the training/competition environment	e.g. Temperature, humidity
Recent growth spurts	Peak height velocity (Balyi and Hamilton 2003)
Unsuitable training and competition facilities	e.g. Playing surface
Poor technique	Even if currently effective and not causing any injury problems
Over-fatigued: local muscle and/or cardiovascular	This is always difficult: the principles of training involve overload. Coaches and physiotherapists must monitor fatigue levels, particularly if this leads to poor technique
Poor foot posture/biomechanics	See Chapter 1.8
Poor general posture	Including right- and left-sided symmetry; unusual postures required for a sport should not be maintained in the athlete's general posture
Poor sports-specific posture	
Asymmetrical mobility, endurance, and strength	Particularly in young athletes who are still developing
Unsuitable endurance/strength/power ratios in opposing groups of muscles	e.g. Concentric agonist:eccentric antagonist ratios
Inadequate rehabilitation from previous injury	Returning to training/competition too early
Compensatory movements	Avoid placing other areas of the body under stress
Unsuitable training drills	Appropriate for the athlete's age (developmental rather than chronological), body type, event
Changes in training methods	Changes need to be instigated progressively
Inadequate rest and recovery	Within the micro- and macro-training cycles (see Chapter 1.7)
Inappropriate opposition	More skilful or just heavier/bigger—a problem in age-related sports
Poor nutrition and hydration	During training and competition
Disregard for the rules of the sport	By the athlete, team mates, opponents

Table 2.8.2 Grading of soft tissue injuries

First degree (mild)	Second degree (moderate)	Third degree (severe)
The result of a mild stretch of ligament or capsular structures, or overstretch or direct blow to muscle	The result of moderate stretch of ligament or capsular structures, or excessive stretch or direct blow to muscle, causing tearing of some fibres	The result of a severe overstretch of ligament, or excessive stretch or direct blow to muscle, causing a complete tear of the injured structure.
Minimal swelling and bruising	Moderate swelling and bruising	Significant swelling and bruising
Mild pain is felt at the end of range of movement or on stretch or contraction of muscle.	Moderate pain felt on any movement that interferes with the ability of the muscle to contract or lengthen	Severe pain even at rest which significantly interferes with function
No joint instability	May be some joint instability with ligament/capsular injuries	Ligament injuries result in gross instability and significant decrease in tensile strength
Minimal muscle spasm	Moderate muscle spasm may result as a reflex response to ligamentous capsular injuries and muscle injuries	Muscle injuries cause severe muscle spasm and 'splinting', and the injured muscle is incapable of exerting force
No loss of function	Because of tearing of some fibres, there is a decrease in the tensile strength of ligament/capsule or a decrease in the contractile strength of muscle, both of which interfere with function	Function is severely impaired

'Pitch-side' assessment of acute injury

For physiotherapists working at the competition venue, the rules regarding when they may enter the field of play and how long they are permitted to assess and treat an injured player vary considerably. In rugby, play may continue whilst the physiotherapist treats a player on the pitch, whilst in field hockey the umpire must stop the game before calling the physiotherapist on.

When the physiotherapist has only a short period of time to make a quick (basic) diagnosis, it is important to follow a set assessment plan to ensure that nothing is missed and that the injury is not exacerbated. The following, taken from the Football Association's Intermediate Treatment and Management of Injuries course provides such a format (www.thefa.com/FALearning).

- ◆ See   the injury happen
- ◆ Ask   for the history
- ◆ Look   signs of inflammation, deformity, etc.
- ◆ Touch   tenderness, numbness, pins and needles
- ◆ Active   patient's own muscular control
- ◆ Passive   range of motion, joint stability, ligaments
- ◆ Strength   (resisted) functional control

Each subsequent stage of the assessment is only continued if the previous section does not raise *any* concerns regarding the underlying pathology or severity of injury. In particular, if an athlete is unable to undertake active movements due to pain, he/she cannot continue to train/compete and passive movements are not required to be tested in the pitch-side situation. Further assessment can take place away from the training/competition area.

As the 'first-contact' person in the sporting situation, it is vital that the physiotherapist is able to cope with the wide variety of injuries which may occur, from grade I soft tissue injuries → fractures → complete joint disruptions → life-threatening incidents. In order to be effective, the physiotherapist must closely observe the event. In some sports this does not mean 'keeping up with play', but rather being slightly behind play. For example, in rugby it is more important to ensure that all the players are injury free following a scrum or maul than it is to watch the ball. The physiotherapist is given some indication of the severity of the injury by observing the injury occur and how the athlete reacts. The second stage of the protocol ('Ask') immediately provides information regarding the ABC of ATLS (Acute Trauma Life Support). Head and spinal injuries are covered elsewhere (Chapters 3.2, 3.4, and 3.7). However, the physiotherapist may be the only person at the venue with medical knowledge and as such must be capable of taking charge of any situation that might occur. Sanchez *et al.* (2005) highlight the need for rapid on-field diagnosis and early stabilization of spinal injuries, and include basic principles to guide the rescuer through the process, including knowledge of the AVPU and/or Glasgow Coma Scales (McNarry and Goldhill 2004).

The importance of the physiotherapist in the 'first-contact' situation cannot be underestimated. An efficient and effective assessment and, whenever possible, a precise diagnosis is vital in order to institute appropriate advice/guidance and treatment regimes. Without a high-quality approach, the athlete's recovery may be delayed and at worst he/she may never fully return to pre-injury levels. In some sports, such as field hockey, rolling substitutions allow a player to leave the field of play and have a more detailed assessment before a decision is made regarding returning to play or not. In sports that do not allow this to occur (e.g. football), the physiotherapist must always err on the side of caution and if in any doubt remove the athlete from the field of play—the most important thing is to protect the player from further, possibly career-threatening, injury.

Whether the athlete continues with the competition or not, there will eventually be time for a more rational assessment. An early examination means that structures can be assessed before joint effusion, soft tissue swelling, or local muscle spasm have time to confuse the assessment.

Subsequent assessment of acute injury in a clinical environment

Assessments of acute soft tissue injuries in the less rarefied atmosphere of a clinical environment follow a basic protocol (Table 2.8.3). The assessment should gather as much information as possible whilst minimizing any further damage to the tissues. The history should be as detailed as possible. For example, a tennis player presents with an effused knee after falling on court. The history suggests that she may have rotated the knee slightly on falling, but the effusion appears more severe than you would have expected. On closer questioning, she recalls resting for several minutes and then resuming the game. Could continuing with the game, rather than the original injury, have a bearing on the amount of joint effusion?

Not all the tests listed in Table 2.8.3 will be performed, either because they are irrelevant to the injured structure or because they would only inflict further pain and injury when a diagnosis has already been arrived at.

The protocol in Table 2.8.3 should be sufficient to fully assess an acute injury, although as treatment and rehabilitation continue it will be important to note any underlying reasons for the acute injury. For example, a high hurdler with acute hamstring strain may have poor eccentric hamstring strength, especially in outer range, which may be a factor underlying the acute injury. Alternatively, there may be an underlying neural component.

Assessment of overuse/chronic injuries

Although similar principles are applied in the subjective and objective assessment of overuse or more chronic injuries, the nature of these injuries tends to mean that the assessment can be more searching with less risk of aggravating the injury. The subjective assessment must refer to the topics in Table 2.8.1 to find any causative factors linked to the injury. This may take time, but is always worthwhile. Most medical practitioners can treat injuries—rest nearly always helps to reduce the pain. However, if the underlying factors are not resolved, the problem will return. The value of a physiotherapist working within sport is the facility to return the injured tissues to their optimum condition and to prevent recurrence.

In some assessments, particularly those of acute injuries, it is too easy to go for the obvious option when providing a diagnosis. An assessment is only completed when the following questions have been fully answered:

- ◆ What other structures could be injured?
- ◆ Have all relevant tests been undertaken to confirm or deny their involvement?

Table 2.8.3 Subjective and objective assessment in acute injuries, using the example of an acute grade II hamstring strain in a footballer assessed within 2–3 hours of the injury

Subjective	
What was happening at the time	Running to chase a ball
The precise position of the injured tissues	Leg fully extended
The actions of team-mates/opposition (if relevant)	Not relevant
An accurate summary of immediate and subsequent treatment – both professional and self-administered	Had to come off pitch. Ice applied pitch-side.
Objective signs	
Posture and quality of movement generally and in more localized tissue	Walking on toes to keep hamstring muscles in a shortened position. Trying to keep weight off affected leg
Pain—When? Where? Intensity? Is it a limitation to movement?	Pain—occurred immediately in posterior of thigh
Deformity; effusion (local or general)	No
Skin colour, temperature, and appearance	Skin—warmer than opposite leg. Would not expect to see bruising within the first few hours
Active RoM: joint and muscle	Pain on active knee flexion and/or hip extension – did not continue with the assessment
Passive RoM: at a joint, this is only tested if active RoM is painfree. If passive joint RoM is painfree, apply overpressure. For a muscle, passive RoM refers to placing the muscle on stretch	Tested with care—placing the muscle on stretch by flexing the hip whilst the knee is extended
Nature of the limitation of movement—reluctance, pain, spasm, tissue tension, tissue compression, muscle weakness	Movement limited by reluctance due to pain
Joint stability	Not relevant
Palpation of injured structures	Pain at musculotendinous junction, medial hamstrings
Muscle strength (isometric, concentric, eccentric)	Not tested—has pain on active concentric movement
Neural tension tests	Not tested
Specific tests, including combined movements	Not required
Functional movements	No heel strike or toe push-off during gait; unequal stride length.

RoM, range of movement.

It is better to avoid giving a definite diagnosis until further tests can be undertaken than to commit to a diagnosis that is not fully proven.

First aid/initial treatment

The importance of accurate diagnosis and appropriate treatment cannot be overestimated. The course of an injury can be significantly affected by appropriate, effective, and timely action. The basis of all first-contact treatment is an understanding of the pathology of inflammation and healing. The physiological mechanisms involved in the first 72 hours post-injury direct the immediate management of injury (Evans 1980; Dyson 1987; Watson 2006).

In 1998, the Association of Chartered Physiotherapists in Sports Medicine (ACPSM) in the UK produced clinical guidelines on the PRICE regime (protection, rest, ice, compression, elevation) for the early management of soft tissue injuries. ACPSM guidelines showed that the modes of application of the individual elements of PRICE did not conform to the traditional 'gold standard' of a randomized control trial and that much of the literature tended to make assumptions about the duration and frequency of application of the elements of PRICE, with authors rarely justifying their selection. The ACPSM guidelines were based on biological bases, consensus and empirical proof. Using more recent research the guidelines were updated in autumn 2010 under the title "Management of Acute Soft Tissue Injury using Protection, Rest, Ice, Compression and Elevation: Recommendations from the Association of Chartered Physiotherapists in Sports and Exercise Medicine" (www.acpsm.org)

For a grade I or II soft tissue injury, it is important to follow the PRICE regime for at least the first 72 hours—the need to keep reassessing the injury during this time has the potential to place more strain on damaged tissues. Treatment modifications in this initial stage should be due to a change in the more obvious signs (e.g. reduced effusion, increased active spontaneous movement) rather than due to a full reassessment of the injury. Grade III soft tissue injuries frequently involve other sports medicine professionals, although using the PRICE regime until these consultations can be made will always stand the athlete in good stead.

Treatment

Physiotherapists working in a sporting environment have several treatment options, ranging from electrotherapy to more manual techniques such as massage and soft tissue therapy, spinal and peripheral joint mobilization, and, when necessary, manipulation and taping.

Table 2.8.4 Subjective and objective assessment in overuse injuries, using the example of a recurring ankle inversion injury of a netballer

Subjective	
When did the first and last incidents occur? How many times has the injury occurred	First incident 6 months ago; latest incident 2 weeks ago 4–5 incidents in between
How did the last injury occur?	During sudden change of direction on court
Is it always the same mechanism of injury?	No, sometimes due to landing badly
The precise position of the injured tissues	Describes inverted and plantarflexed ankle
The actions of team-mates/opposition	Not relevant—never been due to contact
An accurate summary of any treatment—both professional and self-administered	Ice after every episode; has probably resumed playing before regaining full fitness
Objective signs	
Posture and quality of movement generally and in more localized tissue	Protecting ankle and whole lower limb during all movements
Pain—When? Where? Intensity? Is it a limitation to movement?	Sharp pain immediately after each injury; between injuries has nagging pain during any activity
Deformity, swelling (local or general)	Swelling around lateral malleolus, peroneal sheath, and lateral side of forefoot
Skin colour, temperature, and appearance	Some bruising over peroneal sheath and around metatarsal heads; lateral aspect of foot and ankle warm
Active RoM—joint and muscle	Limited ankle mobility, especially dorsiflexion, plantarflexion, and inversion; tight peronei
Passive RoM—tested with care if active RoM is painful. If passive joint RoM is pain free, apply overpressure	Pain on inversion and plantarflexion; restricted movement in subtalar and midtarsal joints
The nature of the limitation of movement—reluctance, pain, spasm, tissue tension, tissue compression, muscle weakness	Movement limited by pain, tissue tension, and athlete apprehension.
Joint stability	Slight laxity into plantarflexion/inversion
Palpation of injured structures	Pain over anterior talofibular ligament and peroneal sheath
Muscle strength (isometric, concentric, eccentric)	General muscle weakness in lower leg and foot; peronei particularly weak, especially in outer range
Neural tension tests	Some neural tension, which may be an underlying cause or be the result of repeated incidents
Specific tests, including combined movements	Check proximal structures, i.e. lumbopelvic control
Functional movements	Gait—poor toe push-off; unequal stride length. Pain on walking over uneven surfaces.

RoM, range of movement.

Electrotherapy

Electrotherapy introduces physical energy into a biological system to produce physiological change(s) for therapeutic benefit. The effects of treatment depend on the modality used (e.g. ultrasound, interferential) and the dose provided. Low-power/energy modalities can enhance the natural ability of the body to stimulate, direct, and control the healing and reparative processes. Recently, the energy levels applied in electrotherapy modalities such as laser, pulsed short wave and ultrasound have been reduced. The low-energy applications aim to stimulate the cells into some higher-activity level and thus use the natural resources of the body to do the work (Watson 2008).

Watson (2007) discusses 'windows of opportunity' where the 'amount' of a treatment is a critical parameter: the same modality applied in the same circumstances but at a different 'dose' produces a different outcome. Watson (2008) provides evidence of an 'amplitude' or 'strength' window: an energy delivered at a particular amplitude has a beneficial effect, whilst the same energy at a lower amplitude may have no demonstrable effect. 'Frequency' windows

are also apparent: a modality applied at a specific frequency (pulsing regime) might have a measurable benefit, whilst the same modality applied using a different pulsing profile does not achieve similar results. Watson (2008) suggests that there is also an energy- or time-based window and another window based on treatment frequency (number of sessions a week or treatment intervals).

The skill of the physiotherapist is to make the appropriate clinical decision regarding the most effective modality, the precise anatomical area, and the correct amplitude and frequency to provide maximum benefit to the athlete.

Massage and soft tissue therapies

Massage and soft tissue therapies, including myofascial release and trigger points, allow the physiotherapist to palpate both normal and abnormal tissues precisely and to use the information to direct further treatment. Manual techniques allow the physiotherapist to be more aware of tissue tension and more able to identify the tissues involved and the type of restriction on movement as well as providing a psychological effect from touch. Not only can massage and soft tissue therapies affect the healing tissues directly, they can also affect the tissues indirectly by influencing fascial, vascular, and neural structures.

The techniques used and the depth to which they are used will depend on the stage of healing of the injured tissues. In the proliferation stage of healing (3–10 days in a grade II injury) it may be more beneficial to massage tissues proximal to the point of injury to assist with pain modification and to reduce oedema by increasing tissue fluid flow, redistributing arterial flow, and increasing lymphatic drainage. Soft tissue techniques can be used in conjunction with elevation, cold therapy, and/or commercial compression garments such as Cryocuff™ or Game Ready™. As with all treatment modalities there are contraindications to be aware of when using soft tissue techniques. Probably the two most common faults are using too deep a technique, particularly over sensitive tissues (e.g. in the early stages of healing or over peripheral nerves). Any sign of infection, common in athletes who frequently walk barefoot in less than clean environments, should also be a cause for concern, as increasing the circulation could exacerbate the problem.

Spinal and peripheral joint mobilizations

Spinal and peripheral joint mobilizations have evolved from passive physiological and accessory techniques applied by the physiotherapist to the concepts of mobilization with movement (MWM) in the extremities and sustained natural apophyseal glides (SNAGS) in the spine with the simultaneous application of physiotherapist-applied accessory and patient-generated active physiological movements. The physiotherapist can often instruct the athlete in self-treatment MWM principles with the athlete providing the glide component of the MWM and their own efforts to produce the active movement (Mulligan 1995).

Taping

Taping, or strapping, can have several different purposes:

- to keep orthopaedic felt and dressings in place
- to provide compression–to assist in reducing bleeding and swelling
- to limit excessive/unwanted movement
- to reduce stress—to allow healing to occur
- to protect from further injury—providing support to ligaments and tendons
- to support injured structure(s) in a functional position during rehabilitation
- to aid proprioceptive feedback
- prophylactically—to enhance confidence
- to prevent injury on return to activity—restricting joint and muscle mobility within safe limits; however, it should not be used to provide support for an athlete who is not fully fit.

Taping should not be used without first fully assessing the injury in order to answer the following questions.

- Which structures are damaged?
- Which tissues need protection and support?

- Do any movements need to be restricted
- Is complete immobilization necessary at this stage?

The large variety of tape available (adhesive, cohesive, stretch, non-stretch) enables the physiotherapist to be adaptable when applying techniques that are suitable for the injured tissues and the purpose. Taping is no substitute for treatment/rehabilitation and should not be used if:

- the injury is not fully assessed or the diagnosis is uncertain, unless it is as a first aid measure before assessment
- the joint is unstable
- there is serious injury
- the area is extremely swollen, irritable, and painful
- there is infection
- there is poor skin sensation and/or circulatory changes—particular care must be taken when treating athletes with a disability.

Taping should be functional and should always achieve its objective whilst avoiding excessive traction on the skin, too many layers of tape, excessive pressure/tension, altered sensation distal to the taping, and skin soreness or skin breakdown with prolonged application. Physiotherapists need to be aware of the effect of exercise on tape fixation and of the rules of competition, which vary from sport to sport and may change from year to year. For example, taping of the knees is prohibited in weightlifting, although knee supports can be used; in gymnastic competitions light brown tape must be used rather than white.

Rehabilitation

Exercise therapy is an important modality for physiotherapists working in sport and has a role to play in many aspects of injury management, injury prevention, and performance enhancement. The following two quotes from Fitzgerald (1997) should inform the planning of any rehabilitation exercise programme.

> The 'best' exercises are those that maximise patients' ability to achieve their goals while minimizing their risk of further injury.
>
> (Fitzgerald 1997, p.1753)

> Should our decision-making schemes be based on how well an exercise simulates the movement and muscle activity characteristics of the target functional activity, or should our strategy be based on how well an exercise can overcome a physical impairment that is believed to be contributing to the functional deficit?
>
> (Fitzgerald 1997, p.1754)

For exercise therapy to have value within the injury management process the physiotherapist needs to be able to progress the exercise safely, making a demand of specific muscles without compromising the healing process or increasing the potential for injury. Once the decision has been made to progress an exercise, it is important to do this in a structured, and preferably quantifiable, way. Table 2.8.5 highlights some considerations when developing a progressive exercise programme, but it is certainly not a definitive list.

The principle components of physical fitness are:

- flexibility
- endurance
- strength

◆ speed/power

◆ skill—balance, control.

Table 2.8.5 Considerations when developing an exercise programme

Levers	Magnitude of the load
Gravity	Joint motion
Buoyancy	Plane of movement
Direction of the force	Muscle action
Fixed/moving boundaries	Motor control
Starting position	Resistance

The relative contribution of each component will depend on the sport. There is not a set time period for the recovery of each component following an injury. When developing an exercise programme each component should be catered for, with the emphasis depending on the stage of healing.

Flexibility

Flexibility exercises should consider joint, muscle, and neural flexibility. Improving one of these aspects to the detriment of the others will ultimately have an untoward effect on functional rehabilitation; increasing joint mobility may be ineffective if the relevant muscles cannot move and work functionally through the new range. Ideally, mobility regimes should reflect sport specificity, encourage left–right symmetry, and use sporting patterns of movement.

Age, gender, somatotype, and existing joint mobility will have an effect on maintaining or improving flexibility. Body types differ and athletes need to concentrate on maintaining or improving mobility levels rather than trying to compete with their peers. Flexibility regimes for young performers take on more significance following growth spurts (also know as peak height velocity (PHV)) (Balyi and Hamilton 2003).

When developing exercises to improve flexibility, it is important to be aware of the risks associated with:

◆ using poor techniques

◆ allowing non-essential structures to become hypermobile

◆ having inadequate strength and control in the new range of movement.

It is important to distinguish between congenital and acquired hypermobility, particular in young performers where flexibility, and even hypermobility, would be deemed an asset in certain sports. The Beighton score and its modifications can be used to score hypermobility in children (Kerr *et al.* 2000).

Hunter (1998) has shown how different sections of a muscle can be placed under more or less stress during flexibility regimes by varying the sequencing of soft tissue mobilization; for example, the fixed point of the muscle can be either the proximal or distal attachment, and using proprioceptive neuromuscular facilitation (PNF) patterns can make demands on muscle flexibility in more than one plane of movement, most importantly by adding a rotatory component.

Endurance

Endurance can refer to local muscle groups or to the body's aerobic system. Rehabilitation programmes must provide suitable cardiovascular exercise for the aerobic demands of the sport. The more general exercises that are used to alleviate boredom during prolonged rehabilitation or to provide rest periods for recuperating injured structures need to use, and make demands of, the energy system(s) required for that particular sport. This requires cooperation between physiotherapists, exercise physiologists, and strength and conditioning coaches to ensure that athletes returning from injury do not spend longer than necessary regaining suitable general and/or local fitness.

During immobilization, type I muscle fibres tend to atrophy more than type II fibres (Paessler and Shelbourne 1995). As athletes progress through a rehabilitation programme, they often regain strength and power (type II muscle fibres) before the muscles concerned with stabilization and control (type I muscle fibres) are fully recovered. It is important that rehabilitation should not be progressed too quickly. An athlete may be capable of throwing a 2 g medicine ball over a distance of 5 m, but poor endurance in the stabilizing muscles will place the non-muscular restrainers of the glenohumeral joint under stress.

Strength

The stimuli for increased muscle strength and hypertrophy involve high force contraction, which cannot be found in most everyday activities.

Before including more functional training, a progressive strength exercise programme needs to address:

◆ correct muscle action with no compensation

◆ sequencing of muscles

◆ non-weighted controlled movement

◆ gradual build-up of skill

◆ range.

Strength training principles involve progressive overload, variability, and specificity, which include combinations of intensity, volume, and frequency of training (Glasgow 2007). The best results come from following a recognized strengthening programme rather than using a light weight for an unsubstantiated set of repetitions, as this rarely results in high force contraction. An understanding of the different forms of resistance training enables physiotherapists to communicate effectively with athletes and strength and conditioning coaches in order to provide successful rehabilitation programmes which not only assist in the rehabilitation of the injured athlete but also maintain or improve the relevant energy systems and muscle type used in the particular sport.

It may depend on the injured tissues, but the easiest strengthening exercises are usually isometric contractions in mid-range. These can be progressed by maintaining isometric contractions in differing parts of the range or by starting eccentric exercises in the inner to mid range. Initially, these may have to be assisted by external support or support from the opposite limb to help the athlete to resume a starting position prior to repeating the eccentric exercise. This type of exercise uses the principles of negative system resistance training (assisted concentric followed by eccentric work) used by strength and conditioning coaches.

Fowler (2008) suggests that the common practice of classifying movements as either 'open' or 'closed' kinetic chains is inappropriate and distracts from the real differences between exercises (Table 2.8.7).

Table 2.8.6 Advantages and disadvantages of strengthening equipment

Free weights/resistance cord	Machines
Require more balance and coordination	Most only allow movement in one plane
Tend to recruit group action of muscle	More controlled environment
Light weights will help to isolate individual muscles	Can measure and isolate individual muscle groups
Allow movement in more than one plane	Have the potential to cause muscle imbalance
Promote joint stability	Can increase the protective participation of healthy limbs/muscle groups

The ability to absorb force requires eccentric muscle work, and is probably more important in regaining function than the ability to produce force. Eccentric exercises allow higher forces to be attained in the muscle, have the lowest energy consumption, and produce greater tension than concentric or isometric exercises. The maximum tension in eccentric muscle contraction is 20–30% higher than in concentric contraction, although eccentric exercises are the most fatiguing. After exercise-induced damage, known as delayed onset muscle soreness (DOMS), the affected muscle fibres degenerate and regenerate, with the new fibres having greater potential for growth. Physiotherapists need to take the effect of DOMS into account when designing rehabilitation programmes, ensuring enough time between exercises, sets, and repetitions, and between rehabilitation sessions, to allow muscles to recover. It is in the rest periods that recovery and super-compensation occur in the tissues.

Eccentric strengthening has become an essential tool in the prevention and rehabilitation of certain tendon pathologies. The strength of tendon is related to its thickness and collagen content, rather than the maximum tension its muscle can exert. The tensile strength in healthy tendon is usually greater than twice the strength of the muscle. Fyfe and Stanish (1992) described a regime of eccentric exercises to prevent and treat tendon injuries. The regime was based on length, load, and speed:

* increasing the length of the muscle tendon unit, thus reducing the strain with joint movement

* increasing the load, resulting in increased tensile strength

* increasing the speed of contraction, thus increasing the force.

Table 2.8.7 Differences between open and closed kinetic chain exercises

Open kinetic chain exercises	Closed kinetic chain exercises
Low resistance forces	Large resistance
Large acceleration	Low acceleration
Distraction and rotatory forces	Greater compressive forces
Promotion of a stable base	Joint congruency
Joint mechanoreceptor deformation	Decreased shear
Concentric acceleration	Stimulation of proprioceptors
Eccentric deceleration	Enhanced dynamic stabilization

Alfredson *et al.* (1998) described a typical eccentric exercise programme for recreational runners with a long duration of Achilles tendinosis which had not responded to rest, non-steroidal anti-inflammatory drugs, changes of shoes or orthoses, physical therapy, and ordinary training programmes. It consisted of loading the calf muscle eccentrically, with the non-injured leg being used concentrically to return to the start position. The patients continued with the exercise even if they experienced pain, but were told to stop if the pain became disabling. When they could perform the eccentric loading exercise without experiencing any minor pain or discomfort, the load was increased by adding weight. After 12 weeks of eccentric calf muscle training, all subjects were back to their pre-injury levels with full running activity.

Alfredson *et al.* (1998) discussed two possible explanations for the positive effects of eccentric training on tendinosis: an effect of stretching, with 'lengthening' of the muscle–tendon unit and consequently less strain during ankle joint motion, or an effect of loading within the musculotendinous unit, with hypertrophy and increased tensile strength in the tendon. Eccentric loading appeared to help with remodelling the tendon, but, unlike Fyfe and Stanish (1992), the authors did not think that this was velocity specific.

Isokinetic machines are set at a particular velocity and designed to encourage voluntary muscle contraction throughout a full range of movement at a preset velocity. Although they are used within rehabilitation settings, it is difficult to design functional and sports specific exercises, particularly as peak torque decreases as speed increases. They are probably more useful when supplying quantitative measurements in order to provide diagnostic evidence or to assess and re-assess progress.

Power/speed

Plyometric ('stretch-shortening') exercises can be used to develop power. They are quick powerful movements which involve pre-stretching of the muscle, the use of the stretch reflex, and the storage of elastic energy, and are based on the principle that activated muscle stores more elastic energy than relaxed muscle. Plyometric exercises rely on the rate of stretch rather than the length of stretch. It is important to keep the exercise sessions short to avoid DOMS, which may develop following a plyometric exercise session.

Muscle reaction times and the time needed to generate peak muscle torque are important components of a rehabilitation programme. Agility training has a beneficial effect on muscle reaction time (Wojtys *et al.* 1996) and is particularly important in sports that require jumping and pivoting. Power exercises require adequate muscle strength, or other compensatory structures will be placed under stress and may 'break down'.

Skill/coordination/technique

Skill/coordination/technique should be an integral part of every stage of a rehabilitation programme—failure to correct an athlete's partial-weight-bearing gait whilst on crutches, and thus allow unequal stride length, may lead to uneven stride length once he/she starts jogging/running/sprinting. Often the athlete has to relearn skills with altered mechanoreceptor information.

Perturbation training uses systems of overload, as applied to all other rehabilitation, to encourage adaptation. As skill acquisition is progressed, the rehabilitation process must include multitasking decisions in order to stimulate reflex and pre-programmed muscle control. Activities should progress from conscious to unconscious motor skills. Initially the athlete should be made aware of what will happen in terms of the amount of force required and the direction of any applied force. As the rehabilitation progresses, the athlete is left unaware of any changes which may take place, i.e. differing force, differing position/direction of force. For example, perturbation training occurs when a netball player has to catch a ball outside her base of support, causing her to be off balance. However, the player is also making demands of motor control systems as she considers the ball (and possibly an opponent) rather than consciously thinking about her balance.

Neuromuscular control can also be progressed by changing commands to move from an internal ('Keep your knee over your foot') to an external ('Keep your eyes level with a fixed point') focus of attention when performing a task.

Glasgow (2007) advises that motor control training should be advanced from neutral positions in the early stages of rehabilitation to increasingly challenging movements performed in less stable positions, and that exercises are performed which simultaneously stimulate sensorimotor function and motor control stability.

Functional rehabilitation

The final stages of rehabilitation should be a progression: using the skills of the sport initially in a controlled fashion and eventually in a manner that reflects the demands that will be placed on the

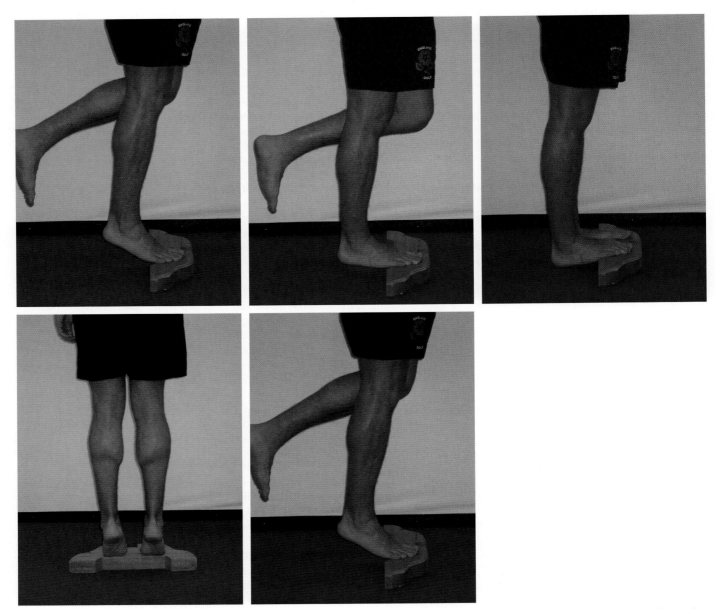

Fig. 2.8.2 A series of photographs showing the progression of eccentric exercises for Achilles tendinosis. The single leg lowers eccentrically and then both calves work concentrically to return to the starting position.

athlete on return to sport. This may be better achieved by using varied practice rather than repetitive practice of one particular element.

The components of fitness are not mutually exclusive: if joint mobility is improved, the muscles which act over that joint, particularly those which pass over more than one joint (e.g. hamstrings, rectus femoris, gastrocnemius, biceps brachii) must also improve their flexibility; if a muscle's flexibility improves it must be strengthened within the new range in order to prevent injury and improve performance.

Functional exercises are developed depending on the demands of the sport—repetitive, explosive, multidirectional, acceleration/deceleration. Just as relevant energy systems need to be stimulated, as rehabilitation progresses the exercises should encourage the type of muscle activation required for the sport.

Functional rehabilitation requires the introduction of specific exercises into a scheme of training to provide controlled stress to the healing tissues. When designing a rehabilitation programme it is important to decide which of the components of fitness you are hoping to target and what is required for the particular sport/event/position, i.e. joint/muscle range, strength type (isometric→ isotonic eccentric → isotonic concentric), power. During all stages of rehabilitation there should be a progressive overload system—neither the exercise frequency nor the force used should be increased too quickly.

Phillips and van Deursen (2008) suggest that functional performance may be associated more with how quickly balance is achieved than with the amount of sway or excursion during quiet standing. In their study, ACL-deficient subjects allowed themselves less freedom of movement, and failed landing and stopping activities rather than trying to recover their balance beyond a threshold point. They suggest that the ACL-deficient subjects demonstrated 'novice' rather than 'expert' motor learning strategies, and that this may account for injured athletes who perform adequately in clinical performance-orientated functional tests but re-injure on return to sports which require temporal and spatial control of deceleration.

Table 2.8.8 lists points which should be considered when commencing or developing running or throwing drills.

Rehabilitation is an ongoing procedure that involves detecting improvement and objectively measuring progress and which ultimately progresses into testing for fitness.

Rehabilitation—return to sport

A physiotherapist's ability to observe and analyse functional (and dysfunctional) movement is put to good effect in the sporting environment, particularly if he/she is in attendance at training and competition. Movements which may be successfully completed within a clinical environment, when the athlete has time to concentrate without any outside distractions (ball, opposition, crowd), may be poorly executed in the sporting arena. It is good use of the physiotherapist's time to observe the demands placed on the athlete, and on particular tissues.

Static and dynamic posture, muscle imbalance, and core and peripheral control (probably a better description than the term 'core stability') can be evaluated and relevant exercise programmes instigated to improve efficiency and economy of movement in sporting techniques. In unilateral sports (e.g. some racket sports) or sports which make different demands on opposite sides of the body (e.g. golf), it is important that the execution of the technique does not start to cause postural changes, for example an elevated left shoulder in right-handed golfers. Gait analysis and the provision of orthotics has been covered elsewhere (Chapters 1.9 and 2.7). However, the physiotherapist is often in a position to observe how an athlete's running gait differs during the execution of his sport compared with that seen when walking in a clinic or running on a treadmill, and hence can provide valuable information to those involved in gait and biomechanical assessment.

To be accomplished within sport requires coordination, proprioception, balance, and muscle control, as well as the accomplishment of technical sporting ability. Control is acquired in sport as a specific skill and it is important that tissues can 'dampen' vibration. Athletes need elasticity, not just stability, and it is important to assess the relative values of mobility and stability. Core control, especially of the lumbopelvic and scapulothoracic areas, must be assessed dynamically and within positions used by athletes for the execution of their sport. It is futile to repeatedly treat a hip adductor strain if the field hockey player does not have adequate control to maintain the correct position of the thigh during a reverse stick shot, when weight is placed on a lunging front leg. Any exercise programmes to correct or enhance core control must take into account the positions and demands placed on athletes during their sport. Observing the demands placed on athletes in their sporting environment allows the physiotherapist to design suitable clinic- and training-based exercises which will provoke the correct response in the appropriate tissues.

Testing for fitness post-injury

Testing for fitness following injury involves making decisions regarding an athlete's participation in a specific game/competition/tour. It should be part of a seamless process if the personnel involved in the testing for fitness have also been involved in the athlete's rehabilitation.

Testing for fitness is a responsible undertaking rather than a 'go and try it' attitude. It should contain objective as well as subjective assessments, and the short- and long-term effects of an athlete undertaking, and subsequently failing, a fitness test should be considered. The activities/sporting actions undertaken in the fitness test and the ensuing decision regarding the athlete's fitness demand mutual trust and respect from all parties concerned, including the athlete, the coach, sport science and medical staff, and, where appropriate, parents.

The components of a fitness test will differ depending on the sport, the athlete's discipline or position within that sport, and the

Table 2.8.8 Points to consider when commencing running or throwing drills

Running drills	Throwing drills
Distance	Distance
Speed	Weight
Stride length	Speed
Incline	Direction
Direction	Type: chest pass/over arm
Rhythm/timing/cadence	Rhythm/timing/cadence

structures being tested, but it is designed to assess the athlete's functional fitness—the ability to complete the physical, technical, and tactical requirements of the sport. The final assessment must be undertaken in the athlete's training or competitive arena. Many acute injuries occur within the last quarter of competition, as athletes become mentally and physically fatigued (Hawkins and Fuller 1999). Fitness tests should include the volume and intensity of work that the athlete has to perform to mimic full training and competition. It is not enough to know that the athlete can cope with 2 minutes of competition if training sessions usually last for 60 minutes.

From a physiotherapy point of view testing for fitness procedures must demonstrate that the injured structure is fully healed and strong enough to withstand more than the demands of the sport. In other words, the tissues have a 'buffer zone' to withstand some element of 'rough tactics'. The test must also show that the athlete has regained his/her aerobic and anaerobic fitness and previous skill levels.

The fitness test should be progressed gradually to avoid unnecessary strain on the repaired tissues or on the athlete generally. Any fitness test that results in the recovering injury being aggravated or further injury occurring has been badly structured. Fitness test procedures are much easier if the physiotherapist involved with the athlete's rehabilitation is also involved with the fitness test. Familiarity with the athlete must not be allowed to cloud the physiotherapist's judgement—awareness of the importance of a successful test to either the athlete or the team must not influence the final decision.

A testing for fitness procedure for an outfield footballer recovering from a strain of the medial collateral ligament (MCL) of the right knee involves analysing the demands of the sport, and the following should be included within the actual test: aerobic and anaerobic energy systems; multidirectional running; quick changes of running pace; acceleration/deceleration in all directions; sudden changes of direction when jogging → sprinting; kicking and trapping a ball; jumping and landing on one or both feet; tackling and being tackled; resisting a 'blocked tackle'; slide tackles (giving and receiving); falling to the ground, with or without close opposition; regaining upright position after falling; balance and control standing on either leg; unexpected contact (ball or opponent) from any direction.

For a footballer, a test procedure needs to last at least 45 minutes (half a game) and should include steady state and interval speed running as well as more specific testing of the injured structures. The tests must be progressed in a structured and controlled manner. For example, the following progressions could be made for the skill of changing direction.

- Jogging forwards in a straight line. Changing to jogging backwards under the player's own volition.

- Jogging forwards in a straight line. Changing to jogging backwards at another's command.

- Gradually increase stride length and/or speed.

- Jogging left and right, remembering that there is potentially more strain on certain tissues depending on the direction moved (e.g. the MCL of the right knee when side-stepping to the left).

- Jogging: change direction (backwards, left, right) under the player's own volition.

- Jogging: change direction (backwards, left, right) at another's command.

- Ensure that the player changes direction by pushing off from either foot rather than the uninjured left one.

- Gradually increase stride length and/or speed.

- Increase the speed of movement during the change of direction, rather than allowing the player to slow down on the change.

- Repeat using a football—use the right leg either to kick the ball or to support the body (when the left foot is kicking).

- Repeat with a football and opposition, changing direction on another's command.

- Shadow/mirror another player who is running and quickly changing direction.

- Add jumping/landing/tackling to any of the previous drills.

If the person organizing the test has not previously seen the player, the steps may have to be as gradual as mentioned above. If the physiotherapist has been involved in the player's rehabilitation, the earlier drills will have been included and the testing for fitness procedures may only require the final two or three stages.

Several sports/squads have developed protocols for determining an athlete's fitness to compete, which include deciding on a follow-up course of action if the test is not completed successfully. The protocols have been designed to provide a robust testing procedure, which will stand up to any potential challenge to the result, and cover the following points:

- Who should lead—coach/medical staff?

- Who should be involved?

- What is being forecast? The athlete's ability to travel, compete today/tomorrow, compete through a scheme of qualifying events/heats/pool groups/finals. How long is the rest period between rounds?

- All those involved must agree on the information which will be made available post-test, to whom the information will be made available, and how the information will be circulated.

- Who decides on the athlete's readiness for testing?

- Does the athlete have the right to insist on a fitness to compete test, even if the medical staff do not think the athlete is ready? The athlete must be informed of the expected content and the potential risks in undertaking an early test.

- When will the test take place? There must be enough time between assessing the athlete's post-test reaction and selection deadlines.

- If the test is successfully completed, is further discussion required regarding the athlete's physical and sports-specific fitness and the risk of re-injury or secondary injury?

- If the test is not successfully completed, is further discussion required regarding further rehabilitation or a possible retest? Is this an unexpected result?

- How are the test, subsequent discussions, and conclusions recorded?

- Who makes the final decision? What if others do not agree with the final decision? Does it matter who the dissenter is—athlete/coach/medical staff?

◆ Disseminating information. Is this only with the athlete's permission? Who informs other relevant personnel, e.g. other athletes, staff, media, national governing body (if this is an elite athlete prior to a major competition)? Does the order in which people are informed matter?

◆ What are the consequences of a failed test—for the athlete, for the staff?

However, it should be remembered that there may be potential problems if the protocols are 'set in stone'.

Warm-up

One of the extended roles of the sports physiotherapist may be to oversee the warm-up prior to training or competition. It is probably more important for the physiotherapist to instruct the athletes about the benefit of good warm-up, and to practise an efficient and effective warm-up with them during training sessions, rather than actually take the warm-up prior to competition, when he/she may have other more pressing demands, e.g. an athlete requiring additional taping.

During the warm-up, athletes should only move joints and muscles through a range they are already capable of achieving. Attempting to improve mobility during the warm-up often results in stiff and sore muscles. Static stretches, when a muscle is positioned at the end of its available range and held for a sustained period of time (recommendations range from 5 to 60 seconds (Roberts and Wilson 1999)) prior to activities where strength and/or power are required (e.g. prior to weight training) are not recommended. Static stretching immediately prior to activity has been shown to reduce vaulting speed in gymnasts (Siatras *et al.* 2003), to have a negative influence on explosive force and jumping performance (Young and Behm 2003), and to impair balance, reaction time, and movement (Behm *et al.* 2004). Stretch-induced impairments have been reported to occur as early as 1 minute post-stretching (Behm *et al.* 2004) and to continue for 120 minutes (Power *et al.* 2004). Conversely, other studies (Larsen *et al.* 2005; Ghaffarinejad et al. 2007) have shown no change or improved joint position sense.

Behm *et al.* (2006) investigated whether the stretch-induced impairments reported in the literature were a training-specific phenomenon. Athletes with a high level of flexibility or tolerance to stretch might be better able to withstand the stress of an acute bout of stretching, or perhaps a musculotendinous unit with greater range, or greater tolerance to stretch, might accommodate the stresses associated with an acute bout of stretching more successfully. Their results showed that an individual's initial level of joint range of movement did not correlate with the stretch-induced deficits and that 4 weeks of flexibility training did not reduce the

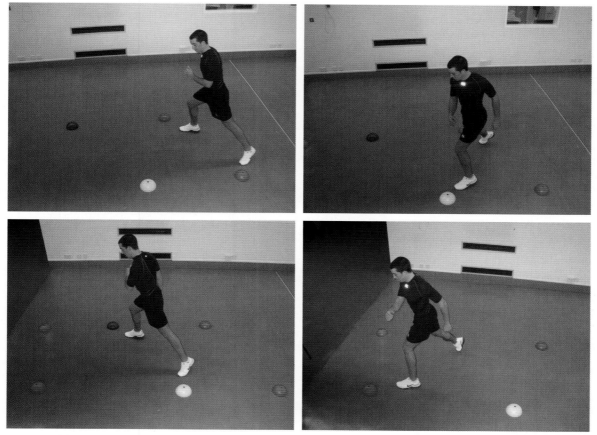

Fig. 2.8.3 Basic running drills to encourage a player to push off either foot.

stretch-induced impairments. They proposed that if individuals hold stretches to the point of personal discomfort, the relative stress will be similar in flexible or inflexible muscles.

Certain elements of the warm-up will be relevant to almost every athlete, but it should also include sport/discipline/position-specific elements. The warm-up routine should follow a set pattern, or at least use routines with which the athlete is fully familiar, enabling the athlete to focus on the event. The time to experiment with new warm-up routines is during training.

Many sports use **dynamic warm-up** in preparation for training/competition. Dynamic warm-up tends to follow a similar pattern and should use the sport's patterns of movement.

◆ Easy aerobic work, e.g. walking, striding, bounding, skipping, and jogging, all performed at low intensity.

◆ As the warm-up session progresses, the exercises move to a higher intensity.

◆ Non-sport-specific full-range ('normal') movement of relevant muscles and joints, e.g. arm circling, leg swinging, rotating the whole body whilst standing—without moving beyond normal range.

◆ Exercises that ensure that all relevant joints and muscles are taken through the largest range of movement that will be required during the sport.

◆ Sport-specific drills at high intensity—skill rehearsal.

There is a difference between exercises used in a dynamic warm-up, when muscles and joints work within their current range, and ballistic stretching exercises (Booth 2006). It is important to stress that athletes using dynamic warm-up still require flexibility work in their general conditioning programmes.

The timing of the warm-up is important. There is no benefit in increasing cardiovascular output, enhancing blood flow to joints and muscles, making demands of neuromuscular pathways, and mentally preparing if the athlete then has to wait before commencing training or competition.

Cool-down/recovery strategies

Good recovery strategies are essential for all athletes. For training adaptations to occur, supercompensation needs to take place in the musculoskeletal and circulatory systems. For this to occur effectively, the body needs the opportunity to recover. In many cases the physiotherapist will be responsible for educating the athletes in cool-down/recovery strategies:

◆ light aerobic exercise post training/competition

◆ long-duration static stretches for all major muscle groups

◆ advice on suitable rehydration and refuelling

◆ the use of contrast techniques (hot/cold showers) or cryotherapy (ice baths, cold whirlpool)

◆ next-day recovery sessions (light cross-training, pool recovery work)

◆ recovery massage.

Psychology and physiotherapists

Apart from the coach, the physiotherapist often has the most regular contact with athletes, especially, but not exclusively, those with injuries. Physiotherapists are often viewed by athletes as being in no-man's land—in the management team but not involved in selection or team tactics. This means that treatment rooms are often seen as safe havens for athletes to discuss any issues, either between themselves or with the physiotherapist. Often the physiotherapist and other medical staff can be privy to confidential/controversial statements about an athlete's fears regarding an injury or issues involving other athletes and/or staff. Physiotherapists and other medical staff can become involved in discussing psychological issues, particularly if there is no sports psychologist attached to the sport (Kolt 2003).

Treating the same athletes, often with similar injuries, over a long period of time means that the physiotherapist has to ensure that athletes are not prejudged. It is not unknown for athletes to use injuries as an excuse to avoid training or as a fallback if a competition does not go as well as they would have hoped. The sports physiotherapist has to tread a fine line between pandering to the athlete's every whim, rather than making them more independent, and missing a real injury problem. Prior to a major competition, would the physiotherapist be justified in treating an imagined injury if it helped to reassure the athlete before the event or does this just compound the problem of making the athlete too dependent?

Whilst respecting athlete confidentiality (British Olympic Association 2000; Macauley and Bartlett 2000), an interdisciplinary approach within the sport allows the physiotherapist to discuss relevant issues with a sports psychologist: how to identify potential (psychological) issues; how a physiotherapist can suggest to athletes that they may benefit from speaking to a sports psychologist; athletes using injury/illness to cope with the demands of training/competing; training and competing whilst denying any injury issues.

References

Alfredson, H., Pietilä, T., Jonsson, P., and Lorentzon, R. (1998). Heavy-load eccentric calf muscle training for the treatment of chronic achilles tendinosis. *American Journal of Sports Medicine*, **26**, 360–6.

Balyi, I. and Hamilton, A. (2003). Long-term athlete development update. *Sports Coach UK*, **20**, 6–8.

Behm, D.G., Bambury, A., Cahill, F., and Power, K. (2004). Effect of acute static stretching on force, balance, reaction time, and movement time. *Medicine and Science in Sports and Exercise*, **36**, 1397–1402.

Behm, D.G., Bradbury, E.E., Haynes, A.T., Hodder, J.N., Leonard, A.M., and Paddock, N.R. (2006). Flexibility is not related to stretch-induced deficits in force or power. *Journal of Sports Science and Medicine*, **5**, 33–42.

Booth, L. (2006). Mobility, stretching and warm-up: application in sport and exercise. *In Touch*, **118**, 12–16.

British Olympic Association (2000). Position statement of athlete confidentiality. *British Journal of Sports Medicine*, **34**, 71–2.

Croisier, J.-L., Forthomme, B., Namurois, M.-H., Vanderthommen, M., and Crielaard, J.-M. (2002). Hamstring muscle strain recurrence and strength performance disorders. *American Journal of Sports Medicine*, **30**, 199–203.

Crossman, J. and Jameson, J. (1985). Differences in perceptions of seriousness and disrupting effects of athletic injury as viewed by athletes and their trainer. *Perceptual and Motor Skills*, **61**, 1131–4.

Dyson, M. (1987). Mechanisms involved in therapeutic ultrasound. *Physiotherapy*, **73**, 116–20.

Evans, P. (1980). The healing process at cellular level: a review. *Physiotherapy*, **66**, 256–9.

Fitzgerald, G.K. (1997). Open and closed kinetic chain exercise: issues in rehabilitation after anterior cruciate ligament reconstructive surgery. *Physical Therapy*, **77**, 1747–54.

Fowler, N. (2008). When chains just don't link up. *sportEX Medicine*, **25**, 18–20.

Fyfe, I. and Stanish, W.D. (1992). The use of eccentric training and stretching in the treatment and prevention of tendon injuries. *Clinics in Sports Medicine*, **11**, 601–24.

Ghaffarinejad, F., Taghizadeh, S., and Mohammadi, F. (2007). Effect of static stretching of muscles surrounding the knee on knee joint position sense. *British Journal of Sports Medicine*, **41**, 684–7.

Glasgow, P. (2007). Sports rehabilitation—principles and practice. *sportEX Medicine*, **32**, 10–16.

Hawkins, R.D. and Fuller, C.W. (1999). A prospective epidemiological study of injuries in four English professional football clubs. *British Journal of Sports Medicine*, **33**, 196–203.

Hoskins, W. and Pollard, H. (2005). The management of hamstring injury. Part 1: Issues in diagnosis. *Manual Therapy*, **10**, 96–107.

Hunter, D.G. and Speed, C.A. (2007). The assessment and management of chronic hamstring/posterior thigh pain. *Best Practice and Research Clinical Rheumatology*, **21**, 261–77.

Hunter, G. (1998). Specific soft tissue mobilisation in the management of soft tissue dysfunction. *Manual Therapy*, **3**, 2–11.

Kerr, A., Macmillan, C.E., Uttley, W.S., and Luqmani, R.A. (2000). Physiotherapy for children with hypermobility syndrome. *Physiotherapy*, **86**, 313–17.

Kolt, G.S. (2003). Psychology of injury and rehabilitation. In: G.S. Kolt and L. Snyder-Mackler (eds), *Physical Therapies in Sport and Exercise*, pp. 165–83. London, Churchill Livingstone.

Larsen, R., Lund, H, Christensen, R., Røgind, H., Danneskiold-Samsøe, B. and Bliddal, H. (2005). Effect of static **stretching** of quadriceps and hamstring muscles on knee joint position sense. *British Journal of Sports Medicine*, **39**, 43–6.

Macauley, D. and Bartlett, R. (2000). Editorial on the British Olympic Association's position statement of athlete confidentiality. *British Journal of Sports Medicine*, **34**, 1–2.

McNarry, A.F. and Goldhill, D.R. (2004). Simple bedside assessment of level of consciousness: comparison of two simple assessment scales with the Glasgow Coma Scale. *Anaesthesia*, **59**, 34–7.

Mulligan, B.R. (1995). *Manual Therapy: 'NAGS', 'SNAGS', 'MWMS' etc.* (5th edn). Plane View Press, Wellington.

Paessler, HH and Shelbourne KD: (1995). Biological, biomechanical and clinical approaches to the follow-up treatment of ligament surgery in the knee. *Sports Exercise and Injury*, **1**, 83–95.

Phillips, N. and van Deursen, R.W. (2008). Landing stability in anterior cruciate ligament deficient versus healthy individuals: a motor control approach. *Physical Therapy in Sport*, **9**, 193–201.

Pieper, H.-G. and Schulte, A. (1996). Muscular imbalances in elite swimmers and their relation to typical sports lesions. *Sports Exercise and Injury*, **2**, 96–9.

Power, K., Behm, D., Cahill, F., Carroll, M., and Young, W. (2004). An acute bout of static stretching: effects on force and jumping performance. *Medicine and Science in Sports and Exercise*, **36**, 1389–96.

Roberts, J.M. and Wilson, K. (1999). Effect of stretching duration on active and passive range of motion in the lower extremity. *British Journal of Sports Medicine*, **33**, 259–63.

Sanchez, A.R., Sugalski, M.T., and LaPrade, R.F. (2005). Field-side and prehospital management of the spine-injured athlete. *Current Sports Medicine Reports*, **4**, 50–5.

Siatras, T., Papadopoulos, G., Mameletzi, D., Gerodimos, V., and Kellis, S. (2003). Static and dynamic acute stretching effect on gymnasts' speed in vaulting. *Pediatric Exercise Science*, **15**, 383–91.

Watson, T. (2006). Tissue repair: the current state of the art. *sportEX Medicine*, **28**, 8–12.

Watson, T. (2007). Modality and dose dependency in electrotherapy. Presented at: 15th International WCPT Congress, Vancouver.

Watson, T. (2008). Current concepts in electrotherapy. Available online at: www.electrotherapy.org

Wojtys, E.M., Huston, L.J., Taylor, P.D., and Bastian, S.D. (1996). Neuromuscular adaptations in isokinetic, isotonic, and agility training programmes. *American Journal of Sports Medicine*, **24**, 187–92.

Young, W.B. and Behm, D.G. (2003). Effects of running, static stretching and practice jumps on explosive force production and jumping performance. *Journal of Sports Medicine and Physical Fitness*, **43**, 21–7.

Surgical issues in sports medicine

Craig Finlayson and Mark Hutchinson

Introduction

Surgical management of the athlete refers not just to the performance of a surgical procedure, but rather to the global perioperative period as a whole. The approach to the surgical patient requires a multidisciplinary team with interaction between the injured athlete, the surgeon, trainers, therapists, coaches, and other physicians in order to achieve an optimal outcome for the patient (Fu *et al.* 2007). Some of the key steps along the pathway are preoperative evaluation, surgical decision-making, surgery, postoperative care, and rehabilitation.

Diagnosis

The importance of making an accurate diagnosis prior to surgery cannot be overemphasized. A well-focused history and physical examination are often enough to diagnose most sports injuries. Appropriate imaging should be obtained to confirm the diagnosis, rule out associated injuries, and facilitate preoperative planning (Ryzewicz *et al.* 2007; Rayan *et al.* 2008). Although surgery is sometimes performed for the purpose of diagnosis, such as diagnostic arthroscopy, the surgeon must make a solid diagnosis or, at the minimum, a focused differential diagnosis prior to undertaking surgery.

Communication and surgical decision-making

Once the diagnosis has been made, it should be communicated to the patient and to any family members, trainers or coaches deemed appropriate in the context of the specific patient–physician relationship. The amount of information disseminated will vary depending on the nature of the relationship between the physician, the patient, and the patient's team or employer. Many collegiate or professional programmes will have a strictly defined communication system which should be respected by the physician (Konin 2007). Many athletes have an awareness of their own body and will expect specific details on the nature of their injury. At the very least, the patient should grasp the functional implications of the injury regarding return to sport and risk of further injury, if not the specific patho-anatomy (Bunch and Dvonch 2004). For example, an injury to the anterior cruciate ligament (ACL) may cause further episodes of instability, thereby increasing the risk of subsequent injury (Fithian *et al.* 2002). After an understanding of the injury has been reached, the discussion should turn to the goals of the patient. For example, is the patient an elite athlete who needs to return to sport as quickly as possible, or is the patient willing to modify his/her sports participation in order to avoid surgery? An elite athlete may opt for surgical fixation of a fifth metatarsal fracture in order to return to sport more quickly than with standard immobilization and protected weight-bearing (Mologne *et al.* 2005), whereas a recreational athlete with ACL deficiency may wish to avoid surgery by eschewing basketball in favour of less rigorous sports (Fithian *et al.* 2002). The type of surgery performed may also influence return to sport and therefore create a conflict of interest for the team physician in terms of the short-term aims of the team and the athlete to return to sport expeditiously versus the long-term health of the patient. For example, debridement of a meniscal tear may allow rapid return to sport but expose the player to risk of accelerated degenerative changes, whereas a meniscal repair will reduce long-term risk of arthritis but exclude the player from competition for an extended period (Dunn *et al.* 2007).

The various treatment options and their relative risks and benefits should be discussed (Bunch and Dvonch 2004). The surgeon should address the implications of both surgical and non-surgical treatment (casting versus surgical repair of the Achilles tendon) as well as distinguishing between various surgical methods (the use of allograft versus autogenous tissues in ACL reconstruction) (Dunn *et al.* 2007). Indications for surgery may be interpreted in a relatively broad or narrow fashion, and it is critical for the patient and physician to determine whether surgical treatment has a high likelihood of achieving the individual goals of the patient with an acceptable level of risk.

In addition to the expected outcome of surgery, the patient should be apprised of any postoperative restrictions or ancillary therapy that will be required. For example, will the patient be required to wear a cast or brace, will weight-bearing or range of motion be restricted, or will a lengthy course of physical therapy be required? Well-executed surgery can be undone by non-compliance, and the treatment plan may need to be modified based on the patient's ability or willingness to comply with certain restrictions (Fisher 1990). Finally, a realistic time-frame for return to competitive sport should also be discussed, but no guarantees should be offered as to if and when preoperative function will be obtained (Bunch and Dvonch 2004).

Specific surgical considerations

In addition to determining whether surgery is indicated, the timing and type of surgery are also critical factors in successful outcomes. Timing may be a matter of simple convenience such as an off-season or school vacation. In many cases, however, the patient will desire surgery as soon as possible in order to return to sport more quickly or to provide a personal sense of closure. Either unnecessary haste or delay may adversely affect surgical results. In the case of acute injury, trauma and swelling of the soft tissue envelope may impair wound healing and predispose to infection. Surgery should be delayed until wrinkles are visible in the skin, and judgement should be exercised when operating in the vicinity of fracture blisters (Tull and Borelli 2003). Surgery may also be delayed when the acute inflammatory phase of an injury causes joint stiffness. This is most commonly discussed in the setting of ACL reconstruction, in which case some authors recommend delaying surgery until a satisfactory range of motion has been achieved (Shelbourne *et al.* 1991). However, delaying surgery by more than 3 months may lead to a higher incidence of meniscal tears (Papastergiou *et al.* 2007).

For a number of biological, technical, and patient-driven factors, increasing attention has been directed to arthroscopic and minimally invasive surgeries (Sperling *et al.* 2007). As arthroscopic technology and experience have improved, outcomes have become equivalent or superior to open methods for many procedures, such as rotator cuff repair (Sauerbrey *et al.* 2005). The decision for arthroscopic or open surgery should be based on surgeon comfort level and training, ability to address pathology adequately through the chosen approach, and patient preference (Gartsman 1998). The possibility that conversion to open surgery may be required based on intra-operative findings or complications should also be discussed.

Many commonly performed sports procedures require reconstruction of injured tissues with transferred or transplanted tissue. The surgeon should discuss the various options with the patient so that he/she can make an informed decision. Autograft tissues carry the risk of donor site morbidity, while allograft tissues bring a risk of disease transmission. Again, the decision will be made based on the preferences of the surgeon and patient, as well as the ability to procure adequate tissue from either the patient or a donor (Bunch and Dvonch 2004).

Preoperative evaluation

Most patients being evaluated for surgery in a sports medicine clinic are relatively young and healthy. Therefore extensive preoperative medical evaluation is not usually required. A focused history and physical examination should be performed to identify patients whot may be at higher risk due to occult cardiac or pulmonary disease, immunocompromise (HIV, immunosuppressive medications), infectious foci (urinary tract, dental), malnutrition, obesity, or other factors. Local factors specific to the surgical site, including dermatitis, psoriasis, arterial/venous insufficiency, lymphoedema, scar, or history of local infection, should also be investigated. Enquiry should be made into current medications (including over-the-counter medicines and supplements), previous surgeries, and any history of prolonged bleeding or drug reactions (DeLee and Drez 2003, Agyros 2005, Lau and Eagle 2008). A validated preoperative screening questionnaire is given in Table 2.9.1.

Table 2.9.1 Suggested preoperative screening questionnaire

1	Have you ever had a heart attack?
2	Have you ever had heart trouble?
3	Have you ever had heart failure?
4	Have you ever had fluid in your lungs?
5	Do you have a heart murmur?
6	Did you have rheumatic fever as a child?
7	Do you ever have chest pain, angina, or chest tightness?
8	Have you ever been treated for an irregular heartbeat?
9	Do you have high blood pressure?
10	Do you ever have difficulty with your breathing?
11	Do you have asthma, bronchitis, or emphysema?
12	Do you cough frequently?
13	Does climbing one flight of stairs make you short of breath?
14	Does walking one city block make you short of breath?
15	Do you now or have you recently smoked cigarettes? If yes, how many packs per day? For how many years?
16	Do you have liver disease, or a history of jaundice or hepatitis?
17	Do you drink more than three drinks of alcohol per day? If yes, how many per week?
18	Do you have indigestion, heartburn, or a hiatus hernia?
19	Do you have a history of thyroid problems?
20	Do you have diabetes?
21	Do you have a kidney problem?
22	Do you have numbness or weakness of your arms or legs?
23	Do you have epilepsy, blackouts, or seizures?
24	Have you had problems with blood clots, or excessive bleeding?
25	Do you have any other important medical problems? Please list.
26	Have you ever had an anaesthetic? If yes, when was your last one?
27	Have you or any member of your family had a reaction to an anaesthetic?
28	Do you have arthritis or pain in your neck or jaw?
29	Do you have dentures, capped or loose teeth?
30	Do you think you may be pregnant?
31	Have you taken **prednisone**, steroid medications, or **cortisone**-like drugs in the past year?
32	Please list any food or medication allergies that you have
33	Please list any medications you are currently taking
34	Please list any operations you have had in the past
35	If this is the day of your surgery, when did you last eat or drink?
36	Age: Weight: Height:

Reproduced from Badner, N.H., Craen, R.A., Paul, T.L., and Doyle, J.A. (1998). Anaesthesia preadmission assessment: a new approach through use of a screening questionnaire. *Canadian Journal of Anaesthesia*, **45**, 87–92.

Because of the low pretest probability of significant medical problems in this population, abnormal laboratory results are often false-positives that lead to unnecessary additional tests and add little to risk estimation. Therefore laboratory tests should be ordered only when indicated based on clinical examination. In healthy patients, laboratory tests can be reliable for up to 4 months provided that there have been no interval medical events (Lau and Eagle 2008). Policies on preoperative laboratory testing vary among institutions, and physicians should be acquainted with these unique policies. Indications for common laboratory tests are given in Table 2.9.2.

Preoperative medications

Medications can have an adverse effect on bleeding and other surgical parameters. However, the potential risks of continuing medications should be weighed against their medical benefits during the perioperative period. In general, cardiac, pulmonary, and psychiatric medications should be continued, including on the day of surgery. Drugs that affect coagulation status should be discontinued for elective surgery if possible. Because of their interference with platelet function, aspirin and clopidogrel should be discontinued a week prior to surgery if possible. NSAIDs may be discontinued a week prior to elective surgery, although no significant increase in blood loss has been shown with their use preoperatively.

Table 2.9.2 Indications for common laboratory tests

Test	Indications
Haemoglobin	Anticipated major blood loss, symptoms of anaemia
White blood cell count	Symptoms suggestive of infection or myeloproliferative disorder, myelotoxic medications
Platelet count	History of bleeding diathesis, myeloproliferative disorder, myelotoxic medications
Prothrombin time	History of bleeding diathesis, chronic liver disease, malnutrition, recent or long-term antibiotic use
Partial thromboplastin time	History of bleeding diathesis
Electrolytes	Known renal insufficiency, congestive heart failure, medications that affect electrolytes
Renal function	Age >50 years, hypertension, cardiac disease, major surgery, medications that affect kidney function
Glucose	Obesity, known diabetes
Liver function tests	No indication; consider albumin for major surgery or chronic illness
Urinalysis	Known diabetes, symptoms of urinary tract infection
Urine pregnancy test	Females of childbearing age
Electrocardiogram	Men >40 years, women >50 years, known coronary artery disease, diabetes, or hypertension
Chest radiograph	Age >50 years, known cardiac or pulmonary disease, symptoms or examination suggesting cardiac or pulmonary disease

Sources: Guss and Bhattacharyya 2006; Lau and Eagle 2008.

Herbal supplements have various potential risks, including bleeding, potentiation, or inhibition of anaesthetic agents, myocardial ischaemia, and cardiac arrhythmia. In general, herbal supplements should be discontinued one week prior to surgery. Patients with adrenal suppression secondary to steroid use should have perioperative corticosteroid treatment. As a rough estimate, a prednisone dose of 5 mg daily long term, 10 mg daily for 1 month, or 20 mg daily for 1 week may cause adrenal suppression. Methotrexate may be continued perioperatively, but newer anti-rheumatoid drugs such as etanercept and infiximab have not been researched specifically and should be withheld (Agyros 2005). Tight blood glucose control has been associated with decreased infection rates in diabetic patients (Olsen *et al.* 2008). Half the usual outpatient dose of insulin should be given on the morning of surgery together with a sliding scale or infusion until the time of surgery. Oral hypoglycaemic agents should be withheld on the day of surgery, and the home drug regimen can be reinstituted when the patient is tolerating a diet. Because of the potential risk of lactic acidosis, some authors recommend withholding metformin for up to a week prior to surgery as well as postoperatively. Perioperative β-blockade is recommended for high-risk patients with a history of ischaemic heart disease, stroke, diabetes, and hypercholesterolaemia (Agyros 2005).

Day of surgery

On the day of surgery, the patient should be met by the surgeon in the preoperative holding area. The surgical site and procedure should be confirmed by the patient, and the surgical site should be marked in indelible ink by the surgeon as specifically as possible (JCAHO 2003). Any last-minute concerns can be addressed at this time, and relevant contingencies should be discussed. For example, a partial meniscectomy versus a meniscal repair may be performed depending upon intraoperative findings, which will in turn impact on postoperative management. The surgeon may remind the patient about what to expect in the immediate postoperative period, such as casts, braces, swelling, or numbness from regional anaesthesia. The patient may also designate a family member, friend, or member of the athletic team with whom the surgeon should speak following the procedure. Plans for postoperative follow-up should be confirmed. Postoperative restrictions (weight-bearing, range of motion), pain management strategies (ice, elevation, NSAIDs, narcotics), home rehabilitation (pendulum exercises, quadriceps sets, continuous passive motion machines), and dressing changes (removal of postoperative dressing or indwelling catheters) should be discussed and the relevant prescriptions provided to the patient. All the above instructions should also be provided in written form.

Once in the operating room, the patient's identity, surgical site, and procedure are confirmed during a 'time-out'. The availability of necessary imaging, implants, or graft tissue should be confirmed. Appropriate antibiotic prophylaxis should be administered prior to inflation of the tourniquet and skin incision (Porucznik 2004). Cefazolin or cefuroxime are preferred for most orthopaedic procedures. Clindamycin or vancomycin may be administered to patients with a history of reaction to β-lactams. Antibiotics may also be tailored to other site- or patient-specific factors, such as a history of methicillin-resistant *Staphylococcus aureus* infection (Agyros 2005). Following surgery, the surgeon should speak with the patient's designated representative and explain the relevant surgical findings and any deviations from the expected plan.

Anaesthesia

Advances in regional anaesthesia have decreased the use of general anaesthesia and endotracheal intubation in extremity surgery. Even when general anaesthesia is administered, supplementary regional anaesthesia can decrease postoperative pain and potentially allow more rapid rehabilitation (Bonnet and Marret 2005; De Ruyter et al. 2006). Although regional anaesthesia is mainly the domain of the anaesthesiologist, the orthopaedic surgeon should be aware of the options and potentially act as advocate for them on behalf of the patient. As with all procedures, there are time requirements and risks of complication with regional anaesthesia, and the ultimate choice of anaesthesia will be a team decision based on the preferences of the patient, anaesthesiologist, and surgeon. Other options available to the surgeon include implantable catheters for continuous administration of local anaesthetic into the surgical field, injection of long-lasting local anaesthetic into the field at the time of wound closure, and thermal dressings that cool the surgical area.

Follow-up and continuity of care

The ability of the patient to be followed up within an appropriate time frame should be established and an appointment scheduled prior to surgery. In the case of transitory patients, such as student-athletes, arrangements for proper postoperative care should be discussed prior to surgery. At the first postoperative visit operative findings and specifics should be discussed with the patient. Postoperative restrictions are again clarified and formal therapy instituted if necessary. Communication and an integrated treatment plan involving the surgeon, patient, and therapists become crucial at this point in order to maximize patient outcome and return to sport.

Complications

Complications can and do occur in sports-related surgery. In the worst case, complications may cause irreversible damage to the patient and even death. Minor complications may prevent an athlete from returning to his/her sport. In addition to the risks associated with anaesthesia, all surgery carries the risk of infection and damage to surrounding osseous and soft tissue structures, including blood vessels, nerves, ligaments, tendon, muscle, cartilage, and skin. Scarring and stiffness from soft tissue damage are important complications of both the initial insult of an injury and surgical treatment. In collision athletes, minor stiffness may be an acceptable trade-off for stability of the shoulder, but a relatively small loss of motion may prevent an elite throwing athlete from returning to sport (Ide et al. 2004).

Venous thromboembolism is a potentially devastating complication, and two points of Virchow's triad may be exacerbated with surgical treatment: endothelial damage and venous stasis. The surgeon should educate the patient regarding prevention and recognition of complications, especially infection and venous thromboembolism, which may be threatening to both life and limb. Pharmacological thromboprophylaxis remains controversial, but is not usually recommended after routine sports procedures. Thromboprophylaxis may be indicated in high-risk patients (history of deep vein thrombosis/hypercoagulable state, polytrauma with expected immobility) or high-risk procedures (knee/hip arthroplasty), but should be weighed against potential complications (Warwick et al. 2008). No benefit has been shown for continuation of postoperative antibiotic prophylaxis beyond 24 hours in complicated procedures (Agyros 2005). At follow-up the surgeon should examine the surgical wound for signs of infection, both lower extremities for signs of deep vein thrombosis, and the extremity distal to the surgical site for signs of neurovascular injury.

Prevention of complications is always the best strategy, but they do occur in the hands of even the most skilled surgeons. Therefore the surgeon must be aware of potential complications and exercise prudent surgical technique and judgement in order to avoid them. Complications should be recognized and addressed as soon as possible with appropriate treatment and communication with the patient.

Postoperative therapy

General therapy protocols for most operative procedures can be established; however, the surgeon may need to modify therapy in accordance with case-specific factors such as associated fractures/ligament damage, bony comminution, nerve injury, and poor fixation of implants or grafts. Postoperative rehabilitation represents a balance between maximizing gains in range of motion and strength and protecting surgically repaired tissue during the healing process. The surgeon must be specific and firm regarding restrictions, but also involve the patient and therapists in a collaborative rehabilitation process (Cascio et al. 2004).

References

Agyros, G. (2005). Perioperative medical management. In: A. Vaccaro (ed.), *Orthopaedic Knowledge Update* (8th edn), pp. 137–42. American Academy of Orthopaedic Surgeons, Rosemont, IL.

Bonnet, F. and Marret, E. (2005). Influence of anaesthetic and analgesic techniques on outcome after surgery. *British Journal of Anaesthesiology*, **95**, 52–8.

Bunch, W.H. and Dvonch, V.M. (2004). Informed consent in sports medicine. *Clinics in Sports Medicine*, **23**, 183–93.

Cascio, B.M., Culp, L., and Cosgarea, A.J. (2004). Return to play after anterior cruciate ligament reconstruction. *Clinics in Sports Medicine*, **23**, 395–408, ix.

DeLee, J. and Drez, D. (2003). Risk assessment. In: *Orthopaedic Sports Medicine: Principles and Practice* (2nd edn), Chapter 7. W.B. Saunders, Philadelphia, PA.

De Ruyter, M.L., Brueilly, K.E., Harrison, B.A., Greengrass, R.A., Putzke, J.D., and Brodersen, M.P. (2006). A pilot study on continuous femoral perineural catheter for analgesia after total knee arthroplasty: the effect on physical rehabilitation and outcomes. *Journal of Arthroplasty*, **21**, 1111–17.

Dunn, W.R., George, M.S., Churchill, L., and Spindler, K.P. (2007). Ethics in sports medicine. *American Journal of Sports Medicine*, **35**, 840–4.

Fisher, A.C. (1990). Adherence to sports injury rehabilitation programmes. *Sports Medicine*, **9**, 151–8.

Fithian, D.C., Paxton, L.W., and Goltz, D.H. (2002). Fate of the anterior cruciate ligament-injured knee. *Orthopedic Clinics of North America*, **33**, 621–36.

Fu, F.H., Tjoumakaris, F.P., and Buoncristiani, A. (2007). Building a sports medicine team. *Clinics in Sports Medicine*, **26**, 173–9.

Gartsman, G.M. (1998). Arthroscopic management of rotator cuff disease. *Journal of the American Academy of Orthopaedic Surgery*, **6**, 259–66.

Guss, D. and Bhattacharyya, T. (2006). Perioperative management of the obese orthopaedic patient. *Journal of the American Academy of Orthopaedic Surgery*, **14**, 425–32.

Ide, J., Maeda, S., and Takagi, K. (2004). Arthroscopic Bankart repair using suture anchors in athletes: patient selection and postoperative sports activity. *American Journal of Sports Medicine*, **32**, 1899–1905.

JCAHO (Joint Commission on the Accreditation of Healthcare Organizations) (2003). *Universal Protocol for Preventing Wrong Site, Wrong Procedure, Wrong Person Surgery*. Joint Commission, Oak Brook, IL. Available online at: http://www.jcaho.org/accredited+org

Konin, J.G. (2007). Communication: the key to the game. *Clinics in Sports Medicine*, **26**, 137–48.

Lau, W.C. and Eagle, K.A. (2008). Medical evaluation of the surgical patient. In: A.S. Fauci, E. Braunwald, D.L. Kasper, *et al.* (eds), *Harrison's Principles of Internal Medicine* (17th edn), pp. 49–52. McGraw-Hill, New York.

Mologne, T.S., Lundeen, J.M., Clapper, M.F., and O'Brien, T.J. (2005). Early screw fixation versus casting in the treatment of acute Jones fractures. *American Journal of Sports Medicine*, **33**, 970–5.

Olsen, M.A., Nepple, J.J., Riew, K.D., *et al.* (2008). Risk factors for surgical site infection following orthopaedic spinal operations. *Journal of Bone and Joint Surgery. American Volume*, **90**, 62–9.

Papastergiou, S.G., Koukoulias, N.E., Mikalef, P., Ziogas, E., and Voulgaropoulos, H. (2007). Meniscal tears in the ACL-deficient knee: correlation between meniscal tears and the timing of ACL reconstruction. *Knee Surgery, Sports Traumatology, Arthroscopy*, **15**, 1438–44.

Porucznik, M.A. (2004). Patient safety tip contest winners announced. *AAOS Bulletin*, **52**, 37. Available online at: http://www.aaos.org/wordhtml/bulletin/apr04/acdnws2.htm.

Rayan, F., Bhonsle, S., and Shukla, D.D. (2008). Clinical, MRI, and arthroscopic correlation in meniscal and anterior cruciate ligament injuries. *International Orthopaedics*, **33**, 129–32.

Ryzewicz, M., Peterson, B., Siparsky, P.N., and Bartz, R.L. (2007). The diagnosis of meniscus tears: the role of MRI and clinical examination. *Clinical Orthopaedics and Related Research*, **455**, 123–33.

Sauerbrey, A.M., Getz, C.L., Piancastelli, M., Iannotti, J.P., Ramsey, M.L., and Williams, G.R., Jr. (2005). Arthroscopic versus mini-open rotator cuff repair: a comparison of clinical outcome. *Arthroscopy*, **21**, 1415–20.

Shelbourne, K.D., Wilckens, J.H., Mollabashy, A., and DeCarlo, M. (1991). Arthrofibrosis in acute anterior cruciate ligament reconstruction: the effect of timing of reconstruction and rehabilitation. *American Journal of Sports Medicine*, **19**, 332–6.

Sperling, J.W., Smith, A.M., Cofield, R.H., and Barnes, S. (2007). Patient perceptions of open and arthroscopic shoulder surgery. *Arthroscopy*, **23**, 361–6.

Tull, F. and Borrelli, J. (2003). Soft-tissue injury associated with closed fractures: evaluation and management. *Journal of the American Academy of Orthopaedic Surgery*, **11**, 431–8.

Warwick, D., Dahl, O., and Fisher, W. (2008). Orthopaedic thromboprophylaxis: limitations of current guidelines. *Journal of Bone and Joint Surgery. British Volume*, **90B**, 127–32.

SECTION 3

Regional Injuries

Ocular sports injuries

Nick Galloway

Introduction

Injuries to the eyes in sport are sufficiently common to have a significant economic impact in terms of loss of working time and cost of treatment, and they are largely preventable. Sometimes the serious nature of an eye injury is not apparent at first glance and it is important that, if damage to the eye is suspected, a proper microscopic examination is arranged without delay. One must not overlook the devastating effect such an injury can have on an individual. Despite the remarkable advances in surgical techniques the results of the treatment of severe injuries are not always satisfactory and prevention is the best approach.

Incidence

Sports injuries have a higher profile now that other types of injury have been greatly reduced by preventive measures. For example, perforating injuries of the eye following road traffic accidents were commonplace in ophthalmic departments prior to the introduction of the compulsory wearing of seat belts, whereas now they are quite rare. Some eye injuries from sport have also become less frequent because of preventive measures (Barr *et al.* 2000), whilst others have increased with an increase in popularity of the sport. Compared with eye injuries in general, sporting injuries have a high incidence of hospital admissions, reflecting their potential to be more severe (Jones 1988).

Between 10% and 25% of all eye trauma is due to sport. The figure varies from centre to centre and is more common in children (Strahlman *et al.* 1990). To date there is no national reporting system in the UK, but useful data are available from the USA and especially Canada. The Canadian Ophthalmological Society has developed a national database, which shows trends and changes with the introduction of rule changes and protective wear. Nevertheless the collection of these data relies on voluntary reporting by ophthalmologists, and the reported cases are likely to be only a small proportion of actual injuries.

The United States Eye Injury Registry (USEIR) has collected and disseminated data on serious eye injuries from sport and recreation since 1988, and although it also probably captures only a small percentage of eye injuries it provides some interesting figures. Between 1988 and 1999, out of a total of 702 serious injuries, 104 were from baseball, 66 from basketball, and 55 from racket sports. A high incidence of fishing injuries illustrates how these figures can vary in different parts of the world depending on the sports pursued locally.

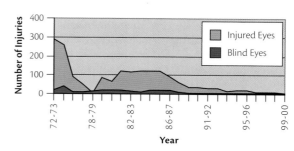

Fig. 3.1.1 Canadian Ophthalmological Society reported ice hockey injuries 1972–2000.

The Canadian Ophthalmological Society has prospectively collected national data for sports injuries (Pashby 2002), and the figures for ice hockey between 1972 and 2000 are of particular interest because of their relation to the rule changes and the introduction of protective wear over this period. They are shown graphically in Fig. 3.1.1. Proper face protection was introduced in 1975.

The pattern of injuries in the UK may be rather different, as can be seen in Table 3.1.1 which records all sports injuries admitted to Manchester Royal Eye Hospital in 1987 (Jones 1988). None of the patients in this series were wearing eye protection, and wearing eye goggles for squash is still not widely recommended in the UK.

Table 3.1.1 Cases of sporting injury admitted to The Manchester Royal Eye Hospital in 1987.

Sport	No. of patients
Football	17
Squash	12
Badminton	10
Tennis	4
Cricket	2
Rugby	2
Golf	2
Hockey	1
Real tennis	1
Darts	1
Total	52

Data from Jones (1988).

Of course football refers to soccer in this case, and there is still a high incidence of injuries from racket sports.

Although national figures may indicate the popularity of a particular sport, they do not tell the individual what their particular risk is when playing. The individual player needs to know exactly what risk they are protecting themselves against when they are being asked to wear possibly cumbersome sportswear, and this in turn may affect their ability to succeed and enjoy the game. Some sporting injuries seem to be less well reported; for example, boxing is recognized by practising ophthalmologists as a high-risk sport but the injuries seem to be under-reported. A questionnaire sent to eye surgeons in the UK, which achieved a 50.35% reply rate, gave a total of 38 cases of retinal detachment in boxers over the previous 5 years (Elkington 1985). Even this figure, which is likely to be under-reported, suggests a higher incidence of retinal detachment than in the general population. The incidence of soccer injuries to the eye has been increasing in many countries, but this could be due to increasing popularity of the game rather than an increase in the risk to the individual player (Capao Filipe 2004).

In the UK squash has been recorded as producing the highest incidence of injuries per playing session as well as the greatest number of hospital admissions (Barrell *et al.* 1981). This figure may have improved recently with the introduction of safety glasses. Protective goggles are mandatory in many clubs in the USA, but not in the UK, although their use is encouraged.

Mechanisms of eye injury

Ocular contusion

The mechanical results of direct contusion depend to some extent on whether the eyelids were open or closed at the time of impact, as well as on the size, speed, and weight of the missile. The squash ball, which measures 40 mm in diameter, is an ideal size for causing compression of the globe, whereas in the case of the larger tennis ball some of the force of impact is cushioned by the surrounding orbital margin. Unfortunately, even a football may mould itself into the orbit and cause contusion of the globe, so that the larger size of ball cannot always guarantee protection. A high-speed missile may contuse the globe through the closed lids, but bruising of the eyelids can be an indication that the globe has had some protection. A squash ball may be travelling at more than 100 mph, and can strike the globe before the blink reflex has had time to occur. In such cases the cornea at the front of the eye tends to be abraded, causing severe sharp pain and photophobia. The more severe effects of such a contusion are due to distortion of the globe. The force of impact is usually upwards and inwards on the lower temporal quadrant. This causes stretching and tearing of the iris root, and may result in rupture of blood vessels. Typically, bleeding into the anterior chamber (Fig. 3.1.2) can occur with an associated iridodialysis or rip of the iris root. The blood forms a red fluid level, which is a sign that specialist advice should be sought immediately. This bleeding may recur more seriously after two or three days in 10% of such patients (Wilson 1980).

If the force of impact is centred more posteriorly, the retina (which is the sensitive lining inside the eye) may be torn. Such breaks may go unnoticed until the retina becomes detached, often after a delay of several weeks or months. These breaks, if spotted in time, can be sealed by laser treatment or cryopexy applied soon after the injury. The distortion of the globe can also cause splitting

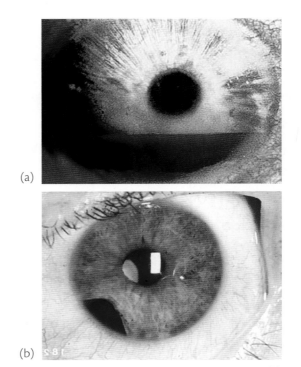

(a)

(b)

Fig. 3.1.2 (a) 'Hyphaema' or fluid level of blood in anterior chamber. (b) Healed contusion: the iris root has been ripped lower left and blood has absorbed.

open of the angle of the anterior chamber, or 'angle recession'. This can affect the drainage of the aqueous humour, causing the intra-ocular pressure to rise, and, if untreated, pressure atrophy of the optic nerve head (secondary glaucoma). Sometimes the sudden stretching produces small tears in the iris sphincter at the inner margin of the pupil, and as a result the pupil may be fixed and dilated. This can cause great concern if a head injury is suspected, but the diagnosis can be clarified easily by proper ophthalmological examination. Contusion of the eye may also cause posterior subcapsular lens opacities (the first signs of cataract), although these may take some days, or sometimes much longer, to develop. After some blows on the surface of the eye there appears to be a 'contra-coup' effect, in that most of the damage is found in the retina and choroid. Bruising of the retina is seen with ophthalmoscopy as grey patches with multiple haemorrhages. This may have a serious effect on visual acuity if the fovea is involved. Distortion of the globe can cause ruptures of the choroid, seen with the ophthalmoscope as circumferential white crescents concentric with the optic disc. One final effect of contusion may be bleeding into the optic nerve sheath. After the impact the player finds that he/she cannot see out of one eye. The physical signs may be minimal, apart from an afferent pupillary defect, despite the fact that the eye is completely blind and usually remains so. After a few weeks the optic disc becomes pale. Early decompression of the optic nerve may be helpful in these cases.

Effect on surrounding structures

It is surprising how often a contused globe is seen as an isolated injury, but other injuries may mask the eye damage. Typically a larger 'missile', such as a knee or fist, may cause a 'blow-out fracture', in which the globe is forced posteriorly, causing fracture of the floor of the orbit and trapping the inferior rectus muscle. The infra-orbital nerve may be injured, causing anaesthesia of the cheek, along with other typical signs such as enophthalmos (posterior displacement of the eye) and limitation of elevation of the eye, with double vision on upward gaze. In the absence of a blow-out fracture, injury to the superior orbital margin may damage the pulley of the superior oblique muscle, which again causes double vision but by a different mechanism.

Ocular perforation

If the globe is severely contused by a blunt object, scleral rupture may occur. More commonly, perforation of the globe is caused by a sharp object and the site of perforation is in the anterior segment of the eye. If the cornea is perforated, aqueous fluid escapes, and the iris shoots forwards to plug the opening. A knuckle of iris may project through the wound, and there is a danger that this could be mistaken for a foreign body by the first aid attendant. Any perforating injury of the eye demands urgent surgical attention because of the risk of infection and disruption of the intra-ocular structures. If the lens of the eye escapes damage, the visual outcome may be good, but once the lens is involved there is an immediate high risk of cataract formation. Cataract surgery may present technical difficulties after injuries, and even the best surgical result leaves the patient with no focusing power. This may be acceptable to the elderly patient with little focusing power before the injury, but may cause handicap to a younger person. If the perforation involves the sclera further posteriorly, there is a high risk of retinal detachment. From this brief description, it can be seen that a perforating injury is a serious risk to the sight of the eye, and may result in the need for repeated operations and time off work. Most people have heard of sympathetic ophthalmia in which the uninjured eye becomes inflamed after a perforating injury. Fortunately, this is very rare indeed, and the risk is largely eliminated by careful reparative surgery.

Injuries relating to particular sports

As one might expect, small high-speed missiles cause the most ocular damage and loss of sight. Pellets from BB guns or airguns nearly always cause serious loss of sight if they strike the eye. Out of 60 cases of airgun pellet injury reported from the UK in 1987, 70% were under the age of 17 and the vision was down to 6/60 or less in 40%. In 18% of cases the injured eye had to be removed (Moore *et al.* 1987). All these injuries occur when the young subject is unsupervised and therefore there would seem to be a strong case for proper supervision and training in the use of these guns. Recently there has been a spate of reporting of injuries from airsoft pellets fired from toy airsoft guns (Saunte and Saunte 2006), and reports suggest that eye injuries from paintball guns are on the increase. Indeed, in a recent review of English language reports, there were 545 cases in 1998 and these increased to 1200 in 2000 (Listman 2004). In a series of 288 sports injuries in Portugal reported in 2003, 29.2% were due to squash balls and 20.8% paintballs (Capao Filipe *et al.* 2003).

Eye injuries from squash balls have a particular importance because of the worldwide popularity of the game. The ball moves at approximately 115–140 mph when the racket head speed is 80–115mph with a forehand shot. It has been estimated that a dedicated squash player playing once or twice a week for 25 years has a 1 in 4 risk of a serious eye injury. It is worth noting that a

proportion of squash injuries are caused by the racket itself. Although wearing protective goggles has now become obligatory for most players in the USA and Canada, this is still not the case in many other countries including the UK. A report of retinal detachments following squash ball injuries from Germany has shown that the results of surgery are less successful than those following non-traumatic cases (Knorr and Jonas 1996).

Injuries from golf balls are less common but nearly always very serious. In one series of eight cases of golfing injuries collected over 8 years from Wisconsin, USA, there were four ruptured globes, and in another series of seven cases from Austria collected over 7 years there were also four ruptured globes and three of these patients had to have the eye removed (Meiler *et al.* 1995).

Unfortunately, there is still a significant injury rate in sports employing a larger ball. In the 1980s cricket ball injuries to the face accounted for 30% of all sporting injuries in New Zealand (Aburn 1990), and a high proportion of soccer eye injuries are caused by the ball. In the latter case where no protective wear is used, there is a 2% risk of eye injury in men over an 8 year period according to National Collegiate Athletic Association (NCAA) figures from the USA. Of some interest and concern is the reported difference between the risk of eye injuries for women and men in lacrosse. Women, who in the past have not worn eye protection, have a greater risk than men, who do wear helmets and masks (Vinger 2005).

Basketball players are at frequent risk of eye injuries not from the ball but from the frequent physical contact with other players. A prospective study of 1092 injuries sustained by basketball players in the USA in the early 1990s revealed that 5.4% of injuries involved the eyes. Most of these were surface abrasions or eyelid lacerations, and most were caused by fingers or elbows. Very few of the eye injury cases were wearing eye protection (Zagelbaum *et al.* 1995).

In the case of boxing the reported injury figures suggest that eye injuries are rare, but in a number of series where groups of boxers have been examined by ophthalmologists the incidence of injuries has been high. This may be because as long as only one eye has been affected the boxer tends to play down or hide his injury, but it may also be because the damaging effect of these injuries may be delayed. Retinal detachments may occur months or even years after the retina has been torn and traumatic cataracts may also take several years to develop.

Certain traditional sports which are played in particular regions or countries, such as hurling in Ireland, shinty in Scotland, or hornussen in Switzerland, have the reputation of causing severe eye injuries, but few cases are reported, reflecting the small numbers who take part in these sports (Flyn *et al.* 2005). One might have expected the sudden rise in venous pressure experienced by bungee jumpers to cause intra-ocular haemorrhages, and this certainly occurs but not very often (David *et al.* 1994). In the UK, darts has been the largest single cause of perforating eye injuries in children, and in a report of 19 dart injuries in 1988, 14 were children (Cole and Smerdon 1988). Following this report, which showed that some of the injuries occurred from the tail of the dart as it was being pulled from the dartboard, recommendations were made to the British Sports and Allied Industries Federation which in turn led to the recommendation that packaging should have a warning against allowing children under 14 to play darts unsupervised.

Eye injuries occur in watersports. Eleven cases of surfing eye injuries were reported from San Francisco in 1998, and nine of these had ruptured globes. An important cause was the way in which the surfer was attached to the board by a lead (Kim *et al.* 1998). At one time swimming goggles in the UK were causing a problem; the wearer pulled the goggles forwards to release water, and the goggles tended to slip from the fingers causing damage when the sharp edge caught the eye (Jonasson 1977). The classical injury suffered by fishermen occurs when casting a dry fly and the fishhook catches the eye. In most cases the hook catches on the eyelid, and the injury occurs to a significant number of observers. A report from Northern Ireland in 2004 described four cases in which the hook caught on the cornea (Knox *et al.* 2004). A successful surgical technique is described in this report.

Economics and prevention of sporting injuries to the eye

The social cost of sporting eye injuries should not be underestimated. Ocular trauma is the most common reason for admission to eye units, and 10–25% of these cases result from taking part in a sport. The cost of treatment and hospitalization has to be added to the cost of lost working time and sometimes the loss of jobs. The important factor is that these injuries are all preventable.

The prevention of injuries involves in the first instance the collection of accurate data and then a study of the mechanism when particular injuries are identified. This leads to consideration of whether the rules of the sport can be modified and whether protective wear is required. The question of training and advice by professionals to those taking up a sport has to be considered. As examples, we now know that spectacle wearers are at a particular risk in racket sports and the wearing of open-type guards around the eye does not prevent a squash ball travelling at 100 mph from causing a contusion. Eye guards with plano or prescription polycarbonate lenses appear to be the safest, and these should be marked to show that they comply with current safety standards (Fig. 3.1.3).

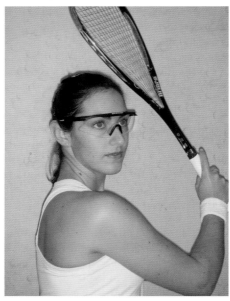

Fig. 3.1.3 Light-weight polycarbonate protective wear for squash.

Pre-existing eye disease or injury

Some people are at special risk when taking part in sport because they have had previous eye surgery. This applies after cataract and corneal graft surgery in particular. Subjects with high myopia (very short-sighted) have a thinner sclera than normal, and this can rupture more easily. They also have a higher risk of retinal detachment after injury. It must be remembered that some high myopes may have undergone refractive surgery, which in itself carries extra risks. Refractive keratotomy, a now largely superseded treatment for myopia, is known to weaken the cornea and has been associated with rupture of the globe. Modern excimer laser treatment for myopia is much safer in this respect, but as with any operation on the eye, surgery to allow better participation in a sport should not be considered without careful consideration of the possible complications.

The patient with only one good functioning eye is at a greater risk of injury, presumably because of the reduced field of vision and distance judgement. Such a patient also has much more to lose if an eye injury occurs. Nonetheless, 'only eyes' are sometimes blinded, and it is very important that those taking up a sport are properly advised about the use of protective glasses and the suitability of different sports before such a tragedy occurs.

First aid management

When a sporting injury involves the eyes, the first aid attendant should make a simple assessment of the vision. If the vision is impaired and cannot be cleared by blinking, immediate referral for specialist treatment is essential. The examiner can test the field of vision by using finger movements in all four quadrants; if the examiner sees his or her own fingers when they are not seen by the injured athlete, referral is indicated. A near-vision test card can be a helpful item in this situation. A simple test of the eye movements in which the athlete is asked to follow the examiner's fingers may reveal damage that needs expert attention. The majority of suspected eye injuries demand prompt referral, but the first aid attendant, if suitably trained, may be able to remove foreign bodies from under the eyelid or assist with the replacement of a contact lens. Many contact lens wearers can replace their own dislodged contact lens if they have a small mirror, and this could be included in the first aid kit together with a pen torch and sterile cotton swabs. A protective eye-shield is also a useful item for taping over the eye if a perforating injury is suspected. A severe eye injury may require immediate surgery under a general anaesthetic, in which case it may be necessary to withhold food and drink as a pre-anaesthetic precaution.

References

Aburn, N. (1990). Eye injuries in indoor cricket at Wellington hospital: a survey January 1987–June1989. *New Zealand Medical Journal*, **103**, 454–6.

Barr, A., Baines, P.S., Desai, P., and MacEwen, C.J. (2000). Ocular sports injuries: the current picture. *British Journal of Sports Medicine*, **34**, 456–8.

Barrell, G.V., Cooper, P.J., Elkington, A.R., MacFadyen, J.M., Powell, R.G., and Tormey, P. (1981). Squash ball to eyeball: the likelihood of squash players incurring an eye injury. *British Medical Journal*, **283**, 893–5.

Capao Filipe, J.A. (2004). Soccer (football) ocular injuries: an important eye health problem. *British Journal of Ophthalmology*, **88**, 159–60.

Capao Filipe, J.A., Roche-Sousa, A., Falcao Reis, F., and Castro-Corriera, J. (2003). Modern sports eye injuries. *British Journal of Ophthalmology*, **87**, 1336–9.

Cole, M.D. and Smerdon, D. (1988). Perforating injuries caused by darts. *British Journal of Ophthalmology*, **72**, 511–14.

David, D.B., Mears, T., and Quinlan, M.P. (1994). Ocular complications associated with bungee jumping. *British Journal of Ophthalmology*, **78**, 234–35.

Elkington, A.R. (1985). Boxing and the eye: results of a questionnaire. *Transactions of the Ophthalmological Societies of the United Kingdom*, **104**, 898–902.

Flyn, T.H., Fennessy, K., Horgan, N., *et al.* (2005). Ocular Injury in Hurling. *British Journal of Sports Medicine*, **39**, 493–6.

Jonasson, F. (1977). Swimming goggles causing severe eye injuries. *British Medical Journal*, **i**, 881.

Jones, N.P. (1988). One year of severe eye injuries in sport. *Eye*, **2**, 484–7.

Kim, J.W., McDonald, H.R., Rubsamen, P.E., *et al.* (1998). Surfing related ocular injuries. *Retina*, **18**, 424–9.

Knorr, H.L. and Jonas, J.B. (1996). Retinal detachments by squash ball accidents. *American Journal of Ophthalmology*, **122**, 260–1.

Knox, F.A., Chan, W.C., McAvoy, C.E., Johnston, S.E., and Bryars, J.H. (2004). Penetrating ocular injuries from fish hooks. *International Ophthalmology*, **25**, 291–4.

Listman, D.A. (2004). Paintball injuries in children. *Pediatrics*, **113**, 1468.

Meiler, W.F., Nanda, S.K., Wolf, M.D., and Harman, J. (1995). Golf related ocular injuries. *Archives of Ophthalmology*, **113**, 1410–13.

Moore, A.T., McCartney, A., and Cooling, R.J. (1987). Ocular injuries associated with the use of airguns. *Eye*, **1**, 422–9.

Pashby T. (2002). Eye injuries in Canadian sports and recreation 1972–2002. *Canadian Journal of Ophthalmology*, **37**, 253–5.

Saunte, J.P. and Saunte, M.E. (2006). Thirty three cases of airsoft gun pellet ocular injuries in Copenhagen 1998–2002. *Acta Ophthalmologica Scandinavica*, **84**, 755–8.

Strahlman, E., Elman, M., Daub, E., and Baker, S. (1990). Causes of pediatric eye injuries. *Archives of Ophthalmology*, **108**, 603–7.

Vinger, P.F. (2005). The eye and sports medicine. In: W. Tasman and E. Jaege (eds), *Duane's Clinical Ophthalmology*, Vol. 5, pp. 1–86. Lippincott–Williams & Wilkins, Philadelphia, PA.

Wilson, F.M. (1980). Traumatic hyphaema. *Ophthalmology*, **87**, 910–19.

Zagelbaum, B.M., Starkey, C., Hersh, P.S., Donnenfeld, E.D., Perry, H.D., and Jeffers, J.B. (1995). The National Basketball Association eye injury study. *Archives of Ophthalmology*, **113**, 749–52.

3.2

Head injuries

John Firth

With the exception of pugilism, head injury is not an intended objective in sport. 'Man is his brain', so deliberate brain injury cannot reasonably be described as 'sport'. Head injury in sport is unnecessary. Avoidable head injury is unacceptable. Therefore a primary objective in sport has to be to eliminate or minimize the opportunities for head injury. This does not have to detract from the excitement and enjoyment of sport. Both can be enhanced (Park and Levy 2008). But it does require those responsible for and participating in sport to have an understanding of the nature of head injury: its mechanisms and effects, and the means for its avoidance, prevention, and attenuation as well as its management.

Head injury mechanisms

Head injury is the injurious application of energy to the head. The key factor in head injury is brain injury (McLatchie and Jennett 1994). Brain injury requires the injurious transfer of that energy from head to brain. The three common brain injury mechanisms are head (i) penetration, (ii) deformation, and (iii) acceleration. Each may be the sole mechanism of injury. Frequently they are combined. Head injury may be 'open', where there is obvious external laceration, or 'closed', where the scalp is intact. Normal external appearances are no guarantee of normality within.

Penetration

Penetration of the skull by missiles or sharp objects scatters bone fragments internally, tears the meninges (the membranes covering the brain), and lacerates the brain itself, together with the brain and meningeal blood vessels.

Deformation

Deformation of the skull causes brain percussion, compression, and mechanical distortion and skull fracture. Fracture may be of the skull vault, the skull base, or both. Skull fracture may disrupt the dura (the brain's outermost tough covering on the inner surface of the skull) of the skull base, allowing a cerebrospinal fluid (CSF) leak, or strip the dura from the inner surface of the skull causing extradural haemorrhage (bleeding). Skull fractures may be 'undisplaced' or 'depressed'. When depressed, areas of fractured skull are driven into the head, reducing its overall volume as well as deforming and tearing meninges, arteries and veins, and the large intradural venous sinuses, as well as the brain itself. Skull fracture is 'compound' when the damage is compounded by overlying scalp laceration, allowing direct access for infection to enter the brain. Such direct access is also provided if there is a continuing leak of CSF through a skull base fracture—a CSF fistula, manifest as a watery salty drip from the nose or down the back of the throat.

Acceleration

Acceleration, the third of the three common head injury mechanisms, is still poorly understood. Debate on its effects has raged since the Paris Academy's consideration of closed head injury in 1766. This confusion is compounded by the fact that as well as the initial, often complex, brain motion imparted by head impact and brain contusion (bruising), that motion unleashes a series of additional injury mechanisms.

1. Transient brain dysfunction expressed as an alteration of consciousness, loss of memory, or impact seizure. While limited in themselves, they may disable the victim for long enough for him/her to drown or asphyxiate.

2. Vasoparesis: local cerebral blood flow autoregulatory failure (Sheinker 1944; Langfitt et al. 1968; Bruce et al. 1981). The associated brain swelling may only cause a headache, but it can kill.

3. Haematoma: bridging vessel disruption causes extracerebral subdural breeding and haematoma (space-occupying clot) formation.

4. Brain shear: the tearing of nervous components and intracerebral blood vessels by differential brain motion of one tissue against another in brain or brainstem. This may cause gross intracerebral haemorrhage, but fine punctate haemorhages are the rule.

5. Cavitation, in which brain tissue is damaged by explosive decompression in the opposite side of the brain—i.e. opposite to the head impact site, the 'contre-coup' phenomenon.

The brain floats like a gelatinous mushroom in the seawater-like CSF within the skull. The CSF is contained within the subarachnoid space between the arachnoid (the second brain-covering membrane, within the dura) and the pia mater (the third rind-like innermost covering of the brain). The brain is anchored imperfectly by blood vessels, cranial nerves, and arachnoidal ligaments which traverse the subarachnoid space. This anchoring is tightest at the skull base and least over the outer convex surfaces of the brain. As a result, the cerebral hemispheres (the 'cap' of the mushroom) have considerable freedom of movement within the head (anteroposteriorly front to back and under rotation or radial acceleration), as has the centre of the brainstem (the 'stalk' of the mushroom) vertically along its axis (allowing 'sleeving' injury).

The injurious force generated by acceleration in any one situation reflects the general equation

$$F = ma$$

where F is the injurious force available to damage the brain, a is the acceleration associated with the accident, and m is the mass involved, often in sport the head itself.

Acceleration is the key to most sporting head injury. It is the rate of change in the velocity of the head (Δv), commonly induced by violent deceleration by head impact. Speed (v) is less important than the actual acceleration imposed ($\Delta v/t$, the change of head velocity in unit time, where Δv is the change in head velocity v in the time t during which that change occurs). Low speed, immediately halted by impact on a hard surface, can generate greater acceleration than the progressive deceleration from high speed of an individual cocooned in a vehicle with a properly arranged safety cage, occupant location by five-point harness, appropriate helmet, airbags, and/or cockpit geometry designed to stabilize the helmet and prevent the head flailing on the body (adding further radial brain acceleration) whilst extending the time for deceleration during the impact sequence (reducing $\Delta v/t$ by extending t).

Apparent anomalies exist, such as heading the ball in soccer (Naunheim *et al.* 2003). Here the art is to match head and ball as a Newtonian couple, with the associated accelerations being undertaken by the ball, not the brain. Unmatched, unintended, and unanticipated ball–head strike can be as lethal as sandbagging (Kirkendall *et al.* 2001).

Transient traumatic brain dysfunction: 'concussion'

Traditionally, 'concussion' describes a transient disturbance of brain function caused by head injury, but presumed to be unaccompanied by brain damage and supposedly entirely reversible without lasting harm, i.e. a physiological rather than a pathological phenomenon. As a term its usefulness is compromised by loose usage (McCrory and Berkovic 2001; Wills and Leathem 2001). It has been tightly tightly defined as a transient trauma-induced alteration of mental state that is not necessarily associated with unconsciousness (Kelly *et al.* 1991). In the literature, concussion is confused with traumatic coma in severe head injury (Cantu 1992). In some cases it may represent a genetic predisposition, express a migrainous trait, or be reflex-based. Whether it is fully reversible is questionable (Bailes and Cantu 2001). Repeated concussion may or may not be cumulative (Guskiewicz *et al.* 2003; Collie *et al.* 2006). However, the more it is investigated (by functional magnetic resonance imaging (fMR)), the greater is the associated brain abnormality found (Chen *et al.* 2008). In practice, concussion is best considered to indicate a significant brain insult, possible lasting injury, and certain vasoparesis with a potential for the second impact syndrome (SIS, see below) if exercise is resumed and head impact repeated before all symptoms and signs have cleared. In the author's view, 'concussion' represents a group 3 head injury profile (see below) with potential for secondary deterioration due to brain swelling, intracranial clot, or both. Rest, recumbency, qualified medical review, and continuous careful observation are indicated until normality is restored and all symptoms have settled.

Vasoparesis and post-traumatic brain swelling

Pure acceleration-induced or impact-related brain motion and brain distortion can cause local cerebrovascular vasoparesis. This is the loss of the normal automatic ability of the brain's terminal arterioles to control local cerebral blood flow (CBF) through the capillary beds they feed. This makes possible a passive expansion in cerebral blood volume (CBV), and hence of brain bulk if combined with a normal or raised blood pressure (Sheinker 1944; Langfitt *et al.* 1968; Bruce *et al.* 1981). This post-traumatic brain swelling may complicate head acceleration alone or compound the effects of intracranial space occupation by haematoma (blood clot). Teleologically, with the skull having a fixed capacity, cerebrovascular autoregulation should be the most hardy of all physiological mechanisms. In fact it is readily abolished by any brain insult, including what may otherwise appear minor injury. As a result, vasoparesis is a major post-traumatic problem in its own right (Langfitt *et al.* 1968). In the past, only one in three of those who died of head injuries had a blood clot in the head (Miller 1979). The remainder died because of raised intracranial pressure caused by vasoparetic brain swelling. This can be controlled, if caught early enough, by manipulating the other mechanisms that control CBF, principally the cerebrovascular carbon dioxide (CO_2) response. The CO_2 response of cerebral arterioles is not abolished when autoregulation is. Blowing-off CO_2 by hyperventilation reduces brain blood flow and hence brain bulk. If necessary, this can be started immediately, at the accident site, by mouth-to-mouth respiration before endotracheal intubation and mechanical ventilation are to hand. ***The significance of this is that cardiopulmonary resuscitation should be available at any sports site where head injury may occur, while resuscitation should be part of the basic training of sports organizers, coaches, linesmen, umpires, and officials alike.***

Second impact syndrome

Although the subject of debate (Cantu 1998a; McCrory and Berkovic 1998b) since its initial definition (Saunders and Harbaugh 1984), SIS is a further manifestation of post-traumatic cerebral vasoparesis (McCrory 2001a). The younger the player, the more likely it is to occur. It represents a hypersensitivity to a second head impact induced by a prior head insult. It may have a migrainous component. The presence of subarachnoid or subdural blood from the first insult may be significant (Mori *et al.* 2006). Typically, the victim is knocked out but makes a rapid recovery, to all appearances complete. All are determined to play on, and do. A second head impact occurs, often apparently trivial, but now catastrophic in outcome. The individual is either knocked out immediately or exhibits a paradoxical inappropriately enhanced impairment by so minor an insult. Rapid deterioration then occurs and all attempts at resuscitation fail. Post-mortem examination reveals a grossly swollen brain. Death is due to raised intracranial pressure. Recovery, where achieved, has been associated with immediate ventilation once deterioration follows the second impact. That this has not been universally successful, as would be expected if vasoparesis were the only culprit, suggests that a second mechanism is also triggered by the first head injury. The adverse effect of youth and the often bizarre effects of post-traumatic vasospasm in children (cerebral blood vessels going into spasm rather than being rendered vasoparetic) makes a migrainous component likely, but this has yet to be confirmed. For the moment, recognition of the phenomenon and prevention are the only sure cure. Hence, the sporting policy that alteration of consciousness is considered a death warrant until proven otherwise. Leave the burden of proof to the hospital doctor.

Traumatic vasospasm

The interaction of migraine with head acceleration may produce bizarre symptoms, particularly in the young. Post-traumatic blindness is a terrifying condition in children. Every investigation is normal. A strong family history of migraine is the clue. Only when vision returns spontaneously, often several days later, can the diagnosis be confirmed.

Vascular disruption and intracranial haemorrhage

In head injury, bleeding may be intra- or extracerebral. If extracerebral, then it may be subarachnoid, subdural, or extradural. Apart from the immediate local tissue and blood vessel damage, bleeding exerts a major deleterious effect through the formation and expansion of space-occupying blood clots (haematomas) within the limited confines of the skull. They take time (minutes or hours) to develop and are a major management concern. They are considered below. Skull base fracture is a hazard to the internal carotid arteries in the carotid canals and cavernous sinuses with the potential for carotico-cavernous fistulae. While neck trauma can cause carotid and vertebral arterial dissection, presenting as stroke (Arnold *et al.* 2009; McCrory 2000).

Shear

Shear in the brain is well described by Holbourn (1943) and Strich (1956, 1961, 1969). As a gelatinous structure under acceleration, the brain's internal complexity induces differential movement between adjacent components of differing structure and density and thereby shear between tissues within the brain itself. The shearing forces so induced disrupt nerve cell axons (the cells' long processes running within the brain and to and from spinal cord), small blood vessels, and dendrites (the multitude of fine connections between adjacent nerve cells which bristle out from each nerve cell body). The resulting disruption, which may be cumulative with repeated head insult, can have a catastrophic effect on brain function, yet with little apparent macroscopic (naked-eye) damage. This was a common finding in multiple repeated head injury—the 'punch-drunk' traumatic encephalopathy of boxing, and the 'lame-brain' jockeys of the days before a series of mandatory safety improvements (including wearing effective head protection to the British Standard Institute's then BS 4472 specification) were introduced to racing under Jockey Club rules (Allen 1976).

Shear is also a problem in the brainstem. Here, the long perforating arteries are at particular risk. They run back from the basilar artery through the brainstem to the floor of the fourth ventricle. Under vertical acceleration along its long axis, the brainstem acts like a column of gelatin. Head acceleration is transferred to the outside of the column, whilst its central core lags behind. Eventually, the core is accelerated, and when the outer surface of the column is halted with the rest of the head the centre continues to surge along the axis of the previous acceleration, producing the phenomenon of brainstem 'sleeving' (Lindgren 1966). The effect is to pull the long perforating vessels off their capillary beds, resulting in multiple punctate brainstem haemorrhages. While not invariably fatal, they give rise to a variety of symptoms, often with few accompanying objective signs. They are one component of the 'post-traumatic syndrome' and may complicate high-Gz aerobatics performed in turbulent conditions, occasioning vector-related vertigo.

Shear occurs within the walls of cerebral vessels causing an arterial dissection—an intimal tear is followed by blood stripping between the layers of the arterial wall. This may lead to occlusion of the artery, local thrombosis, distal embolism and occlusive stroke, fusiform aneurysm formation, and rupture with subarachnoid haemorrhage. Clinically, the most common site in the head is the vertebral artery, associated with its passage through the dura and entry to the posterior fossa through the foramen magnum. More frequently, traumatic vertebral and carotid arterial dissection in the neck, with main vessel occlusion or distal embolism, add focal brain stroke to an already confusing post-traumatic situation.

Cavitation

Under head acceleration, the gelatinous brain lags behind the skull. It behaves much as coffee in a cup when the cup is struck against a wall. Like the skull, the cup comes to an abrupt halt, but the coffee flows on, raising pressure adjacent to the point of impact which causes it to rise up the side of the cup and spill out of it. The rising fluid reflects the increased pressure under the point of impact. At the other side of the cup the coffee level falls as it flows away towards the impact side. Oscillation then follows.

In the intact head, there is a sharp increase in local pressure under the impact point, producing a local percussion insult to the brain, the 'coup' injury of the French Academy. This may just bruise, contuse, or actually disrupt the brain substance. At the opposite side of the head, pressure falls acutely as the brain moves away. Pressure may fall below the tissue vapour pressure of gases in solution in the intracellular fluid in the brain cells, in the extracellular space (which occupies 25% of the brain's volume between brain cells and their blood vessels), and within the blood vessels themselves. If the pressure drops sufficiently, bubble formation occurs, producing an explosive local decompressive lesion, the phenomenon of 'cavitation', opposite the impact site—the 'contre-coup' injury.

As a result, any one impact can cause at least two severe injuries, one at the impact site and the other opposite to it. In practice, a blow to the front of the head produces an impact, percussion, and a coup injury to the frontal poles of the brain and the tips of its temporal lobes. The associated fall in pressure at the back of the head is attenuated, damped by the ability of CSF to move up through the foramen magnum from the elastic spinal thecal sac. (Unlike the dura in the head, which is attached to the inner surface of the skull, the spinal theca covering the spinal cord expands and contracts within the spinal canal with every heart beat, part of the mechanism of the circulation of the CSF.) Therefore frontal impacts produce high-pressure frontal injury. Brain substance may be blown down the nose, through the cribrifom plates in the skull base, to appear as white material at the nostrils. Conversely, occipital impact injury produces little coup (percussion effect under the impact point at the back of the head), again due to the damping effect of the CSF, now moving out of the head through the foramen magnum. No such damping is available at the anterior end the skull. The contrecoup cavitation effect on frontal and temporal poles of occipital injury is devastating. As a result, both frontal and occipital impacts produce frontal injury. Both may be exacerbated further by head rotation and radial brain acceleration. Blows to the side of the head (lateral temporal impact) not only involve the thinnest and most easily fractured part of the skull, with enhanced risk of extradural haematoma formation from tearing of the underlying middle meningeal arteries, but also ensure coup and contre-coup insults to both sides of the brain.

The immediate post-head-injury problem

Once a head injury has occurred, the many agents at work can produce a bewildering series of situations. The immediate priority is to prevent the multiple primary adverse effects of the initial brain injury being exacerbated or compounded by hypoxia and hypotension due to **a**irway obstruction, impaired **b**reathing, and an inadequate **c**irculation (ABC). Having secured the airway, ensured breathing, if necessary by mouth-to-mouth ventilation, and made the best of the circulation, if necessary by external cardiac massage and placing the victim horizontal with legs raised to maximize venous return, all the while being careful for an unstable spine, the individual is left (i) 'concussed' (awake but suffering some degree of brain dysfunction), (ii) unconscious and unresponsive, or (iii) having suffered an impact-induced seizure.

The common index of significance in head injury is whether enough energy has been imparted to the brain to alter consciousness. If it has, this is sufficient for all the other complications of head injury to follow. The most sensitive of all brain structures to head impact is the limbic (memory) system. Its arrangement as two fine looping aerial arrays within the brain ensures its maximum susceptibility to brain acceleration and motion. The crossing of the threshold of significance for later hazard may be manifest in no more than a temporary disorientation, reflecting a disturbed contribution to consciousness from memory and often described as 'concussion'. Greater impact causes immediate loss of consciousness (unresponsive unconsciousness) due to involvement of midbrain pathways in the brain disturbance. Alternatively, the situation may be dominated by impact seizure—an immediate reflex convulsive response to head impact. Persisting unconsciousness is coma. Loss of memory for the immediate 10 minute period before a coma-inducing head injury is commonplace. It probably reflects no more than disturbance of the 'electrical phase' of memory. Loss of pre-traumatic memory of more than 10 minutes indicates actual structural damage to the limbic system. Greater degrees of brain injury are reflected by longer post-traumatic coma, potentially compounded by secondary complication. The extending period of the associated absence of input to memory is the basis of the post-traumatic amnesic interval before continuous memory is restored. The immediate challenge for management is to establish an unobstructed airway and ensure adequate breathing and a satisfactory circulation, to maintain brain oxygenation, while being mindful of an unstable cervical spinal injury, as 'head injury is spinal injury until proven otherwise'. If necessary, airway clearance, mouth-to-mouth ventilation, and external cardiac massage have to be instituted and maintained without disturbing spinal alignment until recovery of consciousness occurs or mechanical ventilation and expert assistance are available.

Early complications of head injury: the first 60 minutes

This is the 'golden hour', in which warranted intervention has the best chance of achieving a good outcome. Primary direct accident injury is now complicated by the potential for secondary insult, starting with an obstructed airway, impaired breathing, and an inadequate circulation—the immediate ABC concerns. Attending to these, with care for coincident spinal injury, provides the opportunity to assess whether this is a 'minor' insult—the victim has not been knocked out—or a 'major' head injury in which the individual has been rendered unconscious. If a rapid recovery to consciousness is made, this is a 'significant' head injury—significant because sufficient energy was delivered to the brain to induce unconsciousness and to establish the circumstances in which secondary deterioration may occur and urgent expert intervention may be necessary. ABC, close observation, and transfer to a competent medical facility are the priority. If a rapid recovery is not made, this is a 'severe' head injury in which primary brain damage is now likely to be compounded by the secondary complications of brain swelling, intracranial haematoma, or both. These are best managed during the first 60 minutes after severe head injury, minimizing the opportunity for secondary brain damage and maximizing that for best recovery—hence the 'golden hour'. Increasing delay progressively increases the risk of worsening secondary injury and residual disability while reducing the opportunity for success. Uncontrolled brain swelling and haematoma expansion displace the brain, and the consequent brain shift eventually leads to the pre-terminal phenomenon of 'coning' (See below).

Brain swelling and its control by hyperventilation is described above. Rapidly expanding post-traumatic haematoma is usually subdural in location, the product of bridging vessel disruption, as described below and is manageable only by prompt surgical evacuation. Meanwhile, unsuspected extradural haematoma development may be about to reverse an initially hopeful situation, ensuring that early improvement cannot be relied upon.

Intracranial haemorrhage

Primary intracerebral haemorrhage

Primary traumatic intracerebral haemorrhage is unusual in sporting injuries, but occurs in contrecoup injury. It may complicate previously unsuspected intracranial abnormality. The possibility of both is covered by the appropriate rapid response to brain swelling and intracranial haematoma, which includes emergency CT scanning on the way to the operating theatre with brain swelling already controlled by hyperventilation and dehydration with intravenous mannitol.

Subarachnoid haemorrhage

Although the centre of much attention, in practice traumatic subarachnoid haemorrhage is a relatively minor problem in sporting injury. If diffuse, it is likely to represent pial disruption, as in subfrontal and temporal polar 'bursting' by cavitation or impact insult. If focal, it may be no more than perimesencephalic venous disruption, but attention should be roused lest this represent an incidental aneurysm, traumatic arterial dissection, or arteriovenous fistula (McCrory et al. 2000).

Subdural haematoma

Rapidly expanding subdural haematoma is a major challenge in all head injury, sports included (Cantu and Mueller 2003). It is the result of continued bleeding following bridging vessel disruption. The prominent parasagittal bridging veins, from brain to intradural venous sinuses, are so arranged so that they are rarely disturbed by an acceleration insult that does not at the same time destroy the fabric of the brain. Therefore they are relatively immune to closed head injury that does not involve depressed skull fracture and their direct rupture. However, although embryologically 'impossible', aberrant blood vessels frequently run from the convex outer surfaces of the cerebral hemispheres to the overlying dura, traversing the subarachnoid and subdural spaces. These may be arteries or veins. Firmly fixed superficially to the dura and the inner surface of the skull, they are also tightly anchored to the surface of the mobile jelly-like brain. Sudden movement or acceleration of the head induces differential motion between skull and brain. A critical vector, which may not cause unconsciousness, can rupture such vessels. Bleeding, which may be arterial, then produces a rapidly expanding haematoma over the surface of the brain in the subdural plane, deep to the dura. Unlike an extradural haematoma (described below), which has to strip the tough dura off the inside of the skull, subdural haematoma expansion is unhindered by any such constraint and may follow apparently trivial head injury. In an all too familiar sporting scenario, recovery from the initial immediate effects of head impact may appear satisfactory, but proves short-lived. It is followed by a rapid secondary deterioration into coma and death. Subdural haematomas are more common in the elderly, but may occur at any age and are a plague of boxing. The 90% mortality of acute traumatic subdural haematoma is staggering for so simple and easily treatable a condition. Subdurals kill by the pace of their expansion, leaving little time for surgical evacuation and no time for delay. The effects of their development are accelerated by their simultaneous disturbance of local brain blood flow control as they distort the adjacent distorted brain. This adds vasoparetic brain swelling to the problem. Management is straightforward: immediate hyperventilation to control the vasoparesis and rapid surgical evacuation of the subdural clot. However, success requires intervention before irreversible brain infarction has occurred. Therefore, if a boxer is still unconscious at the count of 10, he has a subdural haematoma, brain swelling, or both, until proven otherwise. There is no time for delay. Prompt surgical intervention is rarely close at hand. Even when available, it is all too often fatally delayed by failure of the attending medical team to recognize the priorities of the situation. Worse still, the victim's attendants may be lulled into a false sense of security by a transient improvement in conscious level or the apparently minor nature of the initial injury.

Posterior fossa clots are rare, but hydrocephalus adds a further hazard to them. Upward displacement of the midbrain and cerebellum, by the clot, at and through the tentorial hiatus (the aperture in the tough membrane, the tentorium, which separates the posterior fossa from the rest of the inside of the skull) distorts the aqueduct, the narrowest part of the CSF circulatory pathway, and obstructs the CSF circulation to expand the ventricles (the chambers within the brain)—the phenomenon of hydrocephalus.

Coning

Like upward brain displacement through the tentorial hiatus by posterior fossa space occupation, downward brain displacement is caused by supratentorial brain swelling, haematoma expansion, and hydrocephalus forcing midbrain and mesial temporal structures downwards through the tentorial hiatus into the posterior fossa. In its turn, unrelieved rising intracranial and posterior fossa pressure forces the medulla, the lower brainstem, and the adjacent cerebellar tonsils out of the skull, down through the foramen magnum, and into the upper cervical spinal canal. The consequent conical post-mortem appearances of the moulded, displaced, and compressed brain tissues gave rise to the term 'coning' for this terminal process (Robbins *et al.* 1984). While brainstem compression

and coning through the tentorial hiatus produce a progressive deterioration of conscious level with pupillary and vital sign changes, coning of the medulla through the foramen magnum may first be manifest by acute respiratory failure and death, often with little warning of the impending disaster.

Management of coning is by rapid control of brain bulk, reducing the pathologically enhanced CBF by ventilation and hypocapnia (lowering the arterial $paCO_2$), shrinking the brain with the intravenous osmotic agent mannitol, surgical evacuation of the clot, and ventricular drainage if hydrocephaly persists. To achieve this in time to afford the head-injured patient a chance to enjoy his/her days again requires prior planning, detailed preparation, clinical acumen, teamwork, and determined, above all rapid, management. Time is the key—literally a race with death that emphasizes the need for speed once an alteration of consciousness or conscious level has occurred.

Extradural haematoma

Before skull fracture occurs under impact loading, the skull is pliable to a degree. Such distortion can strip the dura off the inner surface of the skull, causing bleeding from meningeal (dural) arteries and providing space and place for a space-occupying haematoma to develop. Likewise, a skull fracture running across the line of a meningeal artery, most commonly the middle meningeal artery deep to the thin temporal region of the skull, can tear dural blood vessels. Both lead to blood clot formation outside the dura, between the dura and the skull (hence extradural haemorrhage and haematoma). Expanding clots strip up more dura, further distorting and displacing the adjacent brain and at the same time compromising local cerebral blood flow control. Once again, loss of local brain blood flow autoregulation, the phenomenon of cerebrovascular autoregulatory failure or 'vasoparesis' (Sheinker 1944; Langfitt *et al.* 1968; Bruce *et al.* 1981), combined with a normal or raised blood pressure increases local CBF, enhances local CBV (the volume of blood in the brain at any one instant), and causes the brain to swell, compounding the danger posed by the expanding haematoma. After a slow start, extradural haematoma may be manifest as a delayed, but now rapid, increase in intracranial pressure (ICP) within the inexpansile skull. With local brain swelling exacerbating pressure gradients within the head, brain shift is accelerated from one side of the head to the other or down through the tentorial hiatus, coning between the supratentorial compartment of the skull and the posterior fossa and on down through the foramen magnum to cone into the spinal canal.

The amount of energy required to fracture the skull and set in train this series of events is less than that required to produce unconsciousness (Gurdjian *et al.* 1950). Therefore, in sport, any loss of consciousness associated with a head injury, however brief, indicates a significant head insult and a brain injury severe enough to lead to meningeal rupture, haematoma formation, brain swelling, and subsequent fatal deterioration. That this deterioration is reversible and death avoidable enhances the cardinal importance of conscious level as the key to head injury management in sport.

Extradural haematoma provides another version of the classical sporting head injury scenario: head impact deforms the skull, percussing the brain and tearing meningeal blood vessels. The victim recovers consciousness, often to apparent normality, only to be overtaken by secondary deterioration as brain swelling complicates the expanding intracranial clot. The initial temporary improvement provides a 'lucid interval'. This lulls the victim and attendants into the false assumption that improvement ensures recovery. A false sense of security then wastes the time on which the apparently recovering victim's life depends. Any individual who has been knocked out remains at risk until proved otherwise by continuous expectant observation in hospital, where scanning and neurosurgery are available.

On the spot

The practical problem, on the spot, is that one cannot determine whether or not such a fatal train of events has been set in motion. Conscious level is the cardinal sign. Once impaired, all else can follow. ABC has to be assured and the victim merits careful observation in an establishment where appropriate intervention can be undertaken immediately, should spontaneous recovery not occur and complications develop. *The key is to recognize the significance of unconsciousness or an alteration in consciousness. It is the threshold for disaster. Once crossed, the need is for speed. Time may be running out, before potential disaster becomes reality.*

Complicating events

Simple ABC, assessment, and rapid transfer to appropriate medical surveillance may be impaired by the practicalities of the situation and by dramatic events. These include impact seizures, stroke, and the ever present risk of cervical spinal injury.

'Impact seizure'—'concussive convulsions': reflex response or epileptic trait?

Facial impact followed by immediate collapse, a tonic phase, and then convulsive movements within a few seconds followed by a rapid recovery is a regular feature of Australian Rules Football (McCrory *et al.* 1997, 1998a). A period of close observation, clearance of all neurological symptoms, normal neuroimaging, and successful completion of a previously practised battery of psychometric tests is taken to indicate sufficient recovery to allow a safe return to the game. SIS has not been a feature of this sporting discipline, in which adult professional players are monitored neurologically and psychometrically. The convulsive movements are similar to those seen in critical basal gangliar perfusion, in syncopal convulsions, and in military aviation during recovery from unconsciousness induced by head-to-foot acceleration in centrifuges (+Gz induced loss of consciousness (GILOC)). It is possible that the instantaneous loss of consciousness is triggered by the same brainstem mechanism that is thought to be responsible for GILOC. The many questions raised by this phenomenon are of undoubted physiological importance and merit further research. In the meantime, there is no indication that such convulsion introduces a risk of later post-traumatic epilepsy.

This invites comparison with the immediate impact-related impact-induced seizure sometimes seen in other head injury. In their turn, these immediate impact-induced seizures do not carry a risk of later post-traumatic epilepsy. This is unlike seizures occurring moments later, after intracranial brain motion has settled. The latter are prognostically indistinguishable from 'early' post-traumatic epilepsy—seizure in the first week following head injury, with a 25% chance of later post-traumatic epilepsy (see below).

Exercise-induced hyperventilation in Australian Rules Football, with all continuously engaged at speed, may induce sufficient hypocapnia to prevent vasoparetic brain swelling. This has made it a factor in the debate as to when, after brain insult, it is reasonable to return to sport. In this, the Australian Rules' experience is of a particular reflex response to facial impact. It does not provide grounds for a general relaxation of the expectant attitude to sporting head insult expressed elsewhere in this chapter. Indeed, on a cautionary note, impact seizure has been reported as the first indication of coincident intracranial mischief, warranting neurological review in this group (Clear and Chadwick 2000).

Post-traumatic stroke

Though timing, focal neurology, and injury detail may provide the diagnosis, stroke complicating head injury can be difficult to distinguish from primary insult and other developing complications in both children and adults. Most frequently the result of carotid or vertebral arterial dissection in the neck and skull base or of the larger intracranial vessels, it is a diagnosis to be considered during imaging of the head, neck, and brain.

'Head injury is also neck injury, until proven otherwise'

This dictum reflects reality (Schneider 1987; Cooper MT *et al.* 2003), especially in children. All head injury should be presumed to be complicated by neck and cervical spinal cord injury until proved otherwise. Even in dedicated head and spinal injury units, neck injury may be difficult to exclude. The hazard that head injury poses to the neck is enhanced by the wearing of helmets and is maximal in the young.

Children are at particular risk from a combination of factors. The anatomy of the paediatric cervical spine with near-horizontal facet joints, lax soft tissues, the carriage of a large head on a relatively small body which imposes greater head–neck dynamic ratios, inexperience, poor balance, and reckless enthusiasm mean that neck dislocation followed by spontaneous reduction is a constant hazard.

These factors combine to ensure that apparently minor head injuries can cause cervical cord insult, yet without neck pain and with cord percussion causing no more than transient sensory symptoms in limbs and trunk. However, that degree of cervical cord percussion is sufficient to render it vasoparetic, as if it were a mini-brain. The cord microcirculation can then no longer autoregulate and maintain spinal cord blood flow at low as well as high systemic blood pressures. The situation is further compounded by percussive or ischaemic compromise of the sympathetic system running down within the cervical spinal cord. Sympathetic function is impaired, and the individual is rendered 'sympathoparetic' and no longer able to maintain normal erect systemic blood pressure. If such a child is allowed to continue to stand or even compete, cervical cord ischaemia induces cervical cord swelling within its tight pial envelope, occasioning venous outflow obstruction and cord infarction.

Therefore a child who complains of 'pins and needles' or any other symptoms in arms, trunk, or legs following accident or injury should be assumed to have sustained a spinal cord insult with established spinal cord vasoparesis. In all cases of head and therefore potential spinal cord injury, children should be questioned for any sensory or motor disturbance, however transient. Again, presume cord injury until proved otherwise as spinal cord percussion may be reported as no more than transient weakness or 'pins and needles' (paraesthesiae). These are all too easily ignored, and the child is allowed to continue standing or even competing until spinal cord infarction occurs.

The child should be managed flat, with the neck stabilized until appropriate assessment can be made by a competent medical practitioner. If the initial symptoms are not reported, or are unsought, overlooked, or dismissed, the result is secondary delayed spinal cord lesion with a rapid-onset tetraparesis; weakness in all four limbs with impaired breathing adds hypoxic insult to the already ischaemic veno-congested cervical cord. By this stage the window of therapeutic opportunity has very nearly closed. Recumbency (lying horizontal) and neck stabilization to optimize cord perfusion, ventilation to reverse hypoxia and to exploit the CO_2 effect on the cord circulation, mannitol to reduce ischaemic oedema, and steroids within 45 minutes of insult may still reverse the situation, but are rarely instituted in time. The best treatment remains recognition of the hazard and its prevention. As in head injury, so in neck injury: prevention is the first priority. When that has failed and head and actual or potential neck injury has occurred, presumption of an unstable spinal cord injury is mandatory.

While one-third of spinal cord injuries are complete and irrecoverable from the moment of injury, two-thirds are not and can recover if further damage and secondary ischaemic insult are avoided. Therefore the greatest care has to be exercised in moving, observing, and transporting individuals with head and spinal injuries because of the probability of further spinal cord insult by the injudicious or thoughtless distortion of an unstable neck or spine. ABC with neck stabilization and horizontal management minimizes the risk of that further insult.

Tertiary problems

A further series of complications provide a 'third row' to the scrum of complications of head injury. They may be early or late, and include the following.

1. CSF leakage in basal skull fractures with CSF rhinorrhoea (CSF running down the back of the nose), later infection, and meningitis.

2. Epilepsy: seizure on head impact, the exacerbation of a prior epileptic trait or later epilepsy in cerebral contusion, haematoma, and skull fracture.

3. Post-traumatic encephalopathy.

4. Hydrocephaly: acute hydrocephalus in posterior fossa lesions, late post-traumatic hydrocephalus, and the phenomenon of post-traumatic encephalopathy and cerebral atrophy, which may be difficult to distinguish from a treatable hydrocephalus.

5. 'Post-traumatic syndromes', including arterial dissection.

Cerebrospinal fluid rhinorrhoea

CSF leak ('fistula': likened to salty seawater dribbling down the nose or back of the throat) through a skull base fracture and the associated risk of ascending infection and hydrocephalus are beyond the scope of this chapter and are properly the business of the hospital doctor. The individual must be questioned for such a leak and this excluded before they return to sport. This makes the possibility of CSF fistula a necessary concern of the individual

sporting discipline and its medical attendants and advisors. Exclusion is essential before flying after head injury. CSF leak may be accompanied by air entry into the head and the formation of an intracranial aerocoele, the effects of which can be exacerbated by ascent to altitude (typically to a cabin altitude of 8000 feet in commercial airline practice). Air in the head can be excluded by a simple horizontal ray lateral X-ray of the head. Any suggestion of CSF leak or air in the head (aerencephaly) requires prompt neurosurgical review.

Post-traumatic epilepsy (PTEP)

'Epilepsy' is the spontaneous recurrence of seizure. The diagnosis depends on the occurrence of a second seizure. The individual can in every other way be normal and meritorious, such as Alexander, Julius Caesar, or Napoleon, and engage normally and competitively in sport, subject to individual neurological review, and fellow participants and supervisors being aware of the potential for seizure and how such seizures should be managed (Fountain and May 2003). However, epilepsy can be caused, as well as exacerbated or elicited, by sporting head injury (Cantu 1998c). A family history of epilepsy or febrile convulsions under the age of 5 years doubles the risk of post-traumatic seizure should head injury occur. A past history of seizure enhances the likelihood of seizure complicating sport, usually on relaxation after effort. Someone subject to seizures should consult their neurologist before engaging in contact sports. All should know the essential management of convulsion: to clear and maintain the airway. With care for head and neck injury, they should be rolled into the recovery position and the patency of the airway maintained until recovery from the seizure occurs. Exercise should not be resumed until the individual's general medical practitioner is satisfied that it is safe so to do.

PTEP may be:

1. 'Immediate', 'impact epilepsy' (as above): immediate seizure-like movements on head impact that are not uncommon. As in the reflex seizure response to facial impact observed in Australian Rules Football, while they indicate a significant brain insult, with the conscious level threshold for major mischief being exceeded, they do not introduce a significant risk of later post-traumatic epilepsy.

2. 'Early' post-traumatic epilepsy: seizure at any time following immediate impact during the first week following injury imparts a 25% hazard of later post-traumatic epilepsy.

3. 'Late' post-traumatic epilepsy is epilepsy related to a head injury but occurring more than a week after insult. This is similar to late-onset epilepsy in the general non-traumatized population. It implies an initial risk of further seizure of at least 16% and potentially a risk of later long-term epilepsy of up to 65%.

In prognostic terms, the risks of later post-traumatic epilepsy are increased by several risk factors. Their presence or absence can be determined after the first week from the head injury has passed. Early epilepsy carries a 25% risk of later post-traumatic epilepsy, as above. Clinically significant intracranial haematoma, which warrants the attention of a neurosurgeon, introduces a 30% later risk. Depressed skull fracture is associated with a variable risk of 6–66%.

This variation reflects the presence or absence of four further factors:

(1) early epilepsy;

(2) focal cerebral hemispheric signs;

(3) a demonstrated tear in the dura covering the brain;

(4) a post-traumatic amnesic interval (period of lost memory following injury) of more than 24 hours (Jennett 1975).

Post-traumatic encephalopathy

The term 'post-traumatic encephalopathy' (PTE) covers a multitude of evils. Strictly, it is a post-mortem pathological diagnosis and is the result of multiple repeated head injuries with widespread shearing damage to the brain. Clinically, it is an alternative term for 'punch-drunkenness' in boxers (Martland 928) and the 'lame brains' once seen in professional jockeys after a career of falls (Foster *et al.* 1976). It can be inferred from the gross anatomy displayed by computed tomography (CT) scanning and the tissue changes evident on magnetic resonance imaging (MRI). It is often used to describe and explain incomplete recovery from severe injury. A concern of medical advisors and selectors alike is whether a previous head injury places a particular individual at enhanced risk of later head injury and PTE (Cantu 2003), and whether retirement from the discipline is appropriate (McCrory 2001b, 2002). Head injury is cumulative and may be compounded by genetic factors (Jordan *et al.* 1997, Jordan 1988). Where the literature is scant, continued participation has often been denied on questionable grounds. With the present social and economic dependency on intellect, decisions and advice have to reflect due caution. However, each individual case is unique. Each requires careful evaluation and the exclusion of a remediable cause, of which post-traumatic hydrocephalus is the most obvious.

Post-traumatic hydrocephalus

This is usually due to either a late CSF resorption block at the arachnoidal level or from basal CSF cistern occlusion. It may be difficult to distinguish from cerebral atrophy, but is demonstrable by lumbar sac infusion testing. The importance of the differential diagnosis is that hydrocephalus is amenable to CSF diversion or 'shunting'.

The post-traumatic syndrome(s)

This is a ragbag term that encompasses a host of chronic physical, emotional, and psychological symptoms, sometimes tinged by litigation. In the sporting world, the syndrome comprises a variable collection of symptoms without signs, each as unique as the individual afflicted. It is an area in which history is paramount. Patterns are discernible. It is important to recognize their origin, however bizarre they may seem. They arise from four principal injury sites: frontal lobes, limbic system, brainstem, and cervical spine, while migraine may contribute to persisting headache (McCrory 2001b).

The frontal lobes differentiate man from monkey. They provide the massive reflex base upon which our emotions, our personality, and our ability to live sociably in harmony with others depends. Frontal injury may persist as anything from a mild alteration of affect or personality, through humour failure, short temper, and intolerance, to incontinence and total asociability. Limbic injury is reflected by continuing memory impairment. Brainstem symptoms after punctate sleeving injury range from no more than vague unsteadiness through to vector-related vertigo. Cervical spine injury is both the most common and the most frequently missed. Current fashionable, slouching, near-Neanderthal, kyphotic posture abuses the neck as well as the lumbar spine. Maximum instability is assured, together with poor paraspinal tonic musculature and intervertebral discs maintained at the compression failure boundary of their viscoelastic hysteretic performance envelope. Athletes are often little better than the general population. Most coaches display little understanding of and less interest in spinal dynamics. All are cervical spinal disasters waiting to happen. Cervical injury is maximized, recovery impeded, and chronicity promoted by continued cervical kyphosis—the sporting prodrome of later cervical spondylosis. The answer lies in symptom recognition, determined restoration and then maintenance of lumbar and cervical lordosis, the rebuilding of the tonic paraspinal musculature, and the achievement of automatic habitual lordotic carriage—'carriage' in the postural sense.

Prevention

The above litany of potential disasters emphasizes the First Law of Head Injury: *Prevention is better than cure*. All sports disciplines need to review their practice continually to define the present incidence and risk of head injury, and to develop their sports either to exclude or at the least to minimize these risks (Mueller 1998; Cantu and Mueller 2003). Sadly, accidents may still happen despite every endeavour and more needs to be done (McIntosh and McCrory 2005).

Protection

Therefore the Second Law of Head Injury is: *If you can't prevent, protect*. The place of head protection should be reviewed carefully, and appropriate head protection worn at all times when the individual is at risk. A cavalier attitude to head injury is inappropriate in today's world, where all have to live by their brains. Likewise, an irresponsible attitude to prevention and protection is likely not only to bring sport into disrepute, as was the case with American college football which was nearly banned by law in the days of Theodore Roosevelt's presidency because of the slaughter it occasioned, but also to attract the attention of lawyers well practised in the extraction of punitive damages from those ignoring simple precautions (Davis and McKelvey 1998).

Major strides have been and continue to be made in head protection (Firth 1994; Levy *et al.* 2004; Hoshizaki and Brien 2004), but again more needs to be done (McIntosh and McCrory 2005; Balendra *et al.* 2008). Where a discipline is such that head injury remains a major hazard, full advantage should be taken of present progress, such as the matching helmets, anti-flailing neck restraints, cockpit margins harness, and safety cages of present Formula 1 motor racing designs. Current specifications are not perfect in any sport, but they reflect the state of the art and therefore should be the minimum acceptable for that sporting activity.

No head injury is necessary in sport; all head injury is potentially preventable, and therefore any head injury has to be unacceptable.

To be effective, protective helmets have to form one unit with the head and skull at impact. Any relative motion between helmet and head may actually exacerbate injury and degrade the helmet's protective performance. Most helmets have an outer shape to provide aesthetic appeal, either a 'hide' or, in riding, 'silk'. Within this is a hard smooth shell to prevent skull penetration and deformation and to facilitate sliding of the helmet along surfaces so as to extend the period of deceleration. Within this 'shell' is an energy-burning acceleration-attenuating 'liner', either an air gap or a 'buffer' material which dissipates energy as it deforms, further extending the time of the deceleration. An air gap is a time-honoured solution to the requirement for energy dissipation. However, it depends for its effectiveness on a very precise relationship between head and shell, with a critical margin for their separation. This must be checked every time that the hat is put on. Buffer materials act by absorbing energy by their own progressive deformation or destruction. They have made possible major improvements in helmet performance. However, once deformed, the buffer's effectiveness is destroyed and the helmet has to be replaced. It will no longer protect from acceleration if it is subjected to a further insult. Within the buffer or air-gap zone is the 'harness', 'cradle', or suspension, which provides the interface between head and helmet. It has to fit snugly, firmly, comfortably, and coolly. It has to ensure that the helmet remains in place under any condition of acceleration, head movement, and impact. It must not be displaced axially or in pitch, roll, or yaw. Maintenance of head–helmet geometry under acceleration usually requires a four-point fixation system with a chin strap. Stabilization forwards and backwards in the sagittal plane conventionally requires two fixation points on each side of the head, four in all. Simple two-point chin straps, even incorporated in complex 'full-face' helmets, still allow helmet loss or separation in violent conditions of head pitch and sagittal plane radial head acceleration, a persisting hazard in motor cycle racing. In single-seat Formula 1 motor racing, progressive developments have positioned the head, body, and limbs within a safety cage, using a five-point harness. Head flailing is restricted by a removable collar, and the helmet–cockpit sill geometry is arranged to allow vision over the sill during normal racing operation with stabilization of the helmet in case of an accident. This simplifies the acceleration environment and extends the head deceleration interval, reducing $\Delta v / t$, as the vehicle progressively collapses about the safety cage. The overall improvement has been spectacular, but helmeted head stabilization remains a major challenge in many disciplines.

In order to satisfy British Standards, European, US, and Australian minimum performance standards, helmet systems:

(1) should be aesthetically attractive, so that all want to wear them, especially the young;

(2) should be mechanically and dynamically effective;

(3) should be comfortable, cool, and light weight;

(4) should be easily, effectively, and conveniently secured, removed, and stored;

(5) should not exacerbate other injury, for instance to the cervical spine or introduce new hazards of their own (Firth 1985).

That these criteria can be met was demonstrated by the commercial introduction of motor cycle 'space helmets' between 1966 and 1968. The protective success of this fashion object can, should, and has been emulated in other sporting disciplines where head protection is appropriate (e.g. BSI 1998). That this can be achieved without increased hazard to the neck, particularly in children, has been confirmed (Macnab *et al.* 2002).

Management strategies

The First Law of Head Injury is to **prevent** and if this fails, the Second Law is to **protect**; if this also fails, the Third Law is to *Prepare for head and spinal injury*. Prudent preparation follows appropriate assessment of the potential for head injury and disaster posed by each sporting discipline. Given such preparation, careful management can then minimize or exclude the secondary and later effects of head injury, if such an accident occurs. In effect, the Third Law of Head Injury can be expanded as *Prepare for the worst, work for the best*.

Having failed to prevent and then to protect the brain, initial assessment is the basis for subsequent successful head and cervical spinal injury management. All head injuries must be assumed to have an unstable cervical spinal injury until proved otherwise. The immediate problem is the infinite combination of head and cervical spinal injury mechanisms available in head injury. The variety of head injury presentation and development creates confusion. Hippocrates (cited by Knight and Rains 1971) noted the poor correlation between initial injury and outcome. A trivial injury can kill, yet a severe initial insult does not guarantee death or a poor outcome, given good management.

Head injury severity

Though head injury is common in sport (MMWR 1997; CDC 1997), serious brain injury is less so. Its comparative rarity ensures that most medical practitioners will be inexperienced in immediate assessment and management when the need arises. The first practical problem following a blow to the head is to assess its significance. This may or may not be obvious.

'Significance' in head insult is best considered as any external sign of head injury and whether sufficient energy has been transferred from head to brain to cause actual brain injury. A significant brain or spinal cord injury is indicated by any neurological symptom or sign, however transient or trivial.

Head injury is 'serious' if sufficient energy has been transferred to the brain to render that individual unconscious, even for a moment, or if his/her mental state is left anything but normal. To be conscious requires the satisfactory function of all parts of the brain. An alteration in conscious level is the best indication of a disturbance somewhere in the brain, that disturbance itself being significant. A disturbance of consciousness, however minor or transient, indicates that sufficient energy was available to fracture the skull, to cause bleeding within the head, to induce autoregulatory failure and vasoparetic brain swelling, and to render that individual a candidate for SIS.

No-one remembers being unconscious. Unconsciousness is accompanied by a longer period of amnesia (loss of memory) both before and after the injury: the pre- and post-traumatic amnesic intervals. The latter is considered to extend until the restoration of continuous memory. It may later be used as an indicator of the severity of that brain insult. Pre-traumatic amnesia of up to 10 minutes is commonplace and may represent disturbance of the initial 'electrical' phase of memory. However, a longer pre-traumatic interval indicates structural brain damage. The fact that many report being 'knocked out' is the result of confabulation, rationalization, and hearsay, often giving rise to a misleading reconstruction of the accident sequence. Independent witnesses should always be sought.

Differential diagnosis

Altered consciousness is not infrequent in sport. Unless the incident is actually observed, an open mind for the differential diagnosis is appropriate. It includes:

(1) sleep, fatigue, and exhaustion;

(2) hypoxia, airway obstruction, pneumothorax;

(3) hypotension, vasovagal faint, cardiac dysrrhythmia, and dehydration;

(4) hyperpyrexia, high fever;

(5) hypoglycaemia;

(6) intoxication (metabolic, electrolytic, or drug-induced);

(7) 'reflex coma'—GILOC in aerobatics or facial impact as in Australian Rules football;

(8) seizure, epilepsy;

(9) narcolepsy (abnormal, day-time somnolence);

(10) fugue (psychiatric);

(11) intracranial catastrophe;

(12) trauma, head injury, with the added hazard of potentially associated spinal injury.

Immediate assessment

Because head and spinal injury go hand in hand, assessment is best made of the whole nervous system. As in all medicine, subsequent successful management depends on the initial assessment. This is based on:

(1) The history to define the details and dynamics, exclude the differential diagnosis, and establish the mechanism of injury and progress since the accident;

(2) physical examination.

In the event, where airway, breathing, circulation, and cervical spine are the priority, the history may have to be brief and expanded later. Yet, however brief, one needs to know the following.

1. Accident: the time, place, circumstances, and details of the accident and injuries.

2. Energy available: the potential for head penetration, deformation, and acceleration, together with that for an associated neck or spinal injury.

3. Conscious level: What is happening to the conscious level? Unconscious at any stage? Still unconsciousness? Unconscious but recovering? Recovered? Recovered but now deteriorating again? Continuous progressive deterioration since the accident? (Fig. 3.2.1)

4. Other neurological symptoms or signs, including arms and legs.

5. Seizure?

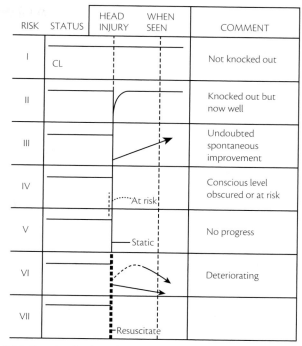

Fig. 3.2.1 Conscious level trends.

The immediate concerns are for ABC.

♦ **Airway.** Ensure that it is clear, get it clear, and keep it clear.

♦ **Breathing.** Is it present and adequate? If not, commence mouth-to-mouth ventilation.

♦ **Circulation, cervical spine, and conscious level:** check that there is a pulse and keep the head and neck straight.

In practice:

1. ABC

2. Position: if airway, breathing, and circulation are satisfactory, leave in the present position or place in the recovery position taking care to maintain head–neck–trunk alignment. If in doubt, lie the victim flat on their back, again with head, neck, and spine moved as one and head–neck–trunk stabilized for fear of neck fracture.

3. Again, check ABC; stop bleeding points with a finger. If ABC satisfactory, continue to watch them until the victim is conscious. If not, proceed as follows.

4. Establish the airway, pulling the jaw and tongue forwards.

5. Commence mouth-to-mouth ventilation and external cardiac massage if adequate breathing or circulation is not demonstrated. With the patient flat, the cerebral circulation is likely to be adequate if there is a carotid, radial, or femoral pulse, provided that venous outflow from the head is not obstructed. Raising the legs together will improve venous return to the heart.

6. If ABC is satisfactory and the patient is cooperative, check whether they can move feet and fingers, legs, arms, and shoulders voluntarily and record what they can and cannot do. If not cooperative, check what they are moving (feet, legs, hands, arms, shoulders). Again, record for the guidance of the hospital team. A suitable form is shown in Table 3.2.3

7. By this stage, conscious level can be defined accurately. It will be apparent whether or not the victim opens their eyes, makes any noise, or moves. These three features—eyes, speech, and movement—provide the most reliable means of recording and communicating conscious level status yet devised, the Glasgow Coma Scale (GCS) (Teasdale and Jennett 1974). Putting numbers on these three features is not easy. In the heat of the moment, many cannot remember the scoring. It is sensible to carry a scoring table (Table 3.2.1) whenever you might encounter injury, and certainly at any and every sporting occasion. The GCS score is re-assessed every 5 minutes and recorded against time. This can be complemented by a limb motor assessment to cover the actual or potential accompanying spinal cord injury. In spinal cord injury, one is concerned for the weakest movement. Power on either side, of foot, leg, hand, arm, and shoulder movement, is best recorded using the Medical Research Council (MRC) motor power (muscle strength) scale (Table 3.2.2). MRC-5 is normal voluntary movement, MRC-0 is no movement, MRC-1 is just detectable, and MRC-3 is able to move against gravity. Recording observations on a sheet greatly aids management. A simple example is given in Table 3.2.3. The importance of timed written observations, together with the history of the injury, for the success of subsequent management cannot be overemphasized. Observation forms can be expanded endlessly, but, to be useful, time, GCS and MRC are the essential minima.

Table 3.2.1 Glasgow Coma Scale score of conscious level

Score	Motor (M)	Conversation (V)	Eye-opening (E)
6	Obeys commands	–	–
5	Localizes pain	Orientated	–
4	Withdraws from pain	Confused	Spontaneous
3	Abnormal flexion	Inappropriate	To speech
2	Extends	Sounds only	To pain
1	Nil	Nil	Nil

Total (M+V+E) =

Table 3.2.2 Medical Research Council movement power score

Score	Movement at joint
5	Normal
4	Strong but not normal
3	Weak but can overcome gravity
2	Movement but not against gravity
1	Movement detected
0	No movement

Table 3.2.3 Observation sheet

Name			
DoB or Age			
Home address and telephone			
Date	Place		
Time and details of accident and injuries			
Observer's name and contact number			
Score	Time		
Motor (M)			
6 Obeys commands			
5 Localizes pain			
4 Withdraws from pain			
3 Abnormal flexion			
2 Extends			
1 Nil			
Conversation (V)			
5 Orientated			
4 Confused			
3 Inappropriate			
2 Sounds only			
1 Nil			
Eye opening (E)			
4 Spontaneous			
3 To speech			
2 To pain			
1 Nil			
GCS Total (M+V+E)			
Pupil size (right, left)			
Limb power (R and L, MRC)	0–5: normal = 5, against gravity = 3, detectable movement = 1, none = 0		
Shoulders			
Arms			
Fingers			
Legs			
Feet/toes			

By using R and L for arms and legs, a single table can be used for both sides. For the pupils, just draw large, small, or equal rings for the pupil size.

Table 3.2.4 Other 'vital signs' for observation sheets, if space allows

Date/Time					
Left pupil					
Right pupil					
Heart rate					
Respiratory rate					
Blood pressure					
Temperature					

8. The 'vital signs': pupillary size and reaction on either side, heart and respiratory rate, blood pressure, and temperature can be added as time and space allow (Table 3.2.4). They are contained in ambulance record sheets.

One or more of these signs will change with the onset of coning at the tentorial hiatus and distortion of the brainstem. This indicates a critical situation at the 'Piccadilly Circus' of the head. The first pupil to enlarge is usually on the same side as the clot and brain swelling causing the cone. Where there is either no scanning available or time is running out, this is a vital indication as to which side requires the first burr hole to start evacuating blood clot and lowering the raised ICP. In sporting head injury, the aim is to have the victim in hospital well before this stage.

Risk status

The assessment of risk is easier if it is based on conscious level once the individual is horizontal with the neck stabilized, ABC established, and an assessment of limb motor function made. Immediate risk is now indicated by conscious level trend once two observations have been made. Progress following head injury falls into one of seven groups, each with its distinctive conscious level trend, each based on improvement or deterioration following the first and subsequent assessments (Table 3.2.5 and Fig. 3.2.1).

Whatever the risk status, all groups need ABC, initial assessment and recorded observation.

- Groups 1–3 need careful observation to ensure that improvement is maintained and that secondary deterioration from swelling, clot, or seizure does not occur. Return to exercise after being knocked out or 'concussed' is foolhardy. It will swell a vasoparetic brain, exacerbate intracranial haemorrhage, and may elicit SIS.

- Group 1 should be put into the care of a responsible adult who can observe the individual for more than 24 hours.

- Groups 2–7 are at risk of the full panoply of post-traumatic complication and merit hospital review.

- Group 4 may need ICP monitoring.

- Groups 5–7 require the immediate control of brain swelling and the exclusion or removal of intracranial clot.

Positioning

Head and spinal injury are more easily managed with the patient horizontal, as long as the airway is clear, breathing and circulation are maintained, and care is taken for an unstable cervical spine with the spinal cord at risk of further injury. However, the supine

Table 3.2.5 Risk groups based on serial assessment.

Risk group	Conscious level profile	Significance
1	Subject to head insult but not knocked out.	Neurological symptoms? If not, unlikely to require assistance.
2	Was unconscious, but has recovered and appears normal by time of assessment.	Potential for intracranial mischief remains. May suffer secondary deterioration. Neurological symptoms? Observe. Hospital.
3	Was knocked out, and still suffering impaired or altered consciousness, though undoubtedly improving.	Recovering, may deteriorate, ABC, observe as 2. Hospital.
4	Difficult to assess because of epilepsy, other injuries sustained, or other treatment in progress.	At risk of every intracranial mischief until proved otherwise. ICP monitoring required. Hospital.
5	Conscious level remains static.	Should be improving, the natural history of recovery following head injury. No improvement means intracranial clot, brain swelling, or both.
6	May have improved initially but is now deteriorating.	*Will die from brain swelling, intracranial blood clot, or both, unless ventilated and clot removed/excluded*
7	Required resuscitation following head injury.	Whole-brain vasoparesis is guaranteed. Immediate ventilation and clot exclusion required.

position requires continuous supervision. ABC observation has to be maintained as the airway is at risk from the tongue falling backwards and obstructing it. If there is no question of head injury and the integrity of the spine is undoubted (as after an uncomplicated spontaneous seizure), the airway can be protected by rolling the individual into the recovery position. However, the essential repeated assessment of the individual's conscious level and limb movements is difficult in the recovery position; ABC has to continue and if there is doubt, they have to be rolled on to their back so that the airway can be restored and maintained, and mouth-to-mouth ventilation and external cardiac massage can be undertaken as necessary.

'Minor' head injury

Where severe injury is present, the ABC requirement and the need for rapid transport on a spinal board to hospital is obvious. 'Minor' head injuries present their own difficulties (Sturmi *et al.* 1998). There may be real uncertainty as to whether or not the conscious level was disturbed. A child or adult under stress may not complain of neurological symptoms—sensory or motor involvement of limbs and body—unless specifically asked for them. Caution is the key and a high index of suspicion is prudent. If the individual is obstreperous, uncooperative, antisocial, or aggressive, this behaviour is itself a sign of frontal lobe injury and reason enough for hospital review. When the individual appears normal, well, and determined to continue the game, the touchstone is altered consciousness. If consciousness was disturbed, then the risk of secondary neurological deterioration can be presumed until such a risk has been judged as remote after an appropriate interval by a properly qualified medical review.

Return to sports after head injury

Though the sporting ethic is to 'press on regardless' in the heroic manner, this otherwise commendable attitude is foolhardy following head injury. Opinion varies as to return after head injury (Cantu 1998b; Sturmi *et al.* 1998). Given the touchstone of an alteration or loss of consciousness, several principles apply in considering when it is reasonable to play or compete again.

1. Early post-traumatic epilepsy may occur at any time during the first week after being knocked out or appearing 'concussed'. It is unwise to risk further brain insult during that period. Two weeks without symptoms is the minimum; a month is prudent.

2. Being knocked out indicates sufficient skull deformation to cause actual skull fracture. Arterial healing cannot be relied on for at least 10 days. Neurosurgeons are not happy about intracranial vascular repair until 6 weeks. The skull takes as long as the femur (thigh bone) to heal and fuse. Unaided, the femur cannot be relied on to bear weight for at least 6 weeks, and 3 months in competition.

3. The incidence of intracerebral haemorrhage into areas of brain contusion is maximum at 10 days; hence the concern over return to competition during the first fortnight following brain insult.

4. The return of cerebrovascular autoregulation (recovery from vasoparesis) cannot be established with certainty by non-invasive means. Transcranial Doppler, NIRSP near infra-red spectrophotometry, and fMR may mislead. A full week, preferably a fortnight, following the cessation of all headache and post-traumatic symptoms is the minimum that can be relied upon.

5. Time and circumstance indicating the cessation of risk for the SIS are debatable. It is unlikely to be less than the 7–14 days for vasoparesis.

6. Persisting symptoms merit neurological review.

7. Individuals with repeated head injury, the effects of which are cumulative but may not yet be obvious to the victim or a lay observer (MMWR 1997; CDC 1997), merit neurological review. In this area of concern for the effects of a too early return to participation or further injury, prepared psychometric protocols are helpful (McCrea *et al.* 1998; Collie *et al.* 2001; Daniel *et al.* 2002).

In practice, the individual should be barred from a return to games or competition until formally assessed by a medical practitioner who is prepared to accept responsibility for the consequences. Once knocked out, even if feeling well, the sportsman or sportswoman should, at least, remain in the care of a responsible adult and their general practitioner directly informed. Return following freedom from symptoms for 2 weeks (Table 3.2.6) and with a letter from one's usual general practitioner (GP) is a reasonable minimum. Skull fracture raises this to 6 weeks.

Communications, back-up, and cover

An on-site, qualified, practised, well-organized, well-led, and motivated medical team with ambulance and/or helicopter back-up for transfer to an alerted trauma unit with neurosurgical cover is the ideal. Whether this is practicable depends on the occasion. At least two Advanced Life Support (ALS) trained individuals on site with telephone communications is a reasonable aim. Provided that ABS and spinal care are available on site and the means to summons an ambulance are to hand, immediate hospital management is available at most accident and emergency departments. However, organizing further investigations and preparing for the removal of intracranial clots takes time. CT head scanning may be required to guide further care. Previous arrangement and prior warning in case of injury allows trauma centre staff and scanners to be prepared and operating theatres to be freed up and made ready. To a degree, this is possible using the ambulance radio network after head injury has occurred. However, a primary requirement in the organization of any sporting event is that the organizers prepare for the worst. This requires liaison, well before an event, with the accident and emergency department within whose catchment area the event is being organized. This is mandatory for an event of any size. Lines of communication can then be established and a plan of disaster management agreed. Without such prior arrangement, opportunities to minimize head injury complication will be lost and questions of neglect of responsibilities of care may be raised.

Sports and head injury overview

Despite best intentions and endeavour, head injuries remain a bane of sport (Cantu 1996). Though head injuries outnumber spinal injury by 10:1, together they cast a shadow over the otherwise welcome increase in participation in and enjoyment of sport, and its contribution to public health. The head injury hazard varies widely between disciplines, but none are immune. Therefore consideration of head injury and cervical spinal cord injury has to be a factor in the following.

♦ Participant selection: the individual's own history is the best guide—based on present symptoms, past history (previous head injury, birth trauma, seizure or febrile convulsions, other neurological conditions, migraine), family history (seizure, head injury, neurological conditions, especially migraine), and

Table 3.2.6 Return to sport after alteration of consciousness

Test	Requirement
History (the most sensitive and specific test)	Personal integrity Reliable observer No symptoms, headache or subjective abnormality
Examination (tests the history)	No physical or neurological signs. No objective abnormality
Investigation (where appropriate)	No abnormality on that appropriate investigation or test
Medical advice	GP letter confirming safe to return (the minimum requirement)
Expert review	Opinion from a specialist, if there is doubt

sporting and social history to date—with examination and a letter from their own GP if in doubt.

◆ Training.

◆ Tactics and their development.

◆ Equipment.

◆ General development of the discipline to reduce hazard while enhancing enjoyment and competitiveness.

◆ Arrangements for assessment and management if head injury occurs.

◆ Criteria for the individual's return to that sport after head injury.

Hopefully, this chapter will be of assistance in addressing these issues.

References

Allen, W.M. (1976). Brain damage in jockeys. *Lancet*, **i**, 1135–6.

Arnold, M., Fischer, U., and Nedeltcher, K. (2009). Carotid artery dissection and sports. *Kardiovasculäre Medizin*, **12**, 209–13.

Bailes, J.E. and Cantu, R.C. (2001). Head injury in athletes. *Neurosurgery*, **48**, 26–46.

Balendra, G., Turner, M., and McCrory, P. (2008). Career-ending injuries to professional jockeys in British horse racing (1991–2005). *British Journal of Sports Medicine*, **42**, 22–4.

Bruce, D.A., Alavi, A., Bilaniuk, L., *et al.* (1981). Diffuse cerebral swelling following head injuries in children. The syndrome of malignant brain oedema. *Journal of Neurosurgery*, **54**, 170–8.

BSI (British Standards Institution) (1998). *PAS 015. Protective Helmets for Equestrian Use*. BSI, London.

Cantu, R.C. (1992). Cerebral concussion in sport. Management and prevention. *Sports Medicine*, **14**, 64–74.

Cantu, R.C. (1996). Head injuries in sport. *British Journal of Sports Medicine*, **30**, 289–96.

Cantu, R.C. (1998a). Second-impact syndrome. *Clinics in Sports Medicine*, **17**, 37–44.

Cantu, R.C. (1998b). Return to play guidelines after a head injury. *Clinics in Sports Medicine*, **17**, 45–60.

Cantu, R. (1998c). Epilepsy and athletics. *Clinics in Sports Medicine*, **17**, 61–9.

Cantu, R.C. (2003). Recurrent athletic head injury: risks and when to retire. *Clinics in Sports Medicine*, **22**, 593–603.

Cantu, R.C. and Mueller, F.O. (2003). Brain injury-related fatalities in American football, 1945–1999. *Neurosurgery*, **52**, 846–53.

CDC (1997). From the Centers for Disease Control and Prevention. Sports-related recurrent brain injuries—United States. *Journal of the American Medical Association*, **277**, 1190–1.

Chen, J.K., Johnston, K.M., Petrides, M., and Ptito, A. (2008). Recovery from mild head injury in sports: evidence from serial functional magnetic resonance imaging studies in male athletes. *Clinical Journal of Sports Medicine*, **18**, 241–7.

Clear, D. and Chadwick, D.W. (2000). Seizures provoked by blows to the head. *Epilepsia*, **41**, 243–4.

Collie, A., Darby, D., and Maruff, P. (2001). Computerised cognitive assessment of athletes with sports related head injuries. *British Journal of Sports Medicine*, **35**, 297–302.

Collie, A., McCrory, P., and Makdissi, M. (2006). Does history of concussion affect current cognitive status? *British Journal of Sports Medicine*, **40**, 550–1. Comment: 40, 802–5.

Cooper, M.T., McGee, K.M., and Anderson, D.G. (2003). Epidemiology of athletic head and neck injuries. *Clinics in Sports Medicine*, **22**, 427–43, vii.

Daniel, J.C., Nassiri, J.D., Wilckens, J., and Land, B.C. (2002) The implementation and use of the standardized assessment of concussion at the U.S. Naval Academy. *Military Medicine*, **167**, 873–6.

Davis, P.M. and McKelvey, M.K. (1998). Medicolegal aspects of athletic head injury. *Clinics in Sports Medicine*, **17**, 71–82.

Foster, J.B., Leiguarda, R., and Tilley, P.J. (1976). Brain damage in National Hunt jockeys. *Lancet*, **i**, 981–3.

Firth, J.L. (1985). Equestrian injuries. In: R.C. Schneider, J.C. Kennedy, and M.L. Plant (eds), *Sports Injuries: Mechanisms, Prevention, and Treatment*, pp. 431–49. Williams & Wilkins, Baltimore, MD.

Firth, J.L. (1994). Equestrian injuries. In: H.U. Fu and D.A. Stone (eds), *Sports Injuries: Mechanisms, Prevention, and Treatment*, pp. 315–31. Williams & Wilkins, Baltimore, MD.

Fountain, N.B. and May, A.C. (2003). Epilepsy and athletics. *Clinics in Sports Medicine*, **22**, 605–16, x–xi.

Gurdjian, E.S., Webster, J.E., and Lissner, H.R. (1950). The mechanisms of skull fracture. *Journal of Neurosurgery*, **7**, 106–14.

Guskiewicz, K.M., McCrea, M., Marshall, S.W., *et al.* (2003) Cumulative effects associated with recurrent concussion in collegiate football players: the NCAA Concussion Study. *Journal of the American Medical Association*, **290**, 2549–55. Comment: 290, 2604–5.

Holbourn, A.H.S. (1943). Mechanics of head injury. *Lancet*, **ii**, 438–41.

Hoshizaki, T.B. and Brien, S.E. (2004). The science and design of head protection in sport. *Neurosurgery*, **55**, 956–67.

Jennett, W.B. (1975). *Epilepsy After Non-Missile Head Injuries* (2nd edn). Heinemann Medical, London.

Jordan, B. (1988). Genetic susceptibility to brain injuries in sports: a role for genetic testing in athletes? *Physician and Sports Medicine*, **26**, 25–6.

Jordan, B., Relkon, N., and Ravdin, L. (1977). Apolipoprotein E epsilon 4 associated with traumatic brain injury in boxing. *Journal of the American Medical Association*, **278**, 136–40.

Kelly, J.P., Nichols, J.S., Filley, C.M., Lillehei, K.O., Rubinstein, D., and Kleinschmidt-DeMasters, B.K. (1991) Concussion in sports. Guidelines for the prevention of catastrophic outcome. *Journal of the American Medical Association*, **266**, 2867–9.

Kirkendall, D.T., Jordan, S.E., and Garrett, W.E. (2001). Heading and head injuries in soccer. *Sports Medicine*, **31**, 369–86.

Knight, G. and Rains, T.J.H. (eds) (1971). *Bailey and Love's Short Practice of Surgery*, p.376. H.K. Lewis, London.

Langfitt, T.W., Marshall, W.J.S., Kassell, N.F., and Schutta, H.S. (1968). The pathophysiology of brain swelling produced by mechanical trauma and hypertension. *Scandinavian Journal of Clinical and Laboratory Investigation, Supplement*, **102**, XIVB.

Levy, M.L., Ozgur, B.M., Berry, C., Aryan, H.E., and Apuzzo, M.L. (2004). Birth and evolution of the football helmet. *Neurosurgery*, **55**, 656–62.

Lindgren, S.O. (1966). Experimental studies on mechanical effects in head injury. *Acta Chirurgica Scandinavica, Supplementum*, **360**, 1–100.

McCrea, M., Kelly, J.P., Randolph, C., *et al.* (1998). Standardized assessment of concussion (SAC): on-site mental status evaluation of the athlete. *Journal of Head Trauma Rehabilitation*, **13**, 27–35.

McCrory, P. (2000). Vertebral artery dissection causing stroke in sport. *J. Clin. Neuroscience*, **7**, 298–300.

McCrory, P. (2001a). Does second impact syndrome exist? *Clinical Journal of Sports Medicine*, **11**, 144–9.

McCrory, P. (2001b). When to retire after concussion? *British Journal of Sports Medicine*, **35**, 380–2.

McCrory, P. (2002). 2002 Refshauge Lecture. When to retire after concussion? *Journal of Science and Medicine in Sport*, **5**, 169–82.

McCrory, P. and Berkovic, S.F (1998a). Concussive convulsions. Incidence in sport and treatment recommendations. *Sports Medicine*, **25**, 131–6.

McCrory, P. and Berkovic, S.F. (1998b). Second impact syndrome. *Neurology*, **50**, 677–83.

McCrory, P. and Berkovic SF (2001). Concussion: the history of clinical and pathophysiological concepts and misconceptions. *Neurology*, **57**, 2283–9.

McCrory, P., Bladin, P.F., and Berkovic, S.F. (1997) Retrospective study of conciussive convulsions in elite Australian rules and rugby leaguefootballers: phenomenology, aetiology and outcome. *British Medical Journal*, **314**, 171–4.

McCrory, P., Berkovic, S.F., and Cordner, S.M. (2000). Deaths due to brain injuries among footballers in Victoria, 1968–1999. *Medical Journal of Australia*, **172**, 217–19.

McIntosh, A.S. and McCrory, P. (2005). Preventing head and neck injury. *British Journal of Sports Medicine*, **39**, 314–18.

McLatchie, G. and Jennett, B. (1994). ABC of sports medicine: head injury in sport. *British Medical Journal*, **308**, 1620–4.

Macnab, A.J., Smith, T., Gagnon, F.A., and Macnab, M. (2002). Effect of helmet wear on the incidence of head/face and cervical spine injuries in young skiers and snowboarders. *Injury Prevention*, **8**, 324–7.

Martland, H.S. (1928). Punch drunk. *Journal of the American Medical Association*, **19**, 1103–7.

Mueller, F.O. (1998). Fatalities from head and cervical spine injuries occurring in tackle football: 50 years' experience. *Clinics in Sports Medicine*, **17**, 169–82.

Miller, J.D. (1979). Intracranial mass lesions. In: A.J. Popp *et al.* (eds), *Neural Trauma*, pp. 173–80. Raven Press, New York.

MMWR (Morbidity Mortality Weekly Report) (1997). Sports-related recurrent brain injuries—United States, **46**, 224–7.

Mori, T., Katayama, Y., and Kawamata, T. (2006). Acute hemispheric swelling associated with thin subdural hematomas: pathophysiology of repetitive head injury in sports. *Acta Neurochirurgica Supplementum*, **96**, 40–3.

Naunheim, R.S., Bayly, P.V., Standeven, J., Neubauer, J.S., Lewis, L.M., and Genin, G.M. (2003). Linear and angular head accelerations during heading of a soccer ball. *Medicine and Science in Sports and Exercise*, **35**, 1406–12.

Park, M.S. and Levy, M.L. (2008). Biomechanical aspects of sports-related head injuries. *Neurologic Clinics*, **26**, 33–43, vii.

Robbins, S.L., Contran, R.S., and Kumar V. (eds) (1984). *Pathologic Basis of Disease* (3rd edn), pp. 1374–7. W.B.Saunders, Philadelphia, PA.

Saunders, R.L. and Harbaugh, R.E. (1984). The second impact in catastrophic contact—sports head trauma. *Journal of the American Medical Association*, **252**, 538–9.

Schneider, R.C. (1987). Football head and neck injury. *Surgical Neurology*, **27**, 507–8.

Sheinker, I.M. (1944). Vasoparalysis of the central nervous systems. A characteristic vascular syndrome. *Archives of Neurology and Psychology*, **52**, 43–56.

Strich, S.J. (1956). Diffuse degeneration of the cerebral white matter in severe dementia following head injury. *Journal of Neurology and Psychiatry*, **19**, 163–85.

Strich, S.J. (1961). Shearing of nerve fibres as a cause of brain damage due to head injury. *Lancet*, **ii**, 443–8.

Strich, S.J. (1969). Pathology of brain damage due to blunt head injury. In: A.E. Walker, W.F. Covaness, and M. Critchicy (eds), *Late Effects of Head Injury*, pp. 501–26. C.C. Thomas, Springfield, IL.

Sturmi, J.E., Smith, C., and Lombardo, J.A. (1998). Mild brain trauma in sports. Diagnosis and treatment guidelines. *Sports Medicine*, **25**, 351–8.

Teasdale, G. and Jennett, W.B. (1974). The Glasgow Coma Scale. *Lancet*, **ii**, 81–4.

Wills, S.M. and Leathem, J.M. (2001). Sports-related brain injury research: methodological difficulties associated with ambiguous terminology. *Brain Injury*, **15**, 545–648.

3.3

Oral and maxillofacial sports injuries

Andrew Gibbons and Neil MacKenzie

Introduction

In sport, the face is frequently the most exposed part of the body. The incidence of sports facial injuries varies hugely around the world, according to the sports played in a particular country. In the USA, approximately 12% of maxillofacial injuries seen in large trauma centres are sports related (Echlin and McKeag 2004). In the UK, a prospective study showed that sports-related maxillofacial trauma accounts for 1% of all attendances at accident and emergency departments (Hill *et al.* 1998), whilst a similar study in Switzerland gave a figure of 1.3% (Exadaktylos *et al.* 2004). Rugby was the sport most commonly associated with injury in the UK, followed by cycling and football. Over 50% of maxillofacial sports injuries in New Zealand are associated with rugby (Antoun and Lee 2008). By comparison, skiing and snowboarding cause the most maxillofacial sports injuries in Switzerland (Exadaktylos *et al.* 2004). Baseball and softball are the leading cases of sports-related facial trauma in the USA (Bak and Doerr 2004).

The UK study showed that most sports-related maxillofacial injuries are soft tissue trauma, which accounts for 80% of patients (Hill *et al.* 1998). Dentoalveolar trauma comprised 11% and only 9% of injuries were facial fractures. Out of 760 patients, the upper third ($n = 257$) and middle third ($n = 201$) of the face were the most frequently injured sites. Injuries to the lip and mouth ($n = 188$) and the mandible area ($n = 124$) were less common. The majority of maxillofacial sports injuries occur in young males between the ages of 18 and 25 (Thomas and Hill 1999). Despite maxillofacial sports injuries being generally less serious than those sustained in road traffic accidents or assaults, fractures remain common, especially in ice and snow sports and cycling (Tanaka *et al.* 1996; Emshoff *et al.* 1997; Bak and Doerr 2004). Le Fort fractures (see section on mechanisms and sites of trauma) are seen more frequently in mountain bike accidents than in many other sports (Gassner *et al.* 1999). Horse-riding and, in particular, horse-kick injuries can lead to severe maxillofacial trauma (Lim *et al.* 1993). Certain sports are related to specific types of facial fractures. Although football (soccer) is a relatively non-violent sport, elbow to head and head to head contact lead to a high proportion of nasal and zygomatic fractures (Cerulli *et al.* 2002). The mandibular angle is a common site of fracture in rugby and football (Mourouzis and Koumoura 2005; Antoun and Lee 2008).

Applied anatomy

The face contains the sensory organs for sight, smell, and taste. At the posterior aspect of the face, the ears communicate with the sensory organs for hearing and balance within the bony cranium. The skin and mucous membranes of the face contribute to the sensation of touch. However, the face contains no organ vital to life apart from the airway. Therefore maintaining the airway is of prime importance in facial injury. When an injury causes significant trauma to the face, adjacent anatomical structures may be damaged. There should be a high index of suspicion of brain or cervical spine injury when there are significant facial injuries.

The face can be divided into three parts. The upper third consists of the forehead over the frontal bone. The mid-face comprises the orbits, nose, zygomatic complexes, and maxilla. The lower third of the face includes the mouth, teeth, and mandible.

Sight is the predominant sense in humans. The eyes are set back in protective eye sockets and the flexibility of the neck and upper torso allow binocular vision to be brought quickly onto an object. With smell a much less important sense and the brain size much larger than other animals, the facial muzzle is placed under the cranium. The face contains the maxillary, ethmoid, frontal, and sphenoid sinuses which help to lighten the weight of the head on the neck. In addition, they humidify air and give resonance to the voice. In facial trauma, the sinuses act as crumple zones to dissipate energy and protect the eyes and the brain.

Struts of dense bone around the orbits, sinuses, nasal and oral airways, and teeth give three-dimensional support to the face (Fig. 3.3.1). The zygomatic arches give the anterior projection of the mid-face. The zygomatic buttresses and the supra- and infra-orbital rims connected centrally by the nasal bones are the horizontal pillars of the mid-face and determine its width. The vertical pillars of the mid-face are the dense bones around the nasal airway, the zygomatic buttresses at the prominence of the cheeks, and the pterygoid plates at the back of the maxilla. These vertical pillars determine the height of the mid-face.

In treating mid-face trauma it is important to position the horizontal and vertical bony pillars precisely. As the bone is dense in the areas of the pillars, they can be held in place by miniplates and screws. The mandibular ramus gives the posterior height of the lower face. The occlusion of the mandibular teeth with the maxillary

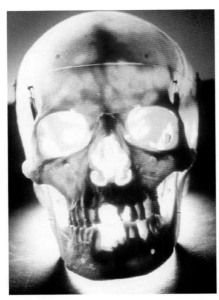

Fig. 3.3.1 Illuminated skull showing the dark areas of dense bone around the orbits, nose, maxillary sinuses, and teeth that support the face.

teeth determines the three-dimensional position of the mandible and lower face. Hence establishing the patient's correct occlusion will accurately reduce most fractures of the lower half of the face.

The facial muscles are important in humans for expression and communication. They are innervated by the five branches of the facial nerve: temporal, zygomatic, buccal, marginal mandibular, and cervical. The proximal ends of these nerves pass deep within the parotid gland and are usually only damaged in severe penetrating or crushing injuries. However, the peripheral branches centrally are more superficial and can be damaged by more superficial trauma.

The trigeminal nerve supplies sensation to the face and movement of the muscles of mastication. It has three main divisions: ophthalmic, maxillary, and mandibular. Sensory nerves of the face are often damaged in facial fractures because many branches pass through the bones and create points of weakness through which fractures often pass. In the upper third of the face the supra-orbital branch of the ophthalmic division may be damaged in frontal sinus trauma, leading to numbness over the ipislateral forehead. In the mid-face, trauma to the orbital floor or the zygomatic complex may damage the infra-orbital branch of the maxillary division. The nerve exits onto the cheek at the infra-orbital foramen just below the orbital rim and is frequently contused in soft tissue trauma to the cheek. If the infra-orbital nerve is damaged an area of numbness may extend from the lateral aspect of the nose to cheek prominence and from the lower eyelid to the upper lip. Damage to branches of the maxillary nerves that cross the thin walls of the maxillary antrum may cause numbness of the upper teeth. This can occur in maxillary or zygomatic complex trauma. The inferior alveolar branch of the mandibular division enters the mandibular foramen within the mandibular ramus and passes through bone to exit at the mental foramen between the roots of the lower premolar teeth. It then supplies sensation to the chin and lower lip. Damage to the inferior alveolar nerve when the mandible is fractured or from bruising where it exits the mandible at the mental foramen will cause numbness to the lip and chin.

The blood supply to the face is mainly supplied from branches of the external carotid artery. The internal carotid artery supplies branches to the forehead and nasal regions via the ophthalmic artery. There is a rich blood supply to the face, with anastomosis between the internal and external carotid systems on both sides and across the midline. The bones of the face can be stripped from periosteum to allow placement of miniplates at fracture sights and still heal extremely well. The common carotid artery and internal jugular vein lie beneath the thick sternocleidomastoid muscle of the neck which to some extent protects them.

Mechanisms and sites of trauma

Penetrating trauma causes most injury along the tract of the inserted object. In contrast, blunt trauma dissipates energy over a wider area. Points of weakness in the facial skeleton lead to classical fracture patterns (Fig. 3.3.2). These types of facial fractures are commonly seen in sports injuries where the majority of trauma is blunt. The mandible often breaks at the parasymphysis at the site of the canine tooth and at the angle through the site of a non-erupted third molar. The long root of the canine and the buried third molar tooth both act as points of bony weakness. In addition, the natural curvatures of the mandible serve to concentrate force in these regions when the mandible is struck by a blunt object. The condylar neck is another weak point in the mandible and is a common site of fracture. The mandible frequently fractures in two places.

At the end of the nineteenth century Le Fort discovered the natural lines of weakness in the mid-face by dropping weights onto the faces of dead convicts. The Le Fort I fracture passes through the base of the nose and the lower aspect of the pterygoid plates and separates the teeth and palate from the mid-face. A high pyramidal fracture (Le Fort II) passes through the maxillary sinus, the floor and medial wall of the orbit and the lower aspect of the nasal bridge, and through the mid-aspect of the pterygoid plates. A Le Fort III fracture passes through the zygomatic arch and the zygomatico-frontal suture, along the lateral and medial orbital walls and the upper aspect of the bridge of the nose, and through the upper aspect of the pterygoid plates. Thus the face is separated from the cranium. Le Fort II and III fractures are frequently associated with

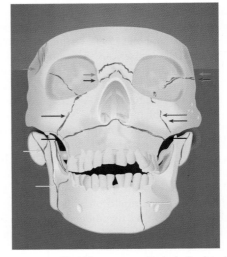

Fig. 3.3.2 Common sites of facial fracture: mandibular (yellow), Le Fort I (black), Le Fort II (blue), Le Fort III (green), and zygomatic (red).

brain damage and can lead to a cerebrospinal fluid leak through the nose. The medial wall and floor of the orbit are naturally weak areas that give way and absorb energy when a blow to the globe of the eye occurs. Cheek bone fractures pass through the outer aspect of the mid-face and involve the combined Le Fort II and III lines of weakness laterally. However, the fracture lines join up in the inferior orbital fissure and do not involve the nose or pterygoid plates.

In blunt soft tissue trauma, splinting of the skin frequently occurs along natural skin creases that act as points of weakness (Langer's lines). These scars often heal well with minimal residual scarring. In penetrating trauma and in blunt trauma with higher energy transfer, skin may be divided along non-anatomical planes. The underlying muscles pull the wound edges apart and tension forces within the skin lead to less aesthetic healing. The resulting scars often require revision to achieve an optimum aesthetic outcome.

Emergency management of facial trauma

The principles of Advanced Trauma Life Support (ATLS) (American College of Surgeons 2004)—airway with cervical spine immobilization, breathing, circulation, neurological deficit treatment—should be applied to all cases of facial trauma. The airway is at risk if the mid-face has been driven backwards in severe Le Fort trauma, if the tongue falls backwards in severe mandibular trauma, and if bleeding, swelling, or fragments of teeth or dentures cause obstruction. If the patient is unconscious, the force may have been sufficient to cause a cervical spine injury. Therefore the cervical spine should be immobilized, and if there are any airway problems simple chin lift or jaw thrust manoeuvres are performed and the mouth cleared of tooth fragments, debris, and blood clots. An airway adjunct such as a Guedel oral airway or nasopharyngeal airway can then be inserted. A definitive endotracheal airway is necessary to definitively protect the airway, but this should only be placed by trained personnel. A conscious patient with airway problems due to facial trauma will try to sit up and lean forward to maintain their airway and spit out debris and blood. A nasopharyngeal airway adjunct is usually well tolerated in the conscious patient but should not be placed with any suspicion of Le Fort II or III fractures as it may inadvertently enter the anterior cranial fossa. The cervical spine should be assessed for signs and symptoms of fracture, and if any exist or the injury has involved a great deal of force, the cervical spine should be immobilized. If no cervical spine injury is detected and the patient requires removal from the field of play on a stretcher, he/she should be placed on their side, if possible, to help keep the airway open.

External and intra-oral bleeding can be treated by applying firm pressure to the area using a gauze square. The patient will be more comfortable sitting up or on their side to help spit blood out and protect the airway. A nosebleed can often be stopped by squeezing the nasal bridge just below the nasal bones at Little's area.

Cold compresses can be applied to the site of the injury and analgesics given with a small sip of water. However, the patient should refrain from eating or drinking until fully assessed by a clinician as a general anaesthetic may be required to treat injuries. Provided that there is no airway problem, a barrel bandage can be placed to support mandibular fractures. Simply applying a wire round adjacent teeth at the fracture site and tightening it may help to reduce and support the fracture enough to treat the pain. A local anaesthetic block (haematoma block) may help with pain in mandibular fractures. Any treatment given must be carefully documented.

Assessment of maxillofacial injuries

Examination for maxillofacial injuries takes place as part of the secondary ATLS survey after life-threatening injuries have been dealt with (Ceallaigh et al. 2006). A systematic assessment is made starting at the cervical spine, proceeding over the scalp and face, and finishing at the neck. All areas are assessed for pain, swelling, bleeding and bruising, lacerations, bony deformity, loss of movement or function, and numbness. It is important to look for bony damage in addition to soft tissue injuries as swelling may mask an underlying fracture.

Once the cervical spine has been assessed, all aspects of the scalp are inspected and palpated from occiput to forehead. Scalp lacerations are commonly missed. The face is most easily examined from top to bottom in a sequential manner. Firstly the forehead is assessed. Then the ears, cheekbones, orbits, and nose are examined on each side. Blood or cerebrospinal fluid leak from the ears or bruising over the mastoid bone may indicate middle cranial fossa trauma. Any indentation or deformity of the cheeks or nose may indicate a fracture. This is best assessed by standing behind the patient looking at the face from above and comparing right with left. Nasal bone fractures are common, but it is important to ask if the patient has had a previous fracture to avoid trying to treat old healed deformities. The nose is also inspected from below, looking for septal haematomas, as these will require early treatment in order to avoid septal cartilage necrosis. Palpation of the zygomatic arches, buttresses, infra-orbital rims, and nose will detect any depressions, steps, or tenderness. Numbness over the cheeks will be due to damage of the infra-orbital nerve and gives a high index of suspicion of orbital floor, zygomatic complex, or Le Fort II fractures. If marked bruising is seen around the eye or on the eye (sub-conjunctival haemorrhage) or if mid-face fractures are detected, there is a chance that some damage has occurred to the globe. Eye movements should be assessed for diplopia, visual acuity recorded with a Snellen chart, and fundoscopy performed. An ophthalmic opinion should also be sought (Gibbons et al. 2004). Orbital floor fractures present with numbness on the cheek due to damage to the infra-orbital nerve and with diplopia and enophthalmos.

The lips are then assessed, followed by the oral cavity. Any missing teeth should be accounted for and if there is any possibility that they may have been inhaled a chest radiograph is required. The oral mucosa and tongue are inspected for cuts and bruises.

A bruise in the floor of the mouth is strongly suggestive of a mandibular fracture. The teeth should be brought together to assess the occlusion. If they do not meet evenly, this frequently indicates a fracture of the mandible or, more rarely, the maxilla. Occasionally a dislocated temporomandibular jaw joint or joint effusion may disrupt the occlusion. Limited mouth opening may be due to bruising of the temporomandibular joint or the muscles of mastication, but is also an important sign of a mandibular fracture. The upper incisors should be grasped between the thumb and fingers of a gloved hand and a gentle but firm attempt made to move them. If Le Fort I fractures are present, the upper jaw can be felt to move at the base of the nose with the other hand. If a Le Fort II fracture is present movement will be felt at the infra-orbital rim. If a Le Fort III fracture is present, slight movement may be detected at the zygomatico-frontal suture on the lateral margin of the orbit. The zygomatic buttress in the buccal sulcus adjacent to the upper first molar will be tender to palpation if zygomatic complex (cheekbone) fractures exist. The mandible is then palpated externally, looking for tenderness. If a fracture runs through any of the teeth sockets a step may be seen by the tooth in the alveolus. By gently grasping the jaw with one hand in front of the suspected fracture and one hand behind and applying mild movement, mobility of parts may be detected confirming the diagnosis. It should be borne in mind that any deep laceration on the face may have a fracture beneath it, especially over the mandible. Numbness of the lower lip or chin indicates bruising to the inferior alveolar nerve and is commonly associated with mandibular fractures. The neck should be inspected for any damage. Neck lacerations deep to the platysma muscle should not be explored. These injuries require treatment in theatre so that if bleeding occurs it can be optimally managed.

After completing a systematic examination of the head and neck, an assessment of the cranial nerves should be performed and the findings recorded.

Radiographs of the face are then ordered to confirm or refute the clinical diagnosis. However, nasal fractures are always a clinical diagnosis and a radiograph is not required to decide if treatment is necessary in simple cases. The mandible can be evaluated using oblique lateral radiographs or orthopentomogram (Fig. 3.3.3), and a postero-anterior view. Using two views at right angles to each other allows the full displacement of fracture ends to be appreciated. The mid-face and zygomatic arches can be assessed by occipito-mental views at 10° and 30°. Isolated fractures of the zygomatic arch are best viewed on a submento-vertex radiograph. Lateral skull views provide additional information in mid-face trauma. Computed tomography (CT) should be used to assess orbital and complex facial trauma. Three-dimensional reconstructions are particularly useful in assessing complex facial trauma (Fig. 3.3.4).

Medical and social histories should be detailed along with a history of the injury event

Particular attention should be paid to any loss of consciousness and the amount of force received in sustaining the trauma. The patient's tetanus status should also be confirmed.

Treatment of facial fractures

Facial fractures that are undisplaced or minimally displaced can often heal without problems provided that there is little movement at the fracture site during function (Fig. 3.3.3). The minimally disrupted periosteum and soft tissues act to splint the fracture and, as no space exists between the fractured bone ends, they interlock together but with reduced load-bearing ability. Where there is

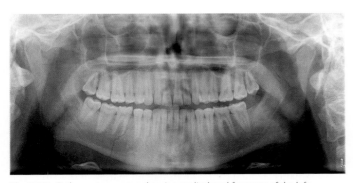

Fig. 3.3.3 Orthopentomogram showing undisplaced fractures of the left mandibular condyle and right mandibular body sustained from a rugby injury that healed uneventfully without active surgical treatment.

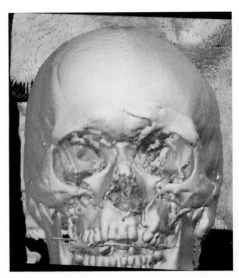

Fig. 3.3.4 Three-dimensional CT reconstruction of severe mid-face and frontal sinus trauma sustained in a motor vehicle accident.

comminution, displacement of bone fragments that is greater than 2 mm, or disruption to the occlusion, active treatment is usually required to gain good functional and aesthetic outcomes. Securing the teeth together locked in occlusion (intermaxillary fixation) will reduce and fix most fractures of the tooth-bearing mandible and is still used as a simple treatment in some cases. However, most facial and mandibular fractures are treated using thin miniplates (Fig. 3.3.5). These are placed directly over fracture sites via open external incisions in aesthetic skin creases or via intra-oral mucosal incisions. As the fracture ends abut together, functional loads from eating and talking are borne by the plate and the bone during healing (load-sharing miniplates). In the mandible, where bone is missing, or in complex comminuted fractures, thicker plates are often used to take all the functional load and support bone grafts (load-bearing reconstruction plates). Orbital wall fractures may be repaired with titanium mesh (Fig. 3.3.5). Patients with fractures involving the antrum, such as zygomatic, Le Fort I or II, or orbital floor fractures, should not blow their nose for 3 weeks whilst the fractures heal to prevent the risks of surgical emphysema and infection.

Treatment of facial lacerations

Lacerations should be thoroughly cleaned to prevent infection and tattooing. Where there is impregnated dirt, scrubbing with a brush and pulsed lavage may be required. The patient's tetanus status must be evaluated and any damage to sensory or motor nerves recorded. Vessels within the face can be freely tied and wound margins only require excision of clearly dead and necrotic tissue. Small flaps of skin and soft tissue with only tenuous blood supplies often heal if carefully sutured. Surgery can often be performed under local anaesthesia, but deep wounds should be explored in theatre under general anaesthetic. The wounds are closed in layers. Deeper tissues are apposed using 3/0 vicryl sutures and the skin closed with fine monofilament sutures such as 5/0 ethilon. Skin sutures should be removed early (after 4 or 5 days) and wound edges supported with adhesive Steri-strips. After a few weeks scars

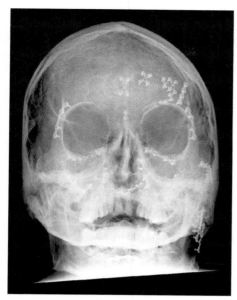

Fig. 3.3.5 Postero-anterior facial radiograph of fracture treatment with miniplates.

frequently appear red and lumpy, but after 6–9 months they fade, flatten, and soften. Patients should be advised to avoid tanning the scars during healing as this may lead to permanent pigmentation in the scar. Nasal septum and ear haematomas should be aspirated or surgically evacuated early to reduce the risk of cartilage necrosis.

Treatment of tooth and dentoalveolar fractures

Patients with broken teeth should see a dental surgeon as soon as possible. Fractures through the enamel or dentine of the tooth crown may be restored with adhesive restorations. If the tooth nerve is damaged, a root canal filling is usually needed. Root fractures often result in the tooth requiring extraction. If the tooth is knocked out it should be washed with clean water and replaced in the tooth socket the correct way round as soon as possible. The root surface should not be handled. If the tooth cannot be replaced, it should be stored in contact lens saline or milk as a transport medium. The tooth should be re-implanted within 2 hours, usually under local anaesthetic, by a dental surgeon. It will then be splinted with wire or a mouth guard for 10 days and a course of antibiotics prescribed. After a few weeks, when the tooth is firm, it will need a root canal treatment.

Rehabilitation, complications, and return to sporting activities

It is important that patients have a balanced and nutritious diet during recovery from facial injuries. This will frequently involve taking a soft diet for 3–6 weeks. It is often easier to take five small meals a day than three large meals. Before discharge from hospital, patients should receive advice from a dietician.

Bruising, swelling, and trismus generally take 3 weeks to resolve depending on the severity of trauma and the treatment. Infection prolongs the healing process and often requires the fracture to be treated with more invasive rigid plating techniques. Numbness of sensory nerves on the face may take up to 18 months to resolve, but some decrease in sensation may be permanent if severe nerve injury has taken place.

In young healthy people fractures of the mandible take 3 weeks to unite to a degree that they do not need support to maintain their position (Banks 1991). However, they usually require at least 4–6 weeks to achieve adequate strength for the patient to return to sporting activities, and this is the period usually advised for facial fractures that have been well treated (Echlin and McKeag 2004; Crow 1991). Some authors recommend 8–12 weeks for mandibular fractures treated with intermaxillary fixation (Tanaka *et al.* 1996). Factors that predispose the patient to take longer to heal include being over 40 years of age, the amount of displacement of the fracture ends, the presence of infection, the number of fractures, and method used to immobilize the fracture. Miniplate immobilization of fractures allows immediate mouth opening and an early return to full function. They also lend mechanical strength to the fracture site in the early stages of healing. Hence, plated facial fractures that heal well allow an earlier return to sporting activities at 4–6 weeks. An assessment of the likelihood of a new blow to the face needs to be made. A longer period of recovery will be required for sports such as rugby and football, where the risk of a repeat blow to the face is high. Nevertheless, after a period of 3–4 weeks, patients with miniplate fixation of fractures can return to exercise. Heavy lifting or weight training often require the teeth to be held firmly in occlusion on excursion, and thus these activities should not be undertaken for at least 6 weeks.

Prevention

Facial protection has decreased injuries to the face in sports such as American football, hockey, and baseball (Crow 1991). Cycle helmets have also become popular, and as well as giving protection to the head they reduce the number and severity of injuries to the upper half of the face. In baseball, a 'C-Flap' polycarbonate and foam guard added to helmets and overlying the temporal and cheek region has proved particularly effective in preventing facial injuries. Mouth guards have had a significant impact on reducing tooth and lip injuries (Hill *et al.* 2003). They protect the teeth, and as they absorb and distribute the force of jaw impacts, they decrease the risk of mandibular fractures (Ranalli 2000). By holding the lips and cheeks away from the teeth they protect against oral lacerations. Mouth guards must be properly fitted, as if they are loose or bulky they will not work properly and may not be worn.

References

American College of Surgeons (2004). *Advanced Trauma Life Support for Doctors. Student Course Manual* (7th edn). American College of Surgeons, Chicago, IL.

Antoun, J.S. and Lee, H.J. (2008). Sports-related maxillofacial fractures over an 11-year period. *Journal of Oral and Maxillofacial Surgery*, **66**, 504–8.

Bak, M.J. and Doerr, T.D. (2004). Craniomaxillofacial fractures during recreational baseball and softball. *Journal of Oral and Maxillofacial Surgery*, **62**, 1209–12.

Banks, P. (1991). Fractures of the tooth-bearing section of the mandible. In: P. Banks (ed), *Killey's Fractures of the Mandible*, pp. 40–79. Butterworth Heinemann, London.

Ceallaigh, P.O., Ekanaykaee, K. Beirne, C.J., and Patton D.W. (2006). Diagnosis and management of common maxillofacial injuries in the emergency department. Part 1: Advanced trauma life support. *Emergency Medicine Journal*, **23**, 796–7.

Cerulli, G., Carboni, A., Mercurio, A., Pergugini, M., and Becelli, R. (2002). Soccer-related craniomaxillofacial injuries. *Journal of Craniofacial Surgery*, **13**, 627–30.

Crow, R.W. (1991). Diagnosis and management of sports-related injuries to the face. *Dental Clinics of North America*, **35**, 719–32.

Echlin, P. and McKeag, D.B. (2004). Maxillofacial injuries in sports. *Current Sports Medical Reports*, **3**, 25–32.

Emshoff, R., Schöning, H., Röthler, G., and Waldhart, E. (1997). Trends in the incidence and cause of sport-related mandibular fractures: a retrospective analysis. *Journal of Oral and Maxillofacial Surgery*, **55**, 585–92.

Exadaktylos, A.K., Eggensperger, N.M., Smolka, K.M., Zimmermann, H., and Lizuka, T. (2004). Sports related maxillofacial injuries: the first maxillofacial trauma database in Switzerland. *British Journal of Sports Medicine*, **38**, 750–3.

Gassner, R., Tull, T., Emshoff, R., and Waldhart, E. (1999). Mountainbiking—a dangerous sport: comparison with bicycling on oral and maxillofacial trauma. *International Journal of Oral and Maxillofacial Surgery*, **28**, 188–91.

Gibbons, A.J., Kittur, M.A., Dhariwal, D.K., Laws, D., and Sugar, A.W. (2004). A form for referral of injured patients between maxillofacial and ophthalmology units. *British Journal of Oral and Maxillofacial Surgery*, **42**, 339–41.

Hill, C.M., Burford, K, Martin, A., and Thomas, D.W. (1998). A one year review of maxillofacial sports injuries treated at an accident and emergency department. *British Journal of Oral and Maxillofacial Surgery*, **36**, 44–7.

Hill, C.M., Eppley, B.L., Thomas, D.W., and Bond S.E. (2003). Etiology prevention of craniofacial trauma. In: P. Ward Booth, B.L. Eppley, and R. Schmelzeissen (ed), *Maxillofacial Trauma and Esthetic Facial Reconstruction*, pp. 3–19. Churchill Livingstone, London.

Lim, L.H, Moore, M.H, Trott, J.A., and David, D.J. (1993). Sports-related facial fractures: a review of 137 patients. *Australia and New Zealand Journal of Surgery*, **63**, 784–9.

Mourouzis, C. and Komoura, F. (2005). Sports-related maxillofacial fractures: a retrospective study of 125 patients. *International Journal of Oral and Maxillofacial Surgery*, **34**, 635–8.

Ranalli, D.N. (2000). Prevention of sports-related traumatic dental injuries. *Dental Clinics of North America*, **44**, 35–51.

Tanaka, N., Hayashi, S., Amagasa, T., and Kohama, G. (1996). Maxillofacial fractures sustained during sports. *Journal of Oral Maxillofacial Surgery*, **54**, 715–19.

Thomas, D.W. and Hill, C.M. (1999). Etiology and changing patterns of maxillofacial trauma. In: P.W. Ward Booth, A.S. Schendel, and J. Hausamen (eds), *Maxillofacial Surgery* Vol. 1, pp. 3–10. Churchill Livingstone, London.

3.4

Regional injuries of the cervical spine: sports-related anatomical, pathophysiological, and clinical perspectives

Ezequiel Gherscovici, Eli Baron,
and Alexander Vaccaro

Introduction

Cervical spine injuries occur infrequently on the athletic field (Dietz and Lillegard 1999). Nevertheless, sporting events have been reported as the fourth most common cause of spinal cord injury (behind motor vehicle collisions, assaults, and falls) (NSCISC 2006). The possibility of catastrophic cervical spine injury exists with involvement in sports, where it can be defined as 'structural distortion of the cervical spinal column associated with actual or potential damage to the spinal cord'. This may result in irreversible neurological injury to the athlete (Banerjee et al. 2004).

The sports most commonly associated with cervical spine injuries include American football, ice hockey, gymnastics, rugby, and diving. Because of their highly regulated nature, organized football, ice hockey, and gymnastics are most amenable to preventative changes that reduce the likelihood of cervical spine injuries. Diving injuries often occur in recreational diving; high-risk behaviour in this setting is more difficult to address (Wetzler et al. 1996; Dietz and Lillegard 1999; Quarrie et al. 2002).

Given the relative infrequency of these injuries, few physicians have experience in the emergency care of serious cervical spine injuries in the sports setting. The equipment typically worn by the player on the field can further complicate the assessment and immobilization processes. Improper handling of the cervical spine on the field or during transport can worsen spinal cord injury and possibly compromise cardiac and respiratory status. Therefore the physician must have specialized training in the care of the injured athlete in this setting (Banerjee et al. 2004).

Definitions and classifications

Minor injuries to the cervical spine

Minor injuries to the cervical spine are those where fractures do not occur or are not readily apparent and significant discoligamentous injury is absent. These are usually classified as soft tissue injuries (Bogduk and Yoganandan 2001).

Cervical strain

A cervical strain is an injury to the cervical musculature (Dietz and Lillegard 1999). There are no bony or neurological injuries with cervical strains. Radiographs show no subluxations or abnormal curves (Cantu et al. 1998).

Cervical sprain

Cervical sprain refers to a ligamentous injury of the cervical spine. Cervical sprains have been subclassified as mild (grade I), i.e. damage to ligamentous structures but no ligamentous lengthening, moderate (grade II), i.e. ligamentous laxity remains after the injury without total disruption, and severe (grade III), i.e. ligamentous disruption. Cervical sprain is rarely an isolated entity. The symptoms of muscle spasm and pain may lead the clinician to diagnose the injured athlete with a cervical strain (Dietz and Lillegard 1999). Dynamic films, as discussed below, may aid the clinician in differentiating cervical sprain from cervical strain.

Whiplash

Whiplash is a soft tissue injury to the cervical spine. Many patients complain of symptoms far beyond a time frame where the injuries would be expected to heal. Minor injuries to the discs, facet joints, and joints of Luschka have been implicated as the patho-aetiology of whiplash (Bogduk and Yoganandan 2001). However, the term whiplash lacks exact definition, and may be used synonymously with cervical sprain syndrome (Sidhu and Fischgrund 2003).

Common cervical spine fractures and dislocations

Upper cervical spine
Jefferson fracture

A Jefferson fracture occurs when the ring of the atlas fails in tension as a result of axial loading. Typically, this results in the ring sustaining three or four vertical fractures. These are commonly seen after diving and striking the head or with falling from a height (Bassewitz and Herkowitz 2003).

Odontoid fractures

Fractures of the odontoid usually result from a blow to the occiput. Clinical presentation is variable and ranges from neck tenderness and spasm to cord compression (Andreychick 2003). Odontoid fractures are subclassified based on fracture location and morphology within the dens; fracture subtype influences treatment in terms of conservative versus surgical management (Grauer *et al.* 2005).

Hangman's fractures

These fractures are variants of traumatic spondylolisthesis of the axis. Their mechanism of injury is quite different from that of judicial hanging. The most common mechanism responsible for this injury is extension combined with axial loading (Hankins *et al.* 2003).

Atlantoaxial rotatory instability

Atlantoaxial rotatory instability is more common in children than in adults. This type of injury may occur as a result of a flexion–extension mechanism coupled with a rotary force. There may be an associated bony fracture. Classically, patients present with neck pain and torticollis (Vaccaro *et al.* 2003).

Lower cervical spine:

Compressive flexion injuries

These fractures are produced by an axial load on a flexed spine. Commonly, this is seen as the result of a shallow dive. In their more severe stages these injuries are classically associated with a large triangular anterior bone fragment with the fracture extending from the anterior surface of the vertebral body to the inferior subchondral plate (Vives *et al.* 2003).

Vertical compression fractures (burst fracture)

These injuries occur as a result of a compressive force with the neck in a neutral position. These injuries tend to be in the lower cervical spine. The posterior vertebral body may be displaced into the spinal canal resulting in neurological deficit (McGuire 2003).

Flexion–distraction injuries

These include a spectrum of injuries including flexion sprain, unilateral facet dislocation, bilateral facet dislocations, and, the most severe, complete translation and distraction of the motion segment (Figure 3.4.1). Flexion in conjunction with rotation can result in these injuries. In athletics this can occur with a blow to the back of the head. Unilateral facet dislocation is associated with a 37% incidence of radiculopathy and a 37% incidence of spinal cord injury. Fewer than 25% of athletes with a bilateral facet dislocation are neurologically intact; complete spinal cord injury occurs with an incidence of 40–90% with this injury (Dekutoski and Cohen-Gadol 2003).

Neurological injuries without obvious bony injury

Stingers and burners

Stingers, also known as burners, are transient upper extremity discomfort/paraesthesiae that occur at the time of injury. They are related to peripheral nerve injuries; controversy exists as to whether

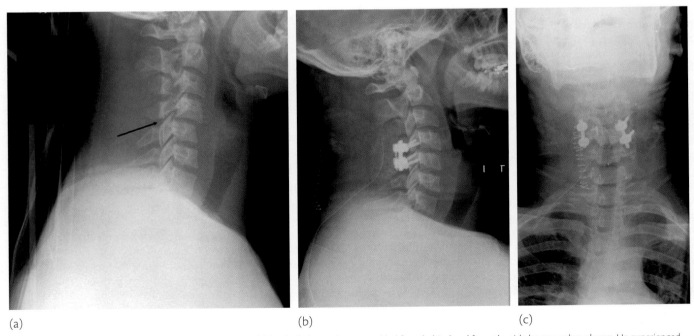

(a)   (b)   (c)

Fig. 3.4.1 (a) Lateral cervical spine radiograph of an 18-year-old football player who was tackled from behind and from the side by two other players. He experienced a sudden onset of neck pain and was noted to be tilting his head to his left side. He was noted to be neurologically intact. Work-up revealed a flexion distraction injury with a unilateral jumped facet (arrow) at C4–5. (b), (c) Traction failed to reduce this athlete's injury and he was taken to the operating room for open posterior reduction and fixation/fusion. Lateral and antero-posterior postoperative films reveal the facet dislocation to be reduced and lateral mass screw and spinous process wire instrumentation.

they are related to cervical nerve root or brachial plexus injury. Symptoms involve only an extremity. Bilateral symptoms are suggestive of cervical cord injury (Weinstein 1998).

Transient quadriplegia/quadriparesis and cervical cord neuropraxia

This occurs most commonly after a hyperextension injury. Transient quadriplegia/quadriparesis is associated with varying degrees of bilateral upper extremity weakness. Similar symptoms can result from spinal cord injury due to cervical fracture or dislocation. Usually symptoms persist for 10–15 minutes; nevertheless residual symptoms may persist for 36 hours. Typically these present as bilateral upper extremity paresthesias with variable weakness in the extremities (Dietz and Lillegard 1999, Vaccaro *et al.* 2002).

Spear tackler's spine

This term originated after careful evaluation of data from the National Football Head and Neck Injury Registry. Permanent cervical cord injury occurred in players using spear-tackling techniques who had coexisting narrowing of the cervical canal, straightening or reversal of the normal cervical lordosis, and pre-existing post-traumatic bony or ligamentous injury (Cantu *et al.* 1998). (In rugby, players may suffer from axial compression injuries to the neck when they are *subjected* to spear tackling, comprising lifting and dropping head first onto the playing surface.)

Spinal cord injury

Spinal cord injuries are classified as complete and incomplete. A **complete injury** occurs when there is absence of sensory or motor function in the lowest sacral segments. An **incomplete injury** occurs when there is preservation of motor or sensory function below the level of injury including the lowest sacral segments. The **motor level** of injury is defined as the most caudal group graded 3/5 or greater with segments rostral to that level being 5/5. The **sensory level** is the most caudal dermatome with normal light touch and pinprick sensation bilaterally. The **neurological level** is the most caudal level where sensation and motor function are intact (Ho *et al.* 2007). The American Spinal Injury Association (ASIA) impairment scale (Table 3.4.1) is commonly used to grade the patient's functional impairment (Tay and Eismont 2003).

Spinal shock

Spinal shock is a controversial term which refers to series of phases occurring after injury to the spinal cord. Depression of all reflexes

Table 3.4.1 American Spinal Injury Association (ASIA) impairment scale

ASIA A (complete injury)	Sensory and motor function absent below the level of injury including the sacral segments
ASIA B (incomplete)	Sparing of sensory function below the injury level with the exception of motor preservation of sacral segments
ASIA C (incomplete)	Motor function is preserved below the level of injury, but more than half of these preserved muscles have a strength of less than three-fifths
ASIA D (incomplete)	Motor function is preserved below the level of injury, but more than half of these preserved muscles have a strength of three-fifths or greater
ASIA E (Normal)	

Adapted from Tay and Eismont (2003).

and withdrawal of impulses from the descending tracts of the spinal cord occurs below the level of the injury. This is followed by a phase of initial reflex return in 1–3 days, followed by a phase of initial hyper-reflexia and a final phase of hyper-reflexia (Ditunno *et al.* 2004). Once the initial phases have resolved and the bulbocavernous reflex returns, examination and grading can proceed with the ASIA impairment scale (Tay and Eismont 2003). Spinal shock should not be confused with the cardiovascular changes that occur in lieu of spinal cord injury.

Intervertebral disc herniation

Cervical disc herniations are less common in the athlete than lumbar disc herniations. They tend to affect older athletes. Disc herniations are classified as either soft or hard. **Soft disc herniation** refers to acute herniation of the nucleus pulposus through a tear in the posterior anulus fibrosis (Zmurko *et al.* 2003). **Hard disc herniation** refers to a more chronic degenerative condition and is synonymous with cervical spondylosis (Baron and Young 2002). Athletes with disc degeneration and/or herniation usually present with varying degrees of arm and neck pain; rarely, a disc herniation will cause cord compression syndromes (Zmurko *et al.* 2003).

Carotid/vertebral artery dissection

Traumatic dissection of the carotid artery may occur in athletics as a result of severe neck hyperextension. Vertebral artery dissection may occur with hyperextension or lateral rotation. The mechanism of this type of vascular injury involves a tear in the intima of the blood vessel, allowing blood to dissect along the blood vessel wall. If untreated, dissection may lead to stroke or even death. Typical presenting syndromes include headache, face/neck pain, Horner's syndrome, and stroke syndromes. Once the diagnosis is made, anticoagulation is usually initiated (Flis *et al.* 2007)

Congenital anomalies of the cervical spine

Various anomalies may have a higher associated risk for cervical spinal cord injury in the athlete. These include odontoid anomalies such as Chiari I malformation, congenital atlanto-occipital fusion, and multilevel Klippel–Feil anomalies (Vaccaro *et al.* 2002). **Chiari I malformation** is a congenital disorder where there is caudal herniation of the cerebellar tonsils through the foramen magnum. Its presence is a relative indication to avoid contact sports in asymptomatic persons; the presence of associated syringomyelia may be a higher risk factor for spinal cord injury (Miele *et al.* 2006). **Os odontoideum** is a condition where the dens is disconnected from the C2 vertebral body. **Ossiculum terminale** is a condition where the tip of the dens fails to fuse with the remainder of the dens; usually it is firmly bound by cartilage. Patients with these anomalies may be at higher risk of C1–2 instability and subsequent spinal cord injury. **Congenital atlanto-occipital fusion**, or occipitalization of the atlas, occurs in approximately 0.25% of the population. It is associated with the development of progressive spinal instability as the atlantoaxial segment may be abnormally stressed. **Klippel–Feil syndrome** was initially described as a triad of short neck, low hairline, and limited neck mobility. The term is commonly used to refer to any fusion of the cervical spine with two or more vertebrae fused. Depending on the radiographic findings, an athlete with Klippel–Feil syndrome may be at higher risk for a spinal cord injury than the general population (Klimo *et al.* 2007).

Epidemiology

Cervical spine injuries account for about 10% of the 10 000 spine injuries seen yearly in the USA (Maroon and Bailes 1996). A better understanding of the epidemiology of sports-related cervical spine injuries can be achieved by looking at individual sports. Most of the data have been collected on injuries related to American football, ice hockey, and diving.

The incidence of (American) football-related cervical spine injuries has decreased significantly over recent decades. This has been attributed to the development of modern helmets and the banning of head-first contact. From 1976 to 1987, spinal cord injuries decreased by 70% at high school level and traumatic quadriplegia decreased by 82% (Banerjee *et al.* 2004). In 2006, cervical cord injuries were reported to occur at rates of 0.53 per 100 000 high school football players and 2.66 per 100 000 collegiate players. The reported range for 2000–2006 has been 0.20–0.60 per 100 000 for high school football player injuries and 0–2.66 per 100 000 players for college football players (Mueller and Cantu 2007).

Tator *et al.* (1998) reported spinal fractures and spinal cord injuries resulting from ice hockey in Canada between 1966 and 1993. A total of 241 injuries were noted, of which 90% involved the cervical spine. Of the 207 athletes with injury whose neurological status was known, 108 (52%) sustained a permanent spinal cord injury, and the cord lesion was incomplete in 52 (25.1%). Although football is associated with a higher total number of non-fatal catastrophic neck injuries per year, the annual incidence of spinal cord damage with paralysis is at least three times greater in Canadian ice hockey than in American football (Banerjee *et al.* 2004). Checking has been identified as a major hockey-related risk factor for cervical spine injury (Tator *et al.* 1998).

Diving injuries are associated with 10–20% of hospital spinal cord injury admissions with over 800 new cases reported annually. They occur most commonly in males under the age of 25 where the diver misjudges the water depth. More than 90% of these accidents result in quadriplegia, and over half are complete injuries. Alcohol consumption is an important risk factor, playing a role in 38–46% of injuries in reported series (Badman and Rechtine 2004). The most common level of injury, as reported by Tator *et al.* (1999), was the C5–6 level. A flexion–compression force acting through the cervical spine is the most common injury mechanism, resulting in burst and/or compression type fractures. However, competitive diving is a relatively safe sport, with no fatalities being reported in the USA over the last 100 years (Badman and Rechtine 2004).

The inidence of spinal cord injury in rugby has also been studied extensively (Quarrie *et al.* 2002; Fuller *et al.* 2007). Although the incidence of spinal cord injuries within rugby is debatable, depending on methodologies used, the best estimates range from 2.3/100 000 to 10/100 000 players per year, depending on the country of origin. Throughout the 1990s a higher rate of injury was associated with tackling, as opposed to scrummaging which was more commonly associated with injury in the 1980s. Ruck and maul injuries are the third most common cause of rugby-related cervical spine injury. The primary mechanism of injury seen in rugby-related cervical spine injury is hyperflexion. Various changes in the rules of the game have been made with the intent of reducing injuries. These include changes in the binding allowed during the scrum, allowing only the substitution of a trained front row player if a trained front row player leaves the field, the increased ability for referees to notice dangerous play, and changes in the procedures of scrum engagement. Nevertheless, the exact impact of these changes on the incidence of cervical spine injuries is hard to interpret (Quarrie *et al.* 2002).

Other sports have also been associated with cervical spine injury. Equestrian sports are associated with significance risk of participant morbidity and mortality, with a rate of injury estimated at 0.5 injuries per 1000 riding hours. Concerning horse-related fatalities, 65.8% were from falls from or with the horse and 34.2% of those who died were not mounted when the fatal injury occurred. A third of all injuries that arise from horseback riding involve the nervous system and/or the spine (Brooks and Bixby-Hammett 1999). Soccer has been associated with a possible increased incidence of decreased range of motion and neck pain/stiffness in its participants. Compression fractures of the lateral masses may also occur (Kirkendall and Garrett 1999). Cervical injuries have also been reported with the martial arts (Birrer 1999), boxing (Place *et al.* 1996; Feinberg 2000), wrestling (Boden *et al.* 2002; Nakagawa *et al.* 2004), basketball (Jordan 1999), baseball (Boden *et al.* 2004), gymnastics (Jordan 1999), rodeo (Jordan 1999), bungee jumping (Louw *et al.* 1998), and hovercraft racing (Cattermole 1997).

Long-term injuries may result from neck overuse in athletes. Recently, in a survey of 164 triathlon athletes, Villavicencio *et al.* (2007) noted a lifetime incidence of neck pain of 47.6 %, with 15.4% possibly being of discogenic origin based on the duration of symptoms (Villavicencio *et al.* 2007). They noted the number of previous triathlons not predictive of neck pain, but that total years in the sport ($p = 0.029$) and number of previous sports-related injuries ($p < 0.0001$) were predictive.

Anatomical considerations

Effective management and understanding of neck injury requires a basic familiarity with the regional anatomy. The cervical spine acts to support the head and protect the neural elements while also allowing for complex movement. The cervical spinal column can be conceptually divided into an upper region and a lower region which differ in terms of anatomical design and function (Banerjee *et al.* 2004).

The upper cervical spine has uniquely shaped C1 and C2 vertebrae. The atlas, or C1, lacks a body and consists of an anterior and posterior arch. Instead of the usual articular processes the atlas has lateral masses that articulate with the occipital condyles of the skull and the second cervical vertebrae alone. Additionally, the arch of C1 has an anterior tubercle to which muscles attach. The axis, or the C2 vertebra, is unique because of the dens which allows rotation between the skull/atlas and axis. Additionally the facet joints of C2 are uniquely configured. The rest of the vertebrae are notable for their small size and the presence of uncinate processes forming the joints of Luschka. Also unique to the cervical spine is the transverse foramen. From C6 upwards the cervical foramina typically contain the vertebral arteries (Hollinshead 1974).

Mercer and Bogduk (1999) noted that the adult cervical disc has a distinct morphology differentiating it from the lumbar disc. The discs have a crescent-shaped anterior anulus fibrosus, are thick anteriorly, and are tapered laterally towards the uncinate process. Cervical discs have a central fibro-cartilaginous core of the nucleus pulposus. Additionally, periosteofascial tissue overlies the uncovertebral area. Cervical discs have a thinner posterior anulus fibrosus than lumbar discs. All of the above characteristics help to determine the structure and shape of the cervical spine and consequently affect its function and movements.

Muscles, ligaments, and cartilaginous structures play an important role in stabilizing the neck. Important static stabilizers include the ligamentous structures such as the anterior longitudinal ligament, posterior longitudinal ligament, ligamentum flavum, facet capsules, and supraspinous ligaments. The discs also serve as static stabilizers. Dynamic stabilization occurs as a result of the surrounding musculature including the strap musculature, the sternocleidomastoid, the trapezius, and the paraspinal muscles (Zmurko et al. 2003).

The cervical spine consists of eight cervical motion segments between the occiput and first thoracic vertebra. Sagittal plane movements occur at each motion segment. Most flexion and extension occurs in the lower cervical spine from C3 to C7. Most rotation occurs in the upper cervical spine at C1–C2. (Bogduk and Mercer 2000). Rotation and lateral flexion occur simultaneously; rotation always accompanies lateral flexion and lateral flexion always accompanies rotation (Ishii et al. 2004a, b). Paradoxical motion may occur at some segments, while the whole cervical spine moves into retraction or protrusion. For example, the upper and lower cervical spine motion segments move in opposite directions while retraction or protrusion occurs (Ordway et al. 1999).

The cervical musculature and the flexibility of the cervical spine are important elements in dissipating energy in high-energy trauma (Dietz and Lillegard 1999). In the presence of normal cervical lordosis, the cervical spine is slightly extended. The forces of an axial load in this situation are effectively dissipated by the ligamentous structures and the paravertebral musculature. When the cervical spine is flexed by approximately 30°, normal cervical lordosis is lost and the spine appears straight. If the spine is axially loaded while in the straight position, soft tissues are unavailable to dissipate energy as they would be in a lordotic cervical posture. In this situation loading forces are transmitted primarily down the through the vertebra and discs (Banerjee et al. 2004). This axial loading mechanism is responsible for most (American) football-related cervical spine injuries (Torg et al. 2002)

The spinal cord, extending downwards from the foramen magnum, is protected circumferentially by the osseoligamentous structures of the cervical spine. At C1 the cord occupies less than half of the canal's cross-sectional area. There is less space caudally between C4 and C7 as progressive narrowing of the bony canal combined with a gradual widening of the spinal cord diameter reduces the space available for the cord. At the lower cervical levels, the spinal cord normally fills approximately three-quarters of the spinal canal (Parke 1988).

Within the subaxial cervical spine the dimensions of the cord remain relatively constant (8–9 mm). However, the size of the vertebral canal in the lower cervical region may vary significantly among individuals (Banerjee et al. 2004). The normal anteroposterior diameter of the subaxial canal is approximately 15 mm; 13 mm or less is considered cervical stenosis (Cantu 1993). Nevertheless, bony measurements alone may be insensitive in detecting actual cord compression. Functional spinal stenosis, where the cerebrospinal fluid cushion around the spinal cord (and/or cord indentation) is decreased, is probably more relevant to the athlete. Athletes with functional stenosis, especially those with symptoms referable to the

cervical cord, have been recommended to discontinue contact sports (Cantu 1993). Although cervical stenosis has been suggested as a risk factor for the burner phenomenon in college football players (Kelly et al. 2000), stingers appear to be a phenomenon related to peripheral nerve injury, and cervical foraminal narrowing may be a more likely cause. Central stenosis does not appear to be a risk factor for stingers(Weinstein 1998).

Aetiology and pathophysiology

Minor injuries

Modern research has demonstrated that whiplash injuries with trauma to the spinal cord occur at impact speeds of approximately 150 m/s. Concurrently, the cervical spine buckles; upper cervical segments are flexed and lower cervical segments extend around an abnormally located axis of rotation, resulting in injury. Previously it had been believed that a cantilever movement was the cause of injury (e.g. extension, flexion). However, numerous studies have demonstrated otherwise (Bogduk and Yoganandan 2001). Chronic symptoms may occur when there is disruption of an intervertebral disc and concurrent facet joint injury. Chronic facet joint injury may be a significant source of chronic pain (Bogduk and Yoganandan 2001).

Serious injuries

Banerjee et al. (2004) identified four entities related to cervical spine trauma which may be associated with catastrophic spinal cord injury: unstable fractures and dislocations, transient quadriplegia, acute central disc herniation, and congenital spinal anomalies. As per White and Panjabi (1990), an osseous or ligamentous injury to the spine is considered unstable when the spine loses its ability to protect the neurological elements, or is likely to develop progressive deformity or pain.

The majority of unstable cervical spine injuries seen in American football and ice hockey occur in the lower cervical spine. Two major patterns of spinal column damage often occur with these sporting activities: compressive-flexion injuries due to a combination of an axial force and a bending moment, and vertical compression fractures (burst fractures) due to a purely compressive vector force. Compressive flexion injuries are considered highly unstable and are frequently associated with a neurological deficit. Retropulsion of collapsed bone in either fracture type may result in neurological deficit (Banerjee et al. 2004). Diving accidents are associated with the top of the head striking the bottom of a pool or a natural body of water. The vector of injury is transmitted axially and results in fracture-dislocations or burst fractures. Most of these injuries occur in the mid-cervical spine (Tator 1999). Flexion–distraction injuries may occur with a bending movement of the cervical spine over the trunk.

Injuries causing instability in the upper cervical spine are less frequently seen. Neurological deficit due to fractures or dislocations involving the upper cervical spine is rare. Cord compression is unlikely in relation to a burst fracture of the atlas (Jefferson fracture) and traumatic spondylolisthesis of the axis (Hangman fracture) because these bony injuries further expand the dimensions of the spinal canal. The traumatic conditions most likely to result in upper cervical cord injury are those that destabilize the atlantoaxial complex, including injury to the odontoid and rupture of the transverse atlantal ligament (Banerjee *et al.* 2004).

Transient quadriplegia may present as temporary bilateral burning, weakness, and paraesthesiae. It usually results from a hyperextension mechanism. Symptoms can last from several minutes to 36 hours. Transient quadriplegia has been associated with cervical stenosis, kyphosis, instability, congenital fusion, and vascular and metabolic aetiologies (Vaccaro *et al.* 2002). The aetiology of spinal cord dysfunction in this condition is thought to be due to a conduction block without anatomical disruption of neural tissue. The tissue is 'post-concussive' and appears unresponsive to stimulation for a variable period of time (Banerjee *et al.* 2004).

Cervical disc rupture may result from high-energy head or neck trauma during collision sport activities. With extrusion of the gelatinous nucleus pulposus through the anulus fibrosus and into the central spinal canal, the space available for the spinal cord is compromised (Banerjee *et al.* 2004). This may result in neck pain, radiculopathy, and transient or permanent cord injury.

Congenital spinal anomalies may also predispose the athlete to spinal cord injury. These include multilevel Klippel–Feil deformity, Chiari malformations, asymptomatic ligamentous laxity, basilar invagination, and congenital stenosis, among others (Vaccaro *et al.* 2002). Systemic conditions such as ankylosing spondylitis and diffuse idiopathic skeletal hyperostosis may also present a higher risk for spinal cord injury.

Investigations

Management of the injured athlete begins on the athletic field. Important field equipment includes instruments to remove facemasks, airway protective equipment, a spine board, and a stretcher. In American football injuries, if the patient is unconscious the helmet is best left in place. The jaw thrust technique is used if intubation is considered. Transportation to a medical facility with the patient immobilized is imperative if the injured athlete has an altered mental status, neurological deficit, neck pain or tenderness, or limited range of motion (McAlindon 2002).

After arriving at an emergency facility attention is directed to the injured athlete's airway, respiratory, and cardiopulmonary status. A neurological examination is then performed followed by plain radiographs of the cervical spine or helical CT of the spinal axis. Administration of high-dose methylprednisolone is considered if a spinal cord injury is suspected (Lee *et al.* 1998).

Computed tomography (CT) provides superior evaluation of bony anatomy and pathology. MRI provides evaluation of soft tissue pathology and directs evaluation of the discs, ligaments, and spinal cord. Dynamic radiography, i.e. flexion–extension plain radiographs, may be useful in the assessment of spinal stability. Because pain and muscle spasm at the time of injury limits range of motion, it is recommended that dynamic studies are performed a week or two after injury (Bagley 2006).

Once a serious injury is excluded a more extensive evaluation can be undertaken. This includes a detailed neurological screen and assessment of range of motion and posture. More specific examination techniques include the upper limb provocation test, the slump test, segmental evaluation of passive accessory and physiological intervertebral motion, and myofascial assessment (Beazell and Magrum 2003). It is also important to assess repeated end range movements or a sustained end range position to investigate

for the presence of the **centralisation phenomenon**. This phenomenon is the process where pain radiating from the spine is sequentially abolished, distally to proximally, in response to therapeutic positions. Its presence as a clinical finding may be a predictor of a good outcome with treatment exercises as well as a predictor of a rapid return to athletic activities (Mckenzie and May 2006; Aina *et al.* 2004; Werneke *et al.* 1999).

Clinical syndromes seen with cervical injuries

Although many clinical syndromes are present with cervical athletic injuries, we will briefly review only the more common ones. Cervical strains, sprains, and contusions are among the most frequently seen cervical injuries which result in varying degrees of neck pain. These injuries tend to overlap. Symptoms may vary from mild pain to instability with facet joint subluxation or dislocation.

A detailed neurological examination and musculoskeletal examination should be performed. Neurological examination should include gross muscle testing of facial musculature, extraocular movements and pupillary assessment, sternocleidomastoid and trapezius musculature, and upper extremity musculature. Additionally, an assessment of upper and lower extremity reflexes should be performed. Asymmetric loss of an upper extremity reflex may suggest radiculopathy; exaggerated lower extremity reflexes may indicate upper motor neuron dysfunction (spinal cord injury). Attempts should also be made to elicit abnormal reflexes such as the Hoffman's sign, sustained clonus, and the Babinski sign. The presence of any of these may suggest spinal cord dysfunction (Cull and Whittle 1995).

Assessment of the cervical spine alignment and a detailed musculoskeletal assessment should also be performed. Normal cervical lordosis is a slight anterior curve. Any kyphosis or posterior head tilt should be noted. These are also visualized on plain radiographs and flexion–extension views.

Palpation of the neck musculature should be performed and any tightness noted. Posterolateral tenderness may be evidence of an upper trapezius strain. Segmental spasm of the muscle may be noted. Tightness of the posterior muscles may be another finding, especially in the setting of a forward head position (Kendall *et al.* 1983). Trigger points may also be noted. These may cause pain at rest. On examination for trigger points, focal tenderness may be noted in addition to the presence of a taut band sensitive to pressure. This may indicate that the affected muscle fibers are continuously contracted (Fischer 2000).

Neck flexors and extensors should be tested. Anterior neck flexors (longus capitis colli and rectus capitis anterior) are tested with the patient supine, elbows bent, and hands besides the head. The patient lifts his/her head from the table and approximates his/her chin towards the sternum. The examiner directs pressure against the forehead in a posterior direction. Note that a patient with flexor weakness may be able to lift his/her head from the table with actions primarily of the sternocleidomastoids. Weakness of the neck flexors would be evident as hyperextension of the cervical spine with subsequent forward head posture.

Assessment of the anterolateral neck flexors (sternocleidomastoid and scalene musculature) should also be performed. These muscles are also tested with the patient supine, elbows bent, and hands besides the head. The patient turns his/her head towards the examiner while the examiner applies pressure in a posterior/oblique direction to the temporal region. Note that a patient with weakness of these muscle groups may be able to provide some head lift by raising his/her shoulders. Thus the shoulders should be kept flat on the table. Posterolateral neck extensors, including the splenius capitis and cervices, semispinalis capitis and cervicis, and cervical erector spinae should also be tested. The patient is examined prone with elbows bent and hands resting overhead on the table. Posterolateral neck extension is tested with the patient's face turned towards the side being tested. The examiner applies anterior pressure against the posterolateral aspect of the head (Kendall *et al.* 1983).

Additional physical examination findings may suggest mechanical injury to the facet joints; an opening or closing restriction pattern may be observed. An opening pattern involves a deviation towards the side of injury when an athlete flexes his neck and limitation of rotation and flexion to the contralateral side. A closing pattern exists when the injured athlete moves his/her neck to the contralateral side on extension and has restricted flexion and rotation on the side ipsilateral to the injury. These movement patterns may be seen with facet capsular injuries and arthritis (Beazell and Magrum 2003). Additional findings may include muscle spasm and loss of the normal cervical lordosis. There may be trigger points in superficial musculature along with decreased range of motion (Cailliet 1991). However, significant midline or paraspinal tenderness should alert the clinician to a possible ligamentous injury (Crowl and Kang 2006). Clinical evaluation includes MRI and dynamic radiography. Typically, these injuries are treated with rest, discontinuation of athletic activity, analgesics, and non-steroidal ant-inflammatory drugs (Zmurko *et al.* 2003). Other treatments that may be useful include acute intravenous steroids, local modalities, physical therapy, mobilization, and possibly careful manipulation (especially for subacute and chronic symptoms) and injection therapy (Conlin *et al.* 2005; Kay *et al.* 2005; Jensen and Harms-Ringdahl 2007; Peloso *et al.* 2007).

As mentioned above, cervical disc herniation typically affects the older athlete. Most often athletes with disc degeneration and/or herniation present with varying degrees of arm and neck pain; rarely, a disc herniation will cause cord compression syndromes. Most treatments are conservative; progressive weakness or symptomatic cord compression may necessitate surgical intervention (Zmurko *et al.* 2003).

Burners and stingers are transient neurological events which consist of unilateral upper extremity pain and paresthesias. The injured athlete may experience numbness, tingling, and burning in a circumferential non-dermatomal distribution. Symptoms may be confined to the neck or radiate to the hand (Castro 2003). These injuries are quite common and may occur in as many as 50% of American football players (Robertson *et al.* 1979). Stingers resolve by themselves; thus no formal treatment is required (Castro 2003). Properly fitting football shoulder pads may be useful in their prevention (Shannon and Klimkiewicz 2002).

Cervical cord neuropraxia or transient quadriparesis/quadriplegia represents a spectrum of clinical entities ranging from mild sensory and/or motor disturbances to frank quadriplegia. It is thought to occur as a result of a pincer mechanism during hyperextension (Castro 2003). Typically, symptoms last for 10–15 minutes but can last as long as 36 hours. After an athlete experiences such an injury, a complete neurological and radiographic work-up should be performed before any decisions regarding returning to sports are made (Vaccaro *et al.* 2002).

Spinal cord injury syndromes are unusual but may be seen in contact sports. **Central cord syndrome** occurs with injury to central portions of the spinal cord. The mechanism of injury is typically extension with a resulting pinching of the cord at a level of preexisting stenosis. Typically patients with a central cord injury will have loss of function in the upper extremities and proximal lower extremity musculature, while the distal lower limbs are spared. **Anterior cord syndrome** occurs with damage to the anterior two-thirds of the spinal cord. This may occur with flexion compression injury to the cervical cord. A patient with this injury will have flaccid paralysis at the level of injury and spastic paralysis below the level of the injury; pressure sense and joint position sense are preserved. **Brown–Sequard syndrome** involves injury to one side of the spinal cord. This results in weakness on one side with spasticity and upper motor neuron signs and loss of pain and temperature sense on the contralateral side (Tay and Eismont 2003).

Returning to sport

Numerous articles have been written concerning return to sport (Torg and Ramsey-Emrhein 1997; Cantu *et al.* 1998; Morganti *et al.* 2001; Vaccaro *et al.* 2002; Morganti 2003,). In summary, an experienced clinician must make the decision for an athlete to return to sport where there is evidence of normal spinal stability (Morganti 2003). In general, the athlete should be pain free. The presence of congenital or acquired anomalies (e.g. congenital stenosis, ankylosing spondylitis, etc) and/or residual deficit are important considerations here. Additionally, playing in an unsafe environment is a contraindication even for an uninjured athlete: appropriate safety measures should be taken and proper safety equipment should be used (Morganti 2003).

Conclusion

Cervical spine injuries can occur in most contact sports. Injuries range in severity from mild cervical sprains to complete spinal cord injury. Cervical injury in the sports setting can be more effectively addressed through preventative measures, such as regulations to reduce incidence of risky behavior, and education of clinicians involved in the care of the injured athlete.

References

Aina, A., May, S., and Clare, H. (2004). The centralization phenomenon of spinal symptoms–a systematic review. *Manual Therapy*, **9**, 134–143.

Andreychick, D. (2003). Odontoid fractures. In: A.R. Vaccaro (ed.) *Fractures of the Cervical, Thoracic and Lumbar Spine*. Marcel Dekker, New York.

Badman, B.L. and Rechtine, G.R. (2004). Spinal injury considerations in the competitive diver: a case report and review of the literature. *Spine Journal*, 4, 584–90.

Bagley, L.J. (2006). Imaging of spinal trauma. *Radiologic Clinics of North America*, **44**, 1–12, vii.

Banerjee, R., Palumbo, M.A., and Fadale, P.D. (2004). Catastrophic cervical spine injuries in the collision sport athlete, part 1: epidemiology, functional anatomy, and diagnosis. *American Journal of Sports Medicine*, **32**, 1077–87.

Baron, E.M. and Young, W.F. (2002). Cervical spondylosis: diagnosis and management. In: W. Nowack, F. Talavera, J.H. Halsey, S.R. Benbadis, and N. Lorenzo (eds), *eMedicine Neurology*. eMedicine, Omaha, NB.

Bassewitz, H L. and Herkowitz, H.N. (2003). Atlas fractures. In: A.R. Vaccaro (ed.) *Fractures of the Cervical, Thoracic and Lumbar Spine*. Marcel Dekker, New York.

Beazell, J.R. and Magrum, E.M. (2003). Rehabilitation of head and neck injuries in the athlete. *Clinics in Sports Medicine*, **22**, 523–57.

Birrer, R.D. (1999). Martial arts. In: W.A. Lillegard, J.D. Butcher, and K.S. Rucker (eds), *Handbook of Sports Medicine: A Symptoms Oriented Approach* (2nd edn). Butterworth Heinemann, Boston, MA.

Boden, B.P., Lin, W., Young, M., and Mueller, F.O. (2002). Catastrophic injuries in wrestlers. *American Journal of Sports Medicine*, **30**, 791–5.

Boden, B.P., Tacchetti, R., and Mueller, F.O. (2004). Catastrophic injuries in high school and college baseball players. *American Journal of Sports Medicine*, **32**, 1189–96.

Bogduk, N. and Mercer, S. (2000). Biomechanics of the cervical spine. I: Normal kinematics. *Clinical Biomechanics*, **15**, 633–48.

Bogduk, N. and Yoganandan, N. (2001). Biomechanics of the cervical spine. III: Minor injuries. *Clinical Biomechanics*, 16, 267–75.

Brooks, W.H. and Bixby-Hammett, D.M. (1999). Equestrian sports. In: W.A. Lillegard, J.D. Butcher, and K.S. Rucker (eds), *Handbook of Sports Medicine: A Symptoms Oriented Approach* (2nd edn). Butterworth Heinemann, Boston, MA.

Cailliet, R. (1991). *Neck and Arm Pain*. F.A. Davis, Philadelphia, PA.

Cantu, R.C. (1993). Functional cervical spinal stenosis: a contraindication to participation in contact sports. *Medicine and Science in Sports and Exercise*, **25**, 316–17.

Cantu, R.C., Bailes, J.E., and Wilberger, J.E., Jr (1998). Guidelines for return to contact or collision sport after a cervical spine injury. *Clinics in Sports Medicine*, **17**, 137–46.

Castro, F.P., Jr (2003). Stingers, cervical cord neurapraxia, and stenosis. *Clinics in Sports Medicine*, **22**, 483–92.

Cattermole, H.R. (1997). Injuries from hovercraft racing. *Injury*, **28**, 25–7.

Conlin, A., Bhogal, S., Sequeira, K., and Teasell, R. (2005). Treatment of whiplash-associated disorders. Part I: Non-invasive interventions. *Pain Research and Management*, **10**, 21–32.

Crowl, A.C. and Kang, J.D. (2006). Cervical spine. In: D.L. Johnson and S.d. Mair (eds), *Clinical Sports Medicine*. Mosby, Philadelphia, PA.

Cull, R.E. and Whittle, I.R. (1995). The nervous system. In: J. Munro and C.R.W. Edwards (eds), *Macleod's Clinical Examination*. Churchill Livingstone, Edinburgh.

Dekutoski, M. and Cohen-Gadol, A.A. (2003). Distractive flexion cervical spine injuries: a clinical spectrum. In: A.R. Vaccaro (ed.) *Fractures of the Cervical, Thoracic and Lumbar Spine*. Marcel Dekker, New York.

Dietz, J.W. and Lillegard, W.A. (1999). Cervical spine injuries. In: W.A. Lillegard, J.D. Butcher, and K.S. Rucker (eds), *Handbook of Sports Medicine: A Symptoms Oriented Approach* (2nd edn). Butterworth Heinemann, Boston, MA.

Ditunno, J.F., Little, J.W., Tessler, A., and Burns, A.S. (2004). Spinal shock revisited: a four-phase model. *Spinal Cord*, **42**, 383–95.

Feinberg, J. H. (2000). Burners and stingers. *Physical Medicine and Rehabilitation Clinics of North America*, **11**, 771–84.

Fischer, A.A. (2000). Trigger point injection. In: T.A. Lennard (ed.), *Pain Procedures in Clinical Practice*. Hanley & Belfus, Philadelphia, PA.

Flis, C.M., Jager, H.R., and Sidhu, P.S. (2007). Carotid and vertebral artery dissections: clinical aspects, imaging features and endovascular treatment. *European Radiology*, **17**, 820–34.

Fuller, C.W., Brooks, J.H., and Kemp, S.P. (2007). Spinal injuries in professional rugby union: a prospective cohort study. *Clinical Journal of Sport Medicine*, **17**, 10–16.

Grauer, J.N., Shafi, B., Hilibrand, A.S., *et al.* (2005). Proposal of a modified, treatment-oriented classification of odontoid fractures. *Spine Journal*, **5**, 123–9.

Hankins, S.M., Quartararo, L.G. and Vaccaro, A.R. (2003). Axis fractures. In: A.R. Vaccaro (ed.) *Fractures of the Cervical, Thoracic and Lumbar Spine*. Marcel Dekker, New York.

Ho, C.H., Wuermser, L.A., Priebe, M.M., Chiodo, A.E., Scelza, W.M., and Kirshblum, S.C. (2007). Spinal cord injury medicine. 1. Epidemiology and classification. *Archives of Physical and Medical Rehabilitation*, **88**, S49–54.

Hollinshead, W.H. (1974). *Textbook of Anatomy*. Harper & Row, Philadelphia, PA.

Ishii, T., Mukai, Y., Hosono, N., *et al.* (2004a). Kinematics of the subaxial cervical spine in rotation in vivo three-dimensional analysis. *Spine*, **29**, 2826–31.

Ishii, T., Mukai, Y., Hosono, N., *et al.* (2004b). Kinematics of the upper cervical spine in rotation: in vivo three-dimensional analysis. *Spine*, **29**, E139–44.

Jensen, I. and Harms-Ringdahl, K. (2007) Strategies for prevention and management of musculoskeletal conditions: neck pain. *Best Practice and Research. Clinical Rheumatology*, **21**, 93–108.

Jordan, B.D. (1999) Neurologic injury in other sports. In: W.A. Lillegard, J.D. Butcher, and K.S. Rucker (eds), *Handbook of Sports Medicine: A Symptoms Oriented Approach* (2nd edn). Butterworth Heinemann, Boston, MA.

Kay, T.M., Gross, A., Goldsmith, C., Santaguida, P.L., Hoving, J., and Bronfort, G. (2005). Exercises for mechanical neck disorders. *Cochrane Database Systematic Reviews*, CD004250.

Kelly, J.D.T., Aliquo, D., Sitler, M.R., Odgers, C., and Moyer, R.A. (2000). Association of burners with cervical canal and foraminal stenosis. *American Journal of Sports Medicine*, **28**, 214–17.

Kendall, F.P., McCreary, E.K., and Provance, P.G. (1983). *Muscle Testing and Function*, Williams & Wilkins, MD.

Kirkendall, D.T. and Garrett, W.E. (1999). Soccer. In: W.A. Lillegard, J.D. Butcher, and K.S. Rucker (eds), *Handbook of Sports Medicine: A Symptoms Oriented Approach* (2nd edn). Butterworth Heinemann, Boston, MA.

Klimo, P., Jr., Rao, G., and Brockmeyer, D. (2007) Congenital anomalies of the cervical spine. *Neurosurgery Clinics of North America*, **18**, 463–78.

Lee, T.T., Manzaon, G.R., and Green, B.A. (1998). Emergency management of cervical spine injuries. In: B.D. Jordan (ed.) *Sports Neurology*. Lippincott–Raven, Philadelphia, PA.

Louw, D., Reddy, K.K., Lauryssen, C., and Louw, G. (1998). Pitfalls of bungee jumping. Case report and review of the literature. *Journal of Neurosurgery*, **89**, 1040–2.

McAlindon, R.J. (2002). On field evaluation and management of head and neck injured athletes. *Clinics in Sports Medicine*, **21**, 1–14, v.

McGuire, R.A. (2003). Vertical compression injuries of the cervical Spine. In: A.R. Vaccaro (ed.) *Fractures of the Cervical, Thoracic and Lumbar Spine*. Marcel Dekker, New York.

McKenzie, R. and May, S. (2006). The Cervical and Thoracic Spine Mechanical Diagnosis & Therapy, 2nd ed. Spinal Publications New Zealand Ltd, Raumati Beach, New Zealand.

Maroon, J. C. and Bailes, J.E. (1996) Athletes with cervical spine injury. *Spine*, **21**, 2294–9.

Mercer, S. and Bogduk, N. (1999). The ligaments and annulus fibrosus of human adult cervical intervertebral discs. *Spine*, **24**, 619–28.

Miele, V.J., Bailes, J.E., and Martin, N.A. (2006). Participation in contact or collision sports in athletes with epilepsy, genetic risk factors, structural brain lesions, or history of craniotomy. *Neurosurgical Focus*, **21**, E9.

Morganti, C. (2003) Recommendations for return to sports following cervical spine injuries. *Sports Medicine*, **33**, 563–73.

Morganti, C., Sweeney, C.A., Albanese, S.A., Burak, C., Hosea, T. and Connolly, P.J. (2001). Return to play after cervical spine injury. *Spine*, **26**, 1131–6.

Mueller, F.O. and Cantu, R.C. (2007). *Annual Survey of Football Injury Research*. National Center for Catastrophic Sport Injury Research, University of North Carolina, Chapel Hill, NC.

Nakagawa, Y., Minami, K., Arai, T., Okamura, Y., and Nakamura, T. (2004) Cervical spinal cord injury in sumo wrestling: a case. *American Journal of Sports Medicine*, **32**, 1054–8.

NSCISC (National Spinal Cord Injury Statistical Center) (2006). *The 2006 Annual Statistical Report for the Model Spinal Cord Injury Systems*. National Spinal Cord Injury Statistical Center, Birmingham, AL.

Ordway, N.R., Seymour, R.J., Donelson, R.G., Hojnowski, L.S., and Edwards, W.T. (1999). Cervical flexion, extension, protrusion, and retraction. A radiographic segmental analysis. *Spine*, **24**, 240–7.

Parke, W.W. (1988) Correlative anatomy of cervical spondylotic myelopathy. *Spine*, **13**, 831–7.

Peloso, P., Gross, A., Haines, T., Trinh, K., Goldsmith, C.H. and Burnie, S. (2007). Medicinal and injection therapies for mechanical neck disorders. *Cochrane Database Systematic Reviews*, CD000319.

Place, H.M., Ecklund, J.M., and Enzenauer, R.J. (1996). Cervical spine injury in a boxer: should mandatory screening be instituted? *Journal of Spinal Disorders*, **9**, 64–7.

Quarrie, K.L., Cantu, R.C., and Chalmers, D. J. (2002). Rugby union injuries to the cervical spine and spinal cord. *Sports Medicine*, **32**, 633–53.

Robertson, W.C., Jr, Eichman, P.L., and Clancy, W.G. (1979). Upper trunk brachial plexopathy in football players. *Journal of the American Medical Association*, **241**, 1480–2.

Shannon, B. and Klimkiewicz, J.J. (2002). Cervical burners in the athlete. *Clinics in Sports Medicine*, **21**, 29–35, vi.

Sidhu, K.S. and Fischgrund, J.S. (2003). Cervical whiplash injuries. In: A.R. Vaccaro (ed.) *Fractures of the Cervical, Thoracic and Lumbar Spine*. Marcel Dekker, New York.

Tator, C.H. (1999). Diving. In: W.A. Lillegard, J.D. Butcher, and K.S. Rucker (eds), *Handbook of Sports Medicine: A Symptoms Oriented Approach* (2nd edn). Butterworth Heinemann, Boston, MA.

Tator, C.H., Carson, J.D., and Edmonds, V. E. (1998). Spinal injuries in ice hockey. *Clinics in Sports Medicine*, **17**, 183–94.

Tay, B. and Eismont, F.J. (2003). Physical examination: ASIA motory/sensory examination and spinal cord injury syndromes.

In: A.R. Vaccaro (ed.) *Fractures of the Cervical, Thoracic and Lumbar Spine*. Marcel Dekker, New York.

Torg, J.S. and Ramsey-Emrhein, J.A. (1997). Management guidelines for participation in collision activities with congenital, developmental, or postinjury lesions involving the cervical spine. *Clinical Journal of Sport Medicine*, **7**, 273–91.

Torg, J.S., Guille, J.T., and Jaffe, S. (2002). Injuries to the cervical spine in American football players. *Journal of Bone and Joint Surgery*, **84A**, 112–22.

Vaccaro, A.R., Klein, G.R., Ciccoti, M., *et al.* (2002) Return to play criteria for the athlete with cervical spine injuries resulting in stinger and transient quadriplegia/paresis. *Spine Journal*, **2**, 351–6.

Vaccaro, A.R., Silber, J.S., Milam, R.A., Bassewitz, H.L., Herkowitz, H.N., and Kubeck, J.P. (2003) Atlantoaxial rotatory instability. In: A.R. Vaccaro (ed.) *Fractures of the Cervical, Thoracic and Lumbar Spine*. Marcel Dekker, New York.

Villavicencio, A.T., Hernandez, T.D., Burneikiene, S., and Thramann, J. (2007). Neck pain in multisport athletes. *Journal of Neurosurgery Spine*, **7**, 408–13.

Vives, M.J., Vaccaro, A.R. and Abibtol, J.J. (2003). Compressive flexion injuries of the cervical spine. In: A.R. Vaccaro (ed.) *Fractures of the Cervical, Thoracic and Lumbar Spine*. Marcel Dekker, New York.

Weinstein, S.M. (1998). Assessment and rehabilitation of the athlete with a 'stinger'. A model for the management of noncatastrophic athletic cervical spine injury. *Clinics in Sports Medicine*, **17**, 127–35.

Werneke, M., Hart, D., and Cook, D. (1999). A descriptive study of the centralization phenomenon. *Spine*, **24**, 676–83.

Wetzler, M.J., Akpata, T., Albert, T., Foster, T.E., and Levy, A.S. (1996). A retrospective study of cervical spine injuries in American rugby, 1970 to 1994. *American Journal of Sports Medicine*, **24**, 454–8.

White, A.A., 3rd, and Panjabi, M.M. (1990). *Clinical Biomechanics of the Spine*. Lipincott, Philadelphia, PA.

Zmurko, M.G., Tannoury, T.Y., Tannoury, C.A., and Anderson, D.G. (2003). Cervical sprains, disc herniations, minor fractures, and other cervical injuries in the athlete. *Clinics in Sports Medicine*, **22**, 513–21.

3.5

Injuries to the shoulder

Cathy Speed and Andrew Wallace

Introduction

The vast majority of shoulder complaints are due to soft tissue lesions, and rotator cuff disorders represent the largest diagnostic category of these. Many shoulder complaints are multifactorial in origin, and articular and extra-articular disorders can coexist. Instability also plays a major role; the shoulder is the most mobile joint of the body, achieving this mobility at the expense of its stability. Loss of the fine balance between optimal mobility of the joint and its stability is a common, albeit frequently subtle, feature of shoulder complaints.

Upper limb injuries in sport are much less common than those affecting the lower limb. Nevertheless they can have a significant effect on performance. Shoulder injuries represent a particular risk in certain sports. In rugby union, most injuries occur during matches and are contact/macrotraumatic in origin during tackling and can result in significant loss of time from training and competition. The most common match injury seen is acromioclavicular joint injury (32%). The most severe is shoulder dislocation and instability (mean severity, 81 days absent), which also causes the greatest proportion of absence (42%) and has the highest rate of recurrence (62%) (Headey *et al.* 2007). Not surprisingly, acute traumatic injuries are also common in American football, ice hockey, and some martial arts. Acute injuries to the shoulder in power-lifting represent over a third of injuries (Keogh et al. 2006).

In contrast to these contact injuries, overuse injuries are particularly common in wheelchair athletes and in sports such as badminton, golf (12% of injuries), tennis, volleyball (10% of overuse injuries), and throwing disciplines. In most sports there is a strong basis for prehabilitation strategies in an effort to minimize the risk of shoulder injury.

Functional anatomy

The shoulder complex is composed of a series of articulations: the glenohumeral, acromioclavicular, and sternoclavicular joints, and the scapulothoracic articulation, where the scapula glides on the rib cage (Fig. 3.5.1). The capsules, ligaments, muscles, tendons, bursae and neurovascular elements complete the framework of the shoulder complex. The particularly remarkable feature of the shoulder is its significant range of motion (RoM). Such mobility is a pre-requisite to playing some sports at a high level. The ability to stabilize such a mobile complex is vital to avoid injury.

Most factors associated with the high RoM of the shoulder complex relate to the glenohumeral joint. In particular, (a) the articular surfaces of the glenohumeral joint are shallow and the area of bony congruity is small, (b) the laxity of many surrounding soft tissue structures such as the joint capsule permits a wide RoM, and (c) combinations of movements through the series of joints within the shoulder complex allow a greater range of movement to be achieved.

The glenohumeral joint stabilizers can be divided into dynamic and static stabilizers (Table 3.5.1). These are discussed further below.

Static stabilizers

The proximal **humerus** consists of the surgical neck, (where fractures usually occur), the anatomical neck (which forms the junction between the articular cartilage and the ligament and tendon attachments) and the head. A ring, consisting of the greater and lesser tuberosities separated by the bicipital groove, provides attachments for muscles and ligaments. The greater tuberosity receives insertions of the muscles of the rotator cuff (with the exception of subscapularis) and acts as a pulley for the deltoid with elevation of the arm below 60°, helping to increase the lever arm of the supraspinatus.

The superiorly inclined head of the humerus is spheroidal and sits slightly retroverted. Only a small area of the head articulates with the relatively shallow surface of the glenoid of the scapula. The diameter of the humeral head is approximately two-thirds larger than the glenoid fossa which, in combination with variations

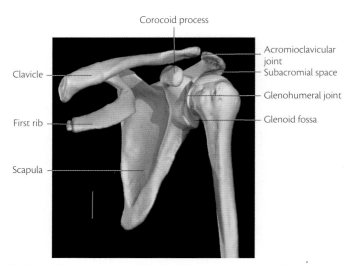

Fig. 3.5.1 The bony anatomy of the shoulder complex (anterior). Copyright © Primal Pictures. Reproduced with permission.

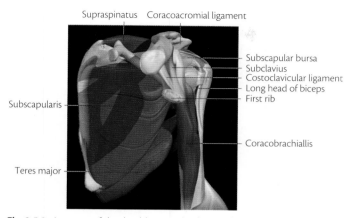

Supraspinatus   Coracoacromial ligament

Subscapular bursa
Subclavius
Costoclavicular ligament
Long head of biceps
First rib

Subscapularis

Coracobrachiallis

Teres major

Fig. 3.5.2 Anatomy of the shoulder complex (anterior). Copyright © Primal Pictures. Reproduced with permission.

Table 3.5.1 Stability of the shoulder complex

Static stabilizers
Joint capsule
Glenohumeral and coracohumeral ligaments
Subscapularis
Slightly negative pressure within the joint
Glenoid labrum
Dynamic stabilizers
Rotator cuff
Deltoid
Teres major

in glenoid morphology and the position of the scapula, may contribute to the inherent instability of the glenohumeral joint (GHJ). Blood supply to the head of the humerus is via branches of the circumflex humeral artery.

The **scapula** is composed of a flattened body with thickened processes where major muscles attach: the coracoid, acromion, spine of the scapula, and glenoid. The lateral border and superior and inferior angles are also thickened for muscle attachments.

Soft tissue structures are also important static stabilizers The **glenohumeral ligaments** are thickened folds of the joint capsule and work to strengthen the anterior capsule (Fig. 3.5.4). The **glenoid labrum**, a fibrous rim that is thicker peripherally than centrally, deepens the glenoid cavity by up to 50%. This increase in surface area for contact with the humeral head creates a buttress, limiting humeral head translation and acting as an attachment for the stabilizing glenohumeral ligaments; the capsule and the superior aspect act as an attachment for the tendon of the long head of the biceps. The labrum is weakest at the 4 o'clock position (Fig. 3.5.5). In some patients the labrum is meniscoid as a normal anatomical variant; on imaging this may be mistaken for a labral tear.

Dynamic stabilizers

Muscles act as the dynamic stabilizers of the GHJ. These can be divided into the outer sleeve formed by the deltoid, teres major, and

pectoralis major; and the inner sleeve, formed by the rotator cuff and the long head of the biceps. The **deltoid**, supplied by the axillary nerve (C5), is composed of three portions: the anterior, middle, and posterior thirds. Loss of deltoid function has a significant functional impact, as it is active in any form of elevation of the arm. It is assisted in the first 60° (and in particular the first 30°) of elevation of the arm by the rotator cuff, specifically the supraspinatus, as the deltoid has its shortest lever arm in this range.

The **rotator cuff** is a complex interweaving of four muscles, the **supraspinatus**, **infraspinatus**, **teres minor**, and **subscapularis**, which have their origins on the blade of the scapula and insert onto the humerus (Fig. 3.5.6). The **long head of the biceps** (LHB) can be considered as the fifth tendon of the cuff, since its tendon is intimately associated with the cuff as it arises from the superoposterior glenoid labrum. Although direct fibres from each rotator cuff tendon have specific sites of attachment, there is considerable interlacing of fibres between the musculotendinous units and with the articular capsule and ligaments. The capsular region between the supraspinatus and subscapularis tendons, containing the superior glenohumeral ligament, is the **rotator interval**. Here the coracohumeral ligament forms connections with the supraspinatus, subscapularis, superior glenohumeral ligament, and glenohumeral joint capsule.

The primary roles of the rotator cuff are to contribute to both mobility and stability, restrain humeral head translation, limit glenohumeral rotation, and control scapulohumeral rhythm and

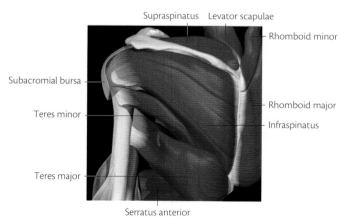

Supraspinatus   Levator scapulae

Rhomboid minor

Subacromial bursa

Teres minor

Rhomboid major
Infraspinatus

Teres major

Serratus anterior

Fig. 3.5.3 Anatomy of the shoulder complex (posterior). Copyright © Primal Pictures. Reproduced with permission.

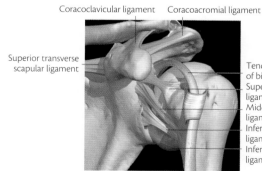

Coracoclavicular ligament   Coracoacromial ligament

Superior transverse
scapular ligament

Tendon of long head
of biceps
Superior glenohumeral
ligament
Middle glenohumeral
ligament
Inferior glenohumeral
ligament (anterior band)
Inferior glenohumeral
ligament (axillary pouch)

Fig. 3.5.4 The stability of the glenohumeral joint is aided by ligaments that behave as static stabilizers. Copyright © Primal Pictures. Reproduced with permission.

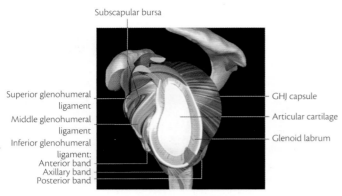

Fig. 3.5.5 The glenoid labrum contributes to stability by deepening the glenoid cavity. Copyright © Primal Pictures. Reproduced with permission.

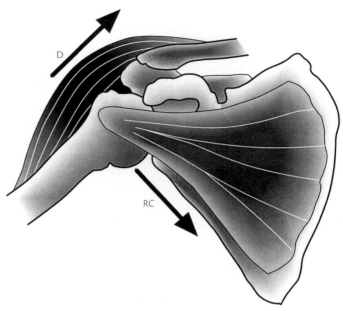

Fig. 3.5.7 The force–couple relationship between the deltoid (D) and cuff (RC) is fundamental to the stability of the shoulder. Copyright © Reproduced from Hazelman, B, Riley, G and Speed, C (ed) (2004). *Soft Tissue Rheumatology*, Oxford Univeristy Press.

position. The muscles of the rotator cuff act synergistically to apply compressive and tensile forces to achieve stable and effective movement of the humeral head. The cuff acts to stabilize and depress the humeral head in the glenoid, counteracting the effect of the deltoid which pulls the humeral head superiorly (Fig. 3.5.7). This force–couple relationship between the deltoid and cuff is fundamental to understanding many shoulder disorders.

Subscapularis is the largest and most powerful of the rotator cuff muscles. It arises from the subscapular fossa and has tendinous insertions on the lesser tuberosity. It extends to form a sheath with the tendon of the LHB, has more insertions along the surgical neck of the humerus, and also interconnects with the tendon of supraspinatus and with the underlying periosteum. It works as an internal rotator of the GHJ and is also a passive stabilizer, since its upper region is rich with dense collagen fibres as it wraps around the humeral head.

Supraspinatus arises from the supraspinous fossa and runs through the supraspinatus outlet. The latter is composed of the acromion and acromioclavicular joint superiorly, coracoid base anteriorly, the spine of the scapula posteriorly, and the superior glenoid and humeral head superiorly. Supraspinatus inserts on the greater tuberosity, and interconnects with the infraspinatus near its insertion and with the coracohumeral ligament at the rotator interval. Active in all movements involving elevation, it creates

maximal effort in 30° of elevation. **Infraspinatus** arises from the scapular infraspinous fossa and inserts on the greater tuberosity, below the supraspinatus. **Teres minor** arises inferolateral to infraspinatus in the midlateral scapula, inserting below infraspinatus on the greater tuberosity. Both these muscles act as external rotators,

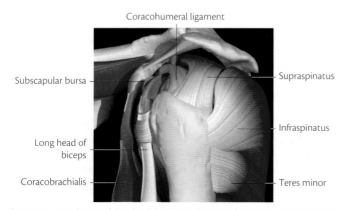

Fig. 3.5.6 Lateral view of the shoulder. The subacromial space and components of the rotator cuff. Copyright © Primal Pictures. Reproduced with permission.

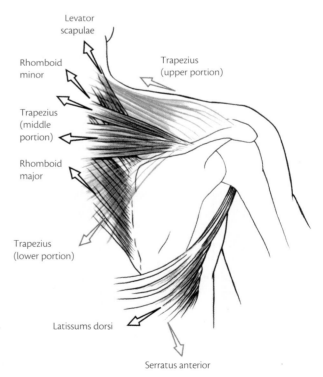

Fig. 3.5.8 Actions of scapulothoracic muscles are vital to normal shoulder movements. Copyright © Reproduced from Hazelman, B, Riley, G and Speed, C (ed) (2004). *Soft Tissue Rheumatology*, Oxford Univeristy Press.

Table 3.5.2 Muscles of the shoulder and scapulothoracic region act together in movement of the arm

Shoulder muscles	Scapular muscles
Flexion (main nerve roots: C5, C6)	
Flexors	Abductor
Anterior deltoid	Serratus anterior
Biceps	
Pectoralis major	
Corachobrachialis	
Lateral rotators	Lateral rotators
Infraspinatus	Serratus anterior
Teres minor	Trapezius
Posterior deltoid	
Abduction (main nerve roots: C5, C6)	
Abductors	Adductor
Deltoid	Trapezius (stabilizes scapula)
Supraspinatus	
Long head of biceps	
Lateral rotators	Lateral rotators
Infraspinatus	Trapezius
Teres minor	Serratus anterior
Posterior deltoid	
Extension (main nerve roots: C5–C8)	
Posterior deltoid	Adductors, medal rotators, elevators
Teres major	Rhomboids
Latissimus dorsi	Levator scapulae
Long head triceps	Pectoralis minor acts to tilt scapula anteriorly
Adduction (main nerve roots (C5–C8)	
Pectoralis major	Rhomboids
Teres major	Trapezius
Latissimus dorsi	
Long head triceps	

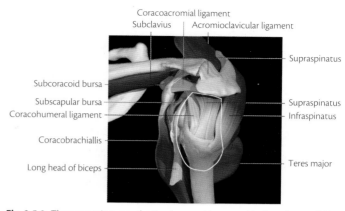

Fig. 3.5.9 The supraspinous outlet & subacromial space with the subacromial/subdeltoid bursa outlined. Copyright © Reproduced from Hazelman, B, Riley, G and Speed, C (ed) (2004). *Soft Tissue Rheumatology*, Oxford Univeristy Press.

Other anatomical features of the shoulder complex.

The **coracoid process** is easily palpable and is an important landmark, since neurovascular structures travel inferomedial to it. It serves as the origin of ligaments, the short head of the biceps and coracobrachialis, and the insertion of pectoralis minor (Figs 3.5.1, 3.5.4, and 3.5.7). Several anomalies have been described, such as a coracoclavicular band or articulation (in 1% of the population).

Acromion morphology, in particular its shape and angle, and any anatomical factors that reduce this space are of clinical relevance in assessing rotator cuff pathologies (Bigliani *et al.* 1986). The coracoacromial ligament makes an important contribution to the roof of the subacromial space and anatomical variations of this ligament complex can reduce the size of the space. The **acromio-clavicular joint** (ACJ) is stabilized by thick ligaments and deltotrapezius thickening, with a fibrous disc separating the articular surfaces and the joint anterosuperiorly. A small amount of motion of the ACJ occurs with glenohumeral elevation and rotation, with the clavicle rotating upward on the sternum at the sternoclavicular joint. The ACJ is narrowed during adduction in the horizontal plane and in elevation above 90°. The posterior component of the joint narrows during extension in the horizontal plane. The morphology of the ACJ has also been divided into three types: vertical (type I), oblique (type II), and more horizontal than vertical (type III), with the former being associated with a greater incidence of ACJ osteoarthritis (OA) (De Palma 1957).

The **sternoclavicular joint** (SCJ) is a synovial joint formed by articulation between the clavicle and sternum and the first rib. It is an incongruent joint, with only up to 50% of the articular surfaces in contact, but an intra-articular disc converts the complex into a congruous unit and additional stability is conferred by surrounding ligaments.

There are several important bursae in the shoulder complex. Clinically, the most important of these, the **subacromial and subdeltoid bursae,** frequently exist as one attached to the undersurface of the coracoacromial ligament and the superior surface of the supraspinatus tendon. These bursae aid the free movement of the rotator cuff beneath the acromion, with a sliding effect occurring between the superior and inferior internal surfaces of the bursa during abduction of the shoulder. It does not communicate with the glenohumeral cavity in the healthy state.

with infraspinatus typically being the greater contributor. LHB runs through the bicipital groove, which is roofed by the transverse humeral ligament. A sling of tendoligamentous structures at the entrance to the groove (the 'rotator interval sling', or 'biceps pulley') acts to constrain the tendon within the groove. It contributes to dynamic stability and depression of the humeral head, functions as a flexor of the forearm in neutral and supination, and contributes to flexion and abduction of the arm.

Other muscles contributing to scapulothoracic motion include the trapezius, rhomboids, levator scapulae, serratus anterior, pectorals, teres major, and coracobrachialis (Table 3.5.2 and Figure 3.5.9)

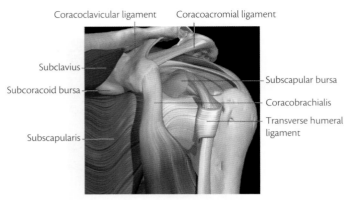

Fig. 3.5.10 Bursae of the anterior shoulder. Copyright © Reproduced from Hazelman, B, Riley, G and Speed, C (ed) (2004). *Soft Tissue Rheumatology*, Oxford Univeristy Press.

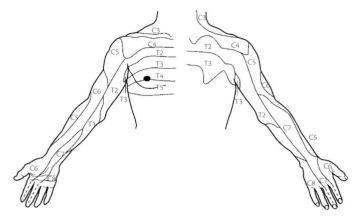

Fig. 3.5.12 Approximate dermatomes of the arm. Copyright © Reproduced from Hazelman, B, Riley, G and Speed, C (ed) (2004). *Soft Tissue Rheumatology*, Oxford Univeristy Press.

The **subscapularis** (or **subcoracoid**) **bursa** usually connects with the GHJ cavity and is found between the upper subscapularis and the neck of the glenoid. Further bursae are located between tendinous insertions of many of the muscles of the shoulder complex, between muscles such as teres major and latissimus dorsi, and beneath coracobrachialis (Figs 3.5.10 and 3.5.11).

Nerves

Nerve trunks from the brachial plexus (C5–T1) pass under the clavicle to divide and form the peripheral nerves of the arm (Fig.3.5.12). The **axillary nerve** (C5) runs with the axillary artery on subscapularis, inferior to the GHJ, and exits the quadrangular space with the posterior circumflex artery. It supplies deltoid and teres minor. The **musculocutaneous nerve** (C5–C7) runs obliquely to enter the corachobrachialis about 5 cm distal to the coracoid process. It also supplies brachialis and biceps. The **suprascapular nerve** (C4–C6) travels posterolaterally beneath the trapezius to the upper border of the scapula, medial to the coracoid process. It passes through the suprascapular notch beneath the transverse scapular ligament and supplies the spinati. The **radial nerve** (C5–C8), which supplies the triceps, brachioradialis, and extensor carpi radialis longus, courses round the humerus in the spiral groove. It passes anterior to the lateral epicondyle and divides into the posterior interosseous and superficial branches in the antecubital fossa. The **ulnar nerve** (C8, T1) gives no branches above the elbow (Table 3.5.3).

Biomechanics of the throwing action

Many overhead activities involve a similar central sequence of actions and muscle recruitment, based on the throwing action, as described in Table 3.5.4 and Figure 3.5.13. The three common elements are cocking (80%), acceleration (2%), and follow-through (18%). However, sports vary in relation to upper limb and body position during the action, and motion analysis of throwing/playing technique needs to be scrutinized by an informed observer as part of the clinical assessment of upper limb injuries. The cocking phase involving wind-up, early cocking, and late cocking starts with winding the shoulder into abduction in external rotation, with the contralateral leg moved quickly in front of the body and the trunk and the pelvis rotated to move the shoulder girdle into position. The arm is then in position to accelerate, bringing the shoulder out of external rotation, and releasing the ball at about 40°–60° of external rotation, with flexion and then extension of the elbow and movement of the wrist from extension to neutral, and with forearm pronation at release of the ball. Follow-through involves significant activation of the pectoralis major and subscapularis (already firing during acceleration to promote internal rotation), and the posterior shoulder–scapular musculature forms a force couple with the biceps. All muscles of the shoulder complex are working to stabilize the GHJ.

There are considerable variations on this theme, depending upon the sport, but in all cases muscle balance must be achieved to prevent injury such as rotator cuff and labral lesions.

Adaptations in the overhead-throwing athlete's shoulder

In a review of the anatomical adaptations of the overhead-throwing athlete's shoulder, Borsa *et al.* (2008) emphasized that throwing athletes frequently have altered RoM patterns in the dominant shoulder which favour increased external rotation and limited internal rotation and a loss of horizontal or cross-body adduction in the throwing shoulder. Posterior shoulder immobility may be due to contraction or reactive scarring of the periscapular soft tissue structures (e.g. posterior capsule and/or cuff musculature). Conversely, glenohumeral translational RoM (laxity) is symmetric between the dominant and non-dominant shoulders of overhead athletes.

The throwing shoulder also has more humeral retroversion than the non-throwing shoulder; this may be due to developmental changes in young pre-adolescent throwers when the proximal

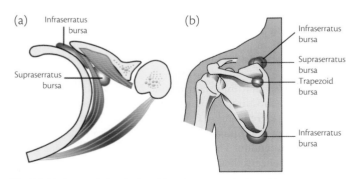

Fig. 3.5.11 Anatomical and adventitious bursae may be found between tendinous insertions of many of the muscles of the shoulder complex. Copyright © Reproduced from Hazelman, B, Riley, G and Speed, C (ed) (2004). *Soft Tissue Rheumatology*, Oxford Univeristy Press.

Table 3.5.3 Motor supply of the arm

Nerve	Roots	Motor supply[a]	Quick motor test
Axillary	C5,6	Deltoid	Shoulder abduction
		Teres minor	
Musculocutaneous	C5–C7	Corachobrachialis, brachialis, biceps	Flexion of supinated forearm
Suprascapular	C4–C6	Spinati	Supraspinatus test, external rotation of shoulder
Radial	C5–C8	Triceps, brachioradialis, ECR longus and brevis, supinator	Elbow extension, supination of extended forearm, wrist extension
Radial nerve branches:	C7, C8	Extensors of wrist/fingers	Wrist extension
Posterior Interosseous			
Superficial radial		—	—
Ulnar	C8, T1	FCU, FDP of ring and little fingers, small muscles of hand except those supplied by median nerve	Abduction little and index fingers, adduction of thumb
Median	C7, C8, T1	Pronator teres, forearm flexors except those supplied by ulnar nerve, 1st and 2nd lumbricals, APB, opponens pollicis, FPB	Pronation of forearm; abduction, opposition of thumb
Median nerve branch anterior interosseus	C7, C8	FDP of index, middle fingers, FPL	Flexion distal phalanx of thumb, index finger

[a] ECR, Extensor carpi radialis; FCU, flexor carpi ulnaris; FDP, flexordigitorum profundus; FPL, flexor pollicis longus; APB, abductor policis brevis; FPB, flexor pollicis brevis.

Table 3.5.4 The phases of throwing

Phase	Description
Wind-up	Body prepares: centre of gravity is raised, shoulder in slight abduction and internal rotation. Little stress on the upper limb.
Early cocking	Arm rotates behind body axis by 15° in abduction, external rotation. Deltoid active early, rotator cuff active later. Elbow flexed, wrist, MCPJs extended, forearm slightly pronated, which continues through late cocking. Ends just before beginning of forward arm and body motion.
Late cocking	Lead leg contacts the ground, ends when arm reaches maximal external rotation. Scapula retracts to stabilize humeral head. Upper arm maintained in ~90°–100° abduction, and humeral head translates progressively posteriorly. External rotators, deltoid, supraspinatus are active early. Subscapularis becomes active at beginning of internal rotation. Elbow extends, wrist and MCPJs flexed. There is a high compression force on the GHJ by the rotator cuff and high valgus torque at the elbow; high stress on UCL and surrounding structures and compressive forces at radiocapitellar joint.
Acceleration	Begins as internal rotation starts, ends at ball release. High angular velocities are generated but little stress through shoulder joint in this phase. In addition to cuff and deltoid, triceps is active early, pectoralis major and latissimus dorsi active later.
Deceleration	Begins just after ball release, ends when humeral internal rotation stops. Scapula protraction and very high load through the rotator cuff with compressive loading on GHJ, and posterior and inferior shear stresses.
Follow-through	Body regains stability. Maximal pronation of forearm. Loads diminish.

MCPJ, metacarpophalangeal joint; GHJ, glenohumeral joint; UCL, ulnar collateral ligament.

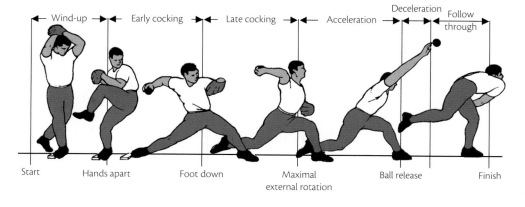

Fig. 3.5.13 Throwing sports vary in their techniques but most involve significant traction on the LHB and labrum. Many throwers also have lax shoulders, imposing greater demands on dynamic stabilizers. Copyright © Reproduced from Hazelman, B, Riley, G and Speed, C (ed) (2004). *Soft Tissue Rheumatology*, Oxford Univeristy Press.

humeral epiphysis is not yet completely fused. The changes, both soft tissue and osseous, will vary according to the individual and their sport. It is possible that altered shoulder mobility in the overhead-throwing athlete is more strongly associated with adaptive changes in proximal humeral anatomy (i.e. retroversion) than with changes in the articular and periarticular soft tissue structures. In addition, this retroversion is thought to account for the observed shift in the arc of rotational RoM in overhead athletes. However, in some athletes, capsulo-ligamentous adaptations such as anterior–inferior stretching or posterior–inferior contracture may make a major contribution. This may ultimately lead to pathological manifestations such as secondary impingement, type II superior labrum from anterior to posterior (SLAP) lesions and/or internal (glenoid) impingement.

Clinical evaluation

History

Symptoms in the shoulder in sports-related complaints can arise because of local structural pathology or in relation to problems at distant sites. Symptoms can also arise in the absence of significant structural abnormality because of dysfunctional movements, or may be referred from elsewhere. Abnormal kinetics is common and may be a cause or an effect of local pathology. The differential diagnosis of shoulder symptoms is wide and causation is often multifactorial (Table 3.5.5).

Assessment starts with a thorough history. Shoulder disorders can vary with respect to their nature and aetiology in different age groups. Hand dominance, past medical history, and a full sporting history should be recorded. The last of these includes details of competition and training patterns, equipment, technical changes, the stage of the competitive season, and the competitive level of the athlete, and everyday demands that are imposed upon the upper limbs which may influence approaches to management and compliance with therapy.

The primary symptom of most shoulder complaints is **pain**. A careful pain history is taken to determine the mode of onset, site, nature, radiation, associated symptoms, exacerbating and relieving features, and the presence of nocturnal symptoms.

The **mode of onset** should be established. Most shoulder disorders arise gradually and are associated with repetitive microtrauma (overuse), particularly with repeated activities during training or play. A history of trauma such as a fall onto the outstretched hand is often given in acute cuff tear and is also frequently reported with an initial dislocation, but subsequent dislocations may occur with seemingly trivial incidents. ACJ sprains may be precipitated by a direct blow or a fall onto the tip of the shoulder or elbow, or an episode of heavy lifting. Rupture of the rotator cuff and/or tendon of the LHB is seen in senior athletes and may appear to occur with minimal trauma, although there is frequently a preceding history of (often minor) shoulder pain. Some disorders arise spontaneously and are not associated with sport, such as primary calcific tendonitis or primary frozen shoulder.

The **site** of the pain is a useful indication of its source, although pain secondary to rotator cuff disease and GHJ and capsular disorders has similar distributions (Fig. 3.5.14). Pain associated with glenohumeral instability may be non-specific and poorly localized. Acromioclavicular and sternoclavicular pain are usually well localized to the joint, and the patient complaining of 'shoulder' pain that is arising from the neck may point to the upper trapezius as the site of their problem. Radiation of pain to the elbow and further distally is suggestive of referred pain from the neck or more peripheral neurological lesions, although it can occur in rotator cuff impingement. Additional neurological and neck symptoms should be sought. The **nature** and **timing** of the pain is also important. Pain that is worse with activity may represent an articular or musculotendinous disorder. Many shoulder complaints give rise to nocturnal pain, particularly when the complaint is severe.

Table 3.5.5 Differential diagnosis of shoulder pain

Site	Lesions
Rotator cuff	Tendinosis, impingement, tears, calcifying tendinitis
Tendon of long head of biceps	Tenosynovitis, subluxation/dislocation, tear/rupture
Capsule	Capsulitis
Joint complex and surrounding musculature	Glenohumeral instabilities, labral lesions
Bursae	Subacromial/subdeltoid bursitis, others
Nerves	Lesions of axillary, suprascapular, long thoracic, musculocutaneous nerves, brachial plexus. Referred pain
Muscle	Muscle injuries, myofascial pain
Joint	Glenohumeral arthritides
Bone	Fractures
Others	Local destructive lesions

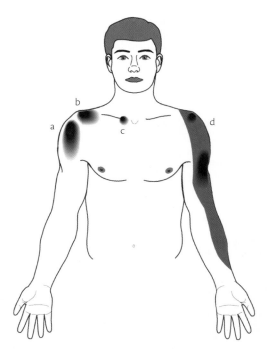

Fig. 3.5.14 Sites of shoulder pain: (a) glenohumeral rotator cuff or capsule; (b) ACJ; (c) sternoclavicular; (d) referred pain from the neck. The darker areas represent more intense pain. Copyright © Reproduced from Hazelman, B, Riley, G and Speed, C (ed) (2004). *Soft Tissue Rheumatology*, Oxford Univeristy Press.

Pain which causes significant nocturnal disturbance, particularly when lying on the affected side, is characteristic of rotator cuff disorders. Pain that is constant, day and night, is typical of the frozen shoulder or underlying systemic disorders, which must always be excluded in presentations of shoulder pain. Pain associated with cervical spondylosis is often better at night once the patient gets their neck into a comfortable position, but referred or radicular pain is not. Neuropathic pain is typically constant, deep and burning in nature, and unaffected by movement.

Exacerbating and relieving features are also noted. Pain with activities involving overhead work is suggestive of subacromial impingement or acromioclavicular pathology. Subacromial or subcoracoid impingement may be associated with pain on movement when the arm is in the forward flexed position. Subscapularis lesions may present with pain when the arm is below shoulder height. Pain when carrying heavy objects is classically associated with ACJ sprains, rotator cuff lesions, or myofascial pain syndromes affecting the scapulothoracic musculature. In 'dead arm syndrome' the athlete reports shooting pains radiating down the arm, with paraesthesiae and temporary weakness of the arm immediately after releasing the ball when throwing or when serving or smashing in tennis. This occurs because of anterior or multidirectional glenohumeral instability with brachial plexus traction during the activity. Pain which is unaffected by movement is often due to referred pain from extrinsic pathologies. A **training history** may reveal a change in use of the affected limb prior to the onset of the complaint; often seemingly minor changes in training or technique may be the issue.

Clicking around the shoulder complex is a common symptom and is frequently long-standing in those who have congenitally lax joints. Clicking is associated with pain and, particularly when unilateral, is more likely to be representative of local pathology such as rotator cuff tendinopathy, tendinopathy, or subluxation or dislocation of the biceps tendon. Clicking and clunking are also symptoms of labral lesions and of instabilities which are more localized when the ACJ and SCJ are involved, and more diffuse when the GHJ is involved. A 'catching' sensation is frequently reported in rotator cuff/subacromial pathology. 'Crunching' on movement can be associated with a variety of pathologies including OA anywhere in the shoulder complex of joints, subacromial bursitis, and rotator cuff pathologies.

Any **previous history** of dislocations should be noted. The direction of the dislocation, its circumstances of onset (mechanism, degree of trauma, additional injuries), and details of subsequent episodes (including the frequency and ease of reduction), symptoms of subluxation, rotator cuff tendinopathy, or any other lesion are all important. Patients may describe apprehension that their shoulder might sublux or dislocate with the arm in certain positions, for example when the arm is in external rotation in abduction in anterior GHJ instabilities. Determining whether recurrent dislocations are voluntary or involuntary is essential for planning appropriate management, although voluntary dislocators may deny that they perform such manoeuvres intentionally.

Weakness may be reported which may be true weakness, pain inhibition, or mechanical restriction. True weakness can result from a significant disruption to the gross structural integrity of tissues of the shoulder complex, usually in the form of a rotator cuff tear. Neurological lesions may also cause weakness.

Swelling of joints of the shoulder complex can occur in relation to arthropathy, infection, or trauma. Swelling of the SCJ is a classical but frequently overlooked presenting feature of an inflammatory arthritis. An insidious onset of restriction or stiffness of the shoulder may be noted in relation to bony constraint such as in GHJ OA, soft tissue restriction such as frozen shoulder, or pain in any local disorder of the shoulder complex.

Enquiry about the presence of systemic symptoms is of paramount importance. Symptoms such as fever, weight loss, and anorexia may suggest sepsis, malignancy, or inflammatory joint disease. The degree of functional disability may be assessed informally by determining the type and degree of activities affected and the number of days lost from work/play, or by the use of a formal assessment score.

Development of a management regime for the complaint requires an assessment of the approaches taken and their effects to date. Medications, physiotherapy regimes, modalities, and interventions of other health professionals, including osteopaths, chiropractors, complementary therapists, etc., should all be listed.

Examination

Assessment of the patient with a shoulder complaint can be complex, but meticulous examination can be very rewarding in reaching an accurate diagnosis.

Inspection

Examination of the patient commences with observation as they enter the consulting room. When the shoulder is very painful, they may support the affected arm with the opposite hand and simple functional tasks such as removing a jacket are difficult. The adequately exposed patient should be inspected from the back, front, and side. Posture should be noted; poor posture can contribute to shoulder pain and postural adjustments as a result of a local complaint are also common. It is normal to hold one shoulder (usually the non-dominant arm) higher than the other. Congenital deformities may predispose to shoulder problems and include a short neck (Klippel–Feil syndrome) and Sprengel shoulder (a congenitally high, poorly developed, and medially rotated scapula).

Inspection continues, starting at the SCJ and working laterally across the clavicle and chest wall to the ACJ, the acromion, the anterior GHJ, biceps, and deltoid, and then moving posteriorly and working medially from the acromion, posterior deltoid, spinati, and other scapulothoracic musculature. The examiner is seeking evidence of muscle wasting or overdevelopment, soft tissue or bony deformity, and swelling, all of which may result in asymmetry. The presence of muscle fasciculation, scars, skin lesions (such as psoriasis), and discoloration should also be noted. The presence of SCJ prominence should be noted; this is associated with underlying inflammatory arthritis, OA, sepsis, or instability. Clavicular deformity is usually secondary to previous fracture or, rarely, congential problems (shortening, pseudarthrosis). ACJ prominence, if bilateral, may be normal, but when unilateral suggests ACJ OA, previous dislocation or fracture, or subcoracoid glenohumeral dislocation. A step deformity at the ACJ is indicative of an acromioclavicular ligament injury.

Muscles which can easily be inspected for wasting and asymmetry are the trapezius, paracervical, deltoid, biceps, and the spinati. Abnormalities of the pectoralis major may be accentuated by the patient placing their hands on their hips and pressing hard inwards. Atrophy of the upper trapezius is associated with spinal accessory nerve palsy, and flattening of the deltoid may be seen with axillary nerve or C5 root pathology or after glenohumeral dislocation.

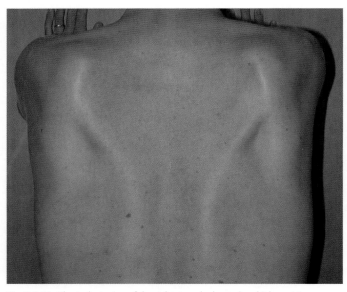

Fig. 3.5.15 Classical winging of the right scapula due to brachial neuritis. Copyright © Reproduced from Hazelman, B, Riley, G and Speed, C (ed) (2004). *Soft Tissue Rheumatology*, Oxford Univeristy Press.

The presence of scapular winging should be sought by standing behind the patient and asking them to push up against a wall. (Figure 3.5.15). Classical winging occurs when the medial border of the scapula moves away from the posterior chest wall. Rotary winging occurs when the inferior angle of the scapula rotates further from the spine than the contralateral scapula (Table 3.5.6). Winging may be due to either structural or neuromuscular causes. Structural winging can occur as a result of deformities of the scapula itself, or deformities of the clavicle, thoracic spine, or ribs, for example thoracic scoliosis with a rotational element. The more commonly encountered form of scapular winging is the functional form, where there is a lack of control of the scapula because of a neuromuscular defect or muscle imbalance.

Palpation

The supraclavicular fossa should be palpated for lymphadenopathy and other masses. Palpation of structures, starting at the SCJ, is performed. Crepitus may be noted when there is localized arthritis or bursitis. Instability of the ACJ or SCJ may be detected through manual pressure. Further instability tests are described below (in the section on special tests). Tender or trigger points may be evident, particularly in fibromyalgia or myofascial pain, respectively.

Table 3.5.6 Causes of winging of the scapula

Structural static winging
Deformity of the scapula, clavicle, thoracic spine, or ribs
Functional (dynamic) winging
Long thoracic nerve palsy
Spinal accessory nerve palsy
Rhomboid weakness
Multidirectional GHJ instability
Voluntary action
Painful shoulder with splinting of the GHJ and reversed scapulohumeral rhythm

Movement

Evaluation of movement commences with inspection of the range, comfort, and rhythm of movement while the patient performs active movements.

Movement in each plane may be restricted due to pain or true restriction. Normal scapulohumeral rhythm involves little or no movement of the scapula in the first 90° of abduction, as this is achieved through glenohumeral movement. The following 70° of abduction is achieved through scapular rotation and the final 20 ° through further movement at the GHJ. Any shoulder disorder can result in a loss of this normal pattern, with premature scapular rotation being a particularly common feature.

Hitching of the shoulder is a common compensatory movement for a restricted or painful shoulder. A painful arc of abduction in mid-range is typical of subacromial pathology which is often eased with supination of the arm, which can reduce mechanical impingement. In some cases a painful mid arc is evident only on slowly lowering the arm from full abduction. A superior painful arc is found with acromioclavicular pathologies, particularly OA (Fig 3.5.16).

Active RoM can be compared with passive RoM. Restriction of both is indicative of GHJ or local/diffuse capsular pathology (e.g. OA or frozen shoulder), whereas good passive RoM in the presence of active restriction indicates either a musculotendinous (usually rotator cuff) or neurological injury. Specific active movements to test strength of the rotator cuff are then tested against resistance provided by the examiner, who notes the presence of pain and

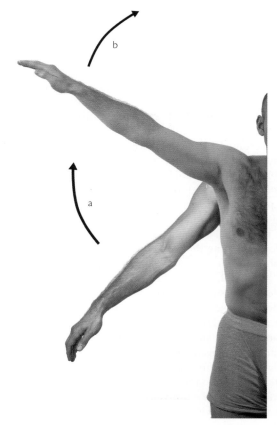

Fig. 3.5.16 A painful arc of abduction indicates (a) subacromial impingement or (b) acromioclavicular disorder. Copyright © Reproduced from Hazelman, B, Riley, G and Speed, C (ed) (2004). *Soft Tissue Rheumatology*, Oxford Univeristy Press.

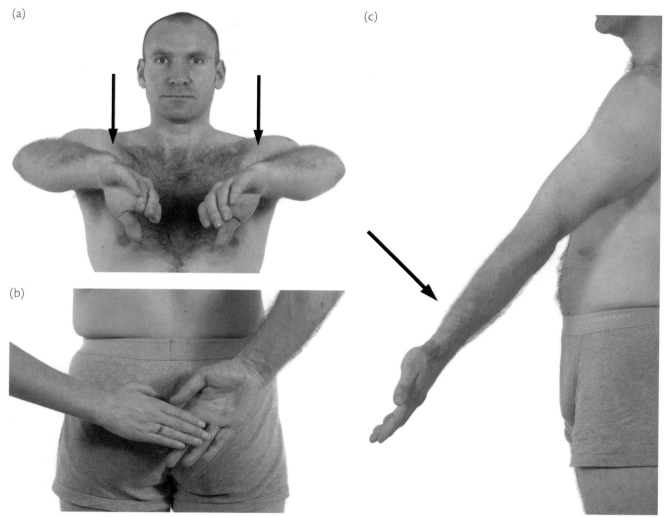

Fig. 3.5.17 Testing the rotator cuff. The examiner applies resistance (indicated by arrows) which the patient resists. Pain and/or weakness indicate pathology: (a) supraspinatus; (b) subscapularis; (c) long head biceps. Infraspinatus and teres minor are tested by resisted external rotation of the shoulder. Copyright © Reproduced from Hazelman, B, Riley, G and Speed, C (ed) (2004). *Soft Tissue Rheumatology*, Oxford Univeristy Press.

weakness and whether the latter is out of proportion to the pain. The components of the rotator cuff and LHB can all be assessed (Fig. 3.5.17).

Special tests
Impingement
Impingement can also be identified when there is pain on passive abduction and internal rotation of the shoulder (Fig. 3.5.18).

Glenohumeral instability
Several tests are helpful in the assessment of glenohumeral laxity and instability. The humeral head can be translated in the glenoid fossa manually by the examiner, to assess laxity of the joint ('load and shift'), with the patient standing and then supine. The first test is with the arm by the patient's side, and then in different positions. For example, with progressive external rotation of the arm with the shoulder in abduction, there should be less translation anteriorly if the inferior glenohumeral ligament (GHL) is intact, as it becomes taut and acts as a restraint. Similarly, by internally rotating the arm, posterior translation is diminished with an intact posterior capsular structure. The **apprehension tests** include tests for

anterior instability (abduction, external rotation) and posterior instability (adduction, internal rotation, and forward flexion). **Jobe's relocation test** is also performed.

Acromioclavicular joint
Pathologies of the ACJ, in particular OA, can be identified by compressing or stressing the joint in adduction across the chest wall anteriorly, or in maximal abduction with the arm behind the head.

SLAP lesions
O'Brien's test for SLAP lesions places the arm in 90° flexion, 20° adduction, full internal rotation, and resisted elevation (Fig.3.5.21). The test is positive if pain is elicited and then relieved on external rotation in the same position (O'Brien *et al.* 1998).

Thoracic outlet syndrome (TOS)
Stress manoeuvres in TOS are widely described but have limited reliability.

Cervical spine
The cervical spine should also be assessed since it is a common source of shoulder pain. This includes evaluation of range of

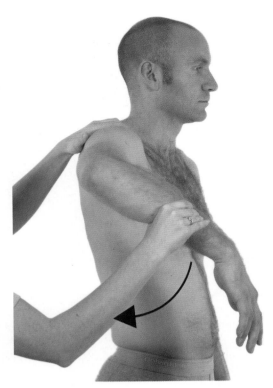

Fig. 3.5.18 A subacromial impingement test. Pain is reproduced with passive internal rotation of the abducted arm. Copyright © Reproduced from Hazelman, B, Riley, G and Speed, C (ed) (2004). *Soft Tissue Rheumatology*, Oxford Univeristy Press.

movement and the surrounding musculature. A full neurovascular assessment of the upper limbs should also be performed.

Investigations

Plain X-rays are useful in the detection of degenerative changes in the shoulder complex, fractures, and after dislocations. Stress views can be helpful in the evaluation of instabilities of the ACJ and SCJ. Diagnostic ultrasound is very sensitive to changes in the rotator cuff and biceps, subacromial/subdeltoid bursa, and joint effusions, and allows dynamic evaluation of the cuff. It is also used for interventions, in particular guided injection. MRI not only demonstrates the rotator cuff elegantly, but also evaluates the surrounding bony anatomy and bone oedema syndromes. MR arthrography (particularly direct) allows accurate assessment of the labrum and articular surfaces. CT is utilized in the evaluation of fractures and detection of loose bodies.

General shoulder pain

Glenohumeral instability

Glenohumeral instability is the symptomatic inability to keep the humeral head centred in the glenoid fossa. It should be distinguished from laxity ('slackness', 'looseness'), which is a variant of the normal joint. Instability may take the form of dislocation when there is complete separation of the articular surfaces or, more commonly, varying degrees of subluxation involving excessive translation of the humeral head on the glenoid without separation of the articular surfaces. This may be very subtle and only provoked by specific activities. Instability is also described according to its

(a)

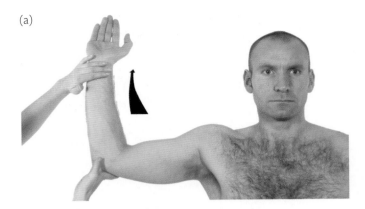

(b)

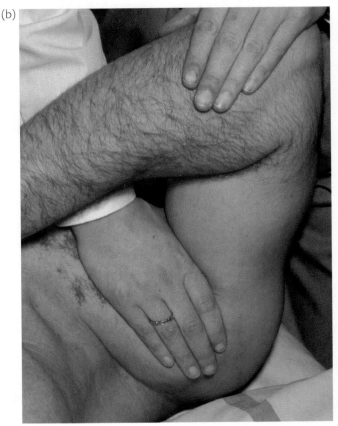

Fig. 3.5.19 Apprehension tests. Anterior glenohumeral instability can be assessed standing, sitting, or supine. (a) As the shoulder is moved passively into abduction and external rotation, the patient becomes apprehensive that the shoulder is going to dislocate anteriorly. (b) Posterior instability can be assessed with the patient supine. The examiner forward flexes and medial rotates the shoulder and applies posterior force on the patient's elbow. The patient reports apprehension that the shoulder is going to dislocate posteriorly. Copyright © Reproduced from Hazelman, B, Riley, G and Speed, C (ed) (2004). *Soft Tissue Rheumatology*, Oxford Univeristy Press.

circumstances of onset, direction, degree, duration, uni/bilaterality, and volition. Determination of these factors is important in planning appropriate management (Table 3.5.8).

Dislocations

Dislocations of the GHJ comprise 45% of all dislocations. Almost 85% of these are in the **anterior direction**. The most common type is subcoracoid, typically after trauma involving forced abduction,

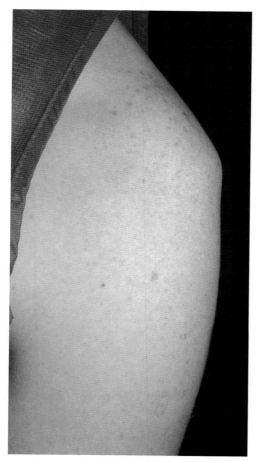

Fig. 3.5.20 The inferior sulcus sign, indicating inferior laxity. Traction is being placed by the examiner on the arm, pulling the humerus inferiorly.
Copyright © Reproduced from Hazelman, B, Riley, G and Speed, C (ed) (2004). *Soft Tissue Rheumatology*, Oxford Univeristy Press.

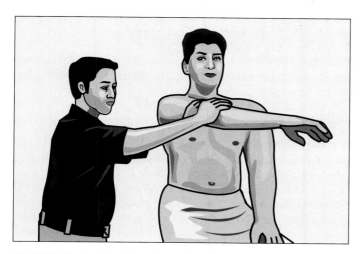

Fig. 3.5.21 The shoulder is placed in 90° of elevation and 30° of horizontal adduction across the midline. Resistance is applied in this position with both full shoulder internal and external rotation (altering humeral rotation against the glenoid in the process). A positive test for labral involvement is when pain is elicited when testing with the shoulder in internal rotation and the forearm in pronation (thumb pointing toward the floor). Symptoms are typically decreased when tested in the externally rotated position or the pain is localized at the ACJ.

Table 3.5.7 Recommendations for radiological investigations in shoulder complaints

Complaint	Investigation	Comments
Shoulder pain	X-ray	Not indicated unless history of trauma, dislocation or calcific tendonitis suspected, or trauma
Impingement	MRI	Impingement is a clinical diagnosis. Imaging to examine state of cuff and contributing pathologies in resistant cases.
	Ultrasound	Allows dynamic imaging.
Instability	MR arthrography, CT arthrography	
Rotator cuff test	Ultrasound, MRI	

extension, and external rotation. The other main mechanism of dislocation is when the patient falls onto the posterior aspect of the shoulder. More rare forms of dislocation, usually in association with severe trauma, associated rotator cuff avulsion, and fracture of the greater tuberosity, include subglenoid, subclavicular, intrathoracic, and retroperitoneal.

The patient usually holds the arm in slight abduction and external rotation. The humeral head may be palpable anteriorly. There is limited internal rotation and adduction. Neurovascular injuries are common and may also occur after reduction, so assessment prior to treatment is mandatory. The axillary nerve is the most commonly injured neural structure, although damage to the radial, musculocutaneous, median, ulnar, or entire brachial plexus may occur. When neurological injury does occur, neuropraxias are the most common; symptoms beyond 3 months have a poor prognosis for recovery. Vascular injury is indicated by a reduced or absent peripheral pulse, an expanding haematoma, pallor, or shock.

Avulsion of the antero-inferior glenohumeral ligaments and capsule from the glenoid rim represent a **Bankart lesion**, a common cause of recurrent instability after previous dislocation. A **Hill–Sachs lesion** often accompanies a Bankart lesion; this is a compression fracture of the posterior surface of the humeral head after impaction against the anterior glenoid rim (Fig. 3.5.22). Rotator cuff tears can coexist, particularly over the age of 40 years. They may be difficult to detect clinically in the acute presentation and a high index of suspicion should be maintained.

Table 3.5.8 Descriptive features of glenohumeral instability

Type	Subluxation/dislocation
Mode of onset	Traumatic/atraumatic
Duration	Acute/chronic
Side affected	Unilateral/bilateral
Direction	Unidirectional (anterior/posterior/inferior)/ multidirectional
Volition	Voluntary/involuntary
Associated features	Congenital laxity/neuromuscular disorder/resulting pathologies (e.g. Bankart, Hill–Sachs lesions)

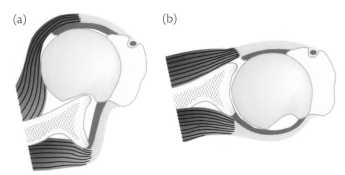

Fig. 3.5.22 (a) A posterolateral defect in the humeral head (Hill–Sachs lesion) and an anterior capsulolabral tear (Bankart's lesion) commonly occur with anterior GHJ dislocation. (b) These persist after reduction of the dislocation. Copyright © Reproduced from Hazelman, B, Riley, G and Speed, C (ed) (2004). *Soft Tissue Rheumatology*, Oxford Univeristy Press.

Table 3.5.9 Sequelae of acute dislocations

Site	Sequelae
Humerus	Anterior: posterolateral defect of the humeral head (Hill–Sachs lesion)
	Posterior: anteromedial compression fracture of the humeral head (reverse Hill–Sachs lesion)
	Fracture of greater tuberosity or more rarely surgical neck
Glenoid	Avulsion fracture of glenoid rim (Bankart lesion)
	Major fractures
Labrum	Tear
Capsule	Anterior calcification
Rotator cuff	Partial or complete tear
Neurological injuries	Most commonly axillary nerve or brachial plexus; other nerves of the upper arm can be affected.
Vascular injuries	Axillary artery

Posterior dislocations occur in relation to trauma but are also a feature of congenital laxity and multidirectional instability. Traumatic dislocations in relation to trauma are mostly subacromial, or rarely subglenoid or subspinous, and frequently are locked. All may arise due to axial loading of the adducted internally rotated arm or by violent muscle contraction. Posterior dislocations are frequently missed, but are indicated by a hollow below the acromion, anterior deltoid flattening, and a palpable humeral head posteriorly. The patient holds the arm in adduction or internal rotation, and there is a lack of active and passive external rotation. Sequelae include fracture of the glenoid rim, fracture of the proximal humerus, and reverse Hill–Sachs lesion (a compression fracture of the humeral head). Rotator cuff and neurovascular injuries are less commonly noted than with an anterior dislocation.

Inferior dislocations may be produced by a significant hyperabduction injury, which levers the humeral head inferiorly out of the glenoid through abutment of the neck of the humerus against the acromion. Such dislocations are locked and, in contrast to posterior dislocations, they are easily identified. Avulsion of one or more portions of the rotator cuff, fracture of the greater tuberosity, and neurovascular damage are all common. Superior dislocation is very rare because of the presence of the cuff and coracoacromial arch, and occurs after a major anterior and upward force on the adducted arm, with multiple injuries of surrounding structures (Table 3.5.9).

Investigations

Plain X-rays are performed in order to confirm a dislocation and to identify associated bony pathologies. Views in at least two planes are obtained, usually an anteroposterior (AP) view in the scapular plane (some recommend that this should be performed with the arm in both external and internal rotation) and a transthoracic lateral view. An axillary view is particularly helpful. Reliance on AP views only may result in a missed fracture or posterior dislocation. Other imaging studies may be necessary to pursue possible sequelae to the dislocation. Ultrasound can assess the integrity of the cuff, as can MRI which will also demonstrate fractures and Hill–Sachs lesions, Bankart lesions, and other labral pathologies. MR arthrography may be necessary, but in the acute case the presence of intra-articular effusion or haemarthrosis may provide sufficient contrast. CT is also useful in the evaluation of bony injuries, and CT arthrography will show contrast extending into an anterior labral tear.

Treatment

Treatment involves early relocation after assessment and plain X-ray. Analgesics, muscle relaxants, and even a general anaesthetic may be necessary. Early reduction is important in order to minimize the effect on the joint and soft tissue structures. A variety of approaches for reduction are advocated, and open reduction may occasionally be necessary. After reduction, neurovascular status and rotator cuff integrity should be reassessed. Traditionally, the arm is then immobilized for 3–6 weeks in the younger patient, but for 1–3 weeks in older individuals as they are more prone to joint stiffness with prolonged immobilization. However, there is no evidence that the direction of immobilization affects the risk of recurrence. The position of the arm during this period depends on the direction of the dislocation; after anterior dislocation the arm is usually maintained in adduction and internal rotation, and posterior dislocations are maintained in slight external rotation, abduction, and extension. Recent studies suggest that immobilization in external rotation for 3 weeks may reduce recurrence in anterior dislocations (Itoi *et al.* 2007). After immobilization, rehabilitation initially involves movement limited to 90° flexion and abduction and no external rotation, isometric strengthening of the rotator cuff and deltoid, and full RoM of the elbow. A progressive cuff and scapular stabilizing programme is then commenced.

Recurrent instability

Recurrent glenohumeral instability forms a spectrum which may vary from repeated dislocations to subtle subluxation and can be broadly classified into two groups (**TUBS** and **AMBRII**), according to some of these features (Thomas and Matsen 1989) at either end of the spectrum. Although an oversimplification of the broad continuum of shoulder laxity, this classification provides a useful clinical approach to shoulder instability.

TUBS: Trauma to any part of the stabilizing complex may precipitate recurrent instability, which is typically reproduced by putting the arm into the position it was in when the trauma occurred. **T**rauma usually results in **u**nilateral instability and there is often other pathology, classically a **B**ankart lesion. Although such cases may respond to a rehabilitation programme, surgery may be necessary. Therefore these lesions are known as **TUBS** lesions.

The patient may present with an overt history of recurrent dislocation, with symptoms suggestive of subluxation and apprehension that dislocation is about to occur with specific movements. Symptoms commonly occur with increasingly trivial provocation. Recurrent dislocation is particularly likely in the younger athlete, especially where additional pathologies are present, in particular labral, glenohumeral ligament, Bankart, or Hill–Sachs lesions or where there is weakness of subscapularis. Recurrence occurs in 80–90% of patients below the age of 20 years, 40–65% of those aged 20–40 years, and 0–15% of those above the age of 40 years (McLaughlin and Cavallaro 1950).

AMBRII: Atraumatic cases (usually those with congenital laxity) typically demonstrate **M**ultidirectional instability that is **B**ilateral. Almost all respond to a **R**ehabilitation programme; the few who do not can be treated surgically by an **I**nferior capsular shift and repair of the rotator **I**nterval. These lesions are termed **AMBRII.**

Recurrent subluxation usually presents in the young patient, in association with activities such as throwing, when there is pain, clicking, clunking, neurological symptoms, and a feeling of instability. Recognizing the AMBRII patient who presents with symptoms of instability or with rotator cuff tendinopathy or impingement is vital to appropriate management. A small proportion of the AMBRII group are voluntary habitual dislocators, who sublux or dislocate the GHJ as a 'party trick' or in association with psychological disorders. Counselling of such patients is of primary importance.

A careful history is taken to document the mechanisms of injury, the degree of trauma involved, associated symptoms and previous injuries, and the degree of functional limitation. Examination includes an assessment for the presence of associated pathologies (such as tendinopathy and impingement), the degree of laxity of the shoulder compared with the unaffected side, response to apprehension stress tests, and the presence of generalized joint laxity.

All individuals should be treated conservatively with an intensive rotator cuff and scapular stabilizing programme, unless associated pathologies are present. Rehabilitation involves neuromuscular training of the muscles of the cuff, deltoid, scapular stabilizers, and pectoralis major. Much of the regime is initially low-intensity endurance exercise and this must be explained to the patient, particularly if he/she is an athlete who frequently prioritizes strength training for power.

Surgical management is considered in those with recurrent instability who fail to respond to an intensive programme, and who continue to experience instability that is interfering with their activities. Those patients who are congenitally lax (AMBRII) often require lengthy rehabilitation and much encouragement. Surgery is discouraged in those who are habitual dislocators. A number of procedures have been described involving repair of the anterior capsular mechanism and other stabilization procedures. Examination under anaesthesia, followed by diagnostic glenohumeral arthroscopy, can often aid decision-making in these patients.

Labral pathologies

Injuries to the glenoid labrum are an importantcause of persisting shoulder pain and instability. They typically occur after an episode of trauma where subluxation or dislocation has occurred, but are also a feature of repetitive microtrauma, usually in throwers. Bankart and SLAP lesions are the most common forms of labral injuries. The aetiology of the Bankart lesion has been described earlier.

SLAP lesions are a spectrum of tears of the superior labrum in the AP direction. They are typically seen in throwers, where there is 'peel-back' traction on the tendon of LHB, which inserts at the superior labrum. Such lesions can also arise in relation to a variety of other activities, including a fall onto an outstretched arm with the shoulder in abduction and slight forward flexion. They also occur with acute traction, or from an abduction–external rotation mechanism. Once a tear of the labrum has occurred, it may propagate anteriorly, posteriorly, or both. The resulting instability can lead to lesions of the rotator cuff and the LHB. In those lesions that are unstable, the majority of the superior labrum and LHB tendon are detached from the glenoid. Snyder *et al.* (1990) proposed a system of classification of SLAP lesions that includes such sequelae (Fig. 3.5.23).

Other forms of labral lesion can also occur, principally in relation to overuse in the overhead athlete, although Bankart lesions after dislocation also fall within this group. Lesions include degenerative

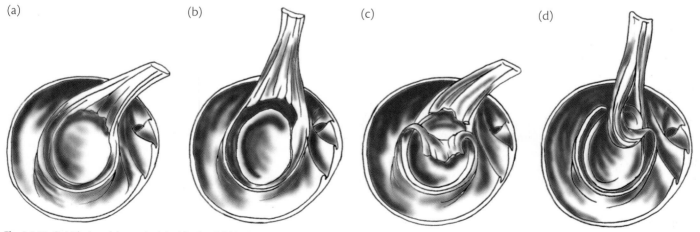

Fig. 3.5.23 SLAP lesions: (a) superior labral fraying; (b) labral amd LHB detachment from the glenoid rim; (c) bucket handle tearing of the labrum; (d) as (c) with extension into the LHB. Copyright © Reproduced from Hazelman, B, Riley, G and Speed, C (ed) (2004). *Soft Tissue Rheumatology*, Oxford Univeristy Press.

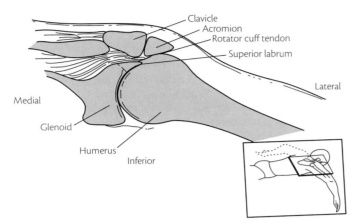

Fig. 3.5.24 Internal impingement of the articular surface of the cuff under the posterior-superior glenoid rim.

lesions and vertical and flap tears. In internal impingement syndromes, the posterosuperior portion of the labrum becomes frayed or torn, and there is an associated undersurface tear of the rotator cuff, usually at the junction of the supraspinatus and infraspinatus (Fig. 3.5.24).

Labral lesions should be considered in any athlete who reports non-specific deep-seated shoulder pain and catching or popping with specific movements. Signs of associated LHB or rotator cuff pathologies may be noted and SLAP tests (described earlier) may be positive, but can be unreliable. There is frequently acquired glenohumeral anterior instability, loss of internal rotation, and some weakness.

Investigations

Diagnosis of labral pathologies can be difficult. Direct MR arthrography is the imaging modality of choice, but many cases require diagnostic arthroscopy. Subtle labral lesions may be noted on imaging of upper limb athletes and may be associated with symptoms such as microinstability, but imaging studies must always be interpreted in the clinical context.

Management

Some patients with more minor lesions may respond to conservative management including analgesia, modification of activities, and a stability programme. However, surgery is frequently necessary and is virtually inevitable for unstable lesions. The torn labrum is resected or repaired, and where necessary the shoulder is stabilized. Many individuals return to full activity after a postoperative rehabilitation programme which addresses instability.

Rotator cuff tendinopathies

Classification

Rotator cuff disorders are the most common complaint affecting the shoulder complex. Lesions can be classified as tendinopathies without tear (tendinosis), isolated tears or global cuff ruptures. Rotator cuff tears can be further classified according to the tendon(s) of the cuff affected—whether they are partial or full thickness, their aetiology, duration, surface area, and additional pathologies. Partial tears may also be described according to their depth, shape, and relationship to the tendon surface (articular surface, bursal surface, intratendinous) (Patte 1990; Ciepela and Burkhead 1996; Fukuda *et al.* 1996).

Rotator cuff tendon tears usually occur in the order of frequency supraspinatus (usually near its anterior insertion), infraspinatus, and subscapularis, with teres minor only rarely affected. The subscapularis tendon may tear first in an anterior dislocation of the glenohumeral joint.

Aetiology/pathogenesis

The pathogenesis of rotator cuff lesions is likely to be multifactorial, but mechanical factors and relative hypovascularity play significant roles. In addition, the presence of cytokines as a response to vibration and repetitive trauma, hypoxic reperfusion mechanisms and the generation of free radicals have been proposed as important. Hyperthermia, a genetic predisposition, underlying chronic disease such as diabetes mellitus, raised subacromial pressure with abduction of the shoulder, and mechanical trauma upon the cuff may also contribute. The latter factors occur with **subacromial impingement**, where the rotator cuff, primarily the supraspinatus, undergoes relative compression at the undersurface of the anterolateral acromion within the coracoacromial arch during elevation of the arm. Subacromial impingement may be primary or may be secondary to numerous factors (Table 3.5.10), many of which cause narrowing of the coracoacromial arch, local friction to the rotator cuff, and/or migration of the humeral head, with resulting abutment on the cuff. Other shoulder pathologies may be present which cause shoulder and scapulothoracic dysfunction and impingement through microinstability weakness, pain, or muscle imbalance. Intrinsic changes within the tendon could themselves cause impingement through swelling or through scapulothoracic dysfunction due to pain.

Other forms of impingement which have been implicated in rotator cuff lesions include internal impingement by the undersurface of the cuff against the undersurface of the glenoid rim (seen in throwing athletes) and impingement between the coracoid and the head of the humerus, particularly in forward flexion and internal rotation.

History

Rotator cuff disorders typically present with shoulder pain, usually anterolateral. A history of macro- or microtrauma may be given. Weakness secondary to a significant tear or more frequently simply due to pain inhibition may be reported. Nocturnal pain is frequently marked, particularly when lying on the affected side, and pain is also usually exacerbated with activity, particularly when working with the arm in the plane of function of the involved muscle tendon unit. Lesions of subscapularis can cause pain with the arm below shoulder level. Symptoms suggestive of associated instability may be reported. Stiffness and/or restriction, which may relate to pain and/or posterior capsular tightness, may be reported. Crepitus may be noted by the patient with a thickened subacromial bursa.

Examination

Muscle imbalances are common, and may be subtle. Atrophy may be noted, particularly in the presence of a significant or long-standing rotator cuff tendon tear. Subacromial impingement may be demonstrated by the presence of painful arc of abduction, usually between 45° and 120°, and a positive impingement test. There is a full passive range of movement of the shoulder (if pain permits), with specific active movements limited by weakness if a significant tear is present. Pain on resisted testing in one or more planes indicates a tendinosis with an intact cuff, whilst significant weakness

Table 3.5.10 Aetiology of rotator cuff tendinopathy

Extrinsic
Macrotrauma
Microtrauma
Foreign bodies
Corticosteroids
Intrinsic
Subacromial impingement:
AC Joint OA
AC Joint instability
Thickened coracoacromial ligament
Narrow subacromial space
Type I or II acromial morphology
Presence of os acromiale
Low acromioscapular angle
Thickening of rotator cuff tendon
Calcification in subacromial space or cuff
Neuromuscular dysfunction
Scapulothoracic
Scapulohumeral
Posterior capsular tightness
Subcoracoid impingement
Internal impingement
Inflammatory arthritis
Diabetes
Hypothyroidism
Hyperparathyroidism
Amyloid
Chronic renal failure

out of proportion to pain and/or crepitus, implies that a tear is present. Associated features, such as ACJ tenderness and deformity (indicative of possible OA) or glenohumeral instability may also be noted. A subacromial injection of local anaesthetic may help to differentiate impingement from other causes of shoulder pain, with improvement in pain and active and passive RoM seen with impingement but not with other disorders (Neer's test).

Imaging the rotator cuff

Ultrasound and MRI are the most helpful imaging modalities in assessing the rotator cuff. Ultrasound is sensitive to even minor changes in the tendons, LHB, and bursae, and demonstrates calcification and neovascularization well. Dynamic evaluation may demonstrate 'bunching up' of the supraspinatus with impingement. MRI evaluates the cuff extremely well, and there is a high degree of correlation between histological changes within the supraspinatus tendon and modifications of its signal on MRI (Shahabpour *et al.* 2008). It also provides information about surrounding structures. Calcifying lesions are not well demonstrated on MRI.

Standard MRI is performed in at least two planes, with a coronal oblique T2- or proton-density-weighted series aligned along the line of the supraspinatus tendon to visualize the supraspinatus and infraspinatus tendons, together with an axially acquired T1-weighted sequence to visualize the subscapularis, LHB, and teres minor. An additional sagittal T2-weighted sequence is sometimes added and provides additional information about the configuration of the acromion and the ACJ in particular.

MRI has been particularly effective in characterizing full-thickness rotator cuff tears. In such cases, a continuous band of fluid that traverses the full thickness of the cuff, retraction of the tendon, and high signal intensity in the cuff on T2-weighted images are the most significant signs. The accuracy of diagnosis of full-thickness tears using MRI is superior to that for partial-thickness lesions and tendinitis/tendinosis. In partial thickness tears, fat-suppressed T2-weighted imaging may increase diagnostic accuracy. In addition, MR arthrography with gadolinium enhancement may help in the detection of articular sided partial-thickness tears.

In long-standing tears, ultrasound and MRI show evidence of fatty infiltration of disrupted muscles of the rotator cuff, which changes little after the repair of the tear. Cuff muscle atrophy has been associated with the degree of tendon retraction and with severe functional impairment and recurrent tear after repair. Such features may play a role in the decision to intervene surgically as, even if repair is possible, function may be poor.

Plain X-rays can indicate calcification and subacromial anatomy, acromial morphology, and degenerative changes in the ACJ and GHJ.

Arthrography may be useful in confirming articular surface tears, but is rarely used now. Subacromial **bursography**, particularly when coupled with helical CT, is also rarely used to assess the bursal side of the rotator cuff and may help in the diagnosis of bursal side lesions, which may be undetected by other imaging methods. **Diagnostic arthroscopy** has the advantage of allowing direct evaluation of the rotator cuff, and has been a significant advance, in particular in the identification of partial-thickness tears and labral pathologies.

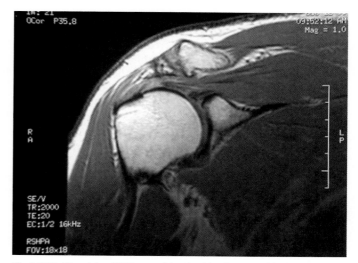

Fig. 3.5.25 T2-weighted MRI scan of the shoulder showing a full-thickness rotator cuff tear and a degenerate AC joint with an inferior osteophyte. Copyright © Reproduced from Hazelman, B, Riley, G and Speed, C (ed) (2004). *Soft Tissue Rheumatology*, Oxford Univeristy Press.

Management of tendinosis with an intact rotator cuff

Standard management of rotator cuff tendinosis commences with control of pain. Relative rest with avoidance of exacerbating activities, regular applications of ice, heat packs to relieve muscle spasm, and the judicious use of a support are all frequently recommended. Non-steroidal anti-inflammatory drugs (NSAIDs), topical glyceryl trinitrate patches, and local modalities, including ultrasound, laser, and electromagnetic field therapy may all assist with pain relief, although evidence for benefit from modalities is limited. Ultrasound-guided subacromial corticosteroid injections are reserved for those individuals with persistent pain which is limiting rehabilitation.

Initial rehabilitation of the rotator cuff focuses upon pain management to allow appropriate mobility and stability work to proceed and to re-establish an optimal kinetic chain. Work commences with RoM exercises, not only at the shoulder but throughout the shoulder girdle, trunk, lumbopelvic region, and lower limb, with additional progressive functional strengthening and stability work. Shoulder-specific work involves scapular stability exercises, and focuses on appropriate scapular and glenohumeral muscle firing patterns to optimize centring of the humeral head on the glenoid.

Surgery is considered in the patient with a tendinosis who fails conservative measures when there are associated structural causes of impingement. Arthroscopic subacromial decompression, resection of the distal clavicle, or excision/debridement of ACJ osteophyte(s) have all been advocated.

Management of rotator cuff tears

Management of the patient with a rotator cuff tear is influenced by their age, activity level, and expectations, the type and extent of the tear, its duration, the mode of onset, and additional pathologies. Rotator cuff tears can be managed conservatively in the same manner as tendinosis. The use of corticosteroid injections in known tears is discouraged because of the potential suppression of collagen synthesis. There is debate about indications for surgery, the most appropriate surgical procedure, and the importance of the size and surface area of the tear in relation to the need for repair.

Surgical options include debridement, subacromial decompression, and excision and repair of the damaged tendon. In some patients who exhibit associated glenohumeral instability, a stabilization procedure may be considered. In full-thickness tears, decompression and repair is the most common surgical approach. Acute traumatic full-thickness tears should be repaired early, but patients with degenerative full-thickness tears should be given a trial of conservative management for 4 months, although this will depend upon the level and expectations of the patient. Surgical intervention is considered if there is progression of symptoms and/or significant functional impairment. The outcome appears to be less satisfactory in older patients and those with large tears, poor active RoM, or weakness preoperatively.

Surgery for a partial-thickness tear is usually reserved for the patient who fails to respond to conservative measures. Debridement may be successful in younger patients with bursal surface tears, but decompression is usually necessary in older patients. Indications for excision and repair of the tendon have not been clearly defined, although surgery may be most appropriate for larger tears.

It has been reported that approximately 40% of cases of articular surface partial-thickness tears respond to conservative management, but that most cases of bursal side and intratendinous tears tend not to heal (Yamanaka and Matsumoto 1994; Breazeale and Craig 1997). Although imaging studies have shown that many partial tears show progression with time, symptoms often improve in these patients. This emphasizes the difficulty in correlating clinical with imaging findings.

Lesions of the tendon of the long head of the biceps

The close relationship between the tendon of the long head of the biceps (TLHB) with the rotator cuff, the labrum, and the rotator interval makes it likely that lesions of the TLHB are commonly associated with pathologies at one or more of these sites. Biceps lesions include tendinopathy without significant tear ('tendinitis' or tenosynovitis), tear (partial/rupture), and instability within the bicipital groove (subluxation or dislocation). These can be classified as shown in Table 3.5.11. Damage to the TLHB at its origin (type I lesions) involves tearing of the biceps–labrum junction at the superior rim of the labrum. These lesions typically occur in throwing athletes and are described further in the section on glenohumeral instability. A rotator interval lesion can be defined as a lesion of the intra-articular portion of the TLHB between the entrance to the bicipital groove and its origin on the superior glenoid, with no cuff pathology.

Biceps tendinosis/tenosynovitis

Tendinopathy affecting the LHB usually occurs in the presence of disease of the rest of the rotator cuff. A primary isolated biceps tendinosis/tenosynovitis is a rare entity in the non-athletic population, but is seen in swimmers, throwers, and weight-lifters, or after an episode of trauma or unaccustomed lifting, and in rotational activities of the upper arm where there is extension of both elbow and shoulder, such as table tennis and karate. Anatomical variations such as a shallow bicipital groove or local osteophytes encroaching

Table 3.5.11 Classification of lesions of the tendon of long head of biceps (TLHB)

Origin of TLHB
Associated with SLAP lesions
Rotator interval lesions
Primary biceps tendinopathy
Isolated rupture
Subluxation
Type I, superior
Type II, at groove
Type III, mal-/non-union of lesser tuberosity fracture
Associated with rotator cuff tear or severe tendinopathy
Tendinopathy
Dislocation
Extraarticular with partial tear of subscapularis
Extraarticular with intact subscapularis
Intraarticular dislocation
Subluxation with cuff tear
Rupture with cuff tear

upon the bicipital groove and causing attrition, indirect or direct trauma, or fracture of the humeral tuberosities may all predispose to bicipital tendon lesions. A proliferative tenosynovitis within the bicipital groove, and ultimately stenosis of the tendon with thickening of the transverse ligament and sheath can occur. However, impingement is the most common cause of LHB tendinopathy and signs of rotator cuff disease are frequently present.

Since bicipital tendinopathies have a varied aetiology and a range of associated lesions, a range of presentations can occur. Typically, LHB tendinosis/tenosynovitis presents in young or middle-aged patients as anterior shoulder and upper arm pain radiating into the biceps muscle belly. It may also radiate proximally or present as impingement. Nocturnal symptoms are variable. The patient may give a history of performing the precipitating activities mentioned above or describe symptoms associated with other pathologies such as rotator cuff tendinosis. There may be a sensation of instability and, where subluxation is occurring, the patient may complain of snapping over the anterior shoulder. Ultrasound may demonstrate fluid in the tendon sheath.

There is tenderness over the bicipital groove which is most easily found with the arm in 10° internal rotation. This tenderness may reduce with further internal rotation of the arm (unlike subacromial impingement). Provocative tests such as Speed's test elicit pain (or weakness in tears). In isolated bicipital tendinopathy there is a full RoM, but in other cases limitation may occur because of other pathologies present.

Management of LHB tendinopathy is similar to that of rotator cuff tendinosis, with ice, analgesics, NSAIDs, and a graduated programme of rehabilitation the mainstays of therapy. A single guided injection of short/moderate-acting corticosteroid into the sheath or joint may help to alleviate pain in more resistant cases.

Biceps tendon subluxation

Subluxation and dislocation of the LHB tendon can be caused by trauma or repetitive microtrauma to the rotator interval sling, through active internal rotation of the arm. Biceps tendon subluxation has been classified into three types (Walch 1963; Habbermeyer and Walch 1996). Superior (type I) subluxation occurs above the entrance to the bicipital groove. It is due to partial or complete tearing of the coracohumeral and superior glenohumeral ligaments, whilst the insertion of subscapularis remains intact. An articular surface partial tear of the tendon of supraspinatus may be associated. Type II subluxation involves medial subluxation at the groove due to a tear of the outermost fibres of subscapularis which usually anchor the TLHB. Type III subluxation occurs secondary to fracture dislocation of the lesser tuberosity with malunion, resulting in loss of the bony restraint of the tendon. Patients may complain of painful clicking or snapping over the bicipital groove, and there may be pain on internal rotation. There is bicipital groove tenderness and Speed's test is positive. It is usually very difficult to feel subluxation of the TLHB, but there may be an audible snap or palpable click as the tendon subluxes when the patient slowly brings the arm down from the passively fully abducted position in external rotation. Dynamic ultrasound is helpful in confirming the diagnosis but arthroscopy may be necessary. Chronic subluxation may lead to tendinopathy and tear due to attrition. Altered transmission of mechanical forces may also occur, resulting in a high incidence of degenerative changes in the anterosuperior portion of the labrum.

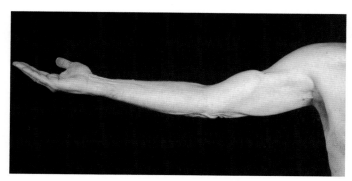

Fig. 3.5.26 Rupture of the long head of biceps: the 'Popeye' sign.

Dislocation of the tendon of the long head of the biceps

Dislocation of the TLHB predominantly occurs in older athletes and tends to involve the dominant arm. It can occur in association with rotator cuff disease or after chronic subluxation of the tendon, most commonly when the rotator interval sling and subscapularis tendon are torn. The tendon may intermittently dislocate with rotation of the arm, or may be permanently displaced from the groove into either an extra-articular or intra-articular position.

The patient complains of shoulder pain and clicking. Signs of a rotator cuff tear are evident and the pain may be worse with flexion and rotation of the arm. Ultrasound and MRI confirm the diagnosis.

Management of subluxation/dislocation

In the symptomatic patient or where the tendon is becoming compromised, arthroscopic or open surgical intervention should be considered. Approaches include reconstruction of the rotator interval sling and/or restoring the tendon to its groove, but the outcome of these procedures is uncertain. Definitive surgical treatment involves tenotomy of the TLHB at the superior glenoid tubercle followed by tenodesis of the tendon into the floor of the bicipital groove (extra-articular). Fixation is usually achieved using implants such as a suture anchor or interference screw. Other pathologies should be addressed, and where significant subacromial impingement is present, decompression is also performed.

Tears of the tendon of LHB

Tears of the tendon of LHB may be partial, complete, or extend to a full rupture. Partial tears may occur in association with any of the causes of tendinitis, in particular impingement, and may present with similar symptoms to those reported with tendinosis/tenosynovitis.

TLHB ruptures

Although certain factors such as osteophytes in the groove have been blamed for tendon ruptures, there is little evidence for this. Ruptures usually occur at the entrance to the bicipital groove where the tendon is exposed to greatest mechanical stresses, resulting in chronic tenosynovitis and attrition. Mechanical impingement is the cause for most cases and additional cuff pathologies are usually present. It appears that the rupture itself may be due to increased stresses on the LHB by rotator cuff dysfunction, and that impingement upon the TLHB is a secondary effect.

Lesions can occur in both the athletic and non-athletic population. They typically occur in the dominant arm of older males and present with a 'Popeye' deformity of the upper arm, often with relatively little pain. There may be a prior history of shoulder or bicipital pain. Significant synovitis of the joint can occur, and the remnant of the attachment of the tendon can become entrapped in the joint with a subsequent chondral lesion of the glenoid or humeral head. Whereas an isolated rupture of TLHB has only a minor impact upon function, when combined with a rotator cuff tear, the effects on upper limb strength are significant.

Management
Rupture of the TLHB can be managed symptomatically, with attention to rehabilitation of the cuff. In cases of painful rupture of the TLHB, a rotator cuff tear and/or SLAP lesion (see above) must be excluded and arthroscopy is useful in this situation. Tenodesis (described above) may be considered in the younger or more active patient with an acute injury. Additional pathologies are managed as appropriate.

Neurological causes of shoulder pain
Axillary nerve lesions
The axillary nerve is closely related to the glenohumeral joint. It supplies the deltoid and teres minor and provides cutaneous innervation to a small area over the lateral deltoid. It is commonly injured in dislocation of the GHJ by direct trauma, and may also be entrapped in the quadrilateral space. The patient presents with shoulder and posterior axillary pain, deltoid wasting, and weakness and associated sensory loss. EMG and nerve conduction studies confirm the lesion. Recovery can be lengthy, and although trick compensatory movements can be learned, deltoid weakness is commonly disabling. If no signs of improvement are noted at 4 months, the nerve should be explored.

Other peripheral nerve complaints
Long thoracic nerve palsy can occur as a brachial neuritis after compression due to prolonged recumbency such as when lying on an operating table or after local surgery to the breast. There is nonspecific shoulder pain, difficulty in elevating the arm, and winging.

The **radial nerve** may be injured in the axilla by trauma, inferior dislocation of the GHJ, local pressure such as under-arm crutches, or pressure from leaning on the back of a chair. There is weakness of the extensor muscles of the arm, with the typical waiter's tip palsy. Electrodiagnostic studies confirm the diagnosis. Removal of the precipitant cause and rehabilitation form the core management, but recovery can be prolonged.

The **musculocutaneous nerve** (C5, 6), though rarely injured, can be damaged when there is open trauma or after surgery for anterior GHJ instability. The result is wasting of the flexor muscles of the upper arm; weakness of forearm supination, loss of the biceps reflex, and sensory loss over a small area on the lateral aspect of the forearm.

Thoracic outlet syndrome is a complex of symptoms that can arise as a result of compression of the neurovascular structures of the thoracic outlet, the brachial plexus, and subclavian artery. The term encompasses other entities, including 'hyperabduction', 'anterior scalene', and 'costoclavicular' syndromes. Local masses and anatomical variations are implicated, including a high first rib or a cervical rib, fibrous bands, anomalies of the scalene muscle, or a transverse process of the seventh cervical vertebra. In the athlete, TOS can occur as a functional entity, seemingly due to overdevelopment of local muscular structures or myofascial tightness in the area.

Symptoms and signs are highly variable and depend upon the structures compressed. Neurogenic symptoms predominate and include dull ache in the entire upper limb, painful paraesthesiae, and weakness and wasting of the small muscles of the hand. Vascular symptoms, usually intermittent cyanosis but rarely trophic skin changes and digital ulceration, are also reported. Symptoms are often exacerbated when carrying heavy objects or working with the arms in the overhead position, and clumsiness and fatigue may be noted in these positions.

As described earlier, numerous clinical tests have been proposed, but the accuracy of such tests is poor. A bruit on auscultation may be noted. A chest X-ray allows evaluation of the outlet, and will demonstrate the presence of a high first or cervical rib and local lung masses. Diagnostic ultrasound can demonstrate local compression of cervical rootlets where a band(s) is present, but is highly specialized. CT or MRI of the thoracic outlet may also be helpful in identifying causative pathology, and angiography, Doppler studies, and venography may be considered necessary where vascular symptoms predominate.

Treatment depends on the cause. In most cases no cause is identified and physiotherapy in the form of RoM and strengthening exercise of the cervical, scapulothoracic, and rotator cuff musculature is advocated. When present, excision of a cervical rib or fibrous band may be necessary in those with severe persisting symptoms.

Scapulothoracic and posterior shoulder pain

Scapulothoracic pain may arise due to neurological lesions, myofascial disorders, or bony injuries, or may be referred from other sites (Table 3.5.12). Myofascial disorders are discussed elsewhere and bony injuries are beyond the scope of this text.

Suprascapular nerve lesions
The suprascapular nerve (C5,6) can be injured as a result of acute trauma to the shoulder complex and can be compressed by tight rucksack straps (backpacker's palsy), a tight transverse scapular ligament, local synovitis (e.g. rheumatoid arthritis), or a ganglion at either the suprascapular or supraglenoid notch. The patient complains of posterior shoulder and scapular pain and there may be wasting of the spinati. Local anaesthetic infiltration into the suprascapular notch should abolish the pain. EMG and nerve conduction studies are necessary to confirm the diagnosis and MRI may be necessary to exclude local pathology. Treatment depends on the cause; local corticosteroid is unhelpful and surgical intervention may be necessary to decompress the nerve.

Snapping scapula
Snapping scapula involves pain and/or palpable snapping at the superomedial edge of the scapula in association with scapulothoracic movement. It can occur spontaneously, after trauma, or after

Table 3.5.12 Differential diagnosis of scapulothoracic pain

Local muscle injury
Myofascial pain syndrome
Subscapular bursitis
Snapping scapula
Suprascapular nerve palsy
Referred pain from cervical or thoracic spine
Bony injury, e.g. fracture or metastatic deposit in scapula

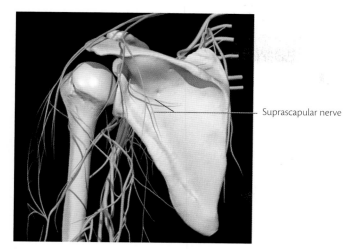

Fig. 3.5.27 The suprascapular nerve can be prone to compression near the suprascapular notch. Copyright © Primal Pictures. Reproduced with permission.

surgical procedures to the shoulder girdle, but most cases are due to abnormal scapular movement patterns, causing the bony margin of the scapula to contact the underlying ribs. In most cases no other cause is found and symptoms are commonly attributed to minor anatomical variations in the medial superior border and the inferior pole of the scapula, and/or neuromuscular imbalance. The snapping may be due to the presence of an exostosis on the undersurface of the vertebral angle of the scapula or local benign soft tissue tumour (elastofibroma dorsi), which rides across the rib cage (Majo *et al.* 2001). The pain has been reported to be the result of inflamed bursae located between the scapula and adjacent thorax or over the scapular exostosis (Carlson *et al.* 1997).

Symptoms usually respond to reassurance, analgesics, and physiotherapy, and surgery is not usually necessary. In the minority of cases where there is localized abnormality, such as an exostosis, this is amenable to resection. Three-dimensional CT will show bony irregularities, and MRI will show bursae and bony changes. Scapulothoracic arthroscopy can be helpful in refractory cases, allowing resection of the bursa and trimming of the superomedial corner of the scapula.

Scapula fractures

Fractures of the scapula are most frequently seen in relation to dislocation of the humeral head or direct trauma after a fall. They may be overlooked in the light of other more serious injuries related to the trauma. They may be graded as (A) acromial, (B) body, (C) coracoid, or (D) involving the scapular neck and glenoid fossa. The latter are the most common in sport. If there is coexistent ACJ separation or clavicular fracture, these should be fixed to confer stability to the complex. Displaced fractures through the glenoid rim require fixation either arthroscopically or by open surgery.

Localized shoulder pain

Acromioclavicular joint disorders.

The ACJ is the sole site of articulation between the scapula and the clavicle. Injures to this joint consist of ligamentous injuries and articular disorders and can be described as scapuloclavicular injuries, since the term illustrates the effects that ACJ disorders can have upon the rest of the shoulder complex.

Ligamentous injuries

The ACJ is stabilized by two major complexes—the coracoclavicular ligaments, providing vertical stability, and the acromioclavicular ligament, which confers horizontal stability. Acromioclavicular **sprains and dislocations** are common injuries in contact sporting activities and other forms of relative trauma. AC dislocations occur predominantly in males, with a 5:1 male-to-female ratio, and the vast majority occur in adolescents and young adult athletes.

ACJ ligament injuries, particularly those that are more severe, usually occur with direct trauma to the point of the shoulder. Indirect mechanisms such as downward traction or upward forces, particularly on the adducted arm, may also be involved. Such injuries can be graded according to either the severity of the ligamentous disruption or the structures involved. (Fig 3.5.28). Significant damage to the deltotrapezius unit, with detachment from the clavicle, is noted in types IV–VI and sometimes in type III. Type VI injuries are catastrophic, usually with major neurovascular damage, and thus are life threatening, but fortunately they are extremely rare.

History

A specific episode of trauma is frequently reported prior to the acute onset of characteristic pain, easily identified as the ACJ since the patient usually points to the joint as the site of pain. There may be radiation to the upper arm. Pain can be severe even in low-grade

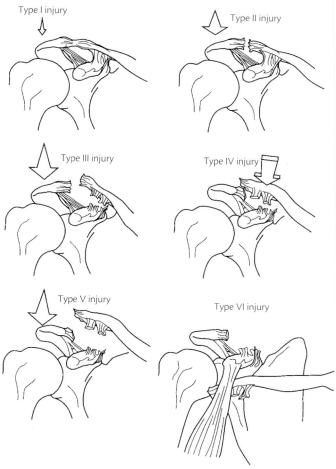

Fig. 3.5.28 The broad range of ACJ injuries. Copyright © Reproduced from Hazelman, B, Riley, G and Speed, C (ed) (2004). *Soft Tissue Rheumatology*, Oxford Univeristy Press.

AC injuries and is typically worse with certain movements, specifically lifting and pushing. Nocturnal pain is common with acute injuries. Symptoms of clicking and grinding may be reported, and some patients have noted the development of a local deformity.

Examination

The patient may hold the arm in the adducted position, supported in slight elevation. In type I injuries, tenderness, swelling, and minor deformity may be noted. Deformity is more obvious in types III to VI. No instability is noted in type I injuries, but horizontal instability occurs in type II injuries. In higher-grade injuries, both horizontal and vertical instability of the ACJ is present. In type III injuries, it should be possible to reduce the dislocation clinically by downward pressure on the clavicle and upward pressure on the elbow. A dimple frequently overlies the outer end of the clavicle in the type IV injury, which increases on attempts to reduce the clavicle downwards. Multidirectional instability of the distal clavicle is clearly evident in the type V injury. In types III–VI associated injuries should be sought, including fracture of the clavicle and/or upper ribs, SCJ dislocation, and brachial plexus traction injuries.

Imaging

Plain X-rays should include routine AP and axillary lateral views. Weight-bearing stress views in the same planes may be useful, particularly to evaluate the more subtle low-grade injuries in the detection and evaluation of instability. The injured and uninvolved sides are compared. AP stress views are taken with the patient holding weights in the standard AP position. Lateral stress views, where the patient thrusts their shoulders forward, assess the placement of the acromion, the AC interval, and the size of the coracoclavicular space (with vertical instability suggested by widening of the latter). They show the acromion to be displaced anteroinferiorly in the unstable ACJ (types III+).

Management

Types I, II, and, in some cases, III are all managed conservatively. Persistent pain with type I and II injuries is not uncommon, although additional pathologies should always be considered (Table 3.5.13).

Relief of pain may be achieved by the regular use of local ice packs, analgesics, and NSAIDs. Support of the injured arm using a sling may be useful in the acute stages until pain is controlled (typically for up to 2 weeks). Reduction of the subluxation in type II injuries has been advocated using manual mobilizations by a therapist or by a variety of braces, taping, supports, harnesses, and traction techniques. It may take many weeks of continuous pressure on the superior clavicle to allow reduction and healing, but the efficacy of bracing techniques is dubious and may cause problems with the overlying skin. Alternatively, the subluxation may be 'skilfully neglected'.

When symptoms allow, RoM exercises should be introduced early (weeks 0–3), beginning with gravity-dependent pendulum exercises, progressing to wall climbing and then active function RoM exercises. Thereafter a progressive rehabilitation programme should be commenced, involving postural and neuromuscular coordination training and strengthening of the cuff and scapular stabilizers. Finally, provided that full pain-free mobility and control has been regained, return to sport-specific training can occur as appropriate (at 4–8 weeks). Heavy lifting and contact sports should be avoided for 12 weeks.

Table 3.5.13 Additional pathologies and complications in ACJ ligament injuries

Torn, entrapped capsular ligaments
Loose articular cartilage
Detached intraarticular meniscus
Rotator cuff injury
Shoulder complex dysfunction, including impingement
Post-traumatic osteolysis of the clavicle
Frozen shoulder
Brachial plexus traction injury
Coracoclavicular ossification
Fractures
Dislocation of SCJ
Non union fracture of the coracoid process
Postoperative complications
ACJ osteoarthritis

Excellent functional outcomes can be achieved by non-surgical management of many patients with type III injuries, but patients should be warned that deformity will persist. However, surgical intervention may be necessary in those who fail conservative approaches, particularly in active patients and those involved in heavy manual work. Some also recommend it for those with type II injuries who fail to settle with conservative approaches, or those with demonstrable additional pathologies such as secondary degenerative joint disease. In such patients, correction of the offending additional pathology, joint debridement, and/or excision arthroplasty may be performed. Surgery for type III injuries, where necessary, may involve primary ACJ or coracoclavicular ligament fixation and excision of the distal clavicle and coracoacromial ligament. Such procedures are performed alone or in various combinations. Surgical approaches are usually employed for the management of types IV, V, and VI injuries.

Sternoclavicular disorders

Fortunately, complaints arising from the SCJ are limited in number to primary articular disorders (osteoarthritis, inflammatory arthritis) and instability.

Instability of the SCJ occurs in two forms, spontaneous or post-traumatic. Traumatic instability of the SCJ, which occurs after dislocation, accounts for 1% of all dislocations of the shoulder girdle. Such injuries involve major trauma to the chest wall; when in the anterior or superior directions they are easily diagnosed by the obvious deformity and can often be reduced by manual pressure. A posterior dislocation may be less evident and may result in airways obstruction or compression of the great vessels—rapid reduction is required.

Spontaneous instability usually occurs in the younger patient, may be bilateral, and occurs with minimal or no trauma. The patient notes a painful or painless clunking of the joint anteriorly or superiorly, which may be followed by swelling and local tenderness. Management is conservative, focusing on scapular positioning and control exercises, and involves reassurance and advice to avoid precipitating activities. Surgical intervention can be a major undertaking and is reserved for those with persistent and disabling symptoms. A number of stabilization techniques have been described.

Clavicular fractures

Fractures of the clavicle are common traumatic injuries in sport, usually secondary to direct contact on the field of play or a fall onto the point of the shoulder. Although painful and unsightly, they usually heal very well over a period of 4–6 weeks. The arm is supported in a figure-of-eight cuff, if they can tolerate it, to prevent overlapping of the fracture ends during healing, which would result in a shortened clavicle with functional consequences. Stiffness is prevented during healing by gentle RoM exercises to up to 90°. Surgery is reserved for those who have cutaneous compromise, comminution, or shortening of the clavicle by more than 1–2cm. Fractures that affect the distal clavicle are less common but can frequently involve AC or coracoclavicular ligament injury. They are more prone to non-union or delayed healing, particularly those situated medial to the ligament attachments. Fractures in the skeletally immature individual generally have a better outcome. Surgery is more likely to be indicated in those injuries medial to the ligaments. Most other cases are managed symptomatically with a sling and gradual RoM exercises.

References

Bigliani, L.U., Morrison, D.S., and April, E.W. (1986). The morphology of the acromion its relationship to rotator cuff tears. *Orthopaedic Transactions*, **10**, 228.

Borsa, P.A., Laudner, K.G, and Sauers, E.L. (2008). Mobility and stability adaptations in the shoulder of the overhead athlete: a theoretical and evidence-based perspective. *Sports Medicine*, **38**, 17–36.

Breazeale, N.M. and Craig, E.V. (1997). Partial-thickness rotator cuff tears. Pathogenesis and treatment. *Orthopedic Clinics of North America*, **28**, 145–55.

Carlson, H.L., Haig, A.J., and Stewart, D.C. (1997). Snapping scapula syndrome: three case reports and an analysis of the literature. *Archives of Physical Medicine and Rehabilitation*, **78**, 506–11.

Ciepela, M.D. and Burkhead, W.Z. (1996). Classification of rotator cuff tears. In: W.Z. Burkhead Jr (ed.), *Rotator Cuff Disorders*, pp. 100–7. Williams & Wilkins, Baltimore, MD.

De Palma, A.F. (1957). *Degenerative Changes in Sternoclavicular and Acromioclavicular Joints in Various Decades*. C.C. Thomas, Springfield, IL.

Fukuda, H., Craig, E.V., Yamanaka, K., and Hamada, K. (1996). Partial thickness cuff tears. In: W.Z. Burkhead Jr (ed.), *Rotator Cuff Disorders*, pp. 174–81. Williams & Wilkins, Baltimore, MD.

Habbermeyer, P. and Walch, G. (1996). The biceps tendon and rotator cuff disease. In: W.Z. Burkhead Jr (ed.), *Rotator Cuff Disorders*, p.142. Williams & Wilkins, Baltimore, MD.

Headey, J., Brooks, J.H., and Kemp, S.P. (2007). The epidemiology of shoulder injuries in English professional rugby union. *American Journal of Sports Medicine*, **35**, 1537–43.

Itoi, E., Hatakeyama, Y., Sato, T., *et al.* (2007). Immobilization in external rotation after shoulder dislocation reduces the risk of recurrence. A randomized controlled trial. *Journal of Bone and Joint Surgery. American Volume*, **89**, 2124–31.

Keogh, J., Hume, P.A., and Pearson, S. (2006). Retrospective injury epidemiology of 101 competitive Oceania power lifters: the effects of age, body mass, competitive standard, and gender. *Journal of Strength and Conditioning Research*, **20**, 672–81.

Majo, J., Gracia, I., Doncel, A., Valera, M., Nunez, A., and Guix, M. (2001). Elastofibroma dorsi as a cause of shoulder pain or snapping scapula. *Clinical Orthopaedics and Related Research*, **388**, 200–4.

McLaughlin, H.L. and Cavallaro, W.U. (1950). Primary anterior dislocation of the shoulder. *American Journal of Surgery*, **80**, 615–21.

O'Brien, S.J., Pagnani, M.J., Fealy, S., McGlynn, S.R., and Wilson, J.B. (1998). The active compression test: a new and effective test for diagnosing labral tears and acromioclavicular joint abnormality. *American Journal of Sports Medicine*, **26**, 610–13.

Patte, D. (1990). Clasification of rotator cuff lesions. *Clinical Orthopaedics and Related Research*, **254**, 81–6.

Shahabpour, M., Kichouh, M., Laridon, E., Gielen, J.L., and De Mey, J. (2008). The effectiveness of diagnostic imaging methods for the assessment of soft tissue and articular disorders of the shoulder and elbow. *European Journal of Radiology*, **65**, 194–200.

Snyder, S.J., Karzel, R.P., Del Pizzo, W., Ferkel, R.D., and Friedman, M.J. (1990). SLAP lesions of the shoulder. *Arthroscopy*, **6**, 274–9.

Thomas, S.C. and Matsen, F.A. (1989). An approach to the repair of avulsion of the glenohumeral ligaments in the management of traumatic anterior glenohumeral instability. *Journal of Bone and Joint Surgery. American Volume*, **71**, 506–13.

Walch, G. (1963). *La pathologie de la longue portion du biceps*. Presented at: Conference d'Enseignement de la SOFCOT, Paris, 1963.

Yamanaka, K. and Matsumoto, T. (1994). The joint side tear of the rotator cuff. A follow up study by arthrography. *Clinical Orthopaedics and Related Research*, **304**, 68–73.

3.6

Injuries to the elbow and forearm

Cathy Speed

Introduction

Elbow injuries in sport can affect any athlete in relation to trauma, but overuse injuries are seen most frequently in overhead/throwing athletes and gymnasts across a wide age spectrum. The consequences of such injuries can be serious and result in loss of time in training and competition. The close interplay between the shoulder and elbow as part of the kinetic chain is well illustrated by the fact that, in those recreational tennis players with a history of lateral epicondylitis, there is a 63% greater incidence of shoulder injury (Priest *et al.* 1980). Seventy-four per cent of male and 60% of female elite tennis players report a history of shoulder or elbow pain that has limited their ability to play (Priest and Nagal 1976). The elbow is a vulnerable region in the skeletally immature athlete, and the high demands that sports such as baseball and gymnastics place on this region can result in serious injury.

Anatomy

Bones

The elbow is a compound synovial joint, composed of a complex of two closely related articulations between the humerus and both the ulna and radius. This is continuous with the superior radio-ulnar joint, which functionally forms part of the elbow complex. The capsule and joint cavity are continuous for all three joints.

The **radiocapitellar joint** is a hinge joint formed by articulation between the hemispherical humeral capitellum and the head of the radius. The **ulnohumeral (trochlear) joint** is formed by the trochlea of the distal humerus and the trochlear notch of the ulna. This modified hinge joint permits 140°–150° of flexion and extension in the normal elbow, with an axis of movement that passes downward and medially, with the elbow travelling through an arc of movement from valgus to varus during flexion. The carrying angle of the elbow, the valgus angle formed by the long axis of the upper arm and forearm when the arm is extended, is typically less than 5° in males and 5–10° in females. Most individuals can straighten their elbow completely (0° full extension/flexion), but hyperextension to −5° is normal particularly in young females.

The side-to-side joint movement necessary for supination and pronation exists because there is incomplete contact between the trochlea and the medial and lateral aspects of the olecranon process in full extension and in full flexion, respectively. Approximately 5° of medial rotation also occurs at this joint during early flexion and 5° of lateral rotation in late flexion. This subtle rotation may account for osteophyte formation on the olecranon, typically seen in activities involving repetitive extension of the elbow, such as throwing.

The forearm can rotate through approximately 165° (80° pronation and 80–85° of supination) through movements at the radio-ulnar joints. The **superior radio-ulnar joint** is a uniaxial pivot joint, where the head of the radius rotates with pronation and supination on the radial notch of the ulna and is held in position relative to the adjacent bones by the annular ligament. In the distal forearm the **inferior radio-ulnar joint**, formed by articulation between the head of the ulna and the ulnar notch of the radius, also allows supination and pronation.

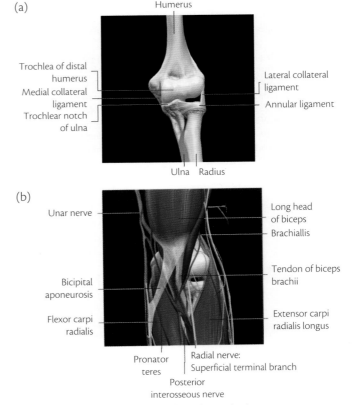

Fig. 3.6.1 The anterior elbow: (a) deep and (b) superficial structures. Copyright © Primal Pictures. Reproduced with permission.

Ligaments

The medial (ulnar) collateral ligament and the lateral (radial) collateral ligament support the humero-ulnar and humeroradial joints respectively. At least 65% of the load to valgus strain is taken up by the **medial collateral ligament** (MCL), and in particular by its anterior bundle, within the range 20°–120° of flexion. This arises from the inferior aspect of the medial epicondyle to insert onto the medial aspect of the coronoid process of the ulna. It divides into an anterior band (tight in extension and therefore resistant to valgus strain in this position) and a posterior band (tight in flexion). The posterior bundle arises from the medial epicondyle to insert onto the medial olecranon. It is taut when the elbow is flexed more than 90°. The transverse bundle has no significant role in the stability of the elbow. The MCL and the flexor carpi ulnaris muscle form the **cubital tunnel,** through which the ulnar nerve travels.

The **lateral collateral ligament** (LCL) consists of three functional components, which provide stability to the elbow against varus stress and, if compromised, can result in a loss of pronation and supination:

(i) the radial collateral ligament, between the lateral epicondyle and inserting on

(ii) the annular ligament which forms a sling for rotation of the radial head

(iii) the lateral ulnar collateral ligament from the lateral epicondyle to the supinator crest of the ulna, which prevents posterolateral rotary movement of the radial head on the capitellum.

Muscles

Four groups of muscles act directly on the elbow: the flexors, flexor–pronators, extensors, and extensor–supinators. The **flexor group** is composed of the biceps brachii, brachioradialis, and brachialis. The **biceps brachii** acts as a primary elbow flexor when the elbow is supinated and is the major contributor to forearm supination when the elbow is flexed. It has two origins. The **long head** arises from the superior glenoid tubercle at the superior rim of the glenoid fossa and the **short head** arises from the coracoid process. They insert onto the posterior aspect of the radial tuberosity and are innervated by the musculocutaneous nerve (C5,6).

The **brachioradialis** functions primarily to flex the arm at the elbow. It originates from the lateral two-thirds of the lateral supracondylar ridge of the humerus and the lateral intermuscular septum distal to the spiral groove to insert on the lateral side of the styloid process of the radius. It is innervated by the radial nerve (C5,6). The **brachialis** flexes the elbow in all positions of the forearm. It arises from the distal half of the anterior aspect of the anterior aspect of the humerus to insert on the ulnar tuberosity and coronoid process. It is innervated by the musculocutaneous nerve (C5,6).

The **flexor–pronator group** consists of the pronator teres, flexor carpi radialis, palmaris longus, flexor carpi ulnaris (FCU), and flexor digitorum superficialis (FDS). All arise directly from, or in close proximity to, the medial epicondyle. The primary role of this group is flexion and pronation of the wrist and hand, while secondarily aiding elbow flexion. All are innervated by the median nerve (C6–8, T1), with the exception of the FCU (ulnar nerve, C8, T1).

The **extensor group** is composed of the triceps and anconeus. The three heads of the triceps arise from the proximal humerus and unite to form the two aponeuroses that join together to form the triceps tendon and insert onto the posterior surface of the olecranon and the deep fascia of the forearm. The triceps is innervated by the radial nerve (C7,8).

The **extensor–supinator group** (brachioradialis, extensor carpi radialis longus and brevis (ECRL and ECRB), supinator, extensor digitorum, extensor carpi ulnaris, and extensor digiti minimi) function primarily to extend and supinate the hand and wrist, while providing dynamic support for the lateral elbow. They originate

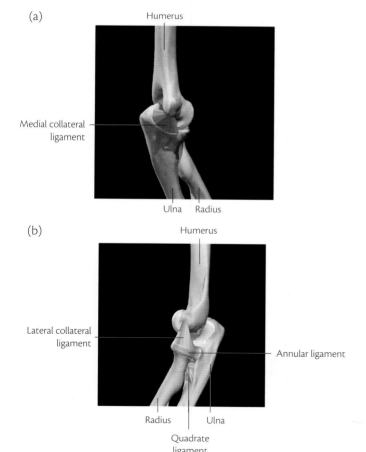

(a)

Humerus

Medial collateral ligament

Ulna Radius

(b)

Humerus

Lateral collateral ligament

Annular ligament

Radius Ulna

Quadrate ligament

Fig. 3.6.2 (a) Medial and (b) lateral ligamentous anatomy of the elbow. Copyright © Primal Pictures. Reproduced with permission.

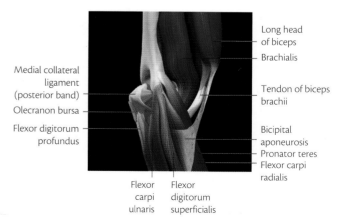

Long head of biceps

Brachialis

Medial collateral ligament (posterior band)

Olecranon bursa

Flexor digitorum profundus

Tendon of biceps brachii

Bicipital aponeurosis

Pronator teres

Flexor carpi radialis

Flexor carpi ulnaris

Flexor digitorum superficialis

Fig. 3.6.3 The medial elbow. Copyright © Primal Pictures. Reproduced with permission.

(a)

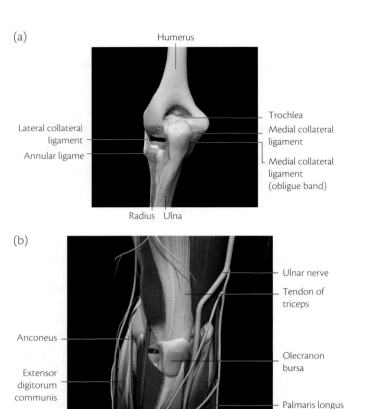

(b)

Fig. 3.6.4 The posterior elbow. (a) deep (b) superficial structures. Copyright © Primal Pictures. Reproduced with permission.

at or near the lateral epicondyle and are innervated by the radial nerve (C5–8, T1).

Nerves

Four nerves are important in function of the elbow (Fig. 3.6.4 and Table 3.6.1).

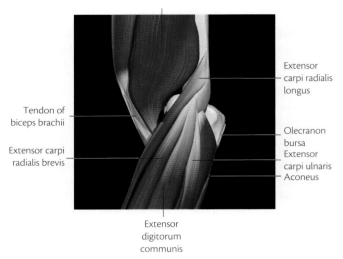

Fig. 3.6.5 The lateral elbow. Copyright © Primal Pictures. Reproduced with permission.

The **musculocutaneous nerve** (C5–7) originates from the lateral cord of the brachial plexus, passes between the biceps and brachialis muscles, and pierces the brachial fascia lateral to the biceps tendon, terminating as the lateral antebrachial cutaneous nerve.

The **median nerve** (C5–8, T1) originates from the lateral and medial cords of the brachial plexus, passes distally over the antero-medial aspect of the arm lateral to the brachial artery, and then crosses the antecubital fossa to lie medial to the biceps tendon and brachial artery. It passes between the two heads of pronator teres and travels down the forearm beneath the FDS. Anomalies in the pronator teres may lead to median nerve compression at this site. The **anterior interosseous nerve** arises from the median nerve at the inferior border of pronator teres and travels along the interosseous membrane to innervate the flexor pollicis longus and the lateral portion of the flexor digitorum profundus (FDP).

The **ulnar nerve** (C8, T1) arises from the medial cord of the brachial plexus and passes distally from the anterior to the posterior compartments of the upper arm through the arcade of Struthers, a fascial raphe between the medial head of triceps and the medial intermuscular septum (approximately 8 cm proximal to the medial

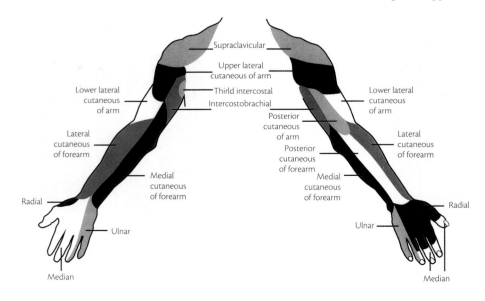

Fig. 3.6.6 Cutaneous supply of the arm by peripheral nerves. Copyright © Reproduced from Hazelman, B, Riley, G and Speed, C (ed) (2004). *Soft Tissue Rheumatology*, Oxford Univeristy Press.

Table 3.6.1 Motor supply of the arm

Nerve	Roots	Motor supply[a]	Quick motor test
Axillary	C5,6	Deltoid Teres minor	Shoulder abduction
Musculocutaneous	C5–C7	Corachobrachialis, brachialis, biceps	Flexion of supinated forearm
Suprascapular	C4–C6	Spinati	Supraspinatus test, external rotation of shoulder
Radial	C5–C8	Triceps, brachioradialis, ECR longus and brevis, supinator	Elbow extension, supination of extended forearm, wrist extension

Radial nerve branches:
  Posterior Interosseous
  Superficial radial
	C7, C8	Extensors of wrist/fingers
		
		—
			Wrist extension
			
			—

Ulnar	C8, T1	FCU, FDP of ring and little fingers, small muscles of hand except those supplied by median nerve	Abduction little and index fingers, adduction of thumb
Median	C7, C8, T1	Pronator teres, forearm flexors except those supplied by ulnar nerve, 1st and 2nd lumbricals, APB, opponens pollicis, FPB	Pronation of forearm; abduction, opposition of thumb
Median nerve branch anterior interosseous	C7, C8	FDP of index, middle fingers, FPL	Flexion distal phalanx of thumb, index finger

[a]ECR, Extensor carpi radialis; FCU, flexor carpi ulnaris; FDP, flexordigitorum profundus; FPL, flexor pollicis longus; APB, abductor policis brevis; FPB, flexor pollicis brevis.

epicondyle). It continues distally behind the medial epicondyle and through the cubital tunnel into the forearm. An articular branch and a branch to the FCU arise at the elbow; there are no branches in the arm.

The **radial nerve** (C6–8) arises from the posterior cord of the brachial plexus and travels laterally down the spiral groove to pass anterior to the lateral epicondyle and posterior to the brachioradialis and brachialis muscles. It then divides into posterior interosseous and superficial radial nerves at the antecubital fossa. The posterior interosseous nerve continues around the posterolateral aspect of the radius and passes between the two heads of the supinator muscle before dividing into terminal motor branches. The superficial branch continues distally to terminate in the hand.

Bursae

Many bursae have been reported to exist. There are three superficial bursae in the elbow region: the olecranon bursa, and the medial and lateral epicondylar bursae. Only the first of these is a common site for pathology. Of several deep bursae, the most significant is the bicipital radial bursa. Intratendinous bursitis, located in the

substance of the triceps tendon near its insertion, may occur with triceps tendinopathy.

The subcutaneous olecranon bursa is a superficial anatomical bursa, situated between the skin and the triceps tendon and olecranon. The bursa is not present in young children but increases in size after the age of 7 years, with that on the dominant side usually being larger. The floor of the bursa adheres to the olecranon. In the healthy state there is no communication between the bursa and elbow joint.

Biomechanics

The elbow is exposed to high stresses during upper limb sports activities. The baseball pitch is often used to describe the motion of the arm during throwing, but a similar action is seen in other sports such as javelin throwing, volleyball, the tennis serve, and throwing in American football. This motion is shown in Fig. 3.6.9. It takes approximately 2 seconds to complete the full motion from wind-up through cocking, acceleration, deceleration,

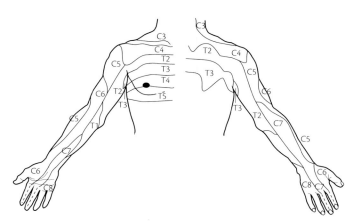

Fig. 3.6.7 Dermatomes of the arm. Copyright © Reproduced from Hazelman, B, Riley, G and Speed, C (ed) (2004). *Soft Tissue Rheumatology*, Oxford Univeristy Press.

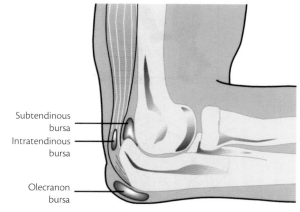

Subtendinous bursa

Intratendinous bursa

Olecranon bursa

Fig. 3.6.8 Some bursae around the elbow. Copyright © Reproduced from Hazelman, B, Riley, G and Speed, C (ed) (2004). *Soft Tissue Rheumatology*, Oxford Univeristy Press.

and follow-through, with 75% spent in the pre-acceleration phases. Angular velocities of the elbow during extension are approximately 220°/s in a baseball pitch, up to 1700°/sec in a tennis serve, and 1900°/sec in a javelin thrust. During the tennis serve, angular velocity of forearm pronation is in the region of 350°/sec and wrist extension is 315°/sec. Range of motion of the elbow during throwing is from 85° of flexion at the time of maximal shoulder rotation at cocking to 20° of extension at ball release.

The ulnar collateral ligament cannot withstand the valgus stresses imposed during throwing alone, and is supported by surrounding musculature. Contraction of the triceps and anconeus may compress the ulnohumeral joint and help to stabilize it during the acceleration phase. At ball release there is a compressive force through the elbow, resisting distraction of the joint. This increases through the throwing motion from the time of contact of the front foot until ball release. Kinematic values for the tennis serve are similar to those seen during overhand throwing.

Clinical evaluation

History

A careful history is obtained to determine the characteristics, mechanisms, severity, and functional consequences of the injury. Hand dominance and the functional impact of the injury in relation to the patient's sport, occupation, and daily activities are noted. The clinician ascertains whether the onset of symptoms was acute or insidious and obtains a clear description of the mechanism of injury, as this can indicate the anatomical structure(s) involved.

The duration and progression of symptoms is an indication of severity of the condition. Pain is the most common symptom and its characteristics should be determined, including its site, nature, radiation, temporal characteristics, and relieving and exacerbating factors. Locking is suggestive of loose bodies within the joint complex. Other symptoms may include swelling, tingling, and numbness, and the characteristics of these symptoms should also be recorded. Symptoms in the proximal arm and neck should be specifically addressed, as elbow symptoms may be referred from these sites. In those patients complaining of stiffness and loss of mobility, the specific movements affected should be ascertained. A full sporting history relating to equipment, technique, and training should be recorded. The treatments used to date should be recorded, and current and past medical history, including previous injuries to the affected arm and neck, obtained.

Examination

Both arms and the neck should be adequately exposed, and both arms should be visualized for comparison.

Inspection

The examiner notes the general appearance of the arms, including soft tissue contour, evidence of wasting or asymmetry of muscle bulk, muscle fasciculation, scars, and swelling. Overdevelopment of the dominant arm is common in upper limb athletes such as throwers and racket sports players. Deformities and alignment should be evaluated. The carrying angle is evaluated with the arm fully extended. The antecubital fossa can be assessed anteriorly for swelling and soft tissue masses.

Inspection of the posterior aspect of the elbow allows the olecranon to be examined. Discrete bursal swelling, or more general swelling suggestive of synovitis or effusion, may be evident. Triceps tendon rupture may appear as an excessively bony prominence, with a gap just above the tip of the olecranon. When dislocation has occurred, it is usually obvious, causing marked distortion of the bony contour, typically with a posteriorly prominent proximal ulna.

If synovitis or a joint effusion is present, all three joints of the elbow complex will be affected since they are continuous. This is usually evident on inspecting the **lateral aspect of the elbow** in the triangular space between the lateral epicondyle, the head of the radius, and the tip of the olecranon. Swelling is also commonly evident on the posterior aspect. The patient usually holds the swollen

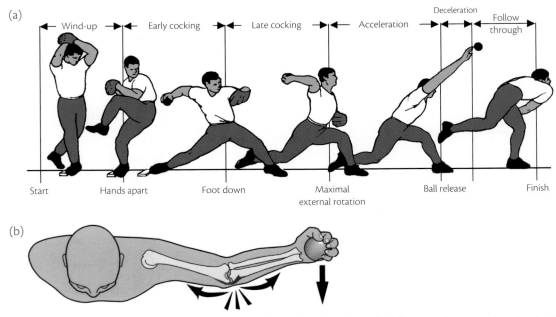

Fig. 3.6.9 The baseball pitch. Note the valgus stress placed on the elbow in the late cocking phase. Copyright © Reproduced from Hazelman, B, Riley, G and Speed, C (ed) (2004). *Soft Tissue Rheumatology*, Oxford Univeristy Press.

elbow in the position of maximum volume (30° of flexion). There may be evidence of subcutaneous atrophy after repeated corticosteroid injections in the region of the lateral epicondyle in patients with chronic lateral elbow pain.

Palpation

Palpation of the bony landmarks is performed with the arm flexed at 90° and includes the medial and lateral epicondyles, the medial supracondylar line of the humerus (prominence of which can be associated with median nerve compression), the lateral supracondylar line of the humerus, the olecranon, and the ulnar border down to the ulnar styloid at the wrist.

In the normal position of function, with the elbow flexed to 90° and the forearm midway between supination and pronation, the olecranon process and the medial and lateral epicondyles will normally form an isosceles triangle. When the arm is fully extended, these points form a straight line. Deformities of any of the involved bones result in loss of these features.

The **olecranon fossa** is best palpated with the elbow in less than 90° flexion, where the ulnar nerve can be evaluated for tenderness and thickening. Where anterior subluxation of the ulnar nerve occurs, it may be evident with flexion and reduced with extension. The **radial head** can be palpated approximately 2.5 cm distal to the lateral epicondyle, just posteromedial to the wrist extensor muscle group. It can be felt with pronation and supination, and may be tender after fracture or with synovitis or osteoarthritis. Dislocation can also occur. In the **cubital fossa** it is possible to palpate several structures. The **biceps tendon** is best differentiated from the **brachioradialis** when the patient makes a fist of the supinated hand, places the hand under the edge of a table, and tries to lift it. Although the insertion is not palpable, the muscle belly and tendon are. The pulse of the **brachial artery** is easily felt, and the **median nerve** lies directly medial to this. The **musculocutaneous nerve** lies lateral to the biceps tendon is not palpable but is located deep under the brachioradialis, 2–5 cm above the elbow joint.

Posteriorly, the **olecranon bursa** may be enlarged, tender, and thick in a bursitis. The triceps tendon can be palpated at its insertion on the tip of the olecranon. Medially, the **ulnar nerve** can be palpated posterior to the medial epicondyle. The **flexor–pronator muscle group** may be tender at its origin with medial epicondylitis. The **MCL** cannot be palpated directly but tenderness in this area, usually after a valgus strain, is indicative of an injury to this ligament.

Laterally, the **LCL** is not directly palpable but the area may be tender if injured, usually after varus stress. The **wrist extensors** are best assessed when the forearm is in neutral position and the wrist relaxed. Local tenderness at or near the epicondyle is indicative of lateral epicondylitis, although the differential diagnosis is wide.

Movement

Passive and active range of motion and movement against resistance are evaluated. The latter is best assessed with the arm flexed to 90°, with the elbow stabilized by one of the examiner's hands around the posterior aspect of the elbow while the other hand grasps the distal forearm.

Flexion: the biceps is tested with the forearm supinated, the brachialis with the forearm pronated, and the brachioradialis with the forearm in mid-position.

Supination and pronation: the patient supinates from a pronated position against resistance and pronation is tested from a supinated position. The triceps is tested against resistance from a position of full flexion.

Neurovascular status is also assessed.

Special tests
Assessment of ligamentous stability

Assessment of ligamentous stability is demonstrated in Fig. 3.6.10. The examiner notes whether pain is provoked and whether there is excessive laxity compared with the contralateral elbow, and if so if a firm endpoint is present. Lack of a firm endpoint indicates total rupture.

Lateral epicondylitis

All tests for lateral epicondylitis aim to reproduce pain at the relevant epicondyle:

1. The ECRB is tested in two positions: Resisted wrist extension is tested with the forearm pronated and the elbow in two positions: firstly extended and then flexed to 90°.

2. The extensor digitorum communis (EDC) is tested when the patient extends the elbow, pronates the forearm, and extends the fingers. The examiner applies downward force to the middle finger.

3. Passive movement of the elbow and forearm from full flexion and forearm supination to extension, forearm pronation, and wrist flexion reproduces pain if there is tightness of the extensor–supinator group.

Medial epicondylitis

All tests for medial epicondylitis aim to reproduce pain at the relevant epicondyle.

1. Resisted wrist flexion with the elbow flexed and forearm supinated reproduces medial elbow pain in medial epicondylitis.

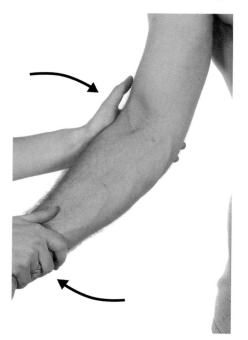

Fig. 3.6.10 Assessment of ligamentous stability of the elbow. Laxity is evaluated on applying valgus then varus stress on the elbow in slight flexion.
Copyright © Reproduced from Hazelman, B, Riley, G and Speed, C (ed) (2004). *Soft Tissue Rheumatology*, Oxford Univeristy Press.

2. Resisted forearm pronation with the forearm extended and in neutral rotation (shaking hands with the examiner) also reproduces pain.

3. Passive movement of the flexed pronated forearm into full flexion and supination with the wrist extended will reproduce pain if there is tightness in the flexor–pronator group.

Tests for neurological dysfunction

Tinel's test at the elbow is often used in suspected nerve compression. It is performed by tapping over the ulnar nerve in the ulnar groove, working from distal to proximal. A positive sign is indicated by tingling in the ulnar distribution of the forearm and hand distal to the point of compression of the nerve. The most distal point at which abnormal sensation is felt is postulated to indicate the limit of nerve regeneration of the sensory fibres of a nerve. However, the test has a low level of sensitivity.

The elbow flexion test is similar to Phalen's test at the wrist but, like Tinel's test, it has poor sensitivity and specificity. The patient sits with the elbows fully flexed for up to 5 minutes. The onset of tingling or paraesthesia in the ulnar nerve distribution of the forearm and hand represents cubital tunnel syndrome.

Ulnar nerve instability can be demonstrated by repeated flexion–extension of the elbow, when the patient will complain of tingling in the distribution of the nerve and pain at the medial elbow. Subluxation of the nerve may be detected.

The presence of **pronator teres syndrome** is tested by extension of the patient's elbow from an initial position of 90° of flexion, while the examiner resists pronation of the forearm. Where the syndrome is present, the patient reports tingling or paraesthesia in the medial nerve distribution of the forearm and hand. Again, the sensitivity of this test is limited.

Wartenberg's sign: the patient sits with his/her hands resting on a table and the examiner passively spreads the fingers apart, instructing the patient to bring the fingers together. An ulnar nerve lesion is indicated by an inability to adduct the little finger.

Froment's sign for ulnar neuropathy is performed by asking the patient to hold an object such as a piece of paper between the thumb and flat of the palm. Inability to hold it in place when the examiner pulls it away, and compensation by flexing the flexor pollicis longis, indicates ulnar nerve dysfunction.

Pinch grip test: the patient attempts to pinch the tips of the index finger and thumb together. Normally there should be tip-to-tip pinch. A pulp-to-pulp pinch indicates an anterior interosseous nerve lesion.

A full neurological assessment is completed and the remainder of the upper limb and neck examined as pain may be referred to the elbow from both proximal and distal sites.

Lateral elbow pain

Lateral epicondylitis

Lateral 'epicondylitis' is in fact a tendinopathy of the common extensor–supinator tendon rather than a true epicondylitis. It is characterized by lateral periepicondylar pain and tenderness that is exacerbated by gripping. When, in 1883, Major noted that this condition commonly affected tennis players, the complaint became popularly known as 'tennis elbow' (Nirschl 1974). Thirteen per cent of elite tennis players and up to 50% of non-elite players have symptoms suggestive of lateral epicondylitis, and approximately

Table 3.6.2 Differential diagnosis of lateral elbow pain

Lateral epicondylitis
Instability
Epicondylar apophysitis (adolescents)
Radiocapitellar bursitis
Forearm compartment syndrome
C6 root pathology
Radial nerve lesions

Radiohumeral joint pathology
    Osteochondritis dissecans
    Osteochondrosis of the radiocapitellar joint
    Instability of the radiocapitellar joint

Fracture/stress fracture
Synovitis of the radiohumeral head

half of these have symptoms for an average duration of 2½ years. Nevertheless, 95% of cases occur in those who do not play tennis and it particularly affects those in manual occupations. The incidence of the complaint is equal among men and women, although in tennis players it may be more common in men. It particularly affects the age group spanning the fourth to sixth decades, with those in the fifth decade four times more commonly affected than at other stages of this span.

Pathology

Degenerative microtears are found in the common extensor–supinator tendon. The tears are likely to be due to repetitive mechanical overload. Typical microscopic features of surgical specimens include hyaline degeneration, fibroblastic and vascular proliferation, and a notable absence of any inflammatory component (Chard *et al.* 1994), although these represent end-stage lesions. The ECRB and the supinator share a common origin at the lateral epicondyle, the joint capsule, and the orbicular ligament. The ECRL arises from the epicondyle and more proximally from the lateral epicondylar ridge, and the EDC also takes part of its origin from the lateral epicondyle. Although the origin of ECRB is most commonly affected, all sites within the complex can be involved.

History

The history is that of epicondylar pain and tenderness, worse with grip and resulting in functional difficulties. Such symptoms may be acute or insidious in onset. There is often a history of overuse, involving repetitive flexion–extension or pronation–supination activity, with overactivation of the extensor carpi in particular. Among tennis players, the backhand appears to be the most commonly implicated stroke in the initiation of the complaint. Less skilled players with a faulty technique are much more likely to sustain the injury, and it is much less common in the experienced player.

Equipment factors frequently play a role, and the patient may give a history of recent change in one or more aspects of equipment, or there may be long-standing errors. These include the tennis racket that is too heavy or too light, string tension that is too tight, and the use of heavy or wet tennis balls. Much has been made of appropriate grip size, although the importance of this is now recognized to be less important than previously considered (Eygendaal *et al.* 2007).

Examination

There is usually tenderness over the ECRB origin at the lateral epicondyle, although the tenderness may be slightly more diffuse over the origins of EDC and/or ECRL. One or more provocation tests, as described earlier, may be positive.

Imaging

Imaging studies are not routinely performed. Features on diagnostic **ultrasound** include swelling, areas of hypoechogenicity, and in some cases neovascularization, which is likely to represent more active severe disease. A local fluid collection may occasionally be seen. In chronic cases there is often dystrophic calcification at the tendon insertion and irregularity of the bone surface. **MRI** may demonstrate increased signal intensity of the extensor tendons close to their insertion on the lateral epicondyle.

Management

The treatment of lateral epicondylitis in the more acute stages involves relative rest, the use of ice (10–20 minutes every 2 hours in the acute stages), analgesia including acupuncture, and short-term use of (preferably topical) NSAIDs. The use of modalities such as ultrasound has no proven benefit, but low-level laser therapy may be helpful. A compression strap or counterforce brace applied distal to the bulk of the extensor mass has been demonstrated to reduce muscle activity in EDC and ECRB with some (but not all) braces on needle EMG studies during isometric contraction of the wrist extensors in healthy subjects (Snyder-Mackler and Epler 1989). Such studies have not been performed in affected individuals and no definitive conclusions can be drawn concerning the effectiveness of these appliances for lateral epicondylitis (Struijs *et al.* 2001). If a brace is used, it is tightened to a comfortable degree of tension with the forearm muscles relaxed, so that a maximum contraction is limited. Constant use of the brace is avoided, as tightness of involved structures can occur. Those who benefit from its use may choose to wear it during periods of significant use of the arm even after symptoms settle.

All these approaches are used in order to allow rehabilitation to commence. Stretching of the forearm extensors and range of motion exercises at the elbow and wrist should start early. Progressive rehabilitation for the strength and endurance forearm extensor–supinator group, and elbow proprioception work, commences as soon as pain

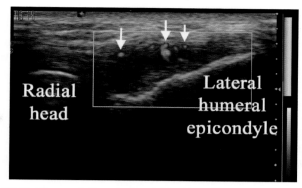

Fig. 3.6.11 Ultrasound of lateral epicondylitis with swelling, neovascularization and areas of hypoechogenicity of the common extensor tendon in a 28-year old tennis player with lateral elbow pain. Longitudinal sonogram demonstrating new vessel formation (arrows) inside the common extensor origin attachment on the lateral humeral epicondyle.

allows. Relative weakness of the extensor carpi radialis or widespread upper limb muscle imbalances may be causative in those with chronic symptoms because of disuse and pain inhibition. The rate of progression depends on the patient's symptoms; if symptoms recur, the patient returns to a lower level of exercise. Ice may be necessary after early rehabilitation sessions to limit an excessive inflammatory response.

Some advocate transverse friction massage in more chronic cases on the basis of breaking down scar tissue at the site but, again, the evidence is lacking and some patients find this aggravating.

The use of corticosteroid injections often provides short-term pain relief, but there is no evidence of benefit over placebo in the longer term (Hay *et al.* 1999). Their use is restricted to those with persistent disability despite the above measures and where ongoing pain is limiting rehabilitation. The patient is counselled on the risk of subcutaneous atrophy, tendon rupture, and other standard risks. A small volume of a short-acting corticosteroid such as hydrocortisone with 0.5–1 ml 2% lidocaine is suitable. A positive response occurs when there is significant reduction in pain lasting for at least 6 weeks. If symptoms recur, the injection may be repeated at a minimum interval of 6 weeks, but the total number of injections should be limited to three. The injection should not be repeated if no response is seen with the first procedure.

Corticosteroid injection has been shown to reduce the hyperaemia of neovascularization noted on ultrasound (Torp-Pedersen *et al.* 2008). Sclerosant therapy of new vessels with sclerosants such as polidocanol under guidance using ultrasound and Doppler may be of some benefit in pain relief and improvement in grip strength. Lidocaine and adrenaline injections into local vessels has also been advocated for the same purpose (Zeisig *et al.* 2008).

In chronic lesions, dry needling can be useful. Ultrasound guided injection of platelet rich plasma (PRP) is increasingly popular, PRP is a promising therapy, but more research is needed.

Extracorporeal shock wave therapy has no role in acute lateral epicondylitis and has mixed results in chronic cases. Therefore it should be reserved for recalcitrant cases where surgery is being considered.

The most common cause of lack of response to the above measures is failure to address the cause of the condition. Even in the athlete, simple aspects of daily activity such as use of a computer or

Table 3.6.3 Extrinsic factors associated with lateral epicondylitis in tennis elbow

Repetitive overuse activities, especially those involving forearm rotation, wrist and forearm flexion/extension
Poor spinal and scapular posture
Thoracic and/or shoulder restriction
Weak wrist extensors
Tennis: technique errors, e.g. leading elbow in backhand, poor body positioning, overuse of forearm extensors
Errors in sporting/work equipment, e.g. heavy/light racket, wrong grip size, strings too loose/tight

manual activities may be the underlying perpetuating factor. In tennis players, technique and equipment factors must be addressed. Proper racket handle size can be estimated by the distance from the mid-palmar crease to the ring finger. Evaluation of technique with the help of a coach may prove beneficial. Improvements may be noted by avoidance of the leading elbow during backhand, ensuring that the forearm is only partially pronated, the forward shoulder is lowered, and the trunk is leaning forward. The patient should also consider reducing string tension to 2–3 pounds less than the manufacturer's recommendations (i.e. 50–55 pounds), using slower and lighter tennis balls, and playing on slower courts.

Surgery should be reserved for those patients with disabling symptoms who fail to respond to all the above measures. Options include repair of the extensor origin after excision of the torn tendon and granulation tissue, and local drilling of the subchondral bone of the lateral epicondyle, with the aim of increasing blood supply. This can be performed under local or general anaesthesia. The elbow is placed in a posterior plaster splint for a week, and then in a lighter splint for 2 weeks, with the elbow in 90° flexion and neutral rotation. Range of motion exercises are commenced thereafter, with a progressive strengthening regime. Light activities can be recommended at 3 months, but the patient can expect to wear a counterforce brace initially.

Other surgical options include reduction of tension on the common extensor origin by fasciotomy, direct release of the extensor origin or lengthening of the ECRB tendon distally. Fasciotomy and complete extensor tendon release can result in loss of strength, and lengthening of ECRB distally appears to be effective only in the minority of cases. Whilst intra-articular procedures such as synovectomy and division of the orbicular ligament have been advocated, these seem inappropriate for an extra-articular condition. Some surgeons advocate decompression of the radial or posterior interosseous nerves on the basis that nerve entrapment is contributing to, or is the primary cause of, chronic symptoms.

Osteochondritis dissecans of the humeral capitellum

This condition occurs after the capitellum has ossified and is the result of trauma—usually microtrauma—to the subchondral bone, typically of the dominant arm. Avascular necrosis of subchondral bone leads to loss of support for adjacent cartilaginous structures. Some cases progress, and these structures separate from the capitellum leading to the development of an osteochondral fragment of articular cartilage on the underlying bone at the superficial surface of the joint. The articulation of the radial head and humeral capitellum provides mobility for a wide range of supination and pronation, as well as flexion and extension. Thus this area is particularly susceptible to the rotary, compressive, axial, and angular forces associated with activities such as throwing. In overhead throwing, articular forces at the radiocapitellar articulation are significant. Progressive pronation, compression, and rotation occur on the anteromedial radial head and the inferior and medial aspects of the capitellum as the elbow is extended. Compressive loads are increased by the valgus orientation of the elbow. In other sports, excessive axial loading to the elbow is also the probable principal factor in development of the condition. The process involves fraying of the articular surface, subchondral bone changes, osteocartilaginous fragmentation, and the development of osteochondritis dissecans.

The condition most commonly occurs in those aged 10–15 years, and is rare in individuals younger than 10 years or older than

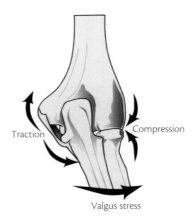

Fig. 3.6.12 Little Leaguer's elbow results from traction on the lateral elbow and compressive forces on the medial side. Copyright © Reproduced from Hazelman, B, Riley, G and Speed, C (ed) (2004). *Soft Tissue Rheumatology*, Oxford Univeristy Press.

50 years. Most cases involve males, and in North America these are usually Little League baseball pitchers. When females are affected, they are usually gymnasts. Other sports that seem susceptible are racket sports and weightlifting. Up to 20% of cases are bilateral.

The patient reports lateral or non-specific elbow pain, worse with use and initially relieved by rest, although with progression there can be nocturnal pain. Initially there may be lateral elbow tenderness, some swelling, and variable limitations in range of motion. In later cases, the patient may report popping, locking, and catching. There is progressive restriction of extension with a fixed flexion deformity. Crepitus, muscle atrophy, and a joint effusion may be present.

Investigations

Plain anteroposterior and lateral radiographs may be normal in early cases, or changes are confined to the humeral capitellum. Flattening, patchy rarefaction consisting of a sclerotic rim of subchondral bone adjacent to the articular surface, irregular ossification, and/or a bony defect adjacent to the articular surface may be seen. Fragmentation may occur and loose bodies may be evident. CT may be necessary to document loose bodies; it also helps to evaluate the level of progression of the condition. T1-weighted MR images show low-signal changes at the surface of the capitellum in early lesions, and can evaluate the size and extent of the lesion and the vascular supply to the area. On T2-weighted images, unstable lesions have pockets of high signal surrounding the displaced fragments. Ultrasound shows localized capitellar bony flattening early, and non-displaced or displaced fragments. Contrast arthrography or arthroscopy may be necessary.

Management

The first line of approach is relative rest and analgesia. Range of motion exercises, progressive strengthening of the upper limb and spine, and attention to technique are all pursued. Surgery is indicated where there is a failure of conservative treatment, progressive joint contracture, partially attached or completely detached fragments, or locking and catching of the joint with extension and/or flexion. Arthroscopy for excision of the loose body and abrasion chondroplasty are preferred, with conversion to an open procedure if necessary. Surgical fixation of the loose body may be attempted; however, most studies show poor results. Radial head excision is recommended in older patients who have a radial head

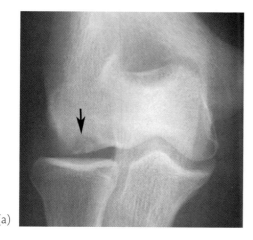

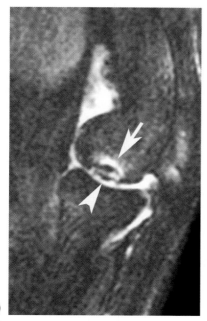

Fig. 3.6.13 (a) Anteroposterior radiograph of elbow shows osteochondritis dissecans lesion of the capitellum (arrow) with a focal well-defined area of subchondral radiolucency. The lesion was unstable at arthroscopy. (b) Sagittal fat-suppressed T2-weighted fast spin-echo MRI scan of the elbow shows osteochondritis dissecans lesion (arrow) as a large area of signal abnormality with a high signal intensity rim and linear bands of high and low signal intensity centrally. Note marked irregularity of articular cartilage overlying osteochondritis dissecans lesion (arrowhead). Reproduced from Kijowski, R. and De Smet, A. (2005). MRI findings of osteochondritis dissecans of the capitellum with surgical correlation. *American Journal of Roentgenology*, **185**, 1453–9.

deformity, radiocapitellar degenerative changes, or limitation of forearm rotation. Anterior capsule release may help to relieve flexion contractures.

Prevention is the best cure: parents and coaches must be educated as to the relative risks of overuse in relevant sports.

Radial head fractures

Fractures of the radial head are common and usually occur following a fall onto the pronated forearm with the elbow extended. They should be suspected if the patient complains of lateral elbow pain, particularly on rotation, although flexion may be well maintained.

A tense haematoma within the elbow joint can be very painful and give rise to a positive 'fat pad' sign on a lateral radiograph.

The radial head is a disc-shaped structure completely covered in hyaline cartilage which rotates within the annular ligament. It is the second most important stabilizer of the elbow joint after the medial collateral ligament. Fractures are classified according to Mason:

type I	undisplaced, stable
type II	displaced (1–2 fragments)
type III	comminuted (>2 fragments)
type IV	associated with ligamentous injury of the elbow or forearm

Type I fractures are stable and can usually be mobilized early with active motion as pain allows. Type II fractures are best managed by open reduction and internal fixation using low-profile screws that can be countersunk below the articular surface, facilitating early motion.

Type III fractures are ideally managed by reconstruction using multiple screws and/or a contoured low-profile plate which provides a buttress for the articular fragments and maintains radial length. If the fracture is unreconstructable and there is no associated ligamentous injury, early excision of the fracture fragments can provide a simple solution, allowing early active motion. However, there is a risk of relative proximal migration of the radius that can alter load transfer at the distal radio-ulnar joint and produce wrist pain.

Type IV fractures are unstable and may be associated with injuries of the collateral ligaments, elbow dislocation, or rupture of the interosseous membrane (the Essex–Lopresti lesion). In these cases fixation of the fracture and ligament repair should be combined so as to allow controlled early motion in an external hinged brace postoperatively. If the fracture is unreconstructable, the radial head should be replaced with a metallic prosthesis after excision of the fragments. In these cases, excision alone is contraindicated. The role of the prosthesis is to maintain radial length and thereby provide stability in both the coronal plane (to varus–valgus loading) and the axis of the forearm (longitudinally). In the past silicone prostheses were used, but these were of insufficient stiffness and frequently led to synovial reactions, osteolysis, and loosening.

Distal biceps tendinopathy

Tendinosis of the distal end of the biceps brachii is a painful and limiting condition that can occur with repetitive supination and

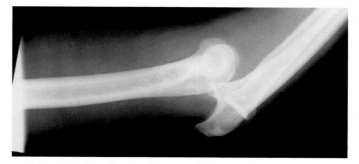

Fig. 3.6.14 Plain X-ray showing dislocation of the elbow after a fall onto an outstretched hand.

pronation activities, including throwing, swimming, weight lifting/training, and racket sports. Pain is felt in the antecubital fossa, and local swelling and tenderness may be noted. Pain is worse with resisted supination. Imaging often includes both MRI and ultrasound to fully evaluate the nature and extent of the lesion. Management involves relative rest, ice, NSAIDs and modification of activities, training strategies (in particular weight-training), and review of technique. Failing to address the problem can ultimately result in rupture.

Rupture of the biceps insertion

Avulsion of the distal insertion of biceps accounts for 3–10% of all biceps tendon ruptures and occurs in association with a single traumatic insult, usually with the elbow in 90° flexion. There is an increased incidence with anabolic steroid use.

The patient notes a sudden tearing pain in the antecubital fossa followed by a deep aching discomfort. There is bruising and considerable functional limitation, with weakness of supination and elbow flexion, and grip strength may also be reduced. The tendon is no longer palpable, having retracted into the forearm as a bulbous swelling. A palpable gap is present. A partial rupture of the tendon produces pain and local crepitus on supination and pronation. Treatment is early surgical repair.

Injury to the musculotendinous junction of biceps brachii and calcifying tendinitis of this unit are both rare.

Radial head bursitis

The deep bursa at the radial head can become inflamed with repetitive pronation/supination and may be confused with distal biceps tendinitis. There is local pain and tenderness in the antecubital fossa and there may be fullness or swelling in this area. Pain is worse with pronation. Ultrasound and/or MRI will confirm the diagnosis. Treatment is symptomatic with modification of activities, ice, and NSAIDs.

Forearm compartment syndrome

A compartment syndrome of the forearm can occur acutely after trauma or, less commonly, may present as a chronic exertional compartment syndrome (CECS). CECS is seen in athletes such as rowers, weight-lifters, or motorcycle riders. The relative frequency of involvement of specific muscle compartments is not known. CECS presents with a history of exertional forearm pain, which quickly subsides with rest. Paraesthesiae in the forearm and hand may be reported. Clinically there may be little to find at rest, although the forearm is usually muscular. The diagnosis may be

Table 3.6.4 Differential diagnosis of medial elbow pain

Medial epicondylitis
Medial apophysitis
Ulnar collateral ligament sprain/instability
Cervical spine radiculopathy
Ulnar neuropathy
Osteochondrosis/Osteochondritis dissecans
Osteoarthritis
Fracture/stress fracture

confirmed by intracompartmental pressure monitoring before and after exercise (normal range 0–8 mmHg), although diagnostic levels for forearm compartment syndrome have not been set. Treatment is fasciotomy of the affected compartments.

Radial nerve lesions

The radial nerve and its branches are vulnerable to compression at the elbow and forearm. Depending upon which portion of the nerve is affected, symptoms may be motor (posterior interosseous nerve (PIN)), sensory (superficial radial nerve), or both. PIN entrapment occurs at five sites, but most commonly at the arcade of Frohse at the proximal edge of supinator, which lies deep to the extensor carpi radialis longus (Fig. 3.6.3). Nerve compression due to synovitis at the radiocapitellar joint, tumours, fractures, vascular anomalies, or other local masses can also occur. The superficial radial nerve can be entrapped alone or in combination with the PIN. The radial nerve can also be entrapped above the level of the elbow, due to a lateral intermuscular septum, although this is rare.

History

The typical patient is one who performs repetitive rotary movements of the forearm, such as those involved in discus throwing and racket sports. The primary symptom is aching pain in the belly of the extensor muscles, of insidious onset, which is worse with forearm pronation and wrist flexion. Pain may be more diffuse over the extensor aspect of the forearm, and exacerbation after exertion and pain at night may be features. Such patients are those often considered to have a 'resistant tennis elbow'.

Examination

Examination reveals tenderness to palpation over the course of the PIN, deep to the extensor muscle belly and just distal to the radial head. Pain may be reproduced with resisted extension of the middle finger with the elbow extended and on resisted supination of the extended forearm.

Investigations

Electromyographic studies are frequently normal, although a decrease in motor conduction velocity in the radial nerve across the entrapment site and changes in the muscles innervated distal to the entrapment site may be noted.

Management

Management is symptomatic in mild cases, with stretching and activity modification. In resistant cases, exploration of the nerve is necessary. Procedures used in the treatment of lateral epicondylitis are often included.

Medial elbow

A range of disorders can result in medial elbow pain (Table 6.3.4).

Medial epicondylitis (flexor–pronator tendinopathy)

Medial epicondylitis is not a true epicondylitis but rather an overuse injury of the common tendinous origin of the flexor–pronator muscle group. This injury commonly occurs as a result of repetitive flexion and pronation and, less commonly, with valgus stresses, resulting in tendinopathy of the flexor carpi radialis and/or pronator teres. Like its lateral counterpart, it is seen most commonly in throwing and racket sports (higher-level tennis players are most

Table 3.6.5 Differential diagnosis of anterior elbow pain

Distal biceps tendinopathies
Forearm compartment syndromes
Lymphadenopathy
C-spine radiculopathy
Median nerve, anterior interosseous nerve, cubital tunnel syndromes
Coronoid fracture/stress fracture

commonly affected) and in golfers ('golfer's elbow'). In throwers, where ulnar collateral ligament injury is common, it may be difficult to distinguish between the two clinically and the conditions may coexist.

History

It presents with an acute or insidious onset of aching pain at the medial elbow and proximal flexor musculature of the forearm. There may be weakness of grip, in particular in association with pain. Some patients report symptoms suggestive of an ulnar neuropathy with paraesthesiae in the ring and little fingers.

Examination

Decreased range of motion at the elbow may be noted, caused by pain with stretching of the flexor–pronator group on full extension. There is tenderness just distal and lateral to the medial epicondyle and symptoms are exacerbated by one or more of the provocation tests described earlier. Pain on resisted pronation of the forearm is almost invariably present. The neck should be examined, as nerve root compression may cause tenderness along the line of the median nerve, and other causes of medial elbow pain considered.

Investigations

Ultrasound will demonstrate similar features noted in lateral epicondylitis, specifically areas of hypoechogenicity, swelling, and neovascularization of the tendon, and more rarely a local fluid collection may be identified. Local dystrophic calcification within the tendon is seen in chronic cases. MRI will show swelling and signal hyperintensity on T2-weighted images of the common flexor origin. It will also demonstrate tears if present.

Management

Medial epicondylitis is considered to be more resistant to treatment than lateral epicondylitis. This may be related to greater difficulty in avoiding stresses imposed on this area during daily activities, characteristics of the tissue that make healing prolonged, or inaccuracy of diagnosis. The diagnosis should be questioned in any patient who fails to respond to standard treatment.

Management follows the same path as has been described with lateral epicondylitis and includes relative rest, ice, analgesics, NSAIDs, and a reverse counterforce brace. Acupuncture and local soft tissue release may help. All aim to allow the patient to commence rehabilitation, including early stretching of the wrist and elbow and a progressive strengthening regime of the wrist flexors and forearm pronators. Return to activities can take place only when there is full pain-free range of movement and strength of grip, forearm pronation, and wrist flexion has returned to at least 80% of normal. Peritendinous corticosteroid infiltrations are used

sparingly and are rarely necessary. PRP injection has been advocated, but evidence is limited and if used it should be reserved for recalcitrant cases. Caution should be exercised when injecting because of the close proximity of the ulnar nerve.

Causative factors must be addressed, including training habits, sporting technique, and equipment. Preventative measures also include adequate conditioning of the forearm, attention to technique, and adequate warm-up, stretching, and cool-down.

Surgical intervention is rarely required and is considered only in the most refractory of cases. Standard approaches include release of the tendinous origin of pronator teres, and usually a portion of the flexor carpi radialis, debridement, and decompression of the ulnar nerve distal to the medial epicondyle. A rehabilitation regime is then commenced postoperatively and is usually continued for 6 months before a return to full activities. Complications of surgery include loss of full elbow extension (up to 5°) in 1% of cases, superficial infection (in less than 1%), and damage to the ulnar nerve and MCL.

Little Leaguer's elbow

Little Leaguer's elbow describes a spectrum of changes that can occur at the elbow of a young individual, in particular in relation to throwing. The term refers to the group in which this condition is seen most commonly, i.e. young baseball pitchers, but it can occur across a spectrum of athletes who participate in sports involving similar action or repetitive loading of the elbow. These changes include a variable combination of a medial apophysitis, MCL injury, and instability and compressive changes at the radiocapitellar joint (discussed earlier).

Medial apophysitis is a true epicondylitis and occurs in the skeletally immature individual when there is traction and inflammation of the growth plate at the medial epicondyle. It is seen in particular in children aged 10–14 years who are involved in throwing and racket sports.

During throwing, repetitive forces secondary to contracture of the flexor–pronator origin at the medial epicondyle can lead to microinjuries of the growth plate. In addition, repetitive valgus stress at the elbow leads to attenuation and microtears of the anterior bundle of the MCL. This can progress to valgus instability of the elbow and subsequent compression of the radiocapitellar articulation laterally, with development of osteochondrosis. In some cases acute or repetitive traction on the MCL may lead to an avulsion injury at the apophysis.

History

The patient typically complains of an insidious onset of aching pain at the medial elbow on a background of the repetitive activities described above. Symptoms may be severe and nocturnal disturbance is common. Weakness of grip is commonly noted, and there may be paraesthesiae in the distribution of the ulnar nerve.

Examination

Examination reveals swelling and tenderness at the medial epicondyle, and bruising and flexion contracture may be evident. Pain is exacerbated with passive extension of the elbow and wrist. A fragment may be palpable if an avulsion injury at the epicondyle has occurred. Stress testing may reveal medial instability or just medial pain. In those who have developed compressive changes, the lateral elbow may be tender, with pain exacerbated on movement and on compression of the joint.

Investigations

Plain X-rays may be normal or may show widening of the physis, fragmentation, or avulsion of the apophysis compared with the other side. Gravity valgus stress views may be necessary. Diagnostic ultrasound will demonstrate hypoechoic areas in the soft tissue structures involved, instability on valgus stressing where a ligament injury coexists, and hyperechoic separated fragments and soft tissue calcification. MRI T1-weighted images will show low signal zones of separation through the epicondylar region and hypointense epicondylar oedema. T2-weighted images will show a variable signal within the medial epicondylar fragment, marrow oedema, and a high signal in the MCL if a tear is present. STIR sequences are sensitive for oedema and may show high signal through involved structures.

Management

Management in the form of relative rest from the causative activities, analgesics, ice, and gentle stretching is usually effective, but healing can be prolonged and the patient, parent, and coach must be counselled with respect to this. Non-compliance may result in chronic apophysitis.

When avulsion has occurred, treatment depends on the degree of displacement. Fragments that are rotated or more than 5 mm in diameter may require open reduction and fixation. Mild displacement is treated with immobilization for 2 weeks followed by progressive rehabilitation.

Medial collateral ligament injury

Acute or chronic MCL injury in adults can occur as a result of repetitive valgus extension overload, most commonly seen in overhand throwers or, much less commonly, with direct trauma.

The throwing action involves specific phases as shown on Fig. 3.6.9. Medial valgus stress on the elbow, in particular during the late cocking and acceleration phases of throwing, results in MCL microtrauma and resulting instability, and a wedging effect of the olecranon into the olecranon fossa with resulting formation of a posterior osteophyte. This in turn can irritate the ulnar nerve.

The late cocking phase of the overhand throw places a marked valgus moment across the medial elbow. This repetitive force reaches the tensile limits of the MCL, subjecting it to microtraumatic injury and attenuation. The anterior bundle of the MCL has been identified as the primary restraint to valgus load and is the focus of reconstruction. Diagnosis of MCL injuries should be suspected in any overhand-throwing athlete with a history of medial-sided elbow pain, decreased control, and reduced throwing velocity. Injury to the MCL can be confirmed by physical examination (moving valgus stress test) and appropriate imaging studies (CT arthrogram and MRI). Reconstructive techniques of the MCL have evolved over time and currently provide superior outcomes, with 80–90% of athletes returning to the same level of competitive play. As our understanding of the patho-anatomy of medial elbow injuries progresses and newer hybrid techniques evolve, our ability to care for the overhand-throwing athlete can be expected to improve.

A history of medial elbow pain in a thrower should immediately raise suspicion of the condition. In the acute injury the patient typically reports a sudden onset of pain during throwing, with an associated 'pop' or 'snap'. In chronic cases, the patient reports progressive medial elbow pain that is functionally limiting and becomes worse during the acceleration phase of throwing. The patient often adapts their throwing technique, usually to an earlier release, but this is less controlled.

Flexion contractures and cubitus valgus deformities are common in throwers. Swelling and local MCL tenderness and instability are present, particularly in the acute injury. Posteromedial osteophytes are occasionally palpable and posterior olecranon tenderness is worsened by bringing the arm into valgus and extension.

Investigations

Plain X-rays may be normal, but in chronic cases commonly demonstrate ectopic bone formation in the MCL, posteromedial osteophyte formation at the olecranon and conoid tubercle, and loose bodies. Stress films can help to confirm medial instability. However, the investigations of choice to assess the lesion most closely are ultrasound and MRI, which will document the degree of ligament injury and coexisting pathologies. CT arthrography is undertaken if necessary to allow full assessment of the MCL and surrounding structures, in particular to assess the possibility of capsular disruption.

Management

The aims of treatment are to settle acute symptoms, where present, and to restore the normal range of motion. Rest from exacerbating activities, ice, analgesics, and NSAIDs may all be helpful. Passive and active range of motion exercises are vital and should be commenced early, and a balanced strengthening regime should be commenced. When full range of motion is regained, throwing activities can be resumed with a programme of progressive velocity and endurance. Surgery is indicated in those who fail to respond and have chronic instability and functional impairment. Excision of osteophytes and local debridement or a straight osteotomy 1 cm proximal to the tip of the olecranon are considered in those with impingement. When instability is a major feature, reconstruction using a tendon graft is recommended, although repair may be performed in the acute rupture.

Prevention of the condition is important through adequate conditioning, warm-up, stretching, and appropriate technique.

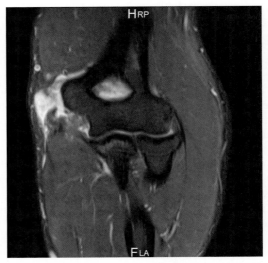

Fig. 3.6.15 MRI scan howing traumatic rupture of the ulnar collateral ligament in a rugby player.

Ulnar neuropathy

The ulnar nerve is vulnerable to trauma, dislocation, and compression during its passage through the cubital tunnel posterior to the medial epicondyle. Individuals with shallow ulnar grooves within the tunnel, with hypermobility or laxity of the soft tissue constraints of the nerve in the tunnel, and who perform repetitive throwing or flexion activities are particularly vulnerable to dislocation or subluxation of the nerve. Recurrent dislocation of the ulnar nerve is reported in 16% of the normal population (Childress 1975). In any individual, the volume of the cubital tunnel decreases as the elbow is flexed, resulting in external compression of the ulnar nerve by the tunnel boundaries, the MCL, and the arcuate ligament. The nerve itself is moved medially by the medial head of the triceps during elbow flexion; scar tissue may tether the nerve and prevent this normal movement. Dislocation or subluxation is most likely during flexion activities, and when this occurs the nerve is particularly at risk of direct trauma. It should be noted that ulnar nerve instability can be an incidental finding.

As has been described, the significant tensile forces at the medial elbow due to repetitive valgus stresses during throwing increase the possibility of a traction neuritis, and this is particularly likely in individuals with MCL instability.

Other aetiological factors can lead to ulnar neuropathy at the elbow. The nerve can become compressed by hypertrophied forearm musculature, the aponeurosis of the flexor carpi ulnaris, a ganglion situated in the cubital tunnel, local bony anomalies, or adhesions within the cubital tunnel.

History

There is sharp deep aching pain at the medial elbow and proximal forearm, which may radiate proximally or distally and may be notable only during flexion and valgus stresses. Neurological disturbances, including paraesthesia, dysaesthesia, and anaesthesia in the ulnar one and a half digits, are usually experienced early in the condition. Whilst clumsiness is frequently reported, true motor weakness is rare since branches within the cubital tunnel to FCU and FDP are situated deep and therefore are frequently spared. Those with recurrent dislocation or subluxation of the nerve may report a popping or snapping sensation prior to the onset of pain and dysaesthesias with elbow flexion and extension.

Examination

Valgus deformity of the elbow, a mild flexion contracture, and MCL instability may be present. Wasting of the small muscles of the hand and hypothenar eminence is a late finding. Soft tissue swelling at the ulnar groove, with tenderness and thickening of the nerve may be evident. Those with ulnar nerve subluxation may be able to demonstrate the phenomenon, and the examiner can frequently dislocate the nerve from the groove. Pressure or percussion may reproduce symptoms, but this is not a sensitive indication of pathology. Symptoms may also be reproduced on sustained elbow flexion (1 minute), particularly when the wrist is extended. Weakness of the small muscles of the hand may be evident. Sensory signs are frequently absent, but in advanced cases evaluation of the ulnar dorsal portion of the hand (supplied by the dorsal cutaneous branch of the ulnar nerve) and ulnar volar forearm (medial antebrachial cutaneous nerve) can indicate whether the nerve injury or compression is in the upper arm, in the cubital tunnel, or at the wrist. A Martin–Gruber anastomosis, where there is communication between the median and ulnar nerves in the forearm, occurs in 15% of people and may confuse clinical findings.

Other causes of ulnar neuropathy should be considered (Table 3.6.6). The cervicothoracic spine should be examined and the patient evaluated for the presence of hypermobility syndrome.

Investigations

Nerve conduction studies classically show reduced conduction velocity across the site of compression compared with the unaffected arm. Although a decline of less than 25% is considered normal, velocities that are reduced by more than 33% are strongly suggestive of neuropathy (Gilliatt and Thomas 1960). Such findings must be considered in the clinical context and cannot be viewed in isolation. Provocative neurophysiology testing with the elbow in flexion is not usually performed because of difficulties in obtaining accurate measurements.

Ultrasound may confirm instability of the nerve and other local soft tissue pathologies. MRI and CT evaluate the local elbow anatomy further. An X-ray of the elbow may also identify associated bony abnormalities (particularly osteophytes).

Management

Ulnar neuropathies may be graded according to symptoms and clinical findings. These do not necessarily correlate with pretreatment electrodiagnostic findings. Mild compression includes those with subjective sensory symptoms only. In moderate compression there is additional weakness and wasting of the interossei and reduced sensation. Severe compression leads to additional wasting of the adductor pollicis and hypothenar muscles and complete or partial anaesthesia of the ulnar innervated portion of the hand (McGowan 1950).

Non-operative management should be pursued in the first instance in most mild to moderate cases (Dellon et al. 1993). Those patients with only sensory symptoms in the absence of motor weakness or wasting are managed conservatively in the first instance. Stress on the ulnar nerve should be avoided by complete rest from exacerbating activities and the use of elbow pads. Splinting the elbow at 30° of flexion may provide symptomatic relief. Ice, NSAIDs, and simple analgesics may be tried but can frequently be unhelpful, whilst modalities are not indicated. If there are signs of local inflammation, a perineural hydrocortisone infiltration under guidance followed by strict rest may be helpful. Gentle range of

Table 3.6.6 Causes of ulnar neuropathy

At the elbow
Fractures/dislocations
Progressive valgus deformity after UCL injury or lateral epicondylar fracture
Pressure on the nerve at the ulnar groove
Entrapment between the two heads of FCU, distal to the medial epicondyle
At the wrist
Compression, e.g. fracture, osteoarthritis, compression against bicycle handlebars, tumours, haemorrhage
Mononeuritis multiplex
Diabetes, vasculitides, sarcoid, amyloid, rheumatoid arthritis, systemic lupus erythemotasus, malignancy

motion exercises are commenced as soon as tolerated. Return to normal activities can commence after full strength is regained, with a progressive strengthening regime of forearm musculature and correction of faulty technique where appropriate.

Prolonged symptom duration, motor and/or sensory deficit, and local joint pathology, in particular MCL instability, are poor prognostic indicators. Half the non-athletic population with mild compression will respond to conservative management. Excellent results have been reported in up to 90% of both athletic and non-athletic patients with mild or moderate compression, with variable results reported in those in whom compression is severe (Dellon *et al.* 1993).

Surgery is considered in those patients who fail to recover with conservative management, those with motor signs, and those with significant MCL instability. In such cases, decompression may be suitable where there is localized compression of the nerve. Surgical options include cubital tunnel decompression or transposition of the nerve in those with nerve subluxation, those with valgus deformity of the elbow, and those in whom decompression has failed. The nerve can be transposed anteriorly with a fascial sling or submuscularly. Medial epicondylectomy has also been advocated, but such a procedure may result in the creation of new sources of nerve pathology. It is recommended that all potential sources of compression of the nerve are explored at operation, even when a specific site of compression has been indicated by electrodiagnostic studies, since more than one site can exist (Kojima *et al.* 1979).

Median nerve compression

Median nerve compression at the elbow or forearm can result in pronator or anterior interosseous syndromes.

The pronator syndrome

Median nerve compression at the elbow and proximal forearm—the pronator syndrome—results in vague aching pain in the proximal volar surface of the forearm. Rarely, there may be dysaesthesias in the distribution of the median nerve in the hand. There is often a history of repetitive strenuous use of the forearm, and thus it is no surprise that the condition is seen in weight-lifters, throwers, and tennis players.

Compression can occur at four sites. The ligament of Struthers, a band between the medial epicondyle and the supracondylar process, is commonly implicated and results in symptoms that are worse with flexion of the elbow against resistance between 120° and 135° flexion. Another fibrous band (the bicipital aponeurosis) can cause indentation of the pronator muscle mass below the medial epicondyle, and symptoms are increased by active and passive forearm pronation. Compression can also occur within the pronator teres due to hypertrophy or tightness of the muscle, when symptoms are worse with resisted pronation of forearm with the wrist in flexion (to relax FDS). Direct pressure over the proximal portion of the pronator teres approximately 4 cm distal to the antebrachial crease, while exerting moderate resistance to pronation, also reproduces the symptoms. Lastly, the nerve can be compressed under FDS, when symptoms are aggravated by resisted flexion of FDS of the middle finger and with passive stretching of finger and wrist flexors.

Tinel's test at possible sites of entrapment is insensitive. Weakness of median nerve innervated muscles is uncommon, but when there is weakness of pinch grip, the condition should be differentiated from anterior interosseous syndrome.

Electrodiagnostic studies help to confirm median nerve latency but may not localize the lesion to the forearm, and exclusion of a carpal tunnel syndrome or double-crush syndrome can be difficult.

Management includes passive stretching of the forearm musculature, NSAIDs, and elbow splinting in neutral rotation. Symptoms may take 2–3 months to improve. Surgical intervention involves exploration of the nerve from 5 cm proximal to the elbow and in the forearm at potential sites of compression.

Anterior interosseous syndrome

Compression of the anterior interosseous nerve results in a pure motor paralysis of the flexor pollicis longus and the index FDP, often in combination with weakness of the pronator quadratus. Those patients with a Martin–Gruber anastomosis may experience weakness of the ulnar intrinsic muscles and/or weakness of the flexor profundus to other fingers. This syndrome is described in individuals lifting heavy weights and where there is cumulative trauma. The patient reports a short episode of pain, which subsides to leave motor weakness. Examination will reveal weakness of pinch grip. After 2–3 weeks, EMG studies will show signs of denervation of affected muscles.

Management involves a course of NSAIDs and relative rest for 8–12 weeks. Those who remain symptomatic are considered for surgery, involving a similar approach to that for pronator syndrome.

Stress fractures of the ulna

Ulnar stress injuries are relatively uncommon but are seen where there is repetitive elbow loading, such as in gymnasts, or loading during extreme contraction of the elbow flexors, such as in overhand throwers and volleyball players, and in lifting weights. Management is relative off-loading, analgesia. and attention to technique, training, and equipment factors.

Posterior elbow pain

Posterior elbow impingement

Posterior elbow impingement is seen particularly in those athletes where high-velocity extension of the elbow is occurring. Impingement may be due to posterior osteophytes, loose bodies, local synovitis, or capsular thickening. The patient points to the posterior elbow as the site of pain and symptoms are reproduced with forced extension. Plain X-rays may show local osteophytes, but MRI and CT are often necessary to assess the condition adequately. Where local synovitis is the only lesion, local injection of corticosteroid may resolve the condition, but in most cases surgery is necessary. Arthroscopic debridement of impingement lesions in the floor of the olecranon fossa, coupled with trimming of the tip of the olecranon, is usually effective. Arthroscopy also facilitates synovial debridement and removal of loose bodies.

Triceps tendinopathies

Triceps tendinopathies, which include tendinosis and rupture, are relatively rare but can occur in sports including throwing, cricket (bowlers), volleyball, and water polo.

Triceps tendinosis

Triceps tendinosis is an overuse injury associated with repetitive elbow extension, and can be associated with the presence of posterior osteophytes or loose bodies in the joint.

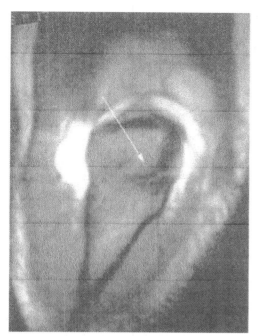

Fig. 3.6.16 MRI scan showing an olecranon stress fracture. Reproduced from Eygendaal. D. and Safran, M.R. (2006). Postero-medial elbow problems in the adult athlete. *British Journal of Sports Medicine*, **40**, 430–4, with permission from BMJ Publishing Ltd.

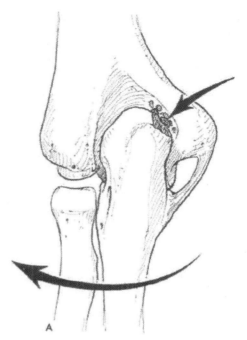

Fig. 3.6.17 Valgus extension overload causing posterior impingement. Reproduced from Eygendaal. D. and Safran, M.R. (2006). Postero-medial elbow problems in the adult athlete. *British Journal of Sports Medicine*, **40**, 430–4, with permission from BMJ Publishing Ltd.

Patients present with posterior elbow pain, which is worse with elbow extension. Examination reveals tenderness at or just proximal to the tendon insertion and pain on resisted elbow extension. X-rays may confirm associated bony pathology. Ultrasound is useful in confirming the diagnosis. MRI or CT may be necessary to evaluate the joint and surrounding structures more closely.

Management is similar to that of lateral epicondylitis and surgical intervention is almost never necessary, although resection of a small part of the triceps insertion has been advocated.

Triceps rupture

Rupture of the triceps occurs much less commonly than that of other tendons such as the long head of the biceps and the Achilles tendon. It typically occurs in men in the fourth and fifth decades. Right and left sides are equally affected, and there appears to be no relation to hand dominance.

The mechanism of injury is usually a fall onto the outstretched hand, with sudden stress upon a contracted triceps. Rarely, the injury may arise after a direct blow to the tendon. As is the case with other tendons, spontaneous rupture with minimal trauma may also occur, usually on the background of a diseased (though frequently asymptomatic) tendon.

Table 3.6.7 Differential diagnosis of posterior elbow pain

Triceps tendinopathies
Triceps avulsion
Traction apophysitis
Olecranon bursitis
C-spine radiculopathy
Fracture/stress fracture

Rupture is usually an avulsion injury of the tendon at the tendo-osseous junction. Rupture at the musculotendinous junction occurs more rarely. Partial ruptures, usually in the central third of the tendon, can also occur. Other injuries may occur simultaneously, including fracture of the radial head. Anabolic steroid use and underlying systemic diseases associated with tendinosis should also be considered. The patient usually describes a mechanism of a fall onto the outstretched hand, a direct blow, or, more rarely, a sudden tear or pop with minimal trauma. Pain, swelling, and weakness of elbow extension result.

Investigations

In the majority of cases lateral **plain X-rays** show flecks of avulsed bone proximal to the olecranon. An additional fracture of the head of the radius should be excluded. **Ultrasound** will confirm tendon rupture.

Management

Conservative management is reserved for the frail patient, in particular when there is a partial tear and some elbow extension is still possible. Otherwise, management is surgical. In the acute rupture, reattachment of the tendon is attempted. In the delayed presentation or in those with an underlying diseased tendon, reconstruction is considered. Results from surgery are reported to be good, with full restoration of strength and normal or near-normal range of motion, although most reports do not focus on the higher-level athlete.

Olecranon bursitis

Olecranon bursitis, which involves inflammatory change in the superficial olecranon bursa, is commonly seen in contact sports where trauma or microtrauma occurs. It is one of the most common sites of bursitis in the body. Bursitis may be acute or chronic, septic or aseptic. Septic bursitis can arise as a result of direct inoculation through local skin breaks that are often seemingly innocuous. Steroid injections precede infections in up to 10% of cases. The most common causative organism is *Staphylococcus aureus*, but group A β-haemolytic streptococci, other staphylococci, *Haemophilus influenzae*, *Pseudomonas*, and, in the immunocompromised patient, fungi, mycobacteria, or anaerobic bacteria may be involved. Bursitis in association with a crystal arthropathy should also be considered (Table 3.6.8).

History

The patient may give a history of direct trauma or repetitive microtrauma to the posterior aspect of the elbow. The initial insult (if identified) is followed by variable degrees of pain and swelling around the olecranon. Sepsis should always be considered.

Examination

There is discrete swelling at the posterior elbow, representing a thickened bursa and/or bursal fluid, or both. The overlying skin is inflamed in the acute and subacute cases and there may be skin breakage. Inclusion nodules, consisting of fibrous tissue formed after significant inflammation within the bursa, may be palpable. A local effusion of the elbow may occasionally be present. Those patients with a septic bursitis may be systemically unwell with a fever and cellulitis, and local lymphadenopathy may be noted. Signs of associated conditions and sepsis elsewhere should be sought.

Investigations

Inflammatory markers (erythrocyte sedimentation rate, C-reactive protein) and white cell count may be elevated in systemic sepsis and crystal-induced bursitis. Whenever there is suspicion of a septic bursitis, blood cultures and sterile aspiration of the bursal fluid with subsequent analysis by Gram stain and culture are essential. Bursal fluid can also be examined for crystals. X-rays are not performed routinely. Calcification and olecranon spurs may also be evident, although this may be coincidental.

Management

Most uncomplicated cases are managed symptomatically with regular ice, NSAIDs, and local protection by an elbow pad or dressing. In acute post-traumatic bursitis, sterile aspiration of blood is indicated to provide symptomatic relief and should be followed by compressive dressing, regular application of ice, and NSAIDs. Repeat aspiration may be necessary. Steroid injections have no role in the management of acute post-traumatic bursitis. Return to contact activities is permitted once the patient is asymptomatic, but a protective elbow pad should be worn initially.

Table 3.6.8 Causes of olecranon bursitis

Trauma (acute or chronic)
Sepsis
Metabolic/crystals
Inflammatory arthritis
Uraemia
Calcific deposits
Idiopathic

In those patients in whom sepsis is confirmed who are systemically well and with little cellulitis, aspiration of the bursa followed by oral broad-spectrum antibiotics is adequate. Intravenous antibiotics are commenced in those who fail to respond and in those with systemic symptoms. Open drainage and lavage may be necessary. Chronic recurrent symptomatic bursitis can be managed surgically, but is best left until the phase of acute infection and surrounding cellulitis has resolved. Surgery can involve simple debridement and excision of the bursal sac. The elbow is splinted in 45°–60° of flexion until the sutures are removed. Range of motion exercises are commenced early. Contact activities should be avoided for at least 6 weeks and an elbow pad worn for several months until all symptoms are settled. Individuals with a history of recurrent bursitis should be advised to wear elbow pads as a preventative measure.

References

Chard, M.D., Cawston, T.E., Riley, G.P., Gresham, G.A., and Hazleman, B.L. (1994). Rotator cuff degeneration and lateral epicondylitis: a comparative histological study. *Annals of the Rheumatic Diseases*, **53**, 30–4.

Childress, H.M. (1975). Recurrent ulnar-nerve dislocation at the elbow. *Clinical Orthopaedics and Related Research*, **108**, 168–73.

Dellon, A.L., Hament, W., and Gittelshon, A. (1993). Nonoperative management of cubital tunnel syndrome: an 8-year prospective study. *Neurology*, **43**, 1673–7.

Eygendaal, D., Rahussen, F.T., and Diercks, R.L. (2007). Biomechanics of the elbow joint in tennis players and relation to pathology. *British Journal of Sports Medicine*, **41**, 820–3.

Gilliatt, R.W. and Thomas, P.K. (1960). Changes in nerve conduction with ulnar nerve lesions at the elbow. *Journal of Neurology, Neurosurgery and Psychiatry*, **23**, 312–20.

Hay, E.M., Paterson, S.M., Lewis, M., Hosie, G., and Croft, P. (1999). Pragmatic randomised controlled trial of local corticosteroid injection and naproxen for treatment of lateral epicondylitis of elbow in primary care. *British Medical Journal*, **319**, 964–8.

Kojima, T., Kurihara, K., and Nagano, T. (1979). A study on operative findings and pathogenic factors in ulnar neuropathy at the elbow. *Handchirurgie*, **11**, 99–104.

McGowan, A.J. (1950). The results of transposition of the ulnar nerves for traumatic ulnar neuritis. *Journal of Bone and Joint Surgery. British Volume*, **32**, 293–301.

Nirschl, R.P. (1974). The etiology and treatment of tennis elbow. *Journal of Sports Medicine and Physical Fitness*, **2**, 308–23.

Priest, J.D. and Nagal, D.A. (1976). Tennis shoulder. *American Journal of Sports Medicine*, **4**, 28–42.

Priest, J.D., Braden, V., and Gerberich, S.G. (1980). The elbow and tennis. Part 1: An analysis of players with and without pain. *Physician and Sports Medicine*, **8**, 81–91.

Snyder-Mackler, L. and Epler, M. (1989). Effect of standard and Aircast tennis elbow bands on integrated electromyography of forearm extensor musculature proximal to the bands. *American Journal of Sports Medicine*, **17**, 278–81.

Struijs, P.A.A., Smidt, N., Arola, H., *et al.* (2001). *Orthotic devices for tennis elbow (Cochrane review). Cochrane Library*, Vol. 2. Update Software, Oxford.

Torp-Pedersen, T.E., Torp-Pedersen, S.T., Qvistgaard, E., and Bliddal, H. (2008). Effect of glucocorticosteroid injections in tennis elbow verified on colour Doppler ultrasound: evidence of inflammation. *British Journal of Sports Medicine*, **42**, 978–82.

Zeisig, E., Fahlström, M., Ohberg, L., and Alfredson, H. (2008). Pain relief after intratendinous injections in patients with tennis elbow: results of a randomised study. *British Journal of Sports Medicine*, **42**, 267–71.

3.7

Injuries to the thoracolumbar spine and thorax

Lyle Micheli and Laura Purcell

Introduction

It can be challenging to make a precise diagnosis in patients with pain in the spinal region and chest wall, not least because demonstrable pathology is not always present. Pain originating from the thoracic spine and the chest wall is relatively uncommon. However, low back pain is very common, both in the general population and in athletes.

Causes of pain in these anatomical regions are somewhat age specific. For instance, scoliosis and Scheuermann's kyphosis are spinal deformities that typically present in adolescents (Schnebel 2000; Singer 2007). Similarly, chest pain in older athletes is more likely to be of cardiac origin. Causes of low back pain in children and adolescents are very different than those in adults (Table 3.7.1) (Micheli and Wood 1995; Brown and Micheli 2001; Kraft 2002; Zetaruk 2007).

In order to make an accurate diagnosis, it is important to have a good working knowledge of the relevant anatomy, a familiarity with the presentation of common disorders in these areas, and a high index of suspicion for unusual causes of pain, particularly in younger athletes.

Epidemiology

Sport-related injuries are increasing over time. More and more people are participating in organized sports and at higher levels of competition, particularly in the younger age groups. Injuries to the trunk, including the chest/thorax, upper back, and lower back, account for only 6.8% of all injuries from all causes (Public Health Agency of Canada 2007; NEISS Statistics). Lower back injuries are much more common in adults than in children, accounting for 4.8% of injuries in adults aged 20–64 years compared with only 1.8% of injuries in children aged 10–14 years and 1.8% in children aged 15–19 years. Upper back injuries account for only 0.7% of all injuries (Public Health Agency of Canada 2007; NEISS Statistics).

Functional anatomy and mechanics

The spine consists of bones, joints, ligaments, and muscles. It is divided into five sections: cervical (seven vertebrae), thoracic (twelve vertebrae), lumbar (five vertebrae), sacral, and coccygeal. The thoracic spine is stabilized by the rib cage and therefore is less flexible. It normally has a kyphosis (concave towards the front), whereas the cervical and lumbar spines assume a lordotic curve (convex towards the front). The five main functions of the spine are (i) support of the head, (ii) support of the abdominal organs and pelvic girdle, (iii) point of attachment of the rib cage, (iv) protection of the spinal cord, and (v) transfer of weight and bending movements of the head and trunk to the pelvis (Schnebel 2000).

The thoracic vertebrae are intermediate in size between the smaller cervical vertebrae and the larger lumbar vertebrae. Each vertebra consists of an anterior body and a posterior arch enclosing the spinal canal. The spinal canal runs through the vertebral foramen. The body of the vertebra is joined to the arch by the pedicle. The posterior arch comprises the transverse processes, the laminae, and spinous process. The vertebrae are joined by joints between the bodies (discs) and the neural arches (facets). The area between the upper and lower facet joints is the pars interarticularis (Fig. 3.7.1).

The intervertebral discs are fibrocartilaginous structures located between the vertebral bodies. They comprise the annulus fibrosus (outer concentric layers of fibrous tissue) and a central springy pulpy zone called the nucleus pulposus (Fig. 3.7.2). The neural components within the spinal canal are the spinal cord from the occiput to L1, the conus medullaris (lower part of the cord) from T11 to L1, and the cauda equina from L1 to the sacrum. The vertebral bodies are connected by two major ligaments, the anterior longitudinal ligament and the posterior longitudinal ligament. Other ligaments are the ligamentum flavum, the interspinous ligaments, and the supraspinous ligaments.

Four groups of muscles act on the spine: (i) the anterior group (interspinal, intertransverse, and levatores costarum); (ii) the middle muscle group (semispinalis, multifidus, and rotators); (iii) the posterior muscle group (erector spinae, iliocostal thoracis, longissimus

Table 3.7.1 Causes of back pain in adolescents and adults

	Adolescents (%)	Adults (%)
Spondylolysis	47	5
Disc-related pain	11	48
Mechanical back pain	26	0
Muscular back pain	6	27
Arthritis/stenosis	0	10

Adapted from Micheli and Wood (1995) and Schnebel (2000).

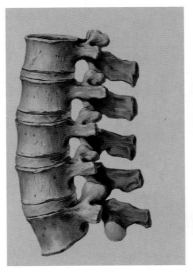

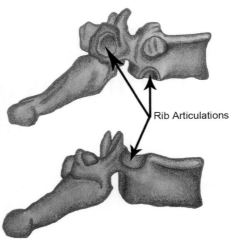

Rib Articulations

Thoracic Vertebrae

Fig. 3.7.1 Thoracic and lumbar vertebrae.

thoracis, and iliocostal lumborum); (iv) accessory muscle group (latissimus dorsi and trapezius).

The ribs are attached to the vertebral bodies and the transverse processes by various ligaments. The costal heads are attached to the intervertebral discs by intra-articular ligaments. The anterior aspects of the rib heads are united with the sides of the vertebral bodies above and below and with the intervening discs by the radiate (stellate) ligaments. The costotransverse joints between the facets on the transverse processes and on the tubercles of the ribs are surrounded by articular capsules and reinforced by costotransverse ligaments (Netter 1991).

Aetiology and pathophysiology

Thoracolumbar spine injuries are more commonly a result of overuse and repetitive microtrauma than acute trauma (Brown and Micheli 2001), particularly in younger athletes. Strenuous physical activity can cause structural abnormalities in the developing vertebrae, including endplate abnormalities (Scheuermann's disease), increased spinal curvatures (Scheuermann's, scoliosis, hyperlordosis), and stress fractures (spondylolysis/spondylolisthesis). Wojtys et al. (2000) showed that there is a significant increase in spinal curvature associated with increased cumulative training time in adolescent athletes (Wojtys et al. 2000). Long-term exposure to repetitive flexion, extension, axial rotation, and compression and shear forces

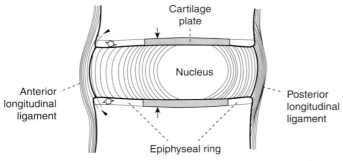

Cartilage plate

Nucleus

Anterior longitudinal ligament

Posterior longitudinal ligament

Epiphyseal ring

Fig. 3.7.2 Intervertebral disc.

through the spine of a growing athlete appears to correlate with altered spinal development (Wojtys et al. 2000; Wood 2002; Ashton-Miller 2004). Athletes participating in gymnastics, American football, hockey, swimming, and wrestling had larger curves than adolescents who participated in other sports or who were not physically active (Wojtys et al. 2000), and they have been shown to have a higher incidence of spinal injuries (Micheli and Wood 1995; D'Hemecourt et al. 2000; Brown and Micheli 2001; Watkins 2002; Wood 2002; Ashton-Miller 2004; Trainor and Trainor 2004; Singer 2007; Zetaruk 2007).

Causes of back pain in children and adolescents are very different from those in adults (Micheli and Wood 1995; Kraft 2002; Trainor and Trainor 2004). Back pain in children is more often a result of a structural problem such as spondylolysis (Micheli and Wood 1995; Kraft 2002), whereas in adults it is more likely to be disc related (Micheli and Wood 1995) (Table 3.7.1).

Conditioning also plays a role in thoracolumbar back injuries. Athletes who are poorly conditioned, particularly at the beginning of their season, as well as athletes who are growing and have lost flexibility in the hamstrings, hip, pelvic, and low back muscles are more prone to spinal injuries (Brown and Micheli 2001; Trainor and Trainor 2004). In addition, abrupt increases in training intensity or duration can precipitate back injuries (Trainor and Trainor 2004). Improper technique and poor equipment can also predispose athletes to injury (Trainor and Trainor 2004).

A high index of suspicion is necessary when athletes present with back or chest pain to avoid missing non-traumatic causes of pain such as infection, neoplasm, metabolic disorders, and cardiac or pulmonary causes.

Investigations

An extensive work-up is not necessary for most athletes presenting with thoracolumbar injuries. Plain films are the most common test ordered to assess possible bony injury. However, X-rays usually add very little to the clinical picture of thoracic back pain. X-rays may show traumatic fractures, endplate abnormalities consistent with Scheurmann's kyphosis, and possibly more sinister abnormalities (neoplasms, infection). For chest wall injuries, X-rays are the first choice to look for fractures as well as injuries to the thoracic organs (lungs, heart, great vessels). Chest X-rays will indicate cardiac size and silhouette, as well as lung abnormalities such as contusion, pneumothorax, or infection. Specific rib views may be necessary to assess rib fractures. In low back pain, X-rays may show congenital abnormalities such as spina bifida occulta, sacralization of lumbar vertebrae, or abnormalities of the sacroiliac joints (Fig. 3.7.3). X-rays of the lumbar spine are recommended to rule out traumatic fractures, spondylolisthesis, stress fracture, or more sinister conditions (neoplasm, infection) (Press 2007).

CT scan can provide more information about specific bone abnormalities, such as stress fractures, but does not give much information regarding other structures in the spine. CT may reveal injuries to the thoracic organs, particularly in cases of acute trauma. MRI can provide information regarding the soft tissues in the spine, including disc abnormalities. However, MRI may show a number of abnormalities that may be clinically insignificant and not contributory to a patient's pain (Press 2007). Bone scan may indicate bony pathology in the presence of negative plain films. Bone scan plus single-photon emission computed tomography (SPECT) is a sensitive test for stress fractures, such as in the ribs and of the pars interarticularis (spondylolysis). Bone scan can also detect infections and neoplasms.

Further investigation is required in patients with atypical pain patterns and in those not responding to conservative management. A higher degree of suspicion is required for children presenting with back pain, and investigations should be considered more frequently (Micheli and Wood 1995; D'Hemecourt *et al.* 2000; Brown and Micheli 2001; Kraft 2002; Zetaruk 2007). Blood tests should be obtained for any patient suspected to have an infectious, malignant, or inflammatory cause for their pain.

Specific conditions

Thoracic pain

Thoracic pain may result from both acute and chronic conditions. Acute injuries may result from trauma and include fractures and muscle strains or contusions. More chronic conditions include disc pathology. Spinal deformities, such as scoliosis and Scheuermann's kyphosis, may present in athletes, particularly in adolescents (Singer 2007).

Scheuermann's kyphosis

The most common cause of excessive kyphosis in adolescents is Scheuermann's disease. The normal curvature of the thoracic spine is approximately 25°–45° (Schnebel 2000). Curvatures greater than 45° are considered abnormal. The excessive kyphosis is thought to be caused by necrosis of the ring apophysis (growth centre of the vertebra). Repetitive trauma is thought to be the causative agent. Scheuermann's kyphosis is seen more often in sports with repetitive movement of the thoracic spine, such as weightlifting, swimming, gymnastics, wrestling, and rowing (D'Hemecourt *et al.* 2000; Schnebel 2000; Wood 2002).

Scheuermann's disease is diagnosed when the presence of abnormal kyphosis is associated with anterior wedging of three or more adjacent vertebrae on X-ray. Other abnormalities seen on X-ray include Schmorl's nodes and endplate irregularities (Fig. 3.7.4). These findings may occur in the thoracolumbar region with a compensatory lumbar hypolordosis. This is called atypical or lumbar Scheuermann's disease.

Most patients are asymptomatic, although some may report fatigue or pain. Cosmetic concern is usually the reason for patients to present for assessment. Clinically, patients present with a roundback deformity which does not correct with passive extension. There is a corresponding hyperlordosis of the lumbar spine and associated tight hip flexors, hamstrings, and lumbar fascia (Brown and Micheli 2001). Treatment consists of physiotherapy to work on postural exercises, as well as core strengthening and stretching of hamstrings, hip flexors, and lumbar fascia. There are no specific sport activity restrictions.

Progression of the deformity is unusual, although rare cases may require bracing (curves greater than 50°) or surgery (curves greater than 70°) (Zetaruk 2007; Brown and Micheli 2001; Hollingworth 1996).

Thoracic disc herniation and prolapse

Thoracic disc herniations are not very common; they represent about 1% of all symptomatic disc herniations (D'Hemecourt

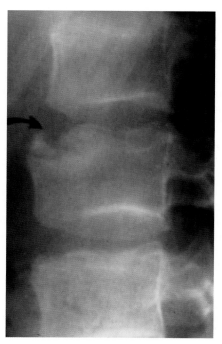

Fig. 3.7.4 Radiographic changes in Scheuermann's kyphosis include anterior wedging, endplate irregularities, and Schmorl's nodes.

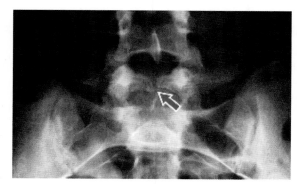

Fig. 3.7.3 Spina bifida occulta.

and Deede 2007). The larger discs of the lower thoracic vertebrae are most often affected. Clinical symptoms include local back pain with radicular pain in the chest or abdomen. However, pain may not be referred in a typical pattern (Singer 2007). Treatment is conservative, as long as there are no progressive neurological symptoms. Back extension strengthening is encouraged as tolerated. The athlete may return to sport when pain has resolved and strength and flexibility are restored (D'Hemecourt and Deede 2007).

Fractures

Typically, fractures are associated with high-energy trauma such as motor vehicle accidents (Brown and Micheli 2001; Trainor and Trainor 2004). Fractures can occur in contact sports such as football, hockey and rugby, although they are uncommon. Compression fractures of thoracic and lumbar vertebrae are associated with axial loading of the spine, usually when it is in flexion. Neurological complications occur less frequently than with cervical vertebral compression fractures. Symptoms include back pain in the area of the injury with or without paraesthesiae (D'Hemecourt *et al.* 2000; D'Hemecourt and Deede 2007). Any athlete suspected of having a vertebral fracture should be immobilized on a backboard and brought to an emergency department for assessment.

X-rays should be obtained for suspected fractures. If a thoracic compression fracture results in less than 25% loss of vertebral body height, it is considered a stable fracture. If a fracture results in 50% or greater loss of height, there is a greater likelihood of involvement of the posterior arch and a CT scan should be obtained. An MRI should be obtained if there are any neurological symptoms, no matter how transient (D'Hemecourt *et al.* 2000; D'Hemecourt and Deede 2007).

For minimal compression fractures with no involvement of the posterior arch, athletes may be treated conservatively with analgesics and activity modification until symptoms resolve (Brown and Micheli 2001). Occasionally, they may require immobilization in a thoracolumbosacral orthosis (TLSO) for 6–12 weeks until pain free (D'Hemecourt *et al.* 2000; Brown and Micheli 2001; D'Hemecourt and Deede 2007). Sport participation should be postponed until the athlete has become pain free and has regained full range of motion and strength. More severe compression fractures, especially if associated with instability and neurological symptoms, may require more prolonged immobilization or surgery. If internal fixation is required, contact sports are contraindicated (D'Hemecourt *et al.* 2000; Brown and Micheli 2001; D'Hemecourt and Deede 2007).

Muscle strain and contusion

Muscle strains and contusions are very common as a cause of acute-onset upper back pain. Initially they can be very debilitating, but most respond to conservative management with anti-inflammatories, massage, rest, and heat. As pain resolves, activity can be resumed. Muscle spasm can sometimes be a sign of underlying spinal injury. If the pain is not resolving or if the patient develops neurological symptoms, further evaluation should be pursued (D'Hemecourt and Deede 2007).

Scoliosis

Scoliosis is a lateral spinal curvature of greater than 10° (Fig. 3.7.5). The aetiology of the majority of scoliosis is unknown and therefore it is called idiopathic scoliosis. Idiopathic adolescent scoliosis occurs in 2–3% of the population and is particularly common in young female athletes. It typically presents between 10 years of age

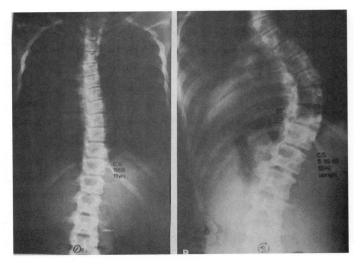

Fig. 3.7.5 Scoliosis is a lateral spinal curvature greater than 10°.

and skeletal maturity (D'Hemecourt and Deede 2007). Minor curves occur with equal frequency in boys and girls; more severe curves have a 4:1 female-to-male ratio. Scoliosis has been reported more frequently in sports such as dance, rhythmic gymnastics, swimming, and serving and throwing sports (D'Hemecourt *et al.* 2000; Wood 2002). Scoliosis typically does not cause pain or functional limitation. If a patient presents with painful scoliosis, a higher degree of suspicion for other entities, such as infection or tumour, must be entertained and appropriately investigated (Brown and Micheli 2001).

Treatment of scoliosis depends on a number of factors, including magnitude of curve at presentation, age, maturity, and Risser score. The Risser score refers to the maturation of the iliac crest apophysis on a plain film of the anteroposterior (AP) pelvis. The iliac crest apophysis matures laterally to medially. A Risser score of 1 indicates an immature ossification of the iliac crest, whereas a score of 5 reflects complete ossification of the iliac crest apophysis with fusion of the apophysis to the ileum (Fig. 3.7.6).

Curves less than 25° are observed with repeat X-rays every 4–6 months. Curves between 25° and 40°, particularly in immature athletes and those whose curves are progressing quickly, are treated with bracing, such as a Boston brace, for 16–23 hours per day. Curves greater than 40°–45° have a high risk of progression and surgery should be considered. There are no specific sport restrictions for scoliosis, although contact sports are contraindicated if instrumentation and fusion are necessary (Fig. 3.7.7) (D'Hemecourt *et al.* 2000; Wood 2002).

Lumbar

Low back pain is extremely common. Possible causes include muscle strain, discogenic pain, sacroiliac joint dysfunction, and stress fractures. Patterns of low back pain in children and adolescents are different from those in adults (Micheli and Wood 1995; Brown and Micheli 2001; Kraft 2002; Zetaruk 2007). A higher degree of suspicion is required in children presenting with back pain and investigations should be considered more often.

Spondylolysis

Spondylolysis is a defect in the pars interarticularis which is seen most often in the lumbar vertebrae. It is a stress fracture resulting

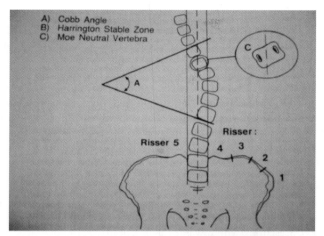

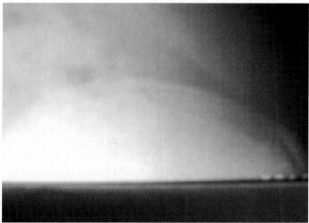

Fig. 3.7.6 The Risser score refers to the maturation of the iliac crest apophysis on a plain film of the AP pelvis.

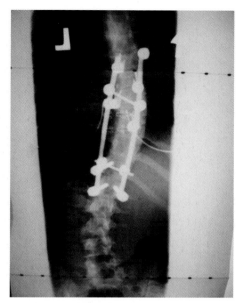

Fig. 3.7.7 Instrumentation and fusion for severe scoliotic curves typically result in restriction from contact sports.

from repetitive hyperextension of the spine. The prevalence of spondylolysis in the general population is 4–6%. The incidence may be much higher in the adolescent athletic population. In one study, almost half (47%) of athletes presenting with low back pain were found to have spondylolysis (Micheli and Wood 1995).

Sports involving repetitive back extension, such as diving, weightlifting, wrestling, gymnastics, high jump, dance, soccer, and American football linemen, are considered high risk and are associated with a higher incidence of spondylolysis (Hollingworth 1996; D'Hemecourt *et al.* 2000; Brown and Micheli 2001; Kraft 2002; McTimoney and Micheli 2003; Zetaruk 2007). Low back pain associated with spondylolysis is usually insidious in onset (Hollingworth 1996; Brown and Micheli 2001; McTimoney and Micheli 2003; Zetaruk 2007). Occasionally it can present following an acute traumatic event. The pain increases with sports activity. Pain is aggravated by hyperextension of the lumbar spine and can be reproduced on physical examination by having the patient hyperextend the spine. A single-leg hyperextension test may be positive. Neurological findings are usually absent.

Investigation should begin with plain radiographs (AP, lateral, ± obliques). Stress fractures may not be detectable on plain films, but they may indicate other abnormalities such as spina bifida occulta (associated with spondylolysis). The lateral view should be inspected for spondylolisthesis. The oblique view may show the

classic lesion of the 'neck of the Scotty dog'. However, there is a significant increase in the amount of radiation involved and therefore obliques are not routinely recommended (D'Hemecourt *et al.* 2000). Following X-rays, bone scan with SPECT is a sensitive test for diagnosing spondylolysis (Fig. 3.7.8). If this is negative, recent spondylolysis is safely ruled out. CT can give more specific information in terms of location of the defect, as well as the potential for the defect to heal. MRI has been studied as a potential adjunct in the diagnosis of spondylolysis, although it is still considered to be inferior to bone scan with SPECT (Campbell *et al.* 2001; McTimoney and Micheli 2003; Masci *et al.* 2006).

Management is conservative, with the aim of relieving pain and achieving healing. Resting from sport until pain free is essential. One retrospective study in adolescent soccer players with spondylolysis showed excellent results (i.e. pain-free return to sport) with a 3 month rest period from sport in more than 95% of cases (Rassi *et al.* 2005). There is some controversy regarding the type of treatment and the length of the rest period. Although not all practitioners recommend bracing, most will start patients in a brace to prevent hyperextension of the spine (D'Hemecourt *et al.* 2000; Brown and Micheli 2001; Kraft 2002; McTimoney and Micheli 2003; Zetaruk 2007). Bracing has been shown to alleviate pain and result in a faster pain-free return to sport (Rassi *et al.* 2005). The brace may be a Boston brace or lumbar corset. It should be worn for 23 hours a day until the patient is pain free. Once the patient is pain free in the brace, sport can be gradually resumed but contact and back extension are initially avoided. Once the patient has resumed full activity while in the brace and remains pain free, he/she can be weaned from it over about 2 months. Physiotherapy with the emphasis on core strengthening and hamstring flexibility is a key component of management (Hollingworth 1996; D'Hemecourt *et al.* 2000; Brown and Micheli 2001; Kraft 2002; Zetaruk 2007).

If patients continue to have pain following a bracing protocol, surgery may be considered. The procedure indicated is a posterolateral transverse process with bone graft. Following surgery, patients

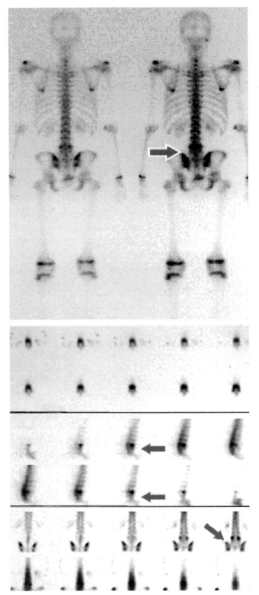

Fig. 3.7.8 A bone scan indicates spondylolysis as a hot spot in the pars interarticularis at L4/5

are immobilized in a brace for 6 months and are restricted from heavy activities for 12 months (D'Hemecourt *et al.* 2000; Brown and Micheli 2001).

Spondylolisthesis

Spondylolisthesis occurs when there is a bilateral pars interarticularis defect at the same level. It refers to slippage, in the sagittal plane, of the vertebral bodies with respect to each other and is graded in terms of severity according to the degree of slippage. Grade 1 slips are less than 25% translation, grade 2 slips are between 25–50% translation, grade 3 slips are 50–75% translation, grade 4 slips are 75–100% translation, and grade 5 slips are >100% translation (spondylotosis). Grades 1 and 2 are monitored with X-rays every 6–12 months until the patient finishes growing. More extensive slips, particularly if symptomatic, should be treated surgically

(McTimoney and Micheli 2003) (figure). Other surgical indications include documented progression of the slip, patients who have failed a 6–12 month course of conservative management, and neurological symptoms (D'Hemecourt *et al.* 2000; Brown and Micheli 2001; McTimoney and Micheli 2003).

For athletes with low-grade slips who are symptomatic, a short period of rest and bracing with a lumbar corset usually resolves their symptoms. Physiotherapy with an emphasis on core strengthening is encouraged. Return to sport in the brace is allowed once pain has resolved, and the brace is gradually weaned (D'Hemecourt *et al.* 2000; McTimoney and Micheli 2003).

Disc herniation and nerve root compression

Discogenic back pain is much more common in adults than in younger patients. One study showed that almost half (48%) of adults presenting with low back pain had disc pathology (Micheli and Wood 1995). In children and adolescents, disc herniation is seen in only about 10% of cases (Micheli and Wood 1995; Trainor and Trainor 2004).

Patients typically present with low back, buttock, or hip pain and radicular symptoms, although the classical radicular pattern may be absent in younger patients (Brown and Micheli 2001; Kraft 2002; Trainor and Trainor 2004; Zetaruk 2007). Patients may have hamstring tightness and antalgic gait. The classic physical examination finding is a positive straight leg raise, which may be absent in younger patients. In younger patients, investigations should be obtained, starting with plain films of the lumbar spine to rule out an osseous injury (Brown and Micheli 2001). If X-rays are negative, MRI should be performed to look for disc pathology, including degeneration or herniation (Brown and Micheli 2001; Watkins 2002; Trainor and Trainor 2004).

Treatment is usually conservative with physiotherapy, anti-inflammatory medication, and rest from sports activities. Prognosis is generally favourable; more than 90% of patients will improve in 4–6 weeks with conservative treatment (Lively and Bales 2005). If symptoms are not improving with conservative measures, MRI should be arranged to look for disc or spinal cord pathology. Once pain has resolved and patients have functionally recovered, they can return to sport.

Epidural injections may be considered in patients not responding to conservative measures (Brown and Micheli 2001; Trainor and Trainor 2004; Lively and Bales 2005). Surgery may be considered if patients fail conservative treatment or in the presence of cauda equina syndrome (D'Hemecourt *et al.* 2000; Brown and Micheli 2001; Watkins 2002; Lively and Bales 2005).

Mechanical low back pain

Mechanical low back pain is also referred to as hyperlordotic back pain (Micheli and Wood 1995) and posterior element overuse syndrome (Zetaruk 2007). This is the most common cause of back pain in athletes (Trainor and Trainor 2004). Mechanical low back pain may result from injury to any of the posterior elements of the spine, including muscle–tendon units, ligaments, joint capsules, and facet joints (Zetaruk 2007). Athletes present with pain related to sport activity, as with other causes of low back pain. On physical examination there is no bony tenderness. Pain may be aggravated with movement in all directions. There may be paraspinal muscle spasm in the lumbar area. Hip and neurological examinations are normal.

Treatment begins with a short period of rest with ice application and anti-inflammatories. Once acute pain has subsided, a trial of physiotherapy with an emphasis on core strengthening should be advised. Pain can be used as a guide when returning to sport. In younger patients, investigations should be considered in any patient with pain for more than 3 weeks (Micheli and Wood 1995; Brown and Micheli 2001; Kraft 2002; Zetaruk 2007).

Sacroiliac joint dysfunction

Low back pain may result from the sacroiliac (SI) joint. Symptoms usually develop insidiously and are aggravated by sports activities. Clinically, patients may present with very similar symptoms to spondylolysis (Kraft 2002; Zetaruk 2007). Patients may be tender to palpation over the affected SI joint with no other bony tenderness. Spine extension is typically more painful than flexion and there may be a positive single-leg hyperextension test. A FABER test (flexion, abduction, and external rotation of the hip) usually reproduces pain in the affected SI joint. A straight leg test is typically negative and there is no hip abnormality. Plain X-rays should be obtained and are usually normal. If there is any suspicion of a pars interarticularis injury, a bone scan with SPECT should be obtained.

Inflammation of the SI joint is associated with various conditions including ankylosing spondylitis, Crohn's disease, and psoriatic arthritis (HLA-B27 seronegative spondyloarthropathies), and infectious conditions such as Reiter's syndrome. If these conditions are suspected, serological screening should be performed, including ESR, CRP, RF, ANA, and HLA-B27 (Zetaruk 2007).

Treatment involves rest from sport, NSAIDs and a rehabilitation program with a physiotherapist. Once pain has resolved, a gradual return to sport is allowed. Occasionally, patients with SI joint pain may require bracing to allow return to sport.

Chest wall pain

Chest pain can result from both acute and chronic injuries. Any significant chest trauma is a medical emergency and may result in significant injuries to the thoracic organs (heart, lungs, great vessels) as well as musculoskeletal injuries, including rib fractures and contusions. Other causes of chest wall pain include sternoclavicular joint disorders, costochondritis, stress fractures of the ribs, and muscle strains. In older athletes, cardiac causes must be considered as a cause of chest pain.

Rib fracture/contusion

Direct trauma to the chest can cause rib injuries ranging from bruising to fractures. Ribs 4–9 are mostly commonly injured (Kerr et al. 2007). Pain is aggravated by deep inspiration or coughing. There will be localized tenderness over the affected rib(s). X-rays will confirm a rib fracture, as well as possible underlying injuries such as pneumothorax (Wong and Ho 2006). Specific rib views may be necessary as rib fractures may not be seen on routine radiographs (Kerr et al. 2007).

Treatment of bruised or fractured ribs is symptomatic. Analgesia is necessary as rib contusions and fractures are quite painful. Patients should be encouraged to do deep breathing exercises to prevent atelectasis (Kerr et al. 2007; Singer 2007). Athletes may return to sport once pain has resolved, typically 3 weeks from the time of injury. Protective padding is recommended for athletes participating in contact sports (Singer 2007).

Complications of rib fractures include pneumothorax and haemopneumothorax. Underlying structures such as the liver, spleen, and kidneys may also be injured as a result of rib trauma. A high index of suspicion should be maintained to rule out these potentially serious complications (Kerr et al. 2007).

Costochondritis

This condition results from inflammation at the joints between the sternum and the ribs and is seen commonly in children and adolescents (Kerr et al. 2007). Pain is activity related, and tenderness to palpation is localized to the costochondral junction. It may be preceded by exercise or upper respiratory tract infection (Kerr et al. 2007). Treatment is conservative with NSAIDs, ice, local physiotherapy, and mobilization of the costochondral joints (Kerr et al. 2007; Singer 2007). Recovery is usually spontaneous, with symptoms typically resolving in 9–12 weeks. In refractory cases, corticosteroid injection to the costochondral junction may help (Singer 2007).

Rib stress fracture

Stress fractures of the ribs are associated with particular sports such as baseball, golf, and rowing (Karlson 1998; Wong and Ho 2006; Singer 2007). The mechanism of injury is thought to be excessive muscle traction at the muscular attachments to the ribs (Karlson 1998; Singer 2007). In rowers, stress fractures of the anterolateral aspect of ribs 5–9 are thought to be due to excessive action of the serratus anterior muscle associated with long-distance training and heavy load per stroke (Karlson 1998; Singer 2007).

The typical history for a rib stress fracture is an insidious onset of pain in the posterior thorax at the spinal border of the scapula. Plain radiographs may initially be negative and diagnosis usually requires a bone scan (Kerr 2007). Treatment consists of relative rest for 4–6 weeks. Athletes may participate in light cardiovascular training while recuperating (Kerr et al. 2007). Rib stress fractures can be avoided by changes to technique and equipment (Karlson 1998).

Sternal fracture

Fracture of the sternum is relatively rare (Wong and Ho 2006). It requires a significant amount of force applied directly to the sternum as in a collision. Pain is localized to the sternum and is aggravated by inspiration and movement. There may be visible or palpable swelling over the sternum (Wong and Ho 2006).

A lateral X-ray of the sternum should demonstrate the fracture. CT may be necessary if the diagnosis is not clear on plain radiographs (Kerr et al. 2007). Blunt cardiac injury is a potential complication of a sternal fracture, as well as other intrathoracic injuries. If there are any arrhythmias, a screening ECG and cardiac troponin should be ordered (Wong and Ho 2006). Chest X-ray can exclude intrathoracic injury. Treatment is conservative and consists of rest and analgesics. Return to sport is allowed when pain resolves, usually in 6–12 weeks (Wong and Ho 2006).

Sternoclavicular joint disorders

Sternoclavicular joint (SCJ) dislocations are extremely uncommon. However, because of the vital structures in the area, such as the great vessels and other structures in the upper mediastinum, injuries to this joint are potentially quite serious and difficult to treat (Bicos and Nicholson 2003). SCJ injuries should be evaluated with CT to determine the extent and direction of SCJ displacement.

Although anterior SCJ dislocations have a tendency to remain unstable, they usually have little long-term functional impact and are generally treated conservatively (Bicos and Nicholson 2003; Singer 2007). Mild sprains are treated with ice and a brief period of immobilization with a sling. More severe sprains (subluxation) require a longer period of immobilization (3–6 weeks). Frank anterior SCJ dislocations can be treated with closed reduction. Surgical intervention is reserved for failure of conservative management or in those with significant cosmetic concerns (Bicos and Nicholson 2003).

Posterior dislocations of the SCJ have more potential for serious neurovascular injury to the vital structures in the mediastinum. Treatment typically requires a closed or open reduction, and once reduced they remain stable (Bicos and Nicholson 2003).

Other causes

More sinister causes of pain in the spinal and chest regions must always be considered in the differential diagnosis. Entities such as discitis, osteoid osteoma, aneurysmal bone cyst, and chondroblastoma must be considered and ruled out, particularly in younger patients.

A history of fever, weight loss, night pain, or malaise is suggestive of a malignant condition, whereas a recent viral or bacterial infection preceding onset of pain may indicate an infectious cause (D'Hemecourt *et al.* 2000; Brown and Micheli 2001; Trainor and Trainor 2004). If any of these red flag symptoms are present, further investigations, including serology, should be done to rule out these entities.

Pain in the low back region may be referred from other areas such as the hip, pelvis or viscera. Bowel pathology, renal disorders, or reproductive organ disease may present as low back pain and must be kept in mind in patients who have unusual symptoms or who are not responding to conservative management. Specialist referral may be required if these conditions are suspected (D'Hemecourt *et al.* 2000; Trainor and Trainor 2004).

References

Ashton-Miller, J.A. (2004). Thoracic hyperkyphosis in the young athlete: a review of the biomechanical issues. *Current Sports Medicine Reports*, **3**, 47–52.

Bicos, J. and Nicholson, G.P. (2003). Treatment and results of sternoclavicular joint injuries. *Clinics in Sports Medicine*, **22**, 359–70.

Brown, T.D. and Micheli, L.J. (2001). Spinal injuries in children's sports. In: N. Mafulli, K.M. Chan, R. Macdonald, R.M. Malina, and A.W. Parker (eds), *Sports Medicine for Specific Ages and Abilities*, pp. 31–44. Churchill Livingstone, London.

Campbell, R.S., Grainger, A.J., Hide, I.G., Papastefanou, S., and Greenough, C.G. (2005). Juvenile spondylolysis: a comparartive analysis of CT, SPECT and MRI. *Skeletal Radiology*, **34**, 63–73.

D'Hemecourt, P. and Deede, J.F. (2007). Cervical and thoracic spine injuries. In: L.J. Micheli and L.K. Purcell (eds), *The Adolescent Athlete: A Practical Approach*, pp. 80–108. Springer, New York.

D'Hemecourt, P.A., Gerbino, P.G., and Micheli, L.J. (2000). Back injuries in the young athlete. *Clinics in Sports Medicine*, **19**, 663–79.

Hollingworth, P. (1996). Back pain in children. *British Journal of Rheumatology*, **35**, 1022–8.

Karlson, K.A. (1998). Rib stress fractures in elite rowers. A case series and proposed mechanism. *American Journal of Sports medicine*, **26**, 516–19.

Kerr H, Curtis C and d'Hemecourt P. Thoracoabdominal injuries. In: L.J. Micheli and L.K. Purcell (eds), *The Adolescent Athlete: A Practical Approach*, pp. 141–64. Springer, New York.

Kraft, D.E. (2002). Low back pain in the adolescent athlete. *Pediatric Clinics of North America*, **49**, 643–53.

Lively, M.W. and Bailes, J.E. (2005). Acute lumbar disk injuries in active patients: making optimal management decisions. *Physician and Sportsmedicine*, **33**, 21.

McTimoney, C.A.M. and Micheli, L.J. (2003). Current evaluation and management of spondylolysis and spondylolisthesis. *Current Sports Medicine Reports*, **2**, 41–6.

Masci, L., Pike, J., Malara, F., Phillips, B., Bennell, K., and Brukner, P. (2006). Use of the one-legged hyperextension test and magnetic resonance imaging in the diagnosis of active spondylolysis. *British Journal of Sports Medicine*, **40**, 940–6.

Micheli, L.J. and Wood, R. (1995). Back pain in young athletes. *Archives of Pediatric and Adolescent Medicine*, **149**, 15–18.

NEISS stats

Netter, F.H. (1991). *The CIBA Collection of Medical Illustrations. Vol 8: Musculoskeletal System*, pp. 2–17. CIBA-Geigy, Toms River, NJ.

Press, J. (2007). Low back pain. In: P. Brukner and K. Khan (eds), *Clinical Sports Medicine* (3rd edn), pp. 352–80. McGraw-Hill, Sydney.

Public Health Agency of Canada (2007). Injury Surveillance Online. Canadian Hospitals Injury Reporting and Prevention (CHIRPP). Distribution of all body parts touched by the injury. Available online at: http://dsol-smed.phac-aspc.gc.ca/dsol-smed/is-sb/chirpp/Final%20BdyPrt.xls (accessed December 12, 2007).

Rassi, G.E., Takemitsu, M., Woratanarat, P., and Shah, S.A. (2005). Lumbar spondylolysis in pediatric and adolescent soccer players. *American Journal of Sports Medicine*, **33**, 1688–93.

Schnebel, B.E. (2000). Spine. In: J.A. Sullivan JA and S.J. Anderson SJ, (eds), *Care of the Young Athlete*, pp. 287–308. American Academy of Orthopaedic Surgeons, Rosemont, IL, and American Academy of Pediatrics, Elk Grove Village, IL.

Singer, K. (2007). Thoracic and chest pain. In: P. Brukner and K. Khan (eds), *Clinical Sports Medicine* (3rd edn), pp. 340–51. McGraw-Hill, Sydney.

Trainor, T.J. and Trainor, M.A. Etiology of low back pain in athletes. *Current Sports Medicine Reports*, **3**, 41–6.

Watkins, R.G. (2002). Lumbar disc injury in the athlete. *Clinics in Sports Medicine* 2002, 21, 147–165.

Wojtys, E.M., Ashton-Miller, J.A., Huston, L.J., and Moga, P.J. (2000). The association between athletic training time and the sagittal curvature of the immature spine. *American Journal of Sports Medicine*, **28**, 490–8.

Wong, T.W. and Ho, H.F. (2006). Thorax, abdomen and genitalia injuries. In: K.M. Chan, L. Micheli, A. Smith, *et al.* (eds), *FIMS Team Physician Manual* (2nd edn), pp. 500–31. CD Concept, Hong Kong.

Wood, K.B. (2002) Spinal deformity in the adolescent athlete. *Clinics in Sports Medicine*, **21**, 77–92.

Zetaruk, M. (2007). Lumbar spine injuries. In: L.J. Micheli and L.K. Purcell (eds), *The Adolescent Athlete: A Practical Approach*, pp. 109–40. Springer, New York.

3.8

Injuries to the pelvis, hip, and thigh

Cathy Speed, Jae Rhee, and Fares Haddad

Introduction and epidemiology

Injuries to the musculoskeletal pelvis and thigh in sport are extremely common. Injury can occur at one or multiple sites of the bony pelvic ring, and in the soft tissues of the groin, abdominal wall, and thigh. Athletes in certain sports are particularly prone to hip injury, especially those involved in running, soccer, hockey, rugby, and dancing. Although recognized as a common region of injury, the true epidemiology is not known, as the spectrum of injury is wide, diagnosis can be complex, and injury classification is still debated in some conditions. Nevertheless, soft tissue injury and dysfunction are the most common forms of injury seen and, indeed, hamstring injury is the most frequent injury in a number of sports, including athletics, soccer, rugby union, and Australian Football League. Hamstring injuries are also the most common recurrent injury in sport.

Pelvic pain arising from the groin, pelvis, and hip has a very wide differential diagnosis, crossing many clinical specialist boundaries (Table 3.8.1). However, other potential causes of groin, pelvic, and even thigh pain include disorders of abdominal and pelvic organs, referred pain from the spine, and neurological complaints. Symptoms can be non-specific and diffuse and may have unusual patterns of referral. Therefore it is not surprising that making a diagnosis can be challenging and a thorough and methodical approach is vital.

The pelvis acts as an important junction in transfer and augmentation of forces between the upper limb and spine and the lower limb. Approximately 2.5% of all sports-related injuries are in the pelvic region (Estanwik *et al.* 1990) and, as mentioned earlier, pelvic injuries are more prevalent in certain types of sport. These include track and field disciplines, ice hockey, fencing, handball, speed skating, cross-country skiing, and football. Hip and groin injuries can account for as much as 7% of all football injuries (Westlin 1997), and more recent reviews have estimated the incidence of hip/groin injury to be 10–18% per 100 football players per year (Ekstrand and Hilding 1999). An incidence rate of 11.5% has been reported for hip injuries in distance runners (Boyens *et al.* 1989), with a strong correlation between the running distance per week and the risk of developing such injuries.

Adductor strains are extremely common, especially in males. For example, they represent 10% of injuries encountered in ice hockey. Groin injuries and hamstring strains are, with anterior cruciate ligament injuries, the most frequent injuries in Australian Football League (Orchard and Seward 2002)

Injuries to the region of the pelvis and thigh can result in significant morbidity, especially with the potential chronicity of such injuries. Although developing improved treatment methods for injuries remains an important goal, prevention and the identification of risk factors have become focal points for current researchers and practitioners. Intrinsic and extrinsic risk factors predisposing to lower limb injuries have been identified, including those around the pelvis (Murphy *et al.* 2003). Intrinsic factors, including increased age, female sex, previous injury, inadequate rehabilitation, and extremes of BMI, have been reported to play some role in increasing tendency for injury, while extrinsic factors include the skill level, the competitive nature of the sport, and the type of playing turf.

The general consensus is that injury risk is greater when participating in competition, playing on artificial playing surfaces, and having had a previous injury at that site, particularly when inadequately rehabilitated.

Functional anatomy

The pelvis serves as a midpoint for the axial and rotary forces that are transmitted through the lumbosacral–pelvis–hip unit. Anatomical features in all parts of this unit are relevant in considering pelvic and thigh injuries in sport (Fig. 3.8.1).

The **hip joint** is a multi-axial ball-and-socket joint—an articulation between the acetabulum and femoral head. The acetabular cavity is formed superiorly by the ileum, anteriorly by the pubis, and posteroinferiorly by the ischium. Stability of the hip joint is afforded by a multitude of factors. The bony acetabulum, which is deepened by the fibrocartilaginous labrum and the transverse acetabular ligament, creates a unique degree of internal stability. Secondly, the fibrous capsule is a strong envelope, adding to the stability of this mobile joint. It attaches proximally to the acetabular rim and distally to the anterior intertrochanteric line and proximal to the intertrochanteric line posteriorly. The Y-shaped iliofemoral ligament reinforces the fibrous capsule anteriorly. The inferior and anterior aspect of the fibrous capsule is reinforced by the pubofemoral ligament. Posteriorly, the ischiofemoral ligament creates stability for the joint.

Table 3.8.1 Differential diagnosis of pain in the hip, groin or thigh

Musculoskeletal causes

Musculotendinous

  Adductor(s): muscle injury, tendinopathy

  Psoas muscle and tendon, snapping psoas, bursitis,

  Trochanteric 'bursitis'

  Hamstrings

Articular

  Pubic symphysis: osteitis pubis, instability

  Hip: arthritides, labral tears, loose bodies, subluxation, 'irritable hip'

  Lumbar spine: 'mechanical' back pain, facet joint dysfunction/arthropathy, spondylolysis, intervertebral disc injury

  Sacroiliac joint: sacroiliitis, instability/dysfunction

Neurological

Nerve entrapment: obturator, ilio-inguinal, lateral cutaneous nerve of the thigh

Abdominal/urological causes

Hernia: clinical (inguinal, femoral), subclinical, and 'sports hernia'

Intrapelvic genitourinary (including testicular) and gastrointestinal disorders

Gynaecological causes

Ovarian, uterine

The muscles play an important role in joint stability. In addition to having powerful action on the hip, they have an inherent role in adding to the stability of the joint.

The motion in the hip joint is in three planes: sagittal, frontal, and transverse, with the greatest motion in the sagittal plane. The normal hip is capable of up to 120° of flexion with the knee in flexion, but only 90° with the knee extended. Hip flexion is largely controlled by iliopsoas and rectus femoris, with smaller contributions from the sartorius, tensor fascia lata, pectineus, adductors, and gracilis. Abduction is normally up to about 45°, contributed by

the action of the tensor fascia lata, gluteus medius, and gluteus minimus. The gluteus maximus has a prime role in hip extension, together with the actions of the hamstrings (semitendinosus, semimembranosus, biceps femoris, and hamstring portion of adductor magnus). The adductors are a powerful group of muscles. Adduction is possible up to 30°, and in addition to the adductor group, the gracilis and pectineus have a small contributory role. Internal rotation (40°) is produced by the gluteus medius and minimus and the tensor fascia lata; external rotation (45°) is produced by the short external rotators (gemelli, piriformis, and obturators), assisted by gluteus maximus. There is considerable variation in range of motion between sports, with dancers and gymnasts generally having greatest mobility.

In the extended position, the hip joint locks. The functional advantage is that the joint can remain in extension (in an upright position) without the need for muscle contraction. In an upright position, the body's centre of mass falls behind the hip joint. Gravity shifts the hip posteriorly into extension, and thus the fibrous capsule (with its spiralling fibres) draws the femoral head into the acetabulum. The iliofemoral ligament also tightens and subsequently screws the femoral head into acetabulum with extension. The ischiofemoral ligament acts similarly to the iliofemoral ligament, but has a much weaker effect. As a result, the head of the femur and the acetabulum are tightly engaged, preventing dislocation and hyperextension of the hip joint (i.e. limiting the femur moving past vertical position). This is an important function in hip stability.

Considerable forces pass through the hip joint, both at rest and on weight-bearing, much of which must be dissipated through the muscular structures surrounding it. For example a third of the body weight passes through the hip when standing on two legs, 2.5 times body weight when standing on one leg, three times body weight when walking up stairs, and 4.5 times body weight when running.

The pubic symphysis is a mobile hyaline cartilaginous joint, joined by thick fibrous bands. The joint is fibrous and allows some movement in a vertical plane. Its nerve supply is from the genitofemoral and pudendal nerves (L1–2 and also S2–4).

The pelvis is joined to the sacrum of the spinal column via the sacroiliac joints. Each sacroiliac joint is fibrocartilaginous in its upper third and is a synovial joint in the distal two-thirds. It is supported by very thick intra-articular ligaments which are extremely important in the stability of the joint. The surfaces of the joint are highly irregular and reduce the scope for movement, but some rotation is possible and laxity is inevitably greater in females.

The muscles arising from the pelvis move the hip and knee joints and support the spinal column. When the anatomy of the abdominal wall is considered, it is understandable that pain in the pelvic region can arise from abdominal muscle pathology. Anteriorly, the abdominal wall has three layers of muscle: from interior to exterior, the transversus, internal oblique, and external oblique. On either side of the midline there is also the rectus abdominis, arising from the symphysis and pubic crest to insert into the fifth to seventh costal cartilages and xiphoid. The external oblique arises from the lower eight ribs and fans to insert into the xiphoid, pubic tubercle, and anterior half of the iliac crest. Internal oblique fibres run at right angles to the external oblique, arising with the transversus from the lumbar fascia, the inguinal ligament, and anterior iliac crest, to insert into the lower three ribs, xiphoid, and symphysis.

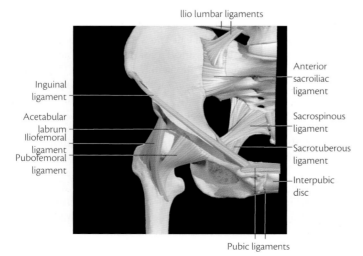

Fig. 3.8.1 Bony anatomy of the pelvis and hip.

lying centrally (Fig. 3.8.2 and Table 3.8.2). These muscles, the deep abdominal wall muscles and several shorter muscles help to control lumbopelvic stability. Muscle actions at the pelvis and hip are described in Table 3.8.3.

The anterior compartment of the thigh

The muscles of the anterior compartment are the sartorius, iliacus, psoas (iliopsoas), pectineus, and quadriceps (Figs 3.8.4 and 3.8.5). The **psoas** muscle arises from the transverse processes of L1–5 and passes across the pelvis where it is joined by the **iliacus**, which arises from the inner blade of the ileum. The **iliopsoas** then passes over the hip joint, to insert into the lesser trochanter of the femur. The function of the iliopsoas is to flex and internally rotate the leg when the hip is extended. When the hip is flexed, the psoas produces external rotation. The tendon of psoas flattens as it crosses the hip joint, separated from the hip joint by the psoas bursa.

The **rectus femoris** and the three **vasti** muscles (**vastus medialis, vastus lateralis**, and **vastus intermedius**) are the four muscles which form the **quadriceps** group, which are powerful extensors of the knee. The vasti arise from the femur. The rectus femoris has two heads of origin and crosses two joints (hip and knee). The straight (direct) head arises from the inferior superior iliac spine, and the reflected (indirect) head from the floor of the groove above the acetabulum. The fibres of the rectus femoris blend with those of vastus intermedius to insert onto the superior pole of the patella. The vastus medialis is composed of two portions, the vastus medialis obliquus (VMO) and the vastus medialis longus. Fibres of the VMO are at an angle of 30°–45° from the long axis of the quadriceps group and prevent lateral subluxation of the patella. The vastus medialis and lateralis insert onto the medial and lateral aspects of the patella respectively and strengthen the capsule of the knee joint. Collectively, these tendons represent the quadriceps tendon, which encloses the patella as a sesamoid bone before inserting into the tibial tuberosity via the patella tendon. Expansions of the insertion are bound to the capsule and the medial collateral ligament of the knee.

The **sartorius**, like the rectus femoris, crosses both the hip and the knee. It arises from the anterior superior iliac spine (ASIS) and inserts onto the medial tibia, forming part of the **pes anserinus** (goose foot). The **pectineus** arises from the pubis and inserts onto the pectineal line of the femur.

The medial compartment of the thigh

The medial compartment consists of the **adductors**, **gracilis**, and **obturator externus**. The adductor muscles (adductors magnus, longus, and brevis) and gracilis (another two-joint muscle) arise from the pubic symphysis and rami to insert along the medial border of the femur, with the gracilis forming part of the pes anserinus inserting onto the tibia. They produce hip adduction and, together

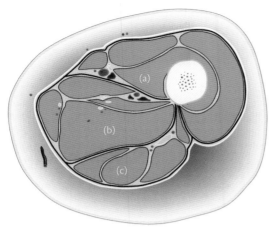

Fig. 3.8.2 Compartments of the thigh: (a) anterior; (b) medial; (c) posterior.

Transversus fibres also arise from the lower six costal cartilages and run horizontally forward to join the internal oblique to form a conjoint tendon which attaches to the inguinal ligament. The inguinal ligament is attached to the fascia lata of the thigh. There are two defects in the muscle layers in the inguinal region, the internal and external rings, which allow the passage of the ilio-inguinal nerve and, in males, structures of the spermatic cord (in females, the round ligament of the uterus is found here). This is a potential area of weakness in males, where inguinal hernias can occur.

Movement between the spine and pelvis occurs with the help of the abdominal muscles. When the pelvis is fixed, the spine moves through actions of the rectus abdominis and the obliques. The obliques laterally flex and rotate the trunk. The rectus abdominis flexes the trunk and stabilizes the pelvis.

Muscles of the gluteal region and the thigh work across the hip to flex, extend, abduct, adduct, and rotate the leg. The thigh is composed of three compartments—anterior, posterior, and lateral—separated by intermuscular septae and with the femur

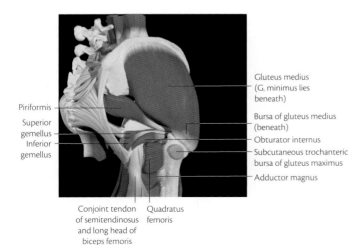

Fig. 3.8.3 The deep gluteal region: lateral view.

Table 3.8.2 Muscles of the gluteal region and thigh

Region	Muscles
Gluteal	Gluteals, piriformis, obturator internus, gemelli, quadratus femoris
Anterior thigh	Quadriceps, sartorius, pectineus, rectus femoris, iliopsoas
Medial thigh	Adductors, obturator internus, gracilis
Posterior thigh	Biceps femoris, semimembranosus, semitendinosus

Table 3.8.3 Muscle actions at the hip

Movement	Muscles		
Hip flexion	Strong: iliopsoas, rectus femoris		
	Weak: adductor longus, gracilis sartorius, pectineus	Hip extension	
	Strong: gluteus maximus, adductor magnus (ischial portion)	Weak: hamstrings, gluteus medius, piriformis	
Hip external rotation (hip and knee flexed)	Gluteus maximus and medius, obturators, quadratus femoris, gemelli, sartorius		
Hip internal rotation	Adductors, gluteus medius and minimus, tensor fasciae lata, pectineus, gracilis		
Hip adduction	Adductors		
Hip abduction	Gluteus medius, gluteus minimus, tensor fasciae latae		
Knee extension	Quadriceps		
Knee flexion	Hamstrings		
Motion of the pelvis at the hip	Anterior pelvic tilt	Hip flexors, trunk extensors	
	Posterior pelvic tilt	Hip extensors, trunk flexors (rectus, obliques)	
	Lateral pelvic tilt	Contralateral hip abductors	

with the sartorius and tensor fascia lata, provide important control of the leg on the pelvis, which has been likened to three guide ropes.

The posterior compartment of the thigh

The **hamstring muscles** consist of the **semimembranosus**, **semitendinosus**, and **biceps femoris** and the **hamstrings portion of the adductor magnus** (Fig. 3.8.6). They share a common origin on the ischial tuberosity, although the semimembranosus can arise as a separate slip in some individuals. The biceps femoris also has a short head, arising from the linea aspera of the femur. The two heads of the biceps femoris form a common tendon, inserting onto the head of the fibula, while the semimembranosus and semitendinosus insert onto the proximal medial tibia, with the latter contributing

to the pes anserinus. The sciatic nerve runs vertically through the hamstring compartment.

The **piriformis** arises from the middle three sacral vertebrae, and extends medially between the anterior sacral foramina so that the sacral nerves and plexus lie upon the muscle. The superior gluteal nerve (L4, 5) and vessels pass over the piriformis and the sciatic nerve lies deep to the muscle, though it may pass through it. Piriformis passes laterally through the greater sciatic notch and crosses the buttock, behind the hip joint, to the apex of the greater trochanter. The muscle acts as a stabilizer of the joint, abducts the flexed thigh, and laterally rotates the extended thigh.

The **iliotibial band** (**tract**) (ITB) represents the most lateral component of the thigh and is external to the three compartments. It is composed of thickened fascia, connecting the ilium with the lateral tibia, and arises from the gluteus maximus and the **tensor**

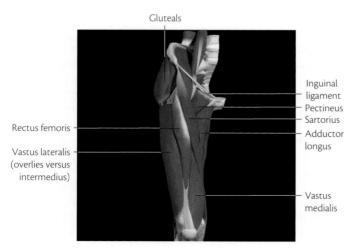

Fig. 3.8.4 The anterior thigh.

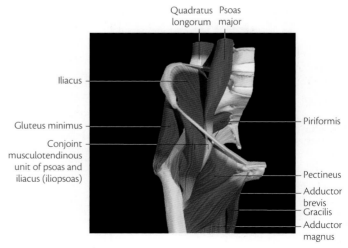

Fig. 3.8.5 Some important muscles of the pelvis and medial thigh.

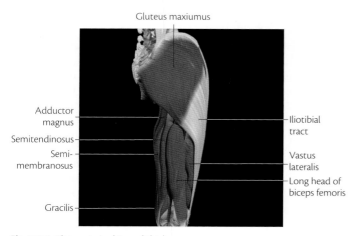

Fig. 3.8.6 The posterior hip and thigh.

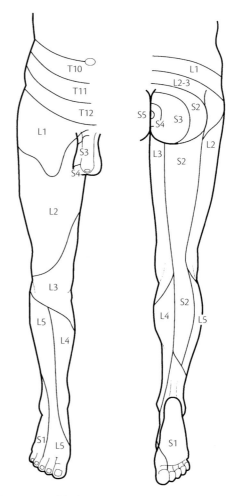

Fig. 3.8.7 Dermatomes of the leg.

fascia lata (TFL), which originates from the anterior iliac crest and lies over the gluteus maximus. The deep fascia of the TFL runs over the greater trochanter of the femur, separated by a bursa which, in thin individuals, is quite superficial. During hip flexion the TFL pulls the ITB forward, while during extension it is pulled backward by the gluteus maximus. The function of the TFL is to brace the iliotibial tract and to abduct and medially rotate the thigh. The ITB has a stabilizing influence on the knee in flexion and extension. Often when standing upright the upward pull of the ITB is the most important factor keeping the knee extended; the quadriceps may be relaxed.

Nerve supply

The pelvis, hip, and thigh are supplied by the lumbosacral plexus via the femoral, obturator, and sciatic nerves. The hip joint itself and its capsule receive sensory innervation from the femoral, obturator, superior gluteal, and sciatic nerves.

The **femoral nerve** (L2–L4) forms behind the psoas, runs down under the inguinal ligament in the femoral canal, and divides into a number of cutaneous and motor branches in the femoral triangle. The nerve supplies the quadriceps and pectineus muscles of the anterior thigh. Skin supplied exclusively by the femoral nerve includes the front and medial side of the thigh and, via the saphenous nerve branch, an area over the medial aspect of the lower leg.

The **sciatic nerve** (L4–S3) emerges from the pelvis through the greater sciatic foramen deep to the piriformis, and then curves around midway between the greater trochanter of the femur and the ischial tuberosity under gluteus maximus. Behind the hip joint, it supplies the long head of biceps femoris and, running over the adductor magnus, supplies the hamstring muscles. In the proximal thigh it divides into the common peroneal and tibial nerves, to supply the hip flexors and muscles of the lower leg. It also provides sensory supply along the posterior thigh.

The **superior gluteal nerve** (L4–5) supplies the gluteus medius and minimus and the TFL. The **inferior gluteal nerve** (L5–S1) supplies the gluteus maximus.

The **obturator nerve** (L2–4) is formed in the psoas muscle and descends within the muscle emerging from the medial border at the brim of the pelvis. The obturator nerve divides in the obturator

notch into the anterior and posterior divisions in the obturator foramen. The anterior division supplies the hip joint and the adductor longus, brevis, and gracilis, with a sensory branch to the medial thigh. The posterior division supplies the obturator internus and adductor magnus. The nerve supplies an area of skin along the middle of the medial thigh.

The **ilio-hypogastric nerve** (L1) pierces the transversus abdominis near the iliac crest and dives into anterior and lateral cutaneous branches. Both pierce the oblique muscles and supply the skin over the inguinal canal.

The **ilio-inguinal nerve** (L1) pierces the transversus abdominis above the anterior part of the iliac crest. It passes through the internal oblique muscle and into the inguinal canal. The nerve leaves the canal through the superficial ring and supplies an area of skin over the medial thigh, and in the male the scrotum and the root of the penis. The **genito-femoral nerve** (L1–2) also supplies part of the scrotal skin and the femoral triangle. The genital branch passes though the pelvis to emerge into the internal ring and pass along the inguinal canal. The femoral branch passes through the femoral sheath lateral to the femoral artery.

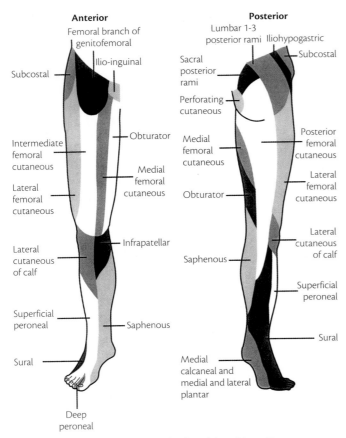

Fig. 3.8.8 Peripheral nerve supply to the skin of the pelvis and leg.

The rectus abdominis is supplied by T7–12. The obliques and transversus are supplied by the lower six thoracic nerves and the ilio-hypogastric and ilio-inguinal nerves.

Vascular supply

Vascular supply to the pelvis is through the internal and external iliac arteries and collateral circulation from the inferior aorta. The hip joint is primarily supplied by the femoral artery and its circumflex branches, with contributions from the artery of ligamentum teres, a branch of the obturator artery. The femoral artery gives rise to the profundus artery to supply the thigh.

Clinical evaluation

History

Symptoms relating to some hip, thigh, and groin injuries can be poorly localized, overlapping, and non-specific. Nevertheless, obtaining a very detailed history of the complaint is imperative in reaching an accurate diagnosis and devising appropriate management strategies.

The age of the patient will indicate different pathology possibilities; younger athletes are more likely to have apophyseal injuries, whereas muscle strains and degenerative intra-articular pathology are more likely in skeletally mature active adults.

Patients may present with an acute injury or, more commonly, with chronic symptoms. Frequently encountered symptoms include clicking, clunking, catching, a feeling of instability,

restriction, limping, and falls. However, the cardinal symptom, as with any soft tissue complaint, is pain. A thorough pain history should be obtained, starting with its nature, principal site(s) and radiation, and provoking and relieving factors. The mechanism of onset of the symptoms should be determined and may include trauma (e.g. a direct blow or twisting injury) or may be related to overuse. A full activity history should also be obtained, including changes in the nature and intensity of activities preceding the onset. The timing of the symptoms and whether they are progressing or improving is also important.

Pain in the groin itself is representative of hip joint pathology, referred pain from the lumbar spine or sacroiliac joints, and pain from localized disorders. Pain from hernias and sports-related abdominal wall syndromes can radiate to the scrotum. Articular pain from the hip can radiate to the thigh, knee, and back. Lumbar and sacroiliac pain can also radiate to the buttock, and typical sciatica can occur with a prolapsed disc or with piriformis syndrome. Exacerbating and relieving factors are noted. Pain worsened with coughing and straining is suggestive of hernias or spinal pathology. Specific movements may aggravate the condition through the range of motion required or due to impact.

The timing of the pain may be relevant. Early morning pain with stiffness that is worse with rest and lessened with activity is suggestive of an inflammatory process. Night pain may be reported. Pain may be localized and alter with sleeping position; for example, the lateral 'hip' pain of gluteal tendinopathy/trochanteric bursitis is worse when lying on the affected side. Most conditions can cause pain on turning over in bed. Pain that is constant through the night regardless of position should raise the suspicion of articular pathology or serious underlying disease, including infection or malignancy. The presence of constitutional symptoms must be directly addressed as a priority.

A history of clicking or clunking when the hip is moved may be due to hip joint pathology, snapping hip syndrome, or a snapping trochanteric bursa. Hypermobile individuals with poor muscular control of the hip girdle also commonly report non-specific clunking.

Neurological symptoms, such as tingling, burning, numbness, and weakness, may indicate a peripheral nerve entrapment and the distribution of such symptoms should be ascertained. For example, obturator nerve entrapment can cause pain in the region of the adductor muscles, and sciatic pain may be induced by entrapment in the pelvis or buttock from an abnormal piriformis or hamstring muscle.

The mode of onset of symptoms is a good indicator of the nature of the injury. Athletes usually remember the first occurrence of symptoms, and the sudden onset of pain that they experienced. Even if they forget the very first onset, the physician must not overlook the possibility of a history of a true traumatic cause. On the other hand, a gradual onset of problems may indicate underlying overuse tendon pathology (e.g. tendonitis), degenerative arthritis, or other differentials for hip pain (e.g. nerve entrapment, hernia, or referred lumbar pain). Patients often recollect the mechanism of injury. This can provide the physician with insight as to the possible injuries the athlete may have suffered.

The location and type of pain must be elicited from the patient. A sharp catching sensation with a history of locking or giving way indicates an underlying mechanical problem such as labral pathology. Localized pain produced with certain movements of the hip can indicate a correlation with a specific muscle–tendon unit or forms of impingement, whereas generalized vague and diffuse symptoms are more likely to be caused by fractures, arthropathy, abdominal wall abnormalities, or referred pain. The latter can implicate a pathology arising from the back, abdominal wall, or inguinal region. Radiation of pain may be a sign of nerve entrapment or any hip pathology that radiates to the knee.

It is important to ask about other associated symptoms. Genitourinary and abdominal symptoms may indicate that the pathology is located in one of these areas instead of the hip. Systemic symptoms such as weight loss, fever, and sweats indicate the possibility of a systemic inflammatory process. A past history of hip trauma or childhood histories of hip problem, such as transient synovitis, slipped capital femoral epiphyses, or Legg–Calvé–Perthes disease, will explain certain predisposition for mechanical hip impingement pathologies. Previous surgery, including past appendicectomy or inguinal hernia repair, can also predispose patients to develop nerve entrapments that will present as hip pain.

Examination

Physical examination should be done in a stepwise systematic way. It should be performed in conjunction with examination of the rest of the lower limb, including the spine. This chapter covers the details of hip examination and the specific tests necessary to elicit signs to aid in diagnosis.

Lumbopelvic muscle function and control can be assessed during simple functional movements such as single-leg dips or lunges. The assessor focuses on (a) the athlete's ability to maintain a neutral lumbar spine (recruitment of the transverse abdominals and gluteals), (b) the ability for the spine to remain upright (good strength in the abdominal, oblique, and spine extensor muscles), and (c) lack of sway of the pelvis (gluteal recruitment) with the front knee remaining aligned with the hip and the foot (recruitment of the gluteus medius and adductor muscles in addition to sufficient flexibility of the ITB and good stability in the front ankle).

Further assessment can include evaluation of the ability to maintain a prone bridge, a lateral bridge, supported back extension, and trunk flexion (Fig. 3.8.9 and Table 3.8.4).

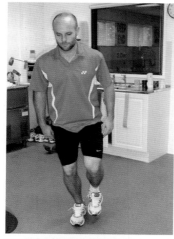

(a)

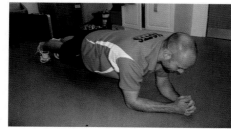

(b)

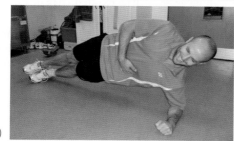

(c)

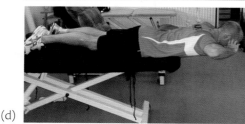

(d)

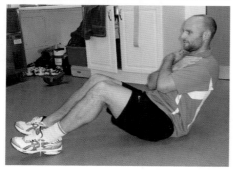

(e)

Fig. 3.8.9 Simple tests of 'core' strength and endurance (a) Single-leg dip. (b) Prone bridge in neutral spine position. Failure occurs when the patient moves into lumbar lordosis with anterior rotation of pelvis. (c) Lateral bridge. Failure occurs with movement of hip from neutral towards the mat. (d) Spinal extension test. (e) Flexion endurance test.

Table 3.8.4 Assessment of core strength and endurance. Mean endurance times (seconds) and appropriate muscle endurance ratios

	Female	Male
Right lateral bridge (RLB)	75	95
Left lateral bridge (LLB)	78	99
Extension	185	161
Flexion	134	136
Ratios:		
Flexion/Extension	0.72	0.84
RLB/LLB	0.96	0.96
RLB/Extension	0.40	0.58
LLB/Extension	0.42	0.50

Adapted from McGill, S. (2002). *Low Back Disorders: Evidence Based Prevention and Rehabilitation*. Human Kinetics, Champaign, IL.

Look

General inspection should include standing posture, evidence of scoliosis and other curvatures of the spine, asymmetries, alignment of the lower limb, muscle bulk, swelling, ecchymosis, atrophy, and masses. A simple assessment of gait is performed, which should involve pain-free smooth movements with an even distribution of weight. Walking involves two basic phases: the stance phase (60% of the normal cycle) and the swing phase (40%). The hip flexors and extensors work phasically in the initiation of gait: this includes eccentric work as the flexors slow and control extension and vice versa. The hip is moved into extension during the stance phase, and the abductors are critical in maintaining the single-limb support phase. The hip moves into flexion during the swing phase, and the pelvis rotates approximately 40° anteriorly around the hip of the supported extremity.

Loss of hip range of motion results in a compensatory increase in motion of the ipsilateral knee and contralateral hip and increased movement of the lumbar spine.

Changes in gait as a result of abnormalities in the region of the hip include an increase in vertical motion of the body's centre of gravity, increased lateral shift of the trunk and pelvis, reduced stride length, and reduced rotation on the symptomatic hip. An **antalgic** gait due to localized pain involves a reduced stride length and a short stance phase, and the gait is slow and deliberate. An **extensor lurch**, due to a weak gluteus maximus, involves a thrust of the trunk backward at stance initiation to try to maintain hip extension and stability. An **abductor lurch**, due to a weak gluteus medius, is the typical **Trendelenburg gait**. The trunk lurches to the involved side to maintain stability by placing the centre of gravity over the affected hip. Bilateral gluteus medius weakness leads to a **waddling gait**. Leg-length inequality leads to a lateral shift to the opposite side, and the pelvis tilts down towards the opposite side.

Standing

The anterior superior and posterior superior iliac spines should be level with the contralateral side and skin creases should be symmetrical. Evidence of bruising, deformity, and discoloration should be sought. The spine is examined with the patient standing to assess posture, and the range and rhythm of lumbar movements and provocation of symptoms may indicate any abnormality that will require more detailed examination.

The **Trendelenburg test** evaluates the stability of the hip and the ability of the hip abductors to stabilize the pelvis on the femur. The patient stands on one limb; normally, the pelvis on the opposite side should rise. If it drops, this normally indicates hip pathology and/or a weak gluteus medius on the weight-bearing leg.

The **sacroiliac joints** (SIJs) are difficult to assess, as pain reproduced by attempts to 'stress' them may be coming from other sites, in particular the lumbar facet joints. Movement at the SIJs is very restricted, but does occur. Numerous tests have been described for evaluation of position, movement, and stress testing of SIJs and the reader is referred to helpful texts in this respect (Fortin and Falco 1997; Slipman *et al.* 1998; van der Wurff *et al.* 2000; Catterley *et al.* 2002; Magee 2008).

The mobility of the SIJs can be measured, with the patient standing or sitting, by comparing relative movement of the posterior superior iliac spine against the sacrum with finger palpation as the hip is flexed (Figure 3.8.11).

Supine

With the patient supine, **leg-length discrepancy** (functional and apparent) can be assessed. The femoral triangle can be palpated. Next, **combined hip movements** are examined, with special attention paid to range of motion and reproduction of symptoms. Combined hip flexion, external rotation, abduction, and adduction are assessed. The capsular pattern of loss of hip mobility is reduced flexion, abduction, and internal rotation, but the order of restriction may vary. Combined flexion and internal rotation may reproduce hip joint pain localized to the groin. Extension of the hip may be best assessed with the patient lying over the end of the couch with one leg flexed, knee to chest. A rectus femoris contracture is evident in this position (see Thomas's test below) and can

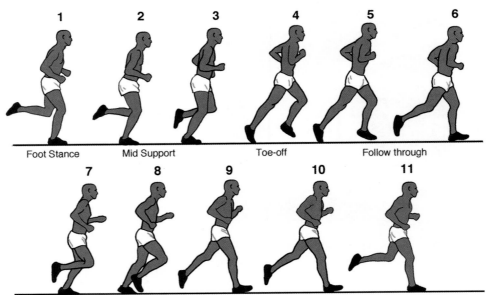

Fig. 3.8.10 The running stride: stance phase, 1–3; swing phase, 4–11.

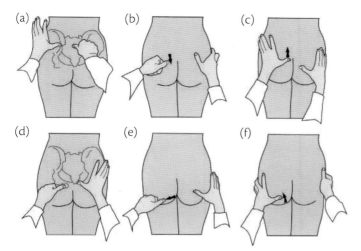

Fig. 3.8.11 Numerous tests to assess the SIJ have been proposed. Here the examiner evaluates for reduced movement relative to the contralateral side. Both the superior (a–c) and inferior (d–f) portions of the joint are evaluated. The examiner's left thumb is placed on the posterior superior iliac spine and the right thumb on a sacral process. The patient lifts the left leg. The examiner's left thumb may move downward (normal, b), or upward if it is fixed (c). For the lower portion of the joint, the left thumb is placed on the ischial tuberosity and the right thumb over the apex of the sacrum. Normally lateral movement of the left thumb occurs.

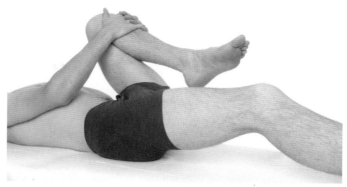

Fig. 3.8.12 Thomas's test assesses for hip flexion contracture. One of the patient's hips is flexed to flatten the lumbar spine. When the straight leg flexes on the table, a contracture is present in that hip. If performed with the knee at 90° over the edge of the table, extension of the knee indicates a probable rectus femoris contracture.

also be demonstrated in the prone position; when the affected knee is flexed, the ipsilateral hip will spontaneously flex. Resisted testing of the musculotendinous structures of the region is then performed.

An iliopsoas lesion can be detected when the patient is lying supine with the pelvis overlying the edge of the couch. The unaffected leg is flexed, knees to chest. The injured leg is extended and the examiner pushes it into further extension. This will reproduce the pain. Asking the patient to flex his/her hip against resistance makes the pain worse. The pain is aggravated by resisting flexion of the hip from a position of extension and external rotation. The patient with a 'snapping hip' may experience pain, clunking, clicking, or snapping on active flexion of the hip and then moving it into abduction and external rotation followed by extension. This moves the psoas tendon over the front of the hip.

The **adductor stretch** is measured by bringing the feet together at the buttock with knees fully flexed and allowing the hips to abduct. In this position, tenderness of the muscle belly and origin can be palpated, together with the pubic symphysis and tubercles. Resisted adduction is assessed. **Hamstring stretch** can be assessed along with the straight leg raise, but is also performed with hip flexion followed by knee extension and tibial rotation as this is thought to have less influence on neural movement than with the leg straight. A positive straight-leg raise with symptoms in the sciatic distribution, including into the foot, and a positive slump test indicate nerve root irritation.

Attempts to stress the SIJs to reproduce symptoms can be made by 'springing' the pelvis, or by flexing the hip and knee and passively adducting the thigh across to the contralateral iliac fossa. **Gaenslen's test** is performed by flexing the hip of the unaffected side and hyperextending the other hip. Unfortunately, such tests are non-specific.

The **hernial orifices** are palpated; in males, invaginating the scrotum with a finger can be a reliable means of detecting a subtle inguinal hernia and an essential examination for conjont tendon rupture. Abdominal and pelvic examinations are performed as indicated.

Many additional tests assess for the presence of contraction of one or more structures of the region. **Thomas's test** evaluates for a hip joint or rectus femoris flexion contracture (Fig. 3.8.12). The patient lies supine and the examiner looks for excess lumbar lordosis, common when the hip flexors are tight. One hip is flexed to flatten the lumbar spine. In the absence of a flexion contracture, the other (tested) leg remains flat on the table, whereas it rises off the table when a contracture is present. A rectus femoris contracture is more likely if palpable tightness is noted.

To assess for an **abduction contracture**, the patient lies supine with the ASIS level. When a contracture is present, the affected leg makes an angle of more than a 90° with the line jointing the ASIS. Typically, there is apparent leg discrepancy.

The **FABER test** (or Patrick's test) assesses for hip or SIJ pathology and iliopsoas spasm (Fig. 3.8.13). The patient lies supine and the test leg is brought into **f**lexion, **ab**duction and **e**xternal **r**otation, with the foot resting on the knee of the opposite leg. The test leg should fall into a position at least parallel with the opposite leg. Failure to do so implies pathology. The examiner may then stress the test leg further in the FABER position to attempt to reproduce the symptoms.

The **Noble compression test** assesses for ITB friction syndrome at the knee. The patient lies supine and flexes the knee to 90° with the hip in some flexion. The patient extends the knee while the examiner applies pressure to the area 1–2 cm above the lateral femoral condyle. Symptoms are reproduced at this site when the knee is 30° from full extension. (Fig. 3.8.14).

A **hamstrings contracture** is evident when there is disparity between the fingers to toes stretch, tested with the patient sitting with legs extended and the contralateral knee flexed to stabilize the pelvis (Fig. 3.8.15).

The **anterior impingement** test involves specific manoeuvres to identify labral tears. The hip is flexed, internally rotated, and adducted. Reproduction of symptoms, including pain and clicking,

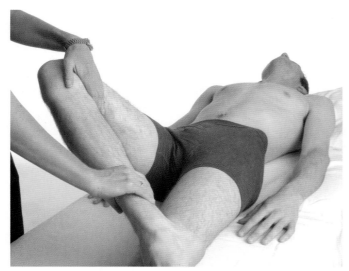

Fig. 3.8.13 The FABER test is a general test for hip, SIJ pathology, or iliopsoas spasm.

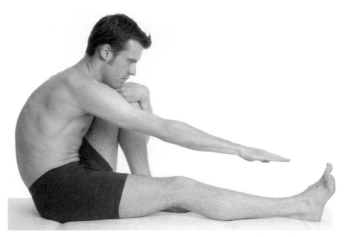

Fig. 3.8.15 A hamstring contracture is evident when there is disparity between the fingers to toes stretch. Hamstring flexibility should also be tested by passive extension of the leg in varying degrees of hip rotation.

indicates a positive anterior impingement. The **posterior impingement** test elicits symptoms with the patient's hip extended, externally rotated, and abducted. Specific functions, including squatting, hopping, and stair-climbing, can then be evaluated in order to reproduce symptoms.

Abdominal wall syndromes may manifest as pain with sit-ups (straight/oblique). When pain is produced by palpation or movement the patient is asked if this reproduces their symptoms.

Finally, neurovascular assessment is performed in the supine position.

Lateral position

Further evaluation continues, with the patient lying on the unaffected side. The greater trochanter can be palpated by following the femur proximally. Local tenderness and reproduction of pain in this area on adducting and flexing the hip may indicate a trochanteric bursitis, although hip joint pain can be referred to this area early in the history of degenerative change.

Ober's test for a tight ITB is performed with the affected leg uppermost. The other leg is flexed at the hip and knee. The examiner then passively abducts and extends the upper leg with the knee extended, and then slowly allows the upper leg to lower onto the couch. Ober initially described the test with the knee of the test leg flexed, but the gluteus medius, the main hip abductor, is tested with the leg in a few degrees of abduction. Pain may be reproduced. Failure to reach the couch indicates a tightness which may be the cause of ITB friction syndrome or trochanteric bursitis (Fig. 3.8.16).

With the patient in the same position, the piriformis test can be performed. With the uppermost knee flexed and the hip flexed to 60°, the examiner applies downward pressure on the knee. Pain in the area of piriformis is reproduced if it is tight. Sciatica may be noted if the piriformis is irritating or compressing the nerve.

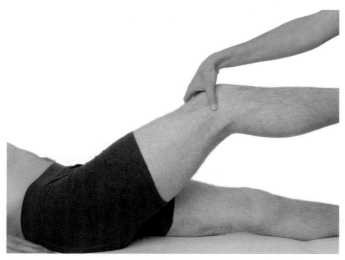

Fig. 3.8.14 The Noble compression test assesses for ITB friction syndrome at the knee.

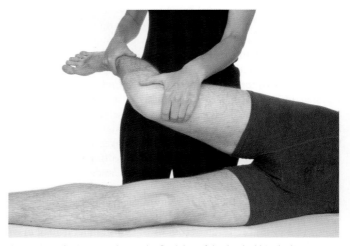

Fig. 3.8.16 Ober's test evaluates the flexibility of the iliotibial band. The ITB is tight if the patient's abducted and extended upper leg remains abducted when slowly released by the examiner.

Prone

The spine and SIJs can be palpated, and the femoral stretch test is performed to assess for nerve entrapment. Gluteus maximus can be tested by resisted hip extension with the knee flexed (to relax the hamstrings). The ischiogluteal region (where a bursa is present) and the hamstring origin can be palpated for tenderness and the muscle group assessed by resisted knee flexion. Active external rotation of the leg during testing helps to isolate the biceps femoris, while internal rotation helps to test semitendinosus and semimembranosus.

Investigations

Diagnostic tools can be used as an adjunct to clinical examination. To aid early diagnosis of injuries, accurate imaging can be a vital tool, allowing appropriate treatment to be started earlier. However, there are no hard and fast rules; rather, the request and use of further investigations is tailored for each individual patient.

X-ray

In acute injuries, plain radiography of the pelvis is required where significant trauma has occurred and where bony/articular damage is suspected. In children and adolescents, plain radiographs are warranted when there is the possibility of an avulsion injury. Plain radiographs of the pelvis may also be indicated in chronic pain in the region, as the pubic symphysis, SIJs, and hip joints are all sources of symptoms. Soft tissue calcification (e.g. at the gluteal enthesis) may be seen. Osteoarthritis (OA) is seen in both young athletes and more senior age groups, but radiographic evidence of OA can be misleading in the interpretation of symptoms. Anteroposterior and lateral views of the joint are obtained routinely. Stork views with the patient standing on alternate legs is used to detect pubic symphysis instability. Radiological changes consistent with osteitis pubis are common in active asymptomatic males.

Ultrasound

Ultrasound is seen by many as an essential extension of the clinical examination. It provides a safe and powerful modality for viewing superficial soft tissue lesions such as bursae and muscle–tendon units (Kalebo *et al.* 1992). It is ideal for identifying soft tissue pathologies and joint and tendon dynamics, as well as intra-articular foreign bodies, synovitis, and effusions. It is useful for assessing sportsman's abdominal wall syndromes, and of course for aspiration and injection. Testicular pathology and intra-pelvic pathology can also be assessed using this imaging modality.

MRI

MRI provides a comprehensive image of both superficial and deep soft tissue structures. It is superior in its contrast differentiation of tissues, and thus is preferred to CT for imaging of soft tissue injuries. Furthermore, following intra-articular administration of gadolinium, it is extremely valuable in the diagnosis of radiographically occult osseous abnormalities as well as soft tissue injuries, such as muscle–tendon unit abnormalities and bursitis (Overdeck and Palmer 2004). Currently, high-resolution direct MR arthrography of the hip provides the best means for evaluating intra-articular pathology. It provides description of labral tears and assessment of cartilage defects, as well as capsule and ligamentous injury and tears of the ligamentum teres, providing prognostic information. A comprehensive imaging strategy requires conventional radiographs and MRI to evaluate intra- and extra-articular sources of pain (Armfield *et al.* 2006).

CT

CT is ideal for further assessment of the bony anatomy and joints, and provides better options for viewing fracture configurations, loose bodies, subtle degenerative changes, and calcifications. Further advantages of CT include image-guided injections into the hip joint or soft tissue structures for diagnostic and therapeutic purposes. However, the radiation dose during a CT scan is considerable, and patient safety should always be considered when requesting this imaging tool.

Isotope bone scans

Although largely superceded by MRI, isotope bone scans are highly sensitive in identifying stress lesion of the bone. Stress fractures are often missed on plain radiographs, but are highlighted as an increased uptake in nuclear bone scan, allowing early diagnosis and treatment. Early OA, as well as other inflammatory joint disorders and bony tumours (benign and malignant), will also be highlighted in a bone scan. Sacroiliac indices are requested where there is the suspicion of inflammatory sacroiliitis.

Hip arthroscopy

Conventional radiographs and MRI may be inadequate, especially in identifying articular, labral, and chondral injuries. A negative imaging study does not exclude important intra-articular pathologies. Direct observation of the joint is beneficial for definitive diagnosis and treatment. With the advent and development of hip arthroscopy, labral tears are increasingly diagnosed. With early diagnosis and treatment, patients are able to return to activities with minimal recovery and rehabilitation, as well as therapeutically preventing future degenerative changes of the hip.

Specific disorders

Anterior hip and groin pain:

Adductor injuries

Adductor injuries are common in the athletic population, particularly in footballers and hurdlers, and may be related to an acute event or to chronic overuse. Injury may occur along the myotendinous junction or the tendon, or at the enthesis, and may be associated with osteitis pubis or symphysis instability. Myotendinous injuries are graded in the same manner as other muscle injuries and usually involve adductor longus.

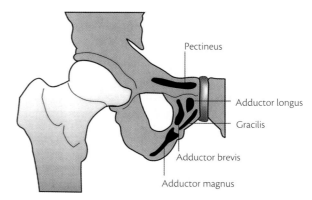

Fig. 3.8.17 Insertions of adductor muscles onto the pelvis.

In the acute injury, the typical mechanism is that of eccentric adductor contraction with the hip in abduction and external rotation, for example a blocked kick in soccer or when changing direction. The pain, adductor spasm, tenderness, and (in the acute injury) swelling can be easily located to the adductor longus, below the pubic tubercle. There is pain on resisted adduction and, in some cases, flexion. Imaging studies are not usually necessary but may be indicated to exclude other causes of groin or thigh pain. In the suspected avulsion fracture, plain radiographs are necessary. MRI and ultrasound will demonstrate tendinopathies and muscle damage, but non-specific intra-tendinous alterations on imaging are common in the active asymptomatic patient.

Management

In the acute stage, the RICE regime is followed, and then a strengthening and stretching programme is commenced before sport-specific rehabilitation starts, as described earlier. Some recommend that acute muscle ruptures are surgically repaired, particularly in the athlete (Sangwan *et al.* 1994). Chronic tendon injuries are treated similarly, but progress may be slow and the patient must be counselled in relation to this in order to prevent premature return to sporting activities. A peritendinous cortisone injection near the insertion, platelet-rich plasma (PRP) injection and/or dry needling may help in resistant tendinopathies. Adductor longus tenotomy may also be considered in those with persistent localized pain (Akermark and Johannson 1992), followed by progressive rehabilitation. Although a decrease in muscle strength may result, this does not seem to be functionally relevant.

Pubic symphysis instability

The phenomenon of instability of the pubic symphysis was first recognized by Hippocrates in relation to post-partum females. It also occurs in athletes (usually male), and may be asymptomatic or associated with a spectrum of symptoms, including local symphysis pain, groin or adductor pain, and clicking. Typically the patient presents with a nagging ache radiating from the midline down into the adductor region and the perineum. Running, and in some cases lifting and cutting, and even walking, aggravates the pain, which persists with rest for some time. X-rays may show signs of osteitis pubis in chronic cases, but such changes are frequently seen in asymptomatic active males. MRI and bone scan will be more sensitive to active osteitis. Stork X-ray views of the symphysis, performed standing on one leg and then the other, may reveal obvious instability across the symphysis. The normal displacement is <0.2mm.

Management involves rehabilitation to regain muscle control with a closely supervised core stability programme, with retraining taking at least 3–6 months. In the female with instability following childbirth, a sacroiliac belt and reassurance are particularly useful. A surgical fusion using autogenous bone graft and plate fixation can be effective (Williams *et al.* 2000), but is only very rarely indicated. Posterior pelvic instability with pain around the SIJs occurring 1 and 5 years postoperatively has been reported (Moore *et al.* 1998).

Osteitis pubis

The term osteitis pubis implies an inflammatory process affecting the pubic symphysis. However, inflammation of the symphysis is frequently not a histological finding in chronic symphysis pain and the term is more commonly used to describe radiological changes at the symphysis, including widening, demineralization, resorption, periosteal reaction, and sclerosis (Harris and Murray 1974). In athletes the cause is usually biomechanical, resulting in excessive movement across the joint. Such biomechanical aberrations may be associated with symphysis instability or relative restriction in joints at other sites around the pelvis. Radiological changes are more common in soccer players and in sports where there is cyclical loading, such as running, when compared with controls, but this may be asymptomatic. Osteitis can also have a range of other causes including osteomyelitis, hyperparathyroidism, sarcoidosis, inflammatory arthritis, and haemachromatosis, all of which should be considered in those presenting with symptoms.

Pain ascribed to osteitis pubis is anterior midline, radiating bilaterally along the adductor muscles and around into the perineum. There may be localized tenderness over the pubic symphysis in the early stages of the condition. In the early stages of osteitis pubis, pain may be bilateral, radiating to the adductor region. In this situation, a flare can be seen on bone scan and MRI shows changes within the pubic rami. Secondly, when the condition reaches the stage where the pubic symphysis is frankly unstable, a midline pain or a dull nagging ache can become sufficiently severe to be disabling.

Where pain ascribed to osteitis pubis is present, the X-ray appearances of osteitis pubis can lag behind the clinical picture and may remain after the symptoms settle with conservative measures. In those with active lesions, technetium-99m scintigraphy will show increased uptake in the joint. However, this has been superseded by MRI, which shows oedema within the pubic symphysis in patients with chronic groin pain. Nevertheless, as emphasized earlier, the findings must be taken in the clinical context.

The recommended treatment of osteitis pubis includes a long period of relative rest, analgesics, and an exercise regime to retrain the weakened pelvic musculature. The core stability programme is central to management, as it is with symphyseal instability. It aims to improve control of the pelvic muscles that control movement of the hip and lower spine, and improve strength and control of the anterior abdominal wall. Symptoms may take 6–12 months or more to settle.

In recalcitrant cases, the use of a guided steroid injection has been advocated. However, there is no convincing evidence that this is of any benefit, and it is more a reflection of the limited options available in a difficult condition.

Sportsman's abdominal wall syndrome

Sportsman's abdominal wall syndrome (SAWS) is a term which helps to express the wide spectrum of soft tissue dysfunction that can affect the abdominal wall and groin in the athlete, typically a male. This can include injuries to the conjoint tendon, inguinal ligament, posterior abdominal wall ('Gilmore's groin' or 'sportsman's hernia') or indeed the pubis at the abdominal wall insertions. Coexistent adductor tendinopathy, symphysis instability or osteitis pubis may occur, emphasising the role that lumbopelvic instability has in the aetiology of the condition.

Sports hernia (Gilmore's groin)

The concept of the sports hernia, also known as Gilmore's groin or sportsman's or footballer's hernia, is reported in males in relation to a number of specific activities, especially soccer.

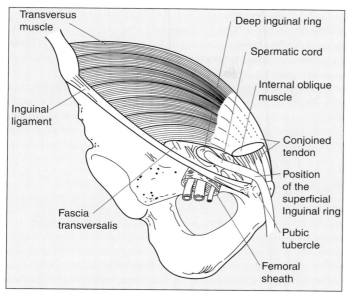

Fig. 3.8.18 The posterior wall of the inguinal canal is formed by the fascia transversalis, which is reinforced in its medial third by the conjoined tendon, the common tendon of insertion of the internal oblique and transversus muscles, which attaches to the pubic crest and the pectineal line (not shown in this anterior view). 'Sports hernia' refers to a spectrum of injuries principally involving the conjoint tendon, inguinal ligament, and fascia transversalis, as well as the internal oblique muscle and the external oblique aponeurosis (not shown here), which form part of the anterior wall of the canal.

Aetiology

The condition is considered to be a generalized distension of the anterior abdominal wall with an incompetence of the posterior inguinal wall. Several theories of causation have been described (Bowerman 1977; Williams 1978; Lloyd-Smith *et al.* 1985; Malycha and Lovell 1992; Polglase *et al.* 1991). According to one theory, a reduction in internal rotation of the hip joint produces a shearing force across the pubic symphysis from continued adductor pull (Williams 1978). Shearing across the pubic symphysis leads to stress on the inguinal wall musculature. The anatomical defects in the wall, i.e. the inguinal rings, may account for the predominance of this condition in the male. The stretching of the conjoint tendon and transversalis, in some cases with true tearing of these structures from the inguinal ligament, accounts for the pain (Bowerman 1977). An alternative theory is that it is simply a chronic stretching of the posterior inguinal wall due to the excess demands of sport (Malycha and Lovell 1992; Gullmo 1980). The condition is rare in females.

History

The groin pain may be of gradual onset or develop after a sudden injury. The initial pain is often described as an ache or stiffness in the adductor region which develops after sport. Early symptoms include pain around the adductor muscles across to the midline and the inguinal region. Pain may spread laterally, proximally into the rectus muscles and distally into the perineum. There may be a history of cough impulse, and testicular pain is a feature in about 30% of cases.

Examination

The findings on examination are also varied. Some clinical features are notably similar to those of osteitis pubis and symphysis instability. By definition, there is no palpable hernia.

There may be adductor spasm with tenderness around the belly and origin of the adductor longus. The ipsilateral pubic tubercle and the symphysis pubis and peripubic area are tender to palpation. There is pain with resisted hip adduction and with sit-ups. The inguinal rings and cough impulse must be assessed via the scrotum. The area around the enlarged external inguinal ring is tender. The mid-inguinal canal is the site of the worst discomfort, and pain is aggravated by coughing, with the cough impulse felt over a wider area. The testes should be formally examined to exclude local pathology.

Other components of SAWS

Conjoint tendon injuries, inguinal ligament defects, external oblique aponeurosis tears, and rectus abdominis tendinopathy/enthesopathy can all result in groin pain in the athlete. As described, these can occur in isolation or in varied combinations.

Investigations

Plain X-rays may show changes consistent with osteitis pubis. MRI and ultrasound findings are varied. Conjoint tendon and inguinal ligament abnormalities may occur as part of the condition or in isolation. Changes consistent with osteitis and/or altered signal within structures of the abdominal wall (e.g. rectus abdominis), adductors, or the perineal region, or a non-specific bulging of the posterior abdominal wall with straining may be demonstrated. Herniography is insensitive and outdated as a form of imaging.

Treatment

In Gilmore's groin or where there is tendinopathy/enthesopathy, conservative management includes a controlled progressive rehabilitation programme. This commences with relative rest and deep tissue massage, adding stretching exercises of the hip/thigh muscles and lumbar spine performed two or three times daily. Light aerobic activity (e.g. static bicycling, aqua jogging, swimming) and then a progressive strengthening programme are introduced, targeting

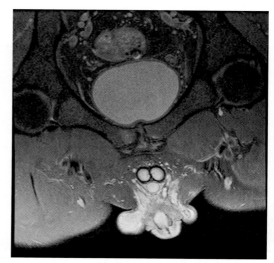

Fig 3.8.19 MRI showing osteitis pubis and associated adductor tendinopathy.

the abdominal muscles, hip flexors, and adductors. In the next stage, functional activities are included and eventually a graduated return to sport is attempted.

Typically, rest settles the pain, but it is reported to return rapidly on resuming sport. When patients fail to settle with conservative treatment, other approaches should be considered. In those with posterior inguinal wall weakness, surgical repair can provide excellent results, with over 80% returning to competition postoperatively (Ingoldby 1977). Thinning or tearing of the conjoint tendon of transversalis and internal oblique muscles and inguinal ligament defects should be repaired. The surgical technique used aims to provide tension to the muscles of the posterior wall of the inguinal canal. Postoperatively, a rehabilitation programme as described earlier is followed, with expected return to sporting activity at 6 weeks.

Rectus abdominis injuries can occur as part of SAWS or, less commonly, as isolated entities. The recti are straplike muscles, each having two tendinous origins; one arising from the anterior surface of the pubis symphysis and a larger head more laterally, originating from the upper border of the pubic crest. Together they form the muscle mass inserting onto the fifth, sixth, and seventh costal cartilages. Nerve supply to the rectus abdominis derives from the lower six thoracic nerves.

Isolated injuries are seen particularly in tennis players, on the non-dominant side, and are due to relative lack of strength and control by other abdominal and core muscle groups, right–left muscle imbalances, and technical issues such as poor body positioning in playing an overhead smash or a kick serve, when the ball is relatively behind the player and the spine is in marked hyperextension.

Hernia

Inguinal hernia

A hernia is defined as the protrusion of a loop or knuckle of an organ through an abnormal opening. An indirect inguinal hernia leaves the abdomen at the internal ring and passes along the inguinal canal, eventually leading to the scrotum. A direct inguinal hernia emerges between the inferior epigastric artery and the edge of the rectus muscle. The direct hernia is often simply a weakness of the wall of the posterior inguinal canal, formed by the internal oblique and transversalis abdominis muscles.

An inguinal hernia may cause pain as a presenting symptom. The patient complains of a dull nagging ache in the inguinal region, frequently prior to the swelling of the hernia becoming apparent (subclinical hernia). Interestingly, once the hernia appears the discomfort often subsides.

A hernia is detected by direct palpation over the inguinal canal and asking the patient to cough. A cough impulse is diagnostic. In males, the palpation is most accurately performed by invaginating the scrotum. A subclinical hernia can be identified using dynamic ultrasonography. Therefore herniography is rarely used. The treatment is a surgical repair where symptoms warrant it.

Snapping hip syndrome

A 'snapping hip' may arise as a result of a number of intra- and extra-articular pathologies (Table 3.8.5). The iliopsoas tendon and its underlying bursa is the most common source, due to tightness, tendinopathy and/or bursitis, when the tendon glides over the lesser trochanter or iliopectineal eminence and snaps as it does so. Other causes of snapping hip include subluxation of the femoral head or flicking of the iliofemoral ligament over it, suction phenomena within the joint, and flicking of either the iliotibial band or the tendon of the gluteus maximus over the greater trochanter. Contributing factors are muscle imbalance and poor flexibility, biomechanical derangements, and training or technical errors.

Acute injury to the tendon or bursa can occur because of a direct blow or overuse, particularly in runners, hurdlers, and soccer players. Iliopsoas bursitis is associated with a number of hip pathologies, including arthritides, sepsis, and osteonecrosis, and such complaints must always be considered in the patient with a bursitis.

History

Deep groin pain is reported, which is worse with activity, particularly climbing stairs. Symptoms may also be aggravated by prolonged sitting, in particular when a bursa is present. A 'click', 'clunk', or snapping sensation is felt deep in the groin when the leg is rotated and flexed, for example as the trail leg crosses a hurdle. The clunk or snap can give rise to a deep ache. When sufficiently large, a bursitis may also present as a painful or painless inguinal mass, or with symptoms related to a compressive effect such as femoral nerve irritation or femoral venous engorgement. A large bursa can even cause compression of the large bowel or bladder.

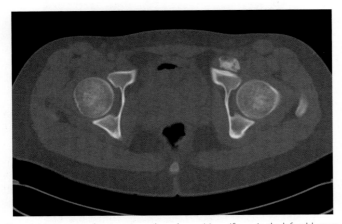

Fig 3.8.20 A cause of groin pain: unilateral myositis ossificans in the left adductors.

Table 3.8.5 Causes of clicking or snapping hip

Extra-articular
Iliopsoas tightness, tendinopathy or bursitis
Tight tensor fascia lata
Trochanteric bursitis
Piriformis syndrome
Articular
Loose bodies within the hip joint
Tear of the acetabular labrum
Subluxing hip joint

Examination

Localized tenderness over the iliopsoas tendon is present. A very large bursa may be palpable. Stretching the psoas tendon and stressing the musculotendinous unit through passive, active, and resisted movements of the hip can reproduce the pain felt by those suffering this injury and are used as diagnostic tests, as described earlier.

Investigation

A plain radiograph is helpful in the initial evaluation to exclude other causes of groin pain, although articular disease and iliopsoas bursitis can coexist. MRI will image the soft tissue and bony structures more clearly, and is particularly useful when coexisting pathologies are likely. Dynamic ultrasonography is frequently diagnostic in a bursitis or tendinopathy. The bursa is typically heart shaped or has an hourglass appearance in the transverse plane due to compression by the iliopsoas tendon. Concomitant effusion of the hip indicates communication between the joint and bursal space, and coexisting hip disease should be suspected. Although the frequency of the communication in the general population is in the region of 15%, it is commonly noted in those with a bursitis, and in particular those with underlying hip disease, which is the primary pathology. The use of ultrasound also provides the opportunity for aspiration of the bursa under direct guidance. Aspiration is mandatory if sepsis is suspected and is also helpful in the relief of acute symptoms. Heterogeneity of iliopsoas fibres in the presence of a tendinopathy can also be demonstrated.

Further investigations, including a white cell count, ESR, uric acid, and blood and bursal fluid cultures, are performed as appropriate.

Treatment

Treatment of both tendinopathy and bursitis initially involves relative rest, non-steroidal anti-inflammatory drugs (NSAIDs), and attention to the underlying cause(s) of the complaint (e.g. overuse, biomechanical abnormalities, or primary hip disease). A stretching programme is usually very successful. The most common reason for failure of stretching is a poor stretching technique or poor compliance, which when corrected gives the desired result. In resistant iliopsoas tendinopathy, surgical division of the tendon may be considered.

In the most resistant cases of bursitis, a local corticosteroid injection (in the absence of sepsis) can be considered, but the physician must note the frequency of communication with the hip joint. When performed, injection under ultrasound guidance is the preferred option.

Surgical intervention is reserved for those intractable cases not responding to conservative measures. Arthroscopy is an option for dealing with intra-articular lesions. A range of operations exist for managing snapping, including the partial resection of the tendon insertion and the underlying bursa, z-plasty and lengthening of the tendon (Provencher *et al.* 2004), or complete tendon release, all with reported promising results (Gruen *et al.* 2002).

Calcific tendinitis of the hip.

Calcification at the site of origin of one or more muscles of the thigh, most commonly the rectus femoris, gluteus maximus, or vastus lateralis, has been described, although it is a rare event. Acute groin pain and limitation of movement (due to pain), without

a history of trauma, are presenting features. Management includes relative rest, analgesics or NSAIDs, ultrasound, shock wave therapy, and if necessary image-guided local corticosteroid injection.

Pain referred from the lumbar spine

Pain referred from the spine may cause groin pain. Associated pathologies include facet joint dysfunction/arthritis, lumbar root pain (irritation or compression from a true disc prolapse) or from a spondylolysis/listhesis. Patients describe a poorly localized, diffuse pain in the anterior pelvis and thigh. Confusingly, there may be no back pain at all. The diagnosis is considered by excluding other causes of groin pain, closely scrutinizing the spine and recognizing that the pattern of pain does not fit any of those described in this chapter.

Investigations

Investigations, such as a plain radiograph and ultrasound, may be necessary to exclude hip pathologies. Lumbar spine X-rays are not performed routinely. However where a spondylolysis/listhesis is suspected oblique radiographs of the lumbar spine are necessary to demonstrate the defect of the pars interarticularis. Bone scan, SPECT scan, or MRI will help determine whether the lesion (usually at L5) is active. A trial injection of local anaesthetic into the pars defect under X-ray control may trigger the patient's pain as the needle enters the pathological area; the pain is then relieved by the local anaesthetic. MRI scanning to assess for a prolapsed disc is performed if the clinical picture warrants it.

Treatment

Treatment of spinal conditions is addressed in other sections of this book. Treatment of spondylolysis initially involves relative rest and analgesics. A polypropylene brace may help to control symptoms. Recommendations for their use range from waking hours to 23 hours per day and from 3 to 6 months. If symptoms persist, surgery (fusion/screw fixation) should be considered.

Ilio-inguinal and genitofemoral nerve entrapment

Ilio-inguinal and genitofemoral neuralgias are characterized by dysaesthesiae and/or burning pain in the appropriate distribution of the nerve. Nerve injury or entrapment in the inguinal fascia can occur after surgery (e.g. herniorrhaphy, appendicectomy, Caesarean section) and has also been described in systemic sclerosis. Local blockade of the ilio-inguinal nerve or paravertebral blocks of L1 and L2 (genitofemoral nerve) can confirm the diagnosis. A tricyclic agent or carbamazepine may reduce symptoms, but if symptoms are severe, neurolysis may be indicated.

Hip joint pathologies

Labral injuries

Acetabular labral tear as a cause for hip pain has received little recognition until recently. Labral tears represent the most common cause for mechanical hip symptoms, and are found to be the cause of groin pain in more than 20% of athletes presenting with hip pain (Lynch and Renstrom 1999). Tears most commonly occur anteriorly and are associated with a range of aetiological factors including degenerative arthropathies, dysplastic hips, trauma following hip dislocation and overload, pivoting, and hyperextension injuries.

Patients present with mainly anterior groin pain that is sharp in nature. Commonly, there is associated clicking, giving way, and a

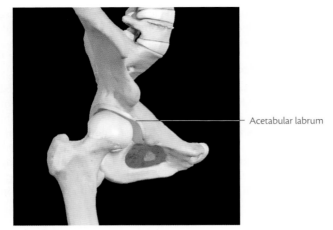

Fig. 3.8.21 The acetabular labrum.

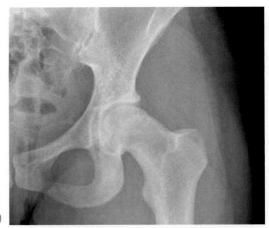

(a)

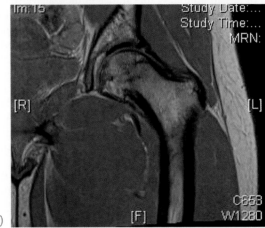

(b)

Fig. 3.8.22 (a) X-ray and (b) MRI of a 25-year-old badminton player showing abnormal left femoral head morphology, with reduction in femoral head, neck offset, and coxa vara deformity. These appearances suggest a chronic slipped upper femoral epiphysis. There are bony impingement changes in the superolateral femoral neck, with subcortical cystic change.

sensation of locking of the hip joint. Examination may reveal a full painless range of motion, but may reproduce the click or locking sensation on extreme movements. An impingement test—a combined movement of flexion and rotation—will cause pain in the groin. More specifically, for anterior labral tears, flexion with internal rotation and adduction will elicit a positive impingement test. Extension with external rotation and abduction will impinge on posterior tears, thus causing pain. Although plain radiographs will identify and exclude any underlying bony abnormalities (such as hip dysplasia and arthritis), they are not considered to be a reliable tool for identifying labral tears. MRI and MR arthrography are more sensitive in identifying labral pathologies (Czerny *et al.* 1996). In recent times hip arthroscopy has increasingly become the gold standard for diagnostic and therapeutic purposes as it allows a comprehensive evaluation of the labral anatomy (McCarthy *et al.* 2003). A period of rest followed by protected weight-bearing can produce good outcome, but labral tears occur on the articular non-vascular edge and may not heal with conservative treatment. Arthroscopic debridement of the torn part of the labrum is the treatment of choice in these patients, who tend be young and active.

Other hip impingement syndromes

Femoroacetabular impingement (FAI) is a cause of hip pain that may be responsible for the progression of degenerative change, and is particularly seen in active young adults or in very flexible hips (Ganz *et al.* 2003). Such impingement within the hip joint is a result of abutment between the bone of the femur and that of the pelvis. The cause of impingement can be developmental, such as Legg–Calvé–Perthes disease, slipped capital femoral epiphysis, or persistent external rotation of the hips or retroversion of the acetabulum. It may also result from post-traumatic or post-osteotomy morphological changes in inclination and anteversion angles of the femoral head.

Two distinct types of FAI have been identified in the literature. Cam impingement is caused by an abnormal femoral head–neck junction, often termed a pistol-grip deformity (Stulberg *et al.* 1975). A reduced head–neck offset results in early abutment against the anterior aspect of the acetabulum, resulting in impingement during flexion, adduction, and internal rotation. The prevalence of

cam impingement is greatest in young athletic men. The second type, pincer impingement, is a result of linear contact between a prominent anterior aspect of the acetabular rim and the femoral head or head–neck junction. This is commonly associated with middle-aged athletic women, occurring as a result of acetabular protrusion or retroversion of the acetabulum (resulting in over-coverage of the femoral head by the prominent anterior aspect of the acetabular rim).

Cam and pincer impingement rarely occur in isolation, and as one epidemiological study identified, most cases of FAI involve a combination of the two mechanisms and are classified as mixed cam–pincer impingement (Beck *et al.* 2005).

Patients present with unilateral activity-related hip/groin pain; many report concurrent mechanical symptoms (clicking, locking, or giving-way) which is indicative of an underlying labral tear or chondral pathology. Clinical examination will often reveal a positive impingement sign, with an otherwise unremarkable hip joint.

Investigation

Plain radiographic assessment is important, as patients with FAI will often have their images reported as normal. Useful images include an anteroposterior and a lateral view of the hip in order to assess the orientation of the acetabulum and the femoral head–neck offset, respectively. CT scans and MR arthrograms are valuable in the assessment of the associated labral injury and articular cartilage delamination, as well as for measuring and quantifying the femoral head–neck abnormality. Furthermore, MRI provides the option of dynamic images to demonstrate real-time imaging of impingement.

Treatment

The management of hip impingement may begin with a trial of conservative measures, including modification of activity, restriction of athletic pursuits, and reduction of excessive motion and burden on the hip. NSAIDs can be useful, especially in the acute phase; however, these may mask ongoing symptoms, leading to further degenerative changes. Definitive treatment requires surgical intervention. Chronicity of signs and symptoms along with radiographic evidence of impingement are clear indications for operative treatment. This involves reconstruction and reorientation of the femoral head–neck offset or acetabulum, as well as addressing associated labral and chondral lesions. Various surgical procedures have been described, including an open procedure with surgical hip dislocation (Ganz *et al.* 2001), an arthroscopic procedure (Crawford and Villar 2005), and a combined hip arthroscopy with a limited open osteochondroplasty. Open operative treatment is the original and best documented method for treatment of FAI, but favourable results have been reported for arthroscopic treatment of FAI and the future for arthroscopic surgery looks promising (Sampson 2005).

Osteoarthritis

OA of the hip is a major cause of disability in the elderly, commonly affecting populations over the age of 55 years. In addition to age, the incidence of hip OA may be increased by a range of other risk factors including hip or acetabular dysplasia, occupational work loads, previous trauma, and joint injuries and obesity (L'Hermette *et al.* 2006). Research has generally shown that, compared with age-matched controls, former elite athletes have an increased risk of developing OA of the hip. The degenerative changes were especially found among those who had played at national or international level. This has been particularly associated with football, where the incidence of OA in former football players has been reported to be up to 49% compared with the

reported incidence of up to 10% in control populations (Turner *et al.* 2000). Other sports predisposing to increased risk of OA include fencing, handball, rugby, and tennis. Patients complain primarily of pain and discomfort. There may be associated altered range of motion and stiffness, especially in relation to flexion and internal rotation. Bone scan and MRI can detect the condition, with evidence of increased uptake and chondral defects, respectively. However, plain radiographs are the first-line imaging modality for OA. Radiographic changes characteristic of OA include cartilage alteration (decreased joint space) and bone response (subchondral sclerosis and cysts, and osteophyte formation). It is important to counsel this group of patients with OA, controlling their symptoms with simple analgesia and NSAIDs, and physiotherapy to strengthen muscles and improve joint stability, thus controlling the progression of the disease. A review of the literature has suggested that properly contracting muscle strength and integrity of joint stability are important factors in the development of this degenerative disease. Thus, proper rehabilitation is important in the prevention of OA progression (Shrier 2004). Ultimately, with severe arthritis, where the pain interferes with activities of daily living, surgery is indicated in the form of resurfacing hip replacement or total joint replacement. With refinement in techniques and the advent of low-wear bearing surfaces, the potential life expectancy of hip replacements has increased.

Bone marrow oedema syndromes of the hip

Bone marrow oedema is a radiological term used to describe those syndromes of the hip where there are areas of signal hyperintensity within the marrow demonstrated on MRI, histologically correlating to a variable degree with interstitial marrow oedema, necrosis, fibrosis, and trabecular bone abnormalities (Vande Berg *et al.* 2007). This can be observed in inflammatory arthritides, infection, avascular necrosis of the femoral head, spontaneous fracture, or stress injury of the femoral head. Additionally it may be associated with transient osteoporosis of the hip or post-traumatic 'bone bruise'—a poorly understood entity which in the absence of other pathology may resolve with time and relative rest. Recommencement of activities is based upon symptoms, not imaging findings, and the time frame is highly variable.

Avascular necrosis

Interruption of blood flow to the bone results in cell death, collapse of the femoral head, bone destruction and subsequent loss of function. Previous childhood history of hip disorders (including Legg–Calvé–Perthes syndrome, slipped capital femoral epiphysis, and congenital dislocated hip), hip trauma, irradiation, steroid use, alcoholism, and vasculitic disorders are a few of the many causes of avascular necrosis (AVN). Early disease is usually asymptomatic, but patients normally present with hip pain and stiffness. With progressive destruction of the femoral head, pain can become very intense with significant deformity and dysfunction. It is important to identify the individuals at risk, and certain sports, including deep sea diving (decompression sickness), can cause AVN. Plain radiographs will reveal degenerative changes, but usually florid changes will be seen at later stages. MRI is the most sensitive at diagnosing and prognostically staging AVN. These patients can be managed conservatively in the early stages. Activity modification and protected weight-bearing may prevent femoral head collapse; however, surgical prevention such as bone marrow decompression can delay the onset of femoral collapse (Mont and Hungerford 1995).

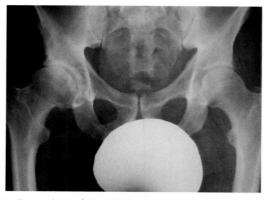

Fig. 3.8.23 Osteoarthritis of the right hip in a 32-year-old footballer.

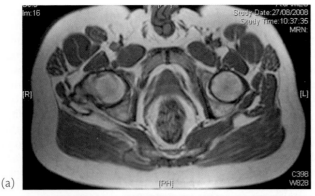

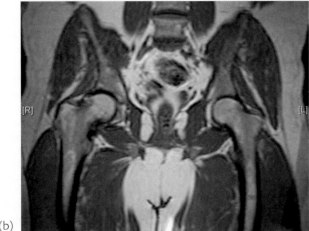

Fig. 3.8.24 MRI of the pelvis in a 25-year-old footballer. There is marked degenerative change within the right hip. There are very large cam lesions bilaterally, more prominent on the right than the left, and there is marked synovitis within the right hip. There is cartilage thinning superolaterally within the acetabulum with subcortical cyst formation.

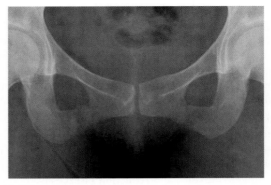

Fig. 3.8.25 Plain X-ray of the pelvis showing a right pubic ramus fracture in a marathon runner.

Other treatment options include free vascular graft and hip replacement surgery in more advanced disease.

Dislocation

Hip fracture–dislocations are commonly associated with high-impact traumatic events. In sporting events, hip dislocations only represent 2–5% of all hip dislocations (Chudik *et al.* 2002). Of these, posterior dislocations are more common. Alpine skiing is an exception, with one study showing higher rates of anterior dislocations in skiers (Matsumoto *et al.* 2003). Mechanism is dependent on the position of the hip at the time of injury and is usually associated with a flexed internally rotated and adducted hip, especially in contact sports. Anterior dislocation, due to a fall with a flexed externally rotated and abducted hip, is more commonly associated with skiers and gymnasts. These patients are in extreme pain, with an inability to weight-bear and move their hips. It is of paramount importance to assess these patients for their neurovascular status, as well as identifying any other injuries. Plain radiographs will identify the dislocation and exclude any concomitant fractures of the femur. The key to treating such dislocations involves the prompt recognition of the injury, assessment for associated neurovascular compromise, and reduction either in a closed or open method. Post-reduction CT and MRI scans may be indicated to assess for soft tissue injuries, and at 6 month intervals to exclude complications such as avascular necrosis of the femoral head. Other complications that a physician needs to be aware of are development of osteoarthritis, instability, and recurrent hip subluxation.

Femoral neck stress fractures

Fractures of the femoral neck are more common in the elderly, and are often associated with a traumatic event. However, stress fractures can occur in young athletes as a result of overuse injuries of bone. They are caused by the repetitive application of stress of less strength than that required to fracture bone in a single load (Peccina and Bojanic 2003). Stress fractures account for approximately 10% of all sports injuries, and commonly occur in the tibia. An estimated 1% of stress fractures occur at the femoral neck (Ha *et al.* 1991). With an insidious onset and generalized symptoms, including vague anterior groin pain which is worse on exertion, diagnosis can be difficult. There may be pain on extreme hip movement, with a positive hop test (the patient attempts to hop on the affected limb). Plain radiographs must be taken, but initial films may be entirely normal. Diagnosis is confirmed with the use of bone scanning or MRI. All such injuries are serious, but those at the superior neck are under tension and more prone to complications. The treatment is initially rest and avoidance of activity, with gradual progression to physiotherapy and gentle exercises. Complications can arise, especially with delayed diagnosis. Such complications include development of a frank fracture and its subsequent consequences such as displacement, delayed healing, avascular necrosis, and symptom recurrence.

Anterior thigh pain

The most common source of anterior thigh pain in sport is injury to the muscles of the thigh in the form of contusions, strains (grades I–III), and delayed-onset muscle soreness (Table 3.8.6). The reader is referred to Chapter 1.2.

Quadriceps strains

Quadriceps strains represent one of the most common injuries in sports such as soccer, football and rugby. The most common site affected is the rectus femoris, which has two heads of origin, the reflected head arising just above the acetabulum and the straight head from the ASIS. It is the most superficial of the quadriceps muscles and, relative to the other components of the quadriceps, is

Table 3.8.6 Grading of muscle injuries [adapted from reference 8].

Grade	Description	Clinical findings (pain, tenderness and bruising can be a feature of all)
I	Microscopic damage to muscle or myotendinous unit	Pain on stretch and stress; bruising may be evident; no/little effect on range of motion and function
II	Partial tear of muscle or myotendinous unit	Pain on stretch and stressing; palpable gap and weakness may be evident; decrease in range of motion and function
IIIA	Rupture of muscle or myotendinous unit	Obvious gap, significant decrease in range of motion and function
IIIB	Avulsion of tendon attachment to bone	

Adapted from Cattley *et al.* (2002).

unprotected from injury in the form of both strain and contusion, particularly as it crosses two joints.

The mechanism of rectus femoris strain is that of forceful stretch of the muscle as a result of resisted flexion of the hip and/or extension of the knee. This occurs with sudden acceleration or a change in speed, but particularly when attempts to kick a ball are met by unexpected resistance (for instance when blocked by an opponent). Contributing factors include overload (e.g. weightlifting), poor flexibility, lack of warm-up, and anabolic steroid intake. Functional imbalance between quadriceps and hamstrings is also a major contributor. The normal quadriceps-to-hamstrings strength ratio is 3:2 (although this may vary between sports), but relative neglect of hamstring strengthening commonly leads to ratios in the range of 5:1. The usual site of strain injuries is the myotendinous junction along the whole course of the muscle.

In the acute setting, the patient presents with a history of acute thigh pain and reduced function and often a sensation of tearing during the acute event. The mechanisms described earlier are usually involved. There is usually swelling, ecchymosis, and a palpable lump or gap with significant injury which may be particularly notable as the bruising begins to settle. Resisted knee extension is painful and weak, particularly in hip extension if the rectus femoris is involved.

In the chronic presentation, the site of pain and clinical signs may be less specific. The role of imaging has been reviewed elsewhere (Chapter 1.2).

Investigations
X-ray is necessary if a bony avulsion injury is suspected.

Treatment
If there is a large haematoma, ultrasound-guided aspiration followed by compression is helpful in reducing pain and speeding recovery. The usual RICE protocol is followed, with restricted range of motion followed by a progressive stretching and strengthening programme with correction of any functional imbalance of quadriceps/hamstrings. Athletes with grade I and II strains usually return to sport in 4–6 weeks, provided that they have full pain-free range of motion and have regained near-normal (90%) strength. Grade III injuries also settle with this regime, although this can take significantly longer. Surgical reconstruction may be necessary in some.

Quadriceps contusions

The quadriceps contusion ('dead leg' or 'Charley Horse') is distinct from a strain, and typically occurs as a result of a direct blow to the quadriceps muscle, causing a deep intra- or intermuscular haematoma. The injury can occur at any site involving the muscle or myotendinous unit, unlike the typical strain, which affects the latter.

Clinical features
There is pain and swelling, and a sympathetic knee effusion may appear in the first 48 hours. Function, in particular knee flexion, is reduced and rarely an acute compartment syndrome can develop

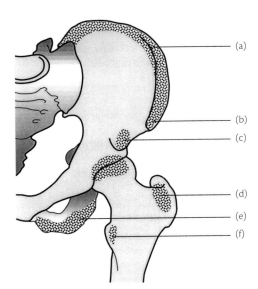

Fig. 3.8.26 Pelvic apophyses are sites of avulsion injuries in adolescents: (a) iliac crest (external obliques); (b) anterior superior iliac spine (sartorius); (c) anterior inferior iliac spine (rectus femoris); (d) greater trochanter (gluteus maximus and medius); (e) ischial tuberosity (hamstrings); (f) lesser trochanter (iliopsoas).

Table 3.8.7 Avulsion injuries within the pelvic region

Site	Muscle
Anterior superior iliac spine	Sartorius
Anterior inferior iliac spine	Rectus femoris
Iliac crest	External oblique
Ischial tuberosity	Hamstrings
Lesser trochanter	Iliopsoas
Greater trochanter	Gluteus medius and minimus
Inferior pubic ramus	Gracilis

with extensive haemorrhage. A dynamic ultrasound scan will reveal the extent and position of the bleeding. If there is extensive trauma, an X-ray to exclude a fractured femur is necessary.

Management

Alerting the patient to the possibility of progressive bleeding into the thigh, with the risk of compartment syndrome, is important. Initial management is aspiration under ultrasound guidance if there is a significant haematoma, followed by ice packs, basic analgesics, and rest with the leg and hip in 30° flexion, mobilizing on crutches if necessary. If the patient can flex the knee to 90° in 48 hours, the prognosis is good. Active knee range of motion exercises are commenced early. When pain-free knee flexion reaches 120°, functional rehabilitation including progressive strengthening is pursued. Return to sport is possible when pain-free range of motion reaches 90% of normal (Ryan *et al.* 1991). The main complications are myositis ossificans and failure to regain strength and flexibility, with a long-term reduction in function (Chapter 1.2).

Myositis ossificans

Myositis ossificans occurs as a complication of a quadriceps contusion when a deep haematoma which involves the periosteum leads

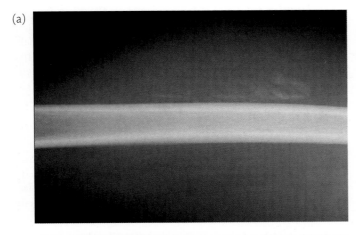

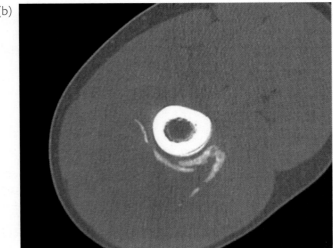

Fig. 3.8.27 (a) Plain X-ray and (b) CT of the thigh showing myositis ossificans.

Table 3.8.8 Radiographic staging of mysositis ossificans

Stage	Plain radiographic changes	
I	X-ray normal (bone scan, ultrasound, MRI show periosteal reaction)	
II	Sandstorm appearance usually around the mid third of the femur	
III	Type A	Stalk: attachment to bone
	Type B	Periosteal: continuity to underlying bone
	Type C	Broad-based: projection into quadriceps with a radiolucent line separating it from the femur
IV	Resorption	

to ectopic ossification. The pathology is poorly understood and some individuals may be predisposed to the development of the condition. Risk factors have been identified and include previous quadriceps injury, prolonged restriction of knee flexion to less than 120°, and/or a delay in treatment.

Clinically, the patient with a quadriceps contusion fails to settle and reports ongoing anterior thigh pain and swelling, often with nocturnal disturbance. The differential diagnosis includes other causes of a mass in the thigh, in particular tumour. The condition is described further elsewhere (Chapter 1.2). Despite radiographic changes, some patients note little loss of function.

Management

Management is symptomatic, with relative rest, analgesics, and graduated active range of motion exercises. Other therapies have been tried without success, including radiotherapy and bisphosphonates. Surgery to remove ectopic bone is rarely necessary and is relatively contraindicated for the first 6 months.

Nerve entrapments

Femoral nerve entrapment

Femoral nerve entrapment is unusual compared with the more common sciatic nerve entrapment. Symptoms include anterior thigh pain with numbness and weakness of the quadriceps. The quadriceps reflex jerk is reduced. The nerve roots are usually entrapped as they leave the spine, or rarely by a massive pelvic tumour.

Obturator nerve entrapment

Obturator nerve entrapment is not well recognized and is considered to be most commonly related to entrapment of the nerve within fascia as it leaves the pelvis. An obturator hernia is another possible cause, along with intra-pelvic masses. The patient complains of pain and dysaesthesia in the medial thigh, together with weakness of the adductor group, worsened by activity. MRI of the pelvis should be performed to assess for muscle hypertrophy or denervation, identify the obturator nerve, and eliminate pelvic masses. Where available, specialized neurophysiological tests or nerve blockade may confirm the diagnosis. Initial management is stretching, lumbopelvic mobilization, and core stability work. Where this proves unproductive, surgical release of the fascia overlying the nerve in the obturator foramen to release the entrapment has been advocated. Neurolysis along the length of the nerve from the obturator foramen to the fascia between the pectineus and adductor longus is required to ensure release (Bradshaw *et al.* 1997).

Meralgia paraesthetica

Meralgia paraesthetica (Greek: *meros* (thigh), *algia* (pain)) occurs when the lateral cutaneous nerve of the thigh (L2–3) becomes entrapped or irritated by scar tissue, or receives a direct blow. The nerve is entirely sensory and supplies an area of skin over the lateral thigh. It runs along the lateral border of the psoas muscle and along the ilium, passing just medial to the ASIS. This is the most common site of entrapment, which may relate to factors such as direct trauma (including surgery in this region), pressure from tight-fitting clothes, weight gain, or pregnancy. The patient complains of a burning pain and dysaesthesiae in the distribution of the nerve. Symptoms may be exacerbated by activity, prolonged standing, or specific postures. Altered sensation of the affected skin is noted and a Tinel test at the site of entrapment may be positive. The diagnosis is usually clinical, although electrodiagnostic studies and nerve blockade with local anaesthetic can also be useful.

Treatment is to address the cause(s) and to control symptoms as necessary. NSAIDs may be helpful, as may local infiltration with corticosteroid and anaesthetic. In severe or intractable cases, surgical release of the nerve by a supra-inguinal approach can be considered (Aldrich and van den Heever 1989).

Posterior hip, buttock, and thigh pain

Hamstring injuries

The hamstrings, and in particular the biceps femoris, are the most commonly injured muscle group in relation to sporting activities. With the exception of the short head of biceps, the hamstrings cross the hip and knee joint, originating on the ischial tuberosity and inserting below the knee on proximal tibia. Anatomical studies show that the musculostendinous junctions of the biceps femoris overlap and in effect span the entire length of the muscle. Therefore any area along the course of the muscle has the potential for injury. Hamstring injury is most likely during fast eccentric loading. The lateral hamstrings (biceps femoris) are most vulnerable during take-off, whereas the medial hamstrings (semitendinosus and semimembranosus) are most likely to be injured during the swing phase of gait, because of the heightened activity in these muscle groups during specific phases of gait. However, the high concentric load through the hamstrings at initial footstrike means that there is also

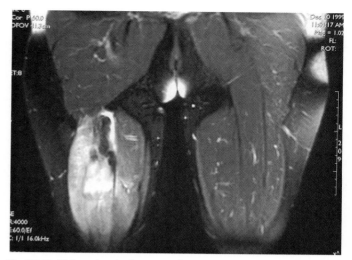

Fig. 3.8.28 T2 fast spin echo fat saturated MRI showing grade III hamstring injury.

high risk of injury at this point. Another consideration is the hybrid nature of the muscle: the semimembranosus, the semitendinosus, and the long head of the biceps femoris are supplied by the tibial branch of the sciatic nerve, whereas the short head of the biceps femoris is supplied by the peroneal branch of sciatic nerve and therefore is essentially a separate muscle. This is relevant not only when considering true hamstrings strains, but also in neurogenic posterior thigh pain.

Injuries include strains, avulsion injuries, and contusions, and occur particularly in those sports that involve high-speed or ballistic movements: gymnastics, sprinting, hurdling, basketball, soccer, and rugby. Injury usually occurs when there has been a sudden hip flexion and knee extension. Poor flexibility, inadequate warm-up, muscle fatigue, muscle imbalance (medial hamstrings/lateral hamstrings or hamstrings/quadriceps), leg-length discrepancy, and previous injury are all predisposing factors. Where injury affects the hamstring muscle, it usually occurs at the myotendinous junction, which spans the whole length of the muscle.

The extent of symptoms and signs is indicative of the severity of the injury. Immediate pain in the posterior thigh with reduced function is noted at the onset, occasionally with a 'pop'. There is ecchymosis and swelling, muscle spasm, and, if rupture has occurred, a palpable lump and associated defect. Where the injury is chronic, symptoms present with a deep dull ache in the thigh and occasionally the buttock. Symptoms are worse with passive or active stretching and frequently with prolonged sitting. Weakness is detectable where there is significant pain and/or disruption. Commonly, a loss of up to 20° of full knee extension in grade I injuries and more than 45° in grade III injuries is noted.

Treatment

Treatment consists of (a) adequate pain management with basic analgesics and modalities such as electrotherapy and ultrasound, (b) stretching and soft tissue mobilization, (c) loading progressing from isometric through to eccentric work, and (d) functional loading (slow return to full sport).

In the acute injury, hourly icing followed by 10 repetitions of 30-second active stretching of the hamstrings through knee extension is followed. If there is excessive inflammation, there is a rationale

Table 3.8.9 Causes of posterior thigh and buttock pain

Musculotendinous
Hamstrings
Gluteals
Neurological
Piriformis or hamstrings syndrome
Mass compressing sciatic nerve
Referred pain from lumbar spine
Other
Referred from pelvic viscera
Sacroiliitis/sacroiliac dysfunction

for NSAIDs during the initial 5 days of an acute injury; otherwise basic analgesics are used. Core stability work starts early, and lumbopelvic mobilizations and neural stretches are used as appropriate to the athlete's needs. Soft tissue release can be started after the initial 5 days and progressive strengthening starts as soon as pain allows.

At least 90% of strength should be regained and the normal quadriceps: hamstrings strength ratio of 3:2 should be set as a goal before a return to sport is permitted. However, this is largely influenced by the nature of the individual's sport and the level of performance. Ruptures can be managed conservatively, but can take 18 months, and functional outcome may be poor. For this reason, some recommend early repair, particularly in proximal hamstring rupture in athletes (Garrett 1996).

Hamstring tendinopathies

Insertion injuries in the adult tend to involve chronic insertional tendinopathies or acute avulsion of the insertion from bone, whereas a bony avulsion injury should be suspected in the child or adolescent with open growth plates.

Hamstring tendinopathies: injuries to the hamstring tendons, tendinopathies, and apophysitis

The gradual onset of activity-related buttock pain in an active adolescent should raise the suspicion of ischial apophysitis, although of course other causes of such symptoms should be considered (Table 3.8.9). Treatment is relative rest, stretching, reassurance and analgesia.

Tendinopathy affecting the hamstrings typically affects active adults. The differential diagnosis is wide, and careful clinical evaluation is mandatory. The typical story is that of a gradual onset of dull ache in the buttock and/or posterior thigh in an active individual. There may be a history of an acute injury. Examination may reveal localized tenderness in the tendon, pain on active and passive stretch, and frequently weakness of hamstring function. Associated factors such as muscle imbalances, hamstring weakness, adverse neurodynamics, lumbar spine dysfunction, and biomechanical gait aberrations should be actively sought and addressed.

Management commences with stretching and soft tissue release, offloading through avoidance of aggravating activities, analgesic and anti-inflammatory approaches, and progressive strengthening through a similar stepwise approach to that advocated for hamstring muscle injuries. Dry needling under ultrasound guidance and/or PRP injection has been advocated to stimulate healing. Corticosteroid injections are also used, but should be avoided where there are severe changes as they may have an adverse effect on tendon integrity.

Bony avulsion injuries

These lesions typically affect adolescents in the age range 12–18 years. There is pain, and in some cases swelling, bruising, and a palpable defect. Some avulsions are subtle but symptomatic. If X-rays do not show a displaced fragment where an acute avulsion injury has occurred, further imaging with ultrasound and/or MRI should be pursued. Rarely, these injuries can also occur in the skeletally mature individual. Management is generally as for grade III hamstring strain injuries. In younger people, non-displaced avulsions can be treated with simple relative rest. If necessary the leg can be protected in knee flexion for 6 weeks using a hip–knee–foot orthosis and monitoring to ensure that there is no further displacement. Displaced avulsions can also be managed conservatively, but

if they are significant, acute surgical reattachment may be necessary. The limitation of conservative management in the younger age group is principally that some athletes can be left with chronic hamstring weakness and/or pain. Where there is a displacement of more than 3 cm, or in any patient where significant hamstring weakness seems likely, surgical reattachment should be considered. Early surgery followed by hamstring rehabilitation is also recommended in the adult athlete.

Piriformis and hamstring syndromes

Posterior thigh pain in the absence of identifiable hamstring pathology or lumbar nerve root compression is a challenge to any sports medicine team. The sciatic nerve can conceivably be compressed or irritated as it travels beneath the pelvic muscles, particularly the piriformis and hamstrings. The 'hamstring syndrome' is considered to be due to neural dysfunction as a result of functional 'compression' beneath the semitendinosus and biceps femoris, pelvic rotation, or lumbar dysfunction. There may be a constricting band in the vicinity of the nerve deep to the associated muscles, although usually none is identified.

Piriformis syndrome is considered to be present when there is sciatic nerve irritation, presumably by a tight piriformis.

Clinical features

In the hamstring syndrome, the patient reports posterior thigh ache, often vague and poorly localized. Symptoms may be present only with certain movement patterns or postures, or may progress to be present at rest. The clinican may find signs of typical hamstring pathology with tenderness (though poorly localized), tightness, and dysfunction of one or more components of the hamstrings. Adverse neurodynamics are usually present, with positive straight-leg raise and slump tests. Lumbopelvic abnormalities such as pelvic rotation should be sought. Gait analysis and dynamic examination to reproduce symptoms are important in identifying the cause, which is most commonly functional rather than structural. Importantly, the cause of the pain may not be related to sport but other lifestyle issues such as prolonged sitting.

Robinson (1947) is credited with introducing the concept of piriformis syndrome, and described six findings:

- a history of trauma to the sacroiliac and gluteal regions

- pain in the region of the sacroiliac joint, greater sciatic notch, and piriformis muscle which usually extends down the limb and causes difficulty with walking

- acute exacerbation of pain caused by stooping or lifting (and moderate relief of pain by traction on the affected extremity with the patient in the supine position)

- a positive Lasègue sign

- a palpable sausage-shaped mass, tender to palpation, over the piriformis muscle on the affected side

- gluteal atrophy, depending on the duration of the condition.

However, many of these findings, particularly the last two, are frequently absent.

Imaging

Imaging studies in the form of ultrasound and MRI are often performed to exclude true hamstring pathology or nerve root compression at the level of the lumbosacral spine. MR neurography is a technique that has been proposed as a useful form of imaging, where the nerve roots are tracked from their origin through the thigh, looking for sites of compression (where the nerve will be enhanced by muscle hypertophy) or signs of denervation of deep pelvic muscles (especially piriformis) or hamstrings due to neural compression. Most commonly, imaging studies are normal.

Management

Treatment of both syndromes involves addressing the adverse neurodynamics through postural work and lumbopelvic mobilizations and strengthening. Typically, hamstring rehabilitation steps as described above are often included in the programme. Epidural injections or selective nerve root blockade may be useful. Of course the cause must be corrected.

Surgical intervention is only very rarely indicated. Benson and Schutzer (1999) described 14 patients with an average age of 38 years, who were managed with an operative release of the piriformis tendon and sciatic neurolysis. All 14 patients had a history of a blow to the buttock, and all had pain in the buttock, intolerance to sitting, tenderness to palpation of the greater sciatic notch, and pain with flexion, adduction, and internal rotation of the hip. Eleven patients had severe radicular pain in the affected lower limb. All 14 patients failed to improve after a prolonged period of conservative treatment with non-steroidal medication or physical therapy, or both. Lasègue's sign is pain in the vicinity of the greater sciatic notch with extension of the knee with the hip flexed to 90° and tenderness to palpation of the greater sciatic notch. Pace and Nagle (1976) described a diagnostic manoeuvre that is now referred to as Pace's sign: pain and weakness in association with resisted abduction and external rotation of the affected thigh.

Spinal referred pain

This overlaps with hamstring and piriformis syndromes. Spinal pain from many sources will refer to the buttock. Facet joints, posterior longitudinal ligament, dura, dorsal root ganglion, and myofascial structures are all recognized as pain-generating tissues. The intervertebral disc also has nociceptive fibres in the outer annulus and may give rise to pain in the distribution described. Examination of the spine aims to reveal signs to confirm the origin of the pain, but investigations such as spinal imaging may be necessary.

Ischial (ischiogluteal) bursitis

Ischial bursitis can occur after a direct blow to the ischial tuberosity, resulting in localized pain and tenderness. There is localized buttock pain and tenderness, although often with a zone of referral. The diagnosis is confirmed on diagnostic ultrasound or MRI. Relative rest, ice, anti-inflammatories, and cushioning are usually effective, but a local guided injection of corticosteroid may be necessary. Surgical excision of the bursa is rarely necessary.

Sacroiliac joint disorders

Sacroiliac problems are common in active individuals but are frequently overlooked and a cause for much debate. The convention is that the joint is extremely stable and, because of its shape and surrounding ligamentous structures, it requires considerable force to disrupt the strong stable construction. Movements are small and complex and there is no single fixed axis of motion, with a combination of flexion/extension, translation, nutation and rotation all contributing. The ilium glides up on the sacrum during extension

with some of the bones anterosuperiorly and the reverse occurs in flexion. However, such movements are very important. During gait the SIJs and ligaments absorb and dissipate stresses developed by twisting of the pelvis due to coupling of flexion of one hip and extension of the other. The results of loss of mobility can include stress injuries or other pelvic injuries such as impingement syndromes of the hip.

Sacroiliac dysfunction is extremely common in females, most commonly in those who have borne children. In the absence of true synovitis, bony reaction or degenerative change pain is presumably due to the stretching of sacroiliac ligaments. Potential mechanisms of onset may include a direct blow to the joint, forceful torsion of the pelvis when rising from the crouched position, or sudden strong contraction of the hamstrings and/or abdominal muscles. However it has been argued that forces upon sacroiliac ligaments are more likely to result in injury to the lumbosacral ligaments.

Pain can be experienced in the buttock, groin, or thigh with activity and, in severe cases, at rest. Stress tests may exacerbate the pain (see examination section).

Investigation

X-rays of the SIJ are usually normal unless there has been longstanding inflammation, or with degenerative change. Bone scans demonstrate sacroiliitis and stress fractures at the ridges of joint surfaces. Where sacroiliitis is demonstrated, the cause must be ascertained, most importantly seronegative arthropathy or pyogenic infection.

Management

Mobilization and manipulation of the joint may help. Muscle imbalances, postural issues, biomechanical irregularities affecting the muscles of the thigh and abdomen, and coexisting abnormalities in the lumbar spine should be addressed. A sacroiliac belt can provide some symptomatic relief. Sacroiliitis as a part of an inflammatory arthritis should be treated with analgesics, anti-inflammatories, physiotherapy, other approaches indicated for the systemic condition, and where necessary local corticosteroid injection under imaging.

Sacral stress injuries

Sacral stress injuries are commonly overlooked in both the general population and the athlete, as they cause vaguely located buttock pain and the diagnosis is often not considered. As with any stress injury, these can be fatigue injuries or due to insufficiency of bone quality. Leg-length discrepancy or local lumbopelvic stiffness or pathology should be pursued. Isotope bone scan or MRI are sensitive imaging techniques. Bone density and bone markers should be considered. In most cases, relative rest is all that is required, but once healed biomechanical assessment should be performed.

Lateral hip and thigh pain

Gluteal enthesopathy and trochanteric bursitis

Enthesopathy of the insertion of gluteus medius and minimus at the trochanter is a common condition, particularly in females, and is often inappropriately termed 'trochanteric bursitis'. The enthesopathy arises as a result of a lack of gluteal strength and the patient may also suffer from lumbar pain.

The aetiological and clinical features of trochanteric bursitis overlap with gluteal enthesopathy, but bursitis is much less common.

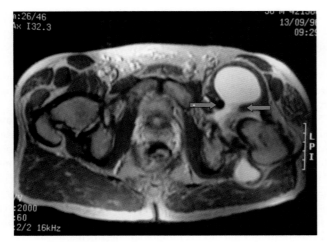

Fig. 3.8.29 T2-weighted spin echo MRI of the pelvis showing an iliopsoas bursa.

The four trochanteric bursae are situated deep to the soft tissues at the lateral hip, protecting them from the bony surface of the greater trochanter. Three of these bursae are constant: the subgluteus minimus bursa lies slightly anterior to the superior surface of the greater trochanter, the subgluteus medius bursa lies anterior to the greater trochanter, and the subgluteus maximus bursa lies posterosuperior and lateral to the greater trochanter. A fourth, unnamed, bursa is also frequently noted. The subgluteus maximus is the largest of the four, and serves as a gliding mechanism to the tendon of gluteus maximus passing over the greater trochanter to insert onto the iliotibial band.

Trochanteric bursitis is also associated with direct trauma, when a blow to the area can cause a haemobursa. Most commonly, however, it is due to overuse. Associated factors include a leg-length discrepancy, lumbar spine disease, and hip pathology, with limitation of internal rotation and reflex tightening of the external rotators. Unaccustomed activity and walking/running on a cambered road may also be reported and are typically associated with a tight iliotibial band.

Investigations

Plain radiography is unhelpful unless articular pathology is suspected, although irregularities of the greater trochanter or calcification within surrounding soft tissues (after trauma) or in the bursa may be noted. Ultrasound may demonstrate irregularities of the gluteal insertions or bursal enlargement, where the differential diagnosis is that of other causes of peritrochanteric fluid collections, namely haematoma, abscess, seroma, or necrotic tumour—all considerably more rare than bursitis.

MRI may demonstrate signal abnormalities in the gluteal tendons, iliotibial band/tensor fascia lata, or the bursae, especially with gadolinium enhancement (Fig. 3.8.29).

Clinical features

Patients report deep aching at the lateral aspect of the hip and proximal lateral thigh, worsened with weight-bearing activities such as walking (particularly walking over uneven ground) and on inclines such as ascending stairs. A snapping, clicking, or clunking over the painful area may also be reported, caused by thickened soft tissues flicking over the greater trochanter. Nocturnal pain when lying on the affected side is commonly noted.

Examination reveals local pain with pressure over the greater trochanter, particularly during passive combined hip flexion and adduction and with resisted active abduction of the hip when lying on the opposite side. In gluteus medius enthesopathy, tenderness often extends to the muscle in the buttock and also in the upper lateral thigh somewhat distal to the greater trochaanter. Gait abnormalities are common but may be cause or effect. Predisposing features include any cause of gait abnormality, including in particular leg-length discrepancy, a tight iliotibial band, coexisting lumbar spine and hip disorders, and other lower limb arthritis.

Treatment

Relative rest, NSAIDs, stretching of the tensor fascia lata and iliotibial tract, and gluteal strengthening are usually effective measures, provided that causative factors are corrected. The efficacy of treatment modalities and massage are unproven.

Infiltration of local anaesthetic and corticosteroid into the bursa or enthesis with or without dry needling can be highly effective. Surgery is the extreme last resort and is rarely indicated. A number of procedures have been described, including the release of the fascia lata, allowing the fascia to heal in a lengthened and tension-free position.

References

Akermark, C. and Johansson, C. (1992). Tenotomy of the adductor longus tendon in the treatment of chronic groin pain in athletes. *American Journal of Sports Medicine*, **20**, 640–3.

Aldrich, E.F. and van den Heever, C.M. (1989). Suprainguinal ligament approach for surgical treatment of meralgia paraesthetica. *Journal of Neurosurgery*, **70**, 492–4.

Armfield, D.R., Towers, J.D., and Robertson, D.D. (2006). Radiographic and MR imaging of the athletic hip. *Clinics in Sports Medicine*, **25**, 211–39.

Beck, M., Kalhor, M., Leunig, M., and Ganz, R. (2005). Hip morphology influences the pattern of damage to the acetabular cartilage: femoroacetabular impingement as a cause of early osteoarthritis of the hip. *Journal of Bone and Joint Surgery. British Volume*, **97**, 1012–18.

Benson, E. and Schutzer, S. (1999). Posttraumatic piriformis syndrome: diagnosis and results of operative treatment. *Journal of Bone and Joint Surgery. American Volume*, **81A**, 941–9.

Bowerman, J.W. (1977). *Radiology and Injury in Sport*, pp. 241–5. Appleton–Century–Crofts, New York.

Boyens, A.M.P., Janssen, G.M.E., Vermeer, H.G.W., Hoeberigs, J.H., Janssen, M.P., and Verstappen, F.T. (1989). Occurrence of running injuries in adults following a supervised training program. *International Journal of Sports Medicine*, **10**, 809–90.

Bradshaw, C., McCrory, P., Bell, S., and Brukner, P. (1997). Obturator nerve entrapment. A cause of groin pain in athletes. *American Journal of Sports Medicine*, **25**, 402–7.

Cattley, P., Winyard, J., Trevaskis, J., and Eaton, S. (2002). Validity and reliability of clinical tests for the sacroiliac joint: a review of literature. *Australasian Chiropractic and Osteopathy*, **10**, 73–80.

Chudik, S., Answorth, A., Lopez, V., and Warren, R.F. (2002). Hip dislocations in athletes. *Sports Medicine and Arthroscopy Review*, **10**, 123–33.

Crawford, J.R. and Villar, R.N. (2005). Current concepts in the management of femoroacetabular impingement. *Journal of Bone and Joint Surgery. British Volume*, **87**, 1459–62.

Czerny, C., Hofmann. S., Neuhold, A., et al. (1996). Lesions of the acetabular labrum: accuracy of MR imaging and MR arthrography in detection and staging. *Radiology*, **200**, 225–30.

Ekstrand, J. and Hilding, J. (1999). The incidence and differential diagnosis of acute groin pain in male soccer players. *Scandinavian Journal of Medicine and Science in Sports*, **9**, 98–103.

Estanwik, J.J., Sloane, B., and Rosenberg, M.A. (1990). Groin strain and other possible causes of groin pain. *Physician and Sportsmedicine*, **18**, 59.

Fortin, J.D. and Falco, F.J. (1997). The Fortin finger test: an indicator of sacroiliac pain. *American Journal of Orthopedics*, **26**, 477–80.

Ganz, R., Gill, T.J., Gautier, E., Ganz, K., Krugel, N., and Berlemann, U. (2001). Surgical dislocation of the adult hip. A technique with full access to the femoral head and acetabulum without the risk of vascular necrosis. *Journal of Bone and Joint Surgery. British Volume*, **83**, 1119–24.

Ganz, R., Parvizi, J., Beck, M., Leunig, M., Notzli, H., and Siebenrock, K.A. (2003). Femoroacetabular impingement: a cause for osteoarthritis of the hip. *Clinical Orthopaedics and Related Research*, **417**, 112–20.

Garret, W.E., Jr (1996). Muscle strain injuries. *American Journal of Sports Medicine*, **24**, 52–8.

Gruen, G.S., Scioscia, T.N., and Lowenstein, J.E. (2002). The surgical treatment of internal snapping hip. *American Journal of Sports Medicine*, **30**, 607–13.

Gullmo, A. (1980). Herniography, diagnosis of hernia in the groin and incompetence of the pouch of Douglas and pelvic floor. *Acta Radiologica Supplementum*, **361**, 229–43.

Ha, K.I., Hahn, S.H., Chung, M.Y., Yang, B.K., and Yi, S.R. (1991). A clinical study of stress fractures in sports activities. *Orthopaedics*, **14**, 1089–95.

Harris, N.H. and Murray, R.O. (1974). Lesions of the symphysis in athletes. *British Medical Journal*, **4**, 211–14.

Ingoldby, C.J. (1997). Laparoscopic and conventional repair of groin disruption in sportsmen. *British Journal of Surgery*, **84**, 213–15.

Kalebo, P., Karlsson, J., Sward, L., and Peterson, L. (1992). Ultrasonography of chronic tendon injuries in the groin. *American Journal of Sports Medicine*, **20**, 634–9.

L'Hermette, M., Polle, G., Tourny-Chollet, C., and Dujardin, F. (2006). Hip passive range of motion and frequency of radiographic hip osteoarthritis in former elite handball players. *British Journal of Sports Medicine*, **40**, 45–9.

Lloyd-Smith, R., Bernard, A.M., Herry, J.Y., and Ramee, A. (1985). Survey of overuse and traumatic hip and pelvic injuries in athletes. *Physician and Sportsmedicine*, **10**, 131–41.

Lynch, S.A. and Renstrom, P.A.F.H. (1999). Groin injuries in sports. *Sports Medicine*, **28**, 187–44.

McCarthy, J.C., Barsoum, W., Puri, L., Lee, J., Murphy, S., and Cooke, P. (2003). The role of hip arthroscopy in the elite athlete. *Clinical Orthopaedics and Related Research*, **406**, 71–4.

Magee, D.J. (2008). *Orthopaedic Physical Assessment*, pp. 617–58. W.B.Saunders, St Louis, MO.

Malycha, P. and Lovell, G. (1992). Inguinal surgery in athletes with chronic groin pain: the sportsmans hernia. *Australian and New Zealand Journal of Surgery*, **2**, 123–5.

Matsumoto, K., Sumi, H., Sumi, Y., and Shimizu, K. (2003). An analysis of hip dislocations among snowboarders and skiers: a 10-year prospective study from 1992–2002. *Journal of Trauma*, **55**, 946–8.

Mont, M.A. and Hungerford, D.S. (1995). Non traumatic avascular necrosis of the femoral head. *Journal of Bone and Joint Surgery. American Volume*, **77**, 459–74.

Moore, R.S. Stover, M.D., and Matta, J.M. (1998). Late posterior instability of the pelvis after resection of the symphysis pubis for the treatment of osteitis pubis. A report of two cases. *Journal of Bone and Joint Surgery. American Volume*, **80A**, 1043–8.

Murphy, D.F., Connolly, A.J., and Beynnon, B.D. (2003). Risk factors for lower extremity injury: a review of the literature. *British Journal of Sports Medicine*, **37**, 13–29.

Orchard, J. and Seward, H. (2002). Epidemiology of injuries in the Australian Football League, seasons 1997–2000. *British Journal of Sports Medicine*, **36**, 39–44.

Overdeck, K.H. and Palmer, W.E. (2004). Imaging of hip and groin injuries in athletes. *Seminars in Musculoskeletal Radiology*, **8**, 41–55.

Pace, J.B. and Nagle, D. (1976). Piriformis syndrome. *Western Journal of Medicine*, **124**, 435–9.

Pecina, M.M. and Bojanic, I. (2003). Stress fractures. In M.M. Pecina and I. Bojanic (eds). *Overuse Injuries of the Musculoskeletal System*, pp. 315–49. CRC, Boca Raton, FL.

Polglase, A.L., Frydman, G.M., and Farmer, K.C. (1991). Inguinal surgery for debilitating groin pain in athletes. *Medical Journal of Australia*, **155**, 674–7.

Provencher, M.T., Hofmeister, E.P., and Muldoon, M.P. (2004) The surgical treatment of external coxa saltans (the snapping hip) by z-plasty of the iliotibial band. *American Journal of Sports Medicine*, **32**, 470–6.

Robinson, D.R. (1947). Piriformis syndrome in relation to sciatic pain. *American Journal of Surgery*, **73**, 355–8.

Ryan, J.B., Wheeler, J.H., Hopkinson, W.J., Arciero, R.A., and Kolakowski, K.R. (1991). Quadriceps contusions: West Point update. *American Journal of Sports Medicine*, **19**, 299–304.

Sampson, T.G. (2005). Arthroscopic treatment of femoroacetabular impingement. *Techniques Orthopediques*, **20**, 56–62.

Sangwan, S.S., Aditya, A., and Siwach, R.C. (1994). Isolated traumatic rupture of the adductor longus muscle. *Indian Journal of Medical Sciences*, **48**, 186–7.

Shrier, I. (2004). Muscle dysfunction versus wear and tear as a cause of exercise related osteoarthritis: an epidemiological update. *British Journal of Sports Medicine*, **38**, 526–53.

Slipman, C.W., Sterenfeld, E.B., Chou, L.H., Herzog, R., and Vresilovic, E. (1998). The predictive value of provocative sacroiliac joint stress maneuvers in the diagnosis of sacroiliac joint syndrome. *Archives of Physical and Medical Rehabilitation*, **79**, 288–92.

Stulberg, S.D., Cordell, L.D., Harris, W.H., Ramsey, P.L., and MacEwen, G.D. (1975). Unrecognised childhood hip disease: a major cause of idiopathic osteoarthritis of the hip. In: *The Hip. Proceedings of the Third Open Scientific Meeting of the Hip Society*, pp. 212–28. C.V. Mosby, St Louis, MO.

Turner, A., Barlow, J., and Heathcote-Elliott, C. (2000) Long term impact of playing professional football in the United Kingdom. *British Journal of Sports Medicine*, **34**, 332–7.

van der Wurff, P., Meyne, W., and Hagmeijer, R.H. (2000). Clinical test of the sacroiliac joint. *Manual Therapy*, **5**, 89–96.

Vande Berg, B., Lecouvet, F., Koutaissoff, S., Simoni, R., Maldague, B., and Malghem, J. (2007). Bone marrow edema of the femoral head. *JBR-BTR*, **90**, 350–7.

Westlin, N. (1997). Groin pain in athlete from southern Sweden. *Sports Medicine and Arthroscopy Review*, **5**, 280–4.

Williams, J.G.P. (1978). Limitation of hip joint movement as a factor in traumatic osteitis pubis. *British Journal of Sports Medicine*, **12**, 129–33.

Williams, P., Thomas, D., and Downes, E. (2000). Osteitis pubis and instability of the pubic symphysis. When nonoperative measures fail. *American Journal of Sports Medicine*, **28**, 350–5.

3.9

Orthopaedic injuries to the hand and wrist

Nicholas Downing

Introduction

Almost any type of hand injury can occur during sport and few, if any, hand-specific injuries occur uniquely during sporting activity. Therefore this chapter will be restricted to injuries that are part of the common spectrum of hand and wrist injuries but are also commonly sustained during sporting activity.

There is a spectrum of severity and complexity of the injuries encountered. Some are minor and simply treated; others are clearly more complex, and require specialist management. Some injuries may appear simple but are not, and require careful specific management if a good outcome is to result. It is important to be able to make an accurate diagnosis and instigate the most appropriate management to return the athlete to optimum function and sporting performance.

The hands of athletes are no different from those of other individuals, but the demands placed on the hand and wrist in the performance of sport may be extreme. This influences the management of injuries and the rehabilitation of the injured athlete's hand and wrist.

Causes of injury

A ball

During ball sports the hand may be struck by the ball which may be hard, like a cricket or hockey ball (Belliappa and Barton 1991), or air-filled (and relatively soft), like a football (Curtin and Kay 1976). The energy imparted to the hand is proportional to the mass and the square of the velocity of the ball. Thus a hard ball of relatively low mass, travelling at high velocity (e.g. a cricket ball) can impart considerable energy to the hand and cause significant damage.

The ball may transmit energy to the bone or joints of the hand, fracturing a bone or dislocating a joint. More damage is caused when, for example, the ball strikes the end of a digit, compressing it longitudinally so that the concave base of one bone is split upon the convex anvil of its proximal partner and the joint surface is disrupted (an intra-articular fracture).

In sports in which the ball is struck with an implement, a hard ball may crush the player's hand between ball and implement, leading to a crush injury with both bone and overlying soft tissue injury.

The ground

During sporting activity players may fall onto an outstretched hand and sustain injury, from a fractured finger to a dislocated shoulder.

Injury is especially common when the sport takes place on a slippery or hard surface, as in skating or skiing. More severe injury occurs when the sports participant is travelling at speed (e.g. in skiing and cycle, motorcycle, or car racing) or falls from a height, as in jumping sports, gymnastics, riding, mountaineering, or flying sports.

The boundary of the playing area

In sports played on confined courts, such as squash, the players may suffer injury by colliding with the wall. This can result in injuries similar to those caused by falling on the outstretched hand; alternatively the impact may be on the back of the hand or wrist, causing a forcible flexion injury and a different injury pattern. In games played on a large field, the player may collide with the boundary fence or an advertising hoarding and be injured.

An opponent

In sports that involve striking the opponent with the hands such as martial arts or boxing, injury is relatively common. Fractures and dislocations may occur (such as fifth metacarpal neck fractures, also known as 'boxer's fracture', though more commonly seen in Saturday night brawlers than in sportsmen). Significant injury to the soft tissues may also occur (e.g. the metacarpophalangeal joint extensor hood injury known as 'boxer's knuckle'). Intentional or unintentional exchanges of blows in non-fighting sports may also lead to injury. In sports involving forceful manipulation of an opponent, such as judo, wrestling, and rugby, digits may be injured by traction and twisting, leading, in particular, to joint injuries.

A finger injury that is frequently overlooked may occur where a player (typically playing rugby) trying to tackle another succeeds only in catching his grasping finger in the opponent's clothing. The opposing extension force ruptures the insertion of the tendon of the flexor digitorum profundus, most commonly in the ring finger.

A sporting implement

Sporting implements are a potent cause of hand injury. A player may be struck accidentally (or on purpose) by an opponent's racket, stick, club, or bat. Injury may also be caused by a sporting implement unexpectedly striking a hard object in mid-swing, as when a golfer's club hits hard ground or a tree root. The force of the impact is amplified by the lever arm of the club and causes the end of the grip to be driven forcibly against the front of the wrist causing a ligament injury or fracture of the hook of the hamate.

Hand injury may occur during shooting sports due to the force of repeated recoil (Jackson and Rayan 2005) or, mercifully rarely, by barrel disruption due to blockage which leads to devastating hand damage.

Assessment of acute injuries to the hand and wrist

As in the assessment of all injuries, it is essential to obtain a detailed history, as the mechanism of the injury will often suggest the nature of the injury.

Clinical examination follows the usual pattern for orthopaedic assessment of an acute injury: look, feel, and move. Bruising, swelling, wounds, and deformity may be seen. In sportsmen seen immediately after the injury, bruising and swelling may not yet have appeared, but careful palpation with the tip of one finger to localize tenderness as precisely as possible is often the most valuable part of the examination.

Palpation of the wrist and hand must be methodical, with reference to the readily palpable bony landmarks. On the dorsum, Lister's tubercle of the radius is used to identify the site of the scapholunate ligament, the ulna styloid, and the insertion of the triangular fibrocartilage. On the palmar aspect, the tubercle of the scaphoid, the hook of the hamate, and the pisiform are readily palpable. The injury may be a fracture of the distal end of the radius or ulna, or the base of a metacarpal. Therefore palpation should start with the distal radius, and progress around the wrist at that level. Subsequent levels of examination are the proximal row of the carpus, the distal row of the carpus, and the bases of the metacarpals.

It is particularly important that care is taken when palpating the region of the anatomical snuff box. It is normally tender there because of pressure on the terminal sensory branches of the radial nerve. Therefore tenderness must always be assessed by comparison with the opposite wrist. The scaphoid is the most common carpal bone to be fractured, but any of the carpal bones may be fractured; all are palpable clinically except the trapezoid. It should not be forgotten that the injury may be to a joint, not a bone; this is especially important because joint injury may not be revealed on the X-ray, and the localization of the tenderness may be the only positive finding. As palpation proceeds along the metacarpals to the digits, it is equally important that tenderness is localized precisely.

The patient is asked to put the part through a full active range of movement. If he can manage a full range, there is probably no serious joint injury. If one is suspected, it is also necessary to examine for abnormal movements (e.g. sideways laxity of finger joints), but it is probably wise, and certainly kind, to defer this until after an X-ray in case there is a fracture.

X-rays are usually necessary, but they support rather than substitute clinical examination. Specific X-rays should be requested; for example, if a proximal interphalangeal joint injury is suspected on clinical examination, an X-ray of that specific joint (rather than an X-ray of the whole hand) will give more accurate information. Similarly, if X-rays of the wrist are requested, standard posteroanterior (PA) and lateral views are taken which often do not reveal a scaphoid fracture, for which specific scaphoid views are needed. In the same way, fractures of the hook of the hamate will be visible only on special views taken for that purpose. Therefore clinical examination is necessary, not only in its own right because of the information which only it can yield, but also to enable the examiner

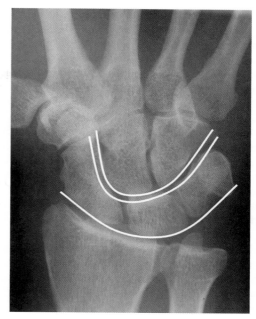

Fig. 3.9.1 A normal PA X-ray of the wrist showing the concentric smooth curved lines of the carpal bones in rows.

to order the appropriate X-ray views without which the diagnosis will not be made.

It is necessary to study the X-rays carefully and methodically otherwise important injuries such as dislocation of the lunate or of the carpometacarpal joints may be overlooked. On the PA view of the wrist, one must look at each bone in turn: radius, ulna, scaphoid, lunate, triquetrum, pisiform, trapezium, trapezoid, capitate, hamate, and each of the five metacarpals. Identifying the concentric curved lines of the proximal and distal carpal rows (Wilson *et al.* 1990) and assessing for disruption of these lines on the PA view will prevent important carpal dislocations and ligament injuries being overlooked (Fig. 3.9.1).

On the lateral view of the wrist (Fig. 3.9.2), one can identify the radius with the proximal pole of the lunate fitting into it, the capitate fitting into the distal pole of the lunate, and the superimposed second to fifth metacarpals, which should be in line with the capitate. At an angle of about 45° to these, one can also see the scaphoid, with

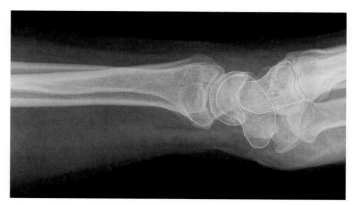

Fig. 3.9.2 A normal lateral X-ray of the wrist. The lunate, capitate, and scaphoid bones are outlined.

its proximal pole overlapping the lunate and its distal pole and tuberosity projecting anteriorly, overlapping the pisiform.

In the fingers, one must not diagnose as a fracture the nutrient artery, the overlapping skin edge of the web between the fingers, an epiphyseal line, or the pseudo-epiphysis sometimes seen at the distal end of the first metacarpal.

After studying the X-rays, re-examination of the patient will give further valuable information. Any doubtful features on the X-ray will be assessed in relation to the clinical findings; a fresh fracture is always tender to palpation. If there are no fractures, the joints should be tested for lateral stability to detect injury to the collateral ligaments. It is especially important to do this after reducing a dislocation.

Occasionally additional specialized imaging will give valuable information not seen on plain X-rays. CT scanning is now readily available and rapid, and can be very useful in diagnosing a fracture suspected clinically but not seen on X-rays such as fracture of the hook of the hamate. In addition, the displacement of scaphoid fractures is better assessed by CT (Lozano-Calderon *et al.* 2006), as is the complexity of many fractures.

Magnetic resonance imaging (MRI) is also a useful tool in diagnosing occult fractures not seen on X-rays but strongly suspected on clinical examination. The presence of bone oedema that occurs in association with a fractured scaphoid is readily appreciated on MRI of undisplaced scaphoid fractures not seen on plain X-rays (Brydie and Raby 2003).

Fractures around the wrist

Fractures of the distal radius and ulna

Fractures of the distal radius in athletes are serious injuries. Usually the bone quality in the athlete is good (unlike in the elderly where distal radius fractures are more common in osteoporotic bone) and so significant energy is required to fracture the bone. This results in greater fracture instability and associated soft tissue damage. The athlete is also likely to put great demands on the wrist, and will desire to regain as near a full range of motion as possible. In addition, an early return to mobilization and training will minimize time away from the sport. Treatment along orthodox lines (Charnley 1950) will require 5–6 weeks of immobilization in plaster of Paris. This management is appropriate for the simpler more stable fracture patterns.

For more complex unstable fractures, more aggressive management by internal fixation facilitates accurate reconstruction of the bone and also enables an early return to motion, minimizing stiffness. Return to contact sports would not be encouraged prior to fracture union, but the athlete could return to training quickly after internal fixation (in approximately 2 weeks).

Many approaches, techniques, and implants are available for internal fixation of distal radius fractures. Recently, the advent of fixed-angle locking plates has enabled most fractures to be reliably fixed through a palmar approach, minimizing soft tissue problems. These devices have revolutionized the management of distal radius fractures (Martineau *et al.* 2007).

Fractures of the scaphoid

Fractures of the scaphoid are fairly common. They usually result from a dorsiflexion injury, they are often missed, and they are prone to develop non-union, even if identified and treated.

Although common and extensively studied, many questions remain about scaphoid fractures. In particular, why some do not unite, the relevance of the blood supply in union, and how they are best treated is not clear. Standard texts are full of dogmatic statements without firm scientific basis, which are passed on to medical students. The scaphoid bone has a peculiar and precarious blood supply that may be compromised when the bone is fractured (Gelberman and Menon 1980), but the precise relevance of this to union is not known (although standard texts will confidently state that this is the cause of non-union and that sclerosis of the proximal pole of the scaphoid indicates avascularity).

In sport, the scaphoid may be fractured by a fall on the outstretched hand, or rarely by a forced dorsiflexion (such as when blocking a powerful shot in football) or hard punch (seen after striking a punch bag more commonly than an opponent).

Clinical signs, apart from tenderness and some pain on movement, may be conspicuous by their absence, and indeed the triviality of the symptoms is the reason why many patients dismiss the injury as a 'sprain' and do not seek medical advice at all—only to re-attend later with a non-united fracture.

Careful examination is important, looking for swelling on the radial side of the carpus, and localized tenderness over the scaphoid (in the anatomical snuff box, palmarly over the tubercle, and dorsally).

X-rays are essential. A sprained wrist should never be diagnosed unless at least one set of adequate X-ray films has been taken. It is frequently said that fractures of the scaphoid are often invisible on the original films, and only become visible a few weeks later after resorption of the bone ends adjoining the fracture. In fact, Leslie and Dickson (1981) found that the fracture was visible on the first X-rays in 98% of cases. However, if a fracture is not seen on the initial films, but the wrist is tender and movement painful, rest for 2 weeks in a splint or plaster of Paris cast, followed by reassessment and further X-rays is reasonable practice. This is good symptomatic treatment for a sprain, and the additional X-rays, often at slightly different angles, may reduce the number of missed fractures. This practice also protects to some degree against claims of negligence for missing a fracture.

Additional imaging modalities are very useful in the management of scaphoid fractures. MRI is very sensitive and specific in the diagnosis of acute fractures. Previously bone scanning was used to investigate the tender and painful scaphoid with apparently normal X-rays. Bone scanning is a very sensitive but non-specific investigation that has been largely superseded by MRI. In the athlete keen to return to sport early accurate diagnosis using MRI is very useful. Further, CT scanning provides accurate images of the anatomy of the scaphoid and gives information regarding fracture displacement not reliably available from X-rays; it is also an excellent imaging modality with which to assess union.

Traditionally, scaphoid fractures have been managed by immobilization in a plaster of Paris cast. The 'scaphoid' plaster is a below-elbow plaster extending to the interphalangeal joint of the thumb, with the wrist slightly extended. There is no convincing evidence that this is any better than the type of cast used for Colles' fractures, in which the thumb is left free (Clay *et al.* 1991). In addition, the lack of thumb immobilization enables more extensive use of the hand whilst in plaster.

There is significant difficulty in deciding when a scaphoid fracture is united, i.e. how long the plaster should be kept on. The bone is too short to test by angular stress, as one would in the tibia. Tenderness is very subjective. It is often very difficult to decide whether the fracture is united or not, even on X-rays taken after 8 or even 12 weeks of immobilization (Dias *et al.* 1988). CT scanning is very useful in this regard and is the most reliable way of assessing fracture union (Bush *et al.* 1987).

When a decision to treat a scaphoid fracture non-operatively has been made, the length of time of immobilization is controversial. The author's current practice is to immobilize fractures of the waist of scaphoid in a Colles' type plaster for 8 weeks and then assess them clinically and radiologically by X-ray. If union is doubtful on either ground, they are assessed by CT scanning. If this shows signs of progression to non-union (e.g. resorption of the fracture edges, developing sclerosis of the fracture edges, or cyst formation), consideration is given to converting to operative management (fixation of the fracture with a headless screw). If there are no adverse signs on the CT scan a further period of 4 weeks in plaster is advised. Following this they are left free to mobilize (i.e. they are never immobilized for longer than 3 months) but are X-rayed 3 months later to assess union. A repeat CT scan may also be useful at 3 months to assess union. The majority of scaphoid fractures will unite when treated by plaster immobilization. In those that develop non-union, a bone-grafting operation may be performed to obtain union, although even this is not invariably successful (Green 1985, Barton 1997).

Clearly, the non-operative management of a scaphoid fracture requires prolonged immobilization in a plaster that will prevent participation in the majority of sports. Therefore there is a wave of enthusiasm for early internal fixation of scaphoid fractures, especially in sportsmen (Rettig and Kollias 1996). A limited ('percutaneous') surgical approach with image intensification guidance, with or without the use of an arthroscope to assess reduction, is employed. This makes it possible to resume sport earlier, as typically no splintage or minimal light-weight splintage for a limited period post-surgery is necessary. Of course, this approach carries the risks of surgery, and in addition it is not clear whether internally fixing acute scaphoid fractures reduces the rate of non-union.

However, it is generally agreed that some scaphoid fractures should be treated operatively, such as displaced acute fractures (best assessed by CT), fractures that are part of a carpal dislocation, and proximal pole fractures (because of their notoriously high non-union rate).

In contrast, fractures of the scaphoid tuberosity are seldom a problem, and need only 4 weeks in plaster.

Other carpal fractures

The most common is a flake of bone pulled off the back of the triquetrum by the distal attachment of the capsule of the wrist joint. It is visible only on a lateral X-ray, where it may look as though it has come from the lunate. This is essentially a ligamentous injury, and 4 weeks in plaster is adequate treatment.

An uncommon injury, which is almost exclusively a sporting injury, is fracture of the hook of the hamate (Walsh and Bishop 2000). It occurs when a golf club, tennis racket, cricket bat, or similar implement hits something in mid-swing and the force is transmitted through the end of the handle to the base of the palm over the hook of the hamate. This lies about 1 cm distal and radial to the pisiform, where it can be felt by deep palpation. If a golf club hits the ground instead of the ball, the impact is severe and such an

injury is likely (Stark *et al.* 1977). It is usually the upper hand which is injured.

This injury is commonly overlooked for two reasons: doctors are not aware of it and ordinary PA X-rays of the wrist are unlikely to show the fracture (Kato *et al.* 2000). A history such as that above, with tenderness localized to the hook of the hamate, suggests the diagnosis. Pain on flexing the ring or little fingers (whose flexor tendons pass alongside the hook) or paraesthesia in those fingers (whose sensory nerves pass over the hook) strengthens the suspicion. The correct X-rays (the carpal tunnel view and a supine oblique view) should be requested to demonstrate the fracture. If pain prevents the patient from dorsiflexing the wrist enough to obtain a satisfactory carpal tunnel view showing all of the hook, the fracture can be readily demonstrated by CT scan, and many consider this to be the imaging modality of choice when this fracture is suspected (Stark *et al.* 1989)

Non-union is treated by excision of the hook of the hamate. The results are excellent, and professional sportsmen can quickly return to full activity (Parker *et al.* 1986). These fractures are rarely diagnosed as fresh injuries and therefore there is little guidance on treatment in the literature. Attachment of the flexor retinaculum to the hook tends to displace it, preventing union even after immobilization in plaster.

Joint injuries of the wrist

A variety of dislocations and fracture–dislocations can occur involving the carpus. All are rare. The least uncommon are the following.

- An anterior dislocation of the lunate which, since it has displaced into the carpal tunnel, may cause acute compression of the median nerve.

- Perilunar dislocation, where the lunate remains in its proper relationship with the radius but everything distal to and around it is dislocated dorsally. It is thought that this is the first stage of the injury described above, after which the carpus moves anteriorly again, pushing the lunate forwards out of place.

- Trans-scaphoid perilunar dislocation (Fig. 3.9.3), in which the scaphoid fractures across its waist and its distal pole displaces with the rest of the carpus, while the proximal pole and lunate remain in the correct position. The dislocation is usually dorsal.

These are rare but serious injuries which may be missed if the X-rays are not studied carefully. The carpus should be realigned as soon as possible. Even if a trans-scaphoid perilunar dislocation is reduced satisfactorily, the scaphoid fracture should be treated by open reduction and internal fixation. Open reduction is required because there may be torn radio-scapho-capitate palmar ligament interposed between the two halves of the scaphoid (Wilton 1987), which would prevent union. This is an unstable injury with a strong chance of non-union, which may be reduced by stable internal fixation with compression. One would also expect carpal instability after these dislocations, which must involve considerable ligamentous damage, but in practice the wrist usually becomes stiff rather than unstable (Panting *et al.* 1984).

Helal (1978) described the condition of chondromalacia of the articular cartilage between the pisiform and triquetral bones in racket sports players—'racket player's pisiform'. The probable

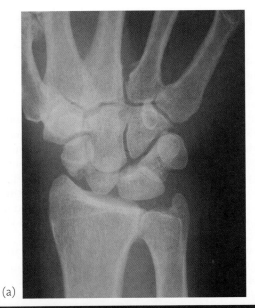

(a)

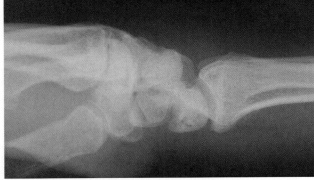

(b)

Fig. 3.9.3   (a) PA X-ray of a transcapho-perilunate carpal dislocation. The displaced fracture of the scaphoid can clearly be seen, and the smooth carpal lines identified in Fig. 3.9.1 are disrupted. (b) Lateral X-ray of a transcapho-perilunate carpal dislocation. The longitudinal axis of the carpus and metacarpals is dorsal to the distal radius. The lunate remains in its normal relationship to the distal radius.

Carpal instability

Damage to the ligaments that stabilize the wrist may lead to abnormal transfer of loads across the wrist and abnormal motion of the wrist. This is known as carpal instability (Linscheid *et al.* 1972). This in turn leads to pain, stiffness, abnormal 'clunking', and a feeling that the wrist will 'give way' when loaded. In the longer term the abnormal biomechanics may lead to premature arthritis of the wrist.

Carpal instability is a complex subject. Simply put, because of the shape of the bones and the ligamentous constraints, the scaphoid naturally tends to flex and the triquetrum tends to extend. The equilibrium of the proximal carpal row is maintained by the ligamentous attachments through the lunate (the 'intercalated segment'). If the attachment of the scaphoid to the lunate (the scapholunate ligament) is disrupted, the scaphoid can flex unhindered and the triquetrum extends the lunate. Hence the radiographic appearance of an extended lunate (dorsal intercalated segment instability (DISI)). The opposite occurs if the attachment of the triquetrum to the lunate (lunotriquetral ligament) is disrupted. The triquetrum is able to extend unhindered, and the scaphoid flexes, pulling the lunate with it into flexion (volar intercalated segment instability (VISI)).

DISI is the most common pattern of carpal instability. In extreme cases, when not only the ligament between the scaphoid and lunate is completely disrupted, but also the other stabilizing ligaments, such as the extrinsic radio-scapho-capitate palmar ligament and the scapho-trapezo-trapezoid ligaments, are torn, a gap appears between these bones (Fig. 3.9.4). Since the instability may only occur when the wrist is loaded, static X-rays may fail to demonstrate it. A series of films with the wrist in various positions is recommended, including a PA view taken with the wrist clenched, thus loading the carpus. Alternatively, the wrist may be screened whilst the patient attempts the movement that provoked pain or

mechanism is a torsional stress on the capsule of the pisotriquetral joint by the sharp and powerful pronation–supination movements at the wrist which occur when wielding a racket, with the racket acting as an additional lever upon the wrist.

Further distally, dislocations and fracture-dislocations of the carpometacarpal joints may occur and are commonly missed (Henderson and Arafa 1987). These injuries are typically caused by punching with a flexed wrist and may be encountered in boxers with poor technique or martial artists. There will be localized tenderness and possibly a palpable step, though this may be obscured by the soft tissue swelling. Careful assessment of PA and true lateral radiographs is essential to make the diagnosis (see Fig. 3.9.2). A pure dislocation may be stable after reduction and be safely treated by immobilization in a Colles' type cast with 15° of wrist extension for 4 weeks. If the injury is a fracture–dislocation (i.e. the dorsal cortex of the hamate bone is fractured), this injury is typically unstable and should be reduced and pinned percutaneously, followed by plaster immobilization.

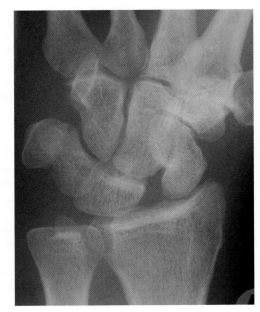

Fig. 3.9.4   PA radiograph of a complete scapholunate dissociation, showing a diastasis between the scaphoid and lunate bones

clicking. If, after X-ray evaluation, clinical suspicion of intercarpal ligament disruption remains, the most accurate way of assessing the carpal ligaments is by wrist arthroscopy (Kozin 1999).

Studies in which injured wrists are routinely examined arthroscopically have revealed an alarming frequency of ligament injury, though the clinical significance of lower-grade injuries has not been clearly established.

The treatment of these instability patterns in the carpus is a complex and controversial subject. It is generally agreed that obvious acute complete injuries should be treated operatively by exploration, reduction, ligament repair, and pinning. The treatment of lesser grades of injury is not so well established. The management of more chronic injuries that are older than, say, 6 weeks (perhaps those missed in the early phase) is not so well established. A variety of techniques for ligament reconstruction have been described (Garcia-Elias *et al.* 2006), but the results of reconstruction are mixed.

Alternative methods of reconstruction include limited or partial arthrodesis (e.g. between the lunate, capitate, hamate, and triquetrum after excising the scaphoid), also with mixed results and usually at the expense of loss of at least half of the range of wrist motion. For further information on this complex subject, the reader is referred to Trail *et al.* (2007), Manuel and Moran (2007), Garcia-Elias (1997), and Garcia-Elias and Geissler (2005).

Some patients complain of pain in the wrist and instability when loading their wrist in sport. A precise diagnosis may be very elusive, even after investigation by MRI arthrogram and wrist arthroscopy. In some cases the symptoms may be due to constitutional ligamentous laxity. It may be impossible to render these patients symptom free during the high demands of their sport. Furthermore, in established carpal instability, even effective treatment may not succeed in allowing the patient to resume top-class sport.

Fractures of the hand

Fractures of the bones of the hand are common, and sport is a common cause. It is probably the most common cause of the end-on blows which result in severe damage to joints.

The essential principles of treatment of hand fractures are the same as for anywhere in the body, and comprise the three Rs of fracture treatment: reduction, retention, and rehabilitation. First, the nature of the fracture is defined by X-ray evaluation. There are many different types and patterns of fracture in the phalanges and metacarpals, each requiring careful assessment and individual management.

Reduction

If the fracture is undisplaced or minimally displaced, it does not need to be reduced. If the fracture is displaced, it may lead to clinical deformity, impede the function of the neighbouring digits and the hand as a whole, and interfere with the function of neighbouring structures such as flexor tendons. In particular, rotational deformity must be corrected, and therefore the finger must be examined specifically to look for this. If pain and swelling allow, the fingers should be seen to flex in parallel, all the tips pointing towards the tubercle of the scaphoid. However, the patient is usually unable to make a fist in the injured hand, and so the fingers of both hands should be studied end-on and the planes of the fingernails compared to assess for abnormal rotation. Unless corrected, the finger will remain rotated permanently, leading to significant

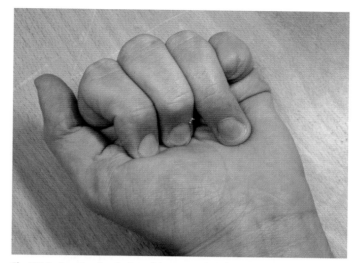

Fig. 3.9.5 Rotational malunion of the proximal phalanx of the ring finger leading to significant deformity and functional disability (although in this case interference with the little finger function is not a problem because of previous little finger amputation).

cosmetic and functional disability (Fig. 3.9.5). Spiral fractures, caused by a rotational force, are particularly likely to have rotational deformity, and subtle rotational deformity will be missed by examination of the X-rays alone.

Some fractures will be reducible closed, but others will not and operative (open) reduction will be necessary.

Retention

Experience is required to determine which fracture patterns are unstable and therefore need external or internal splintage. If a fracture is significantly displaced or multifragmentary, it is likely to be unstable. Stable fractures should be treated by strapping the injured finger to an intact neighbour, which gives some support and protection while allowing movement, with the normal finger acting as a dynamic splint. The strapping must be applied in such a way as to permit, not prevent, movement. If a displaced fracture is reduced closed, its stability should be assessed. If it is stable, it may be treated by neighbour strapping, but if not, reduction will need to be maintained by external splintage or internal fixation.

The hand tends to stiffen with the metacarpophalangeal (MCP) joints extended and the interphalangeal (IP) joints flexed. Therefore, it must always be immobilized in the opposite position, with the MCP joints flexed and the IP joints extended. This position is called the Edinburgh position because it was popularized by Professor J. I. P. James of Edinburgh (James 1970). If the hand is to be immobilized, it is crucial that it is immobilized in the Edinburgh position if permanent stiffness is to be avoided. There are no circumstances in which the IP joints should be immobilized in a flexed position if return to a full range of motion is desired.

External splintage of a single fractured finger can be achieved satisfactorily by a foam-backed malleable aluminium splint. This must be put on correctly, so that the finger is immobilized in the safe position and the fingertip can be inspected end-on to check that there is no malrotation. If more than one finger is fractured, anterior and posterior plaster slabs in the safe position provide the most effective immobilization. A fractured thumb which requires immobilization can be treated in a plaster cast extending almost to the tip of the thumb but leaving the fingers free.

Many fractures of the hand do not need to be immobilized, though clearly the digit should, if possible, be protected from further injury until the fracture has healed.

Fracture union is determined clinically by the loss of fracture site tenderness and pain on stressing the fracture. Radiological union takes a long time, many weeks longer than clinical union.

A small proportion of hand fractures need operative treatment. The indications for operative fixation are debated, and as new systems of small screws and implants are developed, the temptation to fix fractures increases. Well-established indications for operative fixation include the following:

- fractures of the shafts of the phalanges in which good reduction cannot be achieved by closed means; or closed reduction cannot be maintained by splintage (unstable fractures)

- fractures involving joints in which there is either a large fragment carrying a lot of the joint surface (e.g. unicondylar fractures of the proximal phalanx) or a small fragment associated with subluxation of the joint

- multiple fractures within the hand.

The important early management decision is to identify the minority that must be treated by splintage or surgery from the majority where simple strapping to a neighbouring finger is adequate treatment. Failure to do this is likely to result in permanent disability; little delay can be tolerated, as the fracture will begin to unite in the wrong position within a few days.

In the athlete an earlier return to sport or training may be possible by fixing a particular fracture that could be managed adequately by splintage. Each case must be assessed on its own merits, bearing in mind the possible complications of the operative route, including infection and hand stiffness.

Rehabilitation

Rehabilitation is the most important part of treatment. In the hand, rehabilitation should start straight away. In sportsmen, this is usually no problem; on the contrary, the difficulty is to persuade patients with more serious fractures that it is in their interest as sportsmen to accept a period of immobilization in order to achieve a satisfactory long-term result.

In stable fractures, active mobilization within the protective strapping is encouraged. The point when sport can safely be resumed is when tenderness has diminished to an acceptable level. Fractures which have been splinted or operated on may need physiotherapy to help the patient regain a full range of movement. Active exercises should be practised with the hand empty: squeezing a ball or lump of putty should be avoided initially because this promotes redisplacement of the fracture and prevents full flexion. What is required is a full range of movement, so that the finger does not stick out and become injured again; once a full range is regained, power quickly follows.

A detailed account of the management of each type of fracture of the metacarpal and phalanx is available in standard hand surgery texts (Green *et al.* 2005) and so only brief comments on the most common or important types are made below.

Fractures of the phalanges

Fingertip fractures

If the skin has burst or the nailbed is lacerated, the fracture is open and potentially contaminated and must be treated as such. Nailbed lacerations should be carefully repaired with fine absorbable sutures to minimize the risk of future nail deformity. After careful cleansing, the nail may be replaced as a dressing (Henderson 1984). If the fracture is closed and there is a subungual haematoma, it should be released to relieve pain and speed resolution. A paperclip can be opened up so that one end can be heated until it is red-hot and applied to the nail to burn a hole through; this is less painful than trephining and is also sterile.

Large subungual haematomas (more than 50% of the surface area) may indicate a significant tear of the underlying nailbed, and ought to be assessed by removal of the nailplate atraumatically, repair of the nailbed, and return of the nail as a splint (Simon and Wolgin 1987). Generally the fracture will heal uneventfully as long as the soft tissues are treated adequately.

Fractures involving joints

The most common are flake avulsion fractures from the base of the middle phalanx caused by hyperextension injury to the proximal IP joint. The palmar plate that stabilizes the joint in extension is very strong and pulls off its bony attachment rather than tearing itself. The majority of these are small flake fractures and there is no evidence that immobilization improves the outcome. Therefore, provided that the joint is stable, activities can be resumed as soon as pain permits with the protection afforded by strapping the finger to its neighbour (Phair *et al.* 1989).

However, if the fragment is large (and/or comminuted) and the joint is subluxed (Fig.3.9.6), this is a serious injury to the joint and requires very careful treatment. This type of injury is seen in fielders in cricket and in other sports where balls are caught. Typically, the joint can be reduced by traction and flexion in these injuries. In some cases the joint remains reduced in flexion, in which case extension block splinting can be used to treat the injury (Hamer and Quinton 1992). If this technique is not effective in controlling joint subluxation, a variety of alternative operative techniques have been described to treat this difficult injury, including percutaneous pinning (Newington *et al.* 2001), open reduction and internal fixation (Lee and Teoh 2006), and dynamic external fixation (Badia *et al.* 2005). These are serious joint injuries and some degree of permanent joint stiffness is almost inevitable.

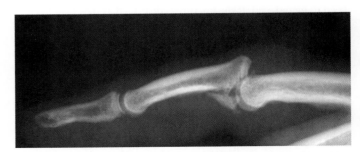

Fig. 3.9.6 Lateral X-ray of an unstable proximal interphalangeal joint fracture/dislocation.

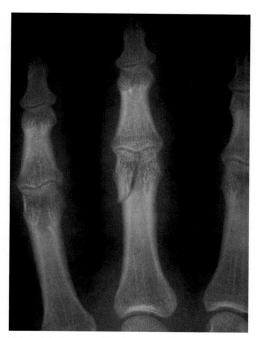

Fig. 3.9.7 Unicondylar fracture of the head of the proximal phalanx. This is a notoriously unstable partial articular fracture that usually requires operative fixation.

Fractures of the head of a phalanx nearly always need internal fixation (McCue *et al.* 1970). The most common are partial articular fractures of the head of the proximal phalanx—unicondylar fractures (Fig. 3.9.7). These fractures are notoriously unstable, and even if minimally displaced initially have a tendency to slip late. Malunion results in significant deformity and functional difficulty that is very difficult to correct. They are best treated by closed reduction and pinning (if reducible) or by open reduction and internal fixation using a lag screw (Weiss and Hastings 1993).

Epiphyseal fractures

In boys, the epiphyses in the hand remain open until the age of 15 or later, and fractures in or near the growth plate are common injuries sustained in sports. A degree of correction of angulation in the flexion–extension plane may be anticipated from the process of remodelling with growth, but it is important to correct lateral angulation near the IP joints and malrotation anywhere because these deformities do not remodel.

Fractures of shafts of phalanges

The palmar aspect of the phalanx is the floor of the tunnel in which the flexor tendon moves. If this is not restored to a smooth bony surface, adhesion of the flexor tendon will result in finger stiffness. The angulation, which is usually into extension, must be corrected, together with any displacement. A skilled manipulation can often achieve the desired reduction. This is performed with the MCP joint flexed to stabilize the proximal fragment: the MCP joint is kept in the flexed position with the IP joints extended while the finger is immobilized. If perfect reduction cannot be achieved or maintained, operative fixation is indicated, especially in the proximal phalanx.

Comminuted fractures

These injuries result from the transfer of a large amount of energy to the digit, and can be the result of crushing injury or very forceful axial loading. Frequently the soft tissues are significantly disrupted. In crushing-type injuries the periosteal envelope around the bone may be intact, so that the fracture is relatively stable and heals surprisingly well with early mobilization. Comminuted fractures of the joint surfaces ('pilon' fractures) are very severe injuries that frequently lead to significant stiffness. External fixation is a very useful technique used in the treatment of these difficult injuries (Hynes and Giddins 2001).

Fractures of the metacarpals

On the whole these cause fewer problems than fractures of the phalanges. Isolated injury of the non-border metacarpals (middle and ring) are stabilized by the deep transverse metacarpal ligaments and the interossei, limiting shortening to a few millimetres and preventing rotation. Metacarpal fractures usually angulate into flexion, and so any permanent loss of movement is loss of extension, which is less likely to result in disability. Malrotation can occur (almost exclusively, and rarely, in the border metacarpals) and, when it does, is serious because there is a greater length of digit distal to the fracture and greater deformity results. Swelling can cause the appearance of rotation (Smith *et al.* 2003), so careful assessment is essential.

When one makes a fist and hits somebody, the impact is taken on the distal end of the metacarpal and commonly causes a fracture at that level (a 'boxer's fracture'), though the force may be transmitted down the shaft to the base of the metacarpal resulting in basal fracture or dislocation of the MCP joint.

Fractures of the metacarpal heads

These are most often seen in the index and middle fingers, and are usually due to fighting. Unless significantly displaced they generally do well with early mobilization. Unfortunately, internal fixation of these fractures usually results in significant joint stiffness. McElfresh and Dobyns (1983) have described 10 different types of fracture of the metacarpal head.

Fractures of the necks of the metacarpals

These are usually the result of fist-fighting, seen in aggressive sports in which fighting is not part of the contest (e.g. rugby).

It is usually the neck of the fifth metacarpal which is fractured, and considerable flexion deformity of this particular fracture is acceptable and compatible with normal function afterwards for the following reasons.

1. Since the fracture is distal, an angulation of, say, 30° produces much less palmar displacement of the metacarpal head and shortening of the bone than would be produced by the same angulation in the mid-shaft or base.

2. The joint between the hamate and the base of the metacarpal of the little finger (fifth carpo-metacarpal joint) normally allows about 30° flexion and extension, as can be observed by clenching one's fist tightly when the fifth metacarpal head moves forward.

3. The head of the metacarpal has articular cartilage over a large part of its surface, and so the joint remains congruous even when the head is flexed.

Any flexion deformity at the neck of the fifth metacarpal can be compensated by extending the joint at the base of the metacarpal. This applies less in the fourth metacarpal, whose basal joint has only about 15° of movement, and not at all in the middle and index fingers, whose basal joints have virtually no movement and therefore cannot compensate for more distal deformity.

Therefore the common fracture of the fifth metacarpal neck invariably does well if treated by neighbour strapping and early motion (Bansal and Craigen 2007). It often takes some weeks to regain full active extension at the MCP joint, but there is hardly ever any permanent disability even in poorly motivated patients (Ford *et al.* 1989). The patient should be warned that the permanent minor cosmetic deformity of a less prominent knuckle will result, but this is only noticeable on making a fist and is of no functional consequence.

Fractures of the shaft of the metacarpals

Often there is little or no displacement, and simple immobilization for 3 weeks is adequate treatment. Marked angulation or displacement may be an indication for surgery, as is true rotation of a border metacarpal. Metacarpal fractures may be treated by a variety of operative techniques, including plate and screw fixation (Fusetti *et al.* 2002) or stabilization using intramedullary wires (Downing and Davis 2006).

Fractures at or near the base of the thumb metacarpal

The most common type is a transverse fracture of the first metacarpal about 1 cm distal to the joint; the metacarpal is angulated into flexion. Since the first metacarpal normally lies in a rotated position compared with the other metacarpals, the injury results in the thumb becoming flexed across the palm, i.e. extension of the thumb

is restricted, and the span between the thumb and the index finger is reduced. Therefore it is important to reduce these fractures. It is usually possible to reduce and hold the fracture in a well-moulded plaster provided that the extension force is applied to the distal end of the metacarpal and not to the phalanges of the thumb (which may merely hyperextend the MCP joint).

Bennett's fracture–subluxation of the first carpometacarpal joint (Fig. 3.9.8) is typically caused by a fall on the thumb or by forced hyperextension and is a relatively common rugby injury. Careful assessment of the X-rays is necessary to avoid missing the injury; the key is the joint subluxation and not the fracture fragment, which may be small. Specific Gedda X-ray views aid in the diagnosis (Billing and Gedda 1952). Although the literature suggests that a surprisingly good functional result may occur despite poor treatment (Cannon *et al.* 1986, Livesley 1990), this cannot be relied upon in the relatively young sporting population. Although traditionally this joint injury has been treated by moulded plaster immobilization, in the author's opinion treatment in all cases should be by either percutaneous pinning and plaster immobilization for 6 weeks or (if the fracture fragment is large) by open reduction and internal fixation (Lutz *et al.* 2003). The latter may allow early mobilization, but not early return to full sporting activity.

Soft tissue joint injuries

Fractures involving the joints have already been considered; the following concerns soft tissue injuries.

Metacarpophalangeal joints

As the thumb protrudes laterally from the hand at the level of the MCP joint, this joint is vulnerable and often injured. Thumb MCP joint injuries are particularly common in skiing, especially on dry slopes where the thumb can easily be caught and wrenched during a fall. If the ulnar collateral ligament of the MCP joint is completely torn, it may displace proximal to the adductor aponeurosis (Stener 1962). It cannot heal with this aponeurosis interposed between the two ends of the ligament, and operative treatment is required. The diagnosis should be made upon the detection of bruising, the absence

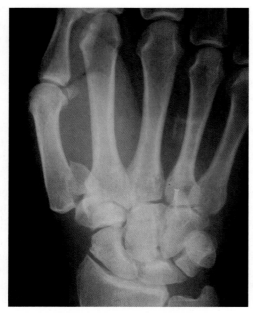

Fig. 3.9.8 Bennett's fracture–subluxation of the thumb carpometacarpal joint. Note that the key element of this injury is the joint subluxation rather than the fracture fragment.

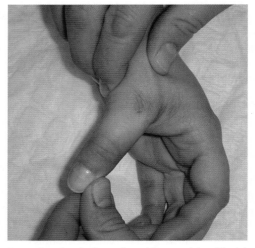

Fig. 3.9.9 A complete thumb ulnar collateral ligament injury. The joint is lax on radial deviation, with no definite endpoint felt.

of fracture on X-ray, and the presence of ligamentous laxity (comparison should be made with the normal thumb) (Fig. 3.9.9). Often the joint is too painful to examine adequately for stability; local anaesthetic injected into the joint will enable accurate stress examination to be undertaken. Ultrasound examination may be helpful in identifying the presence of a Stener lesion (Jones *et al.* 2000).

Occasionally the ulnar collateral ligament avulses its bony origin and a flake fracture is seen on the X-ray. If this is minimally displaced, it indicates that the ligament has not retracted (a Stener lesion is not present) and so the injury can be adequately treated by plaster immobilization for 4 weeks. Of course, if the bony avulsion is displaced proximally, a Stener lesion is present.

Stener lesions must be treated by surgical exploration and repair of the ligament. The adductor aponeurosis is divided to allow reattachment of the ligament. A large bony avulsion fragment (rare) can be fixed with a screw; however, the ligament is generally reattached using a bone suture anchor.

The radial collateral ligament is torn less often. The anatomy is different on that side of the thumb, with little risk of soft tissue interposition, and conservative treatment in a plaster cast is satisfactory except in the more severe cases.

The acute injury (known as 'skier's thumb') is distinct from chronic instability due to an old injury and from 'gamekeeper's thumb' which is not due to a single injury but to gradual attenuation of the ligament over many years while breaking the necks of game (Campbell 1955).

The MCP joints of the fingers are injured less often. Dorsal dislocation of the (usually second or fifth) finger MCP joint is caused by forced hyperextension (Hubbard 1988). This is either easy or impossible to reduce by manipulation. One try is permissible. If it will not reduce, the torn volar plate is probably interposed between the joint surfaces, and this must be dealt with by open operation (Kaplan 1957). Repeated and increasingly forceful attempts to reduce the dislocation are unlikely to be successful, and will probably damage the joint.

Impact to the finger MCP joint during punching may lead to rupture of the extensor hood (usually on the radial side), often with rupture of the underlying joint capsule ('boxer's knuckle') (Arai *et al.* 2002). This injury is seen in boxers, and is frequently overlooked because the X-rays are normal. The patient presents with pain and swelling over the MPJ that does not settle completely with rest. Occasionally the tear in the extensor hood destabilizes the extensor tendon, which subluxes to the ulnar side on making a fist. Acute injuries, if diagnosed early, can be treated by splinting in extension for 4 weeks. Chronic injuries typically require surgical exploration and repair of the defect.

Proximal interphalangeal joints

Dislocation is easy to diagnose clinically and often easy to reduce. It is very tempting simply to reduce the dislocation on the playing field, strap the injured finger, and continue playing. However, it is always wise to obtain an X-ray of the joint because an accompanying fracture makes it a much more serious injury and expert treatment may be required (see above). The usual dorsal dislocation (i.e. with the distal part of the finger displaced dorsally) is easily reduced. The collateral ligaments are often intact, as the base of the middle phalanx has swung round on them like a trapeze artist on his arms, but after reduction the collateral ligaments should be tested by applying radial and ulnar stress to the extended finger. If

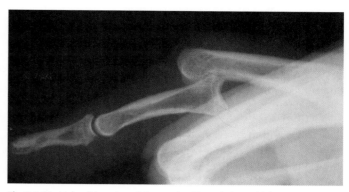

Fig. 3.9.10 Volar dislocation of the proximal interphalangeal joint; a rare injury that must be recognized and treated appropriately or disabling *boutonnière* deformity may result.

the ligaments are intact, it is not necessary to immobilize the finger, and early mobilization, perhaps protected by neighbour strapping, is advised.

Care must be taken during rehabilitation that a fixed flexion contracture does not develop and exercises to maintain full joint extension should be performed.

Volar dislocation of the proximal interphalangeal (PIP) joint is a rare but serious injury (Fig. 3.9.10). There is a high likelihood that the important central slip of the extensor tendon is ruptured. If it is simply reduced and mobilized, it is likely that a boutonnière deformity will develop (see below). This injury should be treated by careful splinting—typically 3 weeks in a static extension splint, allowing distal IP joint flexion (and so lateral band gliding), followed by a spring-loaded dynamic splint that allows flexion but protects extension for a further 3 weeks.

Tears of the collateral ligaments of the PIP joint result from sideways force, for example trying to catch a ball or falling onto the finger. With a complete tear, the instability is usually obvious; in cases of doubt, the finger can easily be anaesthetized by digital block and stress X-rays obtained. Opinions differ as to whether operative repair is required. Provided that the X-ray shows the joint surfaces to be exactly parallel (i.e. the torn ligament is not displaced into the joint) appropriate treatment is to strap the finger to an intact neighbour to prevent further lateral stress but allow flexion and extension.

Sprains are partial tears of the collateral ligament in which lateral stress causes pain but no abnormal lateral angulation. These would appear to be the least serious joint injuries in the fingers, but in practice they are often the most troublesome. Pain may continue for 6 months, and swelling for a year or even more. Eventually they make a full recovery and all that patients need is reassurance.

The **boutonnière injury** is caused by a flexion force which tears the central slip of the extensor mechanism over the back of the PIP joint. This injury is easily overlooked because at first the patient is able to extend the PIP joint using the lateral bands of the extensor mechanism. However, there will be tenderness and pain on extension against resistance and, as the finger is extended from 90° flexion, fixed extension of the distal interphalangeal (DIP) joint (Elson 1986). Treatment is by a splintage regimen as for volar PIP joint dislocation. If the injury is not diagnosed and treated, over the next week or two the lateral bands slip palmarly down the side of the joint and become flexors rather than extensors of the joint as they pass the axis of rotation. A flexion contracture quickly develops, with the joint coming through between the lateral bands like a button through its hole. This is now the boutonnière deformity, which is very difficult to treat particularly when the deformity becomes fixed. Suspicion and early diagnosis is the key to management of this unfortunately frequently overlooked injury (Perron *et al.* 2001).

Distal interphalangeal joint

Dislocation and collateral ligament injuries at this level are uncommon, because there is a short length of finger (and lever arm) distal to the joint.

However, mallet fingers, caused by forcible passive flexion of the DIP joint when the extensor apparatus is contracting, are very common. The injury is not a transverse tear with the ends apart, but internal shredding with the torn ends overlapping but in a lengthened position. The result is a lag in active extension, but full active flexion. An X-ray should be taken as the presence of a fracture may mean that different treatment is required. If there is no fracture, treatment consists of continuous immobilization of the DIP joint in extension for 8 weeks. The type of splint is unimportant, but it must maintain extension of the joint and not be removed for any reason, even briefly.

Stack's moulded polypropylene splint (Fig. 3.9.11), which comes in various sizes, is probably the most satisfactory (Warren *et al.* 1988) and is generally well tolerated. The patient must be compliant with the treatment or it is doomed to fail. There is no place for surgical treatment of the acute injury; the torn tendon is impossible to repair accurately and surgery is hazardous as the overlying soft tissues are thin and prone to wound-healing problems. Late reconstruction is rarely necessary, as even significant extension lag is generally well tolerated and leads to little functional disability. If necessary, the ingenious central-slip tenotomy procedure described by Fowler can be performed under local anaesthetic with predictable satisfactory results (Houpt *et al.* 1993).

If the X-ray reveals an associated avulsion fracture of the insertion of the extensor tendon, the treatment is along similar lines to that of pure tendon rupture except that the duration of immobilization in extension may be shortened to 4 weeks.

Forcible extension of the finger whilst flexing it can cause avulsion of the flexor digitorum profundus (FDP) tendon from its insertion on the palmar aspect of the distal phalanx (Leddy and Packer 1977). This injury is known as 'rugby jersey finger' as it is classically seen in rugby players failing to make a tackle; the digit is caught in the trouser-band of the other player, forcibly extending the finger

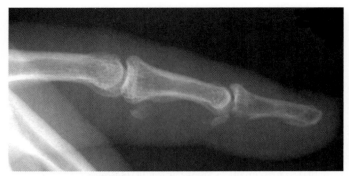

Fig. 3.9.12 Lateral X-ray of an FDP avulsion injury ('rugby jersey finger'). The patient is unable to actively flex to the DIP joint.

against the contracting FDP tendon. Thus the distal end of the FDP tendon, sometimes with a fragment of bone, is avulsed from the distal phalanx (Fig. 3.9.12). It is nearly always the ring finger which is injured. This is often a more severe injury than an open cut of the flexor tendon, because the force of flexion may pull the tendon proximally into the palm, ripping the vincula and filling the empty tendon sheath with blood, which will, if allowed, turn into restrictive fibrous tissue. Therefore primary repair must be performed within a few days of the injury before it is impossible to return the tendon through the flexor sheath and reattach it.

Unfortunately, this injury is commonly diagnosed late, as the initial swollen and stiff finger is dismissed as a 'sprain'. If the opportunity for early surgical repair has been lost, active flexion of the DIP joint can only be restored by a tendon graft, which is an unpredictable procedure. Provided that the patient has full active flexion of the PIP joint (by the intact flexor digitorum superficialis), it may be wise to do nothing and accept lack of flexion at the distal joint. If the DIP joint is flailing and causes problems, tenodesis or arthrodesis of the joint in slight flexion can be offered. Occasionally the avulsed tendon retracts to the palm and causes a painful lump on gripping; it is a simple matter to excise this tendon stump.

Conclusion

Many sports injuries to the hand and wrist are minor and need little treatment or absence from sport. Some, which may at first sight appear to be minor injuries, will cause permanent disability if not treated appropriately. All must be assessed with great care, including X-rays in most cases. It is crucial that the more serious injuries are recognized so that they can be referred to an appropriate hand surgery specialist, ideally within two or three days of injury.

References

Arai, K., Toh, S., Nakahara, K., Nishikawa, S., and Harata, S. (2002). Treatment of soft tissue injuries to the dorsum of the metacarpophalangeal joint (boxer's knuckle). *Journal of Hand Surgery (Edinburgh)*, **27**, 90–5.

Badia, A., Riano, F., Ravikoff, J., Khouri, R., Gonzalez-Hernandez, E., and Orbay, J.L. (2005). Dynamic intradigital external fixation for proximal interphalangeal joint fracture dislocations. *Journal of Hand Surgery*, **30**, 154–60.

Bansal, R. and Craigen, M.A. (2007). Fifth metacarpal neck fractures: is follow-up required? *Journal of Hand Surgery: European Volume*, **32**, 69–73.

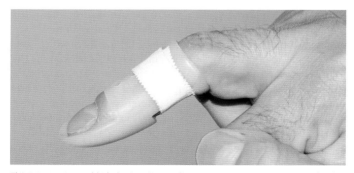

Fig. 3.9.11 A moulded plastic spint used to maintain DIP joint extension for the treatment of mallet injury.

Barton, N.J. (1997). Experience with scaphoid grafting. *Journal of Hand Surgery (Edinburgh)*, **22**, 153–60.

Belliappa, P.P. and Barton, N.J. (1991). Hand injuries in cricketers. *Journal of Hand Surgery (Edinburgh)*, **16**, 212–14.

Billing, L. and Gedda, K.O. (1952). Roentgen examination of Bennett's fracture. *Acta Radiologica*, **38**, 471–6.

Brydie, A. and Raby, N. (2003). Early MRI in the management of clinical scaphoid fracture. *British Journal of Radiology*, **76**, 296–300.

Bush, C.H., Gillespie, T., 3rd, and Dell, P.C. (1987). High-resolution CT of the wrist: initial experience with scaphoid disorders and surgical fusions. *American Journal of Roentgenology*, **149**, 757–60.

Campbell, C.S. (1955). Gamekeeper's thumb. *Journal of Bone and Joint Surgery. British Volume*, **37**, 148–9.

Cannon, S.R., Dowd, G.S., Williams, D.H., and Scott, J.M. (1986). A long-term study following Bennett's fracture. *Journal of Hand Surgery (Edinburgh)*, **11**, 426–31.

Charnley, J. (1950). *The Closed Treatment of Common Fractures*. Williams & Wilkins, Baltimore, MD.

Clay, N.R., Dias, J.J., Costigan, P.S., Gregg, P.J., and Barton, N.J. (1991). Need the thumb be immobilised in scaphoid fractures? A randomised prospective trial. *Journal of Bone and Joint Surgery. British Volume*, **73**, 828–32.

Curtin, J. and Kay, N.R. (1976). Hand injuries due to soccer. *Hand*, **8**, 93–5.

Dias, J.J., Taylor, M., Thompson, J., Brenkel, I.J., and Gregg, P.J. (1988). Radiographic signs of union of scaphoid fractures. An analysis of inter-observer agreement and reproducibility. *Journal of Bone and Joint Surgery. British Volume*, **70**, 299–301.

Downing, N.D. and Davis, T.R. (2006). Intramedullary fixation of unstable metacarpal fractures. *Hand Clinics*, **22**, 269–77.

Elson, R.A. (1986). Rupture of the central slip of the extensor hood of the finger. A test for early diagnosis. *Journal of Bone and Joint Surgery. British Volume*, **68**, 229–31.

Ford, D.J., Ali, M.S., and Steel, W.M. (1989). Fractures of the fifth metacarpal neck. Is reduction or immobilisation necessary? *Journal of Hand Surgery (Edinburgh)*, **14**, 165–7.

Fusetti, C., Meyer, H., Borisch, N., Stern, R., Santa, D.D., and Papaloizos, M. (2002). Complications of plate fixation in metacarpal fractures. *Journal of Trauma*, **52**, 535–9.

Garcia-Elias, M. (1997). The treatment of wrist instability. *Journal of Bone and Joint Surgery. British Volume*, **79**, 684–90.

Garcia-Elias, M. and Geissler, W.B. (2005). Carpal instability. In: D.P. Green, W.C. Pederson, R.N. Hotchkiss, and S.W. Wolfe (eds), *Green's Operative Hand Surgery*, pp. 535–604. Churchill Livingstone, Philadelphia, PA.

Garcia-Elias, M., Lluch, A.L., and Stanley, J.K. (2006). Three-ligament tenodesis for the treatment of scapholunate dissociation: indications and surgical technique. *Journal of Hand Surgery*, **31**, 125–34.

Gelberman, R.H. and Menon, J. (1980). The vascularity of the scaphoid bone. *Journal of Hand Surgery*, **5**, 508–13.

Green, D.P. (1985). The effect of avascular necrosis on Russe bone grafting for scaphoid nonunion. *Journal of Hand Surgery*, **10**, 597–605.

Green, D.P., Pederson, W.C., Hotchkiss, R.N., and Wolfe, S.W. (2005). *Green's Operative Hand Surgery*. Churchill Livingstone, Philadelphia, PA.

Hamer, D.W. and Quinton, D.N. (1992). Dorsal fracture subluxation of the proximal interphalangeal joints treated by extension block splintage. *Journal of Hand Surgery (Edinburgh)*, **17**, 586–90.

Helal, B. (1978). Racquet player's pisiform. *Hand*, **10**, 87–90.

Henderson, H.P. (1984). The best dressing for a nail bed is the nail itself. *Journal of Hand Surgery (Edinburgh)*, **9**, 197–8.

Henderson, J.J. and Arafa, M.A. (1987). Carpometacarpal dislocation. An easily missed diagnosis. *Journal of Bone and Joint Surgery. British Volume*, **69**, 212–14.

Houpt, P., Dijkstra, R., and Storm van Leeuwen, J.B. (1993). Fowler's tenotomy for mallet deformity. *Journal of Hand Surgery (Edinburgh)*, **18**, 499–500.

Hubbard, L.F. (1988) Metacarpophalangeal dislocations. *Hand Clinics*, **4**, 39–44.

Hynes, M.C. and Giddins, G.E. (2001). Dynamic external fixation for pilon fractures of the interphalangeal joints. *Journal of Hand Surgery (Edinburgh)*, **26**, 122–4.

Jackson, T. and Rayan, G.M. (2005). Avulsion fracture of the hamulus from clay gunshot sport: a case report. *Journal of Hand Surgery*, **30**, 702–5.

James, J.I. (1970). The assessment and management of the injured hand. *Hand*, **2**, 97–105.

Jones, M.H., England, S.J., Muwanga, C.L., and Hildreth, T. (2000). The use of ultrasound in the diagnosis of injuries of the ulnar collateral ligament of the thumb. *Journal of Hand Surgery (Edinburgh)*, **25**, 29–32.

Kaplan, E.B. (1957). Dorsal dislocation of the metacarpophalangeal joint of the index finger. *Journal of the Bone and Joint Surgery. American Volume*, **39-A**, 1081–6.

Kato, H., Nakamura, R., Horii, E., Nakao, E., and Yajima, H. (2000). Diagnostic imaging for fracture of the hook of the hamate. *Hand Surgery*, **5**, 19–24.

Kozin, S.H. (1999). The role of arthroscopy in scapholunate instability. *Hand Clinics*, **15**, 435–44, viii.

Leddy, J.P. and Packer, J.W. (1977). Avulsion of the profundus tendon insertion in athletes. *Journal of Hand Surgery*, **2**, 66–9.

Lee, J.Y. and Teoh, L.C. (2006). Dorsal fracture dislocations of the proximal interphalangeal joint treated by open reduction and interfragmentary screw fixation: indications, approaches and results. *Journal of Hand Surgery (Edinburgh)*, **31**, 138–46.

Leslie, I.J. and Dickson, R.A. (1981). The fractured carpal scaphoid. Natural history and factors influencing outcome. *Journal of Bone and Joint Surgery. British Volume*, **63**, 225–30.

Linscheid, R.L., Dobyns, J.H., Beabout, J.W. and Bryan, R.S. (1972). Traumatic instability of the wrist. Diagnosis, classification, and pathomechanics. *Journal of Bone and Joint Surgery. American Volume*, **54**, 1612–32.

Livesley, P.J. (1990). The conservative management of Bennett's fracture–dislocation: a 26-year follow-up. *Journal of Hand Surgery (Edinburgh)*, **15**, 291–4.

Lozano-Calderon, S., Blazar, P., Zurakowski, D., Lee, S.G., and Ring, D. (2006). Diagnosis of scaphoid fracture displacement with radiography and computed tomography. *Journal of Bone and Joint Surgery. American Volume*, **88**, 2695–703.

Lutz, M., Sailer, R., Zimmermann, R., Gabl, M., Ulmer, H., and Pechlaner, S. (2003). Closed reduction transarticular Kirschner wire fixation versus open reduction internal fixation in the treatment of Bennett's fracture dislocation. *Journal of Hand Surgery (Edinburgh)*, **28**, 142–7.

McCue, F.C., Honner, R., Johnson, M.C., and Gieck, J. H. (1970). Athletic injuries of the proximal interphalangeal joint requiring surgical treatment. *Journal of Bone and Joint Surgery. American Volume*, **52**, 937–56.

McElfresh, E.C. and Dobyns, J.H. (1983). Intra-articular metacarpal head fractures. *Journal of Hand Surgery*, **8**, 383–93.

Manuel, J. and Moran, S.L. (2007). The diagnosis and treatment of scapholunate instability. *Orthopedic Clinics of North America*, **38**, 261–77, vii.

Martineau, P.A., Berry, G.K., and Harvey, E.J. (2007). Plating for distal radius fractures. *Orthopedic Clinics of North America*, **38**, 193–201, vi.

Newington, D.P., Davis, T.R., and Barton, N.J. (2001). The treatment of dorsal fracture–dislocation of the proximal interphalangeal joint by closed reduction and Kirschner wire fixation: a 16-year follow up. *Journal of Hand Surgery (Edinburgh)*, **26**, 537–40.

Panting, A.L., Lamb, D.W., Noble, J., and Haw, C.S. (1984). Dislocations of the lunate with and without fracture of the scaphoid. *Journal of Bone and Joint Surgery. British Volume*, **66**, 391–5.

Parker, R.D., Berkowitz, M.S., Brahms, M.A. and Bohl, W.R. (1986). Hook of the hamate fractures in athletes. *American Journal of Sports Medicine*, **14**, 517–23.

Perron, A.D., Brady, W.J., and Keats, T.E. (2001). Orthopedic pitfalls in the ED: acute compartment syndrome. *American Journal of Emergency Medicine*, **19**, 413–16.

Phair, I.C., Quinton, D.N., and Allen, M.J. (1989). The conservative management of volar avulsion fractures of the PIP joint. *Journal of Hand Surgery (Edinburgh)*, **14**, 168–70.

Rettig, A.C. and Kollias, S.C. (1996). Internal fixation of acute stable scaphoid fractures in the athlete. *American Journal of Sports Medicine*, **24**, 182–6.

Simon, R.R. and Wolgin, M. (1987). Subungual hematoma: association with occult laceration requiring repair. *American Journal of Emergency Medicine*, **5**, 302–4.

Smith, N.C., Moncrieff, N.J., Hartnell, N., and Ashwell, J. (2003). Pseudorotation of the little finger metacarpal. *Journal of Hand Surgery (Edinburgh)*, **28**, 395–8.

Stark, H.H., Chao, E.K., Zemel, N.P., Rickard, T.A., and Ashworth, C.R. (1989). Fracture of the hook of the hamate. *Journal of Bone and Joint Surgery. American Volume*, **71**, 1202–7.

Stark, H.H., Jobe, F.W., Boyes, J.H., and Ashworth, C.R. (1977). Fracture of the hook of the hamate in athletes. *Journal of Bone and Joint Surgery. American Volume*, **59**, 575–82.

Stener, B. (1962). Displacement of the ruptured ulnar collateral ligament of the. metacarpo-phalangeal joint of the thumb. *Journal of Bone and Joint Surgery*, **44B**, 869–79.

Trail, I.A., Stanley, J.K., and Hayton, M.J. (2007). Twenty questions on carpal instability. *Journal of Hand Surgery. European Volume*, **32**, 240–55.

Walsh, J.J.T. and Bishop, A.T. (2000). Diagnosis and management of hamate hook fractures. *Hand Clinics*, **16**, 397–403, viii.

Warren, R.A., Norris, S.H., and Ferguson, D.G. (1988). Mallet finger: a trial of two splints. *Journal of Hand Surgery (Edinburgh)*, **13**, 151–3.

Weiss, A.P. and Hastings, H., 2nd (1993). Distal unicondylar fractures of the proximal phalanx. *Journal of Hand Surgery*, **18**, 594–9.

Wilson, A.J., Mann, F.A., and Gilula, L.A. (1990). Imaging the hand and wrist. *Journal of Hand Surgery (Edinburgh)*, **15**, 153–67.

Wilton, T.J. (1987). Soft-tissue interposition as a possible cause of scaphoid non-union. *Journal of Hand Surgery (Edinburgh)*, **12**, 50–1.

3.10

Soft tissue conditions of the hand and wrist

Patrick Wheeler and Nicholas Peirce

Introduction and epidemiology

Hand and wrist injuries represent a considerable challenge for sports physicians and musculoskeletal practitioners. The anatomy is complex and the consequences of minor injury, which are sometimes difficult to assess with routine clinical examination, can have significant impact on function (Hodgkinson *et al.* 1994). Such are the demands of sport that extremes of range of motion, strength, and coordination are required, often in unison. Therefore in hand and wrist injuries close attention should be paid to both the history and the clinical examination as imaging, although improving, may not show functional pathology. This complex structure demands precise diagnosis to ensure that normal function is not lost.

Not surprisingly, musculoskeletal injuries of the hand and wrist are common in sports (Snead and Rettig 2001; Rettig 2003, 2004), with reviews of the literature suggesting that traditional sports including volleyball, netball, basketball and rock-climbing have a high incidence of hand problems (Amadio 1990; Logan *et al.* 2004) (Fig. 3.10.1). Caine *et al.* (1996) found that hand and wrist injuries accounted for 6–36% of fencing injuries, 7–25% of volleyball injuries, 24–29% of diving injuries, and 14–22% of boxing injuries; much smaller numbers occur in cycling and racket sports. These earlier studies suggested that while 27% of all tennis injuries affected the upper limb, only 2% involved the hand and wrist (Hutchinson *et al.* 1995). This compares with 28% of all injuries sustained by rock-climbers affecting the hands and wrists (Logan *et al.* 2004). Not only do different sports have individual patterns of common injuries, but changes in regulations, techniques, and protective equipment change injury profiles within a sport over time (Kujala *et al.* 1995). More recent studies suggest that the incidence is increasing in racket sports such as tennis and also in golf as the forces involved appear to increase (Gosheger *et al.* 2003; Montalvan *et al.* 2006; McHardy and Pollard 2007).

Research in rugby union has shown that wrist injuries occur at a rate of 0.5 per 1000 playing hours, and injuries to the hands and fingers occur at a rate of 4.7 per 1000 playing hours; these figures are for match play with much lower figures for training (Fuller *et al.* 2008). Wrist pain was reported by 56% of gymnasts (33 of 59), with 45% (15 of 33) describing pain of at least 6 months duration. Factors significantly associated with wrist pain included higher skill level, older age, and more years of training. Forty-three per cent of those between 10 and 14 years of age had wrist pain, compared with 44% for those outside of that age range (DiFiori *et al.* 2006).

Injury profiles vary, but common injuries of the hand and wrist include acute fractures seen in football and snowboarding, acute and chronic tendon and pulley injuries seen in climbing, tendinopathies seen in rowing and canoeing, and nerve entrapments seen in cycling. Adolescent gymnasts may sustain physeal injuries and possibly growth arrest (DiFiori *et al.* 2006), whereas veteran athletes

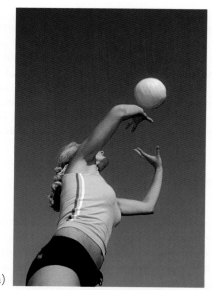

(a)

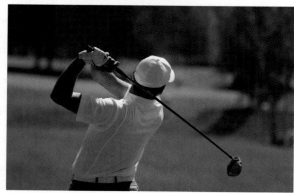

(b)

Fig. 3.10.1 The hands and wrists are vulnerable to injury in many recreational and sporting activities. Part (a) Copyright © Robert Rozbora-Fotolia.com. Part (b) Copyright © photogolfer-Fotolia.com

may suffer from degenerative joint disease. Hand and wrist injuries are also common in wheelchair users, in particular those involved in wheelchair tennis and basketball (Botvin Madorsky and Curtis 1984).

Further evidence of the frequency of hand and wrist injuries comes from attendances at accident and emergency departments, which account for 10–20% of all consultations (Hodgkinson *et al.* 1994; Chan and Hughes 2005), with sports injuries accounting for 15% of these (Hill *et al.* 1998).

In this chapter the common and serious soft-tissue problems that can affect the hand and wrist are discussed along anatomical and structural lines, including important differential diagnoses which should be considered and available management options for treatment.

Functional anatomy

The wrist joint is a synovial joint between the distal radius and the proximal row of carpal bones. The head of the ulna is separated from the proximal carpals by the triangular fibrocartilage complex (TFCC), which also separates the wrist joint from the distal radio-ulnar joint.

In normal subjects the wrist will flex to approximately 80° and extend to about 70° with some of this range of movement being made possible by movement at the mid-carpal joints. As the radial styloid is longer than that of the ulnar, ulnar deviation is greater than that of radial deviation, with normal ranges being 20° for radial deviation and 60° for ulnar. Studies have shown that sports such as baseball and basketball require palmarflexion of 70° and 93°, respectively, and extension (dorsiflexion) of 50° and 32°, respectively (Rettig 2003). The absolute range of motion changes with the expertise of the athlete, and thus accurate assessment demands an understanding of the required range of motion for an individual sport. A spin bowler in cricket has very specific demands on the wrist.

Clinical evaluation

History

As with all clinical assessments, the process starts with a history of the presenting problem with specific attention to age, occupation/ sport and activities, hand dominance, and any previous injuries. Functional limitation should be discussed, including what activities the patient can and cannot do, what provokes, prolongs, or relieves the symptoms, and whether the symptoms are static, intermittent, progressive, or resolving. Certain symptoms may be considered pathognomonic. Understanding the mechanism of injury is vital to an appreciation of the structures that may be damaged and will target the examination and investigations. Unlike deeper joints, the location of pain in the hand is a good indicator as to its source, and although certain neural structures can refer pain into the hand from a variety of sites, these are traditionally thought to be relatively consistent. An understanding of the dynamics of the sport is also vital. Extreme ranges of motion and impact are achieved in some sports and sometimes defy initial perceptions. The ulnar deviation and consequent valgus forces for a pole vaulter, a gymnast, a weightlifter, or a rock-climber are far greater than those experienced during routine sporting hand movements. Sometimes video analysis of the injury is available, and observation

of the techniques and analysis of the forces involved will certainly help in understanding the processes involved, the mechanism of injury, and therefore the requirements for return to sport.

As the wrist forms a vital part of the kinetic chain, it is also important to establish any concurrent or preceding injuries to shoulders, elbows, lumbar spine, or lower limbs. Furthermore, changes in equipment such as rackets, paddles, or rowing blades can all affect the wrist significantly.

Examination

During the initial assessment, and long before a hand is laid on the patient, the examiner should be observing the patient and assessing the use of their hands. Are they appearing to use both hands normally, or are they protecting one with subtle or overt mannerisms? If an initial handshake was performed, this can give useful information, as can a withdrawal from a proffered handshake. This chapter is not meant to be a fully comprehensive examination protocol, but the following can act as a guide.

Look

Inspection can reveal scars, swelling, and bony deformity. Comparison with the opposite hand can reveal subtle muscle wasting. Colour or skin changes can indicate chronic sympathetic nerve dysfunction, and a wide range of systemic illnesses from acromegaly to xanthoma may have features that can be picked up from examination of the hand. Discoloration may also indicate sympathetic nerve dysfunction or, less commonly, arterial occlusion.

Feel

Crepitus (see below) may be palpated or heard. The presence of heat can indicate synovitis, and cool peripheries may be a sign of Raynaud's phenomenon or vascular compromise. Tenderness in the anatomical snuff box can reveal a scaphoid injury, and other bony landmarks that should be examined include the lunate and hook of hamate.

Move

The presence of crepitus on active movement can indicate joint surface damage, but may also be a feature of an acute tendinopathy. Active and passive movements of the hand and wrist can reveal joint surface pathology and ligamentous laxity, but more specific testing will then need to considered. Repeated active movements may be required to highlight an intermittent trigger finger. Resisted movements are used to detect tendon or muscle pathology.

Functional testing

Hand-held dynamometers can measure grip strength, extension, flexion, and ulnar and radial deviation. With improving technology a number of additional functional tests can be considered, including electromyographic studies of forearm or hand muscles (Giangarra *et al.* 1983). These tests can demonstrate peripheral nerve injuries or post-injury weakness/wasting.

Special tests
Watson's test

This is sometimes referred to as the scaphoid shift test, and is a test of scaphoid instability. In the test the examiner fully ulnar deviates and slightly extends the subject's wrist whilst fixing the metacarpals. The examiner then presses onto the distal pole of scapula with their other thumb on the palmar side. Whilst maintaining this pressure, the examiner then radially deviates and slightly flexes the subject's hand. The subject's scaphoid is blocked from flexing by

the examiner's thumb; however, in the presence of scaphoid instability, the dorsal pole of scaphoid subluxes over the dorsal radius
eliciting a click, discomfort, or pain in the subject, indicating a
positive test (Watson *et al.* 1988).

Finkelstein's test

This is a test for De Quervain's syndrome. The examiner asks the
subject to oppose their thumb and then to lightly close their fist.
The examiner then ulnar deviates the wrist reproducing the localized pain in the region of the APL and EPB tendon sheaths at the
radial aspect of the wrist. This can often be uncomfortable in
normal subjects, and comparison with the contralateral side should
be made.

Median and ulnar nerve testing/signs

The median nerve can become compressed in the carpal tunnel at
the wrist. Typical symptoms for this include paraesthesiae in the
median nerve distribution within the hand, typically with sparing
of the fifth finger. Clinical tests for median nerve entrapment
include Tinel's test (tapping over the carpal tunnel) and Phalen's
test, which is performed by passively flexing the wrists and holding
this position for 1 minute. Both tests can be considered positive if
there are paraesthesiae in the lateral three and a half digits. Specific
tests for adverse neural tension can also be performed, with specific
testing for median, ulnar, and radial nerves; positive tests reproduce the patient's symptoms.

The clinical signs for other conditions are dealt with below under
the respective subheadings.

X-rays

In the presence of trauma, AP and lateral X-ray views of the hand
and wrist can sometimes be useful for assessing bony injuries of
either the carpus or the distal ulna and radius. Fractures of the
scaphoid are the most common carpal fracture (Phillips *et al.*
2004), but X-rays are notoriously unreliable in the acute setting
with one study showing 20% of non-fractured scaphoids being
reported as fractures by emergency department staff on initial
X-ray (Dias *et al.* 1990). Specific scaphoid views should be requested
if this diagnosis is considered and can often be normal for at least a
week following injury. To avoid the consequences of a missed fracture the hand may need to be immobilized for 1–2 weeks before
repeat X-rays are obtained. A carpal tunnel view can be carried out
to investigate suspected hook of hamate fractures and the ridge of
the trapezium. Extension and flexion views can also be helpful
when there is a suspicion of ulna instability.

Diagnostic ultrasound

Ultrasound (US) is a useful diagnostic tool for tendon injuries in
the hand and wrist, as well as inflammatory arthropathies. It can be
used in the assessment of injuries to the TFCC, although accurate
detection of traumatic lesions of the TFCC is technically difficult.
US has the advantage of being quick and cheap to perform, and as
it does not require ionizing radiation is thought to be safe. It can
also be performed dynamically, which will potentially give a better
assessment of function. However, it is operator dependent and, as
with all imaging, the results should be placed within the clinical
context. Increasingly US is being used to provide information on
the dynamic properties of ligaments, tendons, and joints. Subtle
changes in the laxity of the ulnar collateral ligament of the wrist
may best be assessed through US, comparing loading of the injured

and non-injured wrist. This is particularly evident in the hand,
where interphalangeal ligaments are very easily imaged and compared. Ganglions and small dorsal impaction cysts are often more
easily visualized on US, and if injections are considered it provides
appropriate precision. Doppler US also allows assessment of neo-
vascularity commonly associated with synovitis and tendinopathy.
This has seen an improvement in the early detection of arthritides,
both inflammatory and osteoarthritic, where additional information is also provided on previously undetected small erosions and
osteophytes.

MRI

It is not uncommon for there to be doubt about the mechanism of
the injury and even for the clinical findings to be uncertain. MRI
provides not only a very effective screening tool, but a diagnostic
tool when directed appropriately. MRI images of the hand and
wrist are improving with better sequences and specific hand and
wrist coils. MRI is a useful investigation for a wide range of conditions that affect the hand and wrist, including ligamentous and
bony injuries, and soft tissue masses. Partial tears of intrinsic ligament structures can be missed on an MRI and there may be a role
for higher-quality 3 T MRI scanners and/or an MRI-arthrogram.
Contrast leakage is often diagnostic for carpal ligament disruption.
Ultimately, wrist arthroscopy is now considered the gold standard
for diagnosis of ligament tears (Fig. 3.10.3).

Specific disorders

Within each sport a high suspicion may be needed for certain
injuries (Table 3.10.1). The pattern of injuries always requires
updating, and newer sports such as snowboarding require attention to trends and new information.

Extensor wrist pain

At the wrist the extensor tendons are in six distinct fascial compartments. They lie as described in Table 3.10.2.

A 'stenosing tenovaginitis' of the first extensor compartment
containing the tendons of abductor pollicis longus and extensor
pollicis brevis was described by Fitz de Quervain in 1895, and it
has borne his name ever since. De Quervain's syndrome is most
commonly seen in middle age, but mothers of young children are
also at risk of developing this condition from carrying babies for a
prolonged period in a relatively supinated wrist position. De
Quervain's syndrome is the most common cause of radial-sided
wrist pain in athletes, affecting tennis players, canoeists, and rowers particularly, as well as the leading hand of golfers. Patients commonly present with discomfort and swelling over the radial aspect
of the wrist at the level of the radial styloid, and in the acute phase
a tendinous crepitus can be also felt. Finkelstein's test (described
above) is typically painful, reproducing their symptoms. Treatments
can include analgesia/NSAIDs, splinting, modification of activities,
corticosteroid injections into the tendon sheath, and rarely surgery.
Differential diagnoses are intersection syndrome and osteoarthritis
of the first carpometacarpal joint, both of which are discussed
elsewhere.

The tendon of the extensor pollicis longus, which lies in the third
extensor compartment, can rupture either acutely in trauma or
more commonly as a consequence of gradual damage from a fracture at the radial styloid such as a minimally displaced Colles' type

Table 3.10.1 Sports-specific wrist and hand injuries

Sport	Common injuries	References
Tennis	FCU rupture/partial tears Triangular fibrocartilage injuries Extensor tendon injuries	Montalvan et al. 2006 Maquirriain et al. 2007
Golf	Hook of hamate fracture/stress fracture TFCC injuries Ulnar neuropathy	Gosheger et al. 2003 McHardy and Pollard 2004 Hsu et al. 2005
Gymnastics	Dorsal impaction syndrome/ganglia Distal radius stress injuries Scaphoid impaction syndrome Scaphoid stress reactions/fractures Capitate avascular necrosis Carpal instability Triangular fibrocartilage complex tears Ulnar impaction syndrome Luno-triquetral impingement	Webb and Rettig 2008 DiFiori et al. 2006
Rock-climbing	Proximal interpahalangeal injuries (23% of all injuries) Digital flexor tendon pulley sheath tears IPJ osteoarthritis Collateral ligament tears of the IPJ	Jones et al. 2008
Rowing, canoeing	Intersection syndrome Exertional compartment syndrome De Quervain's syndrome Tenosynovitis of the wrist extensors	Rumball et al. 2005
Rugby, American football	Distal ulnar/radial fractures Gamekeeper's/skier's thumb' Ulnar collateral ligament injuries	Brophy et al. 2007
Boxing	Widespread IPJ thumb injuries Widespread metacarpal injuries/fractures Boxer's knuckle/disruption of extensor hood	Hame and Melone 2000
Volleyball, basketball	Pisiform stress fractures De Quervain's syndrome	Rossi et al. 2005
Platform diving	Dorsal impaction syndrome Carpal instability	le Viet et al. 1993
Snowboarding, in-line skating, skateboarding	Wrist fractures (25% of all injuries) First MTP injuries (dry ski slope)	Russell et al. 2007 Wilson and McGinty 1993

FCU, flexor carpi ulnaris; TFCC, triangular fibrocartilage complex; IPJ, interphalangeal joint

Table 3.10.2 Location of extensor tendons

Compartment	Tendons
First	Abductor pollicis longus (APL) Extensor pollicis brevis (EPB)
Second	Extensor carpi radialis longus (ECRL) Extensor carpi radialis brevis (ECRB)
Third	Extensor pollicis longus (EPL)
Fourth	Extensor digitorum Extensor indices
Fifth	Extensor digiti minimi
Sixth	Extensor carpi ulnaris (ECU)

fracture. More commonly a tendinopathy can present with features including pain with passive thumb flexion and resisted thumb extension.

The extensor carpi ulnaris (ECU) lies in the sixth extensor compartment, and is a common cause of ulnar-sided wrist pain. It can develop an inflammatory tendinopathy leading to rupture in inflammatory joint diseases such as rheumatoid arthritis, and can develop a degenerative tendinopathy in overuse activities including golf and tennis (Fig. 3.10.2). It presents with pain overlying the ulnar aspect of the wrist, particularly with passive radial deviation in pronation. Other causes of ulnar-sided wrist pain, which will be discussed later, include the inferior radio-ulnar joint and damage to the TFCC or the ulnar collateral ligament. Erosion of the floor of the sixth compartment is a diagnosis of exclusion in chronic ulnar-sided pain (Carneiro et al. 2005).

Carpal instability, scapholunate dissociation, and others

Damage to the scapholunate ligament can often be missed in the acute presentation. It tends to follow a fall onto an outstretched hyperextended wrist, with the brunt of the impact typically borne on the thenar eminence (Beckenbaugh 1984; Tiel-van Buul et al. 1993). However, this is not always the case, as demonstrated in the case report of an atraumatic rupture in an elite rock-climber (Valbuena et al. 2008). Complete ligament rupture can cause scapholunate instability, which if left untreated can progress to a SLAC (scapholunate advanced collapse) wrist, which is a catastrophic consequence with respect to hand function.

Clinical examination for scapholunate instability includes Watson's test, as discussed above. However, while Watson's test is the best known of the clinical tests for scaphoid subluxation, it has a low sensitivity, low specificity, and a false-positive rate of up to 20% (Watson and Black 1987; Watson et al. 1988; Tiel-van Buul et al. 1993).

Plain X-rays may be normal in the early stages, but a stress view, such as the clenched fist PA view, which shows a scapholunate gap of more than 3 mm is suggestive of a rupture of the scapholunate ligament. MRI and MR arthrography may be more sensitive investigations. Early investigation and prompt treatment are required.

Another less common carpal instability is the lunotriquetral instability, which may be caused either by a hyperpronation injury or more often after a hyperextension stress with an impact on the

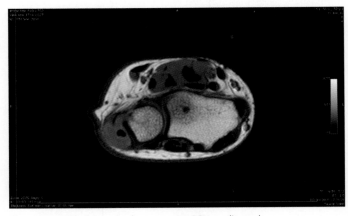

Fig. 3.10.2 MRI of the wrist demonstrating ECU tendinopathy.

ulnar side (Reagan *et al.* 1984; Taleisnik 1988; Pin *et al.* 1989). This injury tends to present with localized ulnar-sided pain, particularly on active pronation–supination against resistance.

A full description of carpal instabilities is beyond the scope of this chapter but can be found in a large number of reviews (http://www.maitrise-orthop.com/corpusmaitri/orthopaedic/dumontier_synth/dumontier_us.shtml).

Triangular fibrocartilage complex injury

The TFCC lies on the ulnar aspect of the wrist between the distal ulna and the carpals, and acts as a main stabilizer of the distal radio-ulnar joint. It is a common site of ulnar aspect wrist pain, and is made up of the triangular fibrocartilage, the ulnar collateral ligament of the wrist, the extensor carpi ulnaris tendon sheath, and various carpal ligaments. The TFCC can be torn by compressive load on the wrist, particularly in any degree of ulnar deviation, and this is more common in sports such as gymnastics, racket sports, golf, and diving. Patients will complain on ulnar-sided wrist pain, as well as pain on resisted ulnar deviation or wrist extension. Examination will often reveal localized pain, particularly on passive ulnar deviation. Investigations can include MRI (Fig. 10.3.3) although partial tears may not be seen. Management options include analgesia, wrist braces, and if necessary arthroscopic surgery and debridement. Subjects with a relatively long ulna compared with the radius are more at risk of a TFCC injury and ulnar impaction syndrome, and may require ulnar-shortening procedures in the event of a TFCC injury.

Synovitis

The hand and wrist are common sites for inflammatory joint disease, and these are important diagnoses that must not be overlooked. Rheumatoid arthritis may present with involvement of the proximal interphalangeal joints (PIPJs), before progressing to the metacarpophalangeal joints (MCPJs). Typically the presentation is insidious and symmetrical, with joint swelling and early morning stiffness being key features. Later laxity of the collateral ligaments of the MCPJs leads to ulnar deviation and joint subluxation. Ultrasound is useful to demonstrate synovitis and erosions, and early and aggressive treatment with disease-modifying drugs is now standard practice.

Dorsal wrist impingement

Dorsal wrist impingement is a spectrum of extensor/dorsal wrist discomfort associated with sports that has also been referred to as scaphoid impingement, dorsal wrist ganglion, and extensor retinaculum impingement. This variety of terminology reflects the diverse nature of the pathological causes of wrist pain with forced/loaded extension. Often the onset is gradual with an absence of an acute injury. Pain is usually reproduced by forced extension, such as floor and vault work in gymnastics, handstands in diving, weightlifting in training, and press-ups. Discomfort is usually palpable over the extensor retinaculum or the proximal carpal row including scaphoid or lunate. Sometimes a small ganglion is palpable or bossing can be present on the impinging carpal bone (Fig. 3.10.4). Occasionally X-rays can demonstrate bony osteophytes, but it is not uncommon for most imaging including US and MRI to be normal. However, MRI will help clarify soft tissue or bony impingement from the alternative diagnoses outlined in Table 3.10.3. Ultrasound demonstrates active inflammation as well as tenosynovitis. It can also exclude tendon rupture.

Management may simply be to explore techniques such as weightlifting alteration, modification of training load, and wrist bracing. Soft tissue conditions may respond well to local cortisone injections. They may occasionally need surgical exploration.

Osteoarthritis of the first carpometacarpal joint

In the early stages, osteoarthritis of the first carpometacarpal (CMC) joint can sometimes be mistaken for De Quervain's tenovaginitis. It presents with pain in the anatomical snuff box and can impair thumb movements and pincer grip, even before progressing

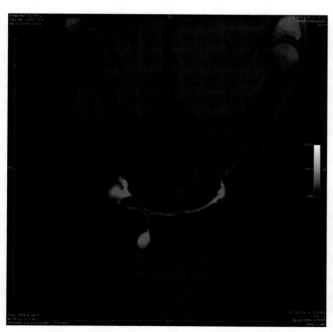

Fig. 3.10.3 Coronal MR arthrogram of the wrist demonstrating a focal TFCC tear.

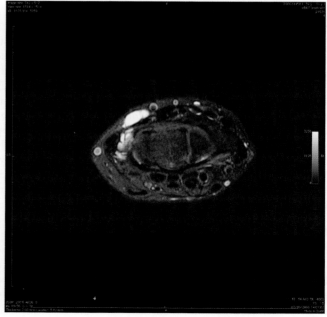

Fig. 3.10.4 MRI of the wrist demonstrating a dorsal wrist ganglion.

Table 3.10.3 Extensor wrist pain

Dorsal wrist impingement
Soft tissue
Dorsal ganglion
Carpal instability
Retinacular impingement
Extensor tenosynovitis
Carpal instability
Radio-ulna instability
TFCC tears
Inflammatory arthropathy/synovitis
Bone
Carpal bossing/osteophytes
Carpal/stress injury
Carpal avascular necrosis
Osteochondral injury
Radial physeal injuries
Carpal impaction
Radial and ulna stress injuries
Ulnar abutment syndrome
Extensor tendinopathy/subluxation

TFCC, triangular fibrocartilage complex

to the classical squared-off appearance. Provocation tests include loading the joint by axially compressing the thumb, which should reproduce their symptoms; care should be taken as this procedure can be very painful. Treatment depends on the functional severity, but can include modified rest, pain relief, splinting, injections, or surgery.

Distal radio-ulnar joint

The radius and ulna articulate proximally and distally, At the wrist, degeneration of the distal radio-ulnar joint will lead to a progressive painful loss of pronation and supination of the wrist. In addition, the distal radio-ulnar joint is vulnerable to dislocation either dorsally, which will inhibit supination, or to the volar side, which blocks pronation. An acute simple dislocation can often spontaneously relocate, or may need simple manipulation followed by immobilization. Chronic and recurrent dislocations can be associated with distal radius malunion or may follow injury. Initially, chronic dislocation is dynamic in nature, but degenerative changes develop later and the dislocation remains static. Surgical intervention may be required.

Keinboch's disease (avascular necrosis of the lunate)

Keinboch's disease ultimately leads to fragmentation and collapse of the lunate. It is rare, occurring most frequently after a trauma to the wrist leading to vascular compromise. This can be classified into four radiographic stages, from a normal radiograph up to fragmentation and secondary degenerative change. There remains a lack of consensus on the most appropriate method of treatment

of the more severe condition, including surgical removal of the lunate and/or fragments and ulnar shortening procedures. Readers are directed to more specific orthopaedic hand surgery textbooks for detailed discussion of this condition,

Lateral wrist pain

De Quervain's tenovaginitis is dealt with above.

Intersection syndrome (also known as 'oarsman's wrist')

Intersection syndrome occurs proximal to the extensor retinaculum at the point where the tendons of the first extensor compartment (APL and EPB) cross those of the second (ECRB and ECRL), causing a supposed bursitis. It presents with pain, swelling, and often crepitus at this location, which is proximal to that of De Quervain's syndrome. Intersection syndrome commonly affects canoeists and rowers. Treatment involves relative rest and modification of training and equipment, with or without an injection of corticosteroid. Conservative treatment is highly successful, but rarely surgical decompression is required.

Superficial radial nerve entrapment, median nerve entrapment, scaphoid impingement, and fractures are dealt with elsewhere.

Flexor wrist pain

Flexor tenosynovitis

The most common flexor tendon to be injured in a sporting group is the flexor carpi ulnaris (FCU), the two heads of which insert via the pisiform into the hook of the hamate and the base of the fifth metacarpal. Problems can arise from repetitive flexion and loading or impact of the wrist such as can be seen in racket sports, cricket and golf. Patients tend to present with pain just proximal to the pisiform, and passive compression of pisiform against triquetral may reproduce their symptoms, as can passive stretching of the FCU by combined wrist extension and radial deviation. The adjacent Guyon canal can also be involved, causing localized compression of the ulnar nerve. Treatments include relative rest and modified activity, wrist braces, or local corticosteroid injections. Partial ruptures of the flexor tendons also appear to be increasing with the increasing forces seen in both golf and tennis. Shot putters may also be at risk of strain to the flexor muscles of the wrist and fingers as a result of wrist hyperextension from the inertia of the shot (Caine *et al.* 1996). In all these diagnoses US and/or MRI will help with an accurate clinical assessment.

TFCC injury, carpal instabilities, median nerve lesion, and fractures are dealt with elsewhere.

Medial wrist pain

FCU tenosynovitis, ulnar neuritis, carpal instability, and fractures are dealt with elsewhere.

Sagittal band rupture and boxer's knuckle

Boxer's knuckle is a tear of the MCPJ capsule which occurs while punching. It is frequently associated with rupture of the sagittal band, which is a portion of the complex retinacular system proximal to the MCPJs (Young 2000). Subsequently, subluxation of the extensor tendons occurs and, as the diagnosis is often delayed, this leads to chronic tendinopathy of the extensor tendons. Therefore, if there is disruption, surgical repair of the extensor hood formed by the capsule and the sagittal band is recommended using either anatomical repair or grafting (Montalvan *et al.* 2006).

Thumb pain

UCL sprain/rupture of first MCPJ

A partial or complete rupture of the ulnar collateral ligament (UCL) of the MCPJ of the thumb is also known as 'gamekeeper's thumb' (when there is chronic attenuation of the ligament) or 'skier's thumb' (following an acute injury). In the acute situation, it is typically caused by forced abduction and extension of the thumb, and is the most common of all injuries in adolescent skiers (Deibert *et al.* 1998). Typically, there is tenderness over the UCL and laxity when compared with the opposite side. If left untreated, it can result in weakness of the pincer grip due to instability of the first MCPJ. Examination reveals laxity of the UCL, with US being helpful in cases of uncertainty.

Treatment is guided by the severity of the instability, from immobilization for minor degrees to surgical repair for a complete rupture (Stener lesion). Even following surgery, splinting may be required on return to sport to minimize the chances of a recurrence.

Bowler's thumb

Radial collateral ligament injuries of the thumb are far less common than those of the ulnar side. Treatment tends to be conservative with immobilization of the joint for 6 weeks to allow healing to occur.

Median nerve lesions, cervical spinal radiculopathy, and fractures are dealt with elsewhere.

Finger pain

Flexor tenosynovitis

A tenosynovitis, or more accurately a stenosing tenovaginitis, of the finger flexors can result in a condition known as trigger finger (or trigger thumb.) In this condition the affected tendon becomes jammed at the level of the A1 pulley, and the finger becomes transiently 'stuck' in a flexed position before releasing into extension with a sudden jolt. In some cases the affected finger can require the use of the other hand to free it or cannot be extended actively. Treatment for flexor tenovaginitis is either local corticosteroid injection or surgical release. Typically, this affects subjects in their middle age, but can follow hand injury. In a sporting environment, injuries to the flexor tendons or pulleys are the most common hand injuries in climbers (Logan *et al.* 2004).

Mallet finger (avulsion of extensor tendon)

This is an avulsion injury of the extensor tendon at the base of the distal phalanx of a finger, and is typically caused by a forced flexion injury. It may be evident on examination by a loss of active extension of the distal phalanx, and if the avulsion has included a piece of bone this may be visible on an X-ray. Treatment is either by splinting the finger in extension within a mallet splint for at least 6 weeks, or by surgical repair.

Jersey finger (avulsion of FDP)

Avulsion of the flexor digitorum profundus (FDP) tendon can occur with a forced extension of the digit during contraction such as during a rugby tackle, and is often called a 'jersey finger'. The subject often feels a 'snap' in the finger, and examination shows that the finger adopts a position of extension at rest compared with the other fingers and a loss of active flexion at the DIPJ. Often the bony attachment of the FDP is avulsed at the same time, rather than a rupture of the tendon, and this is visible on an X-ray. Treatment is by early surgical repair to avoid tendon retraction and ischaemic damage.

Volar plate injury

The volar plate is a fibrocartilagenous structure reinforcing the palmar aspect of the interphalangeal joints. An injury to the fingers at this level can also damage the volar plate and may be missed on X-ray. Treatment can include splinting or occasionally hand surgery.

Boutonnière deformity

This is the consequence of damage to the central slip of the extensor tendon. Initially extension of the finger may still be possible from the remaining two lateral bands; however, over the next few days these can migrate laterally, eventually lying on the flexor aspect of the joint. This results in a flexion deformity, known as a Boutonnière deformity, at the PIPJ from the resting tone of the flexor digitorum superficialis and compensatory hyperextension at the DIPJ from the remaining extensor slips.

Following an acute injury at the level of the PIPJ, any extensor lag of the fingers should highlight the possibility of a rupture of the central extensor slip and consideration should be given to early splinting to avoid future problems.

Nerve lesions

Median nerve

Carpal tunnel syndrome is the most common of the nerve entrapment syndromes of the upper limb. The medial nerve passes through the carpal tunnel in the wrist, which lies between the scaphoid tuberosity and the trapezoid on the radial side, and the pisiform and the hook of the hamate on the ulnar side. It is here that entrapment of the median nerve can occur, giving rise typically to paraesthesiae over the flexor aspect of the radial three and a half digits, typically with sparing of the little finger, and feelings of subjective hand heaviness or clumsiness. Wasting of the thenar eminence is a late sign and should prompt urgent treatment. Symptoms often commence insidiously with gradual worsening over time; nocturnal symptoms are common, as is increased severity of symptoms first thing in the morning. The vast majority of cases of carpal tunnel syndrome are idiopathic, although there are associations with trauma, including distal wrist fractures and disordered bony architecture, pregnancy, diabetes, acromegaly, hypothyroidism, and inflammatory joint diseases including rheumatoid arthritis. Differential diagnosis includes cervical radiculopathy and thoracic outlet syndrome. Diagnostic tests include Phalen's and Tinel's tests, as previously discussed, and in the event of clinical uncertainty nerve conduction studies can be helpful. However, it should be noted that no test has 100% sensitivity.

Treatments of carpal tunnel syndrome include night splints, corticosteroid injection into the carpal tunnel, or surgical decompression. Subjects with thenar wasting should be considered for prompt surgical decompression to avoid further muscle loss.

Other sites of compression of the median nerve are in the proximal forearm:

- pronator syndrome—the median nerve can become compressed by the ligament of Struthers, a musculotendinous band between the two heads of pronator teres, or the flexor digitorus superficialis.
- anterior interosseous syndrome—the median nerve is compressed more distally by either a deep head of pronator teres or an accessory muscle (Gantzer muscle)

In these conditions, while the origin of the compression lies in the forearm, the symptoms are typically felt in the wrist and hand with weakness of thumb flexion and first DIPJ flexion—the so-called 'OK sign' (Cavaletti *et al.* 2005). This can be differentiated clinically from carpal tunnel syndrome by the more proximal symptoms, although nerve conduction studies are diagnostic. Treatment is similar for both conditions: conservative treatment including rest and splints, or surgical exploration and decompression.

Ulnar nerve

Although less common than ulnar nerve entrapment in the cubital tunnel at the medial epicondyle, which is described elsewhere, the ulnar nerve can become trapped at Guyon's canal at the wrist. This level of entrapment will produce similar symptoms of paraesthesia in the ulnar one and a half fingers, as well as generalized weakness of grip caused by impairment of function of the intrinsic hand muscles innervated by the main trunk of the ulnar nerve. In sports medicine this is most commonly seen in distance cyclists, with pressure from handlebars causing irritation of the ulnar nerve, or from racket sports, with the impact of the handle into the hand, as well as karate participants and baseball/softball catchers (Cavaletti *et al.* 2005). Treatment is typically aimed at removing the provoking factor such as poorly set up equipment, although occasionally surgical decompression is required.

Superficial radial nerve

Entrapment of the superficial radial nerve can occur in the distal forearm either from tendons of the brachioradialis or extensor carpi radialis, or from fascial bands. This produces symptoms, including paraesthesia overlying the dorsal aspect of the base of the thumb, which can be provoked by full wrist pronation. Splinting can be helpful in management, although surgical decompression of the entrapment may be necessary.

Digital nerves

The digital nerves, which are terminal extensions of the ulnar and median nerves, can also be directly compressed. After giving branches to the lumbricals, the digital branches divide into digital nerves which pass through the inter-metacarpal tunnel between the superficial and deep transverse metacarpal ligaments. These nerves can be compressed from a local tenosynovitis or local swelling, although they are more commonly injured directly as a forced extension will cause the nerve to be compressed against a rigid metacarpal ligament. Symptoms include pain, numbness, or paraesthesia in one or two fingers, depending on the site of the insult. Treatment is guided by the underlying cause, and can include local injections, splinting, or surgical decompression.

Cervical spine radiculopathy

Sensation to the hand arises from the C6, C7, and T1 dermatomes, and in all cases of paraesthesia it is important to rule out cervical spine radiculopathy, which is dealt with elsewhere in this book (Chapter 3.4).

References

Amadio, P.C. (1990). Epidemiology of hand and wrist injuries in sports. *Hand Clinics*, **6**, 379–81.

Beckenbaugh, R.D. (1984). Accurate evaluation and management of the painful wrist following injury. An approach to carpal instability. *Orthopedic Clinics of North America*, **15**, 289–304.

Botvin Madorsky, J.G.and Curtis, K.A (1984). Wheelchair sports medicine. *American Journal of Sports Medicine*, **12**, 128–32.

Brophy, R.H., Barnes, R., Rodeo, S.A., and Warren, R.F. (2007). Prevalence of musculoskeletal disorders at the NFL Combine: trends from 1987 to 2000. *Medicine and Science in Sports and Exercise*, **39**, 22–7.

Cahalan, T.D. Cooney, W.P., III, Tamai, K., and Chao E.Y.S. (1991). Biomechanics of the golf swing in players with pathologic conditions of the forearm, wrist, and hand. *American Journal of Sports Medicine*, **19**, 288–93.

Caine, D.J., Caine, C.G., and Lindner, K.J. (eds) (1996). *Epidemiology of Sports Injuries*. Human Kinetics, Champaign, IL.

Carneiro, R.S., Fontana, R., and Mazzer, N. (2005). Ulnar wrist pain in athletes caused by erosion of the floor of the sixth dorsal compartment: a case series. *American Journal of Sports Medicine*, **33**, 1910–13.

Cavaletti, G., Marmiroli, P., Alberti, G., Michielon, G., and Tredici, G. (2005). Sport-related peripheral nerve injuries: Part 1. *Sport Sciences for Health*, **1**(2).

Chan, O. and Hughes, T. (2005). Hand. *British Medical Journal*, **330**, 1073–5.

Deibert, M.C., Aronsson, D.D., Johnson, R.J., Ettlinger, C.F., and Shealy, J.E. (1998). Skiing injuries in children, adolescents, and adults. *Journal of Bone and Joint Surgery. American Volume*, **80**, 25–32.

Dias, J.J., Thompson, J. Barton, N.J., and Gregg, P.J. (1990). Suspected scaphoid fractures. The value of radiographs. *Journal of Bone and Joint Surgery. British Volume*, **72B**, 98–101.

DiFiori, J., Caine, D., Malina, R.M. (2006). Wrist pain, distal radial physeal injury, and ulnar variance in the young gymnast. *American Journal of Sports Medicine*, **34**, 840–9.

Fuller, C.W., Laborde, F. *et al.* (2008). International Rugby Board Rugby World Cup 2007 injury surveillance study. *British Journal of Sports Medicine*, **42**, 452–9.

Giangarra, C.E., Conroy, B., Jobe, F.W., Pink, M., and Perry, J. (1993). Electromyographic and cinematographic analysis of elbow function in tennis players using single- and double-handed backhand strokes. *American Journal of Sports Medicine*, **21**, 394–9.

Gosheger, G., Liem, D., Ludwig, K., Greshake, O., and Winkelmann, W. (2003). Injuries and overuse syndromes in golf. *American Journal of Sports Medicine*, **31**, 438–43.

Hame, S.L. and Melone, C.P., Jr (2000). Boxer's knuckle. Traumatic disruption of the extensor hood. *Hand Clinics*, **16**, 375–80.

Hill, C., M. Riaz, Mozzam, A., and Brennen, M.D. (1998). A regional audit of hand and wrist injuries. A study of 4873 injuries. *Journal of Hand Surgery (Edinburgh)*, **23**, 196–200.

Hodgkinson, D. W., Kurdy, N., Nicholson, D.A., and Driscoll, P.A. (1994). ABC of emergency radiology: the hand. *British Medical Journal*, **308**, 401–5.

Hsu, W.C., Chen, W.H., and Oware, A. (2005). Distal ulnar neuropathy in a golf player. *Clinical Journal of Sport Medicine*, **15**, 189–90.

Hutchinson, M.R., Laprade, R.F., Burnett, Q.M., 2nd, Moss, R., and Terpstra, J. (1995). Injury surveillance at the USTA Boys' Tennis Championships: a 6 year study. *Medicine and Science in Sports and Exercise*, **27**, 826–30.

Jones, G., Asghar, A., and Llewellyn, D.J. (2008). The epidemiology of rock-climbing injuries. *British Journal of Sports Medicine*, **42**, 773–8.

Kujala, U. M., S. Taimela, Antti-Poika, I., Orava, S., Tuominen, R., and Myllynen, P. *et al.* (1995). Acute injuries in soccer, ice hockey, volleyball, basketball, and karate: analysis of national registry data. *British Medical Journal*, **312**, 844–5.

le Viet, D.T., Lantieri, L.A., and Loy, S.M. (1993). Wrist and hand injuries in platform diving. *Journal of Hand Surgery*, **18**, 876–80.

Logan, A.J., Makwana, N., Mason, G., and Dias, J. (2004). Acute hand and wrist injuries in experienced rock climbers. *British Journal of Sports Medicine*, **38**, 545–8.

McHardy, A.J. and Pollard, H.P. (2004). Unusual cause of wrist pain in a golfer. *British Journal of Sports Medicine*, **38**, e34.

Maquirriain, J. and Ghisi, J.P. (2007). Stress injury of the lunate in tennis players: a case series and related biomechanical considerations. *British Journal of Sports Medicine*, **41**, 812–15.

Montalvan, B., Parier, J., Brasseur, J.L., Le Viet, D., and Drape, J.L. (2006). Extensor carpi ulnaris injuries in tennis players: a study of 28 cases. *British Journal of Sports Medicine*, **40**, 424–9.

Nagaoka, M., Satoh, T., Nagao, S., and Matsuzaki, H. (2006). Extensor retinaculum graft for chronic boxer's knuckle. *Journal of Hand Surgery*, **31**, 947–51.

Phillips, T.G., Reibach, A.M., and Slomiany, W.P. (2004). Diagnosis and management of scaphoid fractures. *American Family Physician*, **70**, 879–84.

Pin, P.G., Young, V.L.,Gilula, L.A., and Weeks, P.M. (1989). Management of chronic lunotriquetral ligament tears. *Journal of Hand Surgery*, **14**, 77–83.

Rayan, G.M. (1983). Recurrent dislocation of the extensor carpi ulnaris in athletes. *American Journal of Sports Medicine*, **11**, 183–4.

Reagan, D.S., Linscheid, R.L., and Dobyns, J.H. (1984). Lunotriquetral sprains. *Journal of Hand Surgery*, **9**, 502–14.

Rettig, A.C. (2003). Athletic injuries of the wrist and hand. Part I: Traumatic injuries of the wrist. *American Journal of Sports Medicine*, **31**, 1038–48.

Rettig, A.C. (2004). Athletic injuries of the wrist and hand. Part II: Overuse injuries of the wrist and traumatic injuries to the hand. *American Journal of Sports Medicine*, **32**, 262–73.

Rossi, C., Cellocco, P., Margaritondo, E., Bizzarri, F., and Costanzo, G. (2005). De Quervain disease in volleyball players. *American Journal of Sports Medicine*, **33**, 424–7.

Rumball, J.S., Lebrun, C.M., Di Ciacca, S.R., and Orlando, K. (2005). Rowing injuries. *Sports Medicine*, 2005, 35 (6), 537–55.

Russell, K., Hagel, B., and Francescutti, L.H. (2007). The effect of wrist guards on wrist and arm injuries among snowboarders: a systematic review. *Clinical Journal of Sport Medicine*, **17**, 145–50.

Snead, D. and Rettig, A.C. (2001). Hand and wrist fractures in athletes. *Current Opinion in Orthopedics*, **12**, 160–6.

Taleisnik, J. (1988). Current concepts review. Carpal instability. *Journal of Bone and Joint Surgery. American Volume*, **70**, 1262–8.

Tehranzadeh, J. and Labosky, D.A. (1984). Detection of intraarticular loose osteochondral fragments by double-contrast wrist arthrography: a case report of a basketball injury. *American Journal of Sports Medicine*, **12**, 77–9.

Tehranzadeh, G.A., Labosky, D.A., and Gabriele, F. (1983). Ganglion cysts and tear of triangular fibrocartilages of both wrists in a cheerleader. *American Journal of Sports Medicine*, **11**, 357–9.

Tiel-van Buul, M.M., Bos, K.E., Dijkstra, P.E., van Beek, E.J., and Broekhuizen, A.H. (1993). Carpal instability, the missed diagnosis in patients with clinically suspected scaphoid fracture. *Injury*, **24**, 257–62.

Valbuena, S.E., Gasiunas, V., and Roulot, E. (2008). Re: Scapholunate interosseous ligament rupture in an elite rock climber. *Journal of Hand Surgery. European Volume*, **33**, 393–4.

Van Heest, A.E., Luger, N.M., House, J.H., and Vener, M. (2007). Extensor retinaculum impingement in the athlete: a new diagnosis. *American Journal of Sports Medicine*, **35**, 2126–30.

Wang, C., Gill, T.J., IV, Zarins, B., and Herndon, J.H. (2003) Extensor carpi ulnaris tendon rupture in an ice hockey player: a case report. *American Journal of Sports Medicine*, **31**, 459–61.

Watson, H.K., Ashmead, D., 4th, Makhlouf, M.V. (1988). Examination of the scaphoid. *Journal of Hand Surgery*, **13**, 657–60.

Watson, H.K. and Black, D.M. (1987). Instabilities of the wrist. *Hand Clinics*, **3**, 103–11.

Webb, B.G. and Rettig, L.A. (2008). Gymnastic wrist injuries. *Current Sports Medicine Reports*, **7**, 289–95.

Wilson, R.L. and McGinty, L.D. (1993). Common hand and wrist injuries in basketball players. *Clinics in Sports Medicine*, **12**, 265–91.

Young, C. (2000). The sagittal band: anatomic and biomechanical study. *Journal of Hand Surgery*, **25**, 1107–13.

3.11

Injuries to the lower leg

Cathy Speed and Bill Ribbans

The lower leg is one of the most common sites of injury in sport, particularly involving acute and chronic injuries to muscle and bone. For example, almost 50% of stress fractures are seen in the tibia, and over 6% affect the fibula (Matheson *et al.* 1987). Inevitably, sports affected are those usually involving high-impact lower limb activities. Medial tibial stress syndrome is conservatively estimated to affect 13% of runners (Clanton and Solcher 1994), and injuries to the shin or Achilles tendon are reported to occur in 9–32.2% of long distance runners (van Gent *et al.* 2007). Lower extremity injuries in runners, including those to the lower leg, have a higher incidence in females than in males. A higher knee varus angle is associated with a predisposition to shin injuries. However, despite much research on the topic, the overall influence that static biomechanical lower limb alignment has on the predisposition to develop lower limb injuries on the whole remains uncertain (Scott and Winter 1990; van Gent *et al.* 2007).

Although the lower leg is a common site of injury, the epidemiology of specific injuries is not well defined. Many epidemiological studies have evaluated injuries to the lower limb as a whole. In addition, the complexity of evaluation and the overlapping nature of some chronic exertional lower leg pain syndromes can make injury surveillance difficult. As will become clear in this chapter, the lower leg is a prime example of the variable interaction between intrinsic and extrinsic factors that influence the development, chronicity, and recurrence of injury in sport.

Anatomy

The proximal tibiofibular joint communicates with the knee joint It is stabilized by surrounding ligaments, the capsule, and the popliteal tendon, and glides when the ankle comes into dorsiflexion. It dissipates tibial bending moments and torsional loads applied to the ankle and allows distal motion of the fibula with weight-bearing. The interosseous membrane unites the tibia and fibula in the mid-leg, and continues distally as the tibiofibular syndesmosis which acts in combination with four ligaments to unite the bones in the lower aspect of the leg. The tibial tuberosity receives the patellar tendon.

The muscles of the leg are situated within four compartments—the anterior, lateral, and superficial and deep posterior compartments (Fig. 3.11.1).

Anterior compartment

The muscles of the anterior compartment are the tibialis anterior, the extensor digitorum longus (EDL), the peroneus tertius (actually a part of EDL), and the extensor hallucis longus (EHL).

The **tibialis anterior** functions as the most important dorsiflexor of the foot and also assists in adduction and inversion of the foot. It arises from the inferolateral surface of the tibial condyle, the upper two-thirds of the lateral surface of the tibia, and the interosseous membrane. In the upper part of the leg the muscle covers the anterior tibial vessels and the deep peroneal nerve, becoming tendinous in the lower third of the leg. The tendon passes under the extensor retinaculum in front of the ankle joint, travels across the medial side of the foot, and inserts onto the medial and plantar sides of the medial cuneiform and the base of the first metatarsal.

The **EDL** functions to dorsiflex the MTPJs, PIPJs, and DIPJs along with the intrinsic muscles. It arises from the lateral side of the lateral tibial condyle, the proximal two-thirds of the anterior aspect of the fibula, and the anterior intermuscular septum of the leg. It becomes tendinous proximal to the ankle, passing beneath the extensor retinaculum and inserting onto the middle and distal phalanges of the first four toes. The **peroneus tertius** is a part of EDL which inserts onto the base of the fifth metatarsal.

The **EHL** functions as an extensor of the big toe and is also a weak supinator and dorsiflexor of the foot. It arises from the middle three-fifths of the anterior fibula (medial to the origin of EDL) and from the adjacent interosseous membrane. Its proximal half is covered by the EDL and tibialis anterior. Its tendon passes beneath

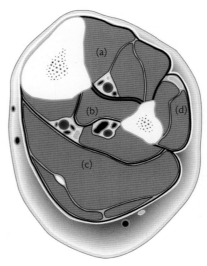

Fig. 3.11.1 Compartments of the lower leg: (a) anterior, (b) deep posterior, (c) superficial posterior, (d) lateral.

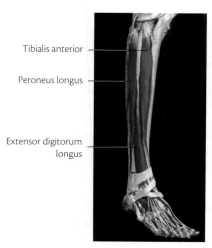

Fig. 3.11.2 The anterolateral leg. EHL arises deep to the tibialis anterior and EDL.

Table 3.11.1 Causes of lower leg pain

Posterior
Chronic compartment syndrome
Gastrocnemius strain/tear
Popliteal artery entrapment syndrome
Muscle/fascial hernia(s)
Common peroneal nerve entrapment
Referred pain
Nerve root compression
Spinal stenosis
Mechanical
Peripheral vascular disease
Anterior/anterolateral
Stress fractures
Medial tibial periostitis
Medial tibial stress syndrome
Muscle/fascial hernia(s)
Superficial peroneal nerve entrapment
Muscle strain (e.g. tibialis anterior)
Tear of interosseous membrane
Syndesmosis injury
Tibiofibular synostosis (rare)
Others
Systemic disease: malignancy, myositis, inflammatory arthropathy
Cellulitis
Deep vein thrombosis
Sepsis

the extensor retinaculum to insert onto the distal (or in some, the proximal) phalanx of the hallux.

The **saphenous nerve** is a sensory nerve which arises from the femoral nerve and enters the adductor canal, dividing into two terminal branches to supply the anteromedial knee and medial leg.

Lateral compartment

The muscles of the lateral compartment of the leg, the peroneus longus and brevis, are separated from the other compartments by intermuscular septae. The **peroneus longus** arises from the lateral aspect of the head and the proximal two-thirds of the body of the fibula. It acts uniquely as a primary plantarflexor of the first ray and also acts as an accessory plantarflexor of the ankle and a weak evertor of the subtalar joint. Its tendon passes around the lateral malleolus behind that of peroneus brevis, underneath the superior peroneal retinaculum to the cuboid notch, and then bends acutely medially and travels to insert onto the medial cuneiform and base of the first metatarsal. The **peroneus brevis** is the strongest evertor of the subtalar joint and is a weak plantarflexor of the ankle. It arises from the lower two-thirds of the lateral fibula and adjacent intermuscular septae and inserts onto the styloid process of the fifth metatarsal. The tendons of the peroneii share a common tendon sheath deep to the peroneal retinaculum behind the lateral malleolus, although they have their own sheaths further distally. Both are also important in maintaining the longitudinal arch of the foot.

The **common peroneal nerve** leaves the lateral popliteal fossa, emerges from between the lateral head of gastrocnemius and biceps, and winds around the neck of the fibula between the origins of peroneus longus to divide into superficial and deep branches.

The deep peroneal nerve pierces the anterior intermuscular septum, passing into the anterior compartment of the leg, supplying its muscles, and entering the foot through the anterior tarsal tunnel. The **superficial peroneal nerve** passes between the peroneus longus and the fibula to travel along the anterior intermuscular septum, supplying the peroneii. It pierces the deep crural fascia approximately 10 cm above the lateral malleolus and divides into cutaneous branches.

The **anterior tibial artery** arises from the popliteal artery and enters the anterior compartment over the proximal interosseous membrane, descending to supply the muscles of the anterior compartment.

Superficial posterior compartment

The gastrocnemius, soleus, and plantaris muscles comprise the muscles of the superficial posterior compartment of the leg. The two heads of the **gastrocnemius** muscle and the **soleus** muscle, collectively termed the **triceps surae** ('three-headed calf muscle'), are vital for propulsion, working as prime movers and stabilizers of the rearfoot.

The two heads of the gastrocnemius arise from the posterior aspects of the femoral condyles and the posterior capsule of the knee. Bursae are situated deep to each head at its origin. The medial head is the larger of the two, whilst the lateral head has a bony sesamoid (fabella) in approximately 11% of individuals. The muscle evolves into a broad tendinous sheet, the Achilles tendon, in the mid-leg (Figure 3.11.3).

The **soleus** arises from the fibula and the posterior aspect of the tibia. It is muscular deep to the Achilles tendon and is adherent to it, which is vital to the vascularity of the Achilles. In the lower third of the leg, the soleus muscle fibres are gradually replaced by tendon, blending with, and becoming part of, the Achilles. When complete,

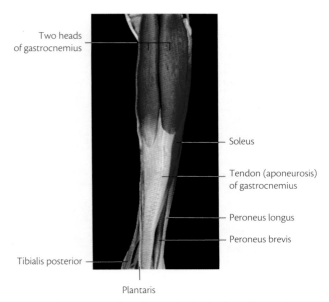

Two heads of gastrocnemius

Soleus

Tendon (aponeurosis) of gastrocnemius

Peroneus longus

Peroneus brevis

Tibialis posterior

Plantaris

Fig. 3.11.3 The Achilles tendon is formed by the blending of the tendon of soleus with the overlying tendon of gastrocnemius.

the inferior fibres of the Achilles tendon twist obliquely in their descent to their insertion onto the posterior aspect of the middle third of the calcaneus. Up to half of the fibres twist in an inferolateral direction around the long axis, with a degree of torsion of 30–150°. This torsion is a phenomenon not seen until the age of 10 years. The lateral fibres rotate to insert superficially (i.e. posteriorly) and the medial fibres insert more deeply (i.e. anteriorly). Localized torque stresses may result and can affect any differential function of the two gastrocnemius heads at the foot. Abnormal talocalcaneal motion places an uneven rotational force upon the fibres, and this is the reason why hyperpronation, by increasing a strain on the medial fibres, is an aetiological factor in Achilles tendinopathies.

The Achilles tendon translates up to four times the power of other crural tendons and may regularly transmit 6–10 times the body weight during gait (Scott and Winter 1990). Forces of 12.5 times body weight have been recorded in the tendon when running at 6 m/sec (Komi *et al.*1992). The strength of the tendon is particularly determined by its size, by the gastrocnemius–soleus muscle mass, and by working through a long moment arm from the ankle. By comparison, all the other tendons acting on the ankle have short moment arms. The thickness of the Achilles tendon shows wide inter-individual variation (up to 25%); hence its strength is also highly variable.

The Achilles tendon is invested by a paratendon consisting of loose elastic connective tissue that is able to stretch with movement of the tendon, allowing the tendon to glide freely.

The paratenon supplies much of the blood supply of the Achilles, since the musculotendinous and osseotendinous junctions are too distant to ensure adequate vascularization of this massive tendon. An intratendinous vascular supply has been demonstrated (Lagergren and indholm 1958) but vascularity in the area 2–5 cm above the insertion, where most ruptures occur, is relatively poor (Carr and Norris 1989). The area around the insertion site is also

relatively hypovascular, which may explain some of the pathologies seen at this site (Schmidt-Rohlfing *et al.* 1992).

Two bursae are associated with the Achilles tendon. The **retrocalcaneal bursa** is a horseshoe-shaped anatomical bursa which is located deeply between the upper third of the posterior surface of the calcaneus and the Achilles tendon. It is located where the tendon potentially rubs against the posterior superior calcaneal process during ankle dorsiflexion. The bursa is filled with 1–1.5 ml of thick synovial fluid and has a synovial lining in the proximal portion where it abuts against the Achilles fat pad. The anterior bursal wall is composed of fibrocartilage laid over the calcaneus, while the posterior wall is indistinguishable from the epitenon of the Achilles tendon. Importantly, communication between the Achilles tendon at its insertion and the retrocalcaneal bursa is not uncommon. The superficial or **subcutaneous calcaneal (retroachilles) bursa** is adventitious and develops as a result of local friction. Where bursitis occurs, the tendon is rarely affected.

An **accessory** or **anomalous soleus muscle** is a rare variant, reported in less than 2% of cases undergoing Achilles tendon surgery. There are two main types: the first and most common form is simply an extension of the muscle more distally along the tendon; the second variant is a separate insertion of soleus into the upper surface of the calcaneum via a separate tendon or insertion of the muscle directly without a tendinous component.

Plantaris, a muscle which is absent in approximately 6% of individuals, arises from the supracondylar line just above the gastrocnemius. It is a rudimentary muscle and is available as a tendon graft. It has a short muscle belly, becoming tendinous whilst in the popliteal fossa and travelling down between the gastrocnemius and soleus to emerge to insert just medial to the Achilles tendon.

Deep posterior compartment

The remaining foot and toe flexors lying deep to the gastrosoleus complex constitute the deep posterior compartment.

The **flexor digitorum longus (FDL)** flexes the distal phalanges of the lateral four toes, assists in plantarflexion at the ankle, and helps to maintain the medial and longitudinal arches. It arises from the posterior aspect of the mid-tibia, becomes tendinous in the lower

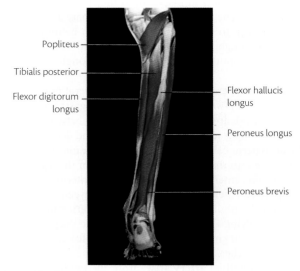

Popliteus

Tibialis posterior

Flexor digitorum longus

Flexor hallucis longus

Peroneus longus

Peroneus brevis

Fig. 3.11.4 The deep posterior and lateral leg.

leg, passes behind the medial malleolus, and enters the foot via the tarsal tunnel. The tendon then separates into four tendons which give origin to the lumbrical muscles and ultimately insert onto the base of the distal phalanx.

The **flexor hallucis longus** (FHL) flexes the distal phalanx of the big toe, assists in plantarflexion at the ankle, and helps to maintain the medial arch. It arises on the posterior aspect of the fibula, and its tendon passes through a fibro-osseous tunnel beneath the sustentaculum tali. It gives variable slips to the second and third toes by crossing fibres with the FDL at the knot of Henry. It inserts into the base of the distal phalanx. In the lower leg it is separated from the Achilles tendon by a fat-filled space and fascial covering. Its proximity is such that it can be used as a tendon graft for the Achilles.

The **tibialis posterior** (TP), the deepest muscle in the calf, arises from the posterior surface of the fibula, the medial posterior tibia, and the intermuscular septa. It becomes tendinous in the lower leg, lies immediately behind the medial malleolus, and enters the foot via the tarsal tunnel at the medial ankle. The TP tendon crosses three joints along its course—the ankle, subtalar, and oblique midtarsal joints—producing specific actions at each joint it crosses through the action of several bands (see Chapter 3.13). It works powerfully at the subtalar and midtarsal joints to invert the heel and supinate the foot. It also plantarflexes the foot at the ankle, plays an important role in maintaining the medial arch of the foot, and contributes to the stability of the foot by its many bony attachments. It has been suggested that tibialis posterior occupies its own osseofascial compartment, distinct from the deep posterior compartment (some term this the 'fifth compartment' of the lower leg).

Neurovascular supply of the posterior compartments

The leg is supplied by branches of the sciatic nerve, which divides into the common peroneal and tibial nerves in the popliteal fossa. The tibial nerve (L4-S3) innervates the muscles of the superficial and deep posterior compartments. It emerges from the popliteal fossa, passing distally with the posterior tibial vessels initially on the tibialis posterior muscle and then on the posterior aspect of the tibia. It winds around the medial malleolus within the tarsal tunnel, terminating beneath the flexor retinaculum by dividing into the medial and lateral plantar nerves.

The medial sural nerve is a cutaneous afferent nerve and originates from the tibial nerve in the popliteal fossa. It runs between

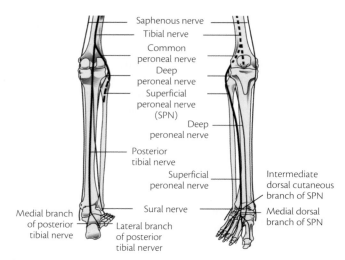

Fig. 3.11.6 Peripheral nerves of the lower leg.

the two heads of gastrocnemius, penetrating the superficial fascia at the junction of the upper two-thirds and lower third of the lateral leg and joining with a branch of the lateral sural nerve in the lower leg to form the sural nerve. This then provides sensation to the lateral aspect of the foot and ankle. It is in close proximity to the Achilles tendon, lying within 2 mm of the lateral border of the tendon at a level approximately 7 cm above the tip of the lateral malleolus.

The posterior tibial vessels and their branches pass with the tibial nerve in the deep compartment, terminating distal to the flexor retinaculum by dividing into the medial and lateral plantar arteries.

Clinical evaluation

History

Many musculoskeletal complaints in the lower leg are activity related. Obtaining a thorough history is important in the clinical assessment of these disorders and will guide subsequent examination and investigations. Be aware that in some complaints related to sport, there is little to find on examination at rest.

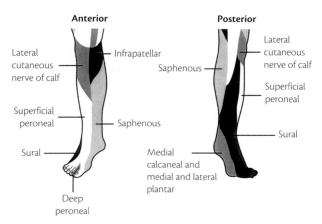

Fig. 3.11.5 Cutaneous supply of the lower leg.

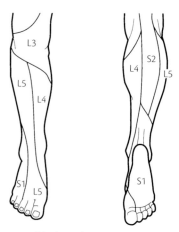

Fig. 3.11.7 Dermatomes of the lower leg.

Acute injuries are rare compared with those of insidious onset. The patient with a spontaneous Achilles tendon rupture or calf muscle tear usually reports a sensation of being kicked in the back of a leg, with difficulty in walking afterwards.

The duration of symptoms, nature of onset, relieving and exacerbating features, and progression should be noted. Pain is the most common symptom and its site, nature, and radiation will help to define the site and nature of the injury. Nocturnal pain is suggestive of a neurogenic origin, severe vascular disease, bony damage, or infective or malignant process. Start-up pain is typical of a soft tissue injury such as Achilles tendinosis.

Pain with stress fractures, medial tibial periostitis, and medial tibial stress syndrome is significantly worse with running or walking, and pain at rest may occur. Symptoms with chronic compartment syndromes develop during specific modes of activity, are localized to one or more compartments, and settle quickly with rest.

Activities and hobbies are highly relevant, with respect to both their nature and any alteration prior to the onset of injury. Overuse is a common precipitant (Table 3.11.2). Surface and equipment factors should also be considered. Has the patient been running on a hard concrete surface? What shoes does the patient wear? The use of orthotics should also be ascertained. Occupational factors, such as standing for long periods, may be relevant.

Swelling, crepitus, and stiffness are common features of Achilles paratendonitis ('peritendinitis' or 'paratendonitis') and tendinosis. Local swelling may also be reported with a stress fracture, and swelling and tightness may occur in relation to a chronic compartment syndrome, settling with rest.

Vascular symptoms such as coldness, colour change, and numbness may indicate a vascular origin, such as popliteal artery entrapment syndrome or a compartment syndrome, but medical causes such as peripheral vascular disease should also be considered, particularly in the older athlete and if symptoms are bilateral. Neurological symptoms raise the possibility of referred pain from the back, nerve entrapment, or chronic compartment syndrome. Bilateral symptoms increase the probability of the former ('two legs equals one back').

Previous injuries should be noted, as this episode may be a recurrence or a 'second injury syndrome'. A medical history should also be recorded.

Examination

The lower leg is not examined in isolation; assessment of the entire lower limb and lumbar spine is included.

Inspection

Inspection begins with observation of the posture and attitude of the leg. Leg length (true and apparent) should be assessed, as leg-length inequality commonly causes lower leg complaints. Those with apparent (or functional) leg-length discrepancies can be further assessed to evaluate the source of the problem. The patient stands in a relaxed position and the examiner palpates the anterior and posterior superior iliac spines (ASIS and PSIS), noting discrepancies in height. The patient is then positioned, standing, with the subtalar joints in a neutral position, with the toes pointing straight ahead. The examiner then palpates the ASIS and PSIS again. If the previously noted discrepancies remain, the leg-length discrepancy is due to changes at the pelvis and sacroiliac joints and these should be further examined. If the differences disappear, the discrepancy is due to changes somewhere in the lower limb.

Many overuse conditions of the lower limbs are associated with biomechanical malalignments. Biomechanical aspects, including femoral anteversion, tibial torsion, and the posture of the foot and ankle, should be assessed. Tibial torsion is evaluated with the patient sitting with the knees over the end of the examination couch. The examiner places the thumb and index finger of one hand on the malleoli and then visualizes the axes of the knee and ankle. The lines usually form an angle of 12°–18°, but internal torsion results in a reduction, and external torsion an increase, of this angle. Femoral anteversion can be assessed by asking the patient to lie flat with the knees still bent over the end of the couch. Passive rotation of the hips should be equal. An increase of internal rotation and decrease of external rotation indicates excess anteversion. An increase in external rotation and decrease in internal rotation indicates a degree of the relatively rarer femoral retroversion.

With the patient lying prone inspection can continue for discoloration, local deformities, swelling, and calf asymmetry. A visible gap may be present after an Achilles tendon rupture.

Integrity of the Achilles tendon is first evaluated by assessing the 'angle of dangle' of the feet over the end of the examining couch with the patient prone. This will be asymmetrical in an Achilles rupture, with the foot hanging vertically with no plantarflexion from the normal gastrocnemius muscle tone. Rupture is confirmed by an absence of plantarflexion of the foot on squeezing the calf. It should be noted that this test can be insensitive, since the long extensors and intact plantaris can assist this function. Other tests have been suggested for Achilles tendon rupture, but are no more sensitive. Diagnostic ultrasound, an extension of the clinical examination, plays a significant role in assessment (see below).

Table 3.11.2 Predisposing factors for overuse injuries

Extrinsic factors	Intrinsic factors
Training errors	Malalignment
Excessive volume	Pes planus
Excessive intensity	Pes cavus
Rapid increase	Rearfoot varus
Sudden change in pattern	Tibia vara
Inadequate recovery	Patella alta
Faulty technique	Genu valgum
Surface	Genu varum
Too hard	Tibial torsion
Too soft	Femoral neck anteversion
Cambered	Leg-length discrepancy
Equipment (shoes)	Muscle weakness/imbalance
Inappropriate	Hypomobility/inflexibility
Worn out	General/local
Environment	Hypermobility
Too hot/cold/humid	Joint instability
Inadequate nutrition	Body composition
Psychological factors	

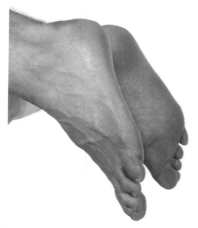

Fig. 3.11.8 Complete tears of the Achilles tendon can be diagnosed by assessing the 'angle of dangle' of the feet over the end of the examination couch.

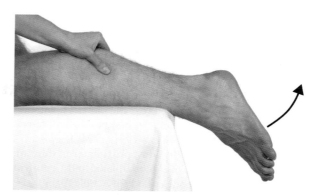

Fig. 3.11.9 Thompson's test. Achilles tendon rupture can be diagnosed if compression of the calf does not cause plantarflexion of the foot.

Palpation

The entire tibial and fibula should be palpated to identify areas of tenderness. Percussion of these areas will often exacerbate pain when stress fracture is present. The soft tissue attachments on the tibia are also palpated and the degree of tenderness compared with that of bone to assist in identifying whether pain is arising from bone or soft tissue. A palpable gap may be present after Achilles tendon rupture or a gastrocnemius tear. Significant pain on squeezing the proximal or distal leg can indicate a syndesmosis injury (see Chapter 3.13). Neurovascular status is also assessed; Tinel's test should be performed over areas of suspected nerve entrapment.

Movement

Inability to perform a single-heel raise test may indicate an Achilles tendon rupture, although pain may limit the ability to undertake this test. Flexibility of the calf musculature and hamstrings should be assessed; tightness of these structures can result in lower limb pain due to the biomechanical problems that result, including hyperpronation.

Special tests

Many of the causes of lower limb pain are present only with exercise ('exertional lower leg pain'), and examination of the patient immediately after exacerbating activities, when symptoms are present, is usually necessary. In addition, compartment studies (described below) may be necessary.

Posterior leg pain

Achilles tendinopathies

The Achilles tendon is the largest and strongest tendon in the human body. It is susceptible to a wide spectrum of acute and chronic injury along its entire length, as a result of its large size and the immense functional demands imposed upon it.

The nomenclature for conditions affecting the Achilles tendon is confusing and often misleading, and does not reflect the underlying tendon disorders. Terms including tendinitis, tendinosis, tendinopathy, peritendinitis, paratendonitis, achillodynia, and insertional tendonitis are often used interchangeably. Any classification scheme should be clinically useful, aiding in treatment, and should be as accurate as possible. A simple and clinically relevant classification encompassing the spectrum of injuries is described in Table 3.11.3.

Paratendonitis, tendinosis, and enthesitis

Most cases of Achilles paratendonitis and tendinosis are related to overuse, although there are some exceptions. Although 25–33% of patients with Achilles tendon problems are reported to be not

Table 3.11.3 Classification of Achilles tendon disorders

Term	Definition	Histology	Clinical[a]
Paratendonitis/ tenosynovitis	Pathology of the paratendon/tendon sheath	Inflammatory cells in paratendon/tendon sheath	Swelling, pain, crepitus, local warmth, dysfunction
Tendinosis	Symptomatic intratendinous degeneration of the tendon	Fibre disarray, ↓cellularity, vascular ingrowth, calcification	Pain, fusiform swelling, palpable nodule
Enthesitis	Inflammatory/degenerative lesion of tendon insertion	Fibre disarray, ↓cellularity, vascular ingrowth, calcification	Localized pain, swelling, erythema, warmth, crepitus
Tear	Disruption of the structural integrity of the tendon	Significant fibre disruption, usually on background of tendinosis	Pain, weakness, palpable gap, poor response to therapy
Haglund's syndrome	Retrocalcaneal bursitis ± enthesitis in the presence of a prominence of the posterior superior portion of the calcaneum	Bursal inflammation, fibrosis, ± enthesis	Localized pain, swelling, erythema, Haglund's deformity

[a]Swelling, warmth, erythema can be minimal

actively involved in sport (Rolf and Movin, 1997), occupational activities may be implicated in their development. Many of the studies of the incidence of injures have focused upon runners, where the incidence is reported to be 6.5-18% (Clement *et al.*1984), increasing to 7–9% in high level runners. Although considered to affect men much more frequently than women, this may be due at least in part to the cohorts studied (e.g. the military), and the variation in injury rates between countries may be due to differences in injury surveillance strategies (Kvist 1991, 1994; Leppilahti *et al.* 1991; Leppilahti and Orava 1998). Approximately a third of elite badminton players, 10–18% of elite triathletes, and 12% of adventure racers will have at least one episode of Achilles pain that limits training.

A number of aetiological factors have been implicated in the development of Achilles tendon lesions. A common thread is one of repetitive impact loading and/or sudden acceleration (ruptures), associated with jumping. The more heavily loaded leg (depending upon the sport) is most likely to be affected. Kvist (1991) assessed 411 players with Achilles tendinopathy and identified one or more anatomical or biomechanical factors in over 50% of cases. Specifically, 21% had calf muscle tightness, 17% hyperpronation, and 15% leg-length inequality greater than 1 cm (Leppilahti *et al.* 1998). No significant relationship was demonstrated between these features and tendon rupture. Fredberg and Bolvig (2002) reported that 11/96 Achilles tendons had asymptomatic abnormalities on pre-season ultrasound assessment, with a 45% risk of developing symptoms during the season; only one of the 85 with normal ultrasound developed symptoms during the season.

Achilles tendon pathology can affect the intrinsic tendon structure (tendinosis), the paratendon (paratendonitis, paratendonitis, or, less appropriately, 'peritendonitis'), or both. Most frequently, the tendinosis is diffuse and typically affects the mid-tendon. Where focal, this is more common on the dorsal surface of the tendon.

The paratendon is frequently underestimated as a source of Achilles pain. It is the most richly innervated structure in the Achilles complex and is vital in providing vascular supply to the tendon proper, which is otherwise poorly supplied. Paratendon involvement with Achilles tendinosis is very common, and in chronic cases it can be difficult to distinguish between the two. In pure paratendon disease the area of thickening and tenderness remains static with dorsiflexion and plantarflexion of the ankle. Acute paratendonitis is usually a result of unaccustomed activity or recent biomechanical changes, such as another injury, or different shoes, training surfaces, or regimes.

Associated features of Achilles tendon complaints reflect the complexity of the pathological processes involved in tendinosis. Much as compromised vascular supply to the tendon is considered to be a primary aetiological factor in tendinosis, neurovascular ingrowth, somewhat paradoxically, is considered to be associated with more severe and painful Achilles tendinosis and is a target for treatment. This hypothesis is supported by the finding that the degree of neovascularization noted on ultrasound Doppler studies correlates with the level of pain (Ohberg *et al.* 2004). Release of

Table 3.11.4 Factors predisposing to Achilles tendinopathies in runners.

Intrinsic factors:
Biomechanical malalignments including gait abnormalities (usually hyperpronation)
Stiff gastrocnemius–soleus complex, tight hamstrings
Leg-length discrepancy
Muscle imbalance
Hyper/hypomobile hindfoot
Haglund's deformity
Spondyloarthritides (enthesopathies)
Extrinsic factors
Overtraining
Training type (e.g. too much heavy weight training)
Poor footwear (too old, poor cushioning, high heel tab, wrong size)
Poor technique
Inappropriate surface
Environment (too hot/cold)
Iatrogenic: fluoroquinolones, corticosteroid injections
Anabolic steroid abuse

Table 3.11.5 Important features to note in the Achilles tendon in the assessment of Achilles tendinosis

Clinical
Site of symptoms
Swelling
Paratendon crepitus
Retrocalcaneal bursal tenderness
Inflammatory signs at insertion (?seronegative enthesopathy)
Heel deformity
VAS and VISA scores
Ultrasound
Site of core tendon involved (insertional vs. mid-tendon)
Degree of swelling
Percentage of cross-sectional area of tendon that is hypoechogenic
Is there partial tear/split
Presence of neovascularization
Paratendon involvement
Retrocalcaenal bursitis
X-ray
Bony/Haglund's deformity
Insertional changes
MRI
Tendon swelling
Signal change
Tearing
Calcaneal deformity
Erosions at enthesis
Bursitis

neuropeptides from the nerves that are closely associated with the new vessels may explain the pain found in pathological tendons. Such neuropeptides may generate a cycle of 'neurogenic inflammation' (Fredberg and Stengaard-Petersen 2008) within the tendon, or the neurovascular bundles may mechanically occupy tendon volume and lead to a compressive effect. Notably however, some patients with neovascularization are not symptomatic (Zanetti *et al.* 2003).

Dystrophic calcification, seen in chronic tendinosis in both midsubstance and insertional tendon injuries, can also contribute to pain, and reflects the dysfunctional behaviour of the tenocyte.

First reported in 1983, oral fluoroquinolones are well recognized as a cause of Achilles tendinopathy and cause a florid inflammatory response (McGarvey *et al.* 1996; Movin *et al.* 1997). By 1992, 100 cases had been reported to French pharmaco-vigilance centres and pharmaceutical companies, including 27 cases of Achilles tendon ruptures. Fifty per cent of ruptures occur within 2 weeks of starting the fluoroquinolone, although they may occur after withdrawal of the drug.

Since fluoroquinolones may be used in bacterial infections in athletes, particularly when travelling, this is of relevance in sports medicine. However, most cases involve the older individual, and other risk factors are usually present such as the use of systemic corticosteroid therapy, renal failure, and advanced age (Szarfman *et al.* 1995). The mean time to symptom onset is 13 days (1–90 days). The adjusted relative risk of Achilles tendinopathy with fluoroquinolones was 3.7 (95% CI 0.9–15.1) and 1.3 (95% CI 0.4- 4.7) for other types of tendinopathy. Achilles tendinitis with ofloxacin had a relative risk of 10.1 (95% CI 2.2–46.0) and an excess risk of 15 cases per 100 000 exposure days.

Hypercholesterolaemia and lipid storage disorders play a role in some cases of Achilles tendinosis.

Haglund's syndrome

Haglund first described a prominence of the posterosuperior lateral calcaneal process in association with a retrocalcaneal bursitis in 1928. Haglund's syndrome is now commonly taken to represent this deformity with a retrocalcaneal bursitis, with an associated Achilles insertional tendinitis (Fig. 3.11.11).

Insertional Achilles pain can be derived from various elements including a prominent calcaneal tuberosity, a retrocalcaneal bursitis, and an insertional Achilles tendinosis, which is of a degenerative aetiology. It is important to distinguish which of these pathologies is present. In addition, a prominent lateral calcaneal ridge ('pump bump'), with or without an overlying superficial bursitis, may be found as a separate distinct clinical entity, particularly in tall thin athletes.

Ruptures

Rupture of the Achilles tendon is the most common form of spontaneous tendon rupture, affecting males more commonly than females, with studies indicating a relative frequency of 2–19 males for every female affected (Zollinger *et al.* 1983; Carden *et al.* 1987). Ninety per cent of ruptures occur during physical activity, with the typical patient being the sedentary middle-aged individual who participates in physical activities at the weekends (the 'weekend warrior'). Twenty per cent are competitive athletes, who are usually younger than those recreational athletes affected. The high incidence of spontaneous ruptures in the sedentary population compares with partial tears, where 76% of the latter are reported in competitive athletes (Josza *et al.* 1989).

Only 10% of all those who rupture have had previous Achilles tendon symptoms, 30% of whom are only mildly symptomatic (Kvist 1991). The left leg is slightly more commonly affected than the right. Rupture most commonly occurs 3–6 cm above the insertion (83%), whilst 12% occur at the musculotendinous junction and 5% at the insertion (Josza 1989). Ruptures of both tendons successively are relatively more common, but simultaneous bilateral rupture is rare.

Several studies suggest an increasing incidence of ruptures, possibly because of an increased participation of the public in sport and to increased rates of consultation and detection.

Angiographic, histological, and surgical evidence supports the hypothesis that rupture occurs in tendons where pre-existing degeneration is present. Poor vascularity, trauma, genetic factors, muscle stiffness, and relative weakening of the tendon are all considered to play a role in rupture, and the degree of force required is often small.

Rarely, a direct contusion (such as that sustained by Achilles himself from the arrow of Paris) can rupture the tendon. In these cases, the tendon is under high tension at impact. Other mechanisms are also described, including (1) rupture with the thrust of the foot against the ground with simultaneous extension of knee, such as coming out of the starting blocks in a race, (2) sudden dorsiflexion of the ankle with the foot planted on the ground (e.g. stumbling into a hole), and (3) enforced dorsiflexion of the foot while it is in plantarflexion (e.g. falling from a height).

Kvist (1991) noted a combination of a high longitudinal arch and an underpronating alignment of the ankle to be significantly higher in patients with ruptures. Iatrogenic causes of Achilles tendon rupture have also been proposed (see Table 3.11.4). No rigorous prospective clinical studies have been performed to address the incidence of rupture after steroid injection. However, there are numerous uncontrolled case reports of Achilles rupture after local corticosteroid injection and there is evidence from animal studies of deleterious effects upon tendon. Crystals have been identified from tendon tissues 6 months after injection (Tomassi 1992), with focal necrosis and foreign body formation around the crystals. Achilles rupture was reported to occur in a range of 0–8% of cases after a corticosteroid injection for Achilles pain (Leppilahti and Orava 1998).

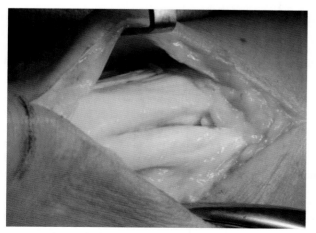

Fig. 3.11.10 A longitudinal tear of the Achilles tendon in a runner with chronic Achilles pain.

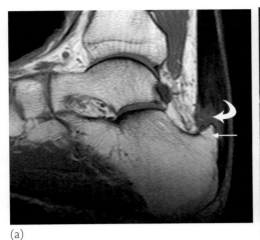
(a)

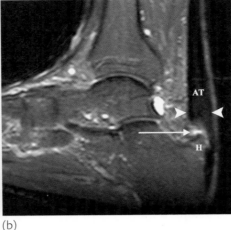
(b)

Fig. 3.11.11 MRI and US of Haglund's syndrome in a 33-year-old male elite marathon runner. (a) Sagittal T1-weighted MRI. Note the prominent posterosuperior process of the calcaneum (Haglund's deformity) (arrow) in association with insertional Achilles tendonitis (curved arrow). (b) Sagittal STIR MRI. The Achilles tendon (AT) is expanded (arrowheads) and there is marked inflammation in the retrocalcaneal bursa (long arrow) associated with a Haglund deformity (H).

The effects of **fluoroquinolones** have been described and tendon rupture may result. **Anabolic steroids** may also play a role in tendon rupture through a direct effect or as a result of increased muscular strength compared with that of the tendon.

History

Symptoms may vary from pain, stiffness, and severe inflammation to a minor ache, depending upon the specific disorder. Pain may be worst at the beginning of the day, with difficulty in putting the foot to the floor on getting out of bed. An acute onset of pain after significant unaccustomed activity raises the possibility of an acute paratendonitis. In acute spontaneous ruptures the history of a loud bang and a feeling as if the patient has been kicked in the back of the leg, with subsequent difficulty in pushing off, is virtually diagnostic. However, pain may be absent and symptoms vague. Perhaps as a result, 25% of Achilles tendon ruptures are missed at initial presentation to a clinician, which can have devastating consequences. Partial tears of the Achilles tendon may occur as a result of a distinct episode or a series of episodes.

Precipitating factors must be sought, including activities, types of footwear and trauma. In the sporting population a careful history must be taken of training patterns, surfaces, equipment use (including shoes), previous injuries, and additional training activities.

In individuals with insertional tendinopathies, a systemic enquiry relating to the possibility of an associated spondyloarthritis is important.

Examination

Paratendonitis, tendinosis, and tears most commonly occur in the mid-third section of the tendon, where the area is particularly hypovascular. Local tenderness, inflammatory signs (consider enthesopathy, paratendonitis, Haglund's syndrome) and/or a palpable tendon nodule (tendinosis) may be evident. Stiffness of the gastrocnemius–soleus complex is common. The tendon may be swollen and generally tender, and there is crepitus in acute paratendonitis.

In acute ruptures swelling and bruising may be evident, whereas in chronic ruptures local thickening of the tendon and paratendon and muscle atrophy are commonly found. Achilles tendon rupture can be detected using a variety of clinical tests, but the easiest is assessment of the 'angle of dangle' of the feet over the end of the

examining couch. Rupture is confirmed by an absence/weakness of plantarflexion of the foot when squeezing the calf (Thompson's test). The patient is unable to perform a single-heel raise and a palpable gap may be present.

Partial tears are often difficult to diagnose; weakness of dorsiflexion and a failure to respond to conservative management should arouse suspicion, but imaging is usually necessary.

Bony deformities should be sought. These can take the form of an exostosis over the lateral aspect of the calcaneus caused by recurrent friction, particularly in association with a hypermobile rearfoot or true Haglund's deformity, which sometimes is evident only with the help of imaging. Insertional tendinitis causes local tenderness, swelling, and hyperaemia at the insertion. It is commonly associated with these deformities, with or without a retrocalcaneal bursitis. In retrocalcaneal bursitis, bursal swelling is often seen on both sides of the Achilles tendon although it is not as obvious in chronic situations. In acute and subacute cases, there is painful swelling and occasionally hyperaemia of overlying skin in the posterosuperior corner of the calcaneus. Plantarflexion of the foot is painful. Features of a spondyloarthritis may be present.

Predisposing anatomical factors should be sought (Table 3.11.4). Gait should be assessed for hyperpronation, leg-length discrepancy, and deformities. Footwear should always be closely examined, specifically inspecting the heel tabs, wear pattern of the sole, and overall condition and suitability for the purpose for which they are being worn.

A VISA score for Achilles tendinopathies is useful in assessment and monitoring of pain and function. This is detailed at the end of this chapter.

Imaging of Achilles tendinopathies.

MRI and ultrasound complement each other in the assessment of the Achilles tendon and its surrounding anatomy. Diagnostic ultrasound is an extremely important part of the clinical examination of any Achilles tendon disorder. It shows the structure of the tendon and paratendon changes in detail, the extent of tendon cross-sectional area involved (hypoechoic areas), and the presence of thickening/swelling or atrophy and important associated features such as neovascularization, dystrophic calcification, and bursitis. The tendon can also be assessed in movement of the foot and ankle to address impingement through Haglund's deformity and to demonstrate sites of adhesions, tears, and of course rupture of the tendon. MRI helps to evaluate the tendon: normal tendons contain high-signal foci on T1-weighted images, but those showing increased signal on fast STIR represent tendinosis. However, the main role of MRI is to assess the surrounding anatomy, including calcaneal deformities. Retrocalcaneal and retro-Achilles bursae are also detected using these imaging modalities (see Fig. 3.11.11).

Plain X-rays may be helpful in the assessment of Haglund's deformity, detecting underlying biomechanical/anatomical abnormalities and bony spurs associated with insertional tendon pain, and excluding posterior impingement osseous problems.

Management of Achilles tendinopathies
Paratendonitis, tendinosis, and enthesitis

Non-surgical management is appropriate in the vast majority of cases, even in severe disease, but the patient must be counselled that progress can be slow. As is the case with so many soft tissue injuries, controlling symptoms to allow rehabilitation to be performed is a central goal. In acute and subacute cases, the PRICES approach (**p**rotection, **r**est, **i**ce, **e**levation, **s**upport) is appropriate. Rest is relative; reducing the intensity, frequency, and duration of loading activities and cross-training through the adoption of alternative modes of activity that do not stress the tendon (swimming, cycling) are encouraged. Whilst heel raises may be useful, they should not be worn constantly. In severe cases, functional casting or, rarely, the use of crutches may be necessary. Initial cryotherapy in the form of ice, cold compresses, or ice immersion is used to control pain and reduce muscle spasm, oedema, and the metabolic demands of tissue, thereby preventing further tissue damage. Cryotherapy can be used for 10–15 minutes at hourly intervals. Ice is also useful for dealing with post-exercise soreness.

NSAIDs may provide pain relief and an earlier return to activities, but the patient should be warned of the masking of symptoms by NSAIDs. Topical NSAIDs are preferable, as high levels in the tendon can be achieved, they have the least risk of side effects, and local massage of the drug into the tendon can itself provide relief. The effects of long-term use on tendon repair are unproven.

In some European countries, local anticoagulant therapy is advocated for early management of acute paratendonitis, with the aim of reducing oedema, fibrin exudate, and resulting adhesions between tendon and peritendinous tissues. Convincing evidence for benefit is lacking, and this approach is not widely advocated elsewhere.

Once the acute symptoms have resolved, the patient is prepared to commence a formal strengthening programme as will be described later. Early stretching of the gastrocnemius and soleus muscles separately, in addition to attention to hamstring stretching, is very important. Heat may be useful later in providing analgesia, reducing muscle spasm, improving tissue extensibility, inducing vasodilatation, and increasing vascular permeability and metabolism. Warm whirlpools, warm packs, hot gels, contrast baths, paraffin wax, and infrared radiaton can all be used for this purpose.

Local modalities, including ultrasound, deep heat, and laser, may be useful but are not applied in isolation and represent a minor component of the treatment programme, if used at all. Soft tissue release of the calf muscles often confers benefit, as does the use of a dorsiflexion night splint. Functional orthotics should be considered, and gradual strength training of the lower leg musculature should be introduced once the patient is pain free. Topical nitrate patches applied over the site(s) of symptoms for 12 hours may help to reduce pain. Their use can be limited by side effects, especially headaches, but low dose patches can help to avoid this.

A rehabilitation programme should be commenced and continued until well after the athlete returns to competitive sport, and ideally should become part of their long-term training programme as a preventative measure to prevent re-injury. The essentials are as follows: (a) it must be progressive in relation to increasing weight or resistance of exercises to progressively overload the muscle–tendon unit to maximize strength gains; (b) it must also use higher repetition and low load exercises to address muscular strength-endurance; (c) the exercises should increase in speed to improve muscle power. Not surprisingly, those who go through a rehabilitation programme without continuing to compete have a better outcome than those who continue to compete whilst rehabilitating.

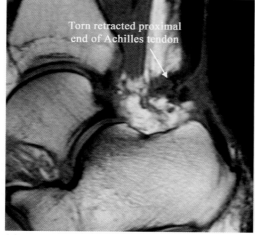

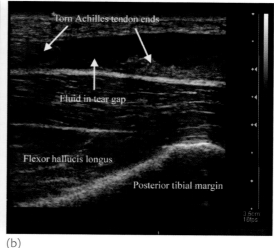

Fig. 3.11.12 MRI and US Achilles tendon tear. A 38-year-old male felt a snap behind ankle whilst playing squash. (a) Sagittal T1-weighted MRI demonstrating a full-thickness Achilles tendon tear. (b) Longitudinal US image. Note the tendon ends with intervening fluid gap.

(a)   (b)

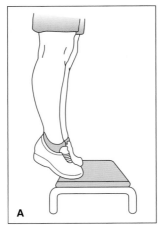
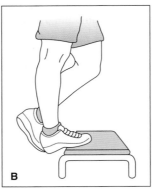

Fig. 3.11.13 Eccentric calf exercise: (a) the patient rises up on the toes over the edge of a step on both legs, and then (b) crosses the opposite leg behind the affected leg and slowly lowers the heel over the edge of the step.

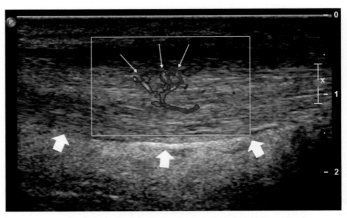

Fig. 3.11.14 Ultrasound Achilles tendinopathy with neovascularization in a 37-year-old fireman and keen amateur runner. Longitudinal ultrasound image demonstrating fusiform expansion of the Achilles tendon (block arrows) with multiple branching vessels within it (long arrows) consistent with non-insertional Achilles tendinopathy.

It is now well established that eccentric exercise programmes represent the cornerstone of Achilles tendinopathy rehabilitation (Kountouris and Cook 2007). There continues to be some debate as to specific aspects of such programmes, including the rate of progression in relation to loading and speed of contraction. Such issues emphasize the need to customize the programme to the needs of the athlete and their sport. The reasons for the high efficacy of eccentric work in alleviating painful Achilles lesions may be related to a reduction in neovascularization (Ohberg and Alfredson 2004) or to improvements in tendon structure (Ohberg *et al.* 2004). Return to activity should be gradual and closely monitored. The key to success is ensuring that the patient has a full understanding of the disorder and that the process of recovery may be lengthy.

Attention to precipitating factors is very important. This may include altering training in terms of intensity, types, and surfaces, addressing biomechanical issues and errors in technique, and changing equipment, particularly footwear, as discussed above. Although shoe design has improved, heel tabs can still be an issue and should be cut down where appropriate to avoid impingement on the tendon.

Recalcitrant tendon pain in the presence of neovascularization may be treated with either intratendinous (Maxwell *et al.* 2007) or targeted new vessel (Alfredson and Lorentzon 2007) sclerosant therapy (e.g. Polidocanol) administered under ultrasound guidance. High success rates are reported (Alfredson and Lorentzon 2007; Maxwell *et al.* 2007), although the long-term effects on the tendon have not yet been established. Alternative regimes include high-volume ultrasound-guided stripping of pathological vessels in the peritendinous space using saline and highly diluted steroids.

In those cases with significant paratendon disease, a minimally invasive paratendon strip using lidocaine or bupivocaine under ultrasound guidance (*Brisement* procedure) may relieve symptoms.

In those cases where a fluoroquinolone is implicated, immediate withdrawal of the offending agent and treatment of the local disorder will have a favourable outcome in the majority of cases, with resolution of symptoms within 2 months. Where the tendinosis is associated with hyperlipidaemic states, hypolipidaemic therapy with a statin is indicated.

Other approaches have been advocated but there is little basis to support their use. For example, glycosaminoglycan polysulphate (GAGPS) resembles the chemical composition of heparin, and the proposed basis for its use is the reduction of fibrin deposition and thrombus formation and inhibition of collagen breakdown. Local injections of GAGPS are of unproven benefit and have potential side effects including haemorrhage, thrombocytopenia, and hypersensitivity (Maxwell *et al.* 1987). It is perhaps because of these side effects that its use is not popular. Corticosteroid injections directly into the tendon have no role to play, as they are usually ineffective and may weaken the tendon with resulting rupture.

Platelet rich plasma injections are showing promise in the treatment of tendinopathies. The basis for their use is enhancement of tendon repair through delivery of natural growth factors by the injection of small volumes of the patient's blood to areas of tendinosis. In Achilles tendinosis specifically, the main concern is the potential for rupture after injection. No adequate randomized controlled trials have been performed.

Numerous surgical treatments have been described, although none have been subjected to rigorous evaluation. These include percutaneous (ultrasound-guided) tenotomy, arthroscopic debridement (tendoscopy), percutaneous paratendon stripping, paratendon stripping with multiple longtitudinal incisions in the area of maximal degeneration (Maffulli *et al.* 1997), open tenotomy and excision of a core of tendinotic material with paratendon stripping, and tendon grafting with FHL tendon transfer. There is a significant potential for complications of surgery in this area, and the reported incidence in such cases is up to 13%. Complications include poor wound healing, local nerve damage, infection, and failure of the repair.

Enthesitis and bursitis

Treatment approaches are similar to those detailed above, with the exception of the use of anticoagulant therapy. As with mid-portion Achilles tendinopathy, an eccentric programme is a mainstay as there is evidence for benefit (Jonsson *et al.* 2008).

Relief of friction between the heel counter and the bursal projection through padding and the modification of the shape, height, and rigidity of the heel counter may help. The height of the heel of the shoe influences symptoms; as the heel is raised, the angle of calcaneal inclination is decreased, bringing projection away from heel counter.

Extracorporeal shock wave therapy (ESWT) can be useful in cases of insertional tendinopathy, particularly where there is calcification or ossification of the Achilles tendon. Rompe *et al.* (2008) showed superior results with shock wave compared with eccentric training programme in one study.

Although corticosteroid injections are recommended by some for the management of insertional tendinopathies, they are usually unnecessary and it is important to remember that the bursa frequently communicates with peritendinous tissue. In acute bursitis with intrabursal fluid, aspiration is performed. Haglund's syndrome may take many months to show signs of improvement with conservative measures.

A seronegative arthropathy should be considered in those patients who have persisting insertional Achilles tendinopathy and/or retrocalcaneal bursitis.

Surgical intervention is reserved for those athletes with recalcitrant retrocalcaneal bursitis or Haglund's syndrome, which may involve debridement of the damaged tendon, resection of the bursa, or (as appropriate) excision of the posterior superior calcaneus (Haglund's deformity). Calcaneal osteotomy has also been advocated, although is considerably more invasive. The overall results for surgical treatment of insertional Achilles pathology suggest a longer recovery period and less overall satisfaction than for non-insertional surgery.

Rupture

Initial treatment of the acute Achilles tendon rupture involves the PRICES regime. The options are then early surgical repair with protective postoperative bracing or bracing for 8 weeks.

In the athlete, surgical intervention is usually pursued, since this results in less calf atrophy, greater range of motion, faster resumption of sporting activities, and fewer subjective complaints (Cetti *et al.* 1993; Popovic and Lemaire 2008). However, non-surgical management may be acceptable in certain circumstances, particularly when the patient is less active or not a good surgical candidate. Primary repair is usually undertaken in the acute phase, although rarely other techniques may be pursued using techniques more associated with chronic repairs.

An aggressive postoperative regimen is commonly followed, with early mobilization and commencement of rehabilitation. Complications of surgery in this region occur at a similar rate to surgery for tendinosis. Re-rupture rate is higher for non-surgical patients (8–21%) compared with surgical patients (2–5%) (Cetti *et al.* 1993; Popovic and Lemaire 2008). However, surgical complications as high as 38% have been reported, including adhesions, sural nerve damage, wound breakdown, deep vein thrombosis/pulmonary embolism, infection, and tendon lengthening.

Chronic tears

The neglected rupture should be treated surgically, as otherwise the functional results can be devastating. Primary repair may be attempted, but additional measures are usually required including (a) gap bridging by primary repair, using autologous tissue (proximal gastrocnemius–soleus complex, or (rarely) fascia lata or bone–tendon graft), synthetics, xenografts, or allografts, or (b) functional augmentation with (most commonly) FHL, plantaris, peroneus brevis, or FDL.

Partial tears

Partial Achilles tears are often classified as tendinosis, particularly when chronic, and are managed in the same way. In the acute stage, management follows the PRICES regime for 4–7 days, with rest to prevent further tearing and the use of a brace support. Surgery is rarely necessary, but those who do not respond to conservative treatment, the high-level athlete, and those with acute large longitudinal splits or substantial tears (more than 50% of circumference) should be considered for primary repair.

Calf muscle tears

The calf is one of the most commonly affected sites of muscle injury, particularly strain injury, in sport. The gastrocnemius is most commonly affected ('tennis leg'). Strain injuries can occur anywhere along the course of the myotendinous junction which spans at least 60% of the muscle length. The proximal third of the muscle, and in particular the medial head, is typically affected, with the injury occurring when it is overstretched with the ankle in dorsiflexion and the knee in full extension. Plantaris tendon rupture may also occur. The patient notes acute searing pain preventing further activity. Extensive swelling and bruising develops quickly and may progress over the subsequent 48 hours. A palpable defect may be present, and there is weakness and pain with resisted ankle plantarflexion.

It is important to exclude deep vein thrombosis, and ultrasound/venography are frequently required. Inappropriate treatment with anticoagulants can lead to further bleeding into the muscle and precipitate an acute compartment syndrome. The latter can also occur in the absence of anticoagulation if the damage is extensive. Ultrasound (US) and MRI are both sensitive methods in the diagnosis of gastrocnemius strain injuries. As with other muscle strain injuries, MRI is superior to ultrasound in the detection of grade I strains, while US is very helpful in assessing grade II and III injuries, and can help to monitor progress and evaluate healing. US can be used to aspirate any large haematomata formed post-injury.

Management involves the PRICES regime. Partial or non-weight-bearing for the first 2–3 days may be necessary. The patient is given a half-inch heel lift for 2 weeks to ease the stretch on the injured muscle. Range of motion exercises are commenced early, and gradual strengthening of the hamstrings and gastrocnemius–soleus complex are introduced when symptoms allow. Ballistic actions are avoided until full range of motion and strength are regained. A pre-exercise warm-up and stretching regime are introduced with the aim of preventing recurrence.

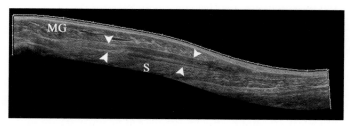

Fig. 3.11.15 Ultrasound of medial gastrocnemius tear in a 25-year-old netball player who felt a tear in the back of the calf during the initial phase of a jump. Longitudinal extended field of view sonogram. There is a tear (arrowheads) of the medial gastrocnemius (MG) at the aponeurosis with soleus (S). This condition has been referred to as 'tennis leg'.

It may take 3 months or longer before a return to full activities is achieved, but the prognosis is excellent and surgical intervention is not usually necessary. An unfortunate consequence of inadequately managed muscle strain injury is the formation of fibrous scarring, demonstrated well on ultrasound, which can result in persistent pain and/or recurrent injury at this site.

Effort-induced venous thrombosis

Although commonly noted in upper extremities, effort-induced venous thrombosis in the lower limb is less well recognized. An acute onset of pain in the calf after exercise is the predominant feature, although symptoms may be felt anteriorly. Examination reveals the typical signs of a deep vein thrombosis—a tight, tender, and usually enlarged calf. An ultrasound scan and a venogram are performed to confirm the diagnosis, and treatment with anticoagulation is commenced immediately.

Anomalous soleus muscle

An anomalous soleus muscle can become painful, and usually presents in adolescence or early adulthood. Symptoms include pain and tenderness in front of the Achilles tendon, and there is evidence of fullness or a bulbous mass at the medial or lateral side of the tendon. Various treatment recommendations exist; stretching, activity modification, a medial heel wedge, and orthotics should all be considered. Surgery in the form of fasciotomy or surgical excision is reserved for intractable cases.

Chronic exertional compartment syndrome

Chronic exertional compartment syndrome (CECS) refers to calf muscle pain as a result of presumed relative ischaemia due to raised intracompartmental pressure during exercise. The raised intracompartmental pressure has been attributed to vascular factors, metabolic factors, and other factors, including fascial hypertrophy, muscular hypertrophy, and tissue oedema. Proposed mechanisms for the development of ischaemia as a result of raised compartment pressure include arterial spasm, obstruction of the microcirculation, arteriolar or venous collapse due to transmural pressure disturbances, or venous obstruction. There is some debate about the existence of tissue ischaemia in CECS. Other explanations for the pain have been proposed, including stimulation of sensory receptors in the periosteum due to elevated pressure or unknown biochemical factors.

History

The patient typically reports dull aching pain and tightness in the lower leg, which typically commences at a defined point in the exercise session and may become progressively severe, frequently necessitating cessation of activity. The symptoms resolve quickly with rest, only to recur when the activity recommences. In some cases there may be residual ache into the next day. The site of the pain varies according to the compartment(s) involved. Most commonly, the anterior compartment is involved, resulting in pain in the anterolateral aspect of the leg. The deep posterior compartment is the next most commonly involved, with pain experienced over the medial shin and/or distal posterior calf that may spread to the medial foot. Superficial posterior compartment syndrome, which gives proximal calf pain, is uncommon, and isolated lateral compartment syndrome is rare, usually being seen in the presence of an anterior compartment syndrome. It is common for more than one compartment to be affected, and symptoms are commonly bilateral although they may be worse in one leg.

Neurological symptoms may occur, varying according to the nerve(s) involved, but typically causing numbness and weakness.

Examination

At rest, clinical examination is normal although the muscles in a compartment may feel rather tense. On standing there may be evidence of small muscle hernias. The patient must be examined when symptomatic, i.e. during and after the onset of symptoms with exercise. At this stage the compartment will be tense, firm, and painful to deep palpation and passive stretch. Neurological impairment may be evident. Anterior compartment syndrome results in deep peroneal nerve compression, with weakness of dorsiflexion and altered sensation over the first web space. Lateral CECS causes superficial peroneal nerve impairment, with sensory signs over the lateral lower leg and dorsum of the foot and weakness of eversion. Deep posterior CECS can result in tibial nerve dysfunction, with sensory changes over the medial arch of the foot and/or cramping of the foot muscles. Distal pulses remain normal. The symptoms and signs will improve, usually over a short period of time during the assessment. Ankle reflexes may be diminished.

Muscle hernias are associated with CECS, particularly at the site where the superficial peroneal nerve exits the deep fascia at the lateral leg. Paraesthesia due to nerve entrapment at the site of the defect is common. Other causes of exertional lower limb pain must be considered during the evaluation.

Investigations: compartment pressure studies

The most useful investigation in suspected CECS is a compartment pressure study. Although high levels on compartment pressure measurements are considered to be necessary for the diagnosis of compartment syndromes, the apparatus, methodologies used, and specific compartment pressure levels for diagnosis of the complaint vary significantly. The accuracy, sensitivity, and specificity of compartment pressure studies are not known.

Apparatus used has varied from needle manometers, side-ported needles, and simple needles to wick catheters, slit catheters, and an infusion or non-infusion technique with an electronic transducer-tipped catheter (Allen and Barnes 1986; Fronek et al. 1987; Bourne and Rorabeck 1989). Pressures can vary considerably with operator experience, apparatus, volume of instilled fluid, leg position, activity type, and timing of measurement(s). Sejersted and Hargens

Table 3.11.6 Diagnostic levels for chronic compartment syndrome

Reference	Criteria
Rorabeck et al. 1988	Pressure >15 mmHg at 15 minutes post-exercise
Bourne and Rorabeck 1989	Elevated post-exercise pressure and delay (>5 minutes) in return to pre-exercise levels'
Fronek et al. 1987	At least 10 mmHg at rest or at least 25 mmHg 5 minutes post-exercise
Pedowitz et al. 1990	Appropriate clinical findings and at least one of: pre-exercise pressure >15 mmHg 1 minute post-exercise pressure >30 mmHg 5-minute post exercise pressure >20 mmHg
Allen and Barnes 1986	Anterior compartment: pressure >15 mmHg Deep posterior compartment: pressure >40 mmHg

(1995) pointed out that intramuscular pressure follows Laplace's law, which means that it is determined by the tension of the muscle fibres, the recording depth, and the fibre geometry (fibre curvature or pennation angle). Such factors will also be sources of variation in the pressure level reading. The patient is tested during the activity which most frequently exacerbates the symptoms, usually running, which is conveniently performed on a treadmill in a laboratory or clinic setting. Measurements are taken at rest and after exercise at specific stages when symptoms are present, including during the recovery.

Wiley *et al.* (1987) performed a meta-analysis of 21 studies (1979–1998) measuring anterior intracompartmental pressures during exercise. They evaluated the type of exercise, the catheter technique, and the diagnostic criteria recommended. Their findings demonstrated that there had been no standardization concerning the type of muscular exertion (isometrics for 5–10 min, exercise on the treadmill between 3.2 and 12 km/h). In eight of the studies the results were attained using the unsuitable Wick catheter technique. There was little or no overlap between teams in the use of suggested criteria for diagnosis, and there were considerable variations (by up to 500%) regarding the recommended parameters. The authors concluded that no uniform recommendation for parameters of diagnostic relevance can be derived.

Positioning of the catheter is important, although it is not usually a problem except in the tibialis posterior and deep posterior compartments. Melberg and Styf (1989) described some of the difficulties associated with pressure recording in the deep posterior compartment, and found that the result of pressure recording depends on which muscle in the deep posterior compartment is investigated and the type of work performed. Ultrasound guidance also has the advantage of placement of the catheter tip into the belly of a specific muscle.

Near-infrared spectroscopy and pre- and post-exercise MRI have also been advocated in the diagnosis of CECS (van den Brand *et al.* 2005). MRI may show an increased T2-weighted signal intensity in the affected compartment(s) which exhibits a delayed (10 minutes) return to normal after exercise (Fig. 3.11.16).

Patients with CECS may undergo a range of other investigations, usually to exclude other causes of exertional lower limb pain.

Management

Beyond stretching, biomechanical modifications, and addressing any equipment or training errors, treatment of chronic compartment syndrome is considered to be either restriction of activity or fasciotomy. Although the latter is claimed to be 'curative' in most cases, neither adequate follow up studies nor randomized controlled trials have been performed.

Although the standard surgery for exertional anterior compartment syndrome is subcutaneous fasciotomy of the anterior compartment through a short incision, some surgeons decompress the lateral compartment at the same time to prevent kinking or entrapment of the superficial peroneal nerve as it exits the lateral compartment. Schepsis *et al.* (1993) suggested that a lateral compartment release is unnecessary when doing a fasciotomy for exertional anterior compartment syndrome alone.

Decompression of the superficial and deep posterior compartments may be performed through a single long incision, protecting the saphenous nerve and long saphenous vein and its tributaries. Fasciotomy under direct vision is safer than blind subcutaneous fasciotomy.

Wallenstein (1983) studied the results of fasciotomy of the affected muscle compartment in eight patients with chronic anterior compartment syndrome and nine patients with medial tibial syndrome (involvement of the deep posterior compartment), all of whom had pain with exercise. In the patients with chronic anterior compartment syndrome, the preoperative intramuscular pressure in the anterior tibial compartment, as measured by the wick-catheter method, was increased to 52 ± 36 mmHg 10 minutes after exercise. After fasciotomy, this pressure was significantly lowered to 4 ± 6 mmHg ($p < 0.01$). In patients with medial tibial syndrome, the preoperative intramuscular pressure in the deep posterior compartment was normal 10 minutes after exercise (8 ± 4 mmHg) and did not significantly change after the fasciotomy (5 ± 6 mmHg). The clinical results after fasciotomy were 'good' in both groups of patients. There was complete relief of pain in all the patients with chronic anterior compartment syndrome and in five of the nine patients with medial tibial syndrome. The other four patients considered their condition to be improved despite some remaining symptoms.

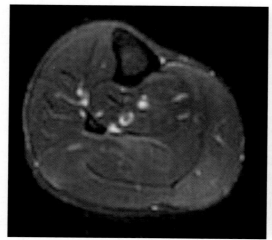
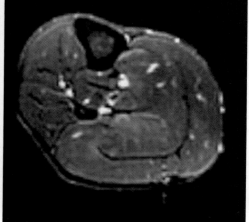

Fig. 3.11.16 MRI of lower leg showing delayed return to normal of an increased T2-weighted signal after exercise: (a) pre-exercise; (b) 15 minutes post-exercise.

(a)

(b)

Rorabeck *et al.* (1988) reported a higher likelihood of recurrence if the deep posterior compartment was involved. Micheli *et al.* (1999) found a lower success rate with operative fasciotomy in young female athletes than the rates generally reported in studies combining male and female patients. The reasons for this are unclear.

Christensen *et al.* (1983) reported normalization of previously elevated compartment pressures in five active middle-aged men with chronic compartment syndrome after 2–3 weeks of diuretic therapy. Rorabeck *et al.* (1988) noted poorer results in patients with deep posterior compartment syndromes, and recommended performance of a formal release of the tibialis posterior at the time of decompression. However, the results of this procedure were not reported.

Closure of muscle hernias is contraindicated and may precipitate a compartment syndrome. Postoperatively, it is essential to commence an exercise programme after 24 hours to maintain muscle tone and bulk and to avoid the fascia from healing without separation.

Popliteal artery entrapment syndrome

Vascular causes are an important cause of exercise-related leg pain but, with the exception of peripheral vascular disease, are rare. However, popliteal artery entrapment syndrome (PAES) is included in the differential diagnosis.

As the artery exits the popliteal fossa, it can become entrapped by the gastrocnemius. Several anomalies have been described, most commonly an abnormal medial head of the gastrocnemius, the accessory part of which may pass behind the popliteal artery. Other anomalies of the medial and lateral heads of the gastrocnemius, accessory tendinous slips, and an abnormal plantaris muscle have also been implicated in this condition. The artery can also become entrapped at the adductor hiatus, and isolated entrapment of the anterior tibial artery as it passes through the interosseous membrane can also occur.

History

The patient complains of an ill-defined deep ache in the calf and/or anterior aspect of the leg with exercise. The severity of symptoms is related to the intensity of the exercise and resolves with rest, typically more quickly than that of chronic compartment syndrome. In addition, unlike chronic compartment syndrome, the pain from PAES is unaffected by exercise the previous day. It should be noted that the conditions can coexist.

Examination

Examination of the patient at rest may reveal a popliteal artery bruit with active resisted plantarflexion or passive dorsiflexion with the knee in extension.

Investigations

Compartment studies are usually performed as clinical differentiation between the two syndromes is often difficult. Duplex ultrasonography of the arterial tree is performed with the ankle being actively and passively plantarflexed and dorsiflexed. If flow is reduced, digital subtraction angiography is performed. MRI angiography is probably the investigation of choice in the young adult with intermittent claudication. This may show displacement and compression of the popliteal artery on axial view.

If angiography shows no evidence of intramural vascular damage, simple division of constricting bands or muscles may be all that is necessary. Otherwise, the abnormal portion of the vessel is bypassed with a reversed vein graft, using the short saphenous vein.

Anterior leg pain

Stress fractures

Stress fractures in the lower leg are extremely common in sport and must be high on any differential diagnosis in an athletic patient with exertional lower limb pain. They are common in all lower limb weight-bearing sports, but are particularly common in runners and military recruits, and in high-impact sports such as basketball, badminton, and gymnastics.

A stress fracture can be defined as a partial or complete fracture of bone caused by an inability to withstand stress that is applied in a rhythmic repeated subthreshold manner. It is a reflection of bone's inability to remodel adequately in response to the mechanical stress placed on it. Those forces include joint reaction forces, muscle forces, and bone contact force on the tibia. Stress fractures represent one end of the spectrum of stress injuries that can affect bone (Table 3.11.7). Injuries can be transverse or, much less commonly, longitudinal.

Stress fractures can be further classified as fatigue fractures, which are due to overloading of normal bone, or insufficiency fractures, produced when physiological stress is applied to bone that has reduced mechanical integrity. Fatigue stress fractures of the tibia and fibula usually occur in relation to running or marching and represent 45% of all stress fractures seen in relation to sport. Since the tibia transmits approximately 83% of body weight, it is the most common site for stress fractures in sport.

Stress injuries of the tibia and fibula can be further classified according to their site. Those affecting the tibia most commonly occur in the proximal or distal thirds of the posteromedial cortex. They may also be seen just distal to the tibial tuberosity in young people. Those just below the tibial plateau may be clinically mistaken for pes anserinus bursitis or a medial collateral ligament sprain. Most lesions occur at sites where bone is under compression stress, but they can also occur at sites of tension, such as the middle third of the tibia on the anterior cortex. Since the bone is under tension at this site, healing is more difficult, with significant risk of non-union or full fracture. Such injuries must be monitored

Table 3.11.7 Imaging of stress reactions: grading system

Grade	Bone scan appearance	MRI appearance
I	Small ill-defined cortical area of mild increased activity	Periosteal oedema: +/++ (T2W) Marrow oedema: absent (T1W, T2W)
II	Better-defined cortical area of moderately increased activity	Periosteal oedema: ++/+++ (T2W) Marrow oedema: present (T2W)
III	Wide to fusiform cortical–medullary area of highly increased activity	Periosteal oedema: ++/+++ (T2W) Marrow oedema: present (T1W, T2W)
IV (stress fracture)	Transcortical area of increased activity	Periosteal oedema: ++/+++ (T2W) Marrow oedema: present (T1W, T2W) Fracture line clearly visible

+ mild, ++ moderate, +++ severe; T1W, T2W, T1- or T2-weighted images.
Sources: Zwas *et al.* 1987; Fredericson *et al.* 1995

particularly carefully, as they are slower to heal and more likely to progress to a complete fracture. Aggressive management, including surgical intervention, may be necessary.

Young athletes with immature skeletal systems are also susceptible, not only in relation to endurance sport but also in relation to sports that involve sudden stops.

Predisposing factors to tibial stress injury are abnormal tibial morphology, in particular having a narrow (i.e. slender) tibia relative to body mass, limitations in aerobic fitness, and menstrual cycle irregularities in females.

History

Symptoms usually commence after a change in one or more of the volume or intensity of activity, training techniques, and equipment (footwear), or after another injury (Table 3.11.2). Menstrual irregularities are often associated with stress fractures in female athletes.

The patient reports a gradual onset of localized dull pain at the site of the injury, usually 2–6 weeks after an increase in training load. The pain is initially noted at a specific stage during exercise, and as symptoms progress the pain occurs earlier during the activity, often leading to a restriction in the volume and/or intensity of the activity. Eventually there is pain at rest, which may disturb the patient at night.

A detailed history is taken of training patterns, surfaces, equipment, technical alterations, diet, and previous injuries, and a menstrual history is taken in females. General health should also be evaluated, in particular in relation to bone health.

Examination

There is local bony tenderness at the site of the stress fracture. Local swelling and warmth may be present and indeed may be the only sign. In more chronic cases, periosteal thickening and/or callus may be palpable. Percussion both close to and distant from the site of the fracture reproduces the symptoms. Exacerbation of pain with the application of therapeutic ultrasound to the symptomatic area is a widely quoted but insensitive test. Intrinsic factors which may predispose the patient to developing a stress fracture must be considered and the patient evaluated appropriately.

Investigations

Plain X-rays have a low sensitivity for the detection of stress fractures and may be normal for up to 12 weeks. However, the specificity is high when changes are evident. Periosteal reaction is the first sign, followed by cortical lucency as osteoclastic resorption occurs. The healing stress fracture will demonstrate thick periosteal new bone formation, endosteal thickening, and cortical hypertrophy. Demonstration of a fracture line is variable. Similar findings may be noted in an osteoid osteoma, osteomyelitis, osteogenic sarcoma, exostoses, or tumours that result in periosteal reaction, peripheral bone reaction or destruction, and Paget's disease.

MRI is now the investigation of choice in the investigation of a suspected stress injury. It has the advantage over isotope bone scanning of lack of radiation exposure, faster imaging time, and demonstration of surrounding anatomy. A combination of T1-weighted sequences that optimize anatomic detail and a sequence that depicts bone oedema (such as STIR, fat-suppressed proton density, and T2-weighted fast spin echo sequences) are required. Fredericson *et al.* (1995) proposed a grading system for MRI in the evaluation of stress lesions, which is clinically useful (Table 3.11.7).

A triple-phase isotope bone scan is highly sensitive (virtually 100%) to stress lesions, with all phases of the triple-phase scan being abnormal within 2 days of onset of the lesion, demonstrating

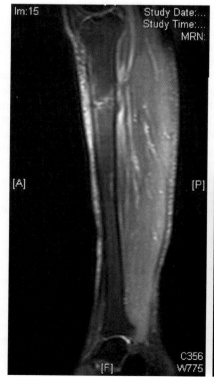
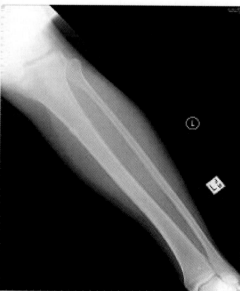

Fig. 3.11.17 MRI and X-ray showing a stress fracture (almost complete) of the proximal tibia.

an increased uptake of radionucleide. A grading system has been developed based on the degree and pattern of tracer uptake (Table 3.11.7). The system reflects a continuum of changes, from the early 'pre-fracture' bone strain through stress reaction, to stress fracture (Zwas *et al.* 1987). The fusiform appearance of an established stress fracture differs significantly from the more diffuse linear uptake seen in medial tibial periostitis.

As healing of the stress fracture progresses, the first (angiogram) phase and subsequently the blood pool images become normal. Delayed images remain abnormal for at least 3–6 (and often up to 12) months. A false-positive rate of 10–20% is reported, and is due to accelerated bone remodelling. Positive scans are also seen at the epiphyses of adolescents.

Stress reactions can be apparent on MRI and scintigrams in the absence of symptoms, as a reflection of bone remodelling in response to mechanical stress. Only a percentage of cases will progress to develop a stress fracture. As with any injury, imaging findings need to be interpreted in the context of the clinical picture.

Computed tomography (CT) can help to differentiate between conditions that can mimic stress fractures, such as osteoid osteoma as described earlier. This mode of imaging is also helpful in demonstrating a fracture line as evidence of a stress fracture as opposed to a stress reaction.

Other investigations include bone densitometry, bone health, bone turnover and endocrine markers, and vitamin D status, as appropriate.

Management

Management depends on the location and severity of the lesion and is based on reducing the stress at the affected site to allow healing to occur. Relative rest by the reduction of loading activities is the cornerstone of management in most cases. Cross-training allows fitness to be maintained to a large extent through activities that involve little or no loading, such as swimming, water running, indoor rowing, and cycling. Strength training can be continued provided that excessive loading of the affected area is avoided.

In the early stages, ice packs and basic analgesics are used for symptomatic relief. The use of a pneumatic brace may also help to relieve symptoms and has been shown to reduce the time taken to return to activity. It probably works through unloading the tibia by compressing the lower leg, redistributing the forces (including to surrounding soft tissue), and decreasing the amount of tibia bowing. Use of low intensity pulsed ultrasound (LIPUS) may speed bone healing (see Chapter 2.4).

Modification of risk factors is vital to prevention of recurrence. Progressive activity is strictly regulated. When the patient resumes full training it is important to ensure that adequate recovery sessions are scheduled between periods of heavy training and that all training errors have been corrected.

Stress fractures of the anterior cortex of the midshaft of the tibia are prone to non-union, delayed union, and complete fracture. If the patient presents late, the plain radiograph may demonstrate the 'dreaded black line' due to bony resorption and indicative of non-union. MRI will confirm with a hyperintense signal with cortical disruption. Isotope bone scan at that late stage may show no abnormality. Management involves avoidance of aggravating load-bearing, whilst using a long pneumatic leg brace and close monitoring, both clinical and radiographic, to ensure that healing is taking place. An initial period of non-weight-bearing for up to 4 weeks may be necessary. Healing may take up to 9 months; failure

to show signs of healing during that time is an indication for consideration of surgical intervention.

Medial malleolar stress fractures are also prone to delayed or non-union. They extend from the tibial plafond proximally in an oblique direction. They are inherently unstable and may require an extensive period of casting. Early internal fixation with screws has been advocated.

Fibular stress fractures usually occur just proximal to the tibiofibular syndesmosis where stress is particularly concentrated during muscle contraction. Less commonly, stress fractures can occur on the neck of the fibula.

Medial tibial periostitis

Several anatomical structures have been proposed to cause traction of the periosteal–fascial junction at the posteromedial tibial border, resulting in medial tibial periostitis. The soleus is the most likely to be involved, since it partially attaches medially to the investing fascia. FDL and the deep crural fascia have also been implicated, as has the tibialis posterior as its origin includes a portion of the lower third of the tibia. The most accepted theory of the aetiology of the condition is that, in some athletes when running, an excessive degree or velocity of pronation increases the eccentric stress on supporting musculature, in particular the soleus. The velocity of pronation may be a more important factor than the actual degree. Stiffness of the gastrocnemius–soleus musculature may also be a contributing factor.

Training errors are reported in 60% of cases. Usually there is an abrupt increase in the frequency, duration, or intensity of training. Training on hard surfaces, hill training, and inappropriate footwear, with inadequate cushioning and/or support, are also common associated factors. The relevance of physical conditioning to the complaint is unclear.

Those who develop the condition acutely after a sudden exposure to high-intensity training (such as in the military) may progress to develop a stress fracture. This is less likely in those with chronic symptoms.

History

The patient complains of dull pain along the posteromedial border of the distal two-thirds of the tibia in association with weight-bearing activity. Symptoms usually commence after a change in one or more of the typical extrinsic factors or may be associated with various intrinsic characteristics associated with overuse injuries. Symptoms appear initially in the early phase of exercise but may disappear if exercise continues, only to return towards the end of the session. At this stage there is no pain at rest. As the condition progresses, symptoms occur earlier in the activity session and when severe can be present during daily activities and finally will disturb the patient at rest (Table 3.11.8).

Examination

The patient should be evaluated for deformities and malalignments of the leg, foot, and ankle. There is diffuse tenderness along the posteromedial border of the distal two-thirds of the tibia, more marked on the bone than on adjacent soft tissue. Local oedema and warmth may be noted. Stretching of the soleus may exacerbate the symptoms. Passive and active movements of the ankle and foot are pain free and normal. Pain will also be exacerbated by progressive loading of the plantarflexor musculature through forced passive dorsiflexion, active plantarflexion against resistance, two-leg

Table 3.11.8 Grading of shin pain in bone stress injuries of the lower leg

Grade	Pain
I	Pain occurs only on extreme exertion and ceases when activity stops
II	Pain occurs with moderate activity, but disappears after a short time; it reappears after cessation of activity and persists for 1–2 hours
III	Pain is present with any activity and may persist for many hours after activity stops
IV	Pain present at rest

standing toe raises, two-leg standing jumps, and maximum stress with one-legged jumps. The condition must be differentiated from other causes of lower limb pain; percussion of the tibia should not cause a local increase in pain and no callus should be palpable. Neurovascular examination is normal.

Gait analysis, looking in particular at rear foot motion, is also performed, in particular to assess the degree of pronation.

Investigation

Plain radiographs are almost always normal; in chronic severe cases there may be evidence of periosteal reaction with new bone formation and cortical hypertrophy at the site of symptoms. MRI may demonstrate periosteal fluid or bone marrow oedema in chronic cases or alteration adjacent to the insertion of the plantarflexor muscles in more acute cases. A triple-phase isotope bone scan will demonstrate diffusely increased uptake on the posteromedial border of the tibia in the delayed phase of the scan. This differs from the more intense focal uptake seen in tibial stress fractures. Medial and lateral views may help to localize the uptake better. Tomographic bone scans (SPECT) may help to identify difficult lesions, although this is rarely necessary.

Management

No intervention will be successful without identification and correction of the underlying causes (Table 3.11.2).

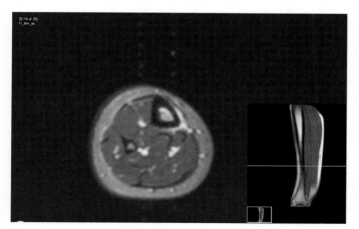

Fig. 3.11.18 Three weeks history of right shin pain in a runner after increased mileage. MRI shows medial tibial periostitis with an underlying tibial stress response.

Relative rest varies according to the severity of the symptoms, and ranges from simply reducing the intensity or volume of training to total avoidance of load-bearing activities. Cross-training, such as cycling, swimming, and water running in a water vest, is helpful for maintaining cardiovascular fitness and muscle strength. Ice and ice massage, local massage, NSAIDs, acupuncture, and stretching are all pursued. Muscle imbalances should be corrected. Orthotics are often useful in this condition; a medial heel post is used for those with hyperpronation, while a medial forefoot post may help those with forefoot varus. Heel pads and cushioned insoles may provide shock absorbency. Cushioned supportive footwear should be recommended, avoiding shoes with a wide heel which can increase the velocity of foot pronation through heel strike.

When the patient is pain free, progressive weight-bearing conditioning commences, supplemented by calf stretching and muscle balance work. Generally the volume can be increased by 10% per week, provided that the patient remains pain free. If symptoms recur, the patient should rest until pain free for 2–3 days and then recommence the programme at a lower level. Ice massage after exercise sessions may help to reduce a reaction. Rehabilitation may be lengthy, and the most common cause of recurrence of symptoms is a premature return to activities. Surgery may rarely be considered in those who fail conservative management and may involve fasciotomy of the posteromedial superficial and deep fascia at the tibia. Some advocate denervation by cauterization of the periosteum along the entire posteromedial border of the tibia in order to achieve scarring and reattachment of the periosteum to underlying bone. Return to light loading activities is then permitted after 4–6 weeks of rest.

Medial tibial stress syndrome

Medial tibial stress syndrome (MTSS) is a diagnosis of exclusion, a term reserved for patients with exertional lower limb pain, in whom all investigations are normal. MTSS and medial periostitis are probably part of a continuum from strain of the muscles that cause traction periostitis to true periostitis. The aetiology and history are the same as described for periostitis, while tenderness may be located to the soft tissue structures adjacent to the bone rather than the bone itself. Investigations are normal. Management of the condition involves the same approaches as for medial tibial periostitis.

Tibiofibular synostosis

Ossification of the interosseous membrane is very rare. It can be congenital or acquired and may be proximal, distal, or diaphyseal. Congenital forms may present in adolescence. Acquired synostosis occurs in relation to repetitive microtrauma or to a single injury, in particular an ankle sprain, where there is tearing of the anterior and posterior tibiofibular ligaments and the lower third of the interosseous membrane. Bone develops from either side as a flat exostosis or across the interosseous membrane, creating a synostosis. Certain individuals appear to be predisposed to this condition, although the specific factors involved are undetermined. The incidence of late calcification in the syndesmosis and distal interosseous membrane may be higher than suspected. In one study, 32% of professional footballers had late calcification in distal tibiofibular syndesmosis (Vincelette *et al.* 1972).

The patient presents with a history of 'spasm' in the anterior leg, worse with weight-bearing and with movement of the ankle.

Symptoms suggestive of ankle instability may be present. There is tenderness over the synostosis and limitation of motion of the ankle, especially dorsiflexion.

A plain X-ray may be normal during the early stages of synostosis formation. An isotope bone scan will show diffuse uptake in the area of the synostosis if the process is active. Later, the bone scan is cold, but radiographic changes are apparent and are also demonstrated on CT. MRI may show signal changes in the tissue.

Treatment involves treating the initial injury (usually ankle sprain), modification of activities and rehabilitation, initially focusing upon flexibility and proprioception, and then a progressive strengthening programme. Further management depends on symptomatology as the long-term effect on ankle biomechanics is unclear. A partial or complete synostosis is compatible with high-level athletic performance in certain individuals (Whiteside *et al.* 1978; Ogilvie-Harris *et al.* 1997). Surgery may be necessary where the patient remains symptomatic, but it is very invasive, involving excision of the synostosis. Recurrence is common.

Nerve entrapment syndromes

Nerve entrapment syndromes in the leg may give rise to pain and sensorimotor symptoms which may be present only during activity. Deep burning pain may be accompanied by shooting pains in the distribution of the nerve. Symptoms can be non-specific and there is considerable inter-individual variation.

When taking a **history**, the location and nature of the pain and associated neurological symptoms should be sought. A history of back pain and the existence of any 'red flags' that may indicate a serious underlying disorder should be specifically sought.

Examination aims to identify the peripheral nerve involved and to exclude other causes of lower limb pain that may mimic nerve entrapment (Table 3.11.1). Neurological symptoms may arise in relation to other complaints affecting the lower leg, such as compartment syndromes.

Investigations: electrodiagnostic tests in the lower limb are used to confirm nerve entrapment but they are often less definitive than those in the upper limb, for a number of reasons. These include protocols having a wider range of normal values, the effects of temperature and local oedema, and the plane of the foot differing from that of the leg, affecting distance measurements. False-positive needle EMG findings are possible for intrinsic muscles of the foot. It is vital to ensure that the clinical features are consistent with the electrophysiological findings. Nevertheless, they are useful; nerve conduction studies may demonstrate a conduction block where localized entrapment is present, and where the lesion is severe or chronic, there may be evidence of denervation.

Abolition of symptoms after infiltration at the site of entrapment with local anaesthetic also helps to confirm the diagnosis.

Common peroneal nerve

The common peroneal nerve (CPN) is vulnerable to injury and compression at the neck of the fibula, for example by a tight leg cast. In addition, activities that cause repetitive pronation and inversion (machine operators, running) may cause traction injuries of the nerve. Compartment syndromes result in dysfunction of the CPN or, more typically its superficial (anterior compartment) or deep (deep posterior compartment) branches.

Superficial peroneal nerve

The superficial peroneal nerve (SPN) is more vulnerable to injury than the deep branch. It can be entrapped or compressed as it exits the crural fascia approximately 10 cm proximal to the lateral malleolus, to divide into its cutaneous branches. Compression by local masses such as a ganglion or lipoma or by callus formation from a previous fracture of the fibula, and traction on the nerve by repeated ankle sprains, can all occur. There is pain and sensory change at the cutaneous distribution of the nerve brought on by exercise, which may be clinically evident with resisted dorsiflexion and eversion, in particular with resisted dorsiflexion and eversion and with passive plantarflexion and inversion of the foot. Even normal increases in compartment pressures can cause impingement of the nerve against the edge of a fascial defect. The SPN is also vulnerable where its terminal branches cross the anterior ankle subcutaneously, particularly when shoe laces are too tight. Electrodiagnostic studies may be necessary to exclude an L5 radiculopathy.

Treatment

Fascial defects must not be closed as this can precipitate an acute compartment syndrome. Conservative management involves appropriate rehabilitation of ankle sprains, including peroneal muscle strengthening, proprioceptive training, and a medial heel wedge to reduce the traction on the nerve. Local infiltration with anaesthetic and corticosteroid may be useful. A tricyclic agent may help to reduce neuralgia. Fascial release and/or neurolysis is the preferred option when surgery is considered.

Deep peroneal nerve

The deep peroneal nerve (DPN) can be compressed with an acute anterior compartment syndrome, and where an anterior tarsal tunnel syndrome (TTS) is present or there are anterior osteophytes on the anterior aspect of the ankle, causing nerve irritation. In the latter two cases, the symptoms are localized to the foot with numbness confined to the dorsum of the first web space. In 22% of individuals, extensor digitorum brevis is innervated by an accessory DPN and therefore weakness may not be present.

In anterior TTS, symptoms may respond to modification of activities and correction of equipment and/or biomechanical factors and padding to protect against further nerve compression. When conservative measures fail or where a compartment syndrome exists, surgery may be necessary to decompress the nerve and deal with any underlying problems such as removing anterior osteophytes.

The sural nerve

Sural nerve entrapment is relatively uncommon, but the nerve may be compressed or entrapped by local mass lesions such as a ganglion, scar tissue, thrombophlebitis, or tight boots or leg casts, or it may be traumatized by surgery or injections. Repeated inversion sprains of the ankle may lead to traction scarring and entrapment. Treatment involves correction of causative factors, footwear modification, protective padding, ankle rehabilitation, and, where necessary, excision of scar tissue or a ganglion where these are implicated in the symptoms.

The saphenous nerve

The saphenous nerve may be injured in the adductor canal in the thigh by trauma, or at the knee, usually relating to surgery. It has also been suggested that repeated knee flexion may stretch the nerve. The patient reports claudicant medial lower leg pain. When the site of entrapment is in the thigh, pain is exacerbated by compression of the nerve in the medial thigh and altered sensation in the cutaneous distribution of the nerve is present. Treatment is symptomatic and may involve the use of a tricyclic agent or, in severe cases, neurolysis.

Tibial nerve entrapment.

The tibial nerve may be entrapped in the popliteal fossa by a local mass such as Baker's cyst, a ganglion, or a popliteal artery aneurysm, but injuries or entrapments affecting this nerve are rare. In contrast, its continuation as the posterior tibial nerve can become entrapped at the ankle in the tarsal tunnel.

VISA score for the assessment of Achilles tendinopathy

IN THIS QUESTIONNAIRE, THE TERM PAIN REFERS SPECIFICALLY TO PAIN IN THE ACHILLES TENDON REGION

1. For how many minutes do you have stiffness in the Achilles region on first getting up?

100 mins |___|___|___|___|___|___|___|___|___|___| 0 mins   POINTS [ ]
      0   1   2   3   4   5   6   7   8   9   10

2. Once you are warmed up for the day, do you have pain when stretching the Achilles tendon fully over the edge of a step? (keeping knee straight)

strong severe pain |___|___|___|___|___|___|___|___|___|___| no pain   POINTS [ ]
             0   1   2   3   4   5   6   7   8   9   10

3. After walking on flat ground for 30 minutes, do you have pain within the next 2 hours? (If unable to walk on flat ground for 30 minutes because of pain, score 0 for this question).

strong severe pain |___|___|___|___|___|___|___|___|___|___| no pain   POINTS [ ]
             0   1   2   3   4   5   6   7   8   9   10

4. Do you have pain walking downstairs with a normal gait cycle?

strong severe pain |___|___|___|___|___|___|___|___|___|___| no pain   POINTS [ ]
             0   1   2   3   4   5   6   7   8   9   10

5. Do your have pain during or immediately after doing 10 (single leg) heel raises from a flat surface?

strong severe pain |___|___|___|___|___|___|___|___|___|___| no pain   POINTS [ ]
             0   1   2   3   4   5   6   7   8   9   10

6. How many single leg hops can you do without pain?

strong severe pain/unable |___|___|___|___|___|___|___|___|___|___| no pain   POINTS [ ]
                    0   1   2   3   4   5   6   7   8   9   10

7. Are your currently undertaking sport or other physical activity?

0   r   Not at all   POINTS [ ]

4   r   Modified training modified ± competition

7   r   Full training ± competition but not at same level as when symptoms began

10 r   Competing at the same or higher level as when symptoms began

8. Please complete **EITHER A, B or C** in this question.
- If you have **no pain while undertaking Achilles tendon loading sports** please complete **Q8a only**.
- If you have **pain while undertaking Achilles tendon loading sports but it does not stop you from completing the activity**, please complete **Q8b only**.
- If you have **pain which stops you from completing Achilles tendon loading sports**, please complete **Q8c only**.

A. If you have **no pain** while undertaking **Achilles tendon loading sports**, for how long can you train/practise?

NIL	1–10 mins	11–20 mins	21–30 mins	>30 mins	POINTS
r	r	r	r	r	[ ]
0	7	14	21	30	

OR

B. If you have some pain while undertaking **Achilles tendon loading sport**, but it does not stop you from completing your training/practice for how long can you train/practise?

NIL	1–10 mins	11–20 mins	21–30 mins	>30 mins	POINTS
r	r	r	r	r	[ ]
0	4	10	14	20	

OR

C. If you have **pain that stops you** from completing your training/practice in **Achilles tendon loading sport**, for how long can you train/practise?

NIL	1–10 mins	11–20 mins	21–30 mins	>30 mins	POINTS
r	r	r	r	r	[ ]
0	2	5	7	10	

TOTAL SCORE (/100) [ ]

% _____

Reproduced from: Robinson, J.M., Cook, J.L., Purdam, C., *et al.* Victorian Institute Of Sport Tendon Study Group. (2001). The VISA—a questionnaire: a valid and reliable index of the clinical severity of Achilles tendinopathy. *British Journal of Sports Medicine*, **35**, 335–41.

References

Alfredson, H. and Lorentzon, R. (2007). Sclerosing polidocanol injections of small vessels to treat the chronic painful tendon. *Cardiovascular and Hematological Agents in Medicinal Chemistry*, **5**, 97–100.

Allen, M.J. and Barnes, M.R. (1986). Exercise pain in the lower leg. Chronic compartment syndrome and medial tibial syndrome. *Journal of Bone and Joint Surgery. British Volume*, **68**, 818–23.

Bourne, R.B. and Rorabeck, C.H. (1989). Compartment syndromes of the lower leg. *Clinical Orthopaedics and Related Research*, **240**, 97–104.

Carden, D.G., Noble, J., Chalmers, J., Lunn, P., and Ellis, J. (1987). Rupture of the calcaneal tendon. The early and late management. *Journal of Bone and Joint Surgery. British Volume*, **69**, 416–20.

Carr, A.J. and Norris, S.H. (1989). The blood supply of the calcaneal tendon. *Journal of Bone and Joint Surgery. British Volume*, **71**, 100–1.

Cetti, R., Christensen, S.E., Ejsted, R., Jensen, N.M., and Jorgensen, U. (1993). Operative versus nonoperative treatment of Achilles tendon rupture. A prospective randomized study and review of the literature. *American Journal of Sports Medicine*, **21**, 791–9.

Christensen, J.T., Eklof, B., and Wulff, K (1983). The chronic compartment syndrome and response to diuretic treatment. *Acta Chirurgica Scandinavica*, **149**, 249–52.

Clanton, T. and Solcher, B. (1994). Chronic leg pain in the athlete. *Clinical Journal of Sport Medicine*, 1994, 13, 743–759.

Clement, D.B., Taunton, J.E., and Smart, G.W. (1984). Achilles tendinitis and peritendinitis: etiology and treatment. *American Journal of Sports Medicine*, **12**, 179–84.

Fredberg, U. and Bolvig, L. (2002). Significance of ultrasonographically detected asymptomatic tendinosis in the patellar and Achilles tendons of elite soccer players: a longitudinal study. *American Journal of Sports Medicine*, **30**, 488–91.

Fredberg, U. and Stengaard-Pedersen, K. (2008). Chronic tendinopathy tissue pathology, pain mechanisms, and etiology with a special focus on inflammation. *Scandinavian Journal of Medicine and Science in Sports*, **18**, 3–15.

Fredericson, M., Bergman, A.G., Hoffman, K.L., and Dillingham M.S. (1995). Tibial stress reaction in runners. Correlation of clinical symptoms and scintigraphy with a new magnetic resonance imaging grading system. *American Journal of Sports Medicine*, **23**, 472–81.

Fronek, J., Mubarak, S.J., Hargens, A.R., *et al.* (1987). Management of chronic exertional anterior compartment syndrome of the lower extremity. *Clinical Orthopaedics and Related Research*, **220**, 217–27.

Jonsson, P., Alfredson, H., Sunding, K., Fahlström, M., and Cook, J,. (2008). New regimen for eccentric calf muscle training in patients with chronic insertional Achilles tendinopathy: results of a pilot-study. *British Journal of Sports Medicine*, **42**, 746–9.

Josza, L., Kvist, M., Balint, B.J., *et al.* (1989). The role of recreational sports activity in Achilles tendon rupture. A clinical, pathoanatomical and sociological study of 992 cases. *American Journal of Sports Medicine*, **17**, 338–43.

Komi, P.V., Fukashiro, S., and Jarvinen, M. (1992). Biomechanical loading of Achilles tendon during normal locomotion. *Clinics in Sports Medicine*, **11**, 521–31.

Kountouris, A. and Cook, J. (2007). Rehabilitation of Achilles and patellar tendinopathies. *Best Practice and Research. Clinical Rheumatology*, **21**, 295–316.

Kvist, M. (1991). Achilles tendon injuries in athletes. *Annales Chirurgiae et Gynaecologiae*, **80**, 188–201.

Kvist, M. (1994). Achilles tendon injuries in athletes. *Sports Medicine*, **18**, 173–201.

Lagergren, C. and Lindholm, A. (1958) Vascular distribution in the Achilles tendon. An angiographic and microangiographic study. *Acta Chirurgica Scandinavica*, **116**, 491–5.

Leppilahti, J. and Orava, S. (1998). Total Achilles tendon rupture: a review. *Sports Medicine*, **25**, 79–100.

Leppilahti, J., Orava, S., Karpakka, J., and Takala, T. (1991). Overuse injuries of the Achilles tendon. *Annales Chirurgiae et Gynaecologiae*, **80**, 202–7.

Leppilahti, J., Korpelainen, R., Karpakka, J., Kvist, M., and Orava, S. (1998). Ruptures of the Achilles tendon: relationship to inequality in length of legs and to patterns in the foot and ankle. *Foot and Ankle International*, **19**, 683–7.

McGarvey, W.C., Singh, D., and Trevino, S.G. (1996). Partial Achilles tendon ruptures associated with fluoroquinolone antibiotics: a case report and literature review. *Foot and Ankle International*, **17**, 496–8.

Maffulli, N., Testa, V., Capasso, G. *et al.* (1997). Results of percutaneous longitudinal tenotomy for Achilles tendinopathy in middle- and long-distance runners. *American Journal of Sports Medicine*, **25**, 835–40.

Matheson, G.O., Clement, D.B., McKenzie, D.C., *et al.* (1987). Stress fractures in athletes: a study of 320 cases. *American Journal of Sports Medicine*, **15**, 46–58.

Maxwell, N.J., Ryan, M.B., Taunton, J.E., Gillies, J.H., and Wong, A.D. (2007). Sonographically guided intratendinous injection of hyperosmolar dextrose to treat chronic tendinosis of the Achilles tendon: a pilot study. *American Journal of Roentgenology*, **189**, W215–20.

Melberg, P. and Styf, J. (1989). Posteromedial pain in the lower leg. *American Journal of Sports Medicine*, **17**, 747–50.

Micheli, L.J., Solomon, R., Solomon, J., Plasschaert, V.F., and Mitchell, R. (1999). Surgical treatment for chronic lower-leg compartment syndrome in young female athletes. *American Journal of Sports Medicine*, **27**, 197–201.

Movin, T., Gad, A., Guntner, P., Foldhazy, Z., and Rolf, C. (1997). Pathology of the Achilles tendon in association with ciprofloxacin treatment. *Foot and Ankle International*, **18**, 297–9.

Ogilvie-Harris, D.J., Gilbart, M.K., and Chorney, K. (1997). Chronic pain following ankle sprains in athletes: the role of arthroscopic surgery. *Arthroscopy*, **13**, 564–74.

Ohberg, L. and Alfredson, H. (2004). Effects on neovascularisationization behind the good results with eccentric training in chronic mid-portion Achilles tendinosis? *Knee Surgery, Sports Traumatology, Arthroscopy*, **12**, 465–70.

Ohberg, L., Lorentzon, R., and Alfredson, H. (2004). Eccentric training in patients with chronic Achilles tendinosis: normalised tendon structure and decreased thickness at follow up. *British Journal of Sports Medicine*, **38**, 8–11.

Pedowitz, R.A., Hargens, A.R., Mubarak, S.J., and Gershuni, D.H. (1990). Modified criteria for the objective diagnosis of chronic compartment syndrome of the leg. *American Journal of Sports Medicine*, **18**, 35–40.

Popovic, N. and Lemaire, R. (1999). Diagnosis and treatment of acute ruptures of the Achilles tendon: current concepts review. *Acta Orthopaedica Belgica*, **65**, 458–71.

Robinson, J.M., Cook, J.L., Purdam, C., *et al.* Victorian Institute Of Sport Tendon Study Group. (2001). The VISA—a questionnaire: a valid and reliable index of the clinical severity of Achilles tendinopathy. *British Journal of Sports Medicine*, **35**, 335–41.

Rolf, C. and Movin, T. (1997). Etiology, histopathology, and outcome of surgery in achillodynia. *Foot and Ankle International*, **18**, 565–9.

Rompe, J.D., Furia, J., and Maffulli, N. (2008). Eccentric loading compared with shock wave treatment for chronic insertional achilles tendinopathy: a randomized, controlled trial. *Bone and Joint Surgery. American Volume*, **90**, 52–61.

Rorabeck, C.H., Fowler, P.J., and Nott, L. (1988). The results of fasciotomy in the management of chronic exertional compartment syndrome. *American Journal of Sports Medicine*, **16**, 224–7.

Schepsis, A., Martini, A.D., and Corbett, M. (1993). Surgical management of exertional compartment syndrome of the lower leg. *American Journal of Sports Medicine*, **21**, 811–17.

Schmidt-Rohlfing, B., Graf, J., Schneider, U., and Niethard, F.U. (1992). The blood supply of the Achilles tendon. *International Orthopaedics*, **16**, 29–31.

Scott, S.H. and Winter, D.A. (1990). Internal forces of chronic running injury sites. *Medicine and Science in Sports and Exercise*, **22**, 357–69.

Sejersted, O.M. and Hargens, A.R. (1995). Intramuscular pressures for monitoring different tasks and muscle conditions. *Advances in Experimental Medicine and Biology*, **384**, 339–50.

Sundqvist, H., Forsskahl, B., and Kvist, M. (1987). A promising novel therapy for Achilles peritendinitis: double-blind comparison of glycosaminoglycan polysulfate and high-dose indomethacin. *International Journal of Sports Medicine*, **8**, 298–303.

Szarfman, A., Chen, M., and Blum, M.D. (1995). More on fluoroquinolone antibiotics and tendon rupture. *New England Journal of Medicine*, **332**, 193.

Tomassi, F.J. (1992). Current diagnostic and radiographic assessment of tendo Achillis rupture. *Journal of the American Podiatric Medical Association*, **82**, 375–9.

van den Brand, J.G., Nelson, T., Verleisdonk, E.J., and van der Werken, C. (2005). The diagnostic value of intracompartmental pressure measurement, magnetic resonance imaging, and near-infrared spectroscopy in chronic exertional compartment syndrome: a prospective study in 50 patients. *American Journal of Sports Medicine*, **33**, 699–704.

van Gent, R.N., Siem, D., van Middelkoop, M., van Os, A.G., Bierma-Zeinstra, S.M.A., and Koes, B.W. Incidence and determinants of lower extremity running injuries in long distance runners: as systematic review. *British Journal of Sports Medicine*, **41**, 469–80.

Vincelette, P., Laurin, C.A., and Lévesque, H.P. (1972). The footballer's ankle and foot. *Canadian Medical Association Journal*, **107**, 872–4.

Wallenstein, R. (1983). Results of fasciotomy in patients with medial tibial syndrome or anterior compartment syndrome. *Journal of Bone and Joint Surgery. American Volume*, **65**, 1252–5.

Whiteside, L.A. (1978). Tibiofibular synostosis and recurrent ankle sprains in high performance athletes. *American Journal of Sports Medicine*, **6**, 204–5.

Wiley, J.P., Doyle, D.L., and Taunton, J.E. (1987) A primary care perspective of chronic compartment syndrome of the leg. *Physician and Sportsmedicine*, **15**, 111–20.

Zanetti, M., Metzdorf, A., Kundert, H.-P., *et al.* Achilles tendons: clinical relevance of neovascularization diagnosed with power Doppler US. *Radiology*, **227**, 556–60.

Zollinger, H., Rodriguez, M., and Genoni, M. (1983). Atiopathegenese und Diagnostik der Achillessehnenrupturen im Sport. In: G. Chapchal (ed), *Sportverletzungen und Sportschaden*, pp. 78–9. Thieme, Stuttgart.

Zwas, S.T., Elkanovitch, R., and Frank, G. Interpretation and classification of bone scintigraphic findings in stress fractures. *Journal of Nuclear Medicine*, **28**, 452–7.

Knee injuries

Henry Colaco, Fares Haddad, and Cathy Speed

Introduction

The knee is a synovial hinge joint which achieves a range of movement of 0°–150° flexion with a complex combination of sliding, gliding, and rolling movements. The three components involved are the medial and lateral compartments of the tibiofemoral joint and the patellofemoral joint. The joint is lined with hyaline articular cartilage and stability is primarily provided by the joint capsule, menisci, ligaments, and muscles.

Knee injuries are among the most common problems facing the sports physician. Therefore a clear understanding of knee anatomy, kinematics, injury mechanisms, and therapeutic possibilities is vital.

Anatomy and biomechanics

Tibiofemoral joint and locking

The tibiofemoral joint is the articulation between the femoral and tibial condyles, where the medial femoral condyle is larger than the lateral femoral condyle. In flexion, the spherical posterior part of the femoral condyles articulates with the tibia. As the knee is moved into extension, the flat anterior part of the smaller lateral femoral condyle comes into contact with the tibia first and stops as the femur rotates medially to accommodate the larger medial femoral condyle. The unique 'screw-home' mechanism of knee locking allows minimal expenditure of muscular energy to maintain a standing position. In this locked position in full extension, the main ligaments are taut and the knee joint is in a stable close-packed configuration which requires no muscular activity, making standing much more comfortable and energy efficient.

Popliteus and unlocking

The knee requires an active unlocking mechanism; the popliteus muscle is unique, with a tendinous origin from the lateral femoral condyle and distal muscle belly at its insertion into the upper part of the posterior surface of the tibia. It unlocks the knee by medially rotating the tibia. The popliteus tendon passes through a hiatus in the coronary ligament, deep to the lateral collateral ligament, and is visualized at arthroscopy. Popliteus also adds to the posterior stability of the knee and resists excessive varus movement and lateral rotation during flexion.

Articular surface

The articular surfaces of the femoral and tibial condyles and the patella facets are lined with hyaline cartilage, which provides a smooth surface for low-friction articulation. It is insensitive and avascular, and therefore exhibits poor healing properties. It consists of a complex layered structure of predominantly type II collagen fibres (10%) and chondrocytes in a proteoglycan matrix, which is 80% water. The configuration of the collagen enables the cartilage to withstand large tensile, shear, and compressive forces of up to 65 times body weight.

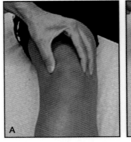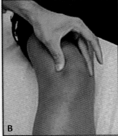

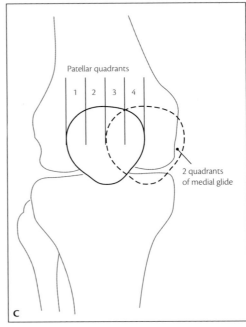

Fig. 3.12.1 Schematic diagram of the right knee, anterior view. Reproduced from Dixit, S., DiFiori, J.P., Burton, M., and Mines, B. (2007) Management of patellofemoral pain syndrome. *American Family Physician*, **75**, 194–202. © 2007 Todd Buck

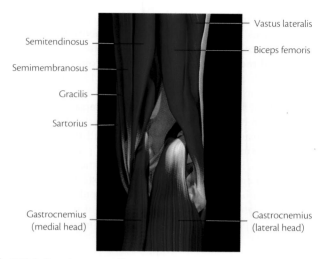

Semitendinosus
Semimembranosus
Gracilis
Sartorius
Gastrocnemius (medial head)

Vastus lateralis
Biceps femoris
Gastrocnemius (lateral head)

Fig. 3.12.2 Posterior aspect of knee.

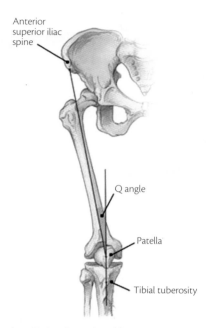

Anterior superior iliac spine
Q angle
Patella
Tibial tuberosity

Fig. 3.12.3 Q angle and VOM. Reproduced from Mark, S. and Juhn, D.O. (1999). Patellofemoral pain syndrome: a review and guidelines for treatment. *American Family Physician*, **60**, 2014. Copyright © 1999 Floyd E.Hosmer

Patella

The patella lies within the quadriceps tendon and is the largest sesamoid bone in the body. It has attachments to the medial and lateral patellofemoral ligaments and the retinaculum. Its major function is to increase the biomechanical advantage to the extensor mechanism across the knee with a secondary protective function. It does this by increasing the functional lever arm of the quadriceps by increasing the distance from the centre of rotation of the knee. The mechanical benefit is maximal at 45° of flexion when the patella is in maximum contact with the femoral condyles. During stair-climbing the force across the patellofemoral joint (PFJ) can be up to three times body weight, and during squats can reach up to eight times body weight. The posterior surface is covered by articular hyaline cartilage, which varies in thickness from 2 to 6 mm and is divided into seven separate articular facets, comprising three medial facets, three lateral facets, and the 'odd' facet. As flexion increases, the area of contact pressure moves from the inferior pole to the superior pole, and the 'odd' facet only contacts the femur in maximal flexion.

The pull of the quadriceps on the patella is in line with the femur, whereas the patellar tendon, which inserts into the tibia, is almost vertical. This discrepancy between these two directions is known as the Q angle, which is defined by a line drawn from the anterior superior iliac spine to the centre of the patella and a line drawn from the centre of the patella through the tibial tubercle (Fig. 3.12.3). Average Q angle values are 14° in men and 17° in women. This angle has important implications for the biomechanics of the patella. In situations where it is increased it gives rise to a greater risk of lateral subluxation or dislocation. The lower oblique fibres of the vastus medialis run at approximately 50° from the vertical. Also known as the vastus medialis obliquus muscle (VMO), they resist the tendency for lateral subluxation. Even minor knee trauma or effusion can trigger reflex inhibition of the VMO, resulting in altered patellofemoral biomechanics and maltracking of the patella. Consequently, exercises for strengthening and recruitment of the VMO are frequently employed in the management of patellar maltracking and anterior knee pain.

The patellar tendon forms part of the extensor mechanism of the knee (quadriceps–patella–patellar tendon–tibial tubercle). It is commonly injured in sport.

Menisci

The menisci are crescent-shaped shock-absorbing fibrocartilagenous structures, which are integral to the normal biomechanics of the knee, aiding joint congruence by deepening the articulation of the femur with the tibia and converting downward force into lateral force, dispersing up to 70% of the axial load (*Wheeless' Textbook of* Orthopaedics, www.wheelessonline.com). They also aid proprioception and distribution of synovial fluid, and limit sagittal glide of the femoral condyles. The menisci are C-shaped in axial view, with a wedge-shaped cross-section. They are attached to the tibia by the peripheral coronary ligaments, and are joined to each other by the small anterior transverse ligament together with a posterior transverse ligament in 20% of the population.

The menisci receive a limited peripheral blood supply from the lateral and medial genicular arteries (Arnoczky and Warren 1982) via the peripheral vascular synovium. The perimeniscal capillary plexus extends 1–3 mm over the articular surface. In adults, only the peripheral few millimetres (10–30% of the medial and 10–25% of the lateral meniscus) is vascular, although the anterior and posterior horns receive a relatively good blood supply. The meniscus can be classified into three zones according to vascularity: zone 1 (peripheral/vascular/red), zone 2 (middle/intermediate), and zone 3 (inner/avascular/white). The peripheral zone has good potential for healing and certain tears in this territory are amenable to repair. Tears more than 5 mm from the outer meniscal rim are generally avascular and have no healing potential, and tears that occur in the middle zone have variable vascularity and less predictable healing properties.

The **medial meniscus**, which covers the concave medial tibial condyle, is larger, thinner, and has a more open C-shape then the lateral meniscus (Fig. 3.12.4). It has an attachment to the deep fibres of the medial collateral ligament, which forms part of the

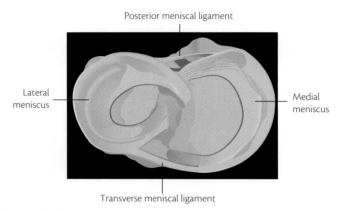

Posterior meniscal ligament

Lateral
meniscus

Medial
meniscus

Transverse meniscal ligament

Fig. 3.12.4 Knee menisci.

medial joint capsule. It is less mobile, sliding 2–5 mm posteriorly only as the knee nears full extension as part of the 'screw-home' mechanism. The relative immobility of the posterior horn of the medial meniscus may explain the high proportion of meniscal tears found in this region. Four variations of the tibial attachment of the anterior horn have been described: type I, flat intercondylar region; type II, downward slope from the medial articular plateau; type III, anterior slope of the tibial plateau; type IV, no bony insertion.

Types III and IV may be unable to resist peripheral extrusion of the loaded meniscus, placing it at risk of anterior subluxation and causing anterior knee pain in specific cases (Berlet and Fowler 1997).

The **lateral meniscus** covers the smaller convex lateral tibial condyle. It is thicker, smaller, and more of a closed C-shape than the medial meniscus. It is more mobile and is not attached to the lateral collateral ligament (LCL) or the lateral capsule. In flexion, it glides 9–11 mm backwards and medially down the slope of the lateral tibial plateau, tightening the anterior and posterior meniscofemoral ligaments which surround the posterior cruciate ligament (PCL). Seventy per cent of the population have either the anterior ligament of Humphrey or the posterior ligament of Wrisberg, with both present in 6% of the population. There is a hiatus posterolaterally in the coronary ligament for the popliteus tendon, which partially separates the lateral meniscus from the capsule.

Major ligaments

The main ligamentous structures are the anterior and posterior cruciate ligaments (ACL and PCL) and the medial and lateral collateral ligaments (MCL and LCL). In addition, support is provided by the quadriceps and hamstring muscle groups as well as the joint capsule, retinaculum, and other ligamentous structures. The popliteus muscle and posterolateral complex provide some resistance to

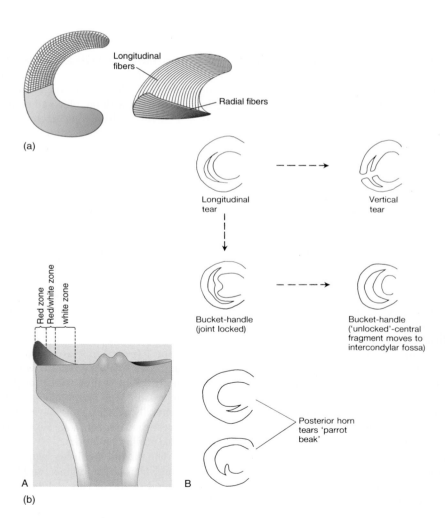

Longitudinal
fibers

Radial fibers

(a)

Longitudinal
tear

Vertical
tear

Bucket-handle
(joint locked)

Bucket-handle
('unlocked'-central
fragment moves to
intercondylar fossa)

Posterior horn
tears 'parrot
beak'

Red zone
Red/white zone
white zone

A   B

(b)

Fig. 3.12.5 Cross-section of menisci.

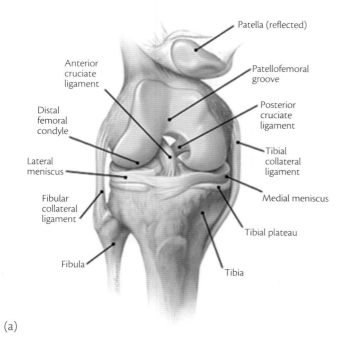

(a)

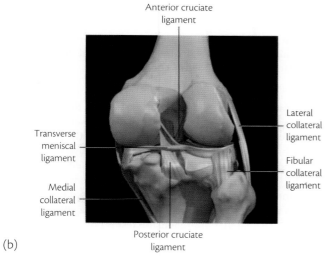

(b)

Fig. 3.12.6 (a) Anterior view of major ligaments. (b) Posterior view of major knee ligaments.

lateral rotation of the tibia during medial rotation of the femur on the tibia while the foot is planted. The joint is surrounded by a series of bursae, including the prepatellar and infrapatellar bursae, which reduce friction between the numerous components. The anterior cruciate ligament limits forward movement and external rotation of the tibia on the femur. The posterior cruciate ligament resists backward movement of the tibia on the femur and prevents hyperextension. The broad medial (or tibial) ligament and round lateral (or fibular) collateral ligament resist valgus and varus stresses, respectively.

Anterior cruciate ligament

The ACL is the primary restraint on anterior tibial translation, accounting for 85% of resistance on the anterior drawer test, and secondarily limits external rotation of the tibia. The femoral attachment is the posteromedial aspect of the medial surface of the lateral femoral condyle in the intercondylar notch.

The ACL is 38 mm long and 10 mm in diameter, with a tensile strength of approximately 2200 N to failure, which is half that of the PCL. It is an entirely intra-articular extrasynovial ligament composed of multiple collagen fascicles grouped into two distinct bundles; anteromedial and posterolateral. The tibial attachment is anterolateral to the anterior spine of the tibia, behind the transverse meniscal ligament. The smaller anteromedial bundle is tight in flexion and limits anterior tibial translation, whereas the larger posterior bundle is tight in extension and also limits external rotation.

Cadaveric studies have shown the bundles to lie parallel in extension and cross in flexion (Amis and Dawkins 1991). Recent *in vivo* studies using three-dimensional MRI reconstructions have not demonstrated this reciprocal movement in either the ACL or, as also proposed, the PCL. The two bundles are shortened and remain parallel in flexion with minimal twist (<5°) (Jordan *et al.* 2007). However, the studies suggest that there is a reciprocal function between the ACL and PCL, with the ACL being more important in low-flexion angles and the PCL in high-flexion angles (Li *et al.* 2004). The ACL receives its major blood supply from the middle genicular artery and innervation from the tibial nerve. It plays an important role in proprioception and accommodates multiple types of nerve endings, which detect motion, speed, and pain.

Posterior cruciate ligament

The PCL is the primary restraint of posterior instability, providing 95% of total restraining force to straight posterior translation of the tibia. It also resists hyperextension, varus, valgus, and external rotation stress. It is taut principally in the mid-range of motion (maximally at 30° flexion). Secondary posterior stabilizers include the posterolateral capsule, the popliteus, the MCL, and the oblique popliteal ligament, which passes laterally upward from the insertion of the semimembranosus. The PCL originates from the anterolateral aspect of the medial femoral condyle and has an extra-articular insertion on to the tibia where it blends with the posterior horn of the lateral meniscus. It is approximately 38 mm long and 13 mm in diameter, and is composed of an anterolateral bundle (65%) which is tight in flexion and a posteromedial bundle (35%) which is tight in extension.

Medial collateral ligament

The MCL is the primary restraint against medial instability and also resists external rotation. The ligament is a broad flat structure 8–9 cm long, composed of a superficial layer and a deep layer. The superficial layer has a proximal attachment at the adductor tubercle of the medial femoral condyle and distal attachment to the tibia

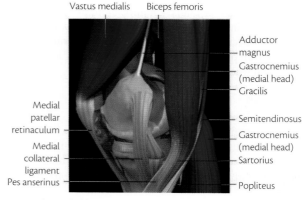

Fig. 3.12.7 The medial knee.

4–6 cm below the joint line beneath the pes anserinus. The anterior fibres are taut when the knee is in 70°–100° flexion; the posterior fibres form the posterior oblique ligament and are taut in the close-packed formation in extension. The strong middle section remains taut throughout most knee movements. The history of a traumatic incident is important as the angle of knee flexion at the moment of injury will give a clue to the area of ligament damage. The deep layer may be separated from the superficial layer by a bursa, and is composed of the meniscofemoral and meniscotibial ligaments which have an attachment to the medial meniscus.

Lateral collateral ligament

The LCL is the primary restraint of lateral instability and also resists internal rotation. The ligament is a round cord 5 cm long, which has no attachment to the joint capsule or the lateral meniscus. It attaches proximally to the lateral femoral epicondyle and distally to the head of the fibula. The distal end of the LCL moves posteriorly in extension and anteriorly in flexion. The LCL forms part of the posterolateral complex with the arcuate ligament, popliteus tendon, and popliteofibular ligament, which is reinforced by the biceps femoris, popliteus, and lateral head of gastrocnemius. The iliotibial band (ITB) also plays a dynamic stabilizing role.

Other important structures

There are several other important structures in and around the knee. The arcuate ligament adds stability to the posterolateral corner, the medial and lateral patellofemoral ligaments stabilize the patella in addition to the retinaculum, and the posterior meniscofemoral ligaments may play a role as secondary restraints on posterior translation of the tibia. The tendons of the pes anserinus (sartorius, gracilis, and semitendinosus) add dynamic stabilization to the medial aspect of the joint and resist varus stress. The proximal tibiofibular joint (PTFJ) is a stable synovial joint with a capsule, which is stronger anteriorly. It is contiguous with the knee joint in 10% of the population and transmits 15% of the axial load and torsional force from the ankle.

History

An accurate history is an essential part of accurate and early diagnosis of sports injuries to the knee. Symptoms at presentation are not always pathognomonic, and delay from the time of injury to presentation can alter the pattern of symptoms. Specific questions to be asked must assess the exact mechanism of injury and the athlete's immediate response: for example, location of pain, inability to continue sporting activity, immediate or delayed swelling, instability, locking, inability to weight-bear, a 'popping' or 'snapping' sensation at moment of injury. Enquire about previous hip, ankle, or foot injuries in addition to pre-existing knee conditions. The patient's age, occupation, expectations, motivation, anticipated compliance with physiotherapy, and level of athletic activity should be considered when planning management.

Examination

The 'look, feel, move' approach of examination can be applied along with specific tests. Full examination must include the hip and spine, which should be excluded as a source of referred pain. Biomechanical assessment, gait analysis, and examination during sport-specific movements is often also necessary in the assessment of chronic symptoms.

Look

The patient's lower limbs should be adequately exposed, ideally wearing mid-thigh-length shorts. With the patient standing, look from the front and inspect for any valgus/varus deformity at the knee, any swellings, erythema, scars, muscle atrophy, or asymmetry, and any deformity of the ankles. Note the size, position, and symmetry of the patellae. Always compare the injured with the uninjured side, and inspect from behind for any posterior swellings. Ask the patient to walk the length of the room and look for any gait abnormality. When the patient is supine, look for any fixed flexion deformity and compare quadriceps bulk with the other side.

Feel

With the patient lying relaxed, supine on a couch, several anatomical structures in the knee can be palpated as much of the joint is subcutaneous. Test for an effusion with the knee in extension (see below). With the knee relaxed, resting in a few degrees of flexion, apply medial and lateral stress to the patella to assess the lateral and medial patellofemoral ligaments. With the knee in 90° flexion and the foot in neutral on the couch, palpate the menisci along the medial and lateral joint lines; this can elicit point tenderness. Palpate the medial and lateral collateral ligaments for tenderness. The lateral collateral ligament is best felt with the leg in the 'figure of four' position with the legs crossed and the ankle resting on the opposite leg. This stresses the ligament, and helps to differentiate it from meniscal tenderness. Finally, palpate behind the knee in the popliteal fossa for any tenderness or swellings.

Move

Normal range of movement is from 0° to 150° flexion. Ask the patient to flex their knee, bringing their heel towards their backside, testing active flexion, and then gently flex the knee further with the hip in flexion to test passive range of movement. During flexion and extension, the palm of one hand is rested on the patella to feel for patellofemoral crepitus. With the patient sitting on the edge of the couch, patellar tracking can be assessed by asking the patient to actively flex and extend the knee, and watching or feeling the patella. The **patellar apprehension test** is positive if the patient cannot tolerate passive flexion of the knee with the patella pushed laterally.

Effusion

Gently ballot the patella in the fully extended knee. A positive **patella tap** denotes a large effusion. A small or moderate effusion can be detected by the **bulge test**, where after emptying the suprapatellar bursa into the joint and sweeping fluid from the medial compartment, a brisk sweep down the lateral compartment will cause a sudden visible 'bulge' of fluid on the medial side.

Medial and lateral collateral ligaments

Apply gentle valgus stress to the knee with the joint in full extension and repeat in 30° of flexion, which tests the superficial fibres of the MCL. Feel for the degree of laxity and a firm endpoint. Apply varus stress in extension and 30° flexion to test the LCL. Palpate for the point of maximum tenderness following an MCL injury to localize the damage to the femoral attachment, midsubstance, or tibial attachment. Opening the joint by 5–8 mm more than the contralateral knee may indicate complete ligament disruption.

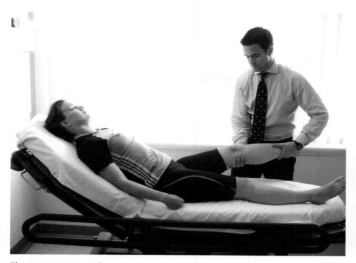

Fig. 3.12.8 Varus–valgus stress test.

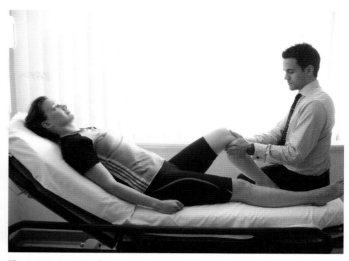

Fig. 3.12.9 Anterior drawer test.

Anterior cruciate ligament

The **anterior drawer test** is performed with knee in 90° of flexion. Relax the hamstrings with the index fingers of both hands and, with thumbs over the tibial tubercle, pull the tibia forwards. The degree of movement can be graded, but is subject to inter-observer variation. The presence or absence of an endpoint is a useful finding. **Lachman's test** works on the same principle but at 30° of flexion; the distal femur is held in one hand while the proximal tibia is held with the other hand and brought forwards. Again, the degree of movement and feel of endpoint can be assessed. In larger patients, it is sometimes easier to fix the femur between the examiner's hand and flexed knee resting on the couch. The **pivot shift test** re-creates anterolateral subluxation of the tibia. The knee is held in full extension with the tibia in internal rotation between the examiner's upper arm and torso, and a valgus stress is applied with one hand. The knee is gently flexed, and if the test is positive, the knee will suddenly reduce at around 20° flexion. The **jerk test** is undertaken the other way round—from flexion to extension, recreating the subluxation.

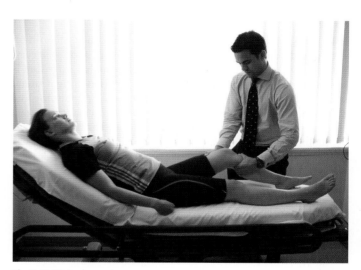

Fig. 3.12.10 Lachmann's test.

Posterior cruciate ligament

The action of gravity will cause a posterior sag of the tibia with the knees flexed at 90°; compare the two sides. This will also help to exclude a false-positive anterior drawer sign in PCL rupture. Posterior drawer is carried out at the same time as anterior drawer, and degree of laxity and endpoint can be assessed. Other tests to be carried out in a suspected PCL injury include the reverse pivot shift test (for posterolateral instability) and the external rotation–recurvatum test detailed in the section on PCL injury.

Menisci

The adapted **Mc Murray's test** attempts to elicit discomfort along the medial or lateral joint line to indicate the injured area. Resting one hand on the patient's knee and using the other hand to hold the patient's foot, bring the knee slowly into extension from a flexed position with the knee in internal rotation, whilst palpating the lateral joint line, and then in external rotation, whilst palpating the medial joint line. The test is most specific for a tear of the posterior horn of the medial meniscus.

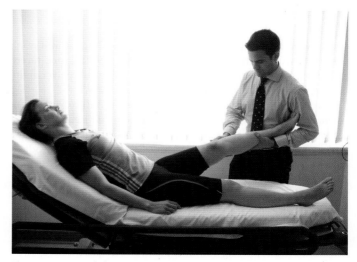

Fig. 3.12.11 Pivot shift test.

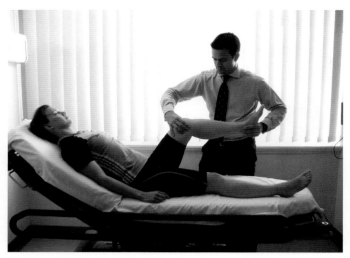

Fig. 3.12.12 McMurray's test.

Patella

Look for VMO bulk, patella alta or baja, and lateral patellar tilt on sitting and standing, in addition to scars of previous surgery. Lateral deviation of the patella as the knee nears full extension is known as the J sign and suggests VMO dysfunction or tight lateral structures. Palpate the retinacular structures surrounding the patella, noting location of any tenderness, in particular the medial patellofemoral ligament. The **Sage sign** or **glide test** assesses patellar mobility: <25% indicates tight lateral structures, and >50% indicates hypermobility, which is commonly seen in adolescent females. The **patellar tilt test** is performed in 20° flexion, with the patella held between the examiner's thumb and index finger. If the patella cannot be lifted upwards laterally above neutral, this suggests tightness of the lateral structures (Kolowich 1990). The **patella apprehension test** is performed by subluxing the patella laterally and flexing the knee; a positive test of pain, reflex muscular contraction, and apprehension indicates previous dislocation. The **patellar compression test** is positive if flexion and extension cause pain while the patella is displaced inferiorly into the trochlear groove by the examiner.

Investigations

Useful investigations include plain radiographs (stress and non-weight-bearing), ultrasound (US), CT scans, MRI scans, rarely arthrography, and diagnostic arthroscopy. There are specific indications for each of these, which are discussed below.

Knee arthroscopy is a minimally invasive procedure, often performed as a day-case, in which a camera is introduced to directly visualize the intracapsular joint structures. A series of portals (most commonly anterolateral and anteromedial) are used to introduce camera, fluid, probe and other instruments. The joint is distended with fluid maintained at a constant pressure to improve the view. Arthroscopy may be performed for diagnostic and/or therapeutic indications. Diagnostic indications include; to confirm the presence of a meniscal tear, ACL tear, osteochondral lesion or loose body, or to elucidate the cause of a haemarthrosis, an unexplained effusion, or unremitting and unexplained knee pain. Therapeutic indications include; to excise or debride a meniscal tear, to remove

Table 3.12.1 Indications for therapeutic arthroscopy

Excise/debride a meniscal tear
Remove loose bodies or osteochondral fragments
Synovial biopsy
Divide/excise a synovial plica
Wash out intra-articular debris
Meniscal repair
Lateral retinacular release
(ACL reconstruction)
(PCL reconstruction)

loose bodies or osteochondral fragments, to perform a synovial biopsy, divide or excise a synovial plica, or wash out intra-articular debris. In addition, arthroscopy is used for meniscal repair, ACL and PCL reconstruction, and lateral retinacular release (Table 3.12.1).

Haemarthrosis

Traumatic haemarthrosis always indicates significant intra-articular trauma, and evolves within the first couple of hours following injury. A serous joint effusion secondary to trauma generally presents later, classically developing overnight and is generally of a smaller volume. An acute knee haemarthrosis causes a tense joint containing up to 100ml of blood. The commonest cause is ACL disruption, found in 72% of cases in a study by Noyes et al. (1980) (Mafulli *et al.* 1993), without significant collateral ligament injury on examination. The other main causes are peripheral meniscus tears and lateral dislocation of the patella causing osteochondral damage and injury to the medial retinaculum.

Less frequent causes include isolated osteochondral injuries, PCL rupture, posterolateral corner injuries, tibial plateau fractures, segond fractures, and avulsion fractures of the tibial insertion of the ACL. Segond fractures occur by forced internal rotation of the tibia in the flexed knee, which places a large force on the middle portion of the lateral capsule, resulting in a tibial avulsion fracture of the lateral capsule attachment. It is an important finding, visible on AP X-ray and is indicative of an associated ACL injury. Tibial plateau fractures are much commoner in non-athletes who suffer a haemarthrosis, and are caused by landing from height or skiing injuries. CT offers high sensitivity and specificity for bony avulsions, as well as high negative predictive value for excluding ligament injury. However, MRI remains necessary for the preoperative detection of meniscal injury (Mui *et al.* 2007). Most PCL and posterolateral corner injuries occur in combination with other ligament injuries (LaPrade *et al.* 2007).

In the acute setting, aspiration will confirm the presence of a haemarthrosis and will provide some pain relief for the patient by relieving the pressure on the sensitive synovium. It may also allow further clinical examination of the knee to assess stability. Haematoma can lead to adhesions and synovitis which can prolong the recovery period and delay rehabilitation. The presence of fat in the aspirate indicates the presence of an intra-articular fracture, and a fat/fluid level may be visible on horizontal beam lateral X-rays (Ferguson and Knottenbelt 1994). CT is the investigation of choice to confirm the presence of a tibial plateau fracture or osteo-chondral damage.

Arthroscopy allows a more accurate diagnosis, but the injury may not be amenable to repair at the time and the patient may require a further arthroscopic procedure. There still exists some controversy as to the indications and timing for arthroscopy (Sarimo *et al.* 2002), but all patients with a traumatic haemarthrosis should be referred to an orthopaedic surgeon for evaluation and follow-up. A definitive diagnosis must be reached rapidly to plan operative and non-operative management, including physiotherapy and rehabilitation to avoid muscle wasting and delayed recovery.

Instability

Knee instability can occur as a result of trauma or overuse, and clinical examination can elicit its direction, which can be defined as one plane, rotatory, or combined (Harries *et al.* 1998).

One-plane instability can occur in isolation or in combination and can be defined as medial, lateral, anterior, or posterior. Medial (or valgus) instability results from damage to the medial structures, which can be divided into thirds: anterior third, only medial joint capsule; middle third, reinforced by superficial and deep fibres of the MCL and attached to the medial meniscus; posterior third, an extension of the MCL—the posterior oblique ligament, the posteromedial capsule, and expansions from the semimembranosus tendon. Dynamic stabilization is provided by the adjacent pes anserinus tendon of sartorius, gracilis, and semitendinosus. The ACL acts as a secondary restraint to valgus stress.

Lateral (or varus) instability results from damage to the lateral structures, which can also be divided into thirds: anterior third, capsule reinforced by patellar retinaculum and expansions from the quadriceps tendon; middle third, support provided by iliotibial band; posterior third, the LCL and arcuate ligament. Additional stabilization is provided by the biceps and popliteus tendons. The ACL also acts as a secondary restraint on varus stress. Posterior instability occurs as a result of damage to the PCL and posterior structures—the arcuate ligament posterolaterally, and the oblique popliteal ligament medially. Popliteus muscle adds stability, particularly in the flexed knee, and dynamic stability is provided by the semimembranosus, gastrocnemius, and biceps. The LCL is a secondary restraint on posterior translation. Anterior instability results from rupture of the ACL. Secondary restraints on anterior translation of the tibia include the ITB, MCL, LCL, menisci, and middle third of the collateral ligaments.

Rotatory instability can be classified as anteromedial, anterolateral (flexion, extension), posteromedial, and posterolateral. Anteromedial instability is due to MCL damage, augmented by ACL damage. Excessive external rotation of the tibia can be tested by repeating the anterior drawer test in external rotation. Anterolateral instability is due to ACL rupture, augmented by damage to lateral joint structures. Excessive internal rotation of the tibia with anterior subluxaion of the lateral tibial condyle (Fig. 3.12.13) can be elicited by the pivot shift test and by repeating the anterior drawer test in internal rotation. Posteromedial instability is most pronounced with a combined PCL and MCL injury, and can be demonstrated as posterior sag with internal rotation. Posterolateral instability indicates insufficiency of the posterolateral corner structures, particularly the arcuate ligament. Abnormal lateral rotation

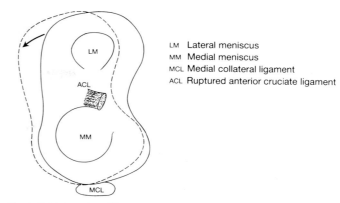

LM Lateral meniscus
MM Medial meniscus
MCL Medial collateral ligament
ACL Ruptured anterior cruciate ligament

Fig. 3.12.13 Anterior subluxation of the lateral tibial plateau occurs in anterolateral (rotatory) instability.

and posterior subluxation of the lateral tibial condyle can be demonstrated by the external rotation–recurvatum or 'big toe test'. In a positive test, when the relaxed lower limb is lifted off the couch by the toes, the knee joint falls into slight varus, hyperextension with external rotation.

Combined instability can be classified as anterolateral–anteromedial, anterolateral–posterolateral, or anteromedial–posteromedial, which can occur as a result of multiple ligament injuries and dislocations of the knee.

Anterior cruciate ligament injury

The ACL is the most commonly damaged knee ligament, accounting for up to 50% of all documented ligamentous knee injuries. ACL tear is also the most common cause of a traumatic haemarthrosis, with an incidence of 63 in 100 000 in North America. In athletes, surgical reconstruction of a ruptured ACL is vital to maintaining high-level performance, but also signals a lengthy time on the sidelines for recovery and rehabilitation. Athletes who continue sports with an ACL-deficient knee have a high incidence of 'giving way' and meniscal and chondral injuries.

The rate of ACL injury is four to eight times more common in women than men. Female athletes who take part in sports involving jumping and 'cutting' movements, such as football, basketball, and gymnastics, are particularly at risk. The aetiology is multifactorial, but includes the wide female pelvis, narrower female intercondylar notch, physiological laxity of the ACL with hormonal influence, and muscle reaction time disparity (Beynnon *et al.* 2005a). Sports-specific neuromuscular training can be employed to reduce the risk of ACL rupture, concentrating on jumping and landing in basketball, and unanticipated cutting movements in football (Cowley *et al.* 2006).

In sporting contexts, ACL rupture will typically occur in a number of mechanisms: athletes who suffer a sudden twisting injury, such as the basketball player who suddenly decelerates and changes direction with the tibia fixed in internal rotation; the football or rugby player who suffers a flexion/valgus/external rotation injury with their boot stuck in the turf; the athlete who lands awkwardly, hyperextending the knee. In older patients, the most common cause is a skiing injury when bindings do not release. Overall, injury is more likely to occur in a non-contact sport.

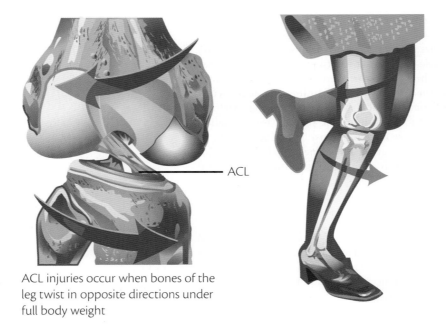

ACL injuries occur when bones of the leg twist in opposite directions under full body weight

Fig. 3.12.14 ACL rupture.

A direct blow on the anterolateral aspect of the knee, such as in a rugby tackle, can also rupture the ACL, commonly associated with MCL rupture and a medial meniscal tear (the 'unhappy triad' of O'Donoghue), resulting in a profoundly unstable knee. An acute haemarthrosis develops rapidly, and in over 50% of cases the patient will hear a 'pop' or feel tearing within the knee and is unable to continue playing sport.

In the acute setting, examination of the knee may be difficult, and the anterior drawer sign, positive pivot shift, and Lachman's tests are more easily demonstrated in the chronic ACL-deficient knee. The initial treatment of an ACL injury is based on reducing pain and swelling, and aspiration of the haemarthrosis may be required for pain relief and to aid examination. Plain X-rays may demonstrate an avulsion fracture at the tibial insertion of the ACL, but an early MRI scan is essential. Tears occur much more commonly in the mid-substance than at the osseoligamentous junctions, which has a higher strain rate.

Acute management and 'prehabilitation'

Avoidance of weight-bearing, elevation, anti-inflammatories, and functional bracing are essential, as is early physiotherapy. Physiotherapy plays a vital role in non-operative management of ACL rupture and 'prehabilitation' prior to planned surgical reconstruction. The aim of 'prehabilitation' is to restore range of movement and strengthen hamstrings and quadriceps muscles. This minimizes the formation of adhesions postoperatively.

Postoperative rehabilitation

In athletes, the aim of postoperative rehabilitation is to restore the knee joint to pre-injury levels of strength, stability, and range of movement to enable them to return to the same level of competitive sport. The graft must also be protected while it is in the vulnerable early phase before revascularization has taken place and it achieves its full strength. The concept of 'accelerated rehabilitation' was introduced by Shelbourne and Nitz (1990) to overcome many of the postoperative complications following ACL reconstruction; prolonged knee stiffness, limitation of complete extension, delay in strength recovery, and anterior knee pain. The protocol emphasizes immediate full range of motion, early full weight-bearing from postoperative day 1, strength training, and an early introduction to closed kinetic chain exercises, which produce the least strain in the graft. The programme follows graduated protocols which are tailored to the patient's needs and progress, and include early range of movement and strength training, with seated isotonic exercises, followed by muscle rehabilitation to increase strength, power, and endurance. The patient can return to activities of daily living unaided after a few weeks, and once quadriceps and hamstring strength has been restored to 70% of the contralateral uninjured side, strength training can be increased. Cycling, swimming, and straight-line jogging are reintroduced gradually before any sport-specific movements are relearned. Finally, cutting movements are practised (Table 3.12.2).

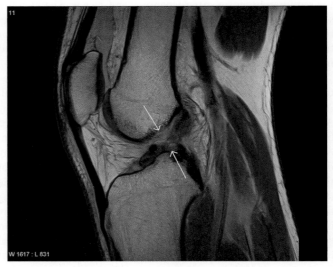

Fig. 3.12.15 Sagittal T1-weighted MRI demonstrating ACL rupture. Reproduced from www.imagingpathways.health.wa.gov.au, with permission.

Table 3.12.2 Modified accelerated ACL rehabilitation protocol.

	Weight-bearing	Brace	Range of motion	Exercise	Precaution
Phase 1 0–2 weeks	WBAT & crutches Working to FWB Off crutches by 10–14 days	No brace if uncomplicated ACL rupture Splint if quads weak Remove bandage after 48 hours	Work to full ext. Hyperext. (R = L), gentle flex. (can use X-bike)	Quads SLR Calf raises or Theraband Hip ext. standing Knee flex, gentle prone	No resisted HS until week 6 postop Wounds clean, dry, covered
Phase 2 2-6 weeks	FWB No crutches		Full ext./ hypertext. (NB swelling tends to restrict full flex.)	Quads closed chain mini Sq2L to lunge to SLSq+leg press Gait re-education Calves two-leg raises Glut. med. work Hamstrings prone Proprioception Pool: no breast troke and straight-leg kick (wounds closed) Scar massage	No resisted HS until week 6 postop Return to work graded as increase pain and swelling
Phase 3 6–12 weeks	FWB Normal gait pattern	No brace	Gain full pain-free	Quads closed chain SLSq + Leg press progress HS resisted X-bike: seat high, no clips Cross trainer/stepper/inclined treadmill walk in preparation for running Proprioception	No running until 3 months postop Phased increases in gym loads Control swelling
Phase 4 3–6 months	FWB	No brace		Running progress time and speed Quads continue leg press progress Start OKCE Agility and gentle impact introduced gradually, progress to sport specific drills and return to training when ready	Paced increases in running
Phase 5 6–9 months				Phased return to sport Training: paced increases in time If all well paced return to games: quarter, half, three-quarters, full	Caution return to training, low impact, non contact initially Phased increase in contact

RoM, range of motion; WBAT, weight bear as tolerated; FWB, full weight-bearing; ext., extension; flex., flexion; SLR, straight leg raise; HS, hamstring; Sq2L, two-leg squat; SLSq, single-leg squat; glut. med., gluteus medius.

Open kinetic chain exercises (OKCEs) involve a single joint (e.g. the knee) and are typically non-weight-bearing where the foot is free to move. Weights can be applied to the leg, and examples include resisted knee extensions and straight-leg raises. OKCEs produce a strong quadriceps contraction, which imparts a large shear force across the joint, placing a large stress on the reconstructed ACL as the tibia is displaced anteriorly. Closed kinetic chain exercises (CKCEs) of the lower limb involve multiple joints and muscle groups. These are typically weight-bearing exercises with the foot planted imparting a compressive force across the joint, using body weight and/or external weights. Examples include front squats, back squats, and lunges. Compared with OKCEs, the movements used are closer to activities of daily living and can be sports specific. Quadriceps contraction is accompanied by co-contraction of the hamstrings, which enhances joint stability and reduces anterior tibial translation, minimizing graft strain and shear force.

Operative management

ACL reconstruction is a successful operation which improves performance in over 90% of patients over a 5 year period. The goals of surgery are to give the patient a stable knee, eliminate the pivot shift, protect the menisci, regain a full range of movement, and to ensure a return to the previous level of sporting activity. The general consensus is that surgery should be deferred until the range of movement in the knee is restored to at least 0°–120°, and the acute inflammatory phase following ACL rupture has resolved. This usually leads to a minimum delay of 6 weeks post-injury even following an intensive physiotherapy protocol. Ability to extend the knee fully and delayed reconstruction significantly decrease the risk of postoperative arthrofibrosis and knee stiffness. The loss of motion caused by arthrofibrosis can be even more disabling than the instability for which the reconstruction was performed, often requiring extensive physiotherapy and/or surgical lysis of adhesions (DeHaven et al. 2003).

There are exceptions when ACL reconstruction is carried out acutely, especially in the presence of other ligament injury (e.g. MCL) or following a traumatic knee dislocation. The presence of an unstable and reparable meniscal lesion combined with ACL insufficiency is a strong indication for early combined ACL reconstruction. Reconstruction of the ACL before further damage has occurred to the knee joint, such as cartilage injury and early osteoarthritic changes, is currently advocated by most surgeons, although as yet no studies have demonstrated a higher incidence of osteoarthritis in non-operatively managed ACL-deficient knees (Jomha *et al.*1999). Intra-articular ACL reconstruction involves the precise placement of tibial and femoral tunnels for the graft to be positioned to replicate the action of the native ligament. There are several options for proximal and distal graft fixation, but the current trend for hamstring graft fixation is to use an 'endobutton' for proximal femoral fixation and a screw for distal tibial fixation, which minimizes trauma to the quadriceps muscles.

Graft selection

There are several options for the graft material for intra-articular ACL reconstruction, but the most commonly used are hamstring tendon and bone–patellar tendon–bone (BPTB) autografts, with excellent results up to 10 years postoperatively (Pinczewski *et al.* 2007). BPTB grafts have a superior tensile strength—2900 N compared with the native ACL, which has a tensile strength of 2200 N. Other options are ITB or quadriceps tendon autografts, allograft using cadaveric BPTB or Achilles tendon, and synthetic materials (Beynnon *et al.* 2005b). A number of factors are involved in graft selection, and the choice is guided by the needs of the individual patient as well as the experience of the surgeon. Hamstring and BPTB grafts are usually harvested from the same side as the ACL-deficient knee, but some surgeons advocate harvesting the graft from the contralateral uninjured lower limb. BPTB grafts should be avoided in patients who participate in jumping sports, such as netball or basketball with much eccentric loading, and patients with pre-existing anterior knee pain or patellofemoral problems. Hamstring grafts are generally avoided in patients with recent medial side injuries or chronic medial side instability. They should also be avoided in heavy patients who need accelerated rehabilitation, or in athletes who need explosive bursts of speed. Hamstring grafts tend to cause fewer harvest site symptoms and a lower incidence of radiographic osteoarthritis (Pinczewski *et al.* 2007). Complications of ACL reconstruction include failure to regain full extension or flexion, most commonly due to malpositioning of the tunnels with resulting impingement.

ITB grafts are effective, but require a long incision and risk herniation of quadriceps and interference with lateral stability. Quadriceps tendon grafts have adequate biomechanical properties, but quadriceps strength is reduced even after a year, and graft harvest is technically difficult and leaves a long scar. BPTB and Achilles tendon allografts are freeze-dried, fresh-frozen, irradiated, or preserved, and are used for revision cases and for specific cases where standard grafts are contraindicated. Synthetic grafts have been made from various materials (carbon fibre, polyester, Dacron) and were in vogue in the 1970s, but none have satisfactory mechanical properties and all suffer from the phenomenon of 'creep', where repetitive cyclical strain results in permanent deformation and elongation of the graft over time.

Double-bundle techniques have been developed using two tunnels to replicate the structure of the native ACL, but although very successful, there is no evidence that the long-term outcome is superior to single-bundle techniques. Tissue engineering offers the possibility of replacing damaged ligaments with specially engineered tissues, and attempts are being made to develop ligament tissues *in vitro* by seeding human ACL and MCL cells onto synthetic biodegradable polymer fibre scaffolds. In addition, there is active research into the use of growth factors to accelerate and promote revascularization of the graft and osseo-integration of the BPTB blocks and hamstring tendon grafts to accelerate healing and rehabilitation to facilitate an earlier return to sport.

Medial collateral ligament injury

MCL damage is the most common knee injury, and is caused by valgus stress and external rotation. Valgus stress caused by a direct blow to the lateral aspect of the knee with the foot planted is a common injury from tackles in rugby and American football. It is more commonly caused by external rotation in Alpine skiing, where a ski caught on the inside edge can confer a large moment of force about the knee. Despite the development of quick-release bindings, MCL injury accounts for up to a quarter of all skiing injuries. Damage can range from a minor sprain to complete rupture, and there are three grades of MCL injury with differing prognosis and management. The knee must be investigated for associated ligament or meniscus damage.

Grade I injury is a sprain of the superficial MCL with no demonstrable laxity. There is minimal or no effusion, with tenderness at the site of injury (usually femoral attachment) and pain on valgus stress of 30° but no instability, and the patient is able to weight-bear. These injuries can be treated with partial or full weight-bearing with supportive strapping, anti-inflammatory therapy, and isometric quadriceps contraction to restore the hamstring-to-quadriceps ratio (Norris 1998).

Grade II injury is a partial tear of the superficial MCL with laxity and intact deep MCL. The presentation varies with time from the injury, with maximal effusion and synovitis on day 2 and restriction of passive flexion to 90°, resolving over 10 days. Application of a valgus stress will demonstrate 10°–15° laxity with a firm painful endpoint in 30° flexion. There will be swelling and tenderness localized to the site of injury (again, usually femoral attachment).

Non-operative management is based on functional bracing and early mobilization, with partial weight-bearing or non-weight-bearing initially. Local measures include ultrasound and friction massage. Range of motion and isometric quadriceps contraction exercises are used until pain-free range of movement reaches 90° flexion (usually 10–14 days post-injury), when flexibility, proprioceptive, and strength training can commence. A supervised functional rehabilitiation plan is followed, slowly increasing strength and confidence with exercises, which gradually introduce rotation, shear, and valgus stress.

Pelegrini–Stieda syndrome is a condition where ectopic calcification (visible on an AP X-ray) develops at the site of injury at the attachment of the ligament to the femoral condyle. This finding may be asymptomatic and there may be no history of trauma, but it can also develop if a grade II injury is not managed acutely with functional bracing. It can cause a chronic mild laxity and intermittent pain, which can be treated with local steroid injection. When it is combined with other ligament injuries, functional instability may ensue and surgical intervention is indicated.

Grade III injury is a complete tear of the superficial and deep layers of the MCL (Fig. 3.12.16). On examination, over 15° laxity may be present and the endpoint has a 'mushy' feel in 30° of knee flexion. This injury may occur in isolation, but is commonly associated with a tear of the medial meniscus and ACL ('the unhappy triad of O'Donoghue'), patella dislocation, or PCL tear. Isolated grade III injuries can be successfully managed non-operatively in a

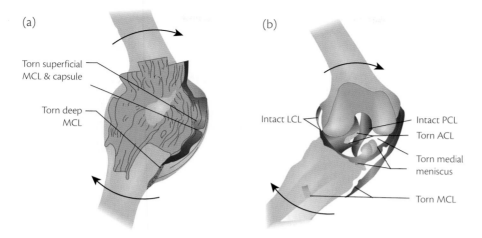

Fig. 3.12.16 (a) Torn superficial and deep components of the MCL and ruptured medial capsule. (b) 'Unhappy triad of O'Donoghue': torn ACL, MCL, and medial meniscus.

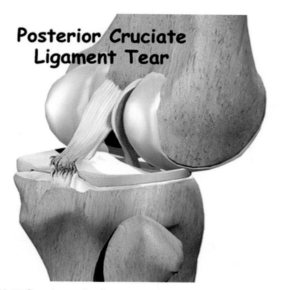

Fig. 3.12.17 Posterior cruciate ligament tear.

brace or cast (Giannotti *et al.* 2006), but primary repair is indicated if there is an associated injury and instability, and can be addressed at the same time as ACL or PCL rupture (Azar 2006), although ACL reconstruction is often delayed until valgus stability has recovered. Associated PCL injury can be treated conservatively, even in elite athletes, although surgical repair of the MCL may still be required, especially if the MCL is avulsed at the tibial attachment.

Posterior cruciate ligament tears

The PCL is the strongest ligament in the knee, and consequently tears are much less common than ACL injuries. PCL tears are most often sustained during direct impact to the anterior aspect of the upper tibia in a flexed knee, such as in a head-on collision at a road traffic accident where the tibia strikes the dashboard at high velocity. In sporting contexts, the most common mechanisms of injury are a fall onto the flexed knee or direct upper anterior tibial trauma from a rugby tackle. In contrast with an ACL injury, the athlete may be able to continue playing and may only experience minimal swelling and posterior knee pain. More commonly, patients present with immediate onset of pain, difficulty in weight-bearing, and early swelling (Bird *et al.* 1997). PCL rupture can be immediately disabling, particularly if sustained as part of a combination injury involving menisci or other ligamentous structures, most commonly posterolateral corner or collateral ligaments. Chronic PCL-deficient knees are not compatible with high-level athletic activities or contact sports.

Patients may present with a chronically PCL-deficient knee and complain of difficulty walking or running. PCL rupture reduces the efficiency of the extensor mechanism by reducing the distance between the patellar tendon and the axis of rotation of the knee, which alters the gait pattern. In the normal gait cycle quadriceps activation occurs after heel strike, but it can occur before heel strike in PCL-deficient athletes. PCL rupture can also lead to onset of early degenerative osteoarthritic changes within 5 years of injury (Keller *et al.* 1993), with maintenance of full muscle strength but significant symptoms including knee pain and limitation of sporting activity.

On examination, the patient may have a posterior sag sign and positive posterior drawer test, and the chronic PCL-deficient knee may hyperextend. The reverse pivot shift test can be used to elucidate posterolateral instability, and is similar to the pivot shift test, but with the tibia held in external rather than internal rotation. The external rotation–recurvatum test and reverse pivot shift test can be performed to detect posterolateral instability, found with combined injuries involving the posterolateral structures. X-rays may demonstrate a posterior intercondylar fracture of the tibia involving the PCL insertion, and urgent surgical opinion must be sought as better outcomes are achieved with acute repair (Kim *et al.* 2001).

Isolated PCL rupture causing unidirectional posterior instability can be managed non-operatively. Non-operative management is based on a structured programme of muscle-strengthening exercises similar to that used following ACL damage. Closed chain exercises with the foot fixed are used to enable co-contraction of hamstrings and quadriceps and improve neuromuscular re-education and proprioception. This minimizes the potentially damaging shear force from early open chain exercises emphasizing isolated hamstring contraction, but open chain quadriceps exercises can be safely incorporated into the rehabilitation of isolated PCL injuries. The programme should progress from exercises to regain full range of knee movement and restore strength to sports-specific exercises which improve power, agility, and coordination, once strength has been restored.

There is debate among surgeons as to the best technique for PCL reconstruction to achieve optimal outcome. Options include a BPTB graft similar to that used for ACL reconstruction, single or double bundle, using transtibial or tibial inlay techniques (McAllister 2002). Recent fully arthroscopic double-bundle techniques have shown encouraging short-term clinical results (Jordan *et al.* 2007b), but long-term follow-up is needed to assess the efficacy fully. Single anterolateral grafts best reproduce the normal PCL force profile, but are relatively lax below 30° of knee flexion. The addition of a second posteromedial graft reduces laxity in this low flexion range but at the expense of higher forces in the posteromedial graft (Markolf *et al.* 2006). Graft materials used include BPTB autograft and BPTB or Achilles tendon allograft.

Posterolateral corner injury

Posterolateral corner injury involves the capsule and ligaments at the posterolateral corner, particularly the arcuate ligament complex (lateral gastrocnemius tendon, lateral collateral ligament, and popliteal tendon). The ITB, LCL, biceps femoris tendon, and lateral meniscus may also be damaged and require surgical repair or reconstruction. The injury is caused by knee hyperextension combined with a varus stress; the most common mechanism is a direct blow to the anteromedial tibia in the hyperextended knee. It occurs most commonly in association with a PCL or ACL tear or as a result of acute knee dislocation, and has been demonstrated in over 9% of acute ligament injuries with haemarthrosis (Ferguson and Knottenbelt 1994).

Examination and recognition of the injury is paramount, as these injuries are frequently missed when combined with PCL or ACL injury. Failure to address posterolateral instability can compromise the reconstructed PCL or ACL. Clinical examination should include external rotation–recurvatum or 'big toe' test where the injured knee moves into hyperextension and the tibia externally rotates on lifting the limb off the couch. The reverse pivot shift test describes the sudden reduction of the posteriorly subluxed lateral tibial plateau at 30° as the knee is held in external rotation and slowly brought from 90° flexion into extension. Plain X-rays may show a Segond fracture or an avulsion fracture of Gerdy's tubercle. Grade I injuries can be successfully managed non-operatively, but Grade II injuries may result in chronic laxity if not addressed surgically. Acute anatomical repair is currently advocated in all grade III and some grade II injuries and produces far superior outcomes compared with chronic reconstructions (Covey 2001).

Lateral collateral ligament injury

LCL injury, which is caused by a varus stress to the knee, is relatively uncommon in sports injuries. Varus instability in 30° of flexion is diagnostic. Isolated LCL damage is rare, and often occurs as part of a combined posterolateral corner injury. If the injury is sustained with the knee in extension, the ACL is often torn and may require reconstruction. In extension, the LCL resists approximately 55% of applied varus stress (25% resisted by the ACL), so significant instability in extension indicates complete LCL rupture with either ACL or PCL tear. Isolated LCL injuries can usually be managed non-operatively with functional bracing and strengthening exercises. There are several surgical options, including anatomical

reconstruction with an autogenous semitendinosus graft, which can be used to treat non-reparable acute or chronic LCL tears in patients with varus instability (Coobs *et al.* 2007).

Meniscal injuries

Meniscal tears are common and can be traumatic or degenerative. Traumatic tears occur classically during twisting forces on the knee in active young people and athletes. Traumatic tears are often vertical longitudinal tears and may be associated with ligament injuries. Meniscal tears can also be caused by minimal trauma, and the patient may not remember a significant injury. Degenerative tears occur as part of a progressive wear pattern in the joint, most frequently in the over-40 age group, and are usually horizontal cleavage tears or flaps which have minimal healing potential. The posterior horn of the medial meniscus is the most commonly damaged area, resulting in pain and sometimes 'locking' of the knee.

Tears can be described as being complete or incomplete, stable or unstable, and of various patterns. Those described include vertical longitudinal (which can develop into a bucket-handle tear as the long thin inner portion can swing into the joint, causing impingement and locking), oblique/parrot-beak/flap, radial, and horizontal tears (Fig. 3.12.18). The majority are either vertical or oblique (80%). The medial meniscus is more commonly affected (75%) than the lateral meniscus (25%). Five per cent of patients will present with tears in both. Most meniscal tears lie within the posterior half of the structure because of the direction of the mechanical forces across the joint. Some types of tear can act as flap valves, leading to formation of a meniscal cyst. ACL injuries are commonly associated with lateral meniscal tears, and less

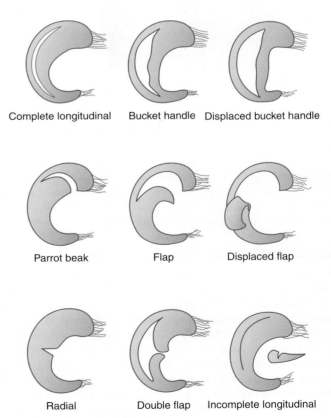

Fig. 3.12.18 Different types of meniscus tear.

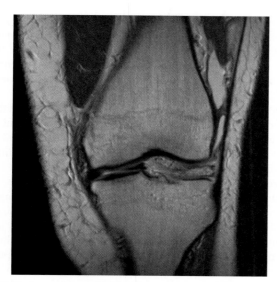

Fig. 3.12.19 Coronal T1-weighted MRI demonstrating medial mediscal tear. Reproduced from www.imagingpathways.health.wa.gov.au, with permission.

frequently with medial meniscal and MCL damage ('unhappy triad' of O'Donoghue).

Patients with chronic tears will give a history of pain on turning, with recurrent episodes of localized pain and a small joint effusion. Acutely, they may present with restricted rotation, particularly external rotation, and a loss of full extension with a springy block, which indicates locking. They may also have tenderness and associated thickening of the coronary ligament at the site of injury. McMurray's and Apley's tests can be used to detect meniscal pathology, although clinical diagnosis is unreliable. MRI is excellent for detection of meniscal tears, but it is only moderately reliable for prediction of meniscus reparability (Matava *et al.* 1999). Diagnostic arthroscopy may be indicated if the cause of symptoms is unclear. Non-operative management can include local steroid injection to the coronary ligament to restore full painless extension, and quadriceps strengthening exercises are commenced immediately. If successful, the meniscus may heal in approximately 8 weeks.

Operative management includes partial meniscectomy and repair, and the decision depends on several factors. Historically, total meniscectomy was performed for symptomatic tears, but this leads to progressive degenerative joint disease, osteochondral damage, and instability (Fairbank 1948; Fauno and Nielsen 1992). The current practice of partial meniscectomy aims to resect the minimum of meniscus involved in the tear, leaving a stable rim. This is carried out arthroscopically under general anaesthetic, often as a day-case procedure.

The indications for meniscal repair are quite specific, and include position and pattern of the tear, the age of the tear, the age of the patient, expected compliance with postoperative instructions, and the nature and level of sporting activities. Classically, repair is reserved for young compliant patients with acute (<8 weeks) peripheral longitudinal tears which lie within the peripheral vascular zone of the meniscus in otherwise stable or concomitantly reconstructed knees. Repair is not indicated if the tear is stable, less than 10 mm long, and less than 3 mm into the joint, or if the tear is in the middle or inner zones (more than 3–5 mm from the meniscal rim).

There are many techniques for meniscal repair and the method chosen will depend on the location of the tear: open repair,

outside-in sutures, inside-out sutures, or (the most recent) all-inside arthroscopic technique (Miller 2008). Open repair has been advocated for vertical tears of the posterior horn of the lateral meniscus, where adequate visualization with an arthroscope is difficult. A range of fixation devices for the all-inside technique have been developed, including arrows, darts, screws, staples, and other tensionable suture devices, which have similar failure rates (Lozano *et al.* 2007). These devices have introduced simpler surgical techniques with potentially shorter operating times, and reduced complication risk, which may have led to a broadening of the indications. Although no overall improvement in clinical success rate has been shown, these devices are accurate and effective, and repair of tears which were previously thought to be irreparable may be attempted (Tuckman *et al.* 2006). As yet, there are no long-term follow-up data. The presence of an unstable and reparable meniscal lesion combined with ACL insufficiency is a strong indication for early combined ACL reconstruction. Meniscal healing has been shown to be more successful in this situation, perhaps because of mediators released following ACL rupture (Barber and Click 1997).

Before repair, the torn edges of the meniscus are debrided of scar tissue, and some surgeons advocate the placement of an exogenous fibrin clot or allow a clot to form *in situ* from the debrided edges to aid repair (Henning *et al.* 1990). Postoperative protocols vary, but the majority of patients will follow a strict rehabilitation programme and will avoid contact sports for 6 months, as opposed to partial meniscectomy when patients can resume normal activities after 2 weeks. Meniscal allograft transplantation was introduced into clinical practice over 20 years ago for the treatment of the post-meniscectomy patient who has not yet developed osteoarthritis. The indications have been fine-tuned, and it is a useful alternative in young patients with severely damaged menisci (Verdonk *et al.* 2007).

Coronary ligament sprain

The coronary (meniscotibial) ligaments are sprained at the time of peripheral meniscal injury, but can also present in isolation, more commonly medially. It presents in the over-40 age group who participate in sports such as golf or squash, which require frequent knee rotation, and the pain can persist for several months even after cessation of the triggering activity. The patient with medial coronary ligament sprain will have discomfort on full extension with localized tenderness and associated thickening along the joint line. Treatment is non-operative and involves local steroid injection and friction massage, which can resolve all symptoms within 3 days. Sport can be resumed after 10 days.

Articular cartilage injuries

Traumatic injuries to articular hyaline cartilage in the knee are common and a frequent cause of pain and loss of function in athletes. Partial-thickness defects are rarely associated with significant symptoms, but even a small defect can alter the biomechanics of the joint, and lead to abnormal weight distribution and ultimately early post-traumatic osteoarthritis. Full-thickness defects constitute a small proportion of total injuries, although the poor capacity for repair presents a great challenge. In the USA, over 40 000 procedures to repair cartilaginous defects are performed each year.

Damage can be due to a single significant impact or repetitive microtrauma, and patients can present with intermittent pain and swelling with locking and 'giving way' if there is a loose osteochondral body. Physiotherapy plays an important role in prevention and treatment: for example. vastus medialis obliquus strengthening for patella maltracking to offload affected areas. Plain X-rays reveal little information, and even extensive lesions can be undetected. MRI scanning shows the osteochondral lesion clearly as well as associated subchondral 'bone bruising', but arthroscopy remains the gold standard. A study of 31 516 diagnostic knee arthroscopies found chondral damage, both partial- and full-thickness defects, in over 60% of cases (Curl et al. 1997).

In selecting the proper management for the individual, one must consider and recognize other injuries to the affected knee such as ligamentous instability, deficient menisci, or malalignment of the extensor mechanism or mechanical axis of the limb (Alford and Coe 2005a). Operative options include traditional methods, such as lavage and debridement, drilling, and microfracture, periosteal and perichondral grafting, as well as the newer methods of osteochondral autografting and autologous chondrocyte implantation (ACI) (Alford and Coe 2005b). Selection criteria for ACI have yet to be fully established, although there are certain prognostic factors associated with favourable outcomes: younger patients, a history of symptoms less than 2 years, a single defect, a defect on the trochlea or lateral femoral condyle, and patients with fewer than two previous procedures on the affected knee (Krishnan et al. 2006). Revision procedures for previous failed ACI produce significantly inferior clinical outcomes.

The original ACI technique involved suturing a tibial periosteum cover to retain the implanted chondrocytes in the defect, although results are similar using a synthetic porcine type I–III collagen cover (ACI-C) (Gooding et al. 2006). Matrix-induced autologous chondrocyte implantation (MACI) produces a more even distribution of chondrocytes by culturing them on a collagen membrane, which is implanted into the defect whole. Clinical, arthroscopic, and histological outcomes are comparable for ACI-C and MACI, and although MACI is technically attractive, further long-term studies are required (Bartlett et al. 2005).

Proximal tibiofibular joint injuries

Acute injuries of the proximal tibiofibular joint (PTFJ) most commonly occur in athletes whose sports involve sudden twisting movements of the knee, such as football or rugby (Lenehan et al. 2006). A fall onto the flexed knee with the leg adducted under the body can disrupt the PTFJ ligaments resulting in subluxation or dislocation and an audible 'pop'. Ogden (1974) described four patterns of instability: atraumatic subluxation, posteromedial dislocation, superior dislocation, and anterolateral dislocation (the most common type). Posteromedial subluxation may be complicated by injury to the common peroneal nerve, causing foot drop (Horan and Quin 2006). Superior dislocation is associated with tibial or fibular fractures (Johnson et al. 2007), as is inferior dislocation, which is a rare injury associated with high-impact trauma and carries the worst prognosis (Nikolaides 2007).

Diagnosis is clinical. Plain X-rays can sometimes demonstrate the dislocation, but CT is the investigation of choice if there is any uncertainty. Atraumatic subluxation presents with non-specific lateral knee pain; examination may reveal tenderness over the fibular head with a subluxing joint and ligament laxity. It is more common in pre-adolescent females and resolves with skeletal maturity. Acute anteromedial dislocation is the most common

type of injury, and the athlete is able to partially weight-bear after the injury. Clinical examination often reveals a prominence in the area of the fibular head; closed reduction with the knee flexed to 90° should be performed at presentation to accident and emergency, and the knee should be assessed for other injuries and instability.

Treatment options depend on the history, pattern of instability, and level of athletic activity of the individual. Atraumatic subluxation is generally managed non-operatively with strapping, gastrocnemius muscle strengthening, or temporary functional bracing. Acute dislocations which are irreducible, closed, or unstable can be stabilized with K-wire fixation, a syndesmosis screw, or repair of the ligaments and capsule. Recurrent dislocation or ongoing pain and symptoms following closed reduction have been managed by arthrodesis or resection of the fibular head, which are largely unsatisfactory, causing abnormal rotational and axial load distribution. Weinert and Giachino reconstruction uses autologous biceps femoris tendon to replace the ligaments. The TightRope method involves the application of two endobuttons with a pre-threaded suture via a percutaneous approach. Stability is achieved without sacrificing the normal anatomical relations of the PTFJ, which allows earlier rehabilitation and results in better outcomes (Thornes et al. 2005).

Bursae

There are a number of bursae around the knee, evident clinically and confirmed on diagnostic ultrasound. The aetiology of bursitis includes direct acute trauma, friction, or overuse and biomechanical discrepancies in lower limb/foot alignment. Sepsis and crystal arthropathies should particularly be considered if the bursa is very inflamed with no other obvious trigger. Treatment is by NSAIDs, addressing the cause where possible, compression, and if necessary aspiration and injection of corticosteroid under ultrasound guidance, provided that no infection is present. Appropriate antibiotics are necessary for septic bursitis. Surgical resection is necessary for the small minority of refractory cases.

Other causes of knee pain in sport

Anterior knee complaints

Patellofemoral pain syndrome

Patellofemoral pain syndrome (PFPS) is a common cause of anterior knee pain in athletes and the general population, accounting for up to 25% of all injuries in runners (Dixit and DiFiori 2007) and over 25% of all presentations to sports medicine clinics (Fagan and Delahunt 2008). The patient complains of knee pain in, underneath, or around the patella, which may be diffuse and bilateral and is aggravated by actions that load the knee joint—running,

Table 3.12.3 Local causes of anterior knee pain

Patellofemoral syndrome
Patellar tendinopathy
Fat pad impingement
Patellar instability
Traction apophysitides
Bursitis

climbing or descending stairs, squatting, and to a lesser extent sitting for prolonged periods (Brushøj *et al.* 2008). The onset is often gradual, and can be associated with an increase in training intensity or a change in training pattern, but can also be caused by an acute episode of trauma.

There are a number of predisposing factors and associations including lateral patella tracking, anatomical abnormalities, lower limb malalignment, patella hypermobility or tight lateral structures, previous knee surgery, poor flexibility, and muscle weakness or dysfunction. As discussed earlier in the chapter, reflex inhibition of VMO resulting in an altered firing pattern and recruitment can result in lateral patella tracking as the pull of the vastus lateralis and vastus intermedius is unopposed. Weak hip external rotator muscles have been found in studies of female athletes with PFPS (Robinson and Nee 2007).

Diagnosis is usually clinical, but imaging can be useful in some cases. AP, lateral, and skyline view X-rays can give useful information about patella position and tilt. CT can also be used to assess patellofemoral alignment at different degrees of flexion, and although MRI is less useful it can demonstrate associated discrete lesions (Fulkerson 2002).

Management is based on addressing the cause, but is generally a programme of rest, avoidance of the triggering joint-loading activity, and a structured rehabilitation programme. Several different protocols involving combinations of both open and closed kinetic chain exercises have been used effectively (Witvrouw *et al.* 2004). There is conflicting evidence regarding the efficacy of taping, but some studies have found it to be useful in reducing pain, perhaps by improving VMO activation and timing (MacGregor *et al.* 2005) and modifying contact areas to offload affected cartilage. Strengthening of weak hip musculature may also be of benefit in female athletes (Tyler *et al.* 2006), although there are no randomized controlled trials supporting this. Braces that pull the patella medially are also used, but there is no evidence that they are better than physiotherapy alone (Lun *et al.* 2005).

A number of different surgical options are used. Lateral release, which is routinely performed arthroscopically, has been used successfully in patients with a tight lateral retinaculum and patellar tilt (Fulkerson 2002) by reducing the pressure on the lateral articular facet of the patella. Proximal realignment or reconstruction of the medial patellofemoral ligament can be used to improve tracking where the medial structures are deficient, but is mainly used in patients requiring stabilization following patellar dislocation (Miller *et al.* 2007). Distal realignment techniques for lateral maltracking include medial (e.g. Elmslie–Trillat procedure) and anteromedial tibial tubercle transfer, which is successful in offloading distal and lateral patellar facet articular cartilage lesions (Pidoriano 1997).

Patellar dislocation

Traumatic dislocation of the patella occurs most commonly in adolescent females, but can also occur in male and female athletes, often in a high-level sporting context. It is usually caused by a valgus stress to the knee or external rotation of the tibia with the knee in slight flexion. Even if the patient appears to have an isolated injury, one or more medial structures will have been damaged in an acute traumatic dislocation, most commonly the medial patellofemoral ligament. This ligament can be ruptured at the femoral or patellar attachment, or even with an avulsion fragment of the medial patella. In addition, there can be associated osteochondral damage to the lateral femoral condyle or posterolateral aspect of

the patella, which predisposes to early PFJ osteoarthritis. Risk factors include patella alta (high-riding patella), increased Q angle, genu valgum, weakness of the VMO, increased femoral anteversion, and external rotation of the tibia.

The patella must immediately be reduced manually, if it has not spontaneously reduced by the time the patient presents to the accident and emergency department. The patient will complain of anterior knee pain and will have a haemarthrosis. There will be bruising and tenderness overlying the medial retinaculum and medial aspect of the patella. The 'patellar apprehension test' will be positive; the patient is apprehensive that further dislocation or subluxation will occur with laterally directed patella pressure with the knee in slight flexion. This test remains positive in chronic patellar instability and recurrent dislocation.

After possible aspiration of the haemarthrosis, initial management of the first episode of traumatic dislocation is non-operative and may require immobilization in a cast or locked brace for up to 4 weeks to allow the medial structures to heal, followed by a strict rehabilitation protocol. The emphasis is initially on isometric muscle contraction (particularly the VMO) and range of motion exercises, as isotonic exercises can predispose the patient to developing chronic patellofemoral pain if introduced too early. AP, lateral, and skyline view X-rays should be taken to look for patella alta, trochlear dysplasia, or acute or chronic patellar osteochondral fracture. CT scans with the knee in different degrees of flexion may also be useful for difficult cases with persistent patellofemoral pain, or where X-rays are inconclusive.

Current operative options include lateral retinacular release, medial retinacular reefing, medial patellofemoral ligament repair or reinsertion, and realignment procedures of the tibial insertion of the patellar tendon. Lateral release can be performed open or arthroscopically, and is only indicated if there is evidence of tightness of the lateral retinaculum. Combined procedures that involve lateral release and medial reefing are commonly performed for recurrent patellar instability, but arthroscopic medial reefing alone is an effective technique for patients with normal patellar alignment (Miller *et al.* 2007).

Patellar tendinopathies

Tendinopathy of the patellar tendon is one of the most common types seen in sport. It typically affects the deep surface of the proximal patellar tendon at the lower pole of the patella and is seen most often in jumping athletes ('jumpers knee').

Clinical features are localized pain and tenderness at the affected site, aggravated by jumping, squatting, and lunging. Severe tendinopathy can result in rest and night pain. Ultrasound findings of swelling and hypoechogenicity, usually with neovascularization in the painful tendon, are typical. Calcification or heterotopic ossification may be seen at the distal patellar pole in long-standing disease. As is the case with other tendons, ultrasonographic abnormalities are common in the asymptomatic athlete and findings do not strongly correlate with symptoms. Cook *et al.* (1998) reported that hypoechoic lesions at the proximal pole of the patellar tendon had an incidence of 22% in asymptomatic elite athletes.

It has been proposed that the mechanism of injury is impingement on the tendon by the lower patellar pole (Johnson *et al.* 1996), although this has been disputed (Schmid *et al.* 2002)

Unilateral tendinopathy has been reported to occur twice as commonly in males as in females (Gaida *et al.* 2004). Bilateral and unilateral patellar tendinopathy appear to have different aetiologies, with anthropometric factors seeming to play a role in unilateral disease. For example, a higher ratio of tibia length to stature in both the affected and non-affected legs, a higher hip-to-waist ratio, and decreased eccentric knee extensor strength have been noted as potential predisposing factors in female basketball players (Malliaris et al. 2007). Higher waist girths are a risk factor in male volleyball players (Cook et al. 2004). Other considerations include greater height and BMI, limitations in quadriceps, hamstring, and calf flexibility, poor core control and calf weakness, and a longer articular surface of the lower pole of the patella (Lorbach et al. 2008).

Ultrasound findings have been described. MRI will demonstrate swelling and increased signal in the affected portion of the tendon. Plain radiography, ultrasound, and CT will show heterotopic bone formation and calcification, and all imaging modalities have the ability to demonstrate an inferior pole osteophyte. Ultrasound can also be helpful in evaluating the patient dynamically for true impingement on the tendon by the patellar pole.

Successful management starts with early recognition of the condition, PRICES and relative off-loading from aggravating activities in the acute phase, and addressing mechanical issues including spinal and posterior leg flexibility, core control, muscle imbalances, and eccentric quadriceps strength. It is well established that controlled eccentric strengthening of the knee extensor complex is a vital element for successful rehabilitation (Jonsson and Alfredson 2005). Eccentric squat training on a decline board has been shown to have a superior therapeutic effect in reduction of pain compared with squatting on a flat surface (Purdam et al. 2004). One-legged squatting, using the decline board, can allow an earlier return to a functional level of sport (Young et al. 2005).

However, where pain limits single-leg work, two-legged eccentric overload training twice a week, using an eccentric overload training device (Bromsman device), may be as efficient and safe as the present standard daily eccentric one-legged rehabilitation–training regimen using a decline board (Frohm et al. 2005). Pain-management strategies to facilitate the rehabilitation process include regular use of ice and/or topical NSAID gel after exercise and basic analgesics prior to rehabilitation.

In those patients with chronic tendinopathy and persistent pain that is limiting progress, further interventions with injections may be considered. These include new vessel sclerosant therapy under guidance, as used in other chronic tendinopathies, with favourable outcomes reported (Alfredson and Lorentzon 2008). Platelet rich plasma injection therapy shows promise. Aprotonin (a broad-spectrum proteinase inhibitor) (Orchard et al. 2008) has also been advocated, although the level of evidence is poor. Corticosteroid injections have no role to play because of the risk of collagen disruption and tendon rupture. As with other tendinopathies, topical glyceryl trinitrate (GTN) patches to enhance blood flow may be useful. Extracorporeal shock wave therapy

may also be useful in alleviating pain (Vulpiano et al. 2007), but again rigorous trials are needed. Low-intensity pulsed ultrasound (LIPUS) has been demonstrated in one study to confer no benefit over placebo (Warden et al. 2008). Surgery is only rarely indicated.

Quadriceps tendinopathy

Quadriceps tendinopathy is relatively rare, and is more likely to occur in older athletes. There is pain and localized tenderness, exacerbated by quadriceps contraction. Imaging findings are similar to those of patellar tendinopathy, and management follows the same principles.

Patellar tendon and quadriceps tendon rupture

Disruption of the extensor mechanism of the knee can occur as a result of tear to the quadriceps tendon, transverse fracture of the patella, or rupture of the patellar tendon. These injuries can be caused by direct trauma, but the most common mechanism is sudden violent contraction of the quadriceps during a fall forwards on to the flexed knee. On examination, the patient will be unable to extend the knee or straight-leg raise, and there may be a palpable gap in the tendon. X-rays must be taken, which may reveal a fracture or characteristic high-riding patella following patellar tendon rupture. Tendon ruptures must be repaired acutely, and the patient will then undergo a graduated programme of strengthening exercises after a period of immobilization. Transverse patella fractures occur more commonly in older patients or due to direct trauma. They can be managed conservatively in plaster, but internal fixation with a tension band wire is preferable as this decreases the rate of non-union and allows earlier mobilization, resulting in less muscle wasting and an earlier return to sporting activity.

Traction apophysitides

These are seen in growing adolescent athletes, seemingly due to stresses through musculoskeletal soft tissues and bone that have disparate growth rates and are being exposed to repetitive loading during sporting activity. Types and features are described in Table 3.12.4. Treatment is counselling of the child and parents, relative rest, ice, flexibility work, and core strengthening. Orthotics may help some patients, particularly where there is pes planus. Symptoms can become chronic and associated tendinopathy can develop in adulthood.

Fat pad impingement

The highly innervated fat pad of the knee can become painful following an acute blow to the knee causing impingement between the lower patellar pole and the femoral condyle, or through chronic irritation. Pain is felt particularly in extension of the knee. Clinical findings are tenderness of the fat pad, particularly if the lower pole of the patella is compressed. Ultrasound may be helpful in demonstrating

Table 3.12.4 Features of traction apophysitides of the knee

Sinding–Larsen–Johansson	Lower pole of patella	Tender lower patellar pole, may be small avulsion	If acute, immobilize in cylinder cast Reduce activity, core and lower limb strengthening, flexibility Address biomechanics
Osgood–Schlatter	Age 13–14 years (M), 10–11 years (F)	Tibial tubercle/patellar tendon insertion	Reduce activity, core and lower limb strengthening, flexibility Address biomechanics

Table 3.12.5 Local causes of lateral knee pain

Iliotibial band syndrome
Iliotibial bursitis
Lateral meniscal injury/degradation
Lateral meniscal cyst
LCL injury
Popliteus injury
Tibiofibular joint injury/ligament sprain
Lateral popliteal nerve injury
Superficial peroneal nerve injury

hypertrophy of the fat pad and dynamic impingement. MRI will show increased signal in the pad on T2-weighted images.

Treatment starts with PRICES, taping the patella to move it forward and offload the fat pad. Attention is given to biomechanics, including lower limb strengthening and flexibility, and orthotics as appropriate.

Lateral knee complaints

Iliotibial band syndrome and bursitis

The ITB is a thick band, an extension of the tensor fascia lata (TFL), inserting onto the tibial tubercle of Gerdy. The TFL–ITB acts as a weak external rotator and extensor of the knee. The ITB lies anterior to the flexion extension axis of the knee when the knee is in extension, moving posterior to the axis when the knee moves into flexion.

ITB 'friction' syndrome is a common condition in sport, particularly in distance runners. Predisposing factors include poor conditioning, overuse, limited core control, tightness of the ITB, quadriceps, and hamstrings, leg-length discrepancy, and lower limb–foot misalignments. Training on hard surfaces, inclines, and/or cambers, equipment issues such as bicycle set-up, and footwear may all also contribute.

The patient typically reports the onset of lateral knee pain, initially like toothache but becoming more severe, to the extent that the runner cannot continue through it. The pain is worse on foot impact, running downhill, and deceleration. Start-up pain after running may also be noticeable (i.e. pain at the same site after, for example, resting in a chair), and pain on stairs is often reported. ITB syndrome is often seen after return to activity after injury, possibly due to alteration in mechanics and fitness.

Examination findings include identification of the predisposing factors listed above, local tenderness of the ITB, and, in the more acute phases, swelling and crepitus. A bursa may be present and palpable. Pain is aggravated by external rotation and extension against resistance, and when the knee moves from 90° flexion through to full extension; pain is reported as the ITB flicks over the femoral condyle at about 30° flexion. Diagnostic ultrasound may show thickening or swelling of the band and will demonstrate a bursa if present.

Management involves ice, NSAIDs (oral/topical), relative rest, and correction of the underlying cause(s). Biomechanical correction may include prescription of orthotics. Injection of corticosteroid is useful in resistant cases. Return to running should be at a slower pace on soft flat terrain over reduced mileage in the initial

phase. Surgery is only very rarely necessary, and involves a z-plasty.

Hamstring tendinopathy

Tendinopathy of the biceps femoris at the lateral knee occurs in sprinting and other rapid stop–start activities. There is localized pain and tenderness, exacerbated by stretch and resisted testing. Ultrasound and MRI will confirm the pathology. Lumbopelvic mechanics (range of motion, core control) should be assessed. Treatment includes progressive strengthening, control and flexibility work, and other interventions for tendinopathies as outlined in relation to patellar tendinopathies and elsewhere in this book.

Popliteus injuries

The popliteus is an important stabilizer of the lateral and posterolateral knee. Injuries to the musculotendinous unit of the polpliteus or the popliteus–arcuate ligament complex can occur, particularly in downhill skiing, acceleration/deceleration activities, and distance running. Typically there is an initial injury to the posterior capsule–arcuate ligament, resulting in increased tibial rotation and traction or overuse of popliteus.

The patient complains of lateral or posterolateral knee pain. Examination may reveal localized popliteus tenderness and pain on resisted knee flexion in external tibial rotation. There may be increased passive and active tibial rotation. Assessment of gait may reveal excessive tibial rotation.

Management includes analgesics or NSAIDs initially, correction of biomechanical aberrations, and strengthening of the tibial rotators and hamstrings.

Gastrocnemius tendinopathy

Tendinopathy of the medial gastrocnemius can develop due to overuse issues in training, equipment factors (bike set-up, shoes), biomechanics (over-pronation in particular), and calf stiffness. There is localized tenderness and pain on resisted knee flexion, calf raise in knee extension, and hopping. Ultrasound and MRI will confirm the pathology.

Management is ice and if necessary NSAIDs early, correction of the underlying cause(s), stretching, strengthening, and if necessary injection of corticosteroid under ultrasound guidance.

Medial knee complaints

Pes anserinus tendinopathy and bursitis

Tendinopathy of the common tendon of sartorius, gracilis, and semimembranosus is common in breaststroke swimmers, cyclists, and runners. It may be related to overuse or problems with equipment or biomechanics. There is localized pain, swelling, and tenderness, and a bursa may be palpable. There is also pain on

Table 3.12.6 Local causes of medial knee pain

MCL sprains
Medical meniscal tear
Degenerate medial meniscus
Osteoarthritis
Medial coronary ligament injury
Medial meniscal cyst

stretching of medial hamstrings and on resisted testing. Ultrasound and MRI confirm the lesion. Flexibility work and hamstring strengthening are important. A local corticosteroid injection may speed effective return to sport.

Osteoarthritis

Medial knee pain due to osteoarthritis is common and is frequently seen in sport. Pain may initially be localized, becoming more global, and is worse with impact activities. There may be post-exercise stiffness. Stretching, lower limb and core strengthening, and reducing high-impact activities are essential components of management. Orthotics or shock-absorbing insoles may help. Oral glucosamine–chondroitin supplementation is popular, and basic analgesics or viscosupplement injections may also help with symptom control. Where necessary intermittent short-term use of oral NSAIDs can be considered, depending upon other medical characteristics of the patient. Topical NSAID gel or capsaicin cream may help with local periarticular pain.

There is conflicting evidence on the benefits of arthroscopic lavage and/or debridement for knee osteoarthritis, and convincing evidence for benefit is lacking.

High tibial valgus osteotomy is another option used in carefully selected young active patients for isolated medial compartment osteoarthritis. This operation results in load transfer to the lateral compartment and can be used to correct anatomical malalignment of the proximal tibia. It also allows preservation of the joint, which facilitates conversion to a total knee replacement (TKR) at a later date. It is most successful in men with low-grade osteoarthritis.

As the indications for knee arthroplasty expand, younger and more active patients are commonly undergoing this procedure. Patients' expectations are increasing, particularly in the younger age group, many of whom wish to return to sporting activities (Healy *et al.* 2001). Mechanical fatigue of the joint-bearing surfaces has been shown to depend on usage not time (Schmalzried *et al.* 2000), and is increased with physical activity and body weight. Combined compressive forces, including muscular and ground reaction forces, across the tibiofemoral joint can exceed four times body weight during walking and eight times body weight when walking downhill (Kuster *et al.* 1997). These forces routinely exceed the yield point of the polyethylene tibial inlays currently used in many implants.

Swimming, cycling, and golf, and to a lesser extent skiing, rowing, and tennis, are recommended following TKR. Squash, running, soccer, rugby, and basketball are not recommended (McGrory *et al.* 1995; Healy *et al.* 2001) because of the repetitive forces involved and the potential for trauma. Fewer patients who undergo TKR surgery return to sporting activity than patients who undergo hip replacement (Huch *et al.* 2005).

Unicompartmental knee replacement is an increasingly used option for the treatment of isolated medial compartment osteoarthritis, and it is successful if used for limited indications. It has several potential benefits over TKR: bone stock, ACL, lateral compartment, and patellofemoral joint preservation, as well as improved kinematics and proprioception. It is relatively easy to revise to a TKR, but is dependent on precise positioning and good surgical technique. The majority of patients return to sporting activities, but the variety of activities and intensity is decreased (Naal *et al.* 2007).

Table 3.12.7 Local causes of posterior knee pain

Popliteal cyst
Popliteal bursa
Semimembranous bursa
PCL injury

Posterior knee complaints

Popliteal cysts

Popliteal (Baker's) cysts can form as an outpouching of the posterior knee. This is not specifically a sport-related injury, and is most evident when disease such as OA is present. They can result in posterior knee pain or can rupture, leaking into the posterior calf, mimicking a deep vein thrombosis. Treatment is focused on the underlying cause; if there is synovitis and effusion of the knee, local aspiration and injection of the knee with corticosteroid can be effective.

Bursae

The two bursae behind the knee can become symptomatic as a rsult of direct trauma or friction. The semimembranus bursa lies between the medial head of the gastrocnemius and the capsule, and when enlarged forms a swelling in the popliteal fossa, enlarging further with repeated flexion–extension of the knee. Unlike a popliteal cyst, it does not communicate with the joint. Aspiration and corticosteroid injection are often effective, but surgical resection may be necessary.

A popliteal bursa arises from the synovial membrane of the knee surrounding the popliteus tendon intra-articulalry. It appears as a rounded swelling at the posterior lateral femoral condyle, underlying the biceps femoris and the ITB. It usually occurs due to overuse. There is local tenderness, including the overlying tendon and the biceps femoris. Treatment is changes to training regime, addressing mechanics, strengthening of surrounding knee musculature, stretching, and local injection with corticosteroid if necessary.

References

Alford, J.W. and Coe, B.J. (2005a). Cartilage restoration. Part 1: basic science, historical perspective, patient evaluation, and treatment options. *American Journal of Sports Medicine*, **33**, 295–306.

Alford, J.W. and Coe, B.J. (2005b). Cartilage restoration. Part 2: techniques, outcomes, and future directions. *American Journal of Sports Medicine*, **33**, 443–60.

Alfredson, H. and Lorentzon, R. (2008). Sclerosing polidocanol injections of small vessels to treat the chronic painful tendon. *Current Vascular Pharmacology*, **6**, 97–100.

Amis, A.A. and Dawkins, G.P. (1991). Functional anatomy of the anterior cruciate ligament. Fibre bundle actions related to ligament replacements and injuries. *Journal of Bone and Joint Surgery. British Volume*, **73**, 260–7.

Arnoczky, S.P. and Warren, R.F. (1982). Microvasculature of the human meniscus. *American Journal of Sports Medicine*, **10**, 90–5.

Azar, F.M. (2006). Evaluation and treatment of chronic medial collateral ligament injuries of the knee. *Sports Medicine and Arthroscopy Review*, **14**, 84–90.

Barber, F.A. and Click, S.D. (1997). Meniscus repair rehabilitation with concurrent anterior cruciate reconstruction. *Arthroscopy*, **13**, 433–7.

Bartlett, W., Skinner, J.A., Gooding, C.R., *et al.* (2005). Autologous chondrocyte implantation versus matrix-induced autologous chondrocyte implantation for osteochondral defects of the knee: a prospective, randomised study. *Journal of Bone and Joint Surgery. British Volume*, **87**, 640–5.

Berlet, G.C. and Fowler, P.J. (1997). The anterior horn of the medial meniscus: an anatomic study of its insertion. *AAOS Annual Meeting Proceedings, February 1997*. AAOS, Rosemont, IL.

Beynnon, B.D., Johnson, R.J., Abate, J.A., Fleming, B.C., and Nichols, C.E. (2005a). Treatment of anterior cruciate ligament injuries: Part 1. *American Journal of Sports Medicine*, **33**, 1579–1602.

Beynnon, B.D., Johnson, R.J., Abate, J.A., Fleming, B.C., and Nichols, C.E. (2005b). Treatment of anterior cruciate ligament injuries: Part 2. *American Journal of Sports Medicine*, **33**, 1751–67.

Bird, S., Black, N., and Newton, P. (1997). *Sports Injuries: Causes, Diagnosis, Treatment and Prevention*. Stanley Thornes, Cheltenham.

Brushøj, C., Hölmich, P., Nielsen, M.B., and Albrecht-Beste, E. (2008) Acute patellofemoral pain: aggravating activities, clinical examination, MRI and ultrasound findings. *British Journal of Sports Medicine*, **42**, 64–7.

Coobs, B.R., LaPrade, R.F., Griffith, C.J., and Nelson, B.J. (2007). Biomechanical analysis of an isolated fibular (lateral) collateral ligament reconstruction using an autogenous semitendinosus graft. *American Journal of Sports Medicine*, **35**, 1521–7.

Cook, J.L., Khan, K.M., Harcourt, P.R., *et al.* (1998). Patellar tendon ultrasonography in asymptomatic active athletes reveals hypoechoic regions: a study of 320 tendons. Victorian Institute of Sport Tendon Study Group. *Clinical Journal of Sport Medicine*, **8**, 73–7.

Cook, J.L., Kiss, Z.S., Khan, K.M., Purdam, C.R., and Webster, K.E. (2004). Anthropometry, physical performance, and ultrasound patellar tendon abnormality in elite junior basketball players: a cross-sectional study. *British Journal of Sports Medicine*, **38**, 206–9.

Covey, D.C. (2001). Injuries of the posterolateral corner of the knee. *Journal of Bone and Joint Surgery. American Volume*, **83**, 106–18.

Cowley, H.R., Ford, K.R., Myer, G.D., Kernozek, T.W., and Hewett, T.E. (2006). Differences in neuromuscular strategies between landing and cutting tasks in female basketball and soccer athletes. *Journal of Athletic Training*, **41**, 67–73.

Curl, W.W., Krome, J., Gordon, E.S., Rushing, J., Smith, B.P., and Poehling, G.G. (1997). Cartilage injuries: a review of 31,516 knee arthroscopies. *Arthroscopy*, **13**, 456–60.

DeHaven, K.E., Cosgarea, A.J., and Sebastianelli, W.J. (2003). Arthrofibrosis of the knee following ligament surgery. *Instructional Course Lectures*, **52**, 369–81.

Dixit, S. and DiFiori, J.P. (2007). Management of patellofemoral pain syndrome. *American Family Physician*, **75**, 194–202.

Fagan, V. and Delahunt, E. (2008). Patellofemoral pain syndrome: a review on the associated neuromuscular deficits and current treatment options. *British Journal of Sports Medicine*, **42**, 489–95.

Fairbank, T.J. (1948) Knee joint changes after meniscectomy. *Journal of Bone and Joint Surgery*, **30B**, 664–71.

Fauno, P. and Nielsen, A.B. (1992). Arthroscopic partial meniscectomy: a long-term follow-up. *Arthroscopy*, **8**, 345–9.

Ferguson, J. and Knottenbelt, J.D. (1994). Lipohaemarthrosis in knee trauma: an experience of 907 cases. *Injury*, **25**, 311–12.

Frohm, A., Halvorsen, K., and Thorstensson, A. (2005). A new device for controlled eccentric overloading in training and rehabilitation. *European Journal of Applied Physiology*, **94**, 168–74.

Fulkerson, J.P. (2002). Diagnosis and treatment of patients with patellofemoral pain. *American Journal of Sports Medicine*, **30**, 447–56.

Gaida, J.E., Cook, J.L., Bass, S.L., Austen, S., and Kiss, Z.S. (2004). Are unilateral and bilateral patellar tendinopathy distinguished by differences in anthropometry, body composition, or muscle strength in elite female basketball players? *British Journal of Sports Medicine*, **38**, 581–5.

Giannotti, B.F., Rudy, T., and Graziano J. (2006). The non-surgical management of isolated medial collateral ligament injuries of the knee. *Sports Medicine and Arthroscopy Review*, **14**, 74–7.

Gooding, C.R., Bartlett, W., Bentley, G., Skinner, J.A., Carrington, R., and Flanagan, A. (2006). A prospective, randomised study comparing two techniques of autologous chondrocyte implantation for osteochondral defects in the knee: periosteum covered versus type I/III collagen covered. *Knee*, **13**, 203–10.

Harries, M., Williams, C., Stanish, W.D., and Micheli, L. (eds) (1998). *Oxford Textbook of Sports Medicine* (2nd edn). Oxford University Press.

Healy, W.L., Iorio, R., and Lemos, M.J. (2001). Athletic activity after joint replacement. *American Journal of Sports Medicine*, **29**, 377–88.

Henning, C.E., Lynch, M.A., Yearout, K.M., Vequist, S.W., Stallbaumer, R.J., and Decker, K.A. (1990). Arthroscopic meniscal repair using an exogenous fibrin clot. *Clinical Orthopaedics and Related Research*, **252**, 64–72.

Horan, J. and Quin, G. (2006). Proximal tibiofibular dislocation. *Emergency Medicine Journal*, **23**, e33.

Huch, K., Müller, K.A.C., Stürmer, T., Brenner, H., Puhl, W., and Günther, K.P. (2005). Sports activities 5 years after total knee or hip arthroplasty: the Ulm osteoarthritis study. *Annals of the Rheumatic Diseases*, **64**, 1715–20.

James, S., Ali, K., Pocock, C., *et al.* (2007). Ultrasound guided dry needling and autologous blood injection for patellar tendinosis. *British Journal of Sports Medicine*, **41**, 518–22.

Johnson, B.A., Amancharia, M.R., and Merk, B.B. (2007). Dislocation of the proximal tibiofibular joint in association with a tibial shaft fracture: two case reports and a literature review. *American Journal of Orthopedics*, **36**, 439–41.

Johnson, D.P., Wakeley, C.J., and Watt, I. (1996). Magnetic resonance imaging of patellar tendonitis. *Journal of Bone and Joint Surgery. British Volume*, **78**, 452–7.

Jomha, N.M., Borton, D.C., Clingeleffer, A.J., and Pinczewski, L.A. (1999). Long-term osteoarthritic changes in anterior cruciate ligament reconstructed knees. *Clinical Orthopaedics and Related Research*, **358**, 188–93.

Jonsson, P. and Alfredson, H. (2005). Superior results with eccentric compared to concentric quadriceps training in patients with jumper's knee: a prospective randomized study. *British Journal of Sports Medicine*, **39**, 847–50.

Jordan, S.S., DeFrate, L.E., Nha, K.W., Papannagari, R., Gill, T.J., and Li, G. (2007a) The *in vivo* kinematics of the anteromedial and posterolateral bundles of the anterior cruciate ligament during weightbearing knee flexion. *American Journal of Sports Medicine*, **35**, 547–54.

Jordan, S.S., Campbell, R.B., and Sekiya, J.K. (2007b). Posterior cruciate ligament reconstruction using a new arthroscopic tibial inlay double-bundle technique. *Sports Medicine and Arthroscopy Review*, **15**, 176–83.

Keller, P.M., Shelbourne, K.D., McCarroll, J.R., and Rettig, A.C. (1993). Nonoperatively treated isolated posterior cruciate ligament injuries. *American Journal of Sports Medicine*, **21**, 132–6.

Kim, S.J., Shin, S.J., Choi, N.H., and Cho, S.K. (2001). Arthroscopically assisted treatment of avulsion fractures of the posterior cruciate ligament from the tibia. *Journal of Bone and Joint Surgery. American Volume*, **83**, 698–708.

Kolowich, P.A., Paulos, L.E., Rosenberg, T.D., and Farnsworth, S. (1990). Lateral release of the patella: indications and contraindications. *American Journal of Sports Medicine*, **18**, 359–65.

Krishnan, S.P., Skinner, J.A., Bartlett, W., *et al.* (2006). Who is the ideal candidate for autologous chondrocyte implantation? *Journal of Bone and Joint Surgery. British Volume*, **88**, 61–4.

Kuster, M.S., Wood, G.A., Stachowiak, G.W., and Gächtner, A. (1997). Joint load considerations in total knee replacement. *Journal of Bone and Joint Surgery. British Volume*, **79**, 109–13.

LaPrade, R.F., Wentorf, F.A., Fritts, H., Gundry. C., and Hightower, C.D. (2007). A prospective magnetic resonance imaging study of the incidence of posterolateral and multiple ligament injuries in acute knee injuries presenting with haemarthrosis. *Arthroscopy*, **23**, 1341–7.

Lenehan, B., McCarthy, T., Street, J., and Gilmore, M. (2006). Dislocation of the proximal tibiofibular joint: a new method of fixation. *Injury Extra*, **37**, 385–9.

Li, G., DeFrate, L.E., Sun, H., and Gill, T.J. (2004). *In vivo* elongation of the anterior cruciate ligament and posterior cruciate ligament during knee flexion. *American Journal of Sports Medicine*, **32**, 1415–20.

Lorbach, O., Diamantopoulos, A., Kammerer, K.P., and Paessler, H.H. (2008). The influence of the lower patellar pole in the pathogenesis of chronic patellar tendinopathy. *Knee Surgery, Sports Traumatology, Arthroscopy*, **16**, 348–52.

Lozano, J., Ma, C.B., and Cannon, W.D. (2007). All-inside meniscus repair: a systematic review. *Clinical Orthopaedics and Related Research*, **455**, 134–41.

Lun, V.M., Wiley, J.P., Meeuwisse, W.H., and Yanagawa, T.L. (2005). Effectiveness of patellar bracing for treatment of patellofemoral pain syndrome. *Clinical Journal of Sport Medicine*, **15**, 235–40.

McAllister, D.R., Markolf, K.L., Oakes, D.A., Young, C.R., and McWilliams, J. (2002). A biomechanical comparison of tibial inlay and tibial tunnel posterior cruciate ligament reconstruction techniques: graft pretension and knee laxity. *American Journal of Sports Medicine*, **30**, 312–17.

MacGregor, K., Gerlach, S., Mellor, R., and Hodges, P.W. (2005). Cutaneous stimulation from patella tape causes a differential increase in vasti muscle activity in people with patellofemoral pain. *Journal of Orthopaedic Research*, **23**, 351–8.

McGrory, B.J., Stuart, M.J., and Sim, F.H. (1995). Participation in sports after hip and knee arthroplasty: review of the literature and survey of surgeon preferences. *Mayo Clinic Proceedings*, **70**, 342–8.

Mafulli, N., Binfield, P.M., King, J.B., and Good, C.J. (1993). Acute haemarthrosis of the knee in athletes. A prospective study of 106 cases. *Journal of Bone and Joint Surgery. British Volume*, **75**, 945–9.

Malliaras, P., Cook, J.L., and Kent, P.M. (2007). Anthropometric risk factors for patellar tendon injury among volleyball players. *British Journal of Sports Medicine*, **41**, 259–63.

Markolf, K.L., Feeley, B.T., Jackson, S.R., and McAllister, D.R. (2006). Biomechanical studies of double-bundle posterior cruciate ligament reconstructions. *Journal of Bone and Joint Surgery. American Volume*, **88**, 1788–94.

Matava, M.J., Eck, K., Totty, W., Wright, R.W., and Shively, R.A. (1999). Magnetic resonance imaging as a tool to predict meniscal reparability. *American Journal of Sports Medicine*, **27**, 436–43.

Miller, J.R., Adamson, G.J., Pink, M.M., Fraipont, M.J., and Durand, P. (2007). Arthroscopically assisted medial reefing without lateral release for patellar instability. *American Journal of Sports Medicine*, **35**, 622–9.

Miller, M.D. (2008). *Review of Orthopaedics* (55th edn). W.B. Saunders, Philadelphia, PA.

Mui, L.W., Engelsohn, E., and Umans, H. (2007). Comparison of CT and MRI in patients with tibial plateau fracture. Can CT findings predict ligament tear or meniscal injury? *Skeletal Radiology*, **36**, 145–51.

Naal, F.D., Fischer, M., Preuss, A., *et al.* Return to sports and recreational activity after unicompartmental knee arthroplasty. *American Journal of Sports Medicine*, **35**, 1688–95.

Nikolaides, A.O., Anagnostidis, K.S., Kirkos, J.M., and Kapetanos, G.A. (2007). Inferior dislocation of the proximal tibiofibular joint: a new type of dislocation with poor prognosis. *Archives of Orthopaedic and Trauma Surgery*, **127**, 933–6.

Norris, C.M. (1998). *Sports Injuries: Diagnosis and Management* (2nd edn). Butterworth Heinemann, Oxford.

Noyes, F.R., Bassett, R.W., Grood, E.S., and Butler, D.L. (1980). Arthroscopy in acute traumatic haemarthrosis of the knee. Incidence of anterior cruciate tears and other injuries. *Journal of Bone and Joint Surgery. American Volume 1980*, **62**(5), 687–695.

Ogden, J.A. (1974). Subluxation of the proximal tibiofibular joint. *Journal of Bone and Joint Surgery. American Volume*, **56**, 145–54.

Orchard, J., Massey, A., Brown, R., Cardon-Dunbar, A., and Hofmann, J. (2008). Successful management of tendinopathy with injections of the MMP-inhibitor aprotinin. *Clinical Orthopaedics and Related Research*, **466**, 1625–32.

Pidoriano, A.J., Weinstein, R.N., Buuck, D.A., and Fulkerson, J.P. (1997). Correlation of patellar articular lesions with results from anteromedial tibial tubercle transfer. *American Journal of Sports Medicine*, **25**, 533–7.

Pinczewski, L.A., Lyman, J., and Salmon, L.J. (2007). A 10-year comparison of anterior cruciate ligament reconstructions with hamstring tendon and patellar tendon autograft: a controlled, prospective trial. *American Journal of Sports Medicine*, **35**, 564–74.

Purdam, C.R., Jonsson, P., Alfredson, H., *et al.* (2004). A pilot study of the eccentric decline squat in the management of painful chronic patellar tendinopathy. *British Journal of Sports Medicine*, **38**, 395–7.

Robinson, R.L. and Nee, R.J. (2007). Analysis of hip strength in females seeking physical therapy treatment for unilateral patellofemoral pain syndrome. *Journal of Orthopaedic and Sports Physical Therapy*, **37**, 232–8.

Sarimo, J., Rantanen, J., Heikkila, I., Hiltunen, A., and Orava, S. (2002). Acute traumatic haemarthrosis of the knee. Is routine arthroscopic examination necessary? A study of 320 consecutive patients. *Scandinavian Journal of Surgery*, **91**, 361–4.

Schmalzried, T.P., Shepherd, E.F., Dorey, F.J., *et al.* (2000). Wear is a function of use, not time. *Clinical Orthopaedics and Related Research*, **381**, 36–46.

Schmid, M.R., Hodler, J., Cathrein, P., *et al.* (2002). Is impingement the cause of jumper's knee? Dynamic and static magnetic resonance imaging of patellar tendinitis in an open-configuration system. *American Journal of Sports Medicine*, **30**, 388–95.

Shelbourne, D.K. and Nitz, P. (1990). Accelerated rehabilitation after anterior cruciate ligament reconstruction. *American Journal of Sports Medicine*, **18**, 292–9.

Thornes, B., Shannon, F., Guiney. A.M., Hession, P., and Masterson, E. (2005). Suture-button syndesmosis fixation: accelerated rehabilitation and improved outcomes. *Clinical Orthopaedics and Related Research*, **431**, 207–12.

Tuckman, D.V., Bravman, J.T., Lee, S.S., Rosen, J.E., and Sherman, O.H. (2006). Outcomes of meniscal repair: minimum of 2-year follow-up. *Bulletin (Hospital for Joint Diseases (New York, NY))*, **63**, 100–4.

Tyler, T.F., Nicholas, S.J., Mullaney, M.J., and McHugh, M.P. (2006). The role of hip muscle function in the treatment of patellofemoral pain syndrome. *American Journal of Sports Medicine*, **34**, 630–6.

Verdonk, R., Almqvist, K.F., Huysse, W., and Verdonk, P.C. (2007). Meniscal allografts: indications and outcomes. *Sports Medicine and Arthroscopy Review*, **15**, 121–5.

Vulpiani, M.C., Vetrano, M., Savoia, V., Di Pangrazio, E., Trischitta, D., and Ferretti, A. (2007). Jumper's knee treatment with extracorporeal shock wave therapy: a long-term follow-up observational study. *Journal of Sports Medicine and Physical Fitness*, **47**, 323–8.

Warden, S.J., Metcalf, B.R., Kiss, Z.S., *et al.* (2008). Low-intensity pulsed ultrasound for chronic patellar tendinopathy: a randomized, double-blind, placebo-controlled trial. *Rheumatology (Oxford)*, **47**, 467–71.

Witvrouw, E., Danneels, L., Van Tiggelen, D., Willems, T.M., and Cambier, D. (2004). Open versus closed kinetic chain exercises in patellofemoral pain: a 5-year prospective randomized study. *American Journal of Sports Medicine*, **32**, 1122–30.

Young, M.A., Cook, J.L., Purdam, C.R., *et al.* (2005). Eccentric decline squat protocol offers superior results at 12 months compared with traditional eccentric protocol for patellar tendinopathy in volleyball players. *British Journal of Sports Medicine*, **39**, 102–5.

3.13

Ankle injuries

Bill Ribbans and Cathy Speed

Introduction

The ankle is the most common region of the body to be injured in sport. However, injuries sustained at this site are commonly neglected, resulting in potentially significant long-term functional and structural sequelae.

Effective prophylactic strategies to minimize ankle injuries in specific sports should be developed. Addressing modifiable risk factors should be an important aspect of conditioning regimes for most sports, and early recognition and management of injuries is vital for preventing the development of chronic pathology limiting the attainment of an athlete's full potential.

Epidemiology

The ankle has been the focus of several sport-, age-, and gender-specific descriptive epidemiological studies (Hootman *et al.* 2007; Nelson *et al.* 2007). Ankle lateral ligament sprains have been identified as the most common injury overall in American collegiate athletes, representing approximately 15% of all injuries across 15 land-based sports (Hootman *et al.* 2007) (Appendix 1). In high-school sports, ankle injuries represent 22.6% of all injuries (5.23 ankle injuries per 10 000 athlete exposures) (Nelson *et al.* 2007). Land-based activities involving running (particularly in close proximity to others), jumping, cutting, and tackling, racket sports, and women's gymnastics are the sports with the highest risk.

Most ankle injuries are more common in competition than in practice (Hootman *et al.* 2007). Ankle sprain injuries in amateur soccer players are primarily contact injuries, occurring mainly in defenders. Injury rates are higher in those with previous sprains and towards the end of a game, and chiefly occur during the first 2 months of the season (Hootman *et al.* 2007). Despite early suggestions of an increased incidence of sprains with artificial turf, this has not been supported by more extensive research, in particular in relation to the later-generation turf (Fuller *et al.* 2007a, b).

Gender comparison studies in relation to ankle injuries in specific sports report conflicting results, with some finding predominance in males, and others in females. Ankle ligament injures have a higher incidence within sports in females, although the degree of female predominance does not appear as marked as seen as ACL injuries (Appendix 1). Injury patterns within different sports must be interpreted with caution, since the nature of the way the sport is played differs between the genders.

Anatomy

Functional anatomy

The ankle (talocrural) joint is a synovial hinge articulation involving the tibia, fibula, and talus. It is described as a mortise, allowing primarily dorsiflexion and plantarflexion. The biomechanics of the ankle are closely linked with those of the other joints of the hindfoot. Most large synovial joints are stabilized by a combination of bony, tendinous, and ligamentous structures. Stability of the ankle is conferred to the mortise through the peroneal muscles, the lateral and medial ligamentous complexes, the syndesmosis, and joint congruity.

Skeletal anatomy

The **talus** is the central component of both the ankle and the hindfoot and has a significant proportion of its surface covered in articular hyaline cartilage. Additionally, it does not have any musculotendinous attachments. These two factors contribute to limiting its blood supply, causing potential problems with healing after injury. The body of the talus forms the distal part of the ankle joint, sitting within the ankle mortise and articulating medially and laterally with the respective malleoli. Superiorly, the **dome** articulates with the **tibial plafond**, which covers 60% of the dome at any joint position. An accessory ossicle, the **os trigonum**, articulates with the posterior talar process and is present in 6–8% of the population in whom it is bilateral in 50%. (See Figs 3.13.1 and 3.13.2)

Ligaments

The **medial**, **spring**, or **deltoid ligament** is a large strong ligament, which only rarely sustains serious injury. It confers significant stability against talar eversion and rotation through five bands, divided into superficial (three bands) and deep (two bands) components. The superficial component originates on the medial malleolus, and has a continuous fan-shaped insertion along the sustentaculum tali to the navicular. The deep component inserts onto the talus.

The **lateral ligament complex** consists of three ligamentous bands, the anterior talofibular ligament (ATFL), the calcaneofibular ligament (CFL), and the posterior talofibular ligament (PTFL).

The **ATFL** runs from the anterior lateral malleolus to the talar neck. It restricts anterior displacement and internal rotation of the talus and is a weak stabilizer of the ankle against inversion stresses. It is the most vulnerable of the three lateral ligaments to injury during inversion.

The **CFL** is anatomically distinct from the ankle capsule. It crosses both the ankle and the subtalar joint. It runs from its origin at the tip of the lateral malleolus deep to (and partly in continuation with)

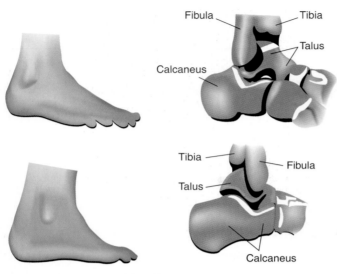

Fig. 3.13.1 Bony anatomy of the ankle.

the peroneal tendon sheaths and inserts onto the calcaneus. This close relationship with the peroneal tendon sheaths explains the significant incidence of peroneal tendon injury in association with CFL tear.

The **PTFL** is both the strongest and the smallest of the three lateral ligaments and lies parallel to the subtalar joint, running from the posteromedial aspect of the lateral malleolus to the lateral talar tubercle. It acts as a restraint on posterior dislocation of the talus but is not stressed during physiological ankle movements. It also restricts external rotation of the talus in the neutral or dorsi-flexed position.

The orientation of the ankle ligaments varies with the position of the foot, such that with the foot in neutral the ATFL and CFL both support the joint, whereas in plantarflexion the ATFL acts almost in isolation to stabilize the ankle against inversion. In dorsiflexion the CFL is the principal stabilizer of the ankle.

The distal **tibiofibular syndesmosis** increases ankle stability against torsional and angular stresses, and is composed of the anterior, posterior, and interosseous tibiofibular ligaments. The latter is in continuity with the interosseous membrane. The joint is most stable with the foot in dorsiflexion. As the ankle moves from

plantarflexion to full dorsiflexion, the intermalleolar distance widens by 1.5 mm, creating greater tension across the syndesmosis.

Retinacula

Five retinacular bands protect and guide the neurovascular bundles and the tendons, which lie within compartments in synovial sheaths (Figures 3.13.3 and 3.13.4). The inferior extensor retinaculum prevents bow stringing of the tendons that run beneath it (i.e. the long extensors of the toes and the tibialis anterior).

The **flexor retinaculum** attaches to the medial malleolus and medial surface of the calcaneal process to form the **tarsal tunnel**. It attaches to and restrains the sheaths of the structures within the tarsal tunnel, which lie superficial to the deltoid ligament and form an arc at the medial malleolus from anteromedial to deep postero-lateral in the order tibialis posterior, flexor digitorum longus, the posterior tibial artery and veins, the tibial nerve and its medial cal-caneal branch, and the flexor hallucis longus. The tibialis posterior and flexor digitorum tendons have their own retinacular compart-ments at the medial malleolus.

Muscles

Posterolateral

The **peroneal muscles** (**peroneus longus** and **brevis**) are important dynamic stabilizers of the ankle joint. The muscles contract in a reflex response to proprioceptive input from the ligaments and capsule, working to counteract the effect of the tibialis posterior which plantarflexes and inverts the foot. The peroneus longus becomes tendinous in the mid-leg and receives muscle fibres until 3–5 cm proximal to the lateral malleolus. The peroneus brevis becomes tend-inous 2–3 cm proximal to the lateral malleolus, lying initially deep to the peroneus longus and then anterior. At the tip of the lateral malle-olus, the peroneus brevis lies superior to the longus. The tendons curve behind the malleolus, usually in a sulcus, and the tendons are secured by a retaining band. The most important part of this reti-naculum is the superior peroneal retinaculum (SPR) which not only restrains the peroneal tendons, but can also act as an accessory CFL. The peroneal tendons run in a common sheath in the retromalleolar region, which subsequently bifurcates at the level of the peroneal tubercle as the course of the two tendons diverges. Both tendons act as plantarflexors of the ankle and evertors of the hindfoot. The per-oneus longus passes medially across the sole of the foot to insert into the base of the first metatarsal and helps to plantarflex the first ray.

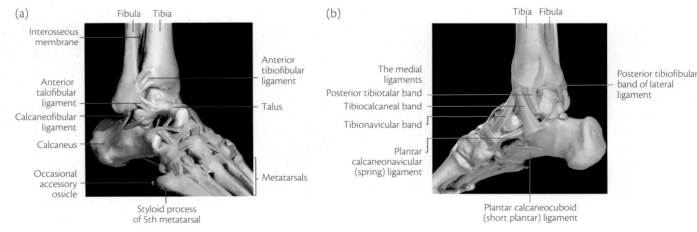

Fig. 3.13.2 Ligamentous anatomy of the ankle: (a) lateral and (b) medial.

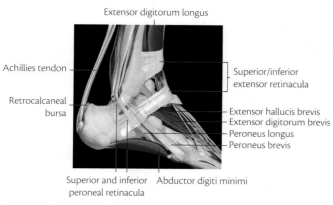

Fig. 3.13.3 The lateral ankle.

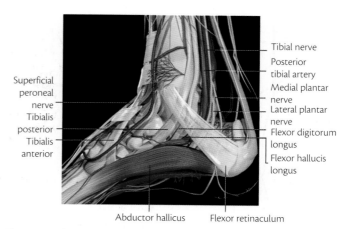

Fig. 3.13.4 The medial ankle.

Posteromedial

The tendons of the posterior compartment (tibialis posterior, flexor digitorum longus, and flexor hallucis longus) pass behind the medial malleolus towards their insertions in the foot.

The **tibialis posterior tendon** (TP) passes inferior to the spring ligament, where a sesamoid may be located. It has insertions on the navicular tuberosity, the medial cuneiform, and the inferior capsule of the navicular–medial cuneiform joint, the second and third cuneiforms, the cuboid and the bases of the middle three metatarsals, and the anterior sustentaculum tali. TP has specific functions at each of the three joints it crosses—the ankle, subtalar, and oblique mid-tarsal joints. TP works powerfully at the subtalar and mid-tarsal joints to invert the heel and supinate the foot. It also plantarflexes the foot at the ankle and plays an important role in maintaining the medial arch of the foot, and contributes to stability of the foot by its many bony attachments.

The **flexor digitorum longus** (FDL) inserts onto the base of the distal phalanx of each of the lateral four toes and acts to flex the lesser phalanges. It is a weak plantarflexor at the ankle. The **flexor hallucis longus (FHL)** inserts into the base of the distal phalanx to assist in plantarflexion of the great toe and assist in flexion of the ankle.

Anterior

From medial to lateral, the tendons of the tibialis anterior, extensor hallucis longus, extensor digitorum longus, and peroneus tertius (a part of EDL) all pass to the foot on the anterior aspect of the ankle. The tendons pass under the inferior extensor retinaculum. The tibialis anterior functions to dorsiflex the ankle and invert the foot. It also actively supports the medial arch.

Posterior

The **Achilles tendon** passes posterior to the ankle joint to insert onto the calcaneal tuberosity. Its anatomical features are described in Chapter 3.11.

Neurovascular supply

The sciatic nerve innervates the ankle and foot through the sciatic nerve via the tibial nerve (medial and lateral plantar nerves), the common peroneal nerve (deep and superficial branches), and the sural nerve. The exception is the saphenous nerve, a branch of the femoral nerve. The **sural** nerve, a branch of the tibial nerve, arises in the posterior superior popliteal fossa and passes down the posterior calf, piercing the deep fascia in the mid-calf. The nerve runs behind and below the tip of the lateral malleolus and forms the cutaneous supply to the inferior part of the lateral malleolus and lateral foot.

Table 3.13.1 Movements and innervation of the ankle and subtalar joint

Action	Muscles involved	Innervation	Nerve root(s)
Plantar flexion of ankle	Gastrocnemius, soleus, FHL, FDL	Tibial nerve	S1–S3
	Tibialis posterior	Tibial nerve	L4–L5
	Peroneus longus and brevis	Superficial peroneal nerve	L5, S1–S2
Dorsiflexion of ankle	Tibialis anterior	Deep peroneal nerve	L4–L5
	EDL, EHL	Deep peroneal nerve	L5–S1
Inversion	Tibialis posterior	Tibial nerve	L4–L5
	FDL, FHL	Tibial nerve	L5–S1
	Tibialis anterior	Deep peroneal	L4–L5
	EHL	Deep peroneal	L5–S1
Eversion	Peronei	Superficial peroneal	L5, S1–S2
	EDL	Deep peroneal	L5–S1

FHL, flexor hallucis longus; FDL, flexor digitorum longis; EDL, extensor digitorum longis; EHL, extensor hallucis longus.

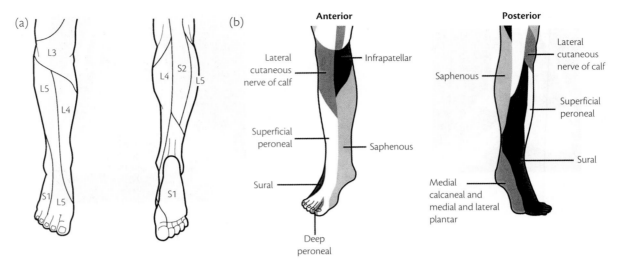

Fig. 3.13.5 Neurological supply around the ankle.

The **superficial peroneal nerve** pierces the fascia to become subcutaneous 10–15 cm above the ankle and provides sensory innervation to the anterolateral ankle and foot.

The **tibial nerve** (from the sciatic nerve) gives off a branch, the medial calcaneal nerve, 2–7 cm above the medial malleolus, and then bifurcates within (or occasionally proximal to) the tarsal tunnel to form the medial and lateral plantar nerves. The medial plantar nerve can occasionally arise from the lateral plantar nerve.

The **medial calcaneal nerve** travels anterior to the Achilles tendon. It divides into anterior and lateral plantar branches, which innervate the sole and the medial aspect of the hindfoot. The **saphenous nerve** arises from the femoral nerve and innervates the ankle, medial malleolus, and medial border of the foot.

The **posterior tibial artery,** arising from the popliteal artery, passes behind the medial malleolus, where it is easily palpated. Through its medial and lateral plantar branches it contributes with the dorsalis pedis to provide the vascular supply to the foot. The **peroneal artery** arises from the posterior tibial artery in the lower leg and divides into branches that supply the ankle.

The branches of the **superficial peroneal nerve** pass superficially across the front of the ankle, in a variable distribution, to supply sensory innervation to the dorsum of the foot. The **deep peroneal nerve** travels with the anterior tibial artery under the inferior extensor retinaculum and lies lateral to the dorsalis pedis artery between the EHL and the EDL on the dorsum of the foot, between the first and second rays. It provides the sensory supply to the first web space through its medial branch, while its lateral branch innervates the extensor digitorum brevis and provides the sensory supply to the mid-tarsal joints and forefoot.

The **anterior tibial artery** is palpated medial to EHL at the anterior ankle. As it passes below the extensor retinaculum it becomes the dorsalis pedis artery and then lies lateral to EHL. It supplies the ankle, the sinus tarsi, and the dorsum of the foot.

Clinical evaluation

History

The history includes details of the injury itself, and past injury, medical, and training histories. Common ankle symptoms are pain, giving way/repeated inversion injuries, swelling, stiffness, clicking, popping, and locking. The timing and mechanism of the onset of such symptoms should be ascertained. Inability to weight-bear immediately after an injury suggests major osseous, articular and/or soft tissue damage. The timing of onset of swelling is important; significant swelling occurring immediately after injury is suggestive of significant structural damage. Swelling is common with chronic injuries.

Giving way of the ankle is typically caused by primary ligamentous instability, tendon subluxation, or pain leading to the sensation of giving way—via a pain reflex. Popping, snapping, or tearing is indicative of ligament, tendon, or cartilage damage. Locking of the ankle joint is a characteristic feature of loose bodies within the joint. Stiffness is common after an acute injury. Chronic stiffness also occurs with a soft tissue injury and degenerative articular complaints. Morning stiffness is suggestive of inflammatory joint disease.

The nature, relationship to activity and rest, intensity and distribution of pain, and exacerbating and relieving features help to determine the structures involved and the severity of the complaint. The presence of neurovascular symptoms should be sought.

Specific details of previous treatment—their timing, compliance, and outcomes—should also be obtained. This includes the use of supports, taping, insoles, and orthotics. Finally, a general medical and musculoskeletal history should be established.

Examination

Evaluation of the ankle may be limited in the acute stage after injury because of pain and swelling. In such situations it may be necessary to review the patient after a period of conservative management of the acute injury with rest, ice and elevation. The old maxim 'look, feel, and move' is followed.

As with other examination areas, it is important to be able to see the patient standing and examine them both prone and supine. Consider the following areas:

- anterior
- posteromedial
- posterolateral
- posterior.

Anterior examination

The important structures to assess passing anterior to the ankle are:

- anterior ankle joint
- extensor tendons and retinaculum
- deep peroneal nerve and dorsalis pedis artery
- superficial peroneal nerve
- dorsalis pedis artery
- saphenous nerve and long saphenous vein.

Anterior ankle joint

The anterior aspect of the ankle joint is a frequent source of pain and pathology. The function of the adjacent inferior tibiofibular joint and syndesmosis has already been discussed. An effusion of the ankle and/or synovitis is frequently seen best at the front of the ankle. Palpate the anterior joint.

Extensor tendons and retinaculum

Four tendons pass across the front of the ankle joint bound down by the extensor retinaculum. From medial to lateral, they are:

- tibialis anterior
- extensor hallucis longus
- extensor digitorum longus
- peroneus tertius.

Tibialis anterior

Tibialis anterior is a powerful invertor and dorsiflexor of the foot and ankle. It attaches principally to the medial cuneiform. It is easily palpated when the patient is asked to dorsiflex their ankle.

Extensor hallucis longus

Lateral to the tibialis anterior tendon is the extensor hallucis longus tendon (EHL). This powerful tendon attaches to the distal phalanx of the great toe and dorsiflexes the digit, and helps the tibialis anterior dorsiflex the ankle. Resisted great toe extension demonstrates the activity and route of this structure.

Extensor digitorum longus

The extensor digitorum longus (EDL) lies lateral to the EHL. It supplies tendons to each of the lesser four toes and extends the MTP and IP joints of these digits. Each tendon is joined from its lateral side by smaller slips from extensor digitorum brevis (EDB) and together they form the extensor hood over the dorsum of the proximal digit to which the intrinsic muscles contribute.

Peroneus tertius

The peroneus tertius is the most lateral and least important of the four tendons of the anterior compartment of the leg. Its tendon passes anterolaterally across the ankle to insert into the dorsum of the base of the fifth metatarsal. It is responsible for dorsiflexion of the ankle and eversion of the hindfoot.

Deep peroneal nerve and dorsalis pedis artery

This nerve is the continuation of the tibial nerve that supplies the anterior compartment of the leg. It passes anterior to the ankle joint deep to the extensor retinaculum between the extensor hallucis longus and extensor digitorum longus tendons. It supplies sensation to the dorsum of the first webspace between the great and second toe.

It may be injured during trauma (including surgical) and can be compressed by dorsal osteophytes (spurs) in the midfoot secondary to degenerative changes in the area. Rarely, the webspace may be rendered numb following an anterior compartment syndrome of the leg (either trauma or exercise induced) causing damage to the nerve.

The dorsalis pedis artery is the continuation of the anterior tibial artery. It accompanies the deep peroneal nerve across the front of the ankle deep to the extensor retinaculum. Feel its pulse as it passes across the dorsum of the midfoot. It terminates by passing deep between the bases of the first and second metatarsals.

Superficial peroneal nerve

This nerve emerges from the peroneal compartment above the ankle joint and passes superficially across the anterolateral aspect of the ankle. In thin individuals, its main trunk and some branches can be seen under the skin, especially if the skin is placed under tension by plantarflexing the ankle and supinating the foot.

The nerve divides into a number of branches which are responsible for supplying sensation to the dorsum of the foot with the exception of the first webspace (deep peroneal nerve territory).

The nerve(s) are at risk from traction damage following injury (e.g. inversion sprains of the ankle) and from injudiciously placed surgical incisions. Look for areas of tenderness and sensitivity along the course of the nerve, and for altered sensation of the dorsum of the foot.

Saphenous nerve and long saphenous vein

The saphenous nerve is a branch of the femoral nerve. It is the only sensory nerve that is not derived from the sciatic nerve below the knee. It passes immediately anterior to the medial malleolus accompanied by the long saphenous vein. It supplies sensation to the medial border of the foot as far as the hallux. It can be damaged by trauma. It may be injured during vein surgery or possibly during an ankle arthroscopy.

The long saphenous vein is the largest of the superficial veins. It drains blood from the medial side of the foot. It passes medial to the knee into the thigh before piercing the cribriform fascia in the groin to enter the femoral vein. Incompetence of the system and its communications with the deep veins of the calf will produce swelling, varicose eczema, and varicosities along its course.

Posteromedial examination

The order of structures lying behind the medial malleolus of the ankle can be remembered by the mnemonic: 'Tom, Dick ANd Harry'. Tom is the Tibialis posterior tendon, Dick is the flexor Digitorum longus tendon, AN represents the posterior tibial Artery, Nerve and veins, and Harry is the flexor Hallucis longus tendon.

Tibialis posterior

The tibialis posterior tendon passes into the foot applied to the posterior aspect of the medial malleolus in its own sheath. It is a strong musculotendinous unit with little excursion on contraction. It attaches to a number of structures in the foot, but principally to the navicular. Failure of this tendon will cause a progressive planovalgus deformity of the foot. It inverts and plantarflexes the foot.

Swelling secondary to synovitis along its course may be seen in the early stages of pathology. Test its function by asking the patient to invert the foot against the resistance of the examiner's hand while the ankle is in slight plantarflexion.

An indication of tibialis posterior dysfunction can be gauged by finding the 'too many toes' sign. When observed from behind, the foot with the incompetent tibialis posterior tendon develops a planovalgus position allowing more toes to be seen lateral to the ankle than the normal side. While the patient is being viewed from the posterior aspect, look for evidence of swelling 'filling in' the sulcus between the medial malleolus and Achilles tendon.

Another useful dynamic test to assess the tibialis posterior function is to ask the patient to undertake tiptoeing. The test should be performed with both feet and legs exposed. Ask the patient to stand in front of a wall and place their hands on the wall for balance. On tiptoeing, the hindfoot should swing into varus as well as plantarflexing since the tibialis posterior tendon is stronger than the peroneal tendons.

Ask the patient to double-stance tiptoe. Can they perform this without pain? Do both hindfeet swing into varus?

Then, in turn, ask the patient to undertake single-stance tiptoe. Is the patient able to lift the heel? Is there a difference between the two feet? Does the hindfoot swing into varus?

Flexor digitorum longus

The FDL lies immediately behind the tibialis posterior tendon in its own sheath. It divides into four tendons to serve digits 2–5. It crosses the EHL tendon at the knot of Henry (see below). It plantarflexes these toes by its insertion into the distal phalanx. Functionally, its loss has little functional effect on the foot and it is used to reconstruct a ruptured tibialis posterior tendon.

Posterior tibial nerve and artery

The posterior tibial nerve and accompanying artery and veins run between the FDL and the FHL. The nerve divides into its terminal branches, the medial and lateral plantar nerves, to supply sensation to the sole of the foot and supply the intrinsic muscles of the sole.

Compression of the nerve on the medial side of the foot produces a tarsal tunnel syndrome similar to a carpal tunnel syndrome in the wrist, albeit much rarer than its upper limb counterpart. Irritation of the nerve may be found by direct palpation. Light tapping (percussion) along the line of the nerve may produce tingling (positive Tinel's test). The nerve gives off medial calcaneal branches to the medial side of the hindfoot that are at risk during surgery to this area.

Flexor hallucis longus

The FHL is the most posterior of these structures. At the ankle it is almost in the midline. It passes medially enclosed in a fibro-osseous tunnel beneath the sustentaculum tali of the os calcis. On the medial border of the foot, it crosses the FDL at the knot of Henry; often fibres between the two tendons interconnect. It inserts into the distal phalanx of the great toe and flexes the hallux.

Test the FHL's function by asking the patient to flex the IP joint of the great toe against resistance. The FHL is a source of posteromedial pain behind the ankle. It can become inflamed and swollen. Occasionally, the entrance into its fibro-osseous tunnel can become stenosed (narrowed) causing restriction of FHL movement and a functional limitation of great toe flexion (hallux saltans).

Medial (deltoid) collateral ligament of the ankle joint

This ligament is less commonly injured than the lateral complex. However, when injured it can occur in association with significant fractures around the ankle. With a diastasis of the joint, the talus moves abnormally laterally tearing the deltoid ligament. The two ends can become folded into the joint, preventing its anatomical reduction.

As the ligament lies deep to the tibialis posterior and FDL, it can be difficult to palpate separately. However, pain and swelling on the medial side of the ankle following injury which involves an element of eversion should raise the suspicion of a deltoid ligament injury.

Posterolateral examination

The important structures to assess behind and below the lateral malleolus are:

- peroneal tendons and sheath
- sural nerve and short saphenous vein.

In addition, the lateral ligament complex of the ankle joint should be considered at this time.

The presence of posterolateral swelling secondary to significant pathology is often best appreciated by observation of both ankles viewed in the standing position from behind.

Peroneal tendons and sheath

The peroneal (lateral) compartment of the leg contains the peroneus brevis and longus tendons. The third peroneal tendon (peroneus tertius) is the most lateral of the tendons in the extensor (anterior) compartment as it crosses the ankle joint.

The two tendons are named according to tendon length. As the tendons curve postero-inferiorly around the lateral malleolus, the longus tendon lies more posteriorly and superficially. The two tendons are contained within the peroneal retinaculum. On the lateral aspect of the foot, beyond the lateral malleolus, the two tendons occupy separate sheaths and are sometimes divided by a prominent bony tubercle, the peroneal tubercle.

The sheath may be swollen secondary to synovitis. This may be caused by injury or a systemic inflammatory condition (e.g. rheumatoid arthritis).

Palpate the tendons along their courses for areas of swelling and tenderness. The brevis tendon is attached to the base of the fifth metatarsal. The longus tendon winds around the lateral border of the foot before disappearing under the cuboid bone until it attaches itself to the base of the first metatarsal. These tendons may sustain splits and tears. The peroneal tubercle is variable in size and may cause discomfort.

Ask the patient to dorsiflex and plantarflex the ankle while observing the tendons in their groove behind and below the lateral malleolus. Deficiencies of the retinaculum, usually due to trauma, can cause the tendons to sublux, or frankly dislocate, over the lateral malleolus. This causes pain and increases the risk of tendon splitting.

Test the function of the tendons by asking the patient to actively evert the foot with and without resistance.

Sural nerve and short saphenous vein

The sural nerve accompanies the short saphenous vein down the back of the calf until they both move laterally to pass behind the lateral malleolus. The nerve innervates the lateral border of the foot. It is a surprisingly large nerve and can be damaged by trauma—including during surgery.

Test sensation over the innervated area. Trace the course of the nerve for signs of tenderness indicative of a neuroma. Percussion of the nerve with the index finger (Tinel's test) may localize the site of a neuroma and cause tingling in the distal distribution of the nerve.

The vein drains the lateral structures of the foot. It passes posteriorly in the calf before piercing the fascia of the popliteal fossa to join the popliteal veins. Incompetence of the system and its communications with the deep veins of the calf will produce swelling, varicose eczema, and varicosities along its course.

Lateral ligament complex of the ankle joint

The lateral ligament complex of the ankle joint comprises three significant structures:

- anterior talofibular (ATFL)
- calcaneofibular (CFL)
- posterior talofibular (PTFL).

Following inversion injury, the ankle can sustain a ligament sprain to these elements.

Usually the ligaments are injured in order from anterior to posterior. Thus the mildest injury would be a grade I (partial) injury to the ATFL and the worst would be a grade III (complete rupture) of all three elements.

In slim individuals CFL can be palpated deep to the peroneal tendons. ATFL is a short structure leading anteriorly from the fibula tip. Following injury, lateral swelling with or without bruising is common. More severe injuries lead to bleeding within the ankle joint (a haemarthrosis). This may cause bruising to become evident on the medial side—an important sign of significant damage following an inversion injury.

Posterior examination

The posterior aspect of the ankle and hindfoot is a frequent source of pathology. It is important to consider the following:

- the Achilles tendon
- the posterior aspect of the calcaneum and related structures
- structures deep to the Achilles.

Achilles tendon and the posterior aspect of the calcaneum

The Achilles tendon is a common source of pain and disability. The patient may present with one or more of the following:

- equinus deformity—lack of ankle dorsiflexion secondary to contracture
- stiffness—especially in the morning and after exercise
- swelling of the tendon itself
- pain
- acute rupture.

With Achilles tendon problems, the first issue to resolve is whether the problem is related to the tendon itself (non-insertional) or to its attachment to the calcaneum (insertional).

The causes of non-insertional Achilles tendinopathy include:

- tendinosis—degeneration of the tendon itself
- peritendonitis—inflammation of the paratenon aroud the tendon
- combination of the above two pathologies
- rupture—full or partial

The causes of insertional Achilles tendinopathy include:

- bursitis
- Haglund's deformity
- insertional Achilles tendinopathy (often biomechanical)
- 'pump bump'—prominent lateral calcaneal ridge
- systemic enthesopathies (e.g. Reiter's disease, ankylosing spondylitis).

An equinus deformity of the ankle joint may be caused by a contracture of the gastrocnemius–soleus complex. It is possible to distinguish between a contracture of the gastrocnemius and the Achilles itself by applying the Silfverskiold test. The patient is examined supine on an examination couch. The knee is initially extended and the degree of loss of ankle dorsiflexion assessed. The knee is then flexed to relax the gastrocnemius, which originates from above the knee joint on the posterior femoral condyles. If this allows the ankle to fully dorsiflex, it can be deduced that the contracture involves the gastrocnemius muscle itself (gastrocnemius equinus). If the restriction of dorsiflexion remains, the problem is a gastrocnemius–soleus deformity, almost certainly from the tendo-Achilles itself.

Structures deep to the Achilles tendon

Patients may present with deep pain in the posterior aspect of the ankle. It is often attributed to Achilles tendon pathology. Frequently, other structures are involved. Posterior impingement of the ankle joint causes:

- deep posterior ankle pain
- restriction of full ankle plantarflexion.

The potential causes of this presentation include:

- inflamed FHL tendon
- large posterior tubercle of the talus
- os trigonum
- Shepherd's fracture of the posterior talar tubercle

Clinical features include:

- swelling behind the ankle, usually medial
- tenderness to deep palpation
- restriction of ankle plantarflexion
- pain reproduced by passive ankle plantarflexion combined with axial compression on the calcaneum (for osseous lesions).

Subtalar varus

Subtalar varus implies that the neutral position of the calcaneus is varus (inverted) in relation to the leg bisection (non-weight-bearing). Subtalar varus or rearfoot varus can affect the function of the rearfoot during gait and may lead to excessive pronation of the foot and delay resupination of the foot during gait.

Abnormal pronation

Abnormal pronation, i.e. excessive subtalar joint pronation during contact phase and/or subtalar joint pronation occurring when the joint should be supinating during midstance and propulsion, is one of the most common disorders of the lower limb. A large degree of frontal plane motion in the foot (due to uncontrolled subtalar joint pronation) is thought to predispose to forefoot pathology and ankle dysfunction, whereas a greater degree of transverse plane tibial rotation is thought to predispose to leg and knee pathology.

The presence of four or more of the following indicates abnormal pronation:

- more than 6° between the relaxed calcaneal stance position (RCSP) and the neutral calcaneal stance position (NCSP)

- medial bulging of the talar head or 'mid-tarsal break', quantified using the navicular drift technique (Menz 1998)

- lowering of the medial longitudinal arch, quantified using the navicular drop technique (Mueller *et al.* 1993)

- more than 4° eversion of the calcaneus

- Helbing's sign (medial bowing of the Achilles tendon)

- abduction of the forefoot at the metatarsal joint (concavity of lateral border of foot)

- apropulsive gait.

Notes on special tests

Assessment of the lateral ankle ligament complex

Assessment of ankle stability involves evaluation of functional and mechanical stability, where the former represents poor ankle control due to weakness and lack of proprioception, whereas the latter represents those ankles that show evidence of instability on stress testing. Of course, the two can coexist. Evaluation of functional stability is described in Chapter 3.8. Proprioception in its simplest form can be assessed by single-leg balance, with the eyes open and then closed, measuring the time the athlete can balance and comparing performance on both legs. The test can be made more difficult by using uneven surfaces, and then further assessing the ability of the athlete (eyes open) to perform progressively more difficult tasks such as throwing a ball.

Mechanical stability of the ankle can be evaluated using the anterior drawer and talar tilt tests. In the **anterior drawer test**, the patient lies supine and relaxed with the knee in approximately 60° of flexion to relieve tension in the gastrocnemius. The examiner stabilizes the tibia and fibula, holds the foot in 20° of plantarflexion and draws the talus forward in the ankle mortise. The examiner subjectively assesses whether there is excessive translation and, if so, whether there is a firm endpoint. A visible dimpling on the anterolateral side of the ankle (the 'suction' sign) helps to confirm excessive translation. Excessive translation and the absence of a firm endpoint indicate rupture of the ATFL. If a firm endpoint is present, the positive drawer may be due to ligamentous laxity, in which case the finding is noted bilaterally.

The **talar tilt test** assesses the integrity of the CFL when the ankle is in neutral or slight dorsiflexion, but also assesses the ATFL if the ankle is in plantarflexion. Alternatively, with the patient supine and the knee flexed to 90° to relax the gastrocnemius–soleus complex, the examiner stabilizes the tibia with one hand and applies an inversion stress at the heel with the other hand. The angle between the talar dome and tibial plafond is evaluated and compared with the unaffected side. An excessive tilt indicates a CFL and/or ATFL tear, depending upon the position of testing. In experienced hands the anterior drawer test is a more reliable indicator of ATFL rupture than talar tilt.

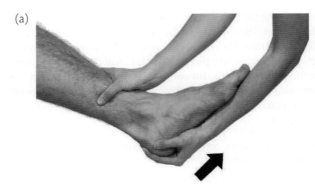
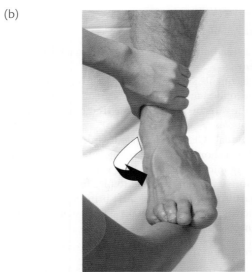

Fig. 3.13.6 (a) Anterior drawer and (b) talar tilt tests.

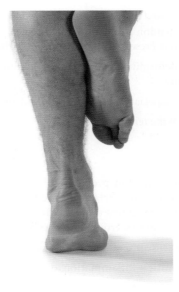

Fig. 3.13.7 Single heel raise test. The examiner takes note of (a) the ability to perform a single heel raise; (b) provocation of pain; (c) heel inversion during heel raise; and (d) fatiguability with repetition. The two feet are compared.

Assessment of the tibiofibular syndesmosis:

The presence of tenderness should be elicited over the anterior aspect of the syndesmosis. Because of intervening structures, it is more difficult to accurately elicit pain from the posterior fibres. The presence of discomfort on proximal palpation superior to the syndesmosis indicates involvement of the interosseous ligament itself and the potential for a more serious injury.

Three specific tests for syndesmotic pathology have been described:

- calf squeeze test
- external rotation test
- Cotton (tibiofibular shuck) test.

A positive **calf squeeze test** is elicited if pain is felt at the syndesmosis when the proximal calf is compressed by manual pressure.

The **external rotation test** is probably the most reliable test for confirming pathology at the syndesmosis. With the knee flexed over the end of the couch, the examiner holds the heel in the palm of the hand. The calf is stabilized with the other hand. The lower hand externally rotates the hindfoot under the tibia. If there is an injury, this manoeuvre will reproduce pain at the syndesmosis.

The **Cotton test** is designed to detect abnormal increased medial and lateral translation within the ankle mortise. The relaxed dependent ankle is grasped in one hand while the leg is stabilized with the examiner's hand. The heel is moved medially and laterally. The amount of translation felt is compared with the other side.

Assessment of **tibialis posterior tendon dysfunction** is described in Chapter 3.14.

Assessment of the **Achilles tendon** has been described in Chapter 3.11.

Imaging

The choice of imaging modalities to assess ankle injuries is determined by the clinical context and provisional diagnosis. Combined imaging may be required.

Plain radiographs

The standard ankle series includes weight-bearing AP, mortise, and lateral views (although the AP view may add little to the mortise view). The mortise view allows clear visualization of the medial and lateral joint space, the presence of loose bodies, or blunting of the talar angles suggestive of an osteochondral lesion. In the fracture patient, evidence of any talar shift should be sought. Weight-bearing radiographs allow assessment of joint-space narrowing and the evaluation of any talar tilt seen in some cases of chronic lateral ligament instability.

The lateral view helps to demonstrate tibiotalar congruity and bony causes of both anterior and posterior impingement. Dorsiflexion–plantarflexion lateral views may demonstrate anterior and posterior osseous impingement problems. A full lateral weight-bearing view of the foot and ankle may demonstrate foot problems which cause secondary ankle pathology (e.g. pes planovalgus deformity) or problems in adjacent joints (e.g. talonavicular pathology).

Stress views, often under fluoroscopic control, to objectively capture abnormal mobility while performing varus and anterior talar drawer stress tests have traditionally been performed in cases of suspected ankle instability, although they are less commonly used now. Radiological assessment of subtalar instability using

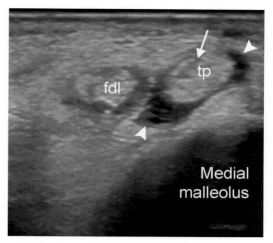

Fig. 3.13.8 Tibialis posterior tenosynovitis in a 32-year-old runner. There is fluid surrounding the tibialis posterior (tp) tendon (arrowheads) consistent with tenosynovitis. Note the presence of a longitudinal split within the superficial aspect of the tendon (arrow). fdl, flexor digitorum longus.

stress views is difficult, although some consider that stress radiographs, with careful positioning and examiner observation, can show both an increased talar tilt and talocalcaneal displacement if there is combined subtalar and ankle instability.

Plain X-rays are sensitive to degenerative changes in the joint.

Ultrasound and MRI

Diagnostic ultrasound is superior in the evaluation of subtle tendon lesions and allows dynamic assessment (e.g. subluxations). Interpretation of pathology is very much operator dependent and experience is required to make the most of this useful imaging tool. As has been described elsewhere, it allows subtle structural changes in muscle, ligaments and tendons in particular to be monitored, assessment of vascularity and neovascularization, and elegantly demonstrates bursae (Figure 3.13.8)

MR imaging (enhanced/unenhanced, or MR arthrography) helps in the assessment of soft tissue structures (e.g. ligaments), impingements, bony and cartilage defects (Fig. 3.13.9)

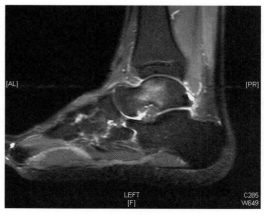

Fig. 3.13.9 A talar osteochondral defect and bone bruising in a cricket bowler.

CT may be necessary for further imaging of possible impingements, loose bodies, and articular pathologies. It is a good method of imaging for subtle diastasis injuires secondary to syndesmotic injuries. Three-dimensional reconstruction aids surgical planning and is a useful educational tool when counselling patients regarding identified pathology.

Isotope bone scanning continues to have a role in the evaluation of stress injuries and conditions such as complex regional pain syndrome type II (CRPS) and bone marrow oedema syndrome.

Specific ankle disorders

Ankle fractures and dislocations

Fractures of the ankle joint occur commonly in sport. The mechanism of injury can be either by a direct impact with another player or object or as a result of an indirect twisting/angulatory injury often on an uneven surface.

The athlete may experience a crack followed by intense pain. The player usually cannot weight-bear. Immediate evaluation should establish whether a deformity suggestive of significant displacement is present. Swelling usually develops quickly. Any footwear should be removed carefully. Circulation and sensation in the foot should be assessed and recorded. The foot and ankle should be splinted to allow safe transportation to a clinic/hospital for further evaluation. However, if the initial examining clinician has sufficient experience, any obvious deformity should be reduced as soon as possible, preferably with adequate analgesia for the athlete. This helps reduce pressure on vulnerable soft-tissues.

Once within an orthopaedic setting further evaluation can begin. Clinical examination should establish the exact sites of tenderness, with care taken to look at the entire leg for evidence of any proximal injury (e.g. a high fibula fracture following a Maisonneuve injury).

Plain radiographs should include AP, mortise, and lateral views. Imaging of the entire leg may be required to exclude proximal bony injury.

Ankle fractures have been classified in a number of different ways, but the most commonly used are the Danis–Weber and Lauge–Hansen systems (Table 3.13.2). Both systems are based on the location and configuration of the fibular fracture. The Danis–Weber system is easier to use.

The treating team have to make the decision as to whether the fracture is undisplaced and, if so, whether it is stable. As a rule of thumb approximately 50% of fractures are undisplaced/minimally

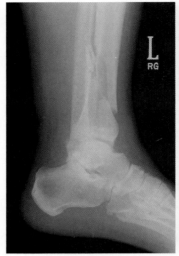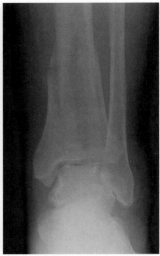

Fig. 3.13.10 X-rays of an ankle fracture.

displaced and stable. These are usually treated conservatively. About 25% are significantly displaced and unstable. These require open reduction and internal fixation. The most difficult group are the 25% which are initially undisplaced or minimally displaced but deemed potentially unstable and thus likely to displace later. In the young athlete, the decision is often taken to operate to ensure an anatomical final outcome and to allow earlier mobilization.

In patients requiring surgery, there is usually a 'golden period' in the first 12 hours before the swelling becomes too severe. Otherwise the patient may have to wait for a number of days with the ankle manually reduced and elevated in a well-padded cast (usually incomplete). Any patient undergoing surgery needs to be informed about the risks including infection, thromboembolic disease, and mal- and non-union. Ankle fractures take a minimum of 6 weeks to heal in an adult, and decisions on mobilization and weight-bearing status vary according to the fracture character and stability. Despite early physiotherapy, stiffness and swelling may persist for months. Disruption of the syndesmosis, requiring reduction and fixation, will delay weight-bearing and probably require removal of metalwork before returning to impact exercise.

Table 3.13.2 Classification systems for ankle fractures

Danis–Weber classification	A	B		C
Fibula fracture position	Below (infra-) the level of the syndesmosis	At the level of the syndesmosis		Above (supra-) the level of the syndesmosis
Lauge–Hansen classification	**Supination–adduction**	**Supination–external rotation**	**Pronation–abduction**	**Pronation–external rotation**
Position of foot at time of injury	Supinated	Supinated	Pronated	Pronated
Direction in which talus exits the ankle mortise	Adduction (internal rotation)	External rotation (eversion)	Abduction	External rotation (eversion)
Further stages of Lauge–Hansen classification	I–II	I–IV	I–III	I–IV

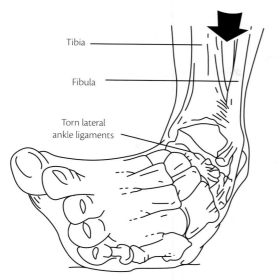

Fig. 3.13.11 Typical mechanism of an inversion sprain of the lateral ligaments.

Table 3.13.3 The Ottawa Ankle Rules

Ankle (inversion) injury
Standard radiograph of the ankle is indicated if the patient has pain near the malleoli and one or more of the following:
Age ≥ 55 years
Inability to weight-bear
Bone tenderness at the posterior edge or tip of either malleolus
Foot injury
Standard radiograph of the foot is indicated if the patient has pain in the midfoot and one or more of the following:
Bone tenderness at the navicular, cuboid or base of the fifth metatarsal
Inability to weight-bear

Source; Stiell *et al.* 1993.

Ankle ligament injuries and instabilities

Acute lateral ankle ligament sprain

As discussed, lateral ankle sprains are the most common injury in sports; they can lead to significant long-term sequelae, with conservative estimates of recurrent instability or prolonged disability occurring in 25–40% of patients.

Mechanism of injury

Lateral ankle sprains usually occur during plantarflexion, adduction, and inversion, as this is the position of least stability for the lateral ankle ligament complex. Partial tears and complete ruptures of the lateral ligaments usually occur in the mid-substance of the tissue, with only 15% of ruptures occurring at the insertion, with or without a bony avulsion. Since the ATFL is the primary lateral stabilizer of the ankle in the position of injury, it is usually the first part of the ligament complex to be injured. As the severity of the stress increases, further injuries to the CFL, joint capsule, and PTFL follow sequentially. Rarely, a pure inversion injury can occur with the ankle in a neutral position. Here the CFL is particularly at risk, although the other two lateral ligaments are frequently involved.

If the inversion is severe, the ligaments of the syndesmosis may be injured in addition. These injuries usually occur with severe external rotation and/or dorsiflexion, since the anterior dome of the talus is wider than its posterior portion, resulting in the tibia and fibula being pushed apart with dorsiflexion. Sixty-five per cent of all ankle sprains involve the ATFL, 20% involve the ATFL and CFL, and 10% also involve the anterior inferior tibiofibular ligament, but only 3% involve the medial (deltoid) ligament. The PTFL is involved only rarely; it plays no role in ankle stability until the ATFL and CFL are both torn.

Since ligaments are stronger than bone in the skeletally immature, the incidence of fractures in children is higher, especially avulsion pull-off injuries to the tip of the fibula. In addition, a number of conditions can present as an ankle 'sprain' in children.

When any child presents with ankle pain, it is particularly important to exclude systemic and other more serious causes, such as infection, tumour, fracture, congenital anomalies such as tarsal coalition, and referred pain.

Classification

Lateral ligament injuries are usually classified according to the degree of tissue disruption, but the resulting morbidity does not necessarily correlate with the extent of tissue damage. Even mild sprains can lead to long-term disability if not correctly managed. A simple approach is as follows.

- Grade I: partial or complete rupture of ATFL.
- Grade II: partial or complete rupture of CFL along with ATFL.
- Grade III: injury to all three ligaments.

It is suggested that additional note should be made of the presence and severity of functional and mechanical instability, swelling, and restriction of range of motion.

History

The history helps to ascertain the severity of the injury and the structures involved. It is also important to ascertain whether this is the first injury. The mechanism may be clearly described and may indicate the specific ligaments involved. However, in repeated sprains the mechanism may be unclear and the degree of trauma trivial.

In the acute inversion sprain, the patient typically reports the onset of lateral ankle pain and may be unable to continue with the sporting activity. The degree of swelling and its timing and progress are indicative of the severity of the injury; significant haemarthrosis in the ankle joint can occur with severe injuries. The onset of swelling, associated with increasing pain, stiffness, and skin discoloration, gradually develops over the following 24 hours, mostly at and distal to the injury. Patients may report symptoms suggestive of functional or mechanical instability of the ankle, with the ankle giving way on weight-bearing.

The presence of a sensation of popping, snapping, or tearing at the time of injury may indicate complete ligament rupture (grade II–III) or associated peroneal tendon injury. An inability to weight-bear immediately after the injury should raise the suspicion of underlying bony injury or other significant pathology. Details should be obtained of any previous injury to either the foot or ankle, all footwear and ankle supports used, and any specific treatments used and their effects. A sporting and occupational history should also be taken.

Inversion sprains of the ankle may result in persistent pain and instability. Instability may be due to true mechanical instability after ligament rupture, or to loss of proprioception and neuromuscular control (functional instability). These forms of instability may occur alone or in combination. Many patients with functional instability have a subjective feeling of instability without the ankle actually moving beyond the normal physiological range.

Examination

The degree of swelling over the first 24 hours after a lateral ligament sprain indicates the degree of the injury. Bruising usually occurs distal to the site of injury; if it is seen proximal to the lateral ligaments after sprain, more extensive injury should be expected. Bruising appearing medially indicates an associated haemarthrosis of the ankle joint.

Examination is performed to evaluate the nature and extent of the injury and to identify additional pathologies. Comparison with the (hopefully) normal unaffected side will establish what is 'normal' for the athlete.

Commence with inspection for the degree and pattern of swelling, discoloration, deformity and the ability to weight-bear. Gently palpate those anatomical areas that may be involved, i.e. the ATFL, CFL, PTFL, malleoli, peroneal tendons, fifth metatarsal, and syndesmosis. If syndesmotic tenderness is present, then palpation of the proximal fibula will determine the likelihood of a high fibular (Maisonneuve) fracture.

Range of movement is usually limited in the early stages because of swelling. Mechanical stability should be assessed, but in many cases this cannot be performed in the acute stage and may need to be delayed. The specificity and sensitivity of delayed physical examination for the presence or absence of a lesion of an ankle ligament have been found to be 84% and 96%, respectively (van Dijk *et al.* 1996). Delayed physical examination gives information of diagnostic quality that is equal to that of arthrography, and causes little discomfort to the patient. The two most important factors are the presence of a haematoma over the ATFL, and the presence of a positive anterior drawer sign (van Dijk *et al.* 1996).

The presence of a syndesmosis injury is indicated by tenderness over the distal tibia and fibula, a positive squeeze test, pain on dorsiflexion and external rotation of the foot, and a positive Cotton test. Peroneal tendon functional testing and a thorough neurovascular assessment should be performed.

Imaging

Plain radiographs may be indicated in some cases (Table 3.13.3). These should include AP, lateral and mortise views. The Ottawa Ankle Rules are very accurate and highly sensitive tools for detecting ankle fractures and help to reduce unnecessary radiation exposure.

Stress radiographs in the acute situation are controversial and offer little that a thorough clinical examination does not. MRI scanning can be helpful in imaging the acute injury, particularly where additional articular pathology is suspected or early surgical repair is considered. Ultrasound is used mainly in the examination of the peroneal tendons.

Treatment

Early diagnosis and aggressive functional rehabilitation are the vital components of management of acute ankle sprains, allowing most patients to return to work and sports. It is usually assumed that the prognosis for untreated ankle ligaments is good; however, patients who are treated functionally do better than those who are not treated at all, or those who are immobilized for 6 weeks. Most consider that surgery is not necessary in the acute setting, unless there is associated pathology such as peroneal tendon injury or an osteochondral fracture. However, Pickenburg *et al.* (2000) showed in a meta-analysis that operative treatment with postoperative functional rehabilitation leads to better results than simple functional treatment. Nevertheless, the decision needs to be taken according to the needs and expectations of the patient and the experience of the treating medical team.

In acute injury the PRICES (protect, rest, ice, compression, elevation) approach is utilized, with the aim of limiting excessive swelling and controlling pain. The use of NSAIDs may assist in controlling these features. Modalities such as ultrasound and interferential stimulation are of unproven benefit. A pneumatic walking boot or ankle brace is helpful in limiting excessive swelling, easing pain, and promoting mobilization. It can be removed to allow application of ice compresses and massage for 15 minutes every 2 hours. Use of crutches in the first 24–48 hours may be necessary, but the patient should be encouraged to mobilize as soon as possible. Range of motion exercises are started immediately, and peroneal and TP strengthening exercises can be commenced as soon as symptoms allow. Once the patient can walk comfortably, the strengthening exercises can be progressively increased and proprioceptive training commenced. This begins with simple exercises performed on the floor, progressing to more difficult balancing tasks and use of a wobble board. Functional activities are also commenced at this stage and depend on the activity levels of the patient. They begin with heel and toe raises, jogging slowly in a straight line, and are followed by progressively more difficult activities at variable speeds and directions and skipping. The use of ice after rehabilitation sessions helps to limit swelling and pain induced in the region of the recently injured tissues.

The use of taping or rigid/semi-rigid braces has been shown to be beneficial in returning patients to activity, because of improved proprioceptive feedback. Supports have the benefit over taping, which may stretch with activity. Of course, such approaches are not a substitute for proprioceptive training. Periarticular hyaluronic acid injection after acute sprain has been reported as helping to reduce pain and facilitate a more rapid return to sport (Petrella *et al.* 2007).

Return to sports should occur only when the patient can perform all the complex actions that their chosen sports involve without provoking any symptoms, although the ability to hop on a single foot is a good indicator of recovery sufficient to return to sport in the outpatient setting. Recovery can take 3 months or longer.

Despite the work of Pickenburg *et al.* (2007), the vast majority of patients with an acute ankle sprain are treated functionally. **Surgery** is indicated in the presence of associated pathologies, such as an osteochondral lesion of the talus, and for those with a diastasis of the tibiofibular joint. In the high-level athlete, consideration should be given to acute repair. Leach and Schepsis (1990) recommended repair in athletes with disruption of both the ATFL and the CFL, a clinical anterior drawer, or a talar tilt of more than 10°. Surgery in the acute setting with significant swelling around the ankle is technically challenging. The presence of specific predisposing anatomical features, particularly a varus hindfoot, should be identified prior to surgical intervention as the outcome of surgery is often poor in such cases unless the heel varus is treated by an appropriate osteotomy.

Surgical repair consists of anatomical repair, which is likely to include bony reattachment of the damaged ligaments, and repair of any significant tear of the anterior capsule. Postoperatively the patient is placed in a cast for 3–4 weeks. This is then changed to an ankle brace and functional rehabilitation is commenced, increasing as tolerated. The brace is worn for sports for up to 6 months.

Chronic ankle instability

Chronic symptoms after an ankle sprain occur in up to 40% of individuals (Gerber *et al.* 1998). Chronic instability is thought to be the result of neural (proprioception, reflexes, muscular reaction time), muscular (strength, power, and endurance), and mechanical (varus hindfoot, posteriorly positioned fibula) mechanisms. Factors influencing proprioception include age, hypermobility, and the presence of other pathologies at the time of the original injury. The clinician should ascertain whether the patient's principal complaint is one of pain, instability, or both. If the primary complaint is of pain, the cause should be determined. In those patients with chronic instability, examination and imaging should be undertaken as outlined above.

Ankle instability after lateral ligament sprain is frequently debilitating. The patient commonly complains of recurrent inversion sprains or 'giving way' of the ankle, when walking on uneven ground or even with minimal or no trauma. Non-specific pain is also commonly reported.

Examination of the patient follows the same pathway as that for an acute ankle sprain. In many cases, rehabilitation has been inadequate in terms of either length of time or expertise. In such cases and in the absence of other obvious pathology, the patient should undergo a trial period of rehabilitation with an experienced practitioner, with the emphasis being placed on peroneal tendon strengthening exercises and proprioceptive training. Use of a brace during training and competition is recommended.

The indications for surgery for pure lateral ligamentous instability are persistent, symptomatic instability in a patient who has failed non-operative treatment. When surgical reconstruction is performed, early functional rehabilitation is important (Kerkhoffs *et al.* 2007). Additional pathologies such as chondral and meniscoid lesions, degenerative changes, and loose bodies within the ankle should be sought by appropriate preoperative imaging and are frequently identified at the time of surgery.

Surgical techniques for reconstruction of chronic lateral ankle ligament instability are numerous, but can be divided into two principal groups:

* 'anatomical' techniques, such as the Brostrum procedure

* tenodesis operations such as the Chrisman–Snook or Colville procedures.

The Brostrum procedure consists of imbricating the ligaments to re-establish their pre-injury length and tension. The repair is often reinforced by reflecting the extensor retinaculum over the reconstructed ATFL (Gould modification). There are numerous eponymously named tenodesis procedures, many utilizing half of the peroneus brevis tendon. There are various concerns with tenodesis procedures, such as postoperative stiffness, overall outcome, and a higher complication rate.

Syndesmosis injuries

Syndesmosis injuries ('high ankle sprains'), involving a syndesmotic sprain or (rarely) rupture, can occur with or without a lateral ankle

Table 3.13.4 Causes of lateral ankle pain

Lateral ligament sprain/rupture
Sinus tarsi syndrome
Peroneal tendinopathy or instability
Impingement
Synovial
Bony osteophyte ('footballer's ankle')
Fibular stress fracture, fracture, or avulsion injury
Superficial peroneal nerve lesion
Complex regional pain syndrome type I
Tumour
Referred pain

Table 3.13.5 Causes of persisting pain after ankle sprain

Articular injury
Chondral/osteochondral fracture
Meniscoid lesion
Bony injury
Fibula
Nerve injury
Superficial peroneal/posterior tibial/sural
Tendon injury
Tibialis posterior (tear, tendinosis)
Peroneal (subluxation/dislocation/tear/tendinosis)
Ligament injury
Mechanical instability due to damage to the lateral ligament, syndesmosis, or subtalar joint
Impingement
Anterior osteophyte/anteroinferior tibiofibular ligament ± anterior soft-tissue impingement secondary to synovitis
Miscellaneous
Failure to regain normal motion (tight Achilles tendon)
Proprioceptive deficit with repetitive sprains (functional instability)

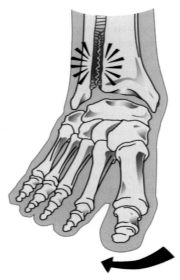

Fig. 3.13.12 Syndesmosis tears usually occur with very severe external rotation and/or dorsiflexion of the ankle.

sprain and reportedly occur in 10% of all ankle sprains. The injury involves the ligaments binding the distal tibia and fibula as part of the inferior tibiofibular joint. Injuries may involve only the anterior or posterior ligamentous fibres in partial injuries or the entire complex in more severe trauma.

The more severe injuries to the syndesmosis occur with dorsiflexion and external rotation of the foot on the leg, for example in pivoting, cutting, or if someone falls on the individual from behind. The torque of external rotation can sequentially tear the anterior inferior tibiofibular ligament, the posterior tibiofibular ligament, and the interosseous membrane, and may result in a high fibular (Maissoneuve) fracture, an injury commonly missed by the inexperienced as routine ankle X-rays miss the more proximal fracture. Rarely, disruption of the peroneal artery can occur, resulting in an acute compartment syndrome. Since injuries to the syndesmosis usually involve significant trauma, avulsion fracture of the medial malleolus or injury to the medial (deltoid) ligament of the ankle is commonly seen. A pure abduction injury, affecting only the syndesmosis, is rare. Severe eversion injuries are rare but can tear the deltoid ligament and disrupt the syndesmosis and interosseous membrane, with resulting distal tibiofibular diastasis. The distal fibula often fractures before the syndesmosis is completely torn. The most frequent mechanism occurs when the athlete has the weight-bearing foot planted and slightly pronated and is struck on the lateral aspect of the leg with the foot fixed. Deltoid ligament injury can also occur in association with a fracture of the proximal or distal fibula.

Injuries are classed as either acute or chronic. Within this classification they can then be divided into simple sprains, syndesmotic injuries that are only unstable on stress testing, and frank diastasis.

Examination

Examination will reveal swelling and discrete tenderness over the anterior tibiofibular ligament. There may be associated tenderness over the deltoid ligament. The squeeze test, where the tibia and fibula are compressed above the syndesmosis, should be performed and may reproduce the pain. Abduction and external rotation stress may also reproduce the pain. The medial side and the entire length of the fibula should be examined for tenderness. Other forms of assessment have been described earlier.

Investigation

A plain AP radiograph of the lower leg and lateral and mortise views of the ankle should be obtained; an increased tibiofibular space may be evident. Harper and Keller (1989) defined the typical radiographic relationship between the tibia and fibula as being (i) at least 6 mm of tibiofibular clear space on AP and mortise views, (ii) at least 6 mm of overlap of the tibia and fibula at the incisura, and (iii) at least 1 mm of overlap between tibia and fibula on the mortise view. Plain X-rays may be normal, and stress views in external rotation and abduction, CT, MRI, or bone scan may be necessary to confirm the diagnosis. Any doubts regarding the presence or absence of a subtle diastasis can be solved by imaging the contralateral ankle with plain radiography or CT (axial images). Calcification or synostosis of the tibia and fibula may be noted on X-ray in chronic injuries.

Management

Sprains of the syndesmosis usually respond to a programme of PRICES, splinting, and a 3 week period of non-weight-bearing, followed by mobilization in a stirrup brace or taping. A rehabilitation programme similar to that for lateral ligament sprain is instituted, although it is important to emphasize that progress is usually slower. A 1 cm heel lift may provide some symptomatic benefit, preventing the anterior talus from irritating the mortise during gait. Injuries that are only unstable on stress testing can be treated either by a period of 4–6 weeks non-weight-bearing, followed by weight-bearing, or surgically. Frank diastasis requires surgical stabilization by transfibular screw fixation 1 cm above the syndesmosis. This is followed by 6 weeks non-weight-bearing with early range of motion exercises after the first 3 weeks and then mobilization in a walking cast. There is great debate regarding removal of the diastasis screw, but most surgeons remove it at 8–12 weeks. Tightrope, an alternative form of fixation using two endobuttons and strong suture material, is gaining in popularity as it does not need to be removed and provides biomechanical support equivalent to a rigid metal fixation.

Delayed diagnosis of a diastasis leads to the rapid onset of degenerate change. As long as the arthritic change is not too advanced, surgical debridement and delayed fixation, using screws or Tightrope, or reconstruction with materials such as free tendon grafts should be considered.

Chronic syndesmosis injuries can be complicated by interosseous ligament ossification. Fortunately, this does not usually limit tibiofibular motion. However, when tibiofibular synostosis does occur, it leads to mortise restriction and anterior ankle pain with dorsiflexion.

Subtalar instability

Subtalar joint instability is a complex entity that can occur in association with subtalar ligamentous damage, including traumatic or degenerative pathology of the interosseous talocalcaneal ligament. It can occur in isolation or, more frequently, after lateral ankle sprain usually involving an inversion injury of the ankle–hindfoot. However, the aetiology and epidemiology of the condition is poorly defined. It has been estimated that subtalar instability is found in 10% of patients with lateral instability of the ankle–hindfoot complex (Yamamoto *et al.* 1998). It can result in chronic hindfoot instability and/or pain along the sinus tarsi or posterior subtalar joint. Clinical findings are non-specific and may simply include typical features of a mechanically unstable ankle–hindfoot. With careful positioning and examiner observation, stress radiographs will show both increased talar tilt and talocalcaneal displacement if there is combined subtalar and ankle instability.

Injection with local anaesthetic can help to confirm that any accompanying discomfort is coming from the subtalar joint as opposed to the ankle. MRI may show synovitis; CT will help to confirm any degenerative changes present.

Best management is poorly defined. Early ice and immobilization, and late bracing and proprioceptive training are often considered effective, but where they are not, stablilization procedures are required. Techniques are similar to those described for lateral ankle instability with the provision that the reconstruction must span both the ankle and the subtalar joint, including reconstruction/repair of the CFL which spans both the ankle and subtalar joint (e.g. the Gould modification of the Brostrum technique), the Colville repair, or the Chrisman–Snook procedure.

Anterolateral impingement syndromes and sinus tarsi pathologies can cause lateral ankle pain and are discussed later in this chapter.

Medial ankle sprain

Medial (deltoid) ligament injuries constitute only 5–6% of ankle sprains, usually in association with other injuries. The patient presents with severe medial ankle pain after an episode of trauma and acute eversion or abduction of the foot and ankle may be described. These injuries may be overlooked because of the presence of other injuries such as a syndesmosis injury, ankle dislocation, or fracture. Examination reveals swelling, discoloration, local tenderness, and pain with eversion of the foot. Other pathologies should be sought, including damage to the syndesmosis, tibia and fibula, other ligaments, the posterior tibial tendon (PTT), the spring ligament, and neurovascular structures. Plain radiographs are usually necessary to exclude bony injury.

Management of an isolated sprain involves relative rest, ice, NSAIDs, and use of an Aircast brace. In cases where other pathologies such as fracture or syndesmosis disruption are present, surgery is necessary. However, even if the deltoid ligament is ruptured it is treated conservatively, unless it is imbricated within the joint and requires open removal to allow reduction. Rarely, chronic medial ankle instability can result from a neglected medial ligament sprain. The patient complains of persistent medial ankle pain and there is progressive ankle and subtalar valgus and development of an adult-acquired flat foot. Associated problems, including PTT and spring ligament dysfunction, can be present.

Weight-bearing AP ankle radiographs and stress radiographs may show valgus instability, and MRI can help to make the diagnosis. However, this is usually a difficult diagnosis to make.

Treatment is with supportive treatment, including physiotherapy, orthoses, and an ankle brace. If these measures fail, surgery can be undertaken with either direct repair of the ligament similar to the Brostrum principle for the lateral ligament injury or reconstruction using a free graft such as a medial hamstring or split tendon transfer locally (e.g. tibialis posterior or FDL).

Peroneal tendinopathies

Peroneus longus and brevis work as important dynamic stabilizers of the ankle. Contraction of the peroneal muscles in an attempt to stabilize the ankle at the moment of injury can result in a spectrum of injuries to one or both tendons, including tenosynovitis, tendinosis, longitudinal tear, rupture, subluxation, and dislocations. Mechanisms of injury include inversion sprains, reflex contraction of the peroneals with either sudden forceful passive dorsiflexion or plantarflexion of the inverted foot, significant trauma such as ankle dislocation or fracture, direct trauma, and, in skiers, indirect trauma occurring when the ski becomes blocked while making a turn. Such lesions are frequently overlooked but should be considered in any patient with lateral ankle pain.

Most cases present with a variable combination of lateral ankle pain, swelling, and instability. Most clinical problems are related to the peroneus brevis and peroneal instability, since the peroneus longus is more protected at the level of the distal fibula. Peroneus longus pathologies are seen more distally and are described further in Chapter 3.14.

Tenosynovitis, tendinosis, and longitudinal tears

Peroneal tenosynovitis around the lateral malleolus is often associated with peroneal tendon instability typically after a sprain, but it can develop after a direct blow.

Chronic peroneus brevis tendon tears are frequently overlooked or misdiagnosed; indeed many seem to be asymptomatic. Degenerative tears in the peroneus brevis are reported with an incidence of 11.3–20.6% in cadaveric studies. However, tears of the peroneus longus, especially without subluxation or dislocation, are rare. Longitudinal tears, or splits, of the peroneal tendons can occur in relation to an acute inversion injury, chronic lateral ankle laxity, intratendinous degenerative change, or rarely after a calcaneal fracture. Mechanical wear in the retromalleolar groove is considered to play a major role in the development of degenerative change and it is at this site that most lesions occur. Local compression of peroneus brevis within the groove, eversion of the foot, subluxation of the peroneal tendons, laxity or rupture of the SPR, and a sharp posterior fibular edge may all contribute to this mechanical wear (Sobel *et al.* 1991).

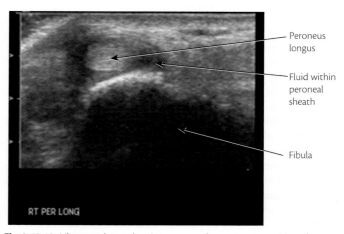

Fig. 3.13.13 Ultrasound scan showing peroneus longus tenosynovitis at the lateral malleolus.

Subluxation usually involves anterior subluxation of the peroneus longus over the inferior surface of the distal fibula. Less commonly, both peroneus longus and brevis may sublux. Occasionally the tendons dislocate and cannot be relocated in the groove. Longitudinal tears of the tendon(s) may subsequently occur. During contraction, the tendon of the peroneus longus is forced anteriorly against that of peroneus brevis, which may splay along the posterior border of the fibula. Partial subluxation of the peroneus brevis over the edge of a sharp posterior border of the fibula will cause further tearing. There are several potential mechanisms, although there may be no obvious precipitant.

There is swelling, localized tenderness, and, with tenosynovitis, crepitus. Pain is exacerbated on passive stretch, by forced plantarflexion and inversion, and on active contraction against resistance. Pain with a combination of eversion and restricted plantarflexion of the first ray indicates peroneus longus involvement, whereas pain only occurs with resisted eversion in peroneus brevis lesions. Ultrasound and MRI may be useful in further assessment.

Where peroneal instability is present, snapping may be reported and instability may be demonstrated by resisted dorsiflexion, eversion, or circumduction of the ankle and hindfoot. Often the patient can demonstrate themselves the manoeuvre causing tendon instability. Ultrasound allows further evaluation. In some cases the tendon is permanently dislocated. Plain AP, lateral, and mortise radiographs of the ankle are helpful in excluding other causes of pain and may reveal a fleck of bone avulsed from the posterolateral fibula, which is pathognomonic of peroneal tendon dislocation. MRI may help to identify anatomical anomalies associated with tendon subluxation (including the shape of the posterior aspect of the distal fibula), to confirm the location of the tendons, and to assess the integrity of the retinacula and tendons.

Management

Treatment of **tenosynovitis** involves relative rest, NSAIDs, ice and ice massage, and use of a lateral heel wedge. Biomechanical aspects and stability must be addressed. The use of local corticosteroids is reserved for recalcitrant cases and only once imaging has established no evidence of an associated tear. Rehabilitation exercises commence early, with flexibility work, gradual strengthening, and an ankle stability programme.

In those with persistent symptoms, a trial of a rocker-bottom walking boot or non-weight-bearing casting can be used. If these approaches fail, surgical exploration should be considered with a view to synovectomy. A careful assessment for peroneal instability and discrete tears (full or partial) should be made.

Similar steps may be taken where a **tear** or **split** is identified, but are frequently ineffective. At surgery any instability should be addressed. The options for tendon repair include primary suture, tubulization of a splayed out tendon, excision of the damaged tendon, or tendon transfer. Krause and Brodsky (1998) advocated resection of the damaged part of the tendon and repair, with or without tubulization, when less than 50% of the tendon was involved. If more than 50% of the diameter of the tendon is involved, excision of the damaged portion of the tendon and a peroneus brevis to longus tenodesis is performed. The occasional cases when both tendons are extensively damaged, or even completely ruptured, are more difficult to treat. The options include mobilization and direct repair, interposition grafting (e.g. with the plantaris tendon), or tenodesis to the lateral wall of the calcaneus. Recovery after surgery is prolonged, but the majority of patients achieve good to excellent function.

Acute peroneal tendon dislocations can be managed conservatively in a below-knee moulded cast, commencing with a 3 week period of cast immobilization with the ankle held in mild plantarflexion and inversion for 3 weeks and then in the neutral position for a further 3 weeks. After cast immobilization, a progressive rehabilitation programme is commenced, beginning with gentle range of motion exercises and stretching followed by gradual introduction of a strengthening programme. Ankle stability exercises are introduced when symptoms permit.

The success rate of non-operative treatment is approximately 50%. Success rates of this level in a young sporting population may be considered unacceptable.

The surgical options described for peroneal tendon instability fall into five groups:

(i)   direct SPR (superior peroneal retinaculum) repair;

(ii)   SPR reconstruction using tendon graft (e.g. with an Achilles tendon sling);

(iii) bone block procedures to produce an osseous barrier to dislocation;

(iv)   retromalleolar sulcus deepening procedures;

(v)   re-routing the tendons under the CFL (Calcaneofibular ligament).

For primary procedures, a direct repair of the SPR, imbricating it and securing it with suture anchors in the fibula, is usually favoured. If the retromalleolar sulcus is shallow, the groove is deepened, attempting to maintain the integrity of the base of the groove where the tendons run. This is achieved by elevating the floor of the groove, removing the cancellous bone from the fibula, and replacing the periosteal flap in its deepened position. Occasionally, further stabilization is required. For example, the tendons are re-routed under the CFL. Any tendon pathology is treated as outlined above.

Osteochondral lesions of the ankle

Chondral and osteochondral (OCD) lesions of the ankle can occur after single trauma, repetitive microtrauma, or ankle sprain. The clinical characteristics are deep exertional ankle pain, anterior joint line tenderness, and swelling. The talar dome is most commonly affected, followed by the medial malleolus and the tibial plafond. Loose bodies can develop subsequent to chondral loosening. Plain X-ray can demonstrate talar angle blunting and loose body formation. Both MRI and CT are used to identify and grade lesions. Arthroscopy should be considered early if a lesion is suspected, but operative findings do not always accord with preoperative imaging.

OCD lesions of the talus were first classified by Berndt and Hardy (1959). Ferkel and Sgaglione (1990) devised a classification based on CT appearances which is useful for determining treatment.

Symptomatic ankles with identified chondral/osteochondral lesions should undergo arthroscopic examination with a view to providing symptomatic relief and where possible some form of healing. The options available are manifold and can be considered under the following headings.

- **Primary repair**: for significant acute fractures, an attempt to reduce and stabilize fragments with internal fixation can be attempted.

- **Palliation:** arthroscopic washout of fragments and debridement of unstable lesions.

- **Late repair:** techniques include abrasion, microfracturing, or drilling.

- **Restoration of defect:** techniques include autologous chondrocyte implantation (ACI) ± a matrix/membrane covering (MACI), osteochondral autograft transfer systems (OATS) or, if multiple, mosaicplasty, and, in large defects, osteochondral allografts.

Anterior ankle pain

Anterior impingement syndromes

Anterior impingement syndromes can be divided into those causing anteromedial and anterocentral ankle pain, which are usually due to a combination of soft tissue and bony impingement, and those resulting in anterolateral ankle pain, which are typically due to soft tissue impingement (Fig. 3.13.14).

Anterolateral impingement can occur due to build-up of impinging synovial and scar tissue. It can occur in particular after a lateral sprain but also in relation to excessive subtalar hyperpronation. When this is accompanied by hyaline degenerative cartilage, it is known as a 'meniscoid' lesion. An abnormal distal slip of the ATFL ('Basset's ligament') can also cause anterolateral impingement by impinging on the talus. Clinical features are anterolateral pain, with or without instability, aggravated variably by eversion/inversion and localized tenderness in the anterolateral gutter. Attention to stability and biomechanics and, if necessary, a local corticosteroid and anaesthetic infiltration, with relative rest from load-bearing activities for 7–10 days, can be useful. If these approaches are unsuccessful, arthroscopic debridement is effective.

Traumatic neuritis of the branch of the deep peroneal nerve that innervates the sinus tarsi (nerve to extensor digitorum brevis) can also cause lateral ankle pain. This may respond to alteration of footwear and orthotics, and/or local corticosteroid injection, but surgical denervation of the sinus has been reported to be effective for recalcitrant cases.

Anteromedial and anterocentral ankle impingement syndromes typically arise in association with osteophytes on the anterior tibia

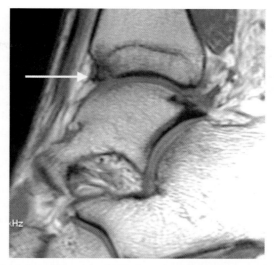

Fig. 3.13.14 Sagittal T1-weighted MRI of anterior ankle impingement in a 22-year-old footballer. There is a prominent osteophyte (arrow) at the anterior margin of the tibial plafond with low-grade surrounding bone oedema consistent with anterior ankle impingement.

and/or superoanterior aspect of the talus at the ankle joint. These are most frequently seen in footballers and dancers and are related to repeated forced dorsiflexion of the ankle in these groups. Impingement of the osteophytes on soft tissue causes pain. The incidence is higher in those with underlying mechanical ankle instability. Although initially presenting with a general activity-related ache, it progresses to more severe localized pain at the anterior ankle joint, with stiffness and reduced range of motion. Examination reveals anterior ankle joint line tenderness, and restriction and pain in dorsiflexion in weight-bearing. Plain lateral ankle X-rays in weight-bearing will confirm osteophytes in most cases, and impingement is shown in non-weight-bearing flexion and extension views. In the early phases the condition may respond to initial relative rest, NSAIDs, ice, a heel raise or orthotic, passive AP mobilization of the ankle joint, and taping. Attention to aspects of ankle stability, where appropriate, is important. In those who do not respond to conservative measures, surgical excision of osteophytes and stabilization procedures may be indicated. This can usually be accomplished arthroscopically, but if the osteophytes are large and emerging from both the talus and tibia an open procedure may be required (O'Donoghue's procedure). Patients should be counselled carefully regarding full resolution of symptoms if the osteophytes form part of a more generalized wear pattern within the joint.

Subtalar joint pathology

The subtalar joint is a complex articulation between the talus and os calcis. It allows inversion and eversion of the hindfoot. The problem of subtalar instability has been dealt with elsewhere in this chapter (pp. 380–1).

Arthritis of the joint can occur in the athlete. Post-traumatic arthritis following os calcis fracture is a disabling and painful condition (see Chapter 3.14). Athletes participating ing high-impact sports over a period of time may develop arthritis in the joint.

Table 3.13.6 Causes of anterior ankle pain

Impingement syndrome ('footballer's ankle')
Anterolateral gutter impingement and sinus tarsi syndrome
Anterior tibial tendinopathy
Extensor hallucis longus tendinopathy
Lateral or medial instability
Syndesmosis injury
Talar dome injury
Tibial plafond injury
Ganglia
Traction neuritis, especially to branches of both the superficial and deep peroneal nerves
Referred pain

Some athletes may have undiagnosed (particularly fibrous) tarsal coalitions (found in 1% of the general population), which can increase the risk of subsequent arthritis. Pain in the hindfoot associated with loss of subtalar mobility should raise the possibility of arthritis. Plain X-rays may show arthritis, particularly in the posterior facet. MRI and CT scan give better information about the health of the subtalar joint. Treatment includes orthotics, avoidance of aggravating activities, and use of NSAIDs or steroid injections. Surgical options include subtalar arthroscopic debridement and, in endstage cases, subtalar arthrodesis.

Sinus tarsi syndrome is characterized by pain emanating from the opening into the sinus tarsi on the lateral side of the hindfoot. It is usually aggravated by exercise. Its existence is controversial and other causes of lateral foot pain should be sought and excluded. Various causes have been described including minor instability, ganglions, pathology related to the talocalcaneal ligament, synovitis, fibrosis, or arthritis.

Clinical examination and plain X-rays may be normal. MRI may show abnormalities such as synovitis and cysts. Injection with local anaesthetic and steroid can be helpful for both diagnostic and therapeutic purposes. Biomechanical abnormalities and technical flaws should be identified and rectified. If all conservative measures fail, either open surgery or arthroscopy can be undertaken. Unless obviously damaged, the intra-osseous ligament is preserved, but any osteophytes, ganglions, fat pad, and/or synovitic tissue is excised.

Synovitis of the ankle joint

Synovitis of the ankle, presenting as pain, swelling, and stiffness (in particular, morning stiffness), can occur as a post-traumatic phenomenon, or as a result of loose bodies, degenerative change, or sepsis, or may be related to an underlying inflammatory arthropathy. The fact that the patient has maintained a sporting profile does not insure them against the development of various arthropathies. In the younger patient, seronegative conditions such as Reiter's syndrome, psoriasis, ankylosing spondylitis, gout, pigmented villonodular synovitis (PVNS), and synovial chondromatosis should be considered in unusual presentations. Plain X-rays may be normal; MRI will confirm synovitis and may demonstrate other pathology. CT is more useful in identifying loose bodies. A blood screen for inflammatory markers, sepsis, and rheumatological diseases should be performed and where necessary synovial fluid or synovium should be sent for microscopy culture and sensitivity and crystal analysis. Management depends on the nature of the underlying condition. Relative rest, ice, and NSAIDs are often effective for simple post-traumatic synovitis.

Osteoarthritis of the ankle joint

Osteoarthritis of the ankle is not uncommon and may present in its early phases as impingement, as detailed above. Chronic instability and/or previous trauma (e.g. fractures) are risk factors. Patients report non-specific aching, stiffness, or swelling of the ankle. Plain X-rays will confirm the diagnosis, although in early cases MRI is more sensitive. Initial management is as for anterior impingement. With later disease, local viscosupplement injections may provide pain relief. Protective orthotics and physiotherapy to maintain mobility, strength, and balance can be helpful. Arthroscopy, similar to knee arthroscopy in similar circumstances, can help with general joint debridement but the patient should be warned that the outcome can be unpredictable and not curative. The athlete should be counselled that high-impact activities are likely to lead to more rapid disease progression.

Tibialis anterior tendinopathy

The tibialis anterior provides 80% of the power of dorsiflexion of the ankle. It works eccentrically after heel strike to control deceleration of the foot to the floor, and then concentrically after toe-off to assist in clearance and ankle dorsiflexion. The tendon is covered in a sheath from 5 cm above the superior extensor retinaculum to the proximal portion of the inferior extensor retinaculum.

Tenosynovitis

Tenosynovitis is most commonly seen in activities involving running/walking downhill and in skiers and skaters with poorly fitting boots or skates. The patient reports pain and swelling over the anterior ankle and difficulty walking up and down inclines. There is evidence of swelling over the anterior ankle, and resisted dorsiflexion of the ankle is painful.

Management involves avoidance of inappropriate footwear, use of local padding and appropriate lacing, anti-inflammatories, and ice and relative rest. A graduated exercise programme can then be commenced.

Tendinosis and rupture

Tendinosis is very rarely symptomatic until an acute rupture of the tendon occurs, a rare event in sport. It is typically seen in men over the age of 60 years or after the administration of steroid injections. There may be a history of a sudden contraction against a plantarflexed ankle, with local pain and swelling or functional difficulty with dorsiflexion of the foot. The usual site of rupture is 1.5–3 cm above the insertion of the tendon, but rupture can also occur anywhere, including at the musculotendinous junction. There may be local swelling on the dorsum of the ankle, a visible and palpable gap, and weakness of ankle dorsiflexion with the toes plantarflexed (which prevents action of the EDL).

In the sportsperson treatment should be operative with either early direct repair or, if there is a defect between the two ends, an EHL transfer, or a sliding graft of the tibialis anterior tendon.

Extensor tendinopathies

The mechanisms of development of tenosynovitis of the extensor tendons of the foot and ankle tenosynovitis are similar to those involved in the development of tenosynovitis of the tibialis anterior.

EDL and EHL tendinopathies

Patients present with pain and swelling over the anterior ankle joint, with pain on resisted testing of the relevant tendons. When rupture has occurred, there may be local swelling and an inability to fully extend the toes depending on the level and tendon involved. Lacerations or blunt trauma are the usual mechanism. Lacerations and ruptures near the ankle are usually repaired, but those more distal to the MTPJ may be treated non-operatively because of the extensor hood, which prevents digit retraction.

Posterior ankle pain

Posterior ankle pain can be noted medically or laterally.

Table 3.13.7 Causes of posterior ankle pain

Posteromedial	Posterolateral
Flexor hallucis longus tendinopathy	Os trigonum/soft tissue impingement
Tibialis posterior tendinopathy	Peroneal tendinopathy
Posteromedial coalition	Fracture of posterior talar process
Soleus syndrome	Pseudomeniscus syndrome

Posterior impingement syndromes

Posterior impingement syndromes may cause posterolateral or posteromedial ankle pain. Pain occurs when there is impingement between the posterior tibial joint surface, soft tissue, and the talus and/or calcaneum. The posterior talus has medial and lateral processes, between which runs the FHL tendon. An os trigonum is seen in 2.7–7% of people and may represent an accessory ossicle, or a non-united fracture of the lateral process of the talus. Those with an unusually large lateral talar tubercle (Stieda's or trigonal process) may also develop this condition. Other causes of posterior impingement include soft issue entrapment (e.g. thickening of the posterior capsule, a synovial plica, pseudomeniscus, or ankle instability) and impingement by osteophytes. Rarely, anomalous muscle may be involved. In posteromedial impingements after ankle sprain, entrapment and contusions of the deep fibres of the medial ligament can occur.

Posterior impingement syndromes can occur due to an acute plantarflexion injury or secondary to overuse in activities involving repetitive plantarflexion of the ankle. They are most commonly seen in dancers because of the repeated extremes of plantarflexion at the ankle. Footballers, cricketers, long jumpers, triple jumpers, trampolinists, gymnasts, and some racket sports players are also frequently affected.

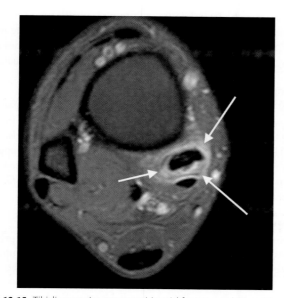

Fig. 3.13.15 Tibialis posterior tenosynovitis: axial fat-saturated T1-weighted MRI post-intravenous gadolinium. There is avid enhancement of the tibialis posterior tendon sheath (arrows) indicating tenosynovitis.

Symptoms typically commence after a lateral ankle sprain or sliding with the ankle in forced plantarflexion. The patient typically complains of posterolateral or posteromedial ankle pain. There may be a history of swelling and catching. Dancers frequently try to compensate for the loss of plantarflexion by placing the foot in an improper position, usually having a more inverted posture *en pointe* ('sickling'). This results in an increased load on the ATFL and hence a higher risk of lateral sprain. Other compensatory postures can lead to more diffuse lower leg, foot, and ankle complaints. On examination there is often tenderness on deep palpation posterolaterally or posteromedially. Pain is exacerbated by extreme passive plantarflexion and forced eversion/inversion in plantarflexion. With the patient prone, a combination of passive plantarflexion and axial heel compression usually reproduces the symptoms, especially with osseous pathology. Infiltration with local anaesthetic, if necessary under ultrasound guidance, may confirm the diagnosis.

Imaging

The accuracy of imaging is contentious. X-ray will help to identify bony abnormalities. Lateral plantarflexion/dorsiflexion films document osseous impingement. MRI may also show bone or soft tissue oedema, localized synovitis, or capsular thickening, confirmed with ultrasound. CT and MR arthrography may allow the most accurate assessment of the capsular recesses. However, some athletes may have normal imaging studies.

Management

Relative rest and modification of activities, ice massage, NSAIDS, and a fluoroscopically guided local anaesthetic corticosteroid injection may be effective in reducing symptoms. A 4–6 week period of casting may be required. A progressive strength training programme is commenced when symptoms permit, and technical factors should be addressed in dancers. Taping can help to prevent excessive plantarflexion when the patient returns to activities.

Surgery should be considered in those with intractable symptoms. The os trigonum can be excised through a lateral, medial, or arthroscopic approach. The advantage of the medial approach is that it allows the FHL tendon to be decompressed. The disadvantage is that great care has to be taken to protect the neurovascular structures, in particular the calcaneal branches of the posterior tibial nerve. Maximum recovery, by whatever approach, should be achieved by 3 months.

Nerve injury and entrapment

Lateral ankle and foot pain commonly arise because of nerve injury or entrapment. Traction injuries to the sural, common peroneal (at the fibular neck), and superficial peroneal nerves are common after inversion sprain or direct impact, although they are frequently overlooked. Neuropraxia (where the axons are not disrupted) and axonotmesis (where they are) can result in burning pain, paraesthesia, dysaesthesia, anaesthesia, shooting pains in the distribution of the affected nerve, and motor weakness. Symptoms can intensify during re-innervation. Specific features depend on the nerve affected and the level of injury. Tinel's test may be positive local to a site of entrapment and can be used to chart the progress of re-innervation during recovery. Temporary resolution of symptoms with local anaesthetic infiltration can help to confirm the diagnosis, as can neurophysiology studies, which help to identify the nature and degree of pathology and evaluate the possibility of

Table 3.13.8 Causes of sural and superficial peroneal nerve injuries

Trauma
Macrotrauma, including surgery, ankle sprain (traction), myositis ossificans, fractures (sural: fifth metatarsal, cuboid, calcaneus; both: fibula)
Microtrauma (overuse)

Compression
Intrinsic: by fascia as the nerve pierces crural fascia, enlarged/scarred Achilles or peroneal tendons, anomalous bands, bony ridge, venous insufficiency, ganglion, neuroma, connective tissue disease, enlarged peroneal tubercle (sural nerve)
Extrinsic: by tight stockings or boots

pathology from the spine. Imaging may be necessary to determine the cause of entrapment where this is suspected.

Management includes treatment of the associated injury, as reduction in local swelling may improve neurological symptoms. Support of the affected limb (e.g. in a boot walker) may be necessary, and in cases where foot drop has developed a night splint in the form of an ankle–foot orthosis can help to prevent gastrocnemius–soleus contractures. Neuralgic pain may respond to measures such as a transcutaneous neural stimulation (TNS) unit, a tricyclic agent, or gabapentin. Neurapraxia usually settles after 2–3 months, but where axonotmesis has occurred recovery commonly can take 6 months to a year.

Lateral ankle pain may also arise from other forms of injury or entrapment of the superficial peroneal and sural nerves in the leg (Table 3.13.8). The superficial peroneal nerve is vulnerable to direct trauma at its origin from the common peroneal nerve at the proximal fibula and is liable to become entrapped or traumatized as it exits the through the deep fascia in the distal leg. Neurophysiology studies may be helpful. If non-operative treatments fail, the occasional patient requires surgical decompression of the nerve and limited fasciotomy.

Medial ankle pain

Posterior tibial tendinopathies

Posterior tibial tendon (PTT) disorders represent a commonly neglected cause of posteromedial ankle and foot pain, with significant consequences in the form of the development of a progressive flat-foot deformity. Amongst other functions, the PTT is a powerful dynamic stabilizer of the hindfoot against eversion, prevents valgus deformity, and is under considerable stress during gait just after heel strike. The PTT brings the hindfoot from loaded eversion into increasing inversion, maximizing the mechanical advantage of the more laterally placed Achilles tendon as the patient rises onto

Table 3.13.9 Causes of medial ankle pain

Posterior tibial tendinopathy
Flexor hallucis tendinopathy
Tarsal tunnel syndrome
Deltoid ligament injury
Referred pain

the forefoot. The tendon also maintains mid-tarsal and forefoot stability through its attachments. The large mechanical stresses applied, relative hypovascularity, and constriction beneath the flexor retinaculum make the PTT particularly vulnerable to injury in its course from the medial malleolus to its insertion on the navicular tuberosity.

The spectrum of disorders that can affect the PTT include dysfunction, tenosynovitis, tendinosis, dislocation, tears, and complete rupture. In the younger age group, an accessory navicular is a common source of TP pain and planovalgus. The hallmark of TP disease is the adult acquired flat foot, in which the medial longitudinal arch collapses, the heel goes into valgus, and the forefoot abducts and becomes supinated (varus). As the disease progresses the spring ligament stretches, and eventually degenerate change occurs in the joints. Various classification systems have been proposed, based on clinical findings, duration of symptoms, or imaging characteristics (see Table 3.13.10).

History

Posteromedial ankle pain and swelling are typical. A gradual flattening of the foot through loss of the longitudinal arch may have been noted. Progressive fatigue with exercise, weakness, and pain on pushing off or standing on tiptoe may also be reported. With late-stage disease symptoms are also associated with degenerative joint disease affecting predominantly the ankle and subtalar joints.

Clinical signs vary according to the stage of disease, but posteromedial ankle tenderness is invariably present. Swelling is variable. Sportspeople are more likely to present early with activity related pain. In those who present later, there may be flattening of the foot with hindfoot valgus which is fixed in later stages of the disease along with degenerative changes of the ankle joint. The single heel raise test (Fig. 3.13.7) elicits pain and fatiguability in early disease, and with progressive disease (late stage II and stage III) the heel fails to invert and finally heel raise becomes impossible. Resisted inversion of the foot in plantarflexion (to isolate the PTT) elicits pain and weakness. On observing the foot from behind, the hindfoot valgus and abduction of the forefoot is noted in later disease, and there may be lateral pain secondary to impingement between the lateral calcaneus and the fibula, with entrapment of the interposed peroneal tendons. The Achilles tendon often becomes progressively tight and fuels the deformity; this should be evaluated.

Imaging

Weight-bearing AP and lateral radiographs are helpful in assessing PTT insufficiency. Additional more specialized views can help in identifying the degree of deformity at the subtalar and ankle levels. They should be inspected for subtalar and mid-tarsal degenerate change.

Ultrasound is sensitive to tendon changes; MRI provides information about the surrounding soft tissue structures and CT can further assess local bony abnormalities.

Management

The aims of treatment are to control the symptoms and prevent progression. Management depends on the stage of the dysfunction and the characteristics and expectations of the patient. In the acute phase, conservative measures include the use of a below-knee walking cast for 4–6 weeks and a medial longitudinal arch support. Simultaneous anti-inflammatory approaches such as ice and NSAIDs may also be of use. In the subacute or chronic stages, a

Table 3.13.10 Posterior tibial tendon disorders

Stage	Pathology	Signs
1A	Tendon normal length. Mild tendinosis/tenosynovitis	No deformity Gastrocnemius–soleus complex is often tight Pain with resisted testing of posterior tibial tendon; single heel raise usually normal but painful Tenderness and swelling along course of tendon
2	Tendinosis of tendon with stretching out of tendon	Correctable valgus hindfoot, abduction of the forefoot, forefoot varus Tenderness, swelling along tendon 'Too many toes' sign and pain with resisted testing Abnormal single heel raise (weak, lack of inversion)
3	Progressive tendinosis and degenerative articular pathology in the foot	Deformities listed above become fixed Poor/absent single heel raise Lateral ankle pain may arise due to impingement
4	Progression of stage 3 with joint pathology now involving the ankle	As stage 3 Ankle deformity (valgus talar tilt with lateral tibiotalar degeneration)

biomechanical analysis, review of training and conditioning, focusing on core control and calf and progressive strengthening of the gastrocnemius–soleus complex and the tibialis posterior, and a custom orthotic are all indicated.

When conservative measures fail, surgery will be required. Persistent synovitis can be treated with either an open or an endoscopic synovectomy. Longtitudinal splits should be openly repaired.

A full rupture can rarely be repaired—some form of reconstruction is usually required. The tendons most commonly used to reinforce the damaged tibialis posterior tendons are the FDL or split tibialis anterior tendon. However, such measures alone are rarely sufficient. Alteration of the hindfoot biomechanics is achieved by either a medial displacement calcaneal osteotomy or lateral column lengthening. Increasingly excessive hindfoot valgus is controlled by placement of a subtalar implant—an arthroereisis procedure. With long-standing valgus heel position, the Achilles tendon frequently becomes contracted and perpetuates the deformity. Occasionally, it is necessary to consider lengthening the gastocnemius–soleus complex.

Flexor hallucis longus (FHL) tendinopathy

FHL functions to plantarflex the IPJ of the hallux and to dynamically stabilize the first MTPJ (and hence the whole forefoot). It is prone to injury in extremes of ankle plantarflexion and MTP dorsiflexion. The spectrum of disorders of the FHL includes tenosynovitis, tendinosis, and tear and rupture of the tendon (Figure 3.13.16).

FHL tenosynovitis at the ankle typically occurs in runners, springboard divers, and, most commonly, dancers. The patient typically complains of posteromedial ankle pain, reproduced by passive, active, and resisted movements of the toe, and swelling. Stenosis may occur, with a palpable nodule present and clicking reported. In dancers the pain is exacerbated by forcing the turn out position, movements on to the ball of the foot (*demipointe*) and onto the tip of the toe (*pointe*), and by the hyperplantarflexion of the *relevé*. The condition can be associated with poor technique, excessive turnout at the hip so that the dancer is not centred over the feet, weakness, and inadequate flexibility of the other soft tissue structures of the lower leg and foot, hard surfaces, excessive training, and poorly fitting and inappropriate shoes.

Management

FHL tenosynovitis in the acute phase is treated by relative rest, anti-inflammatory approaches, and addressing the associated causes, including dancing/sporting technique, where relevant. Biomechanical analysis is important and an orthotic may be effective in non-dancers. A short period of immobilization of 2–3 weeks in a brace may be necessary. There is little role for local corticosteroids in this condition, unless there is a combination of bony and soft tissue pathology, or there is tenosynovitis and it is necessary to maintain an athlete through a competitive season until surgery can be performed.

Surgery is undertaken if conservative measures fail. A medial incision is used to decompress the tendon, and to release any triggering caused by nodules on the tendon. Surgery is often combined with os trigonum excision (see above).

Flexor digitorum longus tendinopathies

FDL tendinopathies are much less common then those affecting FHL. Rarely, tenosynovitis or tendinosis may be seen, particularly in dancers. Lesions occur at two sites: under the flexor retinaculum at the posteromedial ankle, and at the level of the plantar plate. Patients present with similar symptoms to FHL tenosynovitis, but clinically pain is aggravated on resisted flexion of the toes. Treatment is similar to that used in FHL complaints. Most tears or ruptures of the FDL are due to laceration and require primary repair, although patients can function well without an FDL and it is the tendon of choice for transfer in cases of full rupture of the tibialis posterior.

Tarsal tunnel syndrome

Tarsal tunnel syndrome (TTS) refers to entrapment primarily of the tibial nerve within, proximal to, or distal to the flexor retinaculum or within the abductor hiatus. During its course the tibial nerve gives off sensory calcaneal branches, and then medial and lateral plantar branches, which have sensory and motor components.

TTS can be subdivided into proximal TTS, representing entrapment of the PT nerve, and distal TTS, where the medial and/or lateral plantar nerves are involved. TTS has to be differentiated from 'high tarsal tunnel syndrome', where the tibial nerve is entrapped in the leg by a band of tight gastrocnemius fascia. Symptoms are similar, except that tenderness is maximal in the lower calf.

A number of factors within and outside the tarsal tunnel can be involved. Intrinsic lesions include soft tissue masses, synovitis, tenosynovitis, fibrosis, local varicosities, and accessory musculature.

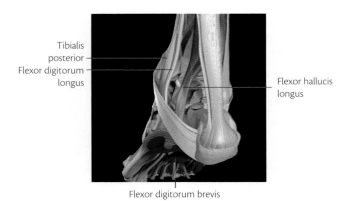

Tibialis posterior
Flexor digitorum longus
Flexor hallucis longus
Flexor digitorum brevis

Fig. 3.13.16 Flexor hallucis longus: 'the beef of the heel'.

Systemic disease, including diabetes and hypothyroidism, should be considered. Structural deformity and congenital abnormalities such as tarsal coalition may contribute. In sport, factors extrinsic to the tunnel are particularly important, in particular foot and ankle biomechanics. Excessive subtalar pronation frequently plays a major role and is often associated with hindfoot valgus and forefoot varus, with stretching of the tibial nerve. Trauma to the medial side of the ankle in the planovalgus foot is also important. Additional stretching of the flexor retinaculum and abductor hallucis muscle causes further compression of the nerve and branches within the abductor hiatus. Trauma (blunt trauma, fracture of ankle mortise, talus or calcaneus, or iatrogenic) may also play a role.

Diagnosis is often difficult as symptoms and clinical signs are variable and electrodiagnostic tests have limitations (see below). The presentation varies according to the cause and site of entrapment. A burning ache or pain around the medial ankle and/or foot is commonly reported, with shooting pains into the plantar aspect of the foot. Paraesthesiae/dysaesthesiae in the same distribution and cramp in the foot are also common. Symptoms may be worse with weight-bearing; removal of tight footwear and rest may help.

Tenderness is found on palpation over the tarsal tunnel and, more notably, proximal and distal to the site of compression (the Valleix phenomenon). A positive Tinel sign and symptoms with deep compression over the tunnel or forced pronation of the foot may be noted. There may be a decrease in two-point discrimination between involved and uninvolved extremities. Late findings include loss of sensation along the medial and/or lateral plantar nerves and atrophy of intrinsic muscles of the foot, resulting in hammer toe deformities. If symptoms are related to activity it is necessary to examine the patient after a period of weight-bearing and/or performing the activity associated with the onset of symptoms. Patients with hyperpronation have increased tibial nerve tension during eversion, dorsiflexion, and cyclic loading with increased internal rotation. Gait analysis should be performed.

The use of neurophysiology studies is controversial and the authors frequently find them insensitive, particularly in athletes.

Management

Successful outcome depends on identification and correction of the cause(s). The patient should have a trial of NSAIDs, and topical applications may provide relief. Regular icing may provide benefit and rest from aggravating activities is important. Orthoses to counteract hindfoot valgus are frequently helpful. Casting for a 3–6 week period may be necessary if symptoms are severe. Local corticosteroid injections are rarely necessary in athletes with the condition. Physiotherapy may include soft tissue release and massage to break down local scar tissue and mobilize the nerve, stretching, and appropriate strengthening exercises where biomechanical factors are involved.

Failure of conservative management is an indication for surgical intervention, which involves identification of the tibial nerve above the level of anticipated compression and its major branches. The nerve is traced distally and any anomalies or compressive features released thoroughly. Judgement of the outcome following surgical release may not be known for several months, and completeness of recovery depends on the duration of symptoms and the extent of intrinsic damage to the nerve.

Appendix 1 Frequency, distribution, and rates of selected injuries (ankle ligament sprains and anterior cruciate ligament injuries) for NCAA Games and Practices Combined for 15 sports, 1988–1989 to 2003–2004

Injury	Frequency	Percentage of all injuries	Injury rate per 1000 athlete exposures	95% CI
Ankle ligament sprains				
Men's baseball	663	7.9	0.23	0.21, 0.25
Men's basketball	3205	26.6	1.30	1.26, 1.35
Women's basketball	2446	24.0	1.15	1.10, 1.20
Women's field hockey	327	10.0	0.46	0.41, 0.51
Men's football	9929	13.6	0.83	0.81, 0.84
Women's gymnastics	423	15.4	1.05	0.95, 1.15
Men's ice hockey	296	4.5	0.23	0.20, 0.26
Women's ice hockey	12	2.8	0.14	0.06, 0.22
Men's lacrosse	698	14.4	0.66	0.61, 0.71
Women's lacrosse	602	17.7	0.70	0.65, 0.76
Men's soccer	2231	17.2	1.24	1.19, 1.29

Appendix 1 Frequency, distribution, and rates of selected injuries (ankle ligament sprains and anterior cruciate ligament injuries) for NCAA Games and Practices Combined for 15 sports, 1988–1989 to 2003–2004 (*Continued*)

Injury	Frequency	Percentage of all injuries	Injury rate per 1000 athlete exposures	95%CI
Women's soccer	1876	16.7	1.30	1.24, 1.36
Women's softball	526	9.9	0.32	0.29, 0.35
Women's volleyball	1649	23.8	1.01	0.96. 1.06
Men's wrestling	715	7.4	0.56	0.52, 0.60
Men's spring football	1519	13.9	1.34	1.27, 1.40
Total ankle ligament sprains	27 117	14.9	0.83	0.82, 0.84
ACL injuries				
Men's baseball	56	0.7	0.02	0.01, 0.02
Men's basketball	167	1.4	0.07	0.06, 0.08
Women's basketball	498	4.9	0.23	0.21, 0.25
Women's field hockey	53	1.6	0.07	0.05, 0.09
Men's football	2159	3.0	0.18	0.17, 0.19
Women's gymnastics	134	4.9	0.33	0.28, 0.39
Men's ice hockey	78	1.2	0.06	0.05, 0.07
Women's ice hockey	3	0.7	0.03	0.00, 0.07
Men's lacrosse	131	2.7	0.12	0.10, 0.15
Women's lacrosse	145	4.3	0.17	0.14, 0.20
Men's soccer	168	1.3	0.09	0.08, 0.11
Women's soccer	411	3.7	0.28	0.26, 0.31
Women's softball	129	2.4	0.08	0.06, 0.09
Women's volleyball	142	2.0	0.09	0.07, 0.10
Men's wrestling	147	1.5	0.11	0.10, 0.13
Men's spring football	379	3.5	0.33	0.30, 0.37
Total ACL injuries	4800	2.6	0.15	0.14, 0.15

Reproduced from Hootman, J.M., Dick, R., and Agel, J. (2007). Epidemiology of collegiate injuries for 15 sports: summary and recommendations for injury prevention initiatives. *Journal of Athletic Training*, 42, 311–19

References

Berndt, A.L. and Harty, M. (1959). Transchondral fractures of the talus. *Journal of Bone and Joint Surgery. American Volume*, **41**, 988–1023.

Ferkel, R.D. and Sgaglione, N.A. (1994). Arthroscopic treatment of osteochondral lesions of the talus: long-term results. *Orthopaedic Transactions*, **17**, 1011.

Fuller, C.W., Dick, R.W., Corlette, J., and Schmalz, R. (2007a). Comparison of the incidence, nature and cause of injuries sustained on grass and new generation artificial turf by male and female football players. Part 1: Match injuries. *British Journal of Sports Medicine*, **41** (Suppl 1), i20–6.

Fuller, C.W., Dick, R.W., Corlette, J., and Schmalz, R. (2007b). Comparison of the incidence, nature and cause of injuries sustained on grass and new generation artificial turf by male and female football players. Part 2: Training injuries. *British Journal of Sports Medicine*, **41** (Suppl 1), i27–32.

Gerber, J.P., Williams, G.N., Scoville, C.R., Arciero, R.A., and Taylor, D.C. (1998). Persistent disability associated with ankle sprains: a prospective examination of an athletic population. *Foot and Ankle International*, **19**, 653–60.

Harper, M.C. and Keller, T.S. (1989). A radiographic evaluation of the tibiofibular syndesmosis. *Foot and Ankle*, **10**, 156.

Hootman, J.M., Dick, R., and Agel, J. (2007). Epidemiology of collegiate injuries for 15 sports: summary and recommendations for injury prevention initiatives. *Journal of Athletic Training*, **42**, 311–19.

Kerkhoffs, G.M., Handoll, H.H., de Bie, R., Rowe, B.H., and Struijs, P.A. (2007). Surgical versus conservative treatment for acute injuries of the lateral ligament complex of the ankle in adults. *Cochrane Database of Systematic Reviews*, CD000380.

Krause, J.O. and Brodsky, J.W. (1998). Peroneal tendon tears: pathophysiology, surgical reconstruction and clinical results. *Foot and Ankle International*, **19**, 271–9.

Leach, R.E. and Schepsis, A.A. (1990). Acute injuries to ligaments of the ankle. In: C.M. Evarts (ed.), *Surgery of the Musculoskeletal System*, Vol 4, pp. 3887–913. Churchill Livingstone, New York.

Menz, H.B. (1998). Alternative techniques for the assessment of foot pronation. *Journal of the American Podiatric Medical Association*, **88**, 119–29.

Mueller, M.J., Host, J.V., and Norton, B.J. (1993). Navicular drop as a composite measure of excessive pronation. *Journal of the American Podiatric Medical Association*, **83**, 198–202.

Nelson, A.J., Collins, C., Yard, E., Fields, S., and Comstock, R. (2007). Ankle injuries among United States high school sports athletes, 2005–2006. *Journal of Athletic Training*, **42**, 381–7.

Petrella, R.J., Petrella, M.J., and Cogliano, A. (2007). Periarticular hyaluronic acid in acute ankle sprain. *Clinical Journal of Sport Medicine*, **17**, 251–7.

Pickenburg, A.C.M., van Dijk, C.N., Bossuyt, P.M.M., and Marti, R.K. (2000). Treatment of ruptures of the lateral ankle ligaments: a meta-analysis. *Journal of Bone and Joint Surgery. American Volume*, **82**, 761–72.

Sobel, M., DiCarlo, E., Bohne, W., et al. (1991). Longitudinal splitting of the peroneus brevis tendon: an anatomic and histologic study of cadaveric material. *Foot and Ankle*, **12**, 165.

Stiell, I.G., McDowell, I., Nair, R.C., *et al.* (1993). Decision rules for the use of radiography in acute ankle injuries. Refinement and prospective validation. *Journal of the American Medical Association*, **269**, 1127–32.

van Dijk, C.N., Lim, L.S., Bossuyt, P.M.M., and Marti, R.K. (1996). Physical examination is sufficient for the diagnosis of sprained ankles. *Journal of Bone and Joint Surgery. British Volume*, **78**, 958–62.

Yamamoto, H., Yagishita, K., Ogiuchi, T., Sakai, H., Shinomiya, K., and Muneta, T. (1998). Subtalar instability following lateral ligament injuries of the ankle. *Injury*, **29**, 265–8.

Injuries to the foot

Bill Ribbans and Cathy Speed

Introduction

Injuries to the foot and ankle are common in sport and considered to represent 10–15% of all sports injuries. The demands of running, jumping, turning, and cutting inevitably take their toll on this complex anatomical region. Even minor injuries can cause significant dysfunction. Adverse biomechanical issues may cause injury to the foot itself and frequently result in injury elsewhere in the lower limb, lumbar, or pelvic regions.

From an epidemiological perspective, foot and ankle injuries are often considered together. There is little information in the literature about the prevalence of injuries specifically in the foot. The ankle is generally considered to be affected more frequently than the foot. However, the foot remains one of the most commonly injured sites during running, and the majority of these injuries are secondary to overuse. Almost a third of injuries to elite gymnasts involve the foot and ankle (Kolt and Kirkby 1999), with significant effects on training and competition. Thirteen per cent of injuries in amateur golfers are to the ankle and foot (McHardy et al. 2007).

Anatomy

The foot can be divided into three regions: hindfoot, midfoot, and forefoot (Fig. 3.14.1). They function together to provide support, stability, flexibility, propulsion, acceleration, and deceleration and to deliver sensory information. This is achieved through a series of arches and chains formed by bones and soft tissues, allowing the foot to transform from a rigid and stable unit to a flexible system.

Bony anatomy

The hindfoot

The hindfoot is composed of the talus, the calcaneus and their attachments.

The **talus** forms three main articulations: the talocrural (ankle), talocalcaneal (subtalar), and talonavicular joints. The head of the talus is located in the depression midway between the medial malleolus and the tuberosity of the navicular.

Although the talus has no musculotendinous attachments, the body and neck of the talus provide attachments for the ligaments and fascia of the ankle and hindfoot. The posterior process of the body of the talus consists of two tubercles, separated by a central groove, through which runs the tendon of flexor hallucis longus (FHL). The lateral tubercle is usually the larger and is particularly vulnerable to fracture because of its position. When it is abnormally large, it is known as Stieda's process. The os trigonum is an accessory ossicle which is associated with the posterolateral tubercle in 2.7–7.7% of individuals (Sarrafian 1983), and when present is commonly bilateral.

The talus receives its vascular supply from branches of the posterior tibial, dorsalis pedis, and peroneal arteries; this supply is easily compromised by injury.

The **sinus tarsi** and **tarsal canal** are located between the talus and calcaneus, lying anterior to the posterior facet of the calcaneus, and giving attachment to a number of structures: the extensor digitorum brevis, the intermediate and medial roots of the extensor retinaculum, the cervical ligament, and the calcaneonavicular and calcaneocuboid ligaments. The structures of the sinus tarsi are taut in inversion.

The **calcaneus** consists mainly of cancellous bone and is highly vascularized. It articulates with the talus in the hindfoot and the navicular and cuboid in the midfoot to form the subtalar and midtarsal joints. Inversion and eversion of the foot take place at these sites.

The posterior calcaneus can be divided into superior, central, and inferior thirds. The Achilles tendon inserts into the central third, with the plantaris (where present) inserting on its medial

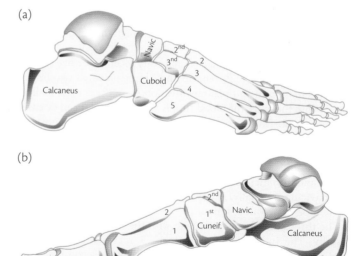

Fig. 3.14.1 Bony anatomy of the foot. (a) Lateral: Chopart's joint is formed by the navicular medially and the cuboid laterally articulating on the calcaneus and the head of the talus. (b) Medial: Lisfranc's joint is formed by articulation of the three metatarsal bases with the three cuneiforms and the cuboid.

aspect. The lengthened posterior section of the calcaneus between the posterior facet and the insertion of the Achilles tendon increases the moment arm of the tendon at the ankle joint, resulting in increased mechanical efficiency.

The superior portion of the calcaneus slopes away from the Achilles tendon, forming a space that is occupied by the retrocalcaneal bursa. The inferior third of the calcaneus forms a tuberosity, the calcaneal process, which divides inferiorly to form the medial and lateral calcaneal processes. These provide attachments for the deep plantar fascia and the first layer of intrinsic plantar muscles. The larger medial process is a common site for plantar fasciitis.

The sustentaculum tali is a shelf that 'sustains' the head of the talus at the medial junction of the subtalar and midtarsal joints. It projects medially from the calcaneus approximately 2.5 cm below the tip of the medial malleolus, and important structures pass close to it. The tendon of tibialis posterior courses above the sustentaculum towards its navicular insertion, the tendon of FHL travels within an osseofibrous tunnel below the sustentaculum, and the tendon of FDL passes around its medial edge. On the lateral surface of the calcaneum there is a small tuberosity, the peroneal tubercle, with the peroneus brevis and longus passing above and below it, respectively.

The **plantar ligaments** also make a major contribution to the stability of the medial longitudinal arch. The long and short plantar ligaments are thick, with strong longitudinally oriented fibres. The **short plantar (plantar calcaneocuboid) ligament** attaches to the anterior tubercle on the plantar surface of the calcaneus, helping to maintain the position of the calcaneus and to support the midtarsal joint inferiorly. Two other ligaments, the **spring (plantar calcaneonavicular) ligament** and the **long plantar ligament,** also contribute. When loaded in gait the calcaneus and these attached soft tissues provide elastic recoil in the arch system.

The midfoot

The bones of the midfoot are the **navicular**, **cuboid**, and **three cuneiforms**, with the **tarsal navicular** (scaphoid) forming the keystone above the longitudinal arch of the foot. (Fig. 3.14.2) The midfoot articulates with the hindfoot through the midtarsal joint (**Chopart's joint**) and with the forefoot through the tarsometatarsal joint (**Lisfranc's joint**).

The medially placed navicular tuberosity receives the insertion of the tibialis posterior (TP) tendon and can be palpated two finger-breadths in a distal and plantar direction from the medial malleolus. As with the talus, the blood supply to the navicular can be easily compromised. The accessory navicular (os tibiale), on the posteromedial aspect of the navicular, is found in up to 11% of individuals and is incorporated into the insertional fibres of the TP tendon.

The **cuboid** articulates with the calcaneus proximally, with the fourth and fifth metatarsals distally, and with the lateral cuneiform and navicular medially. It has a groove on its inferior surface for the tendon of peroneus longus.

The **three cuneiforms** articulate with the first three metatarsals distally. The intermediate cuneiform is recessed compared its medial and lateral counterparts. Consequently the second metatarsal is mortised between the first and third metatarsals, giving an extra element of bony stability to Lisfranc's joint.

The forefoot

The forefoot begins distal to the tarsometatarsal joint and includes the ball of the foot and the toes, all of which have three phalanges,

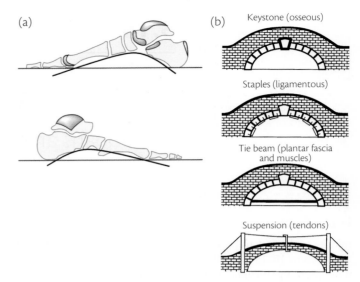

Fig. 3.14.2 The medial arch of the foot is composed of the calcaneus, talus, navicular, three cuneiforms, and the first three metatarsals. The lateral longitudinal arch is composed of the calcaneus, cuboid, and the fourth and fifth metatarsals. The transverse arch (not shown) is composed of the metatarsal bases, the cuboid, and three cuneiforms. All arches are supported by mechanisms similar to those used in bridge construction.

with the exception of the great toe, which has two. The five metatarsals articulate with the proximal phalanges, with the second ray acting as both the pivotal axis and the stiffest portion of the foot. The base of the fifth metatarsal has a palpable styloid at its base where the tendon of peroneus brevis inserts.

Accessory ossicles and sesamoids are commonly found in the foot. The sesamoid complex under the head of the first metatarsal is constant and receives contributions from seven muscles. Sesamoids can also be found in the metatarsophalangeal (MTP) and interphalangeal (IP) joints of other digits. Ossicles can be found, amongst other places, at the posterolateral aspect of the talus (os trigonum), in the tibialis posterior tendon (the accessory navicular) and the base of the fifth metatarsal (os Vesalianum).

The arches of the foot

Since the foot is a segmented structure, it can support weight only if it exists as one or more arches. There are three such arches, the medial and lateral longitudinal and transverse arches, the support of which depends on the shape of the bones and the connections between them.

Soft tissue anatomy

The lateral foot

The **peroneus longus** acts as a primary plantarflexor of the first ray, a unique function that cannot be substituted by other muscles. It also acts as an accessory plantarflexor of the ankle and a weak evertor of the subtalar joint. After passing around the lateral malleolus, the tendon passes underneath the superior peroneal retinaculum to the cuboid notch, bends acutely medially, passes under the inferior peroneal retinaculum, and is guided inferomedially by the peroneal tubercle on the calcaneus. It exits from this retinaculum and turns again to enter the plantar tunnel under the cuboid and fifth metatarsal within a groove on the cuboid tuberosity. In approximately 5% of individuals there is a sesamoid bone within the peroneus longus tendon, which can be a site of pathology. The tendon then inserts into the medial cuneiform and the base of the first metatarsal. Peroneus longus has two sheaths which only rarely communicate with each other; one terminates within the cuboid notch and the second teminates in the sole of foot, extending medially from notch to insertion.

The **peroneus brevis** is the strongest evertor of the subtalar joint and is a weak plantarflexor of the ankle. It emerges from the inferior fibular retinaculum and passes to its broad insertion on the styloid process of the fifth metatarsal. The sheath extends to within 2 cm of its insertion on the base of the fifth metatarsal. Both peroneii are important in maintaining the longitudinal arch of the foot.

The anomalous **peroneus quartus** muscle is present in 13–22% of population. It varies in origin, insertion, and size and its contribution is unclear. It runs behind the lateral malleolus and usually inserts onto an often enlarged peroneal tubercle, the cuboid tuberosity, or the tendon of peroneus longus.

Medial foot and ankle

The **posterior tibial tendon** (TP) works powerfully at the subtalar and midtarsal joints to invert the heel and supinate the foot. It also plantarflexes the foot at the ankle, plays an important role in maintaining the medial arch of the foot, and contributes to stability of the foot by its many bony attachments. It originates from the upper two-thirds of the tibia, intermuscular septum, and fibula. The tendon passes behind the medial malleolus and inferior to the spring ligament, where a fibrocartilaginous or bony sesamoid may be located. The insertion of TP is complex, with the anterior component at the tuberosity of the navicular and other insertions to the bones of the tarsometatarsal joint and to the sustentaculum tali.

The **flexor digitorum longus (FDL)** flexes the distal phalanges of the lateral four toes, assists in plantarflexion at the ankle, and helps to maintain the medial and longitudinal arches. It passes medial to the edge of the sustentaculum tali, then deep to the abductor hallucis and into the central compartment of the foot, crossing the tendon of FHL at the knot of Henry, from which it receives a strong slip and also the insertion of the quadratus plantae muscle. The tendon then separates into four tendons, which give origin to the lumbrical muscles. Each tendon enters the fibrous sheaths of the lateral four toes, perforates the corresponding tendon of flexor

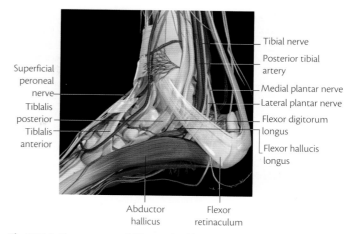

Fig. 3.14.4 The posteromedial foot and ankle.

digitorum brevis (FDB), and inserts onto the base of the distal phalanx.

The **flexor hallucis longus (FHL)** flexes the distal phalanx of the great toe, assists in plantarflexion at the ankle, and helps to maintain the medial arch. The tendon travels below the sustentaculum tali in a fibro-osseous tunnel into the medial compartment of the foot, deep to the FDL, and inserts into the base of the distal phalanx of the great toe. FHL may have a muscle belly which extends as far as the talar tubercles, through which the tendon passes. It is separated from the Achilles tendon by a fat-filled space. The close proximity of these tendons is one reason for the use of the FHL as a tendon graft for the Achilles tendon, just as the close proximity of the FDL is taken advantage of in surgery for tibialis posterior lesions.

Anterior foot and ankle

The tendon of **tibialis anterior** (TA), the long extensors, and the peroneus tertius all pass into the foot on the anterior aspect of the ankle. Medially, TA emerges from beneath the inferior extensor retinaculum to insert into the medial edge of the foot at the first metatarsal base and the first cuneiform. It functions to dorsiflex the ankle, invert the foot, and support the medial arch.

The **extensor hallucis longus (EHL)** acts to extend the great toe. It exits the inferior extensor retinaculum medial to the dorsalis pedis artery, and the deep peroneal nerve, and travels to insert onto the distal phalanx of the hallux or onto the proximal phalanx.

The **extensor digitorum longus (EDL)** functions to dorsiflex the MTPJs, PIPJs, and DIPJs along with the intrinsic muscles. It splits into four slips that pass dorsally to form the extensor hood of the first four MTPJs. Each tendon divides into three slips: the central portion inserts onto the base of the middle phalanx, the slip on the tibial side has a lumbrical insertion, and the extensor hood inserts onto the distal phalanx. The **peroneus tertius** is part of the EDL, which inserts onto the base of the fifth metatarsal.

The **anterior tarsal tunnel** is a narrow space between the fascia overlying the talus and navicular and the Y-shaped inferior extensor retinaculum. The deep peroneal nerve passes through this space between the EHL and the EDL.

The muscles of the **plantar aspect** of the foot can be further divided into four layers, described by their position in relation to the sole (Table 3.14.1 and Fig. 3.14.5). The muscles of the first layer

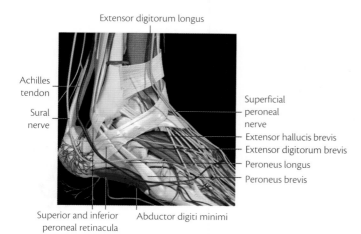

Fig. 3.14.3 The lateral foot and ankle.

Table 3.14.1 The muscles of the plantar aspect of the foot.

Layer	Muscles	Functions
1	Abductor hallucis	Flexion, abduction great toe, braces medial arch
	Flexor digitorum brevis	Flexes lateral four toes, braces both longitudinal arches
	Abductor digiti minimi	Flexion, abduction fifth toe, braces lateral arch
2	Four lumbricals (and FDL, FHL)	Toe extension at IPJs
3	Flexor hallucis brevis	Stabilizes and flexes first MTPJ, supports medial arch
	Adductor hallucis	Flexion, adduction hallux
	Flexor digiti minimi	Stabilizes fifth toe
4	Interossei (and peroneus longus, tibialis posterior)	Abduction, adduction of toes

all arise from the calcaneus and insert onto the proximal phalanges. They play a major role in maintaining the longitudinal arch. The flexor digitorum brevis (FDB) forms four tendons which pierce the fibro-osseous tunnel beneath the metatarsals and divide into two portions, allowing the tendons of FDL to pass between them.

The muscles of the second layer control toe motion. The quadratus plantae muscle inserts onto each of the tendons of the FDL. There are four lumbricals, each a short muscle arising from the segmented tendons of FDL and inserting onto the medial aspect of the extensor hood with the interosseous muscles.

The third layer of muscles is related to the great and little toes. Flexor hallucis brevis (FHB) stabilizes and flexes the first MTPJ, adductor hallucis flexes and adducts the hallux, and flexor digiti minimi helps to stabilize the fifth toe.

The fourth layer is composed of the interossei—four plantar and three dorsal, named according to their function in relation to the second metatarsal. Those moving the toes toward the longitudinal axis of the second metatarsal are adductors, and those moving the toes away from the axis are abductors. The tendons of tibialis posterior and peroneus longus are included in the fourth layer.

The plantar heel pad cushions the foot with each heel strike. It consists of U-shaped fat-filled tissue septae which are reinforced by elastic tissue. Spirals of fibrous fascia are anchored to one another, the calcaneus, and the skin.

Plantar aponeurosis (plantar fascia)

The deep fascia of the foot is thickened to form the flexor retinaculum and the plantar aponeurosis. The latter assists in the maintenance of the arches of the foot, gives firm attachments to the skin, and prevents damage to the underlying structures of the foot. It attaches to the medial and lateral tubercles of the calcaneus and forms a triangular sheet that is thick centrally and thinner in its medial and lateral parts. Distally it divides at the bases of the toes into five slips and then bands, passing superficially to the skin and deep to the toes, and fusing with the fibrous flexor sheath and the deep transverse ligaments. The medial and lateral borders of the thick central aponeurosis are continuous, with the thinner deep fascia covering the abductors of the great and little toes.

The connections between the calcaneus, the ligaments, and the skin allow the plantar aponeurosis to work as a stabilizing **windlass mechanism** (Fig. 3.14.6). When the toes are dorsiflexed as in the last part of stance just prior to toe-off, the aponeurosis is pulled distally and tightens, stabilizing the bones of the foot.

There is continuity between the deep fascia of the foot and that surrounding the ankle and between the deep plantar fascia and the Achilles tendon.

Neurovascular anatomy

The sciatic nerve supplies the majority of the innervation of the foot through the tibial, common peroneal (deep and superficial branches), and sural (the main sensory supply) nerves. The exception is the saphenous nerve, which arises from the femoral nerve and supplies sensory innervation to the ankle, the medial malleolus, and the medial border of the foot.

The arterial supply to the foot arises from branches of the popliteal artery. The anterior tibial artery becomes the dorsalis pedis artery on the anterior aspect of the ankle, giving branches to the ankle, the sinus tarsi, and the dorsum of the foot. It passes into the plantar aspect of the foot, giving off the first plantar metatarsal artery before joining the plantar arch. The posterior tibial artery divides into the medial and lateral plantar arteries after passing behind the medial malleolus. The lateral branch is larger and curves medially at the base of the fifth metatarsal to form the plantar arch. This anastomoses with the dorsalis pedis artery at the proximal end of the first intermetatarsal space, giving off plantar digital arteries along its course. The medial plantar artery supplies the medial side of the great toe.

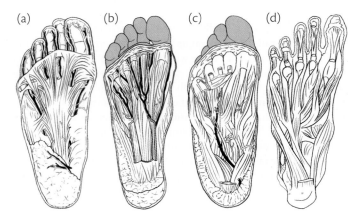

Fig. 3.14.5 The sole of the foot is composed of layers of soft tissue structures, from (a) the thick superficial plantar aponeurosis to (b) the first, (c) the second, and (d) the deep third and fourth layers of muscle. See also Table 3.14.1.

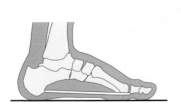
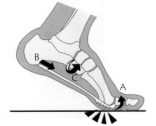

Fig. 3.14.6 The windlass mechanism. When the toes are dorsiflexed just prior to toe-off, the aponeurosis is pulled tight, stabilizing the arches of the foot and allowing its many structures to work as a functional unit.

Clinical evaluation

The foot is a common site for injuries in sport, particularly overuse injuries. Without treatment, even minor complaints involving the foot can lead to protracted pain because of the constant forces of weight-bearing. 'Second injury syndrome', due to the adverse biomechanics that can arise with foot injuries, is common. Conversely, injuries to the foot as a result of abnormalities elsewhere are also frequently seen. In evaluating the individual with a foot injury, it is helpful to consider intrinsic and extrinsic risk factors (Table 3.14.2).

History

The timing and mechanism of onset of symptoms should be ascertained to define whether the condition is acute, acute-on-chronic, or a chronic overuse injury. A history of previous local or distant injury may be relevant as the resulting alteration in gait may lead to further injury. Many injuries are insidious in onset without a clear mechanism. Progression or alteration of symptoms with time should be determined.

The principal modes of presentation of foot problems are pain and deformity. Other symptoms at presentation include stiffness and instability. Since the foot is a complex arrangement of structures, the clinician should aim to work with the patient to localize symptoms precisely.

The nature, intensity, and distribution of pain are noted. Pain may occur in association with swelling, clicking, creaking, and popping. There may be symptoms in the ankle or a previous ankle injury. Exacerbating and relieving features, in particular the relationship of pain to activity, should be determined. Nocturnal pain is suggestive of a significant soft tissue injury, neurogenic pain, an infective process, or a malignant process. Episodic burning pain radiating distally through the foot implies a neurogenic origin and referred pain is common. Whether symptoms are unilateral or bilateral can be a useful clue and should raise the suspicion of referred pain from the spine: 'two feet equals one back'.

A description of events after an acute injury can indicate the extent of the injury. Ability to weight-bear, timing, site and progression of swelling, and the presence of deformity are all relevant.

Stiffness is common after an acute injury, with chronic soft tissue complaints, and with degenerative articular complaints. Significant morning stiffness of 15 minutes or more is characteristic of inflammatory joint disease, and the patient should be questioned about other articular and systemic symptoms in relation to this possibility. Vascular symptoms include pain, coldness, colour change, and

Table 3.14.2 Some intrinsic and extrinsic risk factors for the development of overuse injury of the foot

Extrinsic factors	Intrinsic factors
Overuse (too much, too soon, often, too intense)	Hyper/hypomobility
Equipment: inappropriate footwear	Weakness/easy fatiguability
Surface: too hard/ too soft	Leg-length discrepancy
Technique: technical errors in running	Leg/heel/forefoot malalignment
	Coexisting disease (e.g. diabetes, rheumatoid arthritis)

numbness, and may be due to claudication, Raynaud's phenomenon, or arterial entrapment. Where vascular symptoms are present, the uni/bilaterality of symptoms should be determined and the presence of cardiovascular risk factors ascertained.

Specific details of any treatment approaches used, their timing, compliance, and their effects should be obtained.

A medical history should be established and a comprehensive competition and training history should be obtained, including the specific activities involved, the intensity, frequency, and duration of training sessions, and details of warm-up, stretching, and cool-down periods. Any change in technique, training surfaces, or training pattern prior to the injury may be important. The types, use pattern, and age of footwear and use of socks, supports, taping, insoles, and orthotics should be noted. Knowledge of the specific demands on the foot of the patient's specific sport is important.

Examination

The foot should be examined statically (weight-bearing, non-weight-bearing) and dynamically during gait and other forms of activity, as relevant to the sport. The foot forms one end of the complex kinetic chain of human movement, and overall movement analysis is useful in the assessment of the athlete with a foot injury. The reader is referred to Chapters 1.8 and 1.9 for additional information on this subject.

Inspection: deviations and deformities of the foot and ankle

The foot and ankle should be inspected in a similar manner to any other part of the body. Symmetry (or otherwise) of the feet should be established with regard to size, shape, and the presence of any abnormal features. Ideally, the inspection should begin with the patient standing and the limbs exposed to assess overall alignment and proximal pathology. Problems with the hip and knee region can have secondary affects on the foot and ankle. The limbs should be inspected from all positions. Following this, the patient should be observed supine on an examination couch and, if necessary, prone. Inspection of well-used footwear (both normal shoes and sports shoes) provides additional information on the pattern of weight-bearing during activity.

The clinician should develop a reproducible comprehensive system for initial inspection, which should include the following:

- presence of scars, swelling, ulceration, or skin disease
- pattern of callus formation on the sole of the foot
- evidence of circulatory abnormality—arterial, venous or lymphatic
- deformities of the digits
- midfoot alignment and abnormal bone or soft tissue growth
- ankle and hindfoot alignment, deformity, and swelling
- evidence of wasting of major muscle groups of the lower limb
- general overall angular and rotational alignment of the lower limb.

Posture

In the foot, combined triplanar motion in several joints is often described by a single term.

Pronation of the foot involves eversion of the heel, abduction of the forefoot, internal rotation of the leg relative to the foot, and dorsiflexion of the subtalar and midtarsal joints. It is associated with greater subtalar motion than in the supinated foot. The foot is naturally pronated in infancy, and becomes more supinated as the arches form.

Hyperpronation is common and can result in premature fatigue of the leg muscles since more muscle work is required to maintain stability during gait. An abductory twist at toe-off is often seen, when the foot pivots on the lateral metatarsal head(s) while the rearfoot swings inward toward the midline. Callus formation, plantar fasciitis, arch problems, and joint subluxations are seen. Strain on the anterior and medial knee structures is an association, and low back and sacroiliac joint pain on the side of the trailing leg can occur due to the spine leaning towards this side, with lack of smooth transfer of weight to the leading leg.

Supination of the foot involves a combination of inversion of the heel, adduction at the forefoot, and plantarflexion at the subtalar and midtarsal joints. The leg is externally rotated relative to the foot. The supinated foot is more rigid.

The relationship of the hindfoot to the forefoot

Assessment of the foot when the subtalar joint is in the neutral position allows identification of structural variations. The terminology describing hindfoot–forefoot relationships is complex and, at times, confusing. In assessment of these relationships the hindfoot is evaluated first.

Hindfoot valgus involves angulation of the calcaneus away from the midline and is associated with the flatfoot. The forefoot balances heel valgus by 'supinating' into forefoot varus, where the fifth ray is more plantarflexed than the first.

Hindfoot varus involves calcaneal angulation towards the midline, and is seen in pes cavus, or the 'cavovarus foot'. The forefoot compensates for hindfoot varus by 'pronating' into forefoot valgus, where the first ray is commonly more plantarflexed than the fifth. Failure to compensate leads to excessive weight-bearing on the fifth metatarsal head. These forefoot deviations can be assessed when the hindfoot is brought into neutral.

Pes cavus is defined as a foot with an elevated longitudinal arch and can range from mild to severe. There are many causes and

associations, in particular type 1 hereditary sensorimotor neuropathy (Table 3.14.3); hence careful neurological evaluation is mandatory in this group of patients. Patients with pes cavus have a varus heel, a high arch, excessive plantarflexion of the metatarsals (causing metatarsalgia), and often painful clawing of the toes, particularly at the fifth MTPJ. There may be lateral ankle ligament instability due to the varus heel position.

Pes planus (flat feet): all infants have flat feet up to the age of approximately 2 years because of the presence of a fat pad and incomplete formation of the arches. Its presence in an adult indicates the possibility of a permanent structural deformity, leading to alterations in the tarsal bones and talonavicular joints. The medial longitudinal arch is reduced, and on standing its border comes into contact with the ground. There is calcaneovalgus and forefoot pronation. Although the natural history of the flat foot is unknown, many are asymptomatic and therefore attempts to correct foot posture as a 'preventative measure' can be unproductive and even hazardous.

It is important to establish in the adult patient whether he/she has had 'flat feet' since childhood or whether it has arisen as an adult. Similarly, observe whether the deformity is unilateral or bilateral. Adult-onset unilateral pes planovalgus feet raise the spectre of tibialis posterior tendinopathy and/or spring ligament injury.

There is little substantive evidence to show that shoe modification or orthotic treatment alters the natural history of the flatness of the foot during growth and development.

The toes

Hallux valgus is a deformity of the first MTPJ involving a valgus and rotational deviation of the hallux. The first metatarsal head becomes uncovered and prominent medially. A **bunion** is formed by the combination of a callus which develops over the medial side of the head of the metatarsal, a thickened bursa, and an exostosis.

The normal range of motion at the first MTPJ is 65°–75° dorsiflexion and >20° of plantarflexion. **Hallux rigidus** is a clinical

Table 3.14.3 Associations of pes cavus

Classification	Aetiology
1. Neuromuscular	
(a) Muscle disease	Muscular dystrophy
(b) Peripheral nerve/ spinal root	Hereditary sensory-motor neuropathy type 1
	Spinal dysraphism
	Intraspinal tumour
(c) Anterior horn cell	Poliomyelitis
	Spinal dysraphism
	Diastematomyelia
	Syringomyelia
	Spinal cord tumours
	Spinal muscular atrophy
(d) Central nervous disease	Friedreich's ataxia
	Cerebellar disease
2. Congenital	Idiopathic
	Congenital talipes equino varus
	Arthrogryposis
3. Traumatic	Compartment syndrome sequelae
	Malunion of fracture foot

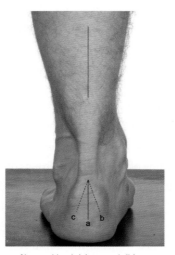

Fig. 3.14.7 Alignment of leg and heel: (a) neutral, (b) varus, and (c) valgus.

diagnosis where there is limited dorsiflexion (extension) of the great toe. It is often bilateral and can be (a) functional, where dorsiflexion of the first MTPJ is limited only when the foot is loaded, or (b) structural, where limitation occurs in both the loaded and unloaded foot (see below).

Considerable confusion exists regarding the terminology for lesser toe deformities. The simplest is a **mallet toe**, in which there is a flexion deformity of the DIPJ. A **hammer toe** consists of a flexion contracture of the PIPJ with or without a deformity of the DIPJ. A **complex hammer toe** deformity adds an extension deformity at the MTPJ. The most complex, and the most common requiring treatment, is a **claw toe**, which has a hyperextension deformity of the MTPJ and flexion deformity of the PIPJ. There is an overlap with the complex hammer toe but the claw toe usually involves all toes to some degree and often has an underlying neurological cause.

Exostoses, often with overlying callus, are found at sites of irritation secondary to trauma, overuse, or pressure. An excessively prominent superior calcaneal process is known as a 'Haglund deformity'; this may be evident only on imaging.

Further inspection and palpation

With the patient adequately exposed, the lower legs and feet are inspected and compared, firstly on weight-bearing and then when non-weight-bearing, from the sides, front, and behind. Leg-length discrepancy and other asymmetries of the lower limbs should be noted. The position of the pelvis, spine, and trunk should also be evaluated. For example, lateral or medial rotation of the hip or trunk can elevate or flatten the medial longitudinal arch of the opposite foot. The presence of deformities, skin lesions, scars, callosities, swelling, and bruising, local and proximal muscle bulk, and any nail changes (e.g. psoriasis, infections, and trauma) are noted.

The posture of the foot (neutral, supinated, or pronated) should be noted in weight-bearing, when the talus is considered to be fixed and compensation for structural and functional abnormalities can be seen. Footprint patterns help to demonstrate the shape of the foot and can easily be obtained by sprinkling talcum powder on the patient's moist feet and asking him/her to stand on some coloured paper (Fig. 3.14.8). More sophisticated standing and gait pattern information can be obtained using portable pressure measurement systems available in many clinics.

Table 3.14.4 Differential diagnosis of the flat foot

Congenital
Asymptomatic flexible
Symptomatic flexible
Rigid associated with tarsal coalition
Accessory navicular
Congenital deformity residual(club foot, vertical talus)
Joint laxity (Ehlers–Danlos syndrome, Marfan's syndrome)
Acquired
Posterior tibial tendon dysfunction
Arthritis (talonavicular, tarsometatarsal joint, Rh A)
Traumatic (calcaneal, midfoot, tarso-metatarsal fracture, spring ligament injury)
Charcot foot (diabetes mellitus)
Neuromuscular (poliomyelitis, cerebral palsy)
Tumour

The longitudinal arches are easiest seen in the medial view. The medial arch should be higher than the lateral. The arches can be assessed further; for example, the **Feiss line** joins the apex of the medial malleolus and the plantar aspect of the first MTPJ when the patient is non-weight-bearing. Then the patient stands and the navicular tuberosity, which should be on or close to the line, is located. The patient has a first-degree flat foot if the tuberosity falls one-third of the distance to the floor, a second-degree flat foot if it falls two-thirds towards the floor, and a third-degree flat foot if it touches the floor (Fig. 3.14.9).

Mobility of a flat foot can be assessed when the patient moves from a normal stance to tiptoes, when the heel should invert, the longitudinal arch should become visible, and the leg should externally rotate. Failure of this mechanism can be the result of tibialis posterior tendon dysfunction, arthritis of the mid- or hindfoot, congenital abnormalities such as a vertical talus, or a tarsal coalition. The 'too many toes' sign refers to the number of toes visible laterally from behind the patient and represents forefoot abduction. The normal number is one to three toes, but the sign is particularly

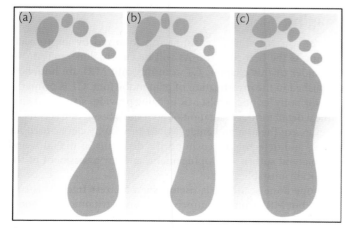

Fig. 3.14.8 Footprints: (a) pes cavus; (b) normal; (c) pes planus.

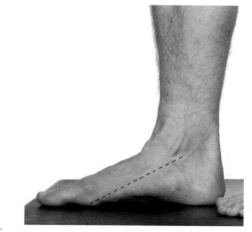

Fig. 3.14.9 The Feiss line.

helpful in unilateral involvement, when the two sides should be compared.

The sole of the foot is examined for skin changes such as calluses and plantar fibromatosis, and for localized areas of tenderness. If the Achilles tendon is symptomatic it may be easier to examine the patient prone.

Evaluation of the foot when the subtalar joint is in a neutral position allows assessment of the relationship between the forefoot and hindfoot. With the knee flexed, and the leg and foot dependent over the side of the couch, the heel is aligned with the longitudinal axis of the leg. The forefoot is then taken in the other hand. The thumb is then placed over the talonavicular joint. The forefoot is then moved to find the position where this joint is reduced, or maximally covered. This is the **subtalar neutral position**. The relative position of the forefoot and hindfoot is then observed (see Chapter 1.8).

To assess **leg–heel alignment,** marks are made over the calcaneus in the midline at the Achilles insertion and 1 cm below this and a connecting line is drawn. A second line connects two points on the lower leg in the midline. With the foot in subtalar neutral the relationship between the two lines is examined (Fig 3.14.10). A normal alignment is seen when the lines are parallel or in 2°–8° of varus. Less than this indicates hindfoot varus (inversion), whilst more than this indicates hindfoot valgus (eversion).

Forefoot–heel alignment is assessed with the patient supine and the feet over the edge of the couch. The foot is maintained in the subtalar neutral position and the relationship between the vertical axis of the heel and the plane of the metatarsal heads is noted. Normally the plane is perpendicular to the vertical axis. If the medial side of the foot is raised, the patient has forefoot varus, and if the lateral side is raised, he/she has forefoot valgus. If preferred, this assessment can be undertaken with the patient prone and the feet over the edge of the couch.

Tibial torsion is assessed in the sitting position with the patient's knees over the edge of the couch. The examiner visualizes the axis of the knee and the ankle. There is normally 12°–18° of external rotation (see Chapter 3.11).

The patient adopts the supine position to allow further inspection and palpation of all aspects of the foot and ankle for sites of specific bony or soft tissue tenderness, swelling, and deformity. Areas of least tenderness are palpated first, progressing towards the more painful sites that the patient has identified.

Movement

Passive, active, and resisted movements should be evaluated, observing for range of motion, reported pain, weakness, and reproduction of subluxation or dislocation of soft tissue structures, in particular the peroneal tendons. Muscles of the foot, and their action and innervation, are detailed in Table 3.14.5.

Pain on resisted testing is indicative of musculotendinous pathology of one or more of the units responsible for that movement. The site of the pathology may be further defined by the notable presence of swelling within a tendon sheath, or tenderness at the tendon insertion for example. Pain may also arise during a resisted movement because of significant intra-articular pathology. Weakness out of proportion to pain indicates rupture or a significant tear of a musculotendinous structure.

Special tests

These include the single heel raise test, the first metatarsal rise sign, the 'too many toes' sign, and assessment of the Achilles tendon. All are described elsewhere (Chapters 3.11 and 3.13).

Pain on direct compression of the calcaneum between the examiner's palms is indicative of a calcaneal stress fracture (the **calcaneal squeeze test**).

Neurovascular examination should be undertaken, including assessment for nerve entrapment. Percussion is performed over the posterior tibial nerve as it travels behind the medial malleolus and the anterior tibial branch of the deep peroneal nerve as it crosses the front of the ankle. The main trunk of the superficial peroneal nerve and its main branches can be seen in slim individuals with the ankle plantarflexed and the hindfoot inverted.

Similar percussion tests over other peripheral nerves are performed as appropriate, with reproduction of tingling, paraesthesia, or pain distally indicating a positive test which implies nerve entrapment or irritation. Neurovascular assessment before and immediately after exercise may be necessary.

Further examination of the patient during gait and other activities, particularly those related to the athlete's particular sport, is imperative in the evaluation of functional status and analysis of any underlying biomechanical factors leading to the patient's specific complaints. Gait analysis is described elsewhere (Chapter 1.9). As has been stated earlier, consideration of the foot as only one end of the complex kinetic chain is essential in considering causation and prevention of injury in sport.

Imaging

As ever, careful clinical examination followed by appropriate imaging is the best practice. As will be clearly illustrated in the remainder of this chapter, CT scanning and MRI are both well established in the investigation of pain in the foot. CT is primarily used for bony lesions, whilst MR imaging provides significant anatomical detail for the evaluation of both the osseous and soft tissue structures of the foot and ankle. MR arthrography can be used for staging and detecting osteochondritis dissecans of the talus and anterolateral soft tissue impingement, and for assessment of the chronically unstable ankle.

Isotope bone scanning is useful when a stress fracture is suspected, but MRI is more routinely used now. Dynamic ultrasonography is increasingly being used in the diagnosis of foot and ankle disorders. It is highly sensitive to structural changes in soft tissues,

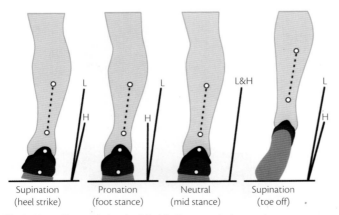

| Supination (heel strike) | Pronation (foot stance) | Neutral (mid stance) | Supination (toe off) |

Fig. 3.14.10 Changes in leg–heel (L–H) alignment during running.

Table 3.14.5 Lower extremity nerve function: preliminary checklist

	Sciatic					Femoral	Obturator	Superior gluteal	Inferior gluteal
Roots	L4–S2					L1–L3	L2–L4	L4–S1	L5–S2
Motor									
Hip						Flexion	Adduction	Abduction, medial rotation	Extension, lateral rotation
	Peroneal		**Posterior tibial**						
	Deep	Superficial		Medial plantar	Lateral plantar				
Roots	L4–S1	L5–S1	L5–S2	S1,S2	S1,S2				
Knee		Flexion				Extension			
Ankle/ subtalar joint	Dorsiflexion	Foot eversion	Plantarflexion, foot inversion						
Toes	Extension great toe	Extensor digitorum brevis	Flexion	Toe flexion, abduction, great toe	Abduction, adduction				
Sensory	1st webspace, dorsum of foot	Dorsum of foot (excluding 1st webspace)	–	Great toe	Small toe	Anterior thigh, medial calf, medial foot	Medial thigh	–	–

and allows dynamic evaluation, serial monitoring, and guided interventions.

Plain radiographs show inter-subject variation in stance, weight distribution, and bony relationships. In our practice we find weight-bearing views more relevant, and a standing AP and lateral plus an oblique view are routinely obtained. AP views provide good views of the forefoot, midfoot, and midtarsal joint. An AP view with 15° of angulation in the sagittal plane gives better visualization of the tarsometatarsal joints. The lateral view shows the posterior facet of the subtalar joint, the talonavicular joint, and first metatarsal–cuneiform articulation.

Specialized views may be required. Examples include the sesamoid view in sesamoid disease, the reversed or medial oblique view in the presence of an accessory navicular, axial views of the calcaneus, and Broden's views of the subtalar joint. In the paediatric patient, since many bones are incompletely ossified, CT or MRI may be needed to provide additional information to assist in the management of congenital and acquired lesions of the foot (Harty 2001).

Lateral foot pain

Stress injuries

Stress injuries are common and can affect any bone in the foot. Any athlete with pain and localized bony tenderness has a stress injury until proven otherwise. Investigations should include plain radiography, isotope bone scanning, MRI, and CT where necessary.

Multiple bone stress injuries of the ankle and foot may occur simultaneously in physically active young adults. Niva *et al.* (2007) performed an 86 month prospective study using MRI to evaluate the incidence, location, and type of bone stress injuries of the ankle and foot in military conscripts with ankle and/or foot pain with negative X-rays. A total of 131 conscripts displayed 378 bone stress injuries in 142 ankles and feet imaged, with the incidence being 126 per 100 000 person-years. This incidence represents the stress injuries not diagnosable with radiographs and requiring MRI. Of the injuries, 57.7% occurred in the tarsal and 35.7% in the metatarsal bones. Multiple bone stress injuries in one foot were found in 63% of the cases. The calcaneus and fifth metatarsal bone were usually affected alone. Injuries to the other bones of the foot were usually associated with at least one other stress injury. The talus and calcaneus were the most commonly affected single bones. High-grade bone stress injury with a fracture line on MRI occurred in 12% of the cases (talus, calcaneus), and low-grade injury presented only as oedema in 88% of the cases.

In the lateral foot, stress fractures of the cuboid are rare, but may be associated with plantar fascia disruption. In comparison, stress injuries to the lateral forefoot are common and are described further below.

Table 3.14.6 Causes of lateral foot pain

Peroneal tendinopathy
Symptomatic os peroneum
Ankle instability
Stress fracture of fifth metatarsal
Avulsion injury at fifth metatarsal
Cuboid instability
Bunionette
Sural nerve injury
Referred pain (S1)

Peroneal tendinopathies

The peroneii are important dynamic stabilizers of the ankle, primary evertors of the foot, and assist in plantarflexion. Injuries to either of these tendons is common in sport both at the ankle, as described in Chapter 3.13, and in the foot, where tenosynovitis, tendinosis, longitudinal tear, rupture, and avulsion occur.

Peroneal pathologies in the foot may present with pain and swelling, clicking, or subluxation/dislocation. Symptoms are worse when walking on uneven surfaces.

Tenosynovitis

Tenosynovitis of the peroneal tendons anywhere along their course is associated with peroneal tendon subluxation at the ankle, hypertrophy of the peroneal tubercle, or the presence of an os peroneum. Stenosing tenosynovitis or tears can develop with time.

The typical presentation is with pain over the peroneal tendons aggravated by exercise. Local swelling, localized tenderness, and crepitus may be present. Pain is exacerbated on passive stretch, by forced plantarflexion and inversion, and also by active contraction against resistance. An antalgic gait may be noted. Differentiation between peroneus brevis and longus involvement is based upon the site of pain, particularly with movement: pain with eversion, with restricted plantarflexion of the first ray, indicates peroneus longus involvement, whereas isolated pain with resisted eversion occurs with peroneus brevis lesions. Tenosynovitis and tears of peroneus brevis may also occur at the insertion, and a stress fracture of the base of the fifth metatarsal must be considered in the differential diagnosis. Similarly, an avulsion fracture of the fifth metatarsal can occur after lateral ankle sprain.

Diagnostic ultrasound will help to confirm tendinopathy and assess the state of the tendon, and will identify an accessory ossicle or avulsion fractures where present. The latter two features will also be confirmed with plain radiographs.

Treatment of peroneal tenosyovitis depends on the cause and location. Peroneal tendon instability is described in Chapter 3.13. The os peroneum syndrome is dealt with below.

Generally, non-operative treatment involves relative rest, NSAIDs, and ice, and short-term use of a lateral heel wedge. Foot biomechanics and footwear must be addressed and a formal orthotic may be indicated. The use of local corticosteroids should be limited, but where significant inflammatory change is seen, short-acting steroid injection under ultrasound guidance followed by strict non-weight-bearing for 7–10 days may be considered. As symptoms settle, a gradual strengthening programme of the peroneii commences.

In those with persisting symptoms, a trial of a rocker-bottom walking boot or even a non-weight-bearing cast is appropriate. If non-operative treatment fails, surgery should be considered. The tendons are exposed and any constriction of the sheath released. An os peroneum or hypertrophied peroneal tubercle should be resected if it is considered to be the cause of the symptoms. Any tears in the tendons are repaired as discussed below.

Tears and rupture of the peroneii in the foot

Tears of the peroneal tendons may either involve the peroneus brevis, peroneus longus, or both. As with tenosynovitis there are three distinct clinical pictures, with pathology occurring at (a) the level of the lateral malleolus, (b) the peroneal tubercle, and (c) the os peroneum. The first group principally affects the brevis tendon, whereas the other two affect the longus tendon. Some tears do not conform to any of the classical pictures, and spontaneous ruptures are described in athletes and non-athletic individuals (in particular

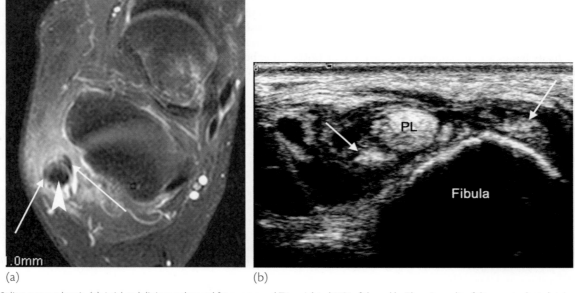

(a)   (b)

Fig. 3.14.11 Split peroneus brevis. (a) Axial gadolinium enhanced fat-suppressed T1-weighted MRI of the ankle. There is a split of the peroneal tendon into medial and lateral limbs (arrows) with the peroneus longus interposed between the two (arrowhead). (b) Axial sonogram. The peroneus brevis tendon has split in two (arrows) with the peroneus longus tendon (PL) interposed between the two. The lateral limb has subluxed over the lateral margin of the fibula.

those with diabetes and rheumatoid arthritis). Incidental finding of a tear of the peroneus brevis tendon during scanning for other problems is surprisingly frequent.

Longitudinal tears of the peroneus brevis occurring at the tendon insertion can be difficult to differentiate from an insertional tendinosis but should be suspected in those cases that fail to settle with conservative measures.

The peroneus longus is guided towards the cuboid by the peroneal tubercle in up to 44% of individuals. An enlarged peroneal tubercle is associated with attrition of the longus tendon.

The os peroneum, which present in about 20% of patients, lies within the substance of the peroneus longus tendon at the level of the cuboid, and may separate or be fractured in an acute ankle sprain or may be injured by direct trauma. This results in tenosynovitis, a partial tear, complete rupture, or simply chronic pain at the os perineum. Examination frequently reveals tenderness along the course of peroneus longus distal to the fibula, pain, and weakness with resisted plantarflexion of the first ray and with active eversion. Patients may report a sensation of walking on a pebble, presumably due to malalignment of the os peroneum on the cuboid.

Plain radiographs (oblique views) may demonstrate disruption of the os peroneum. CT allows assessment of the peroneal tubercle and os peroneum–cuboid articulation. MRI, ultrasound, and bone scanning are all useful in the evaluation of injuries in this area.

Management

Conservative management has little role to play in these injuries, although a trial of cast immobilization and orthotics may be attempted, but is likely to be effective in only up to 20% of patients (Sobel *et al.* 1994; Krause and Brodsky 1998).

An outline of the surgical management of peroneal tendon pathologies at the ankle is given in Chapter 3.13. Excision of a painful enlarged peroneal tubercle should always be accompanied by a careful inspection of the tendons on either side for evidence of degeneration or tears which require attention. The excision of a painful os peroneum requires careful enucleation of the fragment(s) from the peroneus longus tendon. The tendon should be inspected afterwards. It should be repaired or, if too damaged, tenodesed to the adjacent peroneus brevis tendon.

Sinus tarsi syndrome

Sinus tarsi syndrome presents with pain over the sinus tarsi, usually as a result of trauma. Most patients give a history of at least one inversion sprain, although more rarely the syndrome is seen in individuals with arthritides, pes planus, pes cavus, or chronic subtalar instability (Taillard *et al.* 1981). The syndrome is thought to be caused by scarring and impingement of the soft tissues of the sinus tarsi and there may be additional synovitis of the subtalar joint.

The patient complains of lateral ankle and/or foot pain, exacerbated by walking on uneven surfaces or simply with standing. Examination reveals tenderness in the sinus tarsi. The ankle is not usually unstable. Symptoms are relieved temporarily with a local anaesthetic injection into the sinus tarsi. Imaging can be unreliable.

Management

A guided local corticosteroid injection may be effective, but if this fails surgical management is indicated. O'Connor (1958) treated approximately a third of his patients surgically with resection of

the fat pad and the superficial ligamentous floor, with all patients noting that their symptoms improved after surgery. Subtalar arthroscopy and debridement may be utilized. Importantly, Frey *et al.* (1999) found that following arthroscopy the diagnosis was altered in every case. The majority of patients had interosseous ligament tears, but arthrofibrosis and subtalar degeneration were also seen.

Sural nerve entrapment

The sural nerve can be entrapped injured at any point along its course (Table 3.14.7). The nerve may be entrapped as it exits the deep fascia of the middle and distal thirds of the leg, at the ankle, or on the dorsolateral aspect of the foot. Iatrogenic sources (e.g. post-surgery or injudicious injection placement) represent the most common cause.

Although symptoms vary according to the site of entrapment, typically there is burning pain and numbness along the lateral border of the foot. Symptoms may be worse with walking or wearing boots. There is often a history of ankle instability or a sprain. Examination may reveal a positive Tinel's sign at the site of entrapment and evidence of the underlying cause (Table 3.14.7). Relief of pain with infiltration with a small amount of local anaesthetic at the suspected site of entrapment confirms the diagnosis.

Plain radiography, ultrasound, and MRI may all assist in determining the cause of the compression and excluding other pathologies in the differential diagnosis.

Management

Management involves correction, where possible, of the underlying cause(s). NSAIDs, relative rest, ankle support, and massage are commonly recommended, but symptoms are often resistant to simple measures. A trial of a tricyclic agent may be necessary. Surgical intervention is indicated in chronic cases where other measures have failed. The site of compression is identified preoperatively, and the nerve is released. Any bony prominence is smoothed off.

Superficial peroneal nerve injury.

Superficial peroneal nerve entrapment occurs most commonly at one of two sites. Proximally the nerve can be trapped at its origin from the common peroneal nerve at the neck of the fibula. Distal entrapment occurs where the nerve pierces the deep fascia, approximately

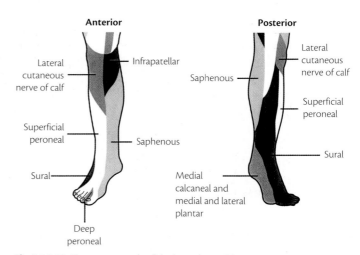

Fig. 3.14.12 Cutaneous supply of the lower leg and foot.

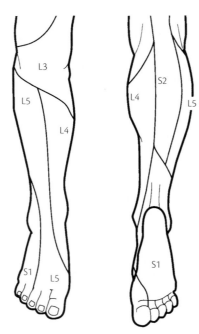

Fig. 3.14.13 Dermatomes of the lower leg and foot.

10–12 cm above the tip of the lateral malleolus, to become superficial and divide into its medial and lateral branches. Typically, the superficial nerve is injured as a result of traction during an inversion sprain or secondary to local trauma.

The patient presents with typical symptoms of nerve compression: burning pain, numbness, tingling, and dysaesthesiae in the distribution of the nerve and its branches. There is local tenderness at the site of compression, and there may be a positive Tinel's test. Sixty per cent of patients have a palpable deficit. Local nerve block is also helpful in making the diagnosis.

NSAIDs, peroneal strengthening exercises, strapping of the ankle, and patience may be all that is necessary in the more acute cases. Where there is chronicity, the aforementioned measures supplemented, if necessary, by local infiltration of hydrocortisone at the site of entrapment should be used before considering surgery. Surgery involves a release of any constriction of the nerve by the fascia. Where there is muscle herniation, a wider fascial release is required to free the nerve.

Cuboid instability

Alternatively known as cuboid syndrome or calcaneocuboid subluxation, cuboid instability is a cause of ill-defined pain on the

Table 3.14.7 Causes of sural nerve entrapment or injury

Trauma	Macrotrauma, including surgery, ankle sprain, fractures of the fifth metatarsal, cuboid, calcaneus, fibula Microtrauma (overuse)
Compression	
Intrinsic	Enlarged or scarred Achilles or peroneal tendons, anomalous bands, bony ridge, enlarged peroneal tubercle, venous insufficiency, ganglion, neuroma, connective tissue disease
Extrinsic	Tight stockings or boots

lateral border of the foot and the lateral plantar surface beneath the cuboid. It is most commonly seen in dancers and others with a hypermobile foot. The pain may arise due to synovial impingement between the cuboid and calcaneum or between the fourth and fifth metatarsal bases and the cuboid. There is tenderness on deep palpation of the cuboid and variably of the base of the fifth metatarsal. Imaging studies are normal, but stress fracture of the fifth metatarsal (or rarely the cuboid) should be excluded. Management involves strapping and manipulation of the cuboid, which typically resolves the pain. Orthotics with some lateral posting are often helpful, although this is difficult in the dancer, and recurrence with the need for further manipulation is common.

Central and lateral forefoot pain

Stress injuries

Stress injuries commonly affect the metatarsals, with only the tibia being more commonly affected. The second metatarsal is most frequently affected, partly due to its fixed position close to the cuneiforms. These injuries are commonly seen in dancers and runners and in other high-impact sports, and predisposing factors include gait and any structural abnormality in the foot and ankle. Those with proximal injuries are more likely to be chronically affected and commonly have tight calves. Those with differences in length of first compared with second metatarsal are more likely to experience multiple stress fractures and exhibit low bone mass. Higher training volumes have been associated with distal injuries (Chuckpaiwong *et al.* 2007).

Investigations are as for other stress injuries; X-rays may demonstrate a radiolucent line or periosteal reaction but may be normal. MRI or isotope bone scan are both sensitive to the lesions.

Management of most stress injuries is straightforward, with a few exceptions which are described below: relative off-loading, varying from strict rest to reducing training activities, addressing biomechanics and training errors, and returning the patient to activities when symptoms allow.

Stress injuries of the fifth metatarsal can be associated with forefoot adduction. Management typically involves non-weight-bearing

Table 3.14.8 Causes of forefoot pain

Metatarsalgia
Metatarsal stress fracture
Synovitis of metatarsalphalangeal joints
Freiberg's disease
Interdigital neuritis/neuromata
Flexor or extensor tendinopathies
Hammer toe
Turf toe
Hallux valgus
Hallux rigidus
Lesser toe deformity
Sesamoiditis
Tarsal tunnel syndrome
Referred pain

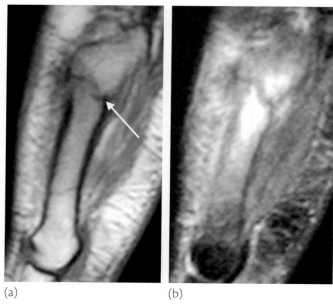

(a)   (b)

Fig. 3.14.14 Metatarsal stress fracture in a 28-year old female runner with pain in midfoot. (a) Sagittal T1-weighted MRI and (b) sagittal STIR MRI illustrating a fracture through the base of the fifth metatarsal.

below-knee cast/boot immobilization for 3 weeks and then 3 weeks or more of weight-bearing immobilization. Healing may still be prolonged.

Fourth metatarsal stress fractures occur less frequently but can be troublesome. They behave like, and should be managed similarly to, fifth metatarsal base fractures, taking longer to heal than other lesser metatarsal fractures and stress fractures (which are typically more distal).

Fractures

Fifth metatarsal fractures

Most fractures of the fifth metatarsal fall into one of three anatomical categories:

◆ proximal

◆ diaphyseal

◆ distal neck.

The four most common forms of fracture are classified as:

◆ tuberosity (zone I)

◆ metaphyseal (zone II) (Jones fracture)

◆ diaphyseal stress (zone III)

◆ neck (dancers' fracture)

Tuberosity fractures are common, caused by avulsion of the peroneus brevis tendon, and usually heal well, although imaging follow-up may show the fracture line to persist for some time after the patient feels clinically recovered. Immobilization in an Aircast boot until the acute symptoms settle is advisable, and the sportsperson should be able to return to activity at 8 weeks or soon after in most cases.

Jones fractures of the metaphysis should be treated more circumspectly. They are more at risk of non-union if not rested adequately

to begin with. Unlike the tuberosity injuries, it is preferable to insist on an initial month of non-weight-bearing followed by a similar period of protected weight-bearing. Internal fixation may be required for high-demand athletes or patients with evidence of delayed union or non-union.

Stress fractures of the diaphysis may seem more benign than the previous fractures. However, conservative management is not universally successful. Patients with a tendency to cavovarus foot, recurrent injuries, non-unions, and high-demand athletes should be considered for internal fixation. Intramedullary screw fixation, supplemented with a bone graft if necessary, is biomechanically the soundest choice for surgical treatment.

Neck fractures are commonly seen in dancers. This fracture can present with a degree of angulation like its counterpart in the hand. It will usually heal soundly, but dancers should be warned they may be away from strenuous dance activities for up to 3 months.

Fractures of the other metatarsals

Fractures of the first to fourth metatarsals may occur as the result of a direct blow or indirect angular or torsional forces. They may occur in isolation or as part of a more extensive injury to the foot and ankle. Non-displaced or minimally displaced fractures simply require protection in a cast or boot until pain diminishes. Healing should occur within 6–8 weeks. Displaced or significantly angulated fractures require reduction and, if unstable, fixation with either K-wires or plates.

Lisfranc injuries (midfoot sprains)

Injuries of the midfoot involving Lisfranc's joint can lead to disabling career- and sports-finishing problems. Lisfranc's joint represents the articulation between the bases of the five metatarsals and the three cuneiform bones and cuboid. The area is stabilized by a series of dorsal and plantar ligaments and the articular configuration, particularly the keying in of the base of the second metatarsal. Lisfranc's ligament itself binds the base of the second metatarsal to the medial cuneiform on the plantar aspect.

Injuries to the area may be due to severe trauma or a relatively innocuous cause. Direct blows or crushes are usually associated with significant soft tissue damage. Indirect injuries, which are more likely to be associated with sporting injuries, usually occur as a result of a twisting or axial loading force on a plantarflexed foot.

The patterns of injury have been classified according to involvement of structures and direction(s) of displacement (Myerson *et al.* 1986). A high index of suspicion should be had for any patient presenting with a painful, tender, and swollen midfoot. The mechanism of injury should be ascertained, and the pattern of bruising, swelling, and tenderness, and any deformity, should be noted.

Plain X-rays should include AP, lateral, and oblique views. Be aware that subtle changes such as widening of the interval between the first and second metatarsal bases may not be apparent on non-weight-bearing views. CT and MRI are far more sensitive at confirming and mapping the extent of such injuries (Fig. 3.14.15).

A mild midfoot sprain without evidence of documented displacement can be treated with immobilization and non-weight-bearing. However, prompt secondary referral should be made to the nearest foot and ankle orthopaedic centre for further evaluation of the benefits of further treatment. Clearly unstable and/or displaced injuries require surgical intervention. Soft tissue swelling

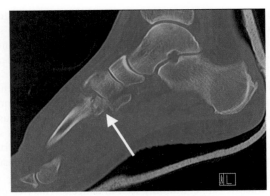

Fig. 3.14.15 A sagittal CT showing a fracture at Lisfranc's level.

can make such surgery difficult, and recovery is prolonged with a high incidence of post-injury stiffness, pain, and later arthritis.

Missed injuries can lead to the development of significant disability and require reduction and arthrodesis of the damaged joints in the long term.

Metatarsalgia

Metatarsalgia is a common presenting symptom in athletes. It simply refers to pain at the level of the metatarsals, principally distally at the MTP level.

Excluding conditions of the first ray, the following list includes the more common problems that may cause metatarsalgia:

- MTP synovitis
- MTP instability—subluxation or dislocation
- problems secondary to digit deformity (e.g. hammer toe, claw toe, mallet toe)
- biomechanical changes secondary to hallux valgus deformity (bunions) or hallux rigidus (first MTP osteoarthrhthirits)
- Morton's neuroma(s)
- bursitis
- inflammatory arthropathy
- stress fracture
- Freiberg's disease
- prominent plantar metatarsal head condyles
- dermatological conditions (e.g verrucae).

Sometimes there is more than one contributing pathology.

The patient reports weight-bearing-related forefoot pain. Where marked morning stiffness is reported, the possibility of an inflammatory arthritis should be pursued. It is important to elicit whether the pain is predominantly plantar or dorsal. Ask whether the pain radiates into the digits and is associated with any altered sensation. Be alert to any possibility of referred pain (e.g. spinal pathology) or neurological condition (e.g. peripheral or compressive neuropathy).

The foot should be inspected for overall alignment and any known predisposing biomechanical derangements (e.g. hyperpronation or pes cavus). Adequacy of peripheral circulation and sensation should be sought. Look for evidence of swelling, either bony or soft tissue. Weight-bearing may demonstrate splaying of digits

indicative of an interdigital swelling and/or MTP instability. Inspection of the sole will indicate a propensity to abnormally load specific areas of the forefoot.

Mobility of each forefoot joint needs assessing with specific regard to any fixed deformities (e.g. hammer toe) or instability (e.g. at the MTP joint). The exact location of the pain should be determined, with particular attention paid to whether the point of maximal tenderness is bony, articular, or in the digital interspaces. Further tests for the presence of Morton's neuromas such as the detection of Mulder's sign should be sought. (Mulder's sign is a palpable click on mediolateral compression of the foot combined with pressure applied to the interdigital web from the plantar aspect.)

X-rays may be normal or may show degenerative changes or erosions consistent with inflammatory arthritis. On viewing the weight-bearing AP films, attention should be paid to the metatarsal cascade or parabola to identify any abnormally long or short metatarsals. A comparison with the other side can often reveal surprising asymmetry.

Ultrasound is the imaging modality of choice for the detection of soft tissue problems, in particular MTP synovitis, bursae, and Morton's neuromas.

MRI will demonstrate synovitis, bursae, and neuromas (Fig. 3.14.16). A bone scan may show increased uptake in the affected areas, although this is rarely necessary.

Management involves correcting the underlying biomechanical cause(s), review of orthotic requirements, and reduction of inflammation with the use of NSAIDs and, if necessary, local corticosteroid injection to address synovitis and swollen interdigital nerves.

In recalcitrant cases, surgery may be required. For instance, unstable joints may need reducing and reconstructing, abnormal metatarsal lengths may need rectifying, underlying biomechanical problems may need correcting, and large painful Morton's neuromas may need excising.

FDL tendinopathies

FDL tendinopathies are rare, and most injuries to the FDL are due to laceration and require primary repair. However, tenosynovitis or tendinosis may be seen in dancers at two sites: under the flexor retinaculum and at the level of the plantar plate. Treatment is relative rest with avoidance of exacerbating activities, local regular icing, NSAIDs, and support.

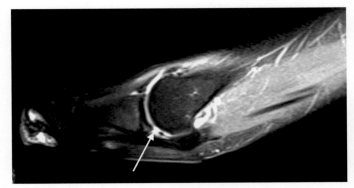

Fig. 3.14.16 MTP joint synovitis. Sagittal fat-saturated T1-weighted MRI after intravenous gadolinium. Note avid enhancement of joint synovium (arrow).

Medial foot pain

Posterior tibial and flexor hallucis longus tendinopathies are described in Chapter 3.13 as common causes of posteromedial ankle pain. Typically symptoms also arise in the midfoot and, in the case of the FHL, under the hallux.

Posterior tibial tendinopathies are described in Chapter 3.13. PTT dysfunction typically causes posteromedial ankle pain, but symptoms may also be noted in the medial arch. In addition, an insertional tendinopathy of the PTT may occur.

Navicular stress injuries

The navicular is one of the most common and potentially serious sites of stress injuries in sport. It is seen in a spectrum of sports, but particularly those involving heavy or repetitive impact loading. Although these injuries are common, a delay in diagnosis is not unusual, which can have devastating effects on the athlete. Predisposing factors, which will need to be identified and addressed as part of the overall assessment, include high training volume on rigid surfaces, a rigid foot, hyperpronation, and other midfoot abnormalities including, rarely, tarsal coalition. The typical presentation is one of a vague midfoot ache, worse on impact and pushing off. Symptoms may settle with rest, but as the condition worsens rest and night pain occurs. There is localized tenderness on palpation of the navicular.

Isotope bone scan will show increased uptake in the navicular and MRI will demonstrate stress reaction within the bone. Careful thin-slice CT scanning with gantry views is necessary to define the injury further. Saxena *et al.* (2000) proposed a CT-based classification system: dorsal cortical break (type I), fracture propagation into the navicular body (type II), and fracture propagation into another cortex (type III). Modifiers were A (**a**vascular necrosis of a portion of the navicular), C (**c**ystic changes of the fracture), and S (**s**clerosis of the margins of the fracture), which was seen particularly in continually symptomatic patients. Type I fractures were more likely to receive conservative treatment ($p = 0.02$) and type III fractures took significantly longer to heal than types I and II ($p = 0.001$ and $p = 0.01$, respectively). Type I and II injuries had an average return to activity of 3.0 months and 3.6 months, respectively, whereas type III injuries required 6.8 months. Saxena and colleagues recommended surgery for patients with these modifiers, particularly with type II and III injuries. Conservative treatment consists of strict non-weight-bearing in a below-knee cast/boot for a minimum of 6 weeks, but this may be prolonged. Assessment of progress is based on clinical grounds, as imaging changes are slow and can correlate poorly with injury status. Persisting tenderness of the navicular should be managed as ongoing stress injury.

Surgery for navicular stress fractures should be considered in the following circumstances:

* displacement and/or comminution
* recurrent injury
* sclerotic fracture margins
* failure to heal after adequate conservative management
* high-demand athletes.

Surgery consists of stabilizing and compressing the reduced fracture using of transversely placed screws. If the fracture appears indolent, it should be opened and freshened, and bone grafted prior to fixation.

The painful accessory navicular

An accessory navicular is a congenital variant, where the navicular tuberosity develops from a secondary centre of ossification. It is seen in up to 14% of the population and is usually asymptomatic, but can occasionally cause medial foot pain. Patients usually present in early adolescence and are generally active individuals.

The patient may present with pain or, in more advanced cases, with progressive PTT dysfunction and flattening of the arch. Radiographs confirm the presence of an accessory bone, although MRI will demonstrate a stress reaction and the health of the distal PTT.

Table 3.14.9 Causes of medial foot pain

Posterior tibial tendinopathy
Symptomatic accessory navicular
Flexor hallucis longus tendinopathy
Tarsal tunnel syndrome
Disorder of lateral plantar nerve or its first branch
Talonavicular arthritis
Navicular stress fracture
Tarsometatarsal arthritis
First ray instability
Great toe
Turf toe
Hallux rigidus
Hallux valgus
Sesamoiditis
Toenail problems

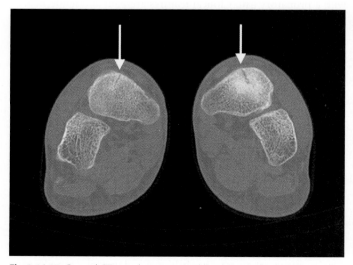

Fig. 3.14.17 Coronal CT scan demonstrating bilateral navicular stress fractures (arrows).

Management

Initial treatment for the significantly symptomatic patient is provision of a medial longitudinal arch support or walking cast, relative rest, and analgesics. Progress may be slow. As pain settles a gradual strengthening regime can be commenced. In those cases where this is not successful, operative intervention may be considered (Grogan *et al.* 1989).

Excision of the ossicle involves enucleating it from the distal posterior tibial tendon. Isolated removal of the bone is rarely sufficient. It is usually necessary to reattach and advance the tendon to the exposed navicular surface (Kidner procedure). Bone anchors allow satisfactory purchase. Reinforcement of the spring ligament helps to support a sagging talo-navicular joint (Chater 1962). The majority of patients have good or excellent results from surgery, but rehabilitation can be prolonged.

Foot conditions in the younger athlete

Like other skeletal regions, the foot is not immune to the development of certain conditions during the growth phases of childhood and adolescence. Sometimes such problems do not manifest themselves until adulthood and, undoubtedly, much goes undetected during life. The conditions clinicians should be aware of are:

- Sever's apophysitis of the calcaneum
- Kohler's disease of the navicular
- accessory navicular (see above)
- Freiberg's disease
- sesamoiditis (see below)
- pes planovalgus
- cavovarus foot
- tarsal coalition.

Calcaneal apophysitis (Sever's disease)

Calcaneal apophysititis, or Sever's disease, is a cause of heel pain at the insertion of the Achilles tendon in young children and adolescents. Like other apophysitides, it is aggravated by activity, and is seen in particular during active phases of growth and is associated with a pronatory gait. Clinical features are pain and tenderness of the posterior and inferior aspects of the calcaneum with or without signs of inflammation. The condition can further be assessed using imaging in the form of plain radiographs which may show delayed fusion and fragmentation of the secondary centre of ossification. Ultrasound confirms these changes and helps to exclude other coexistent lesions such as retrocalcaneal bursitis. An index of suspicion for other paediatric conditions causing heel pain should be maintained for those cases which do not improve with appropriate treatment or whose initial clinical features contain any worrying features. Such conditions in particular include bone injuries (fractures, stress fractures), tumours, and seronegative enthesopathies.

Counselling, restriction of impact activities, hamstring and calf flexibility work, lower limb and core strengthening, a review of footwear, heel raises or orthotics, and post-exercise icing are all helpful.

Kohler's disease of the navicular

This is a true osteonecrosis of the navicular. It is rare, affecting males more than females and with a maximum incidence at age 3–7 years It should be borne in mind in a young dancer or athlete who presents with medial midfoot pain.

Freiberg's disease or infraction

Once again this is a true osteonecrosis of the metatarsal head, most commonly affecting the second metatarsal. It is more common in females, with a peak incidence at age 10–15 years. The patient presents with pain and limitation of movement of the MTP joint. The area is usually thickened. X-rays reveal osteosclerosis in the early stages with later osteolysis and then head collapse. Later images show an abnormally flattened irregular head with new bone formation and occasional fragmentation with loose ossicles.

The initial treatment should be rest from aggravating activities, initially involving immobilization if symptoms dictate. Orthotics to relieve weight-bearing below the damaged head are helpful. Later treatment may include debulking and debridement of the joint, and rarely osteotomies or head excision for advanced arthritic changes.

Pes planovalgus and cavovarus feet

There is no such entity as a 'normal' foot position. Like most biological structures, there is a spectrum of appearances which come within what is accepted as a normal range.

Foot and ankle position causes considerable concern for patients and parents alike. Orthopaedic paediatric clinics have many referrals for such assessments. The world of high athletic endeavour is littered with sports people who have achieved the highest goals despite possessing an exceedingly 'flat foot' or 'high arch'. The importance for the clinician at such an assessment is to identify any red flags which indicate further investigation, for instance:

- foot asymmetry (e.g. unilateral planovalgus or cavovarus foot)
- evidence for recent deterioration in foot position
- excessive pain
- abnormal associated neurology
- stiff hindfoot or midfoot joints
- clawing of digits in association with a cavovarus foot.

For the majority of patients and parents, reassurance is all that is required. Stretching and strengthening programmes can be utilized to prevent deterioration. Advice on appropriate footwear is helpful, and orthotics can improve comfort during activity but are unlikely to improve the overall foot appearance in the long term.

Tarsal coalition

Tarsal coalition represents an abnormal union between two or more tarsal bones. The overall incidence in the population is about 1%. The majority are probably never diagnosed. The three most common coalitions are:

- talo-calcaneal
- calcaneo-navicular
- talo-navicular.

The coalition can be fibrous, cartilaginous, or osseous. The last is more likely to present earlier because of the stiffness and altered mechanics it causes.

Patients can present with what is described as a 'simple ankle sprain' that is not improving. Others may present with pain, stiffness, progressive planovalgus foot, and limited movement. X-rays will frequently demonstrate osseous coalitions, but a normal image does not exclude the diagnosis. CT and MRI will confirm the presence and extent of any coalition. Once the diagnosis has been made, the patient should be referred to a specialist centre for further assessment. Results from surgical interventions are better in the skeletally immature. Once degenerative changes have become established, improvement with simple excision is reduced. Grossly damaged hindfoot joints caused by secondary arthritis may require an arthrodesis.

Midfoot impingement syndromes

Midfoot pain, particularly at the first metatarsal–cuneiform joint, can be caused by mechanically induced joint synovitis or small degenerative osteophytes. This is most commonly seen in those with biomechnical gait abnormalities, either functional or due to structural pathology anywhere in the ankle or foot. Treatment is by biomechanical correction where possible. Local injection with corticosteroid or viscosupplement under imaging guidance can also provide symptomatic relief.

Be aware of the possibility of impingement of the deep peroneal nerve as it passes dorsally towards the first intermetatarsal space. Impingement between an osteophyte and shoewear during activity causes pain and altered feeling in the first webspace.

Surgery to remove osteophytes and, if necessary, decompress the nerve can be undertaken in cases which do not respond to conservative treatment. Patients should be counselled that it will not reverse any pain from degenerative changes from within any joint. Patients with high arched feet (pes cavus) frequently have prominent dorsal bosses of bone. Excision of such prominences does not change the overall shape of the foot and such patients need to be counselled carefully to avoid postoperative dissatisfaction.

Medial arch pain

Distal plantar fascial pain is discussed below.

Medial forefoot pain

FHL tendinopathy

FHL tendon disorders most commonly occur at the entrance to the fibro-osseous tunnel, at the level of the sustentaculum tali. This causes posteromedial ankle pain and crepitus, as described in Chapter 3.13. In the foot, FHL tenosynovitis can occur at the level of the sesamoid complex or proximal to it in the midfoot. Typically occurring in dancers, it is also seen in runners, jumpers, gymnasts, and springboard divers. As in the ankle, tenosynovitis is the most common form of FHL tendinopathy in the foot and may be stenosing in nature. It causes swelling, crepitus, and triggering beneath the first MTPJ. In dancers, symptoms are worse with movements onto the ball of the foot (*demi-pointe*) and onto the tip of the toe (*pointe*).

FHL tendinopathy is associated with overuse, hard surfaces, inappropriate footwear, poor technique, and, in dancers, excessive turnout at the hip so that the dancer is not centred over the feet. Weakness and inadequate flexibility of the lower leg and foot also contribute.

Examination findings include local tenderness and crepitus along the course of the tendon and at the sesamoid complex. In stenosing tenosynovitis (trigger toe), triggering may be described but is difficult to localize, although a palpable nodule and the site of a sensation of popping or snapping felt by the patient may act as a

guide. Symptoms are exacerbated by the movement of the hallux. There is pain with passive, active, and resisted movements of the toe.

Trigger toe, which can be mistaken for a functional hallux rigidus, is associated with an inability to extend the great toe at the metatarsal and interphalangeal joints, usually after forcible flexion of the FHL. The toe can be flexed with ease with the foot in a neutral position but, when the foot is plantarflexed, flexion at the first MTP is not possible. Release is achieved by gentle passive extension of the toe.

Tears of FHL in the foot are less common than tenosynovitis and are usually due to direct trauma, in particular a laceration.

Management

In the acute phase, FHL tenosynovitis is treated by relative rest with avoidance of exacerbating activities, local regular icing and NSAIDs, and the use of an orthotic. The underlying cause must be addressed and the patient advised that recovery may be slow.

When conservative treatment fails, surgical treatment should be considered. This consists of release of the FHL tendon through a posteromedial incision. If the entrapment is associated with posterior impingement, this is addressed through the same incision. If the entrapment occurs in the mid- or forefoot, the tendon is released in the respective area.

Sesamoid injuries

The sesamoid complex of the hallux works to give FHL a mechanical advantage and considerable forces are transmitted through it. Injuries to the complex are often grouped under the term 'sesamoiditis.'

Turf toe

The term 'turf toe' is often used to describe injuries of the first MTPJ. It was initially described by Bowers and Martin (1976) as a dorsiflexion and eversion or inversion injury to the first MTPJ, resulting in a ligamentous sprain of the sesamoid complex. Turf toe was initially most commonly seen in American football, where there is a high incidence, probably as a result of hard playing surfaces and a change in footwear from stiff-soled cleats to more flexible footwear. The injury is also seen in other sports, such as soccer, field hockey, basketball, and track events, along with the occasional episode in the non-sporting individual. Where an additional axial load was present at the time of injury, additional cartilaginous lesions, fractures, or diastasis of a bipartitie sesamoid may be present. Sprains have been classified according to their severity (Table 3.14.10). Although rare, dislocations of the great toe share a

Table 3.14.10 Classification of turf toe

Grade	Description
I	Stretching of capsuloligamentous complex. There is local plantar tenderness, mild swelling, and minimal loss of range of motion, and the athlete is able to bear weight with only mild symptoms.
II	Partial tear of capsuloligamentous complex. Findings include moderate swelling, bruising, and moderate restriction of 1st MTPJ.
III	Complete tear of capsuloligamentous complex with plantar plate/articular injury. Significant swelling, restriction, and disability.

Reproduced from Clanton, T.O. and Ford, J.J. (1994). Turf toe injury. *Clinics in Sports Medicine*, **13**, 731–5.

similar mechanism of injury. The classification in Table 3.14.10 can be extended to include dislocations.

An isolated dorsal dislocation of the first MTP joint should be distinguished from an injury involving additionally the sesamoid ligament and/or a sesamoid fracture. The latter will indicate a more severe injury, likelihood of delayed healing, and long-term disability.

The patient usually presents with a clear description of the mechanism of injury, usually involving aggressive push-off and/or pivoting. There is swelling and tenderness at the first MTPJ, which is worse with movement, particularly on extension of the joint. Stress testing, where possible, will determine the degree of the injury. Additional injuries, in particular a fracture or dislocation of the sesamoid, should be excluded by a series of X-rays including AP, lateral, and, if possible, sesamoid views. The images should be compared with the opposite side. Proximal migration of the sesamoids indicates plantar plate avulsion, confirmed by a lack of movement of the sesamoids from neutral to dorsiflexion on a stress dorsiflexion view. MRI and/or CT may be required to evaluate the lesion clearly.

Management

If plain radiographs are normal, the patient is managed conservatively, with rest in a walking boot for 3 weeks, ice massage, and NSAIDs, until the swelling subsides. Pain and swelling may take many weeks to settle. When symptoms permit, the patient may return to normal activities (including sports) with supportive taping of the hallux in slight plantarflexion and advice to wear stiff supportive shoes.

A total contact functional orthosis with a Morton extension may be necessary in the long term. Surgery is indicated in those patients with a grade III sprain where there are chondral flaps or loose bodies in the joint. If a fracture–dislocation has occurred, surgical reduction is undertaken. Surgical repair of the sesamoid complex is may be indicated.

Sesamoiditis

The aetiology of sesamoid pain can be divided into two groups. Firstly, there is a group of well-characterized diseases causing pain. These include degenerate and inflammatory arthritis, undue prominence of a sesamoid causing plantar keratoses, and, rarely, infection. The second group is seen more commonly in sport, and consists of conditions where there is a debate as to nomenclature and pathology. This group includes sesamoiditis, avascular necrosis, congenital partitism, stress fracture, chondromalacia, and osteochondritis of the sesamoid. The clinical presentation of all of these conditions is identical: pain. As the disease progresses, the surrounding structures, particularly the FHL, become inflamed with associated pain and dysfunction. Sesamoiditis is associated with forefoot valgus, rigid pes cavus (particularly involving an excessively plantarflexed first ray), and the existence of a multipartite sesamoid.

Plain radiographs (AP, oblique, lateral, and axial views) may be necessary to determine if the sesamoid is partite or fractured: a partite sesamoid is regular, with smooth borders and little separation. Diastasis of a partite sesamoid can be demonstrated by a stress view with the hallux dorsiflexed. In the early stages bone scanning is often positive, even if the radiographs are normal. MRI will demonstrate the morphology of the sesamoid complex and will show increased signal intensity if there is sesamoiditis, often on the interface with the first MTPJ where there may be synovitis.

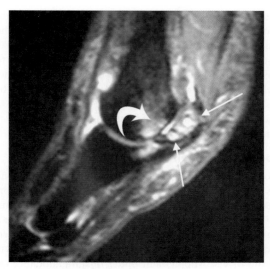

Fig. 3.14.18 Sagittal STIR MRI though the first metatarsophalangeal joint. Note the inflamed medial sesamoid (arrow) with reactive bone marrow oedema in the under-surface of the first metatarsal head (curved arrow).

Differentiating between bipartite and fractured sesamoids can be difficult. The former more frequently affect the medial sesamoid and show smooth margins; in a fracture there is a sharp or hypointense fracture line with bone oedema. CT is helpful in distinguishing between the two pathologies.

Histological examination of sesamoiditis reveals a non-united fracture to be the underlying pathology in the majority of the cases. Avascular necrosis appears to be secondary to the fracture, rather than vice versa.

Management

Management of sesamoiditis is relative rest with activity modification. A change in footwear to shoes with enhanced cushion and support, a total contact orthosis with metatarsal relief, and regular ice and NSAIDs may be enough. In some, a 6-week period of non-weight-bearing in a cast may be necessary. A review of gait mechanics when pain free is vital.

Surgical intervention should be considered for those who fail to respond to conservative treatment. The medial (tibial) sesamoid can be approached medially. Depending on the pathology, the whole sesamoid, or part of it in the case of a bipartite or fragmented sesamoid, can be removed. A particularly bulky sesamoid can be shaved down on its non-articular surface. The patient should be warned that the removal of the whole sesamoid can cause the hallux to drift into valgus.

The lateral (fibular) sesamoid can be approached via a dorsal first webspace incision or more commonly a plantar approach. Sesamoid surgery must respect the FHL tendon, which can easily be damaged during the procedure. Any excessive first-ray plantarflexion can be dealt with by a basal dorsiflexion metatarsal osteotomy.

Hallux valgus

Hallux valgus can be problematic in the sportsperson and causes forefoot symptoms in a number of ways. There may be pain over the 'bunion' area itself, or secondary problems caused by altered forefoot biomechanics such as pain in the second MTPJ secondary to synovitis, clawing of the lesser toes, or formation of Morton's neuromas.

Initial treatment should concentrate on avoidance of those activities exacerbating the symptoms, anti-inflammatory medication, and shoe modification. An orthosis, to be fitted within shoes, should also be considered. A soft medial longitudinal arch support is often helpful. In the presence of lesser toe involvement, metatarsal padding may be required.

Surgical correction is successful in the majority of individuals in the general population. However, in the athlete or dancer, surgery needs to be approached with great caution. There are many surgical options depending on the deformity. However, whatever choice is made, rehabilitation back to sport will be prolonged and foot mechanics will be altered, sometimes in an unpredictable manner. For instance, Mann *et al.* (1992) have shown that the satisfaction rate with a proximal crescentic metatarsal osteotomy was 93%. However, postoperatively the range of dorsiflexion was only 55°, only 59% could wear any shoe that they desired, and only 39% believed that they could perform more activities on their feet than they could preoperatively. Therefore we believe that it is sensible to delay hallux valgus corrective surgery until the symptoms begin to threaten the level of performance in sport or dance, and that the individual should be carefully counselled regarding potential complications.

Osteoarthritis of the first MTPJ

This is not uncommon even in the young athlete. Early osteoarthritis presents with pain and variable swelling, exacerbated at push-off. With progressive disease, the joint becomes stiff and this can have consequences in other areas of the foot. Treatment includes joint mobilization, stretching, an orthotic to enhance forefoot function, analgesia, and, if necessary, viscosupplement or corticosteroid injection.

Surgical options are limited in an active athlete. Significant arthritis in the joint requires careful counselling of the patient with regard to appropriate future sport.

If the patient's symptoms are predominantly dorsal and X-rays demonstrate prominent dorsal osteophytes, a cheilectomy with general joint debridement and sesamoid mobilization can be undertaken. An excessively long first metatarsal can be shortened and plantarflexed with an appropriate metatarsal osteotomy. Dorsiflexion can be regained, at the expense of the less useful plantarflexion, by a proximal phalangeal osteotomy of the Moberg variety.

More severe arthritis requiring some form of arthrodesis or arthroplasty is unlikely to be compatible with high-level impact sport, although patients do return to activities such as golf, tennis, and gentle jogging.

Osteochondral defects and loose bodies in the first MTPJ

Osteochondral defects, leading on occasions to loose bodies, within the first MTP joint can be a cause of pain, swelling, and a feeling of 'locking' for an athlete. Sometimes the patient can feel a loose body on the dorsal surface. Synovitis and swelling can be present.

X-rays may demonstrate early arthritis, a local defect of the first metatarsal head, or a loose body. If the loose body is predominantly chondral it may not be seen easily on X-ray and further imaging with MRI will be required.

Table 3.14.11 Causes of posterior heel pain

Achilles tendinopathies
Retro-achilles bursitis
Retrocalcaneal bursitis
Posterior impingement
Referred pain
(Pain related to Haglund deformity (discuss as aetiological factor))
(Bony injuries: talar dome, os trigonum and calcaneal fractures/stress fractures)

Surgery is aimed at removing any loose bodies, undertaking a synovectomy, and debriding the damaged articular surface. An area of local full-thickness wear of the first metatarsal head can be subjected to microfracturing to encourage some healing with fibrocartilage. Arthroscopy of the joint can be utilized to remove a loose body.

Hindfoot pain

Achilles tendinopathies and associated syndromes have been discussed in an earlier chapter.

Calcaneal stress injuries

These are typically seen in high-impact sports and the military. Stress fractures of the os calcis should be considered in atypical heel pain, particularly in athletes undergoing repetitive impact loading (e.g. long-distance running). Bony pain and tenderness are present, usually aggravated by any attempt to return to sport. Plain X-rays may reveal disruption of the normal bony architecture, but a negative film(s) does not exclude the diagnosis. MRI or technetium isotope scans are required to confirm the diagnosis. Treatment requires rest until symptoms settle. Once the patient is comfortable, a review of training schedules and biomechanical problems and a podiatric assessment are helpful. Nutritional status should be established and, in females, any menstrual irregularities noted. Both may cause osteoporosis and hence increase the risk of stress fractures.

Calcaneal fractures

Calcaneal fractures can be a devastating injury for any athlete. They account for 2.6% of all fractures, but 60% of major hindfoot injuries. The most common mechanism of injury is a fall from a height. The greater the impact, the more likely is a degree of comminution of fracture fragments and displacement. The history should raise the possibility of such a fracture. The patient should be cleared of any concomitant spinal or pelvic injuries. The hindfoot will be tender and swollen. Widening of the heel is often present. Significant swelling can cause a compartment syndrome within the plantar aspect of the foot.

Following clinical evaluation, plain X-rays will confirm the diagnosis. A crucial finding is whether the subtalar joint is involved (56–75% of cases). The leg needs elevating to minimize swelling. If the patient is under consideration for surgery, a CT scan usually clarifies the fracture pattern and aids surgical planning. Involvement of the subtalar joint and/or significant fragment displacement usually requires surgery in the athlete. However, surgery can only take place once the soft tissues allow. It is a prolonged and difficult procedure even in experienced hands.

The athlete may require up to 3 months before full weight-bearing can be allowed, and recovery may take up to 2 years. Some degree of subtalar stiffness, swelling, and heel broadening is expected in intra-articular fractures. The risk of subsequent subtalar arthritis is high. Other potential complications include heel pad disruption, peroneal tendon impingement, and nerve damage.

The likelihood for return to previous levels of sporting excellence is remote following a significant os calcis injury.

Plantar heel pain

The causes of plantar heel pain are diverse and differentiation between the individual causes is difficult. A thorough medical history and clinical evaluation are necessary to identify the specific condition involved. The specific site of the pain and its characteristics help to narrow down the diagnostic possibilities.

Proximal plantar fasciitis

Aetiology

During the gait cycle, the MTPJs dorsiflex and the windlass mechanism of the plantar fascia tightens and raises the longitudinal arch. Repetitive traction can occur at the insertion of the plantar fascia, leading to microtears at the insertion. These microtears may have an inflammatory component in the early stages, progressing to show degenerate changes later. Traction at the insertion of the flexor digitorum brevis muscle leads to the formation of calcaneal spurs over time, which are seen in 50% of patients and 16% of the asymptomatic population.

Entrapment of Baxter's nerve (1st branch of the lateral plantar nerve to the abductor digiti quinti minimi) is difficult to diagnose clinically, and is said to cause heel pain in 20% of cases (Baxter and Pfeffer 1992).

History and examination

The history is of acute or chronic plantar heel pain. Start-up pain due to tightening of the plantar fascia with rest, particularly overnight, is typical. The pain is also worse with prolonged standing

Table 3.14.12 Causes of pain in the sole of the foot: plantar heel pain

Proximal plantar fasciitis
Plantar fascial rupture
Heel bruise syndrome
Heel pad atrophy
Plantar fibromatosis
Nerve lesion:
Tarsal tunnel syndrome
Disorder of lateral plantar nerve or its first branch
Entrapment/irritation/neuroma
Postoperative neuroma of medial calcaneal sensory nerves
Calcaneal stress fracture
Tumour
Medial calaceneal nerve entrapment

Table 3.14.13 Causes of pain in the sole of the foot: midfoot pain

Mid-substance plantar fasciitis
Plantar fibromatosis
Flexor hallucis longus tendinopathy
Spring ligament injury
Peroneus longus or brevis tendinitis ± avulsion fracture of fifth metatarsal base
Cuboid instability
Tarsometatarsal (Lisfranc's) joint sprain
Tarsal stress fracture/fracture
Neurological: tarsal tunnel syndrome, sural nerve, common or superficial peroneal nerve lesions
Referred pain: root lesions

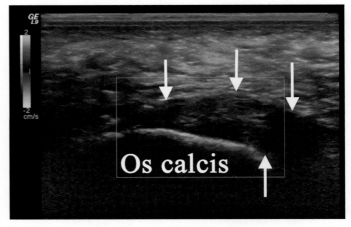

Fig. 3.14.19 Plantar fasciitis in a 42-year-old middle-distance runner. Longitudinal sonogram with transducer placed on heel. Note the markedly thickened plantar fascia (arrows) attached to the medial calcaneal tubercle of the os calcis.

and towards the end of the day. Radiation and neuralgia are unusual and should raise the possibility of an alternative diagnosis.

Examination reveals point tenderness at the medial calcaneal tuberosity, with less marked tenderness 1–2 cm distally. Swelling is absent. Pain on passive dorsiflexion of the toes may be present if the plantar fascia is particularly tight, although this is uncommon. Associated gastrocnemius–soleus tightness should be sought as this can slow response to treatment. It is important to consider associations such as seronegative arthritis and other causes of plantar heel pain (Table 3.14.13).

Typical findings on ultrasonography may include swelling of the fascia, with increased thickness, hypoechogenicity, and insertional irregularity of the plantar fascia (Kane *et al.* 2001). MRI will show thickening and signal alterations at the plantar fascial origin (Berkowitz *et al.* 1991). Additionally, bone oedema in the os calcis close to the site of fascial insertion is commonly noted. Although not routinely used, a delayed technetium-99 bone scan will show localized uptake at medial calcaneal insertion (compared with the diffuse uptake shown with a calcaneal stress fracture).

Management

The cause must be addressed; and weight loss and modification of activity levels are usually necessary. In the sportsperson, reducing training volume, in particular the intensity of exercise, and reducing high impact by running on more forgiving surfaces and resorting to swimming and cycling are beneficial. Care must be taken to avoid a compensatory injury through alteration of gait due to pain.

The use of anti-inflammatory approaches including NSAIDs and regular ice massage are recommended, but are of variable benefit. Provision of supportive cushioned footwear, heel inserts, and in some cases orthoses may all provide symptomatic benefit. Dorsiflexion night splints can help to prevent excessive tightening of the plantar fascia overnight. Stretching of the plantar fascia and calf muscles and a programme of strengthening for the intrinsic muscles of the foot should be commenced early. It is important to address areas of joint stiffness in the ankle and foot.

In chronic resistant cases where the above measures have not been effective over 8–12 weeks and rehabilitation is inhibited by pain, a local corticosteroid injection administered under ultrasound guidance is indicated. Injudicious placement of injection, use of long-acting preparations, and multiple injections can all lead to fat pad atrophy and plantar fascial rupture.

A course of treatment with platelet rich plasma therapy and/or extracorporeal shock wave therapy (ESWT) may help to reduce symptoms. There is little evidence for benefit from the use of other modalities such as conventional therapeutic ultrasound, phonophoresis, iontophoresis, and laser in either early or late plantar fasciitis (Crawford 2001). A period of cast immobilization for 3–6 weeks may be tried.

Surgery

In approximately 95% of patients plantar fasciitis resolves after a period of 12–18 months without operative treatment (Sammaro and Helfey 1996; Crawford 2001). This leaves a small number of patients with recalcitrant, but significant, symptoms.

Many surgical procedures are described ranging from percutaneous release to endoscopic release to open procedures. The structures that are treated surgically include mobilization of abductor hallucis and its superficial and deep fascia, release of the plantar fascia, excision of the calcaneal 'spur', and release of the first branch of the lateral plantar nerve to the abductor digiti quinti minimi (Baxter's nerve). We prefer to perform a partial plantar fascial release and release of Baxter's nerve using an open technique. The reported success rate of such an approach is that 76% of patients have only mild or no postoperative pain. Careful counselling of patients is required since in one study only 49% of patients were totally satisfied with the outcome (Davies *et al.* 1999).

Plantar fascial rupture

Acute plantar fascial rupture presents with the acute onset of proximal heel pain and, in some cases, more diffuse symptoms in the lateral or medial midfoot, often with associated swelling and bruising and inability to continue to weight-bear. Most commonly, the injury occurs at push-off when running, jumping, or lunging. Plantar fascial rupture may also occur after a steroid injection for plantar fasciitis. Less commonly, the injury can occur with acute hyperextension of the midfoot as a result of the foot becoming jammed (e.g. in a pothole) when walking or running.

On examination there is often local bruising and tenderness at the medial calcaneal tubercle, and there may be a palpable defect.

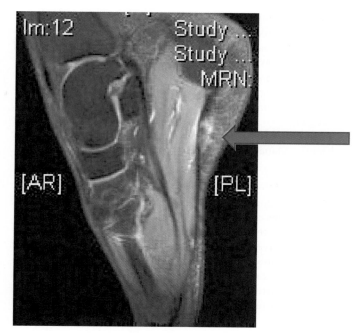

Fig. 3.14.20 MRI showing a mid-substance plantar fascia longitudinal split.

The fascia may be tender more distally and there is diminished tension in the plantar fascia with windlass stretch testing.

Management involves the use of NSAIDs and regular ice, supportive shoes with a medial longitudinal arch support, and, if necessary, a non-weight-bearing cast for 4–8 weeks. Symptoms usually resolve over the course of 6–8 weeks (Ahstrom 1988), although recovery time can be significantly longer in those who have ruptured after a steroid injection (Acevado and Beskin 1998).

Heel fat pad pain

Pain may arise directly from the fat pad in a number of circumstances.

Heel fat pad atrophy

This typically occurs in the older patient, particularly if overweight, who reports heel pain when walking on hard surfaces or wearing hard shoes. Unlike other causes of heel pain, the overlying skin may be inflamed. The fat pad is thin and prominent calcaneal tubercles are easily palpable. Maximum tenderness is located in the central weight-bearing portion of pad.

Management includes the use of analgesics, including NSAIDs, and ice, particularly after activity. Heel cups are usually more useful than in proximal plantar fasciitis. A shock-absorbing insert may also be beneficial and a slight heel elevation may help by shifting the weight anteriorly. High-impact activities should be avoided and obese patients should be instructed to lose weight. There is no place for the use of corticosteroids or surgical intervention.

Painful heel fat pad syndrome

The heel pad can become very painful in individuals without obvious fat pad atrophy, typically in the heavy patient or after high impact, due to bleeding into the fat pad. With the exception of thinning of the pad, the clinical features and management are similar to those with fat pad atrophy.

Piezogenic papules

Piezogenic papules present as white subcutaneous papules which form with the coalescence of the fat chambers. They are associated with degenerative changes in the dermis of the heel pad. The papules develop and appear with weight-bearing. In the majority of cases they are painless, and the patient can be reassured. In rare cases they become painful. It is not clear why they are painful, although it has been suggested that herniation of subcutaneous fat through defects in the dermis due to impact may lead to areas of ischaemia. Management is symptomatic; a heel cup or orthosis may be effective.

Separation of the heel fat pad

Separation of the heel fat pad from its anchor on the plantar aspect of the calcaneus can occur after significant trauma to the region. A cyst forms between the calcaneus and the fat pad; the pad becomes painful and is freely mobile. MRI scanning is diagnostic. Treatment involves aspiration of the cyst and then immobilization in a non-weight-bearing cast. Occasionally surgical resection of the cyst and several millimetres of calcaneus is required. A firm dressing is applied postoperatively. The aim of surgery is to allow the heel pad to reattach.

Other causes of heel pad pain

Rarely, calcification can be seen in the heel pad, presumably following microtrauma and organization of areas of bleeding. Foreign bodies (e.g. thorns and metallic objects) from sporting activities can be a cause of infection, pain, and irritation in the heel pad.

Nerve entrapment

Proximal or distal tarsal tunnel syndrome

Proximal or distal tarsal tunnel syndrome (entrapment of the first branch of the lateral plantar nerve) may cause intractable heel pain or more diffuse symptoms as described above. Entrapment or irritation of the first branch of the lateral plantar nerve (**Baxter's nerve**) is a commonly cited cause of heel pain. The nerve is typically trapped by a well-developed abductor hallucis, and is said to be a factor in 20% of cases of heel pain (Henricson and Westlin 1984). It is particularly common in those athletes whose sport involves substantial activity on their toes, such as sprinters, dancers, figure skaters, and gymnasts.

The nerve is also vulnerable at the medial calcaneal tuberosity. Local inflammation, swelling, fibrosis, and spur formation in and around the flexor digitorum brevis muscle can lead to compression of the nerve against the long plantar ligament. Therefore it is possible that proximal plantar fasciitis can lead to nerve entrapment.

The diagnosis is clinical. Symptoms are a burning or sharp pain in the heel, which may radiate distally into the lateral foot. Pain is noted particularly after prolonged weight-bearing and towards the end of the day, in comparison with the typical morning start-up pain of proximal plantar fasciitis. Some patients note symptoms only when running or in other activities. Tenderness is maximum where the nerve is compressed between the deep taut fascia of the abductor hallucis muscle and the medial caudal margin of the quadratus plantae muscle. As described above, there may also be features suggestive of proximal plantar fasciitis. Although weakness of the abductor digiti minimi is reported, this muscle is not present in all individuals and therefore this is not a helpful clinical sign. There is no sensory deficit and paraesthesia with palpation or percussion is a rare feature.

Neurophysiology studies can be normal, but with the refinement of electrodiagnostic techniques, isolated entrapment of nerves such as the lateral plantar nerve and its branches is possible. Nerve conduction velocities are diminished and there may be prolonged distal motor latencies.

Fortunately, management is similar to that of proximal plantar fasciitis and most cases will settle with such conservative measures. Hyperpronators often benefit from a medial longitudinal arch support. A tricyclic agent such as amitryptiline can be effective in symptom control. The surgical approach is discussed in the section dealing with proximal plantar fasciitis.

Medial calcaneal nerve entrapment

Injury or entrapment of the medial calcaneal nerve, a sensory nerve, can result in burning pain, stabbing pain, itching, or tingling around the medial plantar heel, particularly after a period of weight-bearing. Causes include trauma, including after injection and surgery for proximal plantar fasciitis, a congenital accessory abductor hallucis muscle, overuse, hyperpronation, and compression by local lesions such as a rheumatoid nodule.

Electrodiagnostic studies may be normal but can be helpful in demonstrating delayed conduction velocity through the nerve.

Management is similar to that used for proximal plantar fasciitis and lateral plantar nerve entrapment. The underlying cause(s) are addressed. In the acute phase, a trial of a NSAID and strapping to support the plantar aponeurosis can be made. Stretching of the gastrocnemius–soleus complex and plantar fascia, control of hyperpronation by the use of orthoses, and/or a tricyclic agent may be necessary. Surgical intervention is reported as being successful in the resistant case (Sammarco and Mangone 2000), although the branches are small and sometimes difficult to identify fully amongst the fibrous tissue on the medial side of the heel.

Other causes of plantar heel pain must always be considered. A **glomus tumour** is occasionally found in the heel and is exquisitely painful. Management is surgical removal. **Calcaneal injuries**, in particular stress fracture,s are part of the differential diagnosis, particularly in the runner. A positive calcaneal squeeze test is an indication to obtain an isotope bone scan or (in those with chronic symptoms) a plain radiograph.

Arch pain

Distal plantar fasciitis

Distal plantar fasciitis is rare compared with proximal plantar fasciitis, but is still a significant source of medial foot pain. It presents with pain located in the mid-portion of the plantar fascia, usually of gradual onset. It occurs particularly in individuals with pes planus or pes cavus, as more stress is transmitted through the mid-portion of the plantar fascia. It is also seen in sprinters and middle-distance runners who run on their toes.

The main differential diagnoses are FHL tenosynovitis and plantar fibromatosis, but careful palpation of the structures involved and resisted testing of FHL will help to differentiate between the conditions. Isolated entrapment of the medial plantar nerve at the navicular tuberosity can also occur, and leads to symptoms mimicking distal plantar fasciitis.

Distal plantar fasciitis is often more resistant to treatment than is the proximal condition. Management involves the standard strategy of pain relief (simple analgesics and/or NSAIDs), relative rest, activity modification, appropriate footwear, and regular ice massage. Stretching of the plantar fascia and calf muscles is recommended, although the plantar fascia itself is usually not as tight as in those with proximal plantar fasciitis. Although a medial longitudinal arch support is usually not tolerated as it irritates the affected tissue, a medial heel wedge may be useful. Circumferential taping of the midfoot using 1 inch tape over a non-adhesive elastic wrap may be tolerated and provides short-term relief. Patients can be taught to apply the taping themselves.

Surgery is occasionally indicated in those patients who do not settle with non-operative treatment, and in this case a simple partial plantar fascial release is undertaken.

The authors have encountered a series of ruptures of the fascia in the midfoot region. The medial fascial region is almost always involved. Ultrasound examination will confirm the presence of a partial tear. The mechanism of injury, clinical features (apart from site), and treatment are similar to ruptures at the origin.

Plantar fibromatosis

Plantar fibromatosis is a common benign condition of unknown origin, in which there is nodular proliferation of the medial border of the plantar fascia. It is not sports related but forms part of the differential diagnosis of plantar and medial arch pain. Patients present with painful nodules on the plantar aspect of the foot during weight-bearing. The nodules are usually located on the medial side, just proximal to the first MTPJ. Nodules are usually multiple and less than 2 cm in diameter. Management is symptomatic with reassurance. The acute pain usually settles and surgical resection is required only in rare instances. Recurrence and multiple nodules occur. There is an association with Dupuytren's contractures in the hand and, in males, Peyronie's disease of the penis.

References

Acevado, J.I. and Beskin, J.L. (1998). Complications of plantar fascial rupture associated with steroid injection. *Foot and Ankle International*, **19**, 91–7.

Ahstrom, J.P., Jr (1988). Spontaneous rupture of the plantarfascia. *American Journal of Sports Medicine*, **16**, 306–7.

Baxter, D.E. and Pfeffer, G.B. (1992). Treatment of chronic heel pain by surgical release of the first branch of the lateral plantar nerve. *Clinical Orthopaedics and Related Research*, **279**, 229–36.

Berkowitz, J.F., Kier, R., and Rudicel, S. (1991). Plantar fasciitis: MR imaging. *Radiology*, **179**, 665–7.

Bowers, K.D. and Martin, R.B. (1976). Turf toe: a shoe-surface related football injury. *Medicine and Science in Sports and Exercise*, **8**, 81.

Chater, E.H. (1962). Foot pain and the accessory navicular bone. *Irish Journal of Medical Science*, **37**, 442–71.

Chuckpaiwong, B., Cook, C., Pietrobon, R., and Nunley, J.A. (2007). Second metatarsal stress fracture in sport: comparative risk factors between proximal and non-proximal locations. *British Journal of Sports Medicine*, **41**, 510–14.

Crawford, F. (2001). Plantar heel pain (including plantar fasciitis). *Clinical Evidence*, **6**, 918–26.

Davies, M.S., Weiss, G.A., and Saxby, T.S. (1999). Plantar fasciitis. How successful is surgical intervention? *Foot and Ankle International*, **20**, 803–7.

Frey, C., Feder, K.S., and DiGiovanni, C. (1999). Arthroscopic evaluation of the subtalar joint: does sinus tarsi syndrome exist? *Foot and Ankle International*, **20**, 185–91.

Grogan, D., Gasser, S., and Ogden, J. (1989). The painful accessory navicular: a clinical and histopathological study. *Foot and Ankle*, **10**, 164–9.

Harty, M.P. (2001). Imaging of pediatric foot disorders. *Radiology Clinics of North America*, **39**, 733–48.

Henricson, A.S. and Westlin, N.E. (1984). Chronic calcaneal pain in athletes: entrapment of the calcaneal nerve? *American Journal of Sports Medicine*, **12**, 152–4.

Kane, D., Greaney, T., Shanahan, M., *et al.* (2001). The role of ultrasonography in the diagnosis and management of idiopathic plantar fasciitis. *Rheumatology*, **40**, 1002–8.

Kolt, G.S. and Kirkby, R.J. (1999). Epidemiology of injury in elite and subelite female gymnasts: a comparison of retrospective and prospective findings. *British Journal of Sports Medicine*, **33**, 312–18.

Krause, J.O. and Brodsky, J.W. (1998). Peroneal tendon tears: pathophysiology, surgical reconstruction and clinical results. *Foot and Ankle International*, **19**, 271–9.

McHardy, A., Pollard, H., and Luo, K. One-year follow-up study on golf injuries in Australian amateur golfers. *American Journal of Sports Medicine*, **35**, 1354–60.

Mann, R.A., Rudicel, S., and Graves, S.C. (1992). Hallux valgus repair utilizing a distal soft tissue procedure, and proximal metatarsal osteotomy: a long term follow up. *Journal of Bone and Joint Surgery*, **74**, 124–9.

Myerson, M.S., Fisher, R.T., Burgess, A.R., and Kenzora, J.E. (1986). Fracture dislocations of the tarsometatarsal joints: end results correlated with pathology and treatment. *Foot and Ankle*, **6**, 228.

Niva, M.H., Sormaala, M.J., Kiuru, M.J., Haataja, R., Ahovuo, J.A., and Pihlajamaki, H.K. (2007). Bone stress injuries of the ankle and foot: an 86-month magnetic resonance imaging-based study of physically active young adults. *American Journal of Sports Medicine*, **35**, 643–9.

O'Connor, D. (1958). Sinus tarsi syndrome: a clinical entity. *Journal of Bone and Joint Surgery*, **40A**, 720.

Sammarco, G.J. and Mangone, P.G. (2000). Classification and treatment of plantar fibromatosis. *Foot and Ankle International*, **21**, 563–9.

Sammaro, G.J. and Helfrey, R.B. (1996). Surgical treatment of recalcitrant plantar fasciitis. *Foot and Ankle International*, **17**, 520–6.

Sarrafian, S.K. (1983). *Anatomy of the Foot and Ankle* (2nd edn), pp. 52–3. J.B. Lippincott, Piladelphia, PA.

Saxena, A., Fullem, B., and Hannaford, D. (2000). Results of treatment of 22 navicular stress fractures and a new proposed radiographic classification system. *Journal of Foot and Ankle Surgery*, **39**, 96–103.

Sobel, M., Pavlov, H., Geppert, M., *et al.* Painful os peroneum syndrome: a spectrum of conditions responsible for lateral foot pain. *Foot and Ankle*, **15**, 112–24.

Taillard, W., Meyer, J.M., Garcia, J., and Blanc, Y. (1981). The sinus tarsi syndrome. *International Orthopaedics*, **5**, 117–30.

SECTION 4

Special Considerations

4.1

Sports injuries in older people
Cathy Speed

Introduction

A generally enhanced health status in an increasingly ageing population allows many to maintain high physical activity levels, and competitive masters and seniors events are becoming progressively more popular. This, together with the recognition of the importance of exercise to mitigate or even reverse many age-related changes, means that the physician in sport and exercise medicine requires a high index of awareness of the specific issues that arise in relation to sporting injury in the ageing individual. These issues include not only recognition and management of sports injuries *per se*, but also appropriate prescription of exercise in the older individual who may have underlying musculoskeletal and general medical conditions.

Exercise capacity and ageing

The specific features of biological ageing remain an ongoing area of very active research, complicated by the interactions between ageing and disease. Ageing brings physiological, structural, and psychosocial changes that affect the predisposition and response to injury. In addition to the greater predisposition to general medical problems, individual exercise capacity declines with age, even in the healthy, because of a number of age-related biological changes in different systems. These include a range of cardiovascular, respiratory, renal, metabolic, and neuropsychiatric changes, and profound changes in the musculoskeletal system. Hence there are a number of factors that potentially contribute to the decline noted in maximum attainable workload. There is a decrease in the maximum attainable heart rate, reduced respiratory function during exercise, and decreases in neurotransmitter activity.

Many of the musculoskeletal changes noted are at least in part related to a decline in activity levels, so perhaps the greatest threat to the older person is a sedentary lifestyle. Most research on the ageing soft tissue components of the musculoskeletal system has focused on muscle. 'Sarcopenia' still has no definition that has clear consensus, but can at least be broadly described as loss of muscle mass with age. Sarcopenia can be retarded or even reversed with exercise. However, other changes still occur: there is a decrease in size and number of muscle fibres (especially type II fibres, as opposed to the type I fibre atrophy of disuse), suboptimal contractility properties of muscle, slowing in nerve conduction, and alterations at the neuromuscular junction. Changes in muscle fibre types in older athletes may be more a reflection of training status (endurance versus power events) than ageing (Coggan *et al.* 1992), and active seniors may maintain the fibre distribution seen in

younger people. Decrements in muscle strength with increasing age, in addition to delayed reaction times and prolonged speed of movement, are well documented (Fig. 4.1.1). It is possible that the decline in strength is more related to neural changes than to the muscle itself.

Overall, studies have indicated that (i) the magnitude of the age-related effects is not equivalent for all types and speeds of muscle contraction, (ii) there is evidence to suggest that upper and lower limbs are affected disproportionately, and (iii) different muscle groups exhibit different degrees of change. Factors that predict such changes in skeletal muscle function remain unestablished. Furthermore, the impact that specific changes in muscle function at different sites have upon function remains unclear.

Changes in connective tissues such as ligament and tendon also occur with healthy ageing in active people, with a loss of elastic tissue, reduced collagen turnover, alteration in collagen structure and chemical cross-linking of collagen fibrils to one another, and reduced collagen fibre thickness, water, and glycosoaminoglycan content. The result is increased collagen stiffness and a greater potential for injuries, including tendinosis and rupture of tendons and ligaments. Bony resorption at tendon insertions also increases the susceptibility to avulsion injuries.

The degree to which this can be modified by diet and exercise is not known; some of the changes may be secondary to reduced tensile loading from inactive muscle and/or reduced muscle mass and strength from other causes such as low vitamin D levels. The decline in growth and sex hormones and reduced peripheral blood flow

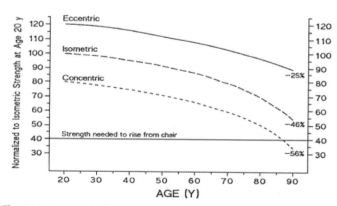

Fig. 4.1.1 An example of the relationship between strength and age. Reproduced from Vandervoort, A.A. (2009). Benefits of warm-up for neuromuscular performance of older athletes. *Exercise and Sport Sciences Reviews*, **37**, 60–5.

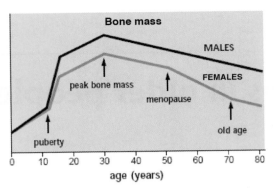

Fig. 4.1.2 Age and bone mass.

may also contribute to the increased tendency to soft tissue injuries—and slower recovery—in older people.

Bone mass also declines with age. Exercise reduces this bone loss, but the decline is associated with an increasing predisposition to bone injury, particularly where there are additional factors present such as altered joint mechanics form arthritic change (Fig. 4.1.2).

A number of additional factors contribute to this susceptibility to musculoskeletal injury. These include slowing in reaction time, postural malalignments, altered balance and proprioception, reductions in neural coordination of sequenced muscle activations and overall cardiorespiratory and muscular endurance, degenerative and inflammatory joint problems, and decline in hearing and/or vision associated with an unsteady gait and cognitive decline.

The effects of these and other changes, and coexistent conditions, results in a decline in exercise capacity with age, even in the fittest. Wright and Perricelli (2008) performed a cross-sectional study of male and female 'Senior Olympians' (>50 years) participating in track and field events at the National Senior Olympic Games in the USA. Demographic and health characteristics and age-related changes in physical performance were determined from mean winning performance times. The performance of senior athletes (male and female) declined by approximately 3.4% per year over 35 years of competition—slowly from age 50 to 75 years and dramatically after age 75 years. Men showed no difference in decline of sprint and endurance events, whereas the decline in sprint events was greater than that in endurance events for women, especially after the age of 75 years.

Epidemiology of sports injuries in older people

Few injury surveillance studies have examined sport-related injury in older people.

Diamond *et al.* (2001) reported that skiing-related head injuries were more common in older people (and children). Ekman *et al.* (2001) reported that the risk of dying due to cycling is about 3.7 times greater among the elderly than among children aged 14 or under. The risk for the elderly being injured or killed is about three times greater than younger adult cyclists, and as much as six times higher for the age group 75–84 years.

McKean *et al.* (2006) performed a retrospective survey of 2886 runners, of whom 34% were masters athletes (>40 years of age). The injury rate for the entire population was 46%. Significantly more masters runners were injured than younger runners ($p < 0.05$).

More masters runners than younger runners suffered multiple injuries ($p < 0.001$). Significantly more masters runners than younger runners ($p < 0.001$) were male, had 7 or more years of running experience, ran more than 30 miles per week, ran six or more times per week, and wore orthotics. The knee and foot were the most common locations of injury for both groups. The prevalence of soft tissue injuries to the calf, Achilles tendon, and hamstrings was greater in masters runners than in their younger counterparts ($p < 0.001$). Younger runners suffered more knee and leg injuries than masters runners ($p < 0.005$). Running more times per week increased the risk of injury for both groups.

Response to injuries in older people

Once an injury has been sustained, recovery time is prolonged. There is a dampening of all three phases (inflammatory, proliferative, and remodelling) of the body's normal response to injury, particularly in soft tissue injuries. Injury in older people can have devastating consequences and may be the determining factor in an individual's degree of independence. Therefore such complaints warrant prompt and thorough attention.

It is important for the physician to be aware of ageism, and to give careful consideration to any injury, avoiding simply attributing musculoskeletal symptoms to ageing. Careful consideration must also be given in planning therapy in older people. Adequate pain relief may be vital in maintaining function, but the use of medications such as NSAIDs is associated with a higher incidence of side effects. The increased incidence of coexisting medical complaints makes interaction with other medications more likely. Tendon rupture after local corticosteroid injection may be more likely because of the presence of degenerative changes, and healing times are prolonged.

Nestorson *et al.* (2000) retrospectively analysed function after Achilles tendon rupture in 25 patients older than 65 years 3 years (1–5 years) after the initial treatment. The median patient age at the time of injury was 71 years (65–86 years). The initial management was surgical in 14 patients and non-surgical (8 weeks immobilization) in 10; one patient was not treated. In both surgically- and non-surgically-treated patients, Achilles function was impaired long term, but the subjective impairment was mild and the patients were able to perform most walking activities. Only nine patients reached their previous activity level. Comorbidity was frequent; 17 patients had other diseases that affected their performance. Five patients sustained a re-rupture (four of these following initial closed treatment with plaster) and nine others had significant complications, but none of these seemed to be age related.

Overall, tendon repairs in older people have poorer outcomes. However, the keen older sportsperson may request surgical intervention despite this risk, given the generally poor outcome if no repair is undertaken. Optimal intervention strategies for significant partial- or full-thickness tendon tears remain an area of research, and decision-taking is based on the individual's needs and expectations.

Rehabilitation programmes must take account of factors that may lead to a reduced capacity to adapt and respond to a treatment programme, including cognitive decline, altered proprioception, expectations, and motivational and psychosocial issues. Such factors can lead to difficulties with compliance, with the patient either expecting 'too much, too soon', or not persevering with the treatment plan.

Table 4.1.1 Interaction between age-related changes in physical function and effects of warm-up

System	Changes with ageing	Effects of warm-up
Muscle	Maximum strength 25–50 years, then decline of 1%/year after 60 years	General body warm-up increases blood flow and body temperature, which speeds up muscle contraction
	↓ No. of motor units	
	↓ No. of muscle fibres	Static and dynamic stretching alters the biomechanical length–tension relationship of shortened tight muscles
	↓ Size of type II fibres	
	Some lean muscle replaced with fat and connective tissue	
Nervous system	Muscle atrophy contributed to by neurological changes	General body warm-up increases blood flow to the brain, which enhances alertness and cognitive function ('getting into the zone')
	37%↓ No. of spinal cord axons	
	10%↓ Nerve conduction velocity in older adults	Dynamic stretching and specific motor rehearsal enhance coordination of muscle activation sequences plus postural control
	↓ Sensory and proprioception function	
	↓ Reflex speed when responding to stimuli	
Skeletal	After third and fourth decade ↓ mineralization of 0.3–0.5%/year	General body warm-up plus static and dynamic stretching gradually increase range of motion for stiffened joints (e.g. shoulders and wrists) to maximum levels needed for full swing
	Over lifetime 35% of cortical and 50% of trabecular bone is lost	
	Men lose only two-thirds of the bone mass that females lose; notable menopause effect	
Connective tissue	Altered proportions and properties of connective components	General body warm-up increases blood flow and body temperature, facilitates elongation of connective tissue
	↑ Stability of cross-links in collagen. ↑ Strength, become non-adaptive	
	↓ Water and ↓ plasticity	Static and dynamic stretching increases the flexibility of the muscle–tendon axis, allowing the golfer to obtain desired biomechanical positions for swing
	Becomes non-pliable, brittle, weak	
	Predisposition to tendon and ligament injury	
Cartilage	Atrophies with age	Weight-bearing activity throughout the warm-up facilitates diffusion of the lubricating fluid into joint space (but need to avoid excessive stresses)
	Proteoglycan subunits smaller	
	↓ Cartilage water content	
	↓ Lubrication of joint	
	Vulnerability to injury	

↑ Increase in variable; ↓ decrease in variable; Gerontological information in the table is based on research summarized in Bellew *et al.*, Nelson *et al.*, Paterson *et al.*, Taylor and Johnson, and Vandervoort.

Reproduced from Vandervoort, A.A. (2009). Benefits of warm-up for neuromuscular performance of older athletes. *Exercise and Sport Sciences Reviews*, **37**, 60–5.

Regardless of age, the most effective strategy for managing injuries is prevention. Patient education on warm-up/down, stretching, posture, aerobic activities (preferably weight-bearing) involving large muscle groups, and a strengthening programme should all be reinforced. Power training may be a more effective strategy in older people than basic resistance strengthening (Porter 2006), but carries at least a theoretically higher risk of injury.

Vandervoort (2009) recommended warm-up prior to an exercise session as a priority in older athletes on the basis of the physiological changes noted in ageing (Table 4.1.1). Warm-up also potentially reduces the cardiovascular risk involved. Further cardiovascular risk reduction involves a full pre-participation assessment in all masters athletes, with peak or symptom-limited exercise testing particularly in those with a moderate to high risk for coronary artery disease, and those who desire to enter vigorous training schedules.

Where the older athlete develops musculoskeletal issues such as osteoarthritis, modification of training patterns is often necessary—in particular, avoiding high-impact activities where possible

and attending to any strength and/or biomechanical issues where appropriate (Table 4.1.2).

Activity after joint replacement

There is an increasing demand by patients to continue sporting activity after lower-extremity total joint arthroplasties. Orthopaedic surgeons frequently recommend participation in low-impact sports, such as swimming, walking, cycling, bowling, and golf, and some recommend avoidance of high-impact sports such as tennis and running postoperatively. This seems to be related to reports in some studies that a higher rate of implant failure occurs with impact activity. However, other studies have reported no negative effects of impact activities. With improving surgical techniques and joint implants, the expectation would be that patients will be able to pursue the activities of their choice without detrimental effect in the future. There is still a need for prospective, randomized controlled studies concerning high activity and its impact on total joint arthroplasty (Seyler *et al.* 2006).

Table 4.1.2 Estimated intensity of joint impact and torsional loading

Joint loading level	Activity	
Low	Recreational swimming	Walking
	Stationary rowing, cycling, or skiing	Water aerobics
	Tai chi	Calisthenics
	Low-impact aerobics	Downhill skiing
	Golf	
Moderate	Bowling	Speed walking
	Fencing	Cross-country skiing
	Cycling	Table tennis
	Rowing	Canoeing
	Ice skating	Hiking
	Rock climbing	Horseback riding
	Doubles tennis	In-line skating
	Weightlifting	
High	Baseball/softball	Lacrosse
	Basketball	Soccer
	Volleyball	Rugby
	American football	Singles tennis
	Handball/racketball	Squash
	Competitive running	

Data from Buckwalter and Martin
Reproduced from Powell, A. (2005). Issues unique to the masters athlete. *Current Sports Medicine Reports*, **4**, 335–40.

Overall, patients do return to sporting activities after joint replacement surgery, but this varies according to the activities involved. Wylde *et al.* (2008) surveyed 2085 patients 1–3 years after joint replacement. They had undergone one of five operations: total hip replacement, hip resurfacing, total knee replacement, unicompartmental knee replacement, or patellar resurfacing. In the 3 years before operation 726 (34.8%) patients were participating in sport, the most common activities being swimming, walking, and golf. A total of 446 (61.4%) had returned to their sporting activities 1–3 years after operation, but 192 (26.4%) were unable to do so because of their joint replacement, with the most common reason being pain. The largest decline was in high-impact sports including badminton, tennis, and dancing. After controlling for the influence of age and gender, there was no significant difference in the rate of return to sport according to the type of operation.

References

Coggan, A., Spina, R., King, D., *et al.* (1992). Skeletal muscle adaptations to endurance training in 60- to 70- year old men and women. *Journal of Applied Physiology*, **72**, 1780–6.

Diamond, P.T., Gale, S.D., and Denkhaus, H.K. (2001). Head injuries in skiers: an analysis of injury severity and outcome. *Brain Injuries*, **15**, 429–34.

Ekman, R., Welander, G., Svanström, L., Schelp, L., and Santesson, P. (2001). Bicycle-related injuries among the elderly—a new epidemic? *Public Health*, **115**, 38–43.

McKean, K.A., Manson, N.A., and Stanish, W.D. (2006). Musculoskeletal injury in the masters runners. *Clinical Journal of Sport Medicine*, **16**, 149–54.

Nestorson, J., Movin, T., Möller, M., and Karlsson, J. (2000). Function after Achilles tendon rupture in the elderly: 25 patients older than 65 years followed for 3 years. *Acta Orthopaedica Scandinavica*, **71**, 64–8.

Porter, M.M. (2006). Power training for older adults. *Applied Physiology, Nutrition and Metabolism*, **31**, 87–94.

Seyler, T.M., Mont, M.A., Ragland, P.S., Kachwala, M.M., and Delanois, R.E. (2006). Sports activity after total hip and knee arthroplasty: specific recommendations concerning tennis. *Sports Medicine*, **36**, 571–83.

Vandervoort, A.A. (2009). Benefits of warm-up for neuromuscular performance of older athletes. *Exercise and Sport Sciences Reviews*, 37, 60–5.

Wright, V.J. and Perricelli, B.C. (2008). Age-related rates of decline in performance among elite senior athletes. *American Journal of Sports Medicine*, **36**, 441–2.

Wylde, V., Blom, A., and Dieppe, P. (2008). Return to sport after joint replacement. *Journal of Bone and Joint Surgery. British Volume*, **90**, 920–3.

Sports injuries in children

Murali Sayana, Chezhiyan Shanmugam, and Nicola Maffulli

Introduction

In the UK, 79% of children aged between 5 and 15 take part in organized sport, and 11% of them are involved in intensive training (Rowley 1989). As a competitive element is introduced, children train harder and longer and participate in sport throughout the whole year. As an undesirable but inevitable consequence, sports-related injuries have increased significantly in children. Approximately 3–11% of schoolchildren are injured annually whilst participating in sport. Twice as many boys as girls sustain sports-related injuries (Crompton and Tubbs 1977; Zaricznyj et al. 1980; Schmidt and Hollwarth 1989; Maffulli and Baxter-Jones 1995).

Children can be divided into three groups depending on age: young children (2–6 years old), older children (6–13 years old), and teenagers (13–19 years old). The growing skeleton in a child is different from the mature skeleton in an adult. A similar mechanism of injury would result in a different injury in a child and and an adult. Therefore the treating physician should take into account the unique features of the paediatric musculoskeletal system when formulating a management plan.

Some of the salient differences between a growing musculoskeletal system and an adult skeleton are as follows.

1. The articular cartilage of growing bone is thicker than that of adult bone.

2. At the junction between the epiphysis and the metaphysis, the physis (growth plate) is vulnerable to disruption, especially from shearing forces. The physis is the weakest of all the structures around a joint in children. Its strength is less than that of bone, capsule, or even the ligaments (Salter and Harris 1963).

3. The tendon and ligament attachment site, or apophysis, is a cartilaginous plate which provides a relatively weak cartilaginous attachment, predisposing to avulsion injuries.

4. The long bones in children have a lower modulus of elasticity and greater plasticity. Paediatric bone is more porous and less dense than adult bone. Thus children tend to suffer incomplete fractures of the greenstick type, buckle fractures, and plastic deformation of bone which do not occur in adults.

5. The strong and thick periosteum of children plays an important role in fracture healing, including remodelling of the bone in the following few years.

6. During rapid growth phases, bone lengthens before muscles and tendons and before the musculotendinous complex develops the necessary strength and coordination to control the newly lengthened bone. This may lead to muscle and tendon injuries (Micheli and Fehlandt 1992), although this is disputed (Feldmann et al. 1999). Growth temporarily reduces coordination (Malina 1994), and this manifests as awkwardness in movement while playing sport.

Children are more likely to injure physis (Fig. 4.2.1), cartilage, and bone or completely avulse an apophysis than to have a significant ligament sprain. Examples of similar mechanisms of injuries resulting in different injuries in children and adults are listed in Table 4.2.1.

In children, traumatic injuries may result in fractures of the long bones or the growth plates. Strong uncoordinated muscle contractions are more likely to lead to an avulsion fracture at the site of attachment of the muscle or tendon rather than a tear of the muscle or tendon itself.

The osteochondroses are another group of conditions affecting children as they involve the growth plates. The aetiology of the osteochondroses is not well understood, and non-articular osteochondroses may well be related to overuse. Detailed discussion of

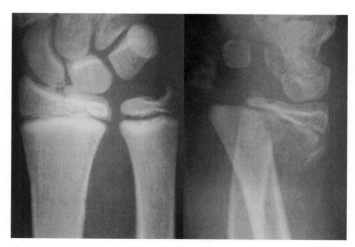

Fig. 4.2.1 Salter–Harris type 2 physeal injury, with positive Thurston–Holland sign.

Table 4.2.1 Comparison of injuries that occur with similar mechanisms in children and adults

Site	Mechanism	Injury in adult	Injury in child
Thumb	Valgus force as in skier's thumb	Sprain of ulnar collateral ligament	Fracture of proximal phalangeal physis (usually Salter–Harris type III)
DIP joint of finger	Hyperflexion injury	Mallet finger	Fracture of distal phalangeal epiphysis (Salter–Harris type II or III)
Hand	Punching injury as in boxing	Fracture of metacarpal head	Fracture of metacarpal epiphysis (Salter–Harris type II)
Shoulder	Fall on point of shoulder	Acromioclavicular joint sprain	Fracture of distal clavicle epiphysis
	Abduction and external rotation force	Dislocated shoulder	Fracture of proximal humeral epiphysis (Salter–Harris type I or II)
Thigh/hip	Acute flexor muscle strain or extensor strain	Quadriceps strain or hamstring strain	Apophyseal avulsion of anterior inferior iliac spine or ischial tuberosity
Knee	Overuse injury	Patellar tendinopathy	Osgood–Schlatter lesion or Sinding-Larsen–Johansson lesion
	Acute trauma (e.g. skiing injury)	Meniscal or ligament injury	Fractured distal femoral or proximal tibial epiphysis, avulsion of tibial spine
Heel	Overuse	Achilles tendinopathy	Sever's apophysitis

every injury is beyond the scope of this chapter. Only the following common paediatric injuries are discussed:

◆ acute fractures

◆ upper limb presentations (shoulder pain, elbow pain, wrist pain)

◆ back pain or postural abnormality

◆ lower limb presentations (hip pain, knee pain, foot pain)

◆ painless abnormalities of gait.

Acute fractures

Three types of fractures can occur in children:

◆ metaphyseal fractures

◆ growth-plate fractures

◆ avulsion fractures.

Metaphyseal fractures

Metaphyseal fractures occur in the forearm and lower leg in particular. The most common type of fracture is buckling of one side of the bone. An incomplete fracture is often referred to as a greenstick fracture. Most fractures of the shaft of long bones that do not involve growth plates can be treated by simple immobilization and will heal quickly, usually within 3 weeks. Occasionally, angular or rotational deformity is present, and may require either closed reduction and casting or open reduction and internal fixation.

Growth-plate fractures

Injury to the growth plate is of particular concern as there is a danger of interruption to the growth owing to injury to the cells in the zone of hypertrophy. Growth-plate fractures are classified according to the Salter–Harris classification (Table 4.2.2). Type I and II fractures usually heal well. Type III and IV fractures involve the joint surface as well as the growth plate and have a relatively high complication rate. If these fractures are not recognized, they could produce permanent injury to the growth plate and the articular cartilage of the joint, resulting in growth disturbance. Therefore an

Table 4.2.2 Salter–Harris classification of physeal injuries

Type	Description
I	Complete separation of the epiphysis and physis (no radiographic changes)
II	Separation of a portion of the physis with the fracture progressing out to the metaphysis (metaphyseal beak or Thurston–Holland sign on radiographs)
III	Fracture through a portion of the physis and out through the epiphysis
IV	Fractures transits longitudinally or obliquely through the epiphysis, physis, and metaphysis
V	Fractures cause a crush injury of the growth plate and are not evident on radiographs at the time of injury.

accurate anatomical reduction must be performed to reduce the possibility of interference in growth and to minimize the possibility of long-term degenerative change. However, occasionally the initial insult can produce permanent growth arrest despite subsequent anatomical reduction. Type V is a crush injury of physis often missed at the time of injury. They will not be evident on the radiographs. This injury may cause growth arrest of the affected bone. They are only suspected at a later stage as a retrospective diagnosis when the growth arrest becomes clinically obvious. The common sites of growth-plate fractures in children with recommended management and potential complications are shown in Table 4.2.3.

It is most important to recognize an epiphyseal fracture. If in doubt, radiographs should be obtained of both limbs (for comparison) if clinical features suggest growth-plate injury. A normal radiograph does not exclude a growth-plate fracture. A history of severe rotational or shear force with accompanying localized swelling, bony tenderness, and loss of function should be regarded as a growth-plate fracture until proven otherwise. If there is any doubt regarding the diagnosis or management of these injuries, specialist orthopaedic referral is mandatory.

Table 4.2.3 Management and possible complications of growth-plate fractures in children

Site	Management	Potential complications
Distal radius fracture	Cast immobilization (3–4 weeks)	Not recognized, growth disturbance
Supracondylar fracture of the elbow	Sling (3 weeks)	Vascular compromise of brachial artery, median nerve damage, malalignment
Distal fibular fracture	Cast, non-weight-bearing (4–6 weeks)	Growth disturbance can occur up to 18 months later
Distal tibial fracture	Cast, non-weight-bearing (4–6 weeks)	Premature closure of physis can lead to angulation and leg-length discrepancy
Distal femur fracture	Anatomical reduction	Greater incidence of growth discrepancies than in other fractures. Salter–Harris type I and II fractures must be observed closely

Avulsion fractures

Avulsion fractures occur when a ligament or tendon pulls off bone from their insertion. An acute rotational injury to the knee may present with the symptoms and signs of an anterior cruciate ligament (ACL) tear. Instead of the intra-substance tear common in adults, the more common injury in children is avulsion of the tibial spine (attachment of the ACL onto the tibial spine) or distal femoral attachment. Radiographs should be performed in all cases of acute knee injuries accompanied by haemarthrosis. Management involves surgical reattachment of the avulsed fragment and ligament.

More commonly, avulsion fractures occur at the apophyseal attachment of large musculotendinous units. The common sites are at the following attachments:

- sartorius muscle to the anterior superior iliac spine
- rectus femoris muscle to the anterior inferior iliac spine
- hamstring muscles to the ischial tuberosity
- iliopsoas tendon to the lesser trochanter of the femur.

Similar force in an adult would result in acute muscle strain. In a child, instead of a tear of the muscle fibres in the mid-substance of the muscle or at the musculotendinous junction, the tendon is pulled away with its apophyseal attachment. This is confirmed on plain radiographs.

Management of avulsion fractures includes measures to reduce pain and swelling, and restoration of full range of motion with passive stretching is initiated. Active range of motion exercises as symptoms settle and a graduated programme of muscle strengthening are started. Any biomechanical abnormalities that may have predisposed the athlete to this injury should be corrected. Reattachment of the avulsed fragment is rarely necessary, although there is a recent trend favouring early open reduction and internal fixation.

Upper limb injuries

Shoulder pain

Acute trauma to the shoulder may result in fracture of the proximal humerus, the clavicle, the acromion, or the coracoid process. Dislocation of the glenohumeral joint is common in teenagers but uncommon in a younger child. It is associated with a high incidence of recurrence and development of post-traumatic instability.

Overuse injuries around the shoulder are common in young athletes involved in throwing sports, swimming, and tennis. A stress fracture of the proximal epiphyseal plate of the humerus is seen in young throwers and has been termed 'Little Leaguer's shoulder'. Radiographs reveal widening of the epiphyseal line, followed at a later stage by new bone formation.

In a young athlete involved in throwing sports, shoulder impingement is usually secondary to atraumatic instability which develops because of repetitive stress to the anterior capsule of the shoulder joint at the end range of movement. Impingement and rotator cuff tendinopathy also occur in swimmers where excessive internal rotation causes a tendency to impinge.

Elbow pain

Delineating injury patterns to the elbow in children can be challenging, given the cartilaginous composition of the distal humerus and the multiple secondary ossification centres which appear and unite with the epiphysis at defined ages. The pitching motion in baseball, serving in tennis, spiking in volleyball, passing in American football, and launching in javelin throwing can all produce elbow pathology caused by forceful valgus stress with medial stretching, lateral compression, and posterior impingement. The valgus forces generated during the acceleration phase of throwing result in traction on the medial elbow structures, and compression to the lateral side of the joint. This may injure a number of structures on the medial aspect of the joint. Injuries include chronic apophysitis of the medial epicondyle, chronic strain of the ulnar collateral ligament (Fig. 4.2.2), or avulsion fracture of the epiphysis (Fig. 4.2.3). The ulnar nerve may also be damaged.

The lateral compressive forces may damage the articular cartilage of the capitellum or radial head. The long-term sequelae of these repetitive valgus forces include bony thickening, loose body formation, and contractures. Flexion contractures can occur because of repeated hyperextension. The majority of these contractures are relatively minor (less than 15°). Significant contractures (greater than 30°) should be treated with active and active-assisted range of motion exercises accompanied by a lengthy period of rest (e.g. 3 months).

Osteochondritis dissecans of the capitellum is more common in gymnasts and less often seen in pitchers. Osteochondritis dissecans

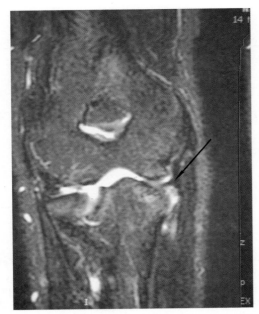

Fig. 4.2.2 MRI—a gold standard tool for confirming ulnar collateral ligament damage.

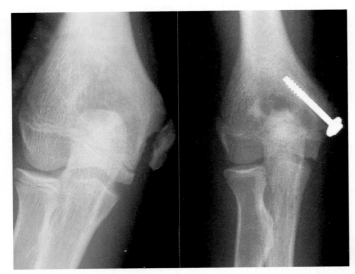

Fig. 4.2.3 Medial epicondyle avulsion fracture sustained while playing rugby fixed with a cancellous screw.

is a localized area of avascular necrosis on the anterolateral aspect of the capitellum. Initially, the articular surface softens and subchondral collapse may occur with resultant formation of loose bodies in the elbow. The early stages of osteochondritis dissecans may respond well to rest. Surgery is required to remove loose bodies. Joint debridement is usually performed at the same time. The results of surgical management of this condition are variable.

Younger children may develop Panner's lesion. This self-limiting condition is characterized by fragmentation of the entire ossification centre of the capitellum. Loose bodies are not seen in Panner's lesion, and surgery is not required. Ensuring that adolescents have

adequate rest between training sessions and that sporting technique is correctly coached and monitored by experts can prevent these injuries.

Wrist pain

Acute wrist pain can occur because of a fracture, and the scaphoid is the most commonly affected bone. Dorsal wrist pain is commonly seen in gymnasts, in whom the pain is aggravated by weight-bearing with the wrist extended. The gymnast complains of tenderness over the dorsum of the hand, and perhaps swelling. Examination findings are usually consistent with local injury. The most likely cause is a stress injury to the distal radial or distal ulnar growth plates. Long-standing injuries are associated with typical radiographic changes, including widening, irregularity, haziness, or cystic changes of the growth plate. Acute growth-plate slippage or fractures of the distal epiphyses are occasionally seen (see Fig. 4.2.1). Other causes of dorsal wrist pain include capsule sprain, tearing of the triangular fibrocartilage complex, and stress fractures.

Kienböck's lesion of the wrist (lunatomalacia) is an osteochondrosis of the lunate bone. It rarely affects young children and most often occurs in young adults between 15 and 40 years of age following a single or repetitive microfractures.

Management of the younger gymnast with dorsal wrist pain includes relative rest, splinting, electrotherapeutic modalities, and NSAIDs. Strengthening of the wrist flexors may also be useful in association with tape and pads to decrease hyperextension of the wrist.

Back pain and postural abnormalities

Older children and teenagers may present with pain and/or postural abnormalities such as 'curvature' of the spine (scoliosis) (Fig. 4.2.4].

Low back pain

Minor soft tissue injuries to the intervertebral disc, the apophyseal joints, and associated ligaments and muscle strains in the paraver-

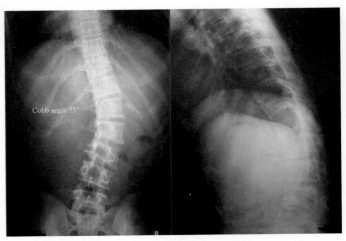

Fig. 4.2.4 Scoliosis may sometimes be a cause of discomfort or even pain in a young athlete.

tebral muscles usually respond well to reduction in activity. Manipulation of these conditions using devices which apply traction forces along the entire spine is contraindicated in adolescent/teenage athletes.

The other causes of low back pain include:

- spondylolysis
- spondylolisthesis
- vertebral endplate fracture
- atypical Scheuermann's lesion (vertebral apophysitis)
- tumour (osteogenic sarcoma)
- infection (discitis).

Stress fractures of the pars interarticularis (spondylolysis) may occur in older children, particularly because of repeated hyperextension and rotational manoeuvres of the lumbar spine. These injuries are typically seen as a result of ballet, gymnastics, diving, volleyball, fast bowling in cricket, and serving in tennis. The amount of hyperextension activity must be reduced and this may involve some alteration in technique.

A painless fibrous union usually develops across the defect, and this is susceptible to repeat injury. There is considerable debate about whether these defects in the pars interarticularis are congenital or acquired. The presence of a pars interarticularis defect does not automatically mean that this is the cause of the patient's pain. An isotopic bone scan or MRI may confirm that the pars interarticularis defect is the site of an acute fracture.

Severe disc injuries and tumours are occasionally seen in the lumbar spine of the adolescent athlete. Biomechanical abnormalities such as leg-length discrepancy, pelvic instability, and excessive subtalar pronation may also indirectly lead to low back pain and require correction if present.

Postural abnormalities

The most common postural abnormality of the spine is excessive kyphosis due to an osteochondrosis (Scheuermann's lesion). This condition typically occurs in the thoracic spine but is also seen at the thoracolumbar junction. Children can present with acute pain. It usually presents in later years as an excessive thoracic kyphosis in association with a compensatory excessive lumbar lordosis. The radiological diagnosis of Scheuermann's lesion is made on the presence of wedging of 5° or more at three adjacent vertebrae.

Management is aimed at preventing progression of the postural deformity and involves a combination of joint mobilization, massage therapy to the thoracolumbar fascia, stretching of the hamstring muscles, and abdominal muscle strengthening. A brace may be worn to decrease the thoracic kyphosis and lumbar lordosis if the kyphosis is less than 70° and is flexible. Surgery may be indicated if the kyphosis is greater than 70° or if signs of spinal cord irritation are present.

Lower limb presentations

Hip pain

Hip pain is a more common presenting symptom in younger athletes than in mature adults. A few important causes of hip pain in children are briefly discussed below.

Apophysitis

A number of large musculotendinous units attach around the hip joint. Excessive activity can result in a traction apophysitis at one of these sites, usually the anterior inferior iliac spine at the attachment of the rectus femoris, the anterior superior iliac spine at the attachment of the sartorius, or the iliopsoas attachment to the lesser trochanter. Management involves a reduction in activity and attention to any predisposing factors such as muscle tightness. These conditions will normally resolve.

Perthes' disease

Perthes' disease is an osteochondrosis affecting the femoral head. It presents as a limp or low-grade ache in the thigh, groin, or knee. On examination there may be limited abduction and internal rotation of the hip. Perthes' disease is usually unilateral. It typically affects children between the ages of 4 and 10 years, is more common in males, and may be associated with delayed skeletal maturation. Radiographs vary with the stage of the disease, but may show increased density and flattening of the femoral capital epiphysis. Management consists of rest from aggravating activity and range of motion exercises, particularly to maintain abduction and internal rotation. The age of the child and the severity of the condition will affect the intensity of the management. Rest and the use of a brace should suffice. Surgery will only be required if the femoral head is not contained within the acetabulum in the neutral position, but is contained in abduction. Recently, arthroscopic chondroplasty and loose-body excision have shown good short-term results (Kocher et al. 2005b).

The condition usually resolves, and return to sport is possible when the athlete is symptom free and radiographs show some improvement. The main long-term concern is the development of osteoarthritis due to irregularity of the joint surface.

Slipped capital femoral epiphysis

A slipped capital femoral epiphysis may occur in older children, particularly those aged between 12 and 15 years. This is similar to a Salter–Harris type I fracture. It occurs typically in overweight boys who tend to be late maturers. The slip may occur suddenly or, more commonly, as a gradual process. There is sometimes associated pain, frequently in the knee, but the most common presenting symptom is a limp.

Examination reveals shortening and external rotation of the affected leg. Hip abduction and internal rotation are reduced. During flexion the hip moves into abduction and external rotation. Radiographs show widening of the growth plate, and a line continued from the superior surface of the neck of the femur does not intersect the growth plate (Fig. 4.2.5). Bilateral involvement is common. Slips are a matter of considerable concern because they may compromise the vascular supply to the femoral head and lead to avascular necrosis. These require orthopaedic assessment. A gradually progressing slip is an indication for surgery. An acute severe slip occurs occasionally. This is a surgical emergency.

Irritable hip

Irritable hip is common in children, but should be a diagnosis of exclusion. The child presents with a limp and pain which may not be well localized. Examination reveals painful restriction of motion of the hip joint, particularly in extension and/or abduction in flexion. In the majority of cases, a specific cause is never identified and the pain settles after a period of bed rest and observation.

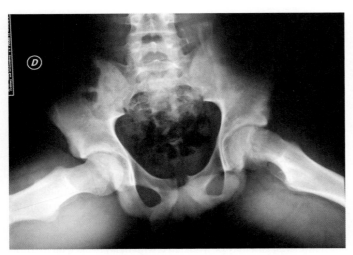

Fig. 4.2.5 Slipped capital femoral epiphysis in a young female athlete.

Radiographs, bone scanning, and blood tests are usually normal, and the child is treated with rest (Maffulli and Bruns 2000).

Knee pain

Knee pain, especially anterior knee pain, is a common presentation in children. The common causes of anterior knee pain are:

- Osgood–Schlatter lesion
- Sinding-Larsen–Johansson lesion
- patellar tendinopathy
- referred pain from the hip
- less common causes of knee pain
- anterior cruciate ligament (ACL) injuries.

Osgood–Schlatter lesion

Osgood–Schlatter lesion is a traction apophysitis of the growth plate of the tibial tuberosity. Repeated contraction of the quadriceps muscle mass may cause softening and partial avulsion of the developing secondary ossification centre. It is extremely common in adolescents at the time of the growth spurt. It is usually associated with sports involving running and jumping, such as basketball, football, or gymnastics. Pain around the tibial tuberosity is aggravated by exercise.

Examination reveals tenderness over the tibial tuberosity. Quadriceps tightness could be an occasional additional finding. Excessive subtalar pronation may be associated with the development of this condition. The diagnosis of Osgood–Schlatter lesion is clinical. In young athletes with severe anterior knee pain with more swelling than expected, a radiograph may be indicated to exclude bony tumour. Although bone tumours are rare, the knee is a relatively common site of osteogenic sarcoma in the 10–30 year age group. Osgood–Schlatter lesion is a self-limiting condition which settles at the time of bony fusion of the tibial tubercle, but symptoms may persist for up to 2 years. Its long-term sequel may be a thickening and prominence of the tubercle. Occasionally, a separate fragment develops at the site of the tibial tubercle.

Management of this condition requires activity modification. While there is no evidence that rest accelerates the healing process,

a reduction in activity will reduce pain. As this condition occurs in young athletes with a high level of physical activity, it may be useful to suggest that they eliminate one or two of the large number of sports they generally play. There is no need to rest completely. Pain should be the main guide to the limitation of activity.

Symptomatic management includes applying ice to the region. A stretching programme and massage therapy to the quadriceps muscle helps counteract the tightness. Muscle strengthening can be introduced as pain allows. Correction of any predisposing biomechanical abnormality, such as excessive subtalar pronation, is necessary. Neither injection of a corticosteroid agent nor surgery is required. Very occasionally, the skeletally mature person may continue to have symptoms because of non-union. The separate fragment should then be excised.

Sinding-Larsen–Johansson lesion

This is a similar condition to Osgood–Schlatter lesion. It affects the inferior pole of the patella at the superior attachment of the patellar tendon. It is much less common than Osgood–Schlatter lesion, but the same principles of management apply.

Patellar tendinopathy

Although symptomatic tendinopathy was thought to be rare in children, there is now evidence that patellar tendinopathy is prevalent in junior basketball players (Cook *et al.* 2000). Management is the same as that outlined for adults, although resolution of symptoms may be quicker in adolescents.

Referred pain from the hip

Conditions affecting the hip, such as a slipped capital femoral epiphysis or Perthes' disease, commonly present as knee pain. Examination of the hip joint is mandatory in the assessment of any young athlete presenting with knee pain.

Less common causes of knee pain

Osteochondritis dissecans may affect the knee. This generally presents with intermittent pain and swelling of gradual onset. Occasionally, an osteochondral lesion may present as an acute painful locked knee associated with haemarthrosis and loose-body formation. Radiographs may reveal evidence of a defect at the lateral aspect of the medial femoral condyle. Osteochondritis dissecans requires orthopaedic referral for possible fixation of the loosened fragment or removal of the detached fragment.

In juvenile rheumatoid arthritis (Still's disease) of the knee, there is persistent intermittent effusion with increased temperature and restricted range of motion. There may be a family history of rheumatoid arthritis. Investigation requires serological examination, including measuring the level of rheumatoid factor and the erythrocyte sedimentation rate, and, if indicated, serological examination of joint aspirate. The child's activity should be adapted to avoid using the painful joints while exercising other body parts and promoting cardiovascular fitness.

A differential diagnosis in paediatric arthritis that is relatively rare but is increasing in the developed world is acute rheumatic fever (Williamson *et al.* 2000). Clinicians may overlook this condition, as there may be no history of sore throat and carditis may be silent. The diagnosis can only be made if the clinician maintains an index of suspicion for this condition. Investigations should include markers of inflammation (erythrocyte sedimentation rate, C-reactive protein), serology for streptococci (anti-streptolysin-O titre, anti-DNase B titres), and echocardiography. Penicillin and aspirin taken orally remain the mainstay of management.

A partial discoid meniscus may cause persistent knee pain and swelling in the adolescent athlete. There is usually marked joint line tenderness. Arthroscopy may be diagnostic and therapeutic. A complete discoid meniscus is characterized by a history of clunking in the younger child (4 years).

Adolescent tibia vara (Blount's disease) is an uncommon osteochondrosis that affects the proximal tibial growth plate. It usually affects tall obese children around the age of 9 years. It is generally unilateral, and radiographs show a reduced height of the medial aspect of the proximal tibial growth plate. Surgery may be required to correct any resultant mechanical abnormality.

Anterior cruciate ligament injuries

Over the last few years there has been an apparent increase in the number of ACL injuries reported in young athletes secondary to higher participation levels, greater awareness, and improved imaging modalities. It is difficult to ascertain the true incidence and prevalence of ACL injuries in young athletes because of the lack of documentation of skeletal maturity and the ambiguity in diagnosis (Paletta 2003). There is a preponderance of these injuries in girls because of the smaller ACL size with a smaller intercondylar notch of the femur, decreased strength and conditioning, different playing mechanisms, and anatomical alignment (Paletta 2003).

ACL injuries usually present with an acute history of a pop in the knee, with an inability to return to play, followed by swelling in the knee within 6–12 hours. Children with chronic ACL insufficiency will present with functional instability in the knee when pivoting. The anterior drawer and Lachmann's tests are usually positive. Caution must be taken in interpreting the findings of these tests given the inherent laxity present in the paediatric knee. Thus, before reaching a clinical diagnosis, the contralateral knee should be examined. MRI scans of the knee should be undertaken to confirm the diagnosis of ACL injuries and to rule out the presence of any associated meniscal tears. MRI is not a substitute for a good history and physical examination, and imaging should only be used to correlate the findings of clinical examination.

The management of ACL injuries in the younger athlete is still controversial. Non-operative management is usually reserved for younger children who have not yet reached skeletal maturity (Tanner stage 1 and 2). Tanner stage 1 and 2 are prepubescent skeletally immature children with wide open physes. Tanner stage 3 and 4 are adolescents in late pubescence. Tanner stage 5 is almost an adult with no growth left. However, non-operative management has a poor outcome (Kannus and Jarvinen 1988; Mizuta et al. 1995). Surgery is usually performed in children who are either non-compliant with conservative management or those demonstrating functional instability with activities of daily living. Surgery is strongly recommended in children with associated meniscal pathology irrespective of their Tanner stage (Paletta 2003). In skeletally immature children, physeal sparing combined intra-articular and extra-articular reconstruction of the ACL using an autologous iliotibial band graft has shown promising results (Kocher et al. 2005a).

Foot pain

Foot pain of gradual onset is a common presenting symptom in the younger athlete. The causes of foot pain are related to either abnormal biomechanics or the development of an osteochondrosis. Examination of younger athletes with foot pain requires precise determination of the site of maximum tenderness.

Sever's lesion

Sever's lesion is a traction apophysitis of the insertion of the Achilles tendon to the calcaneus, which typically occurs between the ages of 7 and 10 years. This is the second most common osteochondrosis seen in the younger athlete after Osgood–Schlatter lesion. As with Osgood–Schlatter lesion, Sever's lesion is often present at a time of rapid growth during which muscles and tendons become tighter as the bones grow longitudinally.

The patient complains of activity-related pain, and examination reveals localized tenderness and swelling at the site of insertion of the Achilles tendon. There may be tightness of the gastrocnemius or soleus muscles, and dorsiflexion at the ankle is limited. Biomechanical examination is necessary. Radiographic examination is not usually required except in persistent cases.

Management consists of activity modification so that the child becomes pain free. The patient should be advised that the condition will settle, usually within 6–12 months, but occasionally symptoms will persist for as long as 2 years. A heel raise should be inserted in shoes. Stretching of the calf muscles is also advisable. Any biomechanical abnormalities should be corrected. Orthoses may be required. Strengthening exercises for the ankle plantarflexors should be commenced when the patient is pain free and progressed as symptoms permit. Corticosteroid injections and surgery are contraindicated.

Tarsal coalitions

Congenital fusion of the bones of the foot may be undetected until the child begins participation in sports. The most common form is a bony or cartilaginous bar between the calcaneus and the navicular. The second most common coalition is between the calcaneus and talus. Calcaneocuboid coalition is the least common form. There is often a family history. The adolescent may present with mid-foot pain after recurrent ankle sprains or after repetitive running and jumping. The pain may be associated with a limp.

Examination reveals restriction of subtalar joint motion. There may be a rigid flat foot deformity. Radiographs taken at 45° oblique to the foot may confirm the diagnosis, but if these are normal and clinical suspicion persists, a CT scan or MRI should be obtained.

Management may require orthotic therapy. Surgical excision may be necessary in a young patient with severe symptoms or after failure of conservative therapy. The bar may recur after surgery.

Köhler's lesion

Köhler's lesion is a form of osteochondrosis affecting the navicular bone which is seen in young children, especially between the ages of 2 and 8 years. The child complains of pain over the medial aspect of the navicular, and often develops a painful limp. Tenderness is localized to the medial aspect of the navicular bone. Radiographs reveal typical changes of increased density and narrowing of the navicular bone. Management in a walking cast for 6 weeks may accelerate relief of the symptoms. Orthoses should be used if biomechanical abnormalities are present.

Apophysitis of the tarsal navicular bone

Pain on the medial aspect of the tarsal navicular in the older child may result from a traction apophysitis at the insertion of the tibialis posterior tendon to the navicular. This condition is often associated with the presence of an accessory navicular bone or a prominent navicular tuberosity. Management involves modification of activity, local electrotherapy, and NSAIDs, with orthoses to control excessive pronation if this is present.

Iselin lesion (apophysitis of the fifth metatarsal)

A traction apophysitis at the insertion of the peroneus brevis tendon to the base of the fifth metatarsal is occasionally seen. Examination reveals local tenderness and pain on resisted eversion of the foot. Management consists of modification of activity, stretching, and progressive strengthening of the peroneal muscles.

Freiberg's lesion

Freiberg's lesion is an osteochondrosis causing collapse of the articular surface and adjacent bone of the metatarsal head. The second metatarsal is most commonly involved (especially in ballet dancers), the third occasionally, and the fourth rarely. It occurs most frequently in adolescents over the age of 12 years.

Standing on the forefoot aggravates pain. The head of the second metatarsal is tender and there is swelling around the second metatarsal joint. Radiographs reveal a flattened head of the metatarsal with fragmentation of the growth plate. However, these changes may lag well behind the symptoms. Isotopic bone scan or MRI are more sensitive investigations.

If Freiberg's lesion is diagnosed early, management with activity modification, padding under the second metatarsal, and footwear modification to reduce the pressure over the metatarsal heads may prove successful. If the symptoms persist, surgical intervention may be necessary.

Painless abnormalities of gait

It is common for a child to present with an abnormal gait. The child is usually brought in by a parent who has noticed an unusual appearance of the lower limb or an abnormal gait while either walking or running. The child may complain of foot pain. However, in many instances, the abnormal gait is painless.

It is not sufficient to say that the child will 'grow out of it'. The child requires a thorough biomechanical assessment, which may reveal a structural abnormality. The most common biomechanical problems in children are rotational abnormalities originating from the hip and the tibia causing either in-toed or out-toed gait.

If the child is asymptomatic and biomechanical abnormalities are not marked, no treatment is indicated. If abnormalities are marked or the child is symptomatic, management may involve the use of braces or night splints when the child is very young. In the older child, orthoses can be used to compensate for the deformity.

Other considerations in the younger athlete

In addition to the musculoskeletal conditions mentioned above, other physiological differences between the younger and the mature athlete may predispose the younger athlete to injury. Depending on their age, lack of motor skills may place them at a greater risk of injury (Baxter-Jones et al. 1993). The adolescent athlete is more susceptible to injury than the prepubescent athlete because of the circulating androgens which result in greater mass, speed, and power. This, combined with the impulsive and reckless attitude typically seen in teenagers, may increase the risk of injury (Adirim and Cheng 2003). Growing children vary greatly in size,

and therefore may not have access to appropriately sized protective equipment.

Prevention

'Prevention is better than cure'. Complications in sports injuries can be prevented by appropriately sized sports gear and addressing safety protection issues. Banning spearing in American football, the use of appropriate head and face guards in ice hockey, breakaway bases in baseball (Janda et al. 2001), appropriate ball selection, limiting repetitive actions such as those in throwing and bowling sports, and appropriate fluid management in hot weather have resulted in a significant reduction in complications. Nonetheless, these interventions are sometimes not entirely successful. For example, despite the use of chest protectors in baseball (Viano et al. 2000), commotio cordis (sudden cardiac arrest from unexpected blunt non-penetrating trauma to the anterior chest resulting in immediate death due to ventricular fibrillation) has still been reported.

References

Adirim, T. and Cheng, T. (2003). Overview of injuries in the young athlete. *Sports Medicine*, **33**, 75–81.

Baxter-Jones, A., Maffulli, N., and Helms, P. (1993). Low injury rates in elite athletes. *Archives of Disease in Childhood*, **68**, 130–2.

Cook, J.L., Khan, K.M., Kiss, Z.S., and Griffiths, L. (2000) Patellar tendinopathy in junior basketball players: a controlled clinical and ultrasonographic study of 268 patellar tendons in players aged 14–18 years. *Scandinavian Journal of Medicine and Science in Sports*, **10**, 216–20.

Crompton, B. and Tubbs, N. (1977). A survey of sports injuries in Birmingham. *British Journal of Sports Medicine*, **11**, 12–15.

Feldman, D., Shrier, I., Rossignol, M., and Abenhaim, L. (1999). Adolescent growth is not associated with changes in flexibility. *Clinical Journal of Sport Medicine*, **9**, 24–9.

Janda, D.H., Bir, C., and Kedroske, B. (2001). A comparison of standard vs. breakaway bases: an analysis of a preventative intervention for softball and baseball foot and ankle injuries. *Foot and Ankle International*, **22**, 810–16.

Kannus, P. and Jarvinen, M. (1988). Knee ligament injuries in adolescents. Eight year follow up of conservative treatment. *Journal of Bone and Joint Surgery. British Volume*, **70**, 772–6.

Kocher, M.S., Garg, S., and Micheli, L.J. (2005a). Physeal sparing reconstruction of the anterior cruciate ligament in skeletally immature prepubescent children and adolescents. *Journal of Bone and Joint Surgery. American Volume*, **87**, 2371–9.

Kocher, M.S., Kim, Y.J., Millis, M.B., et al. (2005b). Hip arthroscopy in children and adolescents. *Journal of Pediatric Orthopedics*, **25**, 680–6.

Maffulli, N. and Baxter-Jones, A.D. (1995). Common skeletal injuries in young athletes. *Sports Medicine*, **19**, 137–49.

Maffulli, N. and Bruns, W. (2000). Injuries in young athletes. *European Journal of Pediatrics*, **159**, 59–63.

Malina, R.M. (1994). Physical growth and biological maturation of young athletes. In: J.O. Holloszy (ed.), *Exercise and Sports Science Reviews*, pp. 389–433. Williams & Wilkins, Baltimore, MD.

Micheli, L.J. and Fehlandt, A.F., Jr (1992). Overuse injuries to tendons and apophyses in children and adolescents. *Clinics in Sports Medicine*, **11**, 713–26.

Mizuta, H., Kubota, K., Shiraishi, M., et al. (1995). The conservative treatment of complete tears of the anterior cruciate ligament in skeletally immature patients. *Journal of Bone and Joint Surgery. British Volume*, **77**, 890–4.

Paletta, G.A. Special considerations. Anterior cruciate ligament reconstruction in the skeletally immature. *Orthopedic Clinics of North America*, **34**, 65–77.

Rowley, S. (1989). *The Effect of Intensive Training on Young Athletes*, pp. 6–7. Sports Council, London.

Salter, R.B. and Harris, W.R. (1963). Injuries involving the epiphyseal plate. *Journal of Bone and Joint Surgery. American Volume*, **45**, 587–622.

Schmidt, B. and Hollwarth, M.E. (1989). Sports accidents in children and adolescents. *Zeitschift für Kinderchirurgie*, **44**, 357–62.

Viano, D.C., Bir, C.A., Cheney, A.K., and Janda, D.H. (2000). Prevention of commotio cordis in baseball: an evaluation of chest protectors. *Journal of Trauma*, **49**, 1023–8.

Williamson, L., Bowness, P., Mowat, A., and Ostman-Smith, I. (2000). Difficulties in diagnosing acute rheumatic fever—arthritis may be short lived and carditis silent. *British Medical Journal*, **320**, 362–5.

Zaricznyj, B., Shattuck, L.J., Mast, T.A. Robertson, R.V., and D'Elia, G. (1980). Sports-related injuries in school-aged children. *American Journal of Sports Medicine*, **8**, 318–24.

Injuries in the female athlete

Cathy Speed

Introduction

Women were banned from competing and even watching events in the ancient Olympics, and were excluded from the first modern Olympic Games. However, with changes in society, participation in sport at all levels has dramatically changed. This has heightened awareness of several important clinical issues relating to women and sport and exercise. In particular, exercise can have positive or deleterious effects on bone health, females are at greater risk of some musculoskeletal injuries, and there is a common need for guidance on exercise in pregnancy and at the menopause.

Menstrual dysfunction and the female athlete triad

The beneficial effects of weight-bearing exercise upon the general health and the skeleton are well recognized (American College of Sports Medicine 2000). However, exercise and training can also have a negative effect on bone and on cardiovascular and gynaecological health. Young female athletes, in particular those participating in lightweight sports such as gymnastics, ballet, figure skating, and endurance events, are at risk of the 'female athletic triad' (Nattiv *et al.* 2007; Speed 2007). This is a complex and poorly understood syndrome, initially described as the triad of osteoporosis, amenorrhoea, and eating disorders. However, this represents only the extreme or endstage of the spectrum, and is more comprehensively described as a syndrome comprising the interrelated features of low bone mass, menstrual dysfunction, and energy deficit (Speed 2007). The last of these is commonly related to an eating disorder, partly influenced by peer pressure and by genetic, neurochemical, and psychodevelopmental factors. Useful definitions are given in Appendix I.

The spectrum of menstrual dysfunction that can affect a female athlete includes amenorrhoea, oligomenorrhoea, or luteal phase dysfunction and is likely to be multifactorial. It has been postulated to be related to hypothalamic inhibition due to physical and/or psychological stress of training and competition, caloric deficiency, low body mass, low body fat, inadequate leptin levels, or relative hyperandrogenism. Genetic influences may also play a role. It can occur independently of low body weight. Girls who start intense exercise before the onset of menstruation have an increased chance of delayed menarche and subsequent menstrual dysfunction.

The incidence of secondary amenorrhoea varies between sports (Redman and Loucks 2005). It is reported to occur in up to 65% of distance runners (Abraham *et al.* 1982; Dusek 2001), 44% of women in the general population who exercise vigorously, and over 22% of divers, cheerleaders, and gymnasts, compared with 1–5% of the general population (Petterson *et al.* 1973; Loucks and Horvath 1985; De Cree 1998; Nattiv *et al.* 2007). Athletes who present with amenorrhoea are at the severe end of the spectrum of exercise-related menstrual dysfunction. Subtle menstrual disturbances are more common, occurring in nearly four-fifths of very active women (De Souza 2003). The impact of this on bone mineral density (BMD) is unclear (De Souza *et al.* 1997, 2003) and there is no evidence that women whose menstrual function recovers develop chronic infertility.

No specific threshold at which exercise or energy deficit leads to menstrual dysfunction has been defined because contributing physiological and psychological factors produce considerable individual variation. However, women who run more than 50 miles each week have a significantly increased incidence of amenorrhoea (Cumming and Rebar 1983).

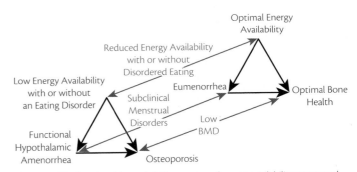

Fig. 4.3.1 The female athlete triad. The spectra of energy availability, menstrual function, and bone density in female athletes. An athlete's condition moves along each spectrum at a different rate. Energy availability, defined as energy intake minus expenditure, affects bone health via metabolic hormones and effects on menstrual function and therefore oestrogen. Reproduced with permission from Nattiv, A., Loucks, A., Manore, M., Sanborn, C., Sundgot-Borgen, J., and Warren, M. (2007). ACSM position stand. The female athlete triad. *Medicine and Science in Sports and Exercise*, **39**, 1867–82.

Table 4.3.1 Menstrual dysfunction in female athletes

Condition	Comment
Delayed menarche	
Amenorrhoea	Primary
	Secondary
Oligomenorrhoea	Due to annovulation, or low oestrogen and progesterone
Luteal phase dysfunction	May have regular menses

Abnormal menstrual cycles, with chronically low ovarian hormones, may lead to a reduced BMD and increase the risk of fracture. Bone mineral loss in athletes who have been amenorrhoeic for more than 6 months resembles that seen after the menopause, and may occur not only in the axial skeleton but also in the appendicular weight-bearing sites. However, athletes in weight-bearing sports usually have a BMD that is 5–15% higher than that of non-athletes (Risser *et al.* 1990; Robinson *et al.* 1995; Nattiv *et al.* 2007) and therefore the influence of loading through exercise may result in a different pattern of bone loss peripherally. Of necessity, reference groups for comparing BMD in premenopausal athletes use age- and sex-matched controls from the general population rather than healthy athletes.

The consequences of the female athlete triad involve the musculoskeletal, gastrointestinal, renal, cardiovascular, and central nervous systems.

Assessment

Those who present with amenorrohea should be assessed thoroughly and investigated appropriately. A detailed history should be obtained, including a general systemic enquiry, dietary, gynaecological, and sexual histories. Previous fractures and stress fractures, family history of gynaecological disorders and osteoporosis, training regimes, medications and supplements, and recent weight loss should all be recorded. A social history, including conflicts and support systems, is also relevant. A thorough examination includes assessment of height, weight, stigmata of Turner's syndrome, fundi and visual fields, Tanner stage, signs of androgen excess and other endocrine disease, and a gynaecological examination.

Standard investigations, as in the general population, include a pregnancy test, thyroid-stimulating hormone (TSH), follicle-stimulating hormone (FSH), luteinizing hormone (LH) (and LH/FSH ratio, which is raised in polycystic ovary syndrome), prolactin, oestradiol, and a progesterone challenge test (medroxyprogesterone acetate 10 mg/day for 7–10 days) as an indirect assessment of oestrogen status. A positive response indicates adequate oestrogen levels.

If a hypothalamic lesion is suspected an MRI of the head is indicated, and if polycystic ovary syndrome is suspected a pelvic scan is organized.

If androgen excess is suspected, free testosterone and dehydroepiandrosterone sulphate levels should be measured. Mild elevation of serum cortisol may be seen in functional hypothalamic amenorrhoea, compared with very high levels in Cushing's syndrome. Karyotype should be determined in young women with elevated FSH and ammenorhoea, or in those with an absent uterus. Luteal phase dysfunction is associated with a poor LH surge, inadequate LH pulse, and low progesterone production. Where there is any uncertainty input from a gynaecologist is recommended.

An ECG should be obtained, as arrhythmias and long QT syndrome can occur, even in the absence of electrolyte abnormalities.

Where a low bone mass is suspected a DEXA scan is performed, including PA lumbar spine and hip (femoral neck and total hip). In those less than 20 years of age, PA spine and whole body are preferred sites (Khan *et al.* 2004). Scans should be obtained, preferably also including peripheral sites such as tibias and forearm. Re-evaluation at 12 months is recommended in those with persistent triad disorders (Nattiv *et al.* 2007).

Management

Preventative strategies include education of the patient, parents, and coaches and heightening awareness of the problem and its potential sequelae. Management aims to restore normal menstrual function through alteration of training programmes, dietary counselling to ensure a positive energy balance, and adequate calcium and vitamin D intake. In some females, a small alteration in the training programme can result in a return of menstrual function, indicating that a 'training threshold' exists. However there is high inter-individual variability in where the threshold lies in relation to training, energy balance, and weight changes in particular.

Eating disorders present a management challenge, and a multidisciplinary approach involving the patient, coaches, family, and health professionals is fundamental to success. Counselling, not only from the nutritional perspective but also emotional and psychological counselling, including cognitive behavioural and family

Table 4.3.2 Some consequences of the female athlete triad

Musculoskeletal injuries	
Bone	Risk of stress fracture 2–4× greater in amenorrhoeics
	Probably slower healing
	Loss of BMD may not be reversible
Soft tissue	Increased incidence and slower repair
Reduced perfusion of working muscles	
Impaired skeletal oxidative metabolism	
Vaginal dryness	
Infertility	
Vitamin and mineral deficiencies	
Psychological associations of eating disorders	E.g. anxiety, depression
Dehydration, renal dysfunction	
Bloating, malabsorption, reflux	Eating disorders
Cardiovascular problems (including dyslipidaemia prolonged QT interval, arrhythmias, etc.)	

Table 4.3.3 Assessment and management of the amenorrhoeic athlete

- ◆ **Assess**
  - Thorough history and examination
- ◆ **Investigate**
  - Pregnancy test
  - TSH, FSH, LH, prolactin, oestradiol, progesterone challenge test
  - Free testosterone and dehydroepiandrosterone suphate levels
  - Pelvic ultrasound (if androgen excess).
- ◆ **Manage**
  - Education and counselling of patient, parents, and coaches
  - Optimize nutrition and energy balance
  - Modify training schedules
  - Address other stressors

Table 4.3.4 Typical features in functional hypothalamic amenorrhoea

Test	Result
Gonadotrophins	Low
Oestradiol	Low
Prolactin	Normal
Thyroid function	Normal TSH
Serum cortisol	Slightly raised or normal
Progesterone challenge test	Withdrawal bleed in some; may not occur in severe cases

therapy, is often indicated. Antidepressants may be useful, as in other cases of eating disorders.

If menstrual function does not return, oestrogen–progesterone supplementation may help to maintain bone density. The optimal dosing schedule has not been determined and, although supplementation with low-dose oral contraceptive pills has been associated with a small increase in BMD, their use to preserve bone loss remains controversial. Bisphosphonates do not appear to be indicated in this group, as their effects in the premenopausal individual are as yet unproven and their long half-life in bone makes them a potential risk to a developing fetus during pregnancy.

The effects of exercise-related menstrual dysfunction on long-term fertility are not clear, but there is no evidence of long-term infertility in those who recover menstrual function.

The influence of menstrual cycle on predisposition to injury

Considerable research has been focused on the influence of the menstrual cycle on performance in sport and predisposition to injury (Moller-Nielson and Hammer 1989; Myklebust *et al.* 1998; Wojtys *et al.* 1998; Arendt *et al.* 1999, 2002; Agel *et al.* 2006; Wojtys and Huston 2000; Slauterbeck *et al.* 2002).

Findings from these studies are mixed: some indicate that most injuries occur just before or at the onset of menses (Moller-Nielson and Hammer 1989; Arendt *et al.* 2002), some just before or just after menses (Myklebust *et al.* 1998), some during the ovulatory phase (Wojtys *et al.* 1998; Wojtys and Huston 2000), and others have noted no relationship (Agel *et al.* 2006). The irregularity of menstrual cycles in the female athlete, limitations in the reliability of a spectrum of approaches to accurate monitoring (and variability between studies in this respect), and the relatively low incidence of specific injuries in study cohorts make this a difficult area of research.

Musculoskeletal and other soft tissue injuries

Females are considered to be at increased risk of specific musculoskeletal injuries including anterior cruciate ligament (ACL) injuries, ankle sprains, and stress injuries. A number of reasons for this have been proposed, including hormonal issues, morphometry, and mechanics. Females have narrower shoulders and wider pelvises, greater valgus angles of the elbows and knees, and greater varus angle of the hips. Increased joint laxity, the effects of hormones and hormonal cyclical variations, altered proprioception, and reduced neuromuscular control are also considered to be significant contributors.

There remain uncertainties as to the relative inter-gender incidences and severity of many injuries in specific sports. Undoubtedly the risk factors for specific injuries differ between the sexes, and differences in exposures to different sports also make it difficult to be confident in inter-gender comparisons. However, ACL injuries of the knee provide the strongest example of an injury with a significantly higher incidence in the female athlete (Table 4.3.5). The non-contact ACL injury is two to ten times times higher in female athletes than in their male counterparts, occurring in sports such as skiing, lacrosse, netball, hockey, and soccer (Griffin *et al.* 2000; Harmon and Ireland 2000; Silvers *et al.* 2005). Neuromuscular factors undoubtedly play a role, and injuries are usually sustained in deceleration, landing, or cutting, particularly with the knee extended, the foot flat, or the body off balance. As has been discussed, the relative impact of a variety of other potential risk factors, including phase of the menstrual cycle, has yet to be established. However, it has been demonstrated that ACL laxity is greatest at peak oestrogen and progesterone levels during the menstrual cycle (Heitz *et al.* 1999). In a select athletic college-age population, a combination of increased body mass index (BMI), narrow notch width, and increased joint laxity were directly correlated with ACL injury (Silvers *et al.* 2005).

Preventative strategies commence with athlete and coach education. Neuromuscular training programmes can significantly reduce the incidence of severe ACL injuries in the female athlete. A prophylactic training programme that focuses on developing neuromuscular control of the lower extremity though strengthening exercises, plyometrics, and sport-specific agilities may address the proprioceptive and biomechanical deficits that are demonstrated in the high-risk female athletic population (Griffin *et al.* 2000; Harmon and Ireland 2000).

Other soft tissue injuries

Current epidemiological evidence relating to inter-gender comparisons of the relative incidence of specific sports injuries is mixed. However, it appears that females may have an increased incidence of some injuries such as ankle sprains and concussion (Table 4.3.5). It can be postulated that inversion ankle injuries are more common in females for similar reasons to those proposed for the higher frequency of ACL injuries, but more research is needed on this subject. Prophylactic bracing or taping and neuromuscular/balance exercise programmes should be utilized in females in at-risk sports for ankle injuries, such as those indicated in Table 4.3.5.

The breast is also a common site of injury. Although significant trauma to the breast is rare, blunt trauma can result in tenderness and bruising, fat necrosis, fibrosis, and calcification. Nipple abrasion due to friction against a bra or shirt can also occur. The athletic bra should have seamless cups over the nipple area and should support the upper portion of the breast in particular, preventing discomfort due to motion.

Stress fractures

Women are reported to be at a significantly increased risk of sustaining stress injuries of bone, including stress fractures (Reinker and Ozburne 1979; Pester and Smith 1992; Fredericson *et al.* 1995; Arendt *et al.* 2003; Milner *et al.* 2006).

This increased predisposition is likely to be multifactorial in origin. The tibia is the most frequently researched site in the study of

Table 4.3.5 Frequency, distribution, and rates of selected injuries (ankle ligament sprains and anterior cruciate ligament injuries) for NCAA Games and Practices Combined for 15 sports, 1988–1989 to 2003–2004

Injury	Frequency	Percentage of all injuries	Injury rate per 1000 athlete exposures	95% CI
Ankle ligament sprains				
Men's baseball	663	7.9	0.23	0.21, 0.25
Men's basketball	3205	26.6	1.30	1.26, 1.35
Women's basketball	2446	24.0	1.15	1.10, 1.20
Women's field hockey	327	10.0	0.46	0.41, 0.51
Men's football	9929	13.6	0.83	0.81, 0.84
Women's gymnastics	423	15.4	1.05	0.95, 1.15
Men's ice hockey	296	4.5	0.23	0.20, 0.26
Women's ice hockey	12	2.8	0.14	0.06, 0.22
Men's lacrosse	698	14.4	0.66	0.61, 0.71
Women's lacrosse	602	17.7	0.70	0.65, 0.76
Men's soccer	2231	17.2	1.24	1.19, 1.29
Women's soccer	1876	16.7	1.30	1.24, 1.36
Women's softball	526	9.9	0.32	0.29, 0.35
Women's volleyball	1649	23.8	1.01	0.96. 1.06
Men's wrestling	715	7.4	0.56	0.52, 0.60
Men's spring football	1519	13.9	1.34	1.27, 1.40
Total ankle ligament sprains	27 117	14.9	0.83	0.82, 0.84
ACL injuries				
Men's baseball	56	0.7	0.02	0.01, 0.02
Men's basketball	167	1.4	0.07	0.06, 0.08
Women's basketball	498	4.9	0.23	0.21, 0.25
Women's field hockey	53	1.6	0.07	0.05, 0.09
Men's football	2159	3.0	0.18	0.17, 0.19
Women's gymnastics	134	4.9	0.33	0.28, 0.39
Men's ice hockey	78	1.2	0.06	0.05, 0.07
Women's ice hockey	3	0.7	0.03	0.00, 0.07
Men's lacrosse	131	2.7	0.12	0.10, 0.15
Women's lacrosse	145	4.3	0.17	0.14, 0.20
Men's soccer	168	1.3	0.09	0.08, 0.11
Women's soccer	411	3.7	0.28	0.26, 0.31
Women's softball	129	2.4	0.08	0.06, 0.09
Women's volleyball	142	2.0	0.09	0.07, 0.10
Men's wrestling	147	1.5	0.11	0.10, 0.13
Men's spring football	379	3.5	0.33	0.30, 0.37
Total ACL injuries	4800	2.6	0.15	0.14, 0.15

Reproduced with permission from Hootman, J.M., Dick, R., and Agel, J. (2007). Epidemiology of collegiate injuries for 15 sports: summary and recommendations for injury prevention initiatives. *Journal of Athletic Training*, 42, 311–19.

causes of stress fracture, since it is the most commonly affected site. Although bone structure has been demonstrated to be a significant predisposing factor in males with tibial stress fractures, this has not been demonstrated in females. Therefore other factors must play a role, including limitations in bone health, hormonal factors, bone density, and soft tissue laxity during pregnancy and the post-partum period (when sacral stress injuries can be a particular concern), vertical and peak ground reaction forces during running (Milner *et al.* 2006), gait mechanics, and other biomechanical issues that have been listed above.

Scoliosis

The incidence of scoliosis in females over the age of 8 years is 4.6 per 1000 compared with 0.2 per 1000 in boys, with females tending to have larger curves compared to males. Sports that are associated with a delay in menarche are those where scoliosis is more likely to be seen (e.g. gymnasts and dancers). Others that seem predisposed are taller thinner athletes.

Nevertheless, when a female athlete complains of back pain and has a scoliosis, other causes should be considered, including spondylolysis and posterior element/facet syndromes. Gymnasts and dancers are at particular risk of such conditions.

Curves that are greater than 5° should be radiographically assessed. Scolioses should be clinically monitored during growth, and management is influenced by the age of the patient and the severity and progression of the curve (Omey *et al.* 2000).

Exercise and pregnancy

Regular physical activity during pregnancy may confer several advantages to both mother and fetus. The mother should experience improvements in aerobic fitness and psychological well-being, reduced discomforts of pregnancy such as swelling, leg cramps, fatigue, and dyspnoea, less overall weight gain, improved glucose tolerance during pregnancy, lower diastolic blood pressure for those at risk of hypertensive disorders, and possible beneficial effects on labour and delivery. There is a decreased risk of large infant size and an association with advanced early neurodevelopment (Clapp 1996; Clapp *et al.* 1999).

In general, healthy women with uncomplicated pregnancies do not have to restrict their exercise for fear of adverse effects, but they are at potential risk. Alterations in coordination and balance make falls more likely, and increased ligamentous laxity in pregnancy may result in a higher risk of musculoskeletal injuries—a particular risk in those with pelvic instability. Although occupational studies suggest an increased risk with bending and standing for prolonged periods, exercise studies suggest that no increased risk is associated with exercise during pregnancy, and indeed it may result in a reduced risk of spontaneous abortions. Increased heat exposure due to rises in core temperature is a theoretical risk, although thermoregulatory responses to exercise help to reduce this risk.

Recommendations for exercise in pregnancy are based on clinical consensus as there is a relative lack of large clinical studies. Women who already participate in regular exercise can continue without major modifications, although they may choose to modify it for comfort or specific symptoms. Those who have not previously exercised regularly should begin only after medical approval, with low-intensity low-impact activities recommended

Table 4.3.6 Recommendations for exercise in pregnancy

In the absence of medical or obstetric contraindications
◆ 30 minutes or more of moderate exercise per day on most or all days of the week
◆ Avoid exercise in the supine position after the first trimester
◆ Stop exercise if fatigued and do not exercise to exhaustion
◆ Non-weight-bearing exercise is likely to help to reduce the risk of musculoskeletal injury
◆ Avoid any exercise where there is a risk of trauma
◆ Ensure that there is an adequate diet to compensate for additional energy exposure
◆ Augment heat dissipation by wearing appropriate clothing; ensure adequate hydration and alter environment as necessary
◆ Many of the physiological changes persist for 4–6 weeks post-partum, and return to pre-pregnancy higher-intensity regimes should be gradual

Source: American College of Obstetricians and Gynecologists 2003.

Table 4.3.7 Absolute contraindications to exercise in pregnancy

- ◆ Pregnancy induced hypertension
- ◆ Preterm membrane rupture
- ◆ History of preterm labour during current or prior pregnancy
- ◆ Incompetent cervix
- ◆ Persistent second or third trimester bleeding
- ◆ Intrauterine growth retardation

Source: American College of Obstetricians and Gynecologists 2003.

Table 4.3.8 Exercise recommendations for menopause

Type	Frequency
Flexibility	Daily: spinal, upper and lower limbs
Resistance training	Three times weekly: upper and lower limbs
Aerobic activities 60–80% of maximum heart rate	20–60 minutes (continuous or intermittent) on most days of the week

(Table 4.3.6). Where medical conditions such as chronic hypertension or endocrine, cardiac, or pulmonary disease is present, the advising physicians are likely to modify these recommendations.

Exercise and the menopause

The menopause is associated with well-recognized increases in the risk of cardiovascular disease, osteoporosis, vasomotor instability, low mood and insomnia, weight gain, and age-related declines in muscle mass and strength. All such changes are at least partly reversible through appropriate exercise regimens, which should include flexibility work, resistance training, and aerobic activity, as in younger populations.

Maintenance of an appropriate osteogenic activity programme throughout life, and in particular in the menopausal years, is important for bone health. Surprisingly, such programmes are still poorly defined, but information from multiple small randomized controlled trials and epidemiological studies suggests that the exercise prescription should include weight-bearing endurance activities, activities that involve jumping, and resistance exercise (weightlifting).

These should be performed at a moderate to high intensity in terms of bone-loading forces, the specific magnitudes of which are as yet undefined. However, a higher-intensity loading would be, for example, jumping off a 12 inch step. It is not currently possible to easily quantify exercise intensity in terms of bone-loading forces, particularly for weight-bearing endurance activities. Weight-bearing endurance activities should be performed three to five times per week, and resistance exercise two to three times per week, totalling at least 60 minutes per session (Kohrt *et al.* 2004).

Conclusions

There are several issues relating to the participation of females in sports and exercise. Many of these impact, directly or indirectly, on the predisposition to specific injuries. Most can be prevented by adequate education of females, their coaches, and their families in the earliest stages of participation.

Appendix I

Appendix 1 Useful definitions. From: ACSM position stand. The female athlete triad. Medicine and Science in Sports and Exercise. 39, 1867–1882. With permission.

Female athlete triad	relationships among energy availability, menstrual function, and BMD that may have clinical manifestations including eating disorders, functional hypothalamic amenorrhea, and osteoporosis.
Energy availability (EA)	dietary energy intake (EI) minus exercise energy expenditure (EEE) normalized to fat-free mass (FFM), i.e., EA = (EI − EEE)/FFM, in units of kilocalories or kilojoules per kilogram of fat-free mass. For example, for a dietary energy intake of 2000 kcal·d^{-1}, an exercise energy expenditure of 600 kcal·d^{-1}, and a fat-free mass of 51 kg, EA = (2000 − 600)/51 = 27.5 kcal·kg^{-1} FFM·d^{-1}.
Exercise energy expenditure	strictly, the energy expended during exercise training in excess of the energy that would have been expended in nonexercise activity during the same time interval. Neglecting the adjustment for non-exercise activity causes EA to be underestimated by a few kcal·kg^{-1} FFM·d^{-1}, which is a negligible error for most purposes.
Disordered eating	various abnormal eating behaviors, including restrictive eating, fasting, frequently skipped meals, diet pills, laxatives, diuretics, enemas, overeating, binge-eating and then purging (vomiting).
Eating disorder	a clinical mental disorder defined by DSM-IV (8) and characterized by abnormal eating behaviors, an irrational fear of gaining weight, and false beliefs about eating, weight, and shape.
Eumenorrhea	menstrual cycles at intervals near the median interval for young adult women. In young adult women, menstrual cycles recur at a median interval of 28 d that varies with a standard deviation of 7 d.
Oligomenorrhea	menstrual cycles at intervals longer than 35 d, i.e., greater than the median plus one standard deviation.
Luteal suppression	a menstrual cycle with a luteal phase shorter than 11 d in length or with a low concentration of progesterone.

Anovulation	a menstrual cycle without ovulation.
Amenorrhea	absence of menstrual cycles for more than 90 d.
Low BMD*	bone mineral density Z-score** between −1.0 and −2.0.
Osteoporosis*	bone mineral density Z-score** ≤ −2.0 together with secondary risk factors for fracture (e.g., undernutrition, hypoestrogenism, prior fractures).

* These definitions apply to physically active and athletic premenopausal women and children.

**A Z-score compares the bone mineral density of an individual to those of age, race, and sex-matched controls.

References

Abraham, S.F., Beumont, P.J., Fraser, I.S., and Llewellyn Jones, D. (1982). Body weight, exercise and menstrual status among ballet dancers in training. *British Journal of Obstetrics and Gynaecology*, **89**, 507–10.

Agel, J., Bershadsky, B., and Arendt, E.A. (2006). Hormonal therapy: ACL and ankle injury. *Medical Science in Sports and Exercise*, **38**, 7–12,.

American College of Obstetricians and Gynaecologists (2003). Exercise during pregnancy and the postpartum period. *Clinical Obstetrics and Gynecology*, **46**, 496–9.

American College of Sports Medicine (2000). Benefits and risks associated with exercise. *Guidelines for Exercise Prescription* (6th edn), pp. 3–21. Lippincott–Williams & Wilkins, Philadelphia, PA.

Arendt, E.A., Agel, J., and Dick, R. (1999). Anterior cruciate ligament injury patterns among collegiate men and women. *Journal of Athletic Training*, **34**, 86–92.

Arendt, E.A., Bershadsky, B., and Agel, J.A. (2002). Periodicity of non-contact anterior cruciate ligament injuries during the menstrual cycle. *Journal of Gender Specific Medicine*, **5**, 19–26.

Arendt, E., Agel, J., Heikes, C., and Griffiths, H. (2003). Stress injuries to bone in college athletes: a retrospective review of experience at a single institution. *American Journal of Sports Medicine*, **31**, 959–68.

Clapp, J.F. (1996). Morphometric and neurodevelopmental outcome at age five years of the offspring of women who continue to exercise regularly throughout pregnancy. *Journal of Paediatrics*, **129**, 856–63.

Clapp, J.F., 3rd, Simonian, S., Lopez, B., Appelby-Wineberg, S., and Harcar-Sevcik, R. (1998). The one year morphometric and neurodevelopmental outcome of the offspring of women who continue to exercise regularly through pregnancy. *American Journal of Obstetrics and Gynecology*, **178**, 594–9.

Cumming, D.C. and Rebar, D.W. (1983). Exercise and reproductive function in women: a review. *American Journal of Industrial Medicine*, **4**, 113.

De Cree, C. (1998). Sex steroid metabolism and menstrual irregularities in the exercising female. A review. *Sports Medicine*, **25**, 369–406.

De Souza, M.J. (2003). Menstrual disturbances in athletes: a focus on luteal phase defects. *Medical Science in Sports and Exercise*, **35**, 1553–63.

De Souza, M.J., Miller, B.E., Sequenzia, L.C., et al. (1997). Bone health is not affected by luteal phase abnormalities and decreased ovarian progesterone production in female runners. *Journal of Clinical Endocrinology and Metabolism*, **82**, 2867–76.

De Souza, M.J., Van Heest, J., Demers, L.M., and Lasley, B.L. (2003). Luteal phase deficiency in recreational runners: evidence for a hypometabolic state. *Journal of Clinical Endocrinology and Metabolism*, **88**, 337–46.

Dusek, T. (2001). Influence of high intensity training on menstrual cycle disorders in athletes. *Croatian Medical Journal*, **42**, 79–82.

Fredericson, M., Bergman, A.G., Hoffman, K.L., and Dillingham, M.S. (1995). Tibial stress reaction in runners: correlation of clinical symptoms and scintigraphy with a new magnetic resonance imaging grading system. *American Journal of Sports Medicine*, **23**, 472–81.

Griffin, L.Y., Agel, J., Albohm, M.J., et al. (2000). Noncontact anterior cruciate ligament injuries: risk factors and prevention strategies. *Journal of the American Academy of Orthopedic Surgeons*, **8**, 141–50.

Harmon, K.G. and Ireland, M.L. (2000). Gender differences in noncontact anterior cruciate ligament injuries. *Clinics in Sports Medicine*, **19**, 287–302.

Heitz, N.A., Eisenman, P.A., Beck, C.L., and Walker, J.A. (1999). Hormonal changes throughout the menstrual cycle and increased anterior cruciate ligament laxity in females. *Journal of Athletic Training*, **34**, 144–9.

Khan, A.A.,Bachrach, L., Brown, J., et al. (2004). Standards and guidelines for performing central dual-energy X-ray absorptiometry in premenopausal women, men, and children. *Journal of Clinical Densitometry*, **7**, 51–64.

Kohrt, W.M., Bloomfield, S.A., Little, K.D., Nelson, M.E., and Yingling, V.R. (2004). American College of Sports Medicine Position Stand: physical activity and bone health. *Medical Science in Sports and Exercise*, **36**, 1985–96.

Loucks, A.B. and Horvath, S.M. (1985). Athletic amenorrhea: a review. *Medical Science in Sports and Exercise*, **17**, 56–72.

Milner, C.E., Ferber, R., Pollard, C.D., Hamill, J., and Davis, I.S. (2006). Biomechanical factors associated with tibial stress fracture in female runners. *Medical Science and Sports Exercise*, **38**, 323–8.

Moller-Nielson, J. and Hammer, M. (1989). Women's soccer injuries in relation to the menstrual cycle and oral contraceptive use. *Medical Science and Sports Exercise*, **21**, 126–9.

Myklebust, G., Maehlum, S., Holm, I., and Bahr, R. (1998). A prospective cohort study of anterior cruciate ligament injuries in elite Norwegian team handball. *Scandinavian Journal of Medicine and Science in Sports*, **8**, 149–53.

Nattiv, A. Loucks, A., Manore, M., Sanborn, C., Sundgot-Borgen, J., and Warren, M. (2007). ACSM position stand. The female athlete triad. *Medicine and Science in Sports and Exercise*, **39**, 1867–82.

Omey, M.L., Micheli, L.J., and Gerbino, P.G. (2000). Idiopathic scoliosis and spondylolysis in the female athlete: tips for treatment. *Clinical Orthopaedics and Related Research*, **372**, 74–84.

Pester, S. and Smith, P. (1992). Stress fractures in the lower extremities of soldiers in basic training. *Orthopedic Review*, **21**, 297–303.

Petterson, F., Fires, H., and Nillius, S.J. (1973). Epidemiology of secondary amenorrhea: incidence and prevalence rates. *American Journal of Obstetrics and Gynecology*, **117**, 80–6.

Redman, L.M. and Loucks, A.B. (2005). Menstrual disorders in athletes. *Sports Medicine*, **35**, 747–55.

Reinker, K. and Ozburne, S. (1979). A comparison of male and female orthopedic pathology in basic training. *Military Medicine*, **144**, 532–6.

Risser, W.L., Lee, E.J., Leblanc, A., Poindexter, H.B., Risser, J.M., and Schneider, V. (1990). Bone density in eumenorrheic female college athletes. *Medical Science and Sports Exercise*, **22**, 570–4.

Robinson, T.L., Snow-Harter, C., Taaffe, D.R., Gillis, D., Shaw, J., and Marcus, R. (1995). Gymnasts exhibit higher bone mass than do runners despite similar prevalence of amenorrhea and oligomenorrhea. *Journal of Bone and Mineral Research*, **10**, 26–35.

Silvers, H., Giza, E., and Mendelbaum, B. (2005). Anterior cruciate ligament tear prevention in the female athlete. *Current Sports Medicine Reports*, **4**, 341–3.

Slauterbeck, J.R., Fuzie, S.F., Smith, M.P., et al. (2002). The menstrual cycle, sex hormones, and anterior cruciate ligament injury. *Journal of Athletic Training*, **37**, 275–80.

Speed, C.A. (2007). Exercise and menstrual function. *British Medical Journal*, **334**, 164–5.

Wojtys, E.M. and Huston, L.J. (2000). Longitudinal effects of anterior cruciate ligament injury and patellar tendon autograft reconstruction on neuromuscular performance. *American Journal of Sports Medicine*, **28**, 336–43.

Wojtys, E.M., Huston, L.J., Lindenfeld, T.N., Hewett, T.E., and Greenfield, M.L.V.H. (1998). Association between the menstrual cycle and anterior cruciate ligament injuries in female athletes. *American Journal of Sports Medicine*, **26**, 614–19.

4.4

Disability sport

Nick Webborn

Introduction

Disability sport is the term used for any sport undertaken by someone with a disability and in this respect is all encompassing. The word 'Paralympic' is the term applied to elite sport competition for people with disabilities who have physical or visual impairments. It is derived from the Greek word 'para' meaning 'alongside' and the word 'Olympic', i.e. it is 'parallel to the Olympics'. The International Paralympic Committee was formed in 1989 and is the overall body that organizes the summer and winter Paralympic Games. There are 20 summer Paralympic sports and five winter Paralympic sports. Reference to injuries in these sports will be discussed in this chapter rather than injuries in disability sport in general which is too broad a topic.

Five major impairment groups are currently represented within the Paralympic Games: visual impairment, spinal-cord-related disability (congenital or acquired), limb deficiencies (congenital or acquired), cerebral palsy and Les Autres. The Les Autres group includes those physical impairments that do not fit into the other impairment groups. Athletes with an intellectual disability have been included in previous Paralympic Games, but their current participation is suspended while further refinement of the classification of intellectual disability is agreed and implemented. They may be included at the London 2012 Games, but for the purposes of this chapter athletes with an intellectual disability but without any physical impairment are likely to have the same patterns of injury that would be seen in an able-bodied athlete and, as such, readers may refer to other sport-specific chapters.

This chapter will aim to describe the different Paralympic sports (Table 4.4.1) and how they are similar, or different, to sports undertaken by their able-bodied counterparts. Readers can refer to the individual sport chapters for further information where required. Where information relates to the sports rules or regulations, this may be quoted directly from the sport rules to ensure accurate compliance. The IPC website is acknowledged as a major source of the sport-specific information (www.paralympic.org) and is commended to the reader.

Published data on injuries in Paralympic sport are relatively sparse and the majority of these are not sport specific. Published papers often describe, for example, injuries to elite wheelchair athletes across multiple sports which gives little insight into sport-specific injury patterns. However, there is some useful information within these papers to which the reader is referred for further examination (Ferrara and Davis 1990; Wilson and Washington 1993; Ferrara and Buckley 1996; Ferrara and Peterson 2000; Ferrara et al.

2000; Nyland et al. 2000). A full review of papers is given by Webborn (2009).

Archery

Archery has a founding place in Paralympic sport. The first Stoke Mandeville games were an archery competition on the front lawns of the hospital between 16 wheelchair competitors from the spinal unit and a disabled ex-servicemen's home in London. This took place in July 1948 on the opening day of the Olympic Games in London and started the first Stoke Mandeville Games which then became an annual event. Four years later four Dutch paraplegic ex-servicemen made the journey to England and the first International Stoke Mandeville Games was held. It has developed into a highly technical sport with disabled archers competing against non-disabled archers in many competitions. A Paralympic archer, Antonio Rebollo, lit the flame for the Barcelona Olympics and Paralympics by firing a flaming arrow.

Governing body FITA (transferred governance from IPC in 2007)

First appearance in Paralympic Games 1960

Competing nations 37 countries in 2006

Distances A 70 m distance is used in Paralympic competition, but in general outdoor competitions the target is placed at different distances ranging from 30 to 90 m.

Events There are individual and team events. The target for team competition is 122 cm in diameter at a distance of 70 m for both men's and women's events. In team events, an end consists of nine arrows (or three per team member) and one match consists of 27 arrows or three ends. All three archers on a team will be required to finish shooting before the prescribed time limit (currently 3 minutes). The archers may shoot in any sequence and may shoot one, two, or three arrows each time they are on the shooting line, but only one member of a team may be shooting at any one time.

Sport equipment Two types of bow are shot in international competition: the recurve bow and the compound bow. However, only the recurve bow is currently used at Paralympic Games. Competition arrows are made of carbon graphite with an inner tube of aluminium. An arm guard, bracer, and finger tabs can be used for protection.

Disability groups The sport is open to athletes with a physical disability (including spinal injury, cerebral palsy, amputee, and

Table 4.4.1 Paralympic sports

Summer Paralympic sports				Winter Paralympic sports
Archery	Football (five-a-side)	Rowing	Volleyball (sitting)	Alpine skiing
Athletics	Football (seven-a-side)	Sailing	Wheelchair basketball	Biathlon
Boccia	Goalball	Shooting	Wheelchair fencing	Cross-country skiing
Cycling	Judo	Swimming	Wheelchair rugby	Ice sledge hockey
Equestrian	Powerlifting	Table tennis	Wheelchair tennis	Wheelchair curling

les autres) in three functional classes in standing and wheelchair competitions.

Classification Three different classes based upon a bench test of muscle function, coordination, and/or joint mobility, and then a shooting test.

◆ *Archery Standing (ARST)* Archers in the Standing Class have no disabilities in the arms. The legs show some degree of loss of muscle strength, coordination, and/or joint mobility. Archers in this class may choose to compete sitting in an ordinary chair with their feet on the ground or standing.

◆ *Archery Wheelchair 1 (ARW1)* Archers in the ARW1 class have a disability in their arms and legs (tetraplegia). They have limited range of movement, strength, and control of their arms, and poor or non-existent control of the trunk. The legs are considered non-functional because of amputation and/or similar limitations of movement, strength, and control. These athletes compete in a wheelchair.

◆ *Archery Wheelchair 2 (ARW2)* Archers in the ARW2 class have paraplegia and limited mobility in the lower limbs. These athletes require a wheelchair for everyday use and compete in a wheelchair.

Physiological and biomechanical demands

These are essentially the same as for Olympic archery for performance of the sport. Impaired trunk control and upper body strength may make the task harder, but performance capabilities may be similar in terms of scores achieved. Very limited data exist on the physiological characteristics of elite Paralympic archers (Gass and Camp 1979; Veeger et al. 1991).

Injury epidemiology

No published data on specific injury types are available. Six out of ten (60%) British archers presented with injuries during the Barcelona Paralympics, but the injury types were unspecified (Reynolds et al. 1992). Athletes with a spinal cord injury are more susceptible to heat injury, and prolonged exposure in a hot environment can occur in archery by the nature of the competition.

Athletics

Wheelchair racing was first introduced at the 1952 Stoke Mandeville games with competitors using their standard hospital chairs, and other athletics events have evolved over time. Since then athletes with all disabilities have been included and great advances in technology and training have resulted in outstanding performance levels.

Examples of these exceptional performances include wheelchair marathon world record of 1:20:14 for men and 1:38:29 for women, 100 m time of 10.91 seconds for a bilateral amputee, and a high jump of 2.10 m for a single-leg amputee (correct in April 2008).

Governing body IPC Athletics

First appearance in Paralympic Games 1960

Gender Male and female

Competing nations 107

Events

Track events:

◆ sprint (100 m, 200 m, 400 m)

◆ middle distance (800 m, 1500 m)

◆ long distance (5000 m, 10 000 m)

◆ relay races (4 × 100 m, 4 × 400 m)

Road event:

◆ marathon

Jumping events:

◆ high jump

◆ long jump

◆ triple jump

Throwing events:

◆ discus

◆ shot put

◆ javelin

Combined events:

◆ pentathlon (track and road events, jumping events, and throwing events, depending on the athlete's classification).

Disability groups The sport is open to athletes with a physical disability including spinal injury, cerebral palsy, amputee, and les autres, and also to those with a visual impairment. The impairment classes compete independently of one another, in contrast with swimming, for example, where different physical impairment groups compete against each other.

Classification

◆ Classes 11, 12, and 13 cover the different levels of visual impairment.

◆ Class 20 covers athletes with an intellectually disability (not currently in Paralympic competition).

◆ Classes 32–38 cover athletes with different levels of cerebral palsy, both wheelchair (32–34) and ambulant (35–38).

◆ Classes 40–46 cover ambulant athletes with different levels of amputations and other disabilities, including les autres (e.g. dwarfism).

◆ Classes 51–58 cover wheelchair athletes with different levels of spinal cord injuries and amputations.

Sport equipment

Wheelchairs have been modified for track athletics, incorporating cycling technology materials and design for lightness and aerodynamics. The dimensions and features of wheelchairs are clearly specified in the IPC Athletics rules, which include, for example, restrictions on wheel diameter and chair height, and forbid the use of gearing or mirrors. The wearing of helmets is compulsory in all individual and team track races of 800 m and over, including the 4 × 400 m relay, and in all road races. Gloves may be used for protection of the hands during wheelchair propulsion to prevent blisters and skin abrasions.

For field events, the maximum height of the throwing frame, including the cushion used as a seat, must not exceed 75 cm and must not have any articulation or joints that might assist the thrower.

Prosthetic devices may be used by amputees to assist in sport performance. Technology has improved over time with a 'flexible foot' imparting stored energy back to the ambulant athlete using a leg prosthesis. A bilateral lower limb amputee athlete has reached the performance levels of elite able-bodied athletes. However, the IAAF have ruled that these devices gave an advantage to the athlete and decided that these prosthetic blades, known as 'cheetahs', should be considered as technical aids in contravention of IAAF Rule 144.2. As a result, the athlete was deemed ineligible to participate in competitions organized under IAAF Rules. This decision is subject to appeal. IPC rules require the use of leg prostheses in track events; however, the use of prostheses in field events is optional.

Visually impaired athletes may use a small tether to the guide runner, although the guide must not lead the athlete. Acoustic devices (or a sighted 'caller') may be used to indicate take-off in jumping events, throwing target areas, etc.

Physiological and biomechanical demands

Physiologically, wheelchair athletic performance differs from that of able-bodied athletes in that wheelchair athletes are competitive across a wider range of events. Athletes who have won marathon races have also been competitive at an elite level in sprint events. Clearly, different levels of disability influence performance, but average power output in quadriplegic athletes is around 40 W whereas in paraplegic athletes the average power is 100–150 W. Peak aerobic power in quadriplegic athletes gives Vo_2 peak values of up to 1.43 L/min compared with over 3 L/min in paraplegic athletes.

As wheelchair design has evolved over time, so has the pushing technique and the biomechanical demands. From the more upright sitting position of a standard wheelchair, athletes have now adopted a 'tucked-up' position with the legs underneath them. This means that there is a lot of spinal flexion and extension but a limited amount of shoulder abduction. This reduces the potential for shoulder impingement previously implicated as a common cause of injury in the wheelchair athlete (see below). However, application of force to the push rim of the chair has injury implications for the upper limb.

For the athlete with a lower limb unilateral prosthesis there will be a leg-length discrepancy to allow the prosthetic limb to swing through more easily without catching the ground. This may have biomechanical implications for injury further up the kinetic chain.

Injury epidemiology

The literature in this area is fairly limited with different qualities of study. In one paper on junior athletes, all the athletes reported some form of injury but this included skin abrasions, blisters, etc. In a study of British wheelchair athletes 70% reported an injury over a 1 year period, with 60% of these being overuse injuries (Taylor and Williams 1995). Interestingly, there was no relation between the distance pushed or the number of training sessions undertaken and the risk of injury. Although shoulder pain is commonly reported in wheelchair athletes, it appears to be a less common symptom than in wheelchair users who are non-athletes and therefore the physical conditioning may have a protective effect on the shoulder. Most studies have been of self-reported diagnosis and this has led other authors to suggest that the source of the shoulder pain may commonly come from the cervical spine rather than primary shoulder joint pathology. Given the biomechanics of wheelchair propulsion, this seems a reasonable conclusion. However, the upper limb is the most commonly injured region in the wheelchair athlete, particularly hand injuries including carpal tunnel syndrome.

Boccia

This is a sport for athletes with severe cerebral palsy or related neurological conditions and is similar to the game of boules where players throw a ball trying to get as close as possible to the 'jack' ball. A 'throw' is the term used for propelling a ball onto court and can include throwing, kicking, or releasing a ball with an assistive device such as a ramp. It has no Olympic equivalent. It is also known as bocce, and its name is derived from *bottia* the Latin word for ball.

Governing body International Boccia Commission, a committee of the Cerebral Palsy International Sports and Recreation Association (CPISRA)

First appearance in Paralympic Games 1984

Competing nations 42

Gender Mixed gender

Court The court is a flat smooth surface, usually a wooden gymnasium floor. An area of 12.5 m × 6 m is marked out with tape; this includes the throwing area which is divided into six throwing boxes. On the court is a V-shaped line over which balls must cross for the throw to be valid. A cross marks the position where the jack must be placed if it touches or crosses the boundary line or in the case of a tie break.

Events Individual and pairs events consist of four ends with or without a tie-break. Team competition consists of six ends with or without a tie-break.

◆ Individual BC1–4

◆ Pairs BC3 and BC4

◆ Team BC1 and BC2

Sport equipment A set of boccia balls consists of six red, six blue, and one white jack. The balls must weigh 275 ± 12 grams and be 270 ± 8 mm in circumference. A ramp can be used to guide the ball onto the court but must not contain any other assistive device to aid propulsion or aiming of the ball.

Disability groups Wheelchair-using athletes with severe cerebral palsy or related neurological conditions.

Classification

Players with cerebral palsy classified as CP1 or CP2 athletes as well as athletes with other severe physical disabilities (e.g. muscular dystrophy) are eligible to compete in boccia. Players are classified into four classes depending on their functional ability.

- BC1: For both CP1 throwers and CP2 foot players. Athletes may compete with the help of an assistant, who must remain outside the athlete's playing box.

- BC2: For CP2 throwing players. Players are not eligible for assistance.

- BC3: For players with a very severe physical disability. Players use an assistive device and may be assisted by a person, who will remain in the player's box but who must keep his/her back to the court and eyes averted from play.

- BC4: For players with other severe physical disabilities. Players are not eligible for assistance.

Physiological and biomechanical demands

Boccia is a target sport requiring high degrees of accuracy and concentration. The nature of the disabilities involved mean that altered muscle tone and impaired coordination and strength make this a challenging sport for the individual. There is no great physiological demand but high heart rates have been observed in players in simulated competition, reflecting possibly both psychological factor and the effect of recurrent muscle contraction with tremor. All players are wheelchair users and in most cases use their normal day chair for competition. It is important to have a stable position within the chair if trunk control is impaired.

Injury epidemiology

No data are available.

Cycling

Cycling is a relatively new Paralympic sport, first appearing in 1988 with visually impaired cyclists. It has evolved with different impairment groups, including the introduction of hand-cycling for the first time as a medal event in the 2008 Beijing Games.

Governing body International Cycling Union (UCI—Union Cycliste Internationale)

First appearance in Paralympic Games 1988 Seoul

Competing nations 40 +

Events

Track events

- Tandem sprint race (men and women)

- Team sprint race (men) – 500 metre time trial (women)

- 1000 m time trial (men)

- Individual pursuit (men and women).

Road events

- Individual time trials (men and women)

- In-line events (men and women)

Sport equipment Depending on their disability and functional ability, athletes use a bicycle, tricycle (cerebral palsy where balance is poor—road events only), or tandem (for the visually impaired). Athletes who are wheelchair users and are unable to ride a standard racing bicycle, or tricycle, because of severe lower limb disabilities compete in road events only using three-wheeled hand-cycles. During competition, athletes must wear a hard shell protective helmet to a recognized international standard. The helmet colour is standardized depending on the class of the athlete (red, blue, green, or white).

Disability groups The competitions comprise four impairment groups: blind and partially sighted riders, cerebral palsy sufferers, locomotor handicaps, and hand-cycle riders.

Classification A total of 14 functional classes for men and women in all the age categories defined by the UCI. Riders are placed in the appropriate category in the light of their functional capacity which is assessed during a medical examination.

- Locomotor disabilities: LC 1–4

- Cerebral palsy: CP 1–4

- VI: men, women and mixed. Cyclists with a visual impairment compete on the rear of tandem bicycles with a sighted pilot. A tandem pilot may not be registered with a UCI trade team or must not have been registered as a trade team cyclist for a period of three calendar years although they can work as a coach, manager, mechanic, or physiotherapist.

Physiological and biomechanical demands

The quest for improved performance has the lead to optimization of many aspects of the bicycle set-up. Many Paralympic athletes will have unique bicycle configurations to adapt for their disability. Researchers found that relatively simple adjustments in the seat height and fore–aft positions could produce a reduction in the rider's frontal-surface height by 0.22 m without compromising power output. (Burkett and Mellifont 2008). Hand-cycling will produce typically lower Vo_2 peak values as a result of using the upper limbs only for propulsion. However, values up to 53.7 ml/min/kg have been observed in elite hand-cyclists (Knechlte et al. 2004).

Injury epidemiology

In a report of injuries from the Great Britain team in the 1992 Paralympic Games, 17% of athletes were injured during training and competition in cycling compared with 50–90% of all athletes in 15 different sports ranges (Reynolds et al. 1994). However, at the next Paralympic Games the same nation reported that up to 70% of the cycling team were treated for injuries. It is clear that there are issues relating to reporting of what counts as an injury which were not defined by Reynolds et al. (1994) Furthermore, athletes have the opportunity to access medical services more readily in the Games situation than they might do in their normal training environment, which will increase the reporting rate. The injury patterns appear to be similar to Olympic cycling—impact injuries from crashes, overuse injuries from training, and postural-related spinal pain from maintaining the cycling position, but there is little detail on incidence. The introduction of hand-cycling is likely to see the development of further injury patterns related to the shoulder. For further information see www.uci.ch/ and www.paralympic.org/release/Summer_Sports/Cycling

Equestrian competition

Horse riding for people with a disability is long established as a means of rehabilitation and enjoyment, but it was it was not until the 1970s that equestrian events developed as a sport for athletes with a disability. International dressage competitions began in 1984 with the first World Championships in 1987 in Sweden. In the Paralympic Games competition consists only of dressage events, although other disciplines such as carriage driving and show jumping occur outside the Paralympics.

Governing body FEI—Para-Equestrian

First appearance in Paralympic Games 1996

Competing nations 40+

Gender Mixed gender

Event arena 20 m × 40 m arena (20 m × 60 m for Grade IV competitions). Markers in the form of a letter are placed at set locations around the arena. The test movements are defined by letter sequences. For example 'HEK medium walk' means that starting at H and going past E to K the horse must demonstrate medium walk. Letters (D, X, and G) indicate positions on the marked centre-line of the arena.

Events Dressage events consist of the following.

- Championship Test of set movements (a set of movements).
- Freestyle Test to music (which has to include some compulsory movements). The movement with music highlights the unity between horse and rider
- Team Test for three or four riders per team. Teams consist of three or four riders from the same country. At least one of the athletes must be Grade I or II (see classification). The team's final score is based on the sum from the best three performances in the Team Test and the individual Championship Test. If a team consists of four riders, the least successful total score is excluded from the final score.

Disability groups Multi-disability; physical and visual impairments.

Classification Classification of riders is undertaken by two accredited classifiers who perform an assessment of the rider's impairments and observe the rider in training and competition. The gradings include both physical and visual impairments and range from Ia to IV. For example, Grade I is described as 'Mainly wheelchair users with poor trunk balance and/or impairment of function in all four limbs or no trunk balance and good upper limb function'. The classification is important because it not only grades the impairment level but also sets the requirements for competition.

- Grade Ia – At this level the rider will ride a walk-only test.
- Grade Ib – At this level the rider will ride walk with some trot work excluding medium trot.

- Grade II – At this level the rider will ride a novice-level test excluding canter.
- Grade III – At this level the rider will ride a novice-level test.
- Grade IV – At this level the rider will ride an elementary/medium-level test.

Grade III includes riders who are blind and Grade IV includes riders who are partially sighted. These riders require alternative methods to orientate themselves within the arena and may use 'callers', whistles, or other sound systems.

Sport equipment

Riders

The rider's basic items of clothing must include a riding hat of international safety standard and riding boots or stout riding shoes with heels. Other items of clothing are specified for appearance rather than safety or sport performance (e.g. shirt, jacket, and tie). However, riders are permitted compensating aids that they may use, such as a whip instead of a leg, ladder reins, elastic bands, or special stirrups. Any compensating aid used must allow the rider to fall free of the horse if necessary for safety reasons.

Horse

The saddle is adapted to suit the individual rider to help maintain balance. The inner saddletree which is made of steel, glass fibre, or wood, and the external part of the saddle is usually made of leather, with padding between the two. The regulations say that riders may not be tied to the saddle and there must be at least 3 cm between any means of support and the rider's trunk.

Physiological and biomechanical demands

With the use of adaptations to equipment, riders with quite severe disabilities can participate in equestrian competition. There are no data exist on the physiological requirements of dressage in riders with a disability, but each event is completed in a matter of minutes and does not require significant aerobic fitness. Balance and coordination skills help, but people with even quite severe disabilities are able to participate using aids.

Injury epidemiology

There are no data for Paralympic dressage, but the number of injuries during competition is thought to be low. Injuries can occur when handling the horses (e.g. from kicks). Two falls (causing only ligament strains) were reported in the World Dressage Championships in 2007. However, the risk of injury remains with the unpredictability of horses causing injury and the potential for a fall to cause head or spinal injury. For further information, see www.ipec-athletes.de and www.fei.org/Disciplines/Para-Equestrian/Pages/Default.aspx

Football (five-a-side and seven-a-side)

Two versions of football are played at Paralympic Games involving two disability groups (Table 4.4.2). The seven-a-side version evolved in the 1970s for people with cerebral palsy, while the five-a-side version developed later and is for people with visual impairment. The versions are slightly different but have the same aim of scoring the highest amount of goals.

Table 4.4.2 Versions of football played at the Paralympic Games

	Five-a-side	Seven-a-side
Governing body	International Blind Sports Association (IBSA)	Cerebral Palsy International Sports and Recreation Association (CPISRA)
First appearance at Paralympics	2004	1984
No. of countries participating	21	22
Gender	Male	Male
Disability group	Visually impaired	Cerebral palsy
Classification	Out-field players B1–B3 Goalkeepers may be partially sighted B2–B3 or sighted but must not have been registered with FIFA in the previous 5 years	Ambulant classes C5–C8, e.g. C5: difficulties when walking and running, but not when standing or kicking the ball C8: mild hemiplegia, diplegia, athetosis, or monoplegia
Pitch size	38–42 m × 18–22 m A wall 1–1.2 m high surrounds the entire area	70–75 m × 50–55 mNo surround wall
Surface	Natural or synthetic grass	Natural or synthetic grass
Goalposts	3 m × 2 m	5 m × 2 m
Duration	2 × 25 min 10 min half-time	2 × 30 min15 min half-time
Competition schedule	Six teams play each other and then first and second teams play off for the final, and third and fourth play off for bronze	Two groups of four teams with four teams proceeding to knockout stages
Ball	Ball has sound system inside so that players can locate it	Standard ball
Equipment	All outfield players wear an eye-shield to ensure equality	Standard equipment
Rule adaptations	No throw-ins No offside rule Penalties are awarded if: a player touches their eyeshade the goalkeeper steps outside their area a player kicks or pushes an opponent Each team has a guide behind the opponent's goal to direct the players when they shoot.	No offside rule Throw-ins may be made with only one hand At least one C5 or C6 class athlete per team must play throughout the match

Physiological and biomechanical demands

The sport is technically similar to 11-a-side football but the shorter duration means that the physiological demands are less. In five-a-side football players aim to keep the ball under close control, and lofted passing and heading is not a feature of the game.

Injury epidemiology

There are no data specific to Paralympic football, but similar injuries to those in the able-bodied game can be anticipated, with twisting injuries to the knee and ankle and contact injuries, particularly in the visually impaired athletes where accidental collisions will occur to the head. Several players with cerebral palsy will have had Achilles lengthening procedures and tendon problems seem to be more prevalent. Quadriceps tightness is common, particularly where there is generally increased tone (personal communication, Patrick Wheeler).

Goalball

Goalball was devised in 1946 as an activity for blind war veterans and was introduced to the Paralympics in 1976 in Toronto as a demonstration sport. It has been an official Paralympic sport since 1980. Now more than 112 countries participate in the sport worldwide. It is one of the sports unique to the Paralympics rather than an adaptation of an able-bodied sport and involves a team of three players defending a goal against a ball thrown by the opposing team. The ball contains a bell so that the defenders can hear the ball and throw themselves in the way to defend their goal. Spectators must be silent during play to enable the players to hear the ball.

Governing body IBSA

First appearance in Paralympic Games 1980

Competing nations 50+

Gender Male and female competitions

Disability groups Visually impaired athletes only

Classification Although competition is open to any of the visually impaired classes B1–B3 as detailed below, all athletes must wear blackout goggles which eliminate any vision.

- B1: Total absence of perception of the light in both eyes, or some perception of the light but with inability to recognize the form of a hand at any distance and in any direction.

- B2: From the ability to recognize the form of a hand to a visual acuity of 2/60 and/or a visual field of less than 5°.

- B3: From a visual acuity of above 2/60 to a visual acuity of 6/60 and/or a visual field or more than 5° and less than 20°.

Events Paralympic Games

- Men: 12 teams in two pools of six.

- Women: eight teams in one pool—round robin.

Event duration Two 10 minute halves with a 3 minute break in between. In the case of a tie at the end of the regular time, two additional overtime periods of 3 minutes each are played. If the match is still tied at the end of overtime, free throws are taken.

Event arena The court used for goalball is a rectangle 18 m × 9 m. Areas for each team and a cental 'neutral' area are marked out with all markings being tactile to enable player orientation.

Sport equipment

- **Goals** Regulation goals measure 9m (equal to the width of the court) x 1.3m high.

- **Ball:** The ball used for goalball competition is made of rubber and weighs 1.25 grams with a circumference of approximately 76 cm. It has eight holes and noise bells inside.

- **Clothing** Players can wear padded clothing to protect themselves from injury as they dive about to prevent the ball entering the goal. However, the padding may not extend more than 10 cm from the body.

- **Eyeshades:** All competitors must wear eyeshades at all times on the court. At all major competitions, all players shall have their eyes covered by gauze patches under the supervision of the IBSA Goalball Technical Delegate. Penalties are given if a player touches the eyeshade during play.

Sport-specific rules:

There are three basic rules concerning the manner of throwing.

- A thrown ball must touch the floor of the court before passing over the highball (or centre) line, which is the line 6 m from the goal line at the thrower's end.

- A throw must take place within 8 seconds of coming under the control of the defending team. Passing can take place within the 8 seconds, and players may move about the court to adopt favourable positions.

- No player may take more than two consecutive throws for his team.

Medical time out

In the case of injury or illness, a medical time out shall be called by a referee and the ten (10) seconds timer closest to the injury player shall start a clock to record the forty-five (45) seconds. An audible warning will be given to the referee at the expiration of the forty-five (45) seconds. If the injured player is not prepared to play at the expiration of forty-five (45) seconds or if any member of the team enters the court, that player must be replaced until the end of that half of play.

Medical treatment

During any half of play if it is necessary for any player to leave the field of play for medical attention or equipment adjustment, the player can leave only at an official stoppage in play and may not return to the field of play until the expiration of that half.

Blood rule

Should at anytime during a game a player receive an injury where blood is observed by the referee the player will be immediately removed from the court and may not be permitted to return to the court unit the following has taken place:

- bleeding must be stopped

- the open wound covered

- if there is an excessive amount of blood on the uniform, it must be changed.

Physiological and biomechanical demands

The sport requires fast reactions and explosive movements to detect and block the incoming ball. A powerful throwing arm will increase the speed of the ball and reduce the opponent's reaction time.

Injury epidemiology

There are no data in the literature, but injuries will occur from collisions with team mates, the ball, or the floor or from twisting to react quickly to the ball.

Judo

Judo is the only Paralympic sport that originated in Asia. It was used as an activity for developing motor skills, self-control, and independence for people with a visual impairment. It evolved into a competitive sport and had its first international tournament in 1987. It was introduced to the Paralympic programme in Seoul in 1988.

Governing body IBSA

First appearance in Paralympic Games 1988

Competing nations 45

Gender Male and female

Weight categories

- Male: <60 kg, <66 kg, <73 kg, <81 kg, <90 kg, <100 kg, and >100 kg

- Women <48 kg, <52 kg, <57 kg, <63 kg, <70 kg, and >70kg

Disability groups Visually impaired only

Classification B1–B3 (see previous descriptions, but the athletes compete together).

Event arena As for standard judo: The *tatami* or mat measures 10 m × 10 m with a danger area of 1 m and an outer safety area of 3–4 m. In most competitions the mat is green with a red danger area.

Event duration Male and female, 5 minutes effective fighting time.

Technology and equipment To aid identification for the referee B1 athletes have a red circle 7 cm in diameter sewn on the outer part of both sleeves. If an athlete is also deaf, a small blue circle 7 cm diameter is attached to the back of the judogi on the upper right hand of the bib.

Rules As for judo except at the commencement of combat when athletes take a grip on each other and are forbidden to release this before the referee calls *hajime* (start). In the case of an athlete who is also deaf the referee will raise his arms for the *kumi kata* (grip) and when announcing *hajime* (start) will tap him/her once on the shoulder blade.

Physiological and biomechanical demands

Judo demands great upper body strength, balance, and agility. The visually impaired athlete particularly needs great proprioceptive awareness of body position to maintain control while the opponent is trying to throw him off balance.

Injury epidemiology

Visually impaired athletes have similar patterns of injury to able-bodied athletes. Injuries to the upper limb including fractures and dislocations are common, particularly fracture of the clavicle, acromioclavicular joint injury, shoulder dislocation, and forearm fractures. Twisting injuries to the knee and ankle are also frequent. It is very important for the visually impaired athlete to fall correctly to avoid injury. Learning to fall also gives a life skill that is applicable in daily activities where falls are more common. Athletes learn techniques of falling to the side or front and avoid being thrown onto the back, which would give their opponent victory in a competition.

Powerlifting

Powerlifting, which consists of a bench press performed from a flat platform, is described as the ultimate test of upper body strength. In Beijing 2008 a lift of 169 kg was made in the under 48 kg weight category—over three times body weight! In the over 100 kg weight category a lift of 265 kg was made to win the gold medal. Powerlifting made its debut at the Paralympic Games in 1964 as 'weightlifting'. Initially only men with spinal injuries participated, with slightly different rules than are used today, but it has expanded to include other disability groups. The sport evolved and became known as powerlifting when it incorporated rules identical to those of able-bodied powerlifting. Women entered the sport for the first time in Sydney 2000. Powerlifting is one of the world's fastest growing Paralympic sports with more than 5500 male and female lifters in the ranking lists. Unfortunately it is also the Paralympic sport with the highest number of doping offences, including the use of anabolic steroids.

Governing body IPC Powerlifting

First appearance in Paralympic Games Male, 1964; female, 2000

Competing nations 115 male; 60 female

Gender: Male and female

Disability groups Cerebral palsy, spinal injuries, amputees (lower limb amputees only), and les autres who meet minimal disability criteria.

Classification Athletes with a minimum disability must be at least 14 years of age and must have the ability to fully extend the arms with no more than a 20° loss of full extension on either elbow when making an approved lift according to the rules for their body weight.

Event arena A bench for the lifting is placed on an accessible platform.

Events

Men: <48 kg, <52 kg, <56 kg, <60 kg, <67.5 kg, <75 kg, <82.5 kg, <90 kg, <100 kg and >100kg divisions.

Women: <40 kg, <44 kg, <48 kg, <52 kg, <56 kg, <60 kg, <67.5 kg, <75 kg, <82.5 kg and >82.5 kg divisions.

Sport equipment

Standardized equipment is used for all powerlifting competitions organized under the rules of the IPC Powerlifting. Competition is performed lying on a bench. The official bench is 2.1 m long. The main part of the bench is 61 cm wide. At the end of the bench and towards the head, the bench narrows down to 30 cm. The height of the bench varies between 45 and 50 cm from the ground.

Rules

The weigh-in

All athletes must be weighed prior to competing and this cannot start until 2 hours before the event. The weigh-in period itself will last 1.5 hours. Each lifter is weighed once unless their bodyweight is heavier or lighter than their category limits. They are allowed to make the weight and be reweighed during the 1.5 hours allocated for the weigh-in or they are eliminated from the competition for that bodyweight category.

The lift

Athletes are given three lift attempts and the winner is the athlete who lifts the highest number of kilograms. The athlete lies on the bench and assumes a position with head, trunk (including buttocks), legs, and both heels extended and must maintain this position during the complete lift. An exception may be accepted for medical reasons. From the moment the the athlete is announced with name, country, attempt, and weight on the bar, the competitor has 2 minutes to complete the attempt. Competitors must lower the bar to the chest, hold it motionless on the chest, and then press it upwards to arms' length with locked elbows. Three referees assess the success of each attempt by choosing the white or red light. The lifting order within each round will be determined by the lifter's choice of weight for that round and the weights must be a multiple of 2.5 kg with the exception of a new record. Between the first and second attempt, and between the second and third attempt, there must be a minimum increase of 2.5 kg.

Physiological and biomechanical demands

To achieve lifts of up to 265 kg huge forces must be generated using pectoral, deltoid, and triceps muscles predominantly as prime movers, although shoulder and trunk stabilizers also have a significant role to play. These muscles are strengthened through high load resistance exercises but also technical refinement such as grip placement or optimizing the path of the bar can have significant impact on performance.

Injury epidemiology

There are no published data on injuries in Paralympic powerlifting, but injuries to the shoulder, elbow, and wrist joints including dislocation, rotator cuff tears, and long head of bicep injuries can be expected in addition to muscle tears in the major groups. Powerlifting has the highest incidence of positive tests for anabolic steroids in Paralympic sport and so the sports physician should consider this possibility in assessment of the injured athlete.

Rowing

Adaptive rowing was first introduced in 1975 as a sport for people with disabilities, but it was not until the 2008 Beijing Paralympic Games that it entered the Paralympic programme. The term 'adaptive' refers to the fact that the equipment is adapted to enable athletes to compete rather than the sport being adapted to the disability. In 2002 FISA introduced Adaptive Rowing at its World Rowing Championships in Seville, Spain, where 38 athletes competed in the single sculls and the coxed four and have extended this since to four events.

Governing body FISA—Fédération Internationale des Sociétés d'Aviron (in English, International Federation of Rowing Associations)

First appearance in Paralympic Games Beijing 2008

Competing nations 24 countries

Gender Male and female. Mixed gender in coxed fours and double sculls. Separate male and female single sculls.

Event arena 1000 m straight course

Events

- LTA4+ (legs, trunk and arms: coxed fours)
- TA2× (trunk and arms: double sculls)
- AW1× (arms only: women's single)
- AM1× (arms only: men's single)

Disability groups Adaptive rowing permits competition from a number of disability groups who meet the minimum disability requirements, including amputees and those with neurological impairments including cerebral palsy. In the LTA group it combines athletes with a physical disability and those with visual impairment. From 2009 athletes with an intellectual disability are also included in FISA events but this is not yet confirmed for the London 2012 Paralympics.

Classification The process involves a 'bench test' by a medically qualified classifier, an 'ergometer test' by a technical classifier, and an 'on-water observation' by both classifiers during training and competition.

- LTA class: for rowers with a disability who have functional use of their legs, trunk, and arms for rowing, and who can utilize the sliding seat.
- TA class: for rowers who have functional use of the trunk and who are not able to use the sliding seat.
- AS class: for rowers who have no or minimal trunk function (i.e. shoulder function only).

Sport equipment

The hulls of adaptive rowing boats are identical to those of standard rowing boats but athletes use a fixed or sliding seat, depending on the disability, along with different degrees of support in the seat. Pontoons for stability can be used in single and double sculls.

Visually impaired rowers must wear approved eyewear at all times when on the water during training, warm-up, cool-down, and competition from the opening day of the course until completion of the final race of their competition. The eyewear completely blocks all light to ensure no advantage for partially sighted athletes.

Physiological and biomechanical demands

Events will vary in duration from around 3.5 minutes for an LTA4 crew completing the 1000 m course to 5.5–6 minutes for a top female single sculler. Local muscle fatigue may occur earlier than central fatigue in an 'arms-only' rower when only the upper limbs are used for propulsion.

Injury epidemiology

No data are available.

Sailing

Sailing has been a sport for people with disabilities for many years and disabled sailors have circumnavigated the globe. The International Handicap Sailing Committee was first established in 1988 and later became the International Foundation for Disabled Sailing. It was recognised by the International Sailing Federation in 1991. Competitive Paralympic sailing started following a successful demonstration event at the Atlanta Paralympic Games and was introduced to the full Paralympic programme in Sydney 2000.

Governing body International Foundation for Disabled Sailing

First appearance in Paralympic Games Sydney 2000

Competing nations 34 member nations of IFDS

Gender Mixed

Event course A course is set which aims to have a race lasting for 50–75 minutes. There is an overall time limit for each race which is 1 hour and 45 minutes for the first boat to finish. In Paralympic Games a total of 11 races are carried out in each class with points awarded for each race and the winner determined by overall placement.

Events: There are competitions in three classes of boat.

- 2.4mR: single-person keelboat
- SKUD18: two-person keelboat
- Sonar: three-person keelboat

Disability groups People are eligible if they have a permanent physical impairment that limits their ability to compete equitably in elite sport with athletes without a disability as determined by classification. Athletes with a visual impairment are also eligible.

Classification

In sailing the classification system examines the individual's ability to perform the main functions of sailing which are defined as:

- operating the control lines and the tiller (hand function)
- ability to see whilst racing (vision)
- compensation for the movement of the boat (stability)
- ability to move about in the boat (mobility).

These are examined by:

- a physical examination (Functional Anatomical Test (FA))

◆ observation of standardized simulated sailing functions (Functional Dock Test (FD))

◆ Observation of the sailor during competition and/or training and/or out of competition (Functional Sail Test (FS))

Any assistive devices or adaptations such as prostheses or orthotics must be worn during the classification process.

Points are awarded for the level of disability (1–7) and in the three-person Sonar boat a combined score of 14 or less is required which ensures that people with more severe disabilities are included. In the two-person boat only one sailor with the minimum disability may be included in each crew.

Sport equipment

◆ **International 2.4mR** A single-handed keelboat, 4.1 m long and weighing 260 kg. The design allows the helmsperson to sit amidships holding all the instruments for controlling the boat and navigating.

◆ **Sonar** This boat has a crew of three, a fixed keel, a length of 7 m, and a weight of 950 kg. In Paralympic competition the crew uses just a mainsail and jib. A crew of varying disabilities is required and the boat allows different adaptive aids for those sailors with more severe disabilities.

◆ **SKUD 18** This is a two-person keelboat with a length of 5.8 m, a minimum weight of 380 kg, and three sails (one mainsail, one jib, and one spinnaker). Sailors are seated on the centre-line for Paralympic events. The helmsperson can transfer manually and steer with tillers, or be in a fixed seat on the centre-line using a manual joystick, push–pull rods, or a servo assist joystick with full control of all functions.

Physiological and biomechanical demands

Although events are aimed to last around an hour, several hours may be required out on the water for getting ready, racing, and returning to shore. Thus environmental conditions can play a role—either trying to stay cool and hydrated in the heat or trying to maintain body temperature in the cold. Upper body strength is required for managing the control lines and trunk stability helps maintain position in the boat.

Injury epidemiology

A survey of sailors in the International Foundation for Disabled Sailing World Championship 1999, with 24 teams and multiple disability types, showed an injury prevalence of 6.34% (Allen 2003).

Shooting

Shooting is another long-established target sport which challenges the athlete's control and accuracy. In its earlier years it used a disability-specific classification system with five classes, but has changed to a functional system combining disability groups and reducing the number of classes to three.

Governing body The International Shooting Committee for Disabled represents the International Paralympic Committee

First appearance in Paralympic Games Toronto 1976

Competing nations 59 countries in 2008

Gender Mixed and separate male and female events

Event arena Shooting range

Events 10 m, 25 m, and 50 m individual and team events in pistol and rifle.

Disability groups Physically and visually impaired athletes

Classification

Shooting moved to a functional classification system for physical impairments which enables athletes from different disability classes with similar abilities to compete together, either individually or in teams. There are two classes for athletes with a physical impairment: those who require support of their arm (a shooting stand) (SH2) and those who do not (SH1). The SH3 class is for athletes who are visually impaired.

There are minimum disability requirements for all classes. For SH3 athletes this is a visual acuity no higher than 6/60 with best correction and/or visual field limitation less than 20°. Each visually impaired competitor is allowed to have one assistant during competition but they may not coach.

◆ SH1: Pistol and rifle competitors that do not require a shooting stand.

◆ SH2: Rifle competitors who have no ability to support the weight of the firearm with their arms and therefore require a shooting stand.

◆ SH3: Rifle competitors with visual impairment.

Sport equipment

◆ **Weapons** Athletes use 22 calibre rifles and air guns.

◆ **Bullets** For 10 m events held with an air rifle or air pistol, bullets with a diameter of 4.5 mm are use. For 25 m pistol events, and 50 m pistol and rifle events, 5.6 mm bullets are used.

◆ **Target** For the Paralympic Games, five different targets are used depending on the type of gun. These targets are electronic for increased accuracy.

◆ **Shooting chair** This can be a wheelchair, stool, or seat that an athlete may use. There are limitations on the level of support it can provide which are outlined in the sport technical manual.

◆ **Shooting table** For sitting classes this may be attached to the shooting chair or may be free standing and must meet the sport technical specifications.

◆ **Sights for visually impaired** SH3 athletes uses a sight that emits a light and the reflection from the target is converted into an audible tone

Additional rules: epilepsy

It is imperative that epilepsy is stable and under control. During classification the certification of a neurological doctor must be handed over to the classification panel to certify that the epilepsy is stable and what type of epilepsy it is. It is evident from the perspective of safety on the shooting range that temporal partial epilepsy is a contraindication for shooting.

Physiological and biomechanical demands

As a target sport, strength and stability are key components in performance. However, aerobic fitness is also beneficial as this lowers resting heart rate, producing a longer period of diastole during which firing normally takes place.

Injury epidemiology

No data are available.

Swimming

Swimming has been a method of rehabilitation for a long time and it is little wonder that competitive swimming was introduced into the Stoke Mandeville Games at a relatively early stage. It is a very accessible sport and has worldwide participation. It is also one of the largest Paralympic sport programmes with 141 medal events at the Beijing Games in 2008. It is also a popular spectator event with 200 000 people watching over the nine-day Paralympic swimming programme in Sydney.

Governing body IPC Swimming

First appearance in Paralympic Games Rome 1960

Competing nations Sydney 2000—62 competing nations

Gender Male and female

Event arena A FINA standard eight-lane 50 m pool

Events In Paralympic Games the following events take place but other events may be included at other championships (see classification for class details):

* 50 m and 100 m freestyle: class S1–S10
* 200 m freestyle: class S1–S5
* 400 m freestyle: class S6–S10
* 50 m backstroke: class S1–S5
* 100 m backstroke: class S6–S10
* 50 m butterfly: class S1–S7
* 100 m butterfly: class S8–S10
* 50 m breaststroke: class SB1–SB3
* 100 m breaststroke: class SB4–SB9
* 150 m individual medley: class SM1–SM4
* 200 m individual medley: class SM5–SM10
* 4 × 50 m freestyle relay and 4 × 50 m medley relay
* 4 × 100 m freestyle relay and 4 × 100 m medley relay

Disability groups Swimmers with physical disabilities of a wide range and also swimmers with a visual impairment. Swimmers with intellectual impairment were included in the Sydney 2000 Games and may be reinstated in the London 2012 Games.

Classification

Swimming employs a functional classification system for assessing physical impairments that uses a 'bench test' of physical measures alongside an assessment of swimming performance including starts and turns. This allows swimmers with widely different causes of physical impairment to compete against each other based upon swimming ability. For example, two swimmers may have no ability to move their legs on the bench test but in the swimming assessment, one swimmer's legs may float high in the water while the other swimmer's legs do not, adding considerable drag resistance. Swimmers may also start a race in the water, sitting, or standing depending on their impairment.

After the assessment is completed, athletes are classified as follows, with the lowest number indicating the severest impairment:

* ten classes (S1–S10) in freestyle, backstroke, and butterfly
* ten classes (SM1–SM10) for individual medley
* nine classes (SB1–SB9) in breaststroke.

Swimmers with a visual impairment are assessed ophthalmologically for visual acuity and visual field and categorized according to the International Blind Sports Association (IBSA) criteria, and classes B1, B2, and B3 are matched to S11, S12, and S13 for swimming. Swimmers with a B1 class have no purposeful sight and for complete equality across the group are required to wear a 'black-out' goggle for competition. To indicate that they are nearing the pool end a person, known as a 'tapper', will tap them on the head or shoulder using a pole with a rounded end.

Sport equipment

There have been many adaptations to swimsuit design over the years and to ensure fair competition based upon swimming ability IPC Swimming has adopted the new FINA regulations on the swimsuit (Dubai Charter) implemented in 2009.

Physiological and biomechanical demands

The physiological demands of swimming depend on both distance and disability. The lactate profiles of athletes in the higher classes, i.e. with less disability, are similar to those of able-bodied swimmers. However, as the degree of impairment increases, there may be different patterns. For example, a paraplegic only using the upper limbs may experience local fatigue rather than central fatigue as a limiting factor in longer events because of the small amount of muscle mass. Individual variations in lactate accumulation also occur, particularly where there is increased tone with conditions such as cerebral palsy. Biomechanical assessment of Paralympic swimmers has proved very valuable, with the Great Britain swim team using underwater video footage. The work is unpublished, but individual assessment of the athlete's stroke pattern, streamlining, starts, and turns can have significant performance advantages.

Injury epidemiology

Paralympic sports injury reporting is often collective of sports rather than itemized. A two-year prospective study by Ferrara and Buckley (1996) of 319 multi-disability athletes in summer Paralympic sports produced an overall injury rate of 9.3 per 1000 hours of exposure; however, no details on specific sports were provided. This compares with results for non-elite swimmers reported by Wilson and Washington (1993), who found that 91% self-reported injuries. Whilst the shoulder is commonly cited as the source of pain in swimmers (Ferrara and Davis 1990), Webborn and Turner (2000) found that the cervical and thoracic spine was the source of the shoulder pain more frequently than the shoulder itself. This related to multiple factors including existing spinal pathology and habitual postural changes.

Table tennis

Table tennis was introduced as a sport for rehabilitation to help improve balance and coordination as well as providing competition for people with a spinal cord injury. It was included in the Stoke Mandeville Games and has been on the Paralympic programme since 1960. In the 1970s the sport was governed under the International Stoke Mandeville Games Federation before other disability groups were gradually included, and it has finally passed governance from the disability organization to the international sports federation (ITTF).

Governing body International Table Tennis Federation Para-Table Tennis. This has recently been transferred to ITTF from IPC Table Tennis.

First appearance in Paralympic Games Rome 1960 (wheelchair), Toronto 1976 (amputee and les autres), Arnhem 1980 (cerebral palsy)

Competing nations 104

Gender Male and female

Event arena A table tennis arena meeting ITTF standards. A separate ventilated gluing area is provided for players to glue new rubber surfaces to their bats prior to competition.

Events Individual, doubles, and team events. A match consists of the best of five sets, each being played to 11 points.

Disability groups Athletes with a physical impairment over a wide range including wheelchair and standing players.

Classification Athletes are classified into 11 classes TT1–TT11. Classification includes a physical examination and a functional assessment including balance in the wheelchair, if used, and the ability to handle the racket.

◆ Classes TT1–TT5: wheelchair athletes

◆ Classes TT6–TT10: standing athletes.

Class TT11 is for intellectually disabled athletes according to the INAS-FID/IPC definition, but this class is currently not included in Paralympic competition.

Sport equipment All equipment used is standard ITTF approved equipment, but the tables should have legs at least 40 cm from the end for wheelchair players to manoeuvre without restriction.

Rules adaptations It is not permitted to serve off the side of the table in wheelchair classes, but otherwise the rules are the same as for standard table tennis.

Physiological and biomechanical demands

Table tennis, particularly for standing players, is a very demanding sport physically, requiring stamina, speed, and agility as well as skill. There is reduced requirement for movement for wheelchair players, but the chair position needs to be controlled while playing. There are no physiological data for Paralympic table tennis.

Injury epidemiology

No data.

Volleyball (sitting)

Sitting volleyball is an adaptation of volleyball played from a sitting position in a reduced court with a lower net. The aims of the game are similar, i.e. to get the ball to touch the floor in the opponent's court area using your own team of six players to keep the ball in play on your side before playing the ball over the net. Only three contacts or passes are permitted on one side of the net, not including blocks. At all times players must have their pelvis in touch with the floor. It evolved in Holland in the 1950s from a combination of volleyball and *sitzball*, a game played in Germany. As it developed internationally it came under the governance of the International Sports Organization for the Disabled and made its first appearance in the Paralympic programme in 1980.

Standing volleyball was developed in Great Britain, initially for amputees, and later for other disabilities, but is no longer on the Paralympic programme.

Governing body World Organization Volleyball for Disabled

First appearance in Paralympic Games Arnhem 1980

Competing nations About 50

Gender Male and female competition.

Event arena The playing area is a court floor 10 m × 6 m with an extended area or 'free zone' extending out to the sides and rear. The playing area has a dividing line 2 m back from the net separating offensive and defensive zones. The net is 1.15 m high for men and 1.05 m for women, and is stretched between two post supports.

Events Teams have a maximum of twelve players of which six may be on court at one time. They play the best of five sets with the first four sets up to twenty-five points. The final set is to fifteen points, with a difference of at least two points over the opposing team.

Disability groups Athletes with physical impairments are eligible to play provided that they meet the minimum disability requirements.

Classification Athletes are eligible to participate as long as they have a physical impairment that meets the minimum disability requirements. For example in the upper limb this is:

◆ amputation of the first two fingers on two hands

◆ amputation of seven fingers or more on two hands

◆ amputation on one hand between the MPJ and the wrist.

Sport equipment 'The ball has a circumference of 65–67 cm and its weight varies from 260 to 280 grams, and can be of a single colour or a combination of several colours. Both its component materials and colour must be in compliance with the rules and regulations of WOVD.'

Physiological and biomechanical demands

No specific information is available, but upper limb strength and trunk control are required to move around the court and play the ball.

Injury epidemiology

No data specific to sitting volleyball are available, but injuries to the upper limb predominate and particularly the fingers and shoulders.

Wheelchair basketball

Wheelchair basketball is one of the fastest developing and most exciting Paralympic sports. It first developed in 1946 in the USA among injured servicemen who had formerly played basketball. The game crossed the Atlantic and became an integral part of the International Stoke Mandeville Games, and it entered the

Paralympic programme in 1960. Although it evolved as a game for people with a spinal cord injury, people with other physical impairments were attracted to the sport which became faster and more competitive as a consequence.

Governing body International Wheelchair Basketball Federation

First appearance in Paralympic Games Rome 1960

Competing nations More than 80

Gender Male and female competition

Event arena A standard basketball court with a hard surface 28 m long and 15 m wide. The basket and backboards are at the standard height.

Events A team consists of five players on court at any time and seven substitutes. A match consists of four periods of 10 minutes with 1 minute breaks after the first and third periods and a fifteen minute break in the middle. The competition format for men in the Paralympic Games is two groups of six teams, with the top four in each group progressing to a knockout stage. For women there are two groups of five teams with the top four teams progressing to the knockout stage.

Disability groups Physical impairments such as spinal cord injury or lower limb amputee.

Classification

Basketball uses a functional assessment based upon sport-specific tests of shooting, passing, rebounding, pushing, and dribbling, and allocates the player to one of eight classes using a point system from 1 to 4.5 in half-point graduations. In competition a team may only include a maximum total of 14 points amongst the five players on court, thus ensuring that a spread of physical impairment levels are included. Examples include the following:

- A 2 point player would typically be someone with T8–L1 paraplegia or post-polio paralysis without control of lower extremity movement.

- A 4.5 point player may be a single below-knee amputee or a player with extensive orthopaedic involvement of hips, knees, or ankles or post-polio paralysis with minimal (ankle/foot) involvement on one or both sides

Sport equipment

The basketball equipment is standard, but the chairs have been adapted over time to provide a combination of speed, stability, and turning ability. The chair is considered to be part of the player and is subject to certain restrictions. For example, the maximum height from the floor to the top of the cushion must not exceed 63 cm for 1.0–3.0 point players or 58 cm for 3.5–4.5 point players. The main wheels are cambered to provide easy turning and also reduce fingers clashing together. Anti-tip castor wheels are used to improve stability and high-pressure tyres to improve speed. Players may use a variety of strapping techniques to secure themselves within the chair and protective taping on their fingers or wrists.

Physiological and biomechanical demands

Wheelchair basketball is a highly demanding physical game requiring sprint endurance using the upper limbs. Peak Vo_2 peak values vary from 3.66 L/min in 4.5 point players to 2.07 L/min in 1 point players (Goosey-Tolfrey 2005).

Injury epidemiology

Several multi-sport studies have identified wheelchair basketball as a relatively high-risk sport for injury and this was borne out in the basketball-specific study by Burnham and Higgins (1994). This was a questionnaire study collected over nine tournaments in 1990 and examined training loads, equipment, and injury. Eighty-two per cent of athletes reported an injury in the previous year, with nearly one in five of these causing significant time loss from sport. Eighty-seven per cent of injuries were to the upper limb and, although injuries to the hands, including blisters and abrasions, were the most common, it was the injuries to shoulders, elbow, and wrist that caused more time loss. These injuries were also associated with more training days per week. Curtis and Black (1999) found that shoulder and upper limb pain was present in 90% of forty-six female wheelchair basketball players.

Wheelchair fencing

Wheelchair fencing commenced in Stoke Mandeville Hospital in the UK in 1953. Initially the sport was for spinal-injured persons and the wheelchairs were not fixed in position. Sometimes an assistant would hold and stabilize the chair. As the sport has evolved, other disability groups have take up the sport and the chairs are now fixed in a frame.

Governing body International Stoke Mandeville Wheelchair Sports Federation–International Wheelchair Fencing Committee

First appearance in Paralympic Games 1960

Competing nations 24

Gender Male and female

Event arena The wheelchairs are fixed in place by metal frames. The chair is preferably clamped to both sides of the frame to keep it from tipping. The length of the playing area (distance between the two chairs) is decided by the fencer with the shortest arms. This person decides if the distance will be at his distance (of reach) or that of his opponent. The chairs must be fixed at a 110° angle to the central bar.

Events Foil and épée for men and women. Sabre events are limited to men. There are three divisions of competition, with divisions based upon disability classification. There are individual and team events for men and women.

Disability groups At the Seoul Paralympic Games in 1988, a new system of integrated classification for wheelchair fencing was introduced which allows athletes with different disabilities (amputee, polio, cerebral palsy and paraplegia) the opportunity to compete together.

Classification Athletes who use wheelchairs are eligible to compete in wheelchair fencing. Classification is based upon functional tests and 'bench' assessments of muscle. Functional tests are performed in the wheelchair with a variety of movements with and without the use of a weapon.

Sport equipment

Standard fencing equipment and weapons are used with some additions. The athlete uses his/her own chair which may be specifically adapted for use in fencing. The inside rear wheel should be covered by metal detachable shields. The chair may have a cushion between 5 and 10 cm in height. If the athlete has significant loss of grip function, the weapon may be attached to the hand with taping or binding. Fencers must wear protective clothing, including a mask, a jacket, a vest, and a glove covering the sleeve opening. In foil events, a protective cover is placed on the wheelchair to prevent hits on the chair from being recorded. In épée, a metal covering (an 'apron') must be placed over the athlete's legs for added protection.

Rules

The targets for foil and sabre competitions are exactly the same as in able-bodied competition. In épée competition, the target is everything above the waist, with an apron being worn below the waist to aid in cancellation of these touches. Feet must remain on the footrest and the fencer must remain seated (no space between the fencer's buttocks and the seat of the chair).

In preliminary individual events, each bout lasts 4 minutes. The winner is the first to score five hits (or the greatest number of hits) in the bout. This is followed by a knockout system where athletes compete in three 3 minute rounds with a 1 minute break between rounds. The winner is the first to score 15 hits (or the greatest number of hits). In the case of a tie, extra 1 minute bouts are played and the first to score a hit is the winner. Athletes are connected electronically to a signal box which records the touches of the weapon. A point is awarded each time a fencer touches the opponent in the target area.

Physiological and biomechanical demands

There are no published data on this sport. Speed of movement, quick reactions, and dexterity are required, and certainly a good degree of upper body strength is necessary for the sabre.

Injury epidemiology

No published data are available but injuries occur from contact by the opponents weapon and upper limb overuse injuries in the dominant arm. For further information see www.iwfencing.com and www.paralympic.org/release/Summer_Sports/Wheelchair_Fencing/

Wheelchair rugby

Athletes with tetraplegia found that opportunity to participate in wheelchair basketball reduced as the sport evolved with increased participation by other disability groups. As the most impaired players, the tetraplegic athletes had reduced involvement and their importance in basketball diminished. As a consequence, in the 1970s a group of players in Canada developed a new game for tetraplegic athletes, originally termed 'murderball', which developed into the sport of wheelchair rugby. It takes components from different games, but the object of the game is to carry the ball across the opposing team's goal line to score a point. The ball can be passed forward and collision between chairs is permitted even with a non-ball carrier to produce an exciting tactical game. It made its way onto the Paralympic programme as a demonstration sport in Atlanta 1996 and onto the full medal programme in Sydney 2000.

Governing body International Wheelchair Rugby Federation under the International Wheelchair and Amputee Sports Federation

First appearance in Paralympic Games Sydney 2000

Competing nations 28

Gender Mixed

Event arena A standard basketball court is used, but the basketball key area is replaced by a wheelchair rugby key area 8 m wide and 1.75 m deep. The part of the end-line within the key is called the goal-line, and it is marked with a cone or pylon at each end to mark the goal.

Events Each team consists of up to 12 players of mixed genders, four of whom can be on court at one time. Each match consists of four 8 minute quarters with a 2 minute break between the first and third quarters, and a 5 minute break at half-time. In the Paralympic Games the competition consists of two groups and then progresses to a knockout stage.

Disability groups To be eligible to play, individuals must have a disability which affects both the arms and the legs. They must also be physically capable of propelling a manual wheelchair with their arms. Athletes with neurological disabilities must have at least three limbs with limited functions; athletes with non-neurological disabilities must have limited function in all four limbs. The majority of players have a spinal cord injury.

Classification Players are classed into one of seven classes: 0.5, 1.0, 1.5, 2.0, 2.5, 3.0, and 3.5, where 0.5 indicates the most severe impairment. The classification is based on the player's functional ability in a series of bench, functional, and on-court assessments that include functional movement tests (e.g. pushing, turning, stopping, starting, dribbling, and passing). During the game, the total value of all the players on the court for a team cannot exceed 8 points, ensuring that mixes of athletes of all functional levels participate.

Sport equipment

- Ball: An official size and weight volleyball is used for play that must weigh 280 grams and be white in colour.

- Gloves: Athletes may wear gloves to improve their grip on the ball, to improve pushing efficiency, and for protection. A tacky substance may also be applied to the glove or push-rim to improve contact when pushing.

- Wheelchair: The sport can be quite brutal in collisions and the chairs must be strong enough to withstand this force. They may also have defensive bars or bumpers to protect it or for offensive moves. The wheels have spoke guards to protect them. However, the chair also needs to be light enough to be manouevrable. The regulations for wheelchair design are strictly governed by the International Federation.

Physiological and biomechanical demands

Wheelchair rugby is essentially an intermittent sprint sport with short bursts of high-intensity upper body activity, but it also requires static strength to maintain blocking positions. The system of rolling substitutions in match play allows fatigued players to be replaced for rest periods. The high-intensity activity, particularly in tetraplegic athletes, makes them susceptible to rises in core temperature which may result in impaired performance or heat injury. Goosey-Tolfrey *et al.* (2006) assessed the aerobic capacity and peak power output of elite quadriplegic rugby and tennis players.

Peak power output over a 5 second sprint was 220 ± 62 W and mean Vo_2 peak was 0.96 ± 0.17 L/min.

Injury epidemiology

No published data purely on wheelchair rugby player is available but upper limb injuries predominate as one would expect with shoulder joint and muscle injuries common. Collisions also cause sudden jarring which particularly may affect the cervical spine in athletes with a previous spinal injury.

Wheelchair tennis

Wheelchair started in the 1970s in the USA and as it developed an international governing body was founded in 1988—the International Wheelchair Tennis Federation. Ten years later, the IWTF was integrated into the International Tennis Federation and a worldwide tour of competitions takes place with over 130 competitions from January to December. It can be played on all court surfaces, with full medal events now introduced at the Wimbledon Championships. It is a sport that wheelchair players can play against or alongside able-bodied players, making it a fun and integrated recreational sport as well.

Governing body International Tennis Federation

First appearance in Paralympic Games Barcelona 1992

Competing nations 90+

Gender Male and female. Mixed gender competition in the quad division.

Event arena Standard tennis court size. Tennis competitions are played on all surfaces but on hard courts for Paralympic Games.

Events Singles and doubles. Best of three sets with tie-breaks.

Disability groups Athletes with physical impairments that meet the minimum disability criteria.

Classification

◆ Open division: The minimum eligibility requirement for men's and women's events is a permanent substantial or total loss of function in one or both legs due to conditions such as spinal injury, ankylosis, amputation, or other lower limb disability.

◆ Quad division: The eligibility criteria require that a player has a disability in three or more limbs. An off-court physical assessment and on-court functional assessment are performed to determine eligibility.

Sport equipment Standard tennis rackets and balls are used but a quad division player may also tape the racket to the hand for racket control. Tennis wheelchairs have developed and adapted over the years to meet the needs of the sport. Rapid changes in direction, stability, and light weight are key. The main wheels are cambered to assist turning, and rear anti-tip castor wheels are used to prevent overbalancing when leaning backwards.

Rule adaptations The ITF rules are applied exactly apart from two exceptions.

◆ The wheelchair tennis player is allowed two bounces of the ball. The player must return the ball before it hits the ground a third time. The second bounce can be either in or out of the court boundaries.

◆ The wheelchair is considered part of the body and all applicable rules, which apply to a player's body, shall apply to the wheelchair. For example, if the ball hits the player's chair on the full outside the court area then the opponent wins the point.

Physiological and biomechanical demands

Physiologically, tennis is an intermittent sprint sport, but the players must use the upper limbs for propulsion as well as to hold the racket and play the shots, placing increased demands on the upper limb. The physiological performance of quad players is discussed in the section on wheelchair rugby.

Injury epidemiology

No sport-specific data have been published on wheelchair tennis. However, as can be anticipated upper limb injuries will predominate but spinal problems can also occur. The dominant hand is relatively overloaded as it is used to push the chair with the racket still in the hand and to hit the ball. The tetraplegic player with poor finger function can use the base of the hand to apply force to the wheel, which may result in wrist joint injuries or nerve compression injuries at the wrist.

Winter Sports

Alpine Skiing

Alpine skiing developed initially for people with visual impairment and amputations with the first documented competition held in Badgastein, Austria, in 1948. It was not until the 1970s, with the development of the sit-ski, that people with spinal cord injury and bilateral amputations were able to participate. In the first Winter Games in 1976 there were only slalom and giant slalom events, with downhill added in 1984 in Innsbruck. The sport has grown rapidly since. Now there is an IPC Alpine Skiing World Cup with events over the season in Australia, Japan, Korea, North America and Europe and an annual world championship competition.

Governing Body IPC Alpine Skiing

First appearance in Paralympic Games Örnsköldsvik, Sweden 1976

Competing nations 39

Gender Male and Female

Event arena Alpine ski slope. Typically the Olympic women's downhill course is used for Paralympic events, but the course for each event is determined by the vertical drop

Events Downhill, Super-G, Giant Slalom, Slalom and Super-combined

Disability Groups Athletes with a physical impairment such as spinal injury, cerebral palsy, amputation, Les Autres conditions and athletes with a visual impairment

Classification Athletes are classified into 3 main categories with sub-divisions:

Visually Impaired

◆ B1 - Totally blind participants up to light perception/hand movement

◆ B2 - visual acuity of 2/60 and/or visual field of less than 5 degrees

◆ B3 - visual acuity above 2/60 to 6/60 and/or visual field of more than 5 degrees and less than 20 degrees

Standing Athletes

- LW 1 - double above knee amputation
- LW 2 - single above knee amputation
- LW 3 - double below knee amputation/cerebral palsy
- LW 4 - single below knee amputation
- LW 5/7 - double arm amputation
- LW 6/8 - amputation or other disabilities in one arm
- LW 9 - one upper limb and one lower limb disability

Sitting Athletes

- LW 10 - no functional sitting balance
- LW 11 - fair sitting balance
- LW 12 - good sitting balance, incomplete paraplegic/amputation of the lower limb/s

Sport equipment In general the sport equipment is identical apart from a few adaptations listed below. Helmets are compulsory for safety.

Athletes in standing classes requiring extra balance assistance e.g. a single leg amputee may use an adaptation to the ski-pole called an out-rigger. This has a small ski fitted to the end of an extended pole similar to a crutch.

Athletes is sitting classes use a sit-ski or mono-ski which has a customized seat attached to the ski, usually incorporating a suspension device. Athletes in sit-skis also use a form of out-rigger.

Athletes in B1 class of visual impairment wear black-out goggles to ensure all athletes in this class are equal.

Rule adaptations: Visually impaired athletes are guided down the course following a sighted guide who gives verbal instructions. This can be called out or via a headset and microphone system.

Physiological & Biomechanical demands

Each event takes a few minutes to complete and place similar physiological demands as able-bodied skiing. Athletes in sit-skis require more upper body strength.

Injury epidemiology

Comparative data of injury rate by sport from two Winter Paralympic Games (2002 & 2006) found similar injury incidences at both Games in alpine skiing (13% & 12% respectively). Athletes in seated classes have more injuries to the upper limb whereas athletes in standing classes have similar injury patterns as able-bodied skiers e.g. ACL ruptures (Webborn AD 2007). Injuries to the head in alpine skiing appear to be more common than in summer sports due to the high speeds and collision potential (Webborn N et al. 2006). The authors also found an incidence of wrist fractures in sit-skiers relating to heavy landing on the out-riggers, which may have an implication for equipment design.

Ice Sledge Hockey

Ice sledge hockey is the Paralympic version of ice hockey played by people with impairments in lower limb function that cannot play ice hockey. It developed in Sweden in the 1960s with the players sitting on an adapted sledge with a skate fixed beneath. It slowly developed over a couple of decades and was first introduced to the Paralympic programme in 1994. It has become one of the most exciting spectacles of the winter games with high-speed collisions and spectacular goals.

Governing Body IPC Ice Sledge Hockey

First appearance in Paralympic Games Lillehammer 1994

Competing nations 12 (2006)

Gender Mixed gender (approved for Vancouver 2010)

Event arena Ice sledge hockey is played on a standard ice hockey rink – maximum size 61m long x 30 m wide and minimum 56m long x 26m wide. There are rounded corners and a board surround 1.17m-1.22m in height above the ice. At the lower part of the board is a stiff kick plate 15-25cm in height. Protective glass along the sides and ends is fitted above the boards for spectator safety.

Events At Paralympic Games it is an eight-team tournament with two pools of four. The top two and bottom two teams in each group then play off in a knockout to determine the final positions 1-8.

Disability Groups Sledge hockey has a minimal disability system of eligibility (see classification) that enables a wide range of people with physical impairments to participate.

Classification The rules state that to compete an athlete must have a permanent impairment in the lower part of the body that is obvious and easily recognisable and makes ordinary skating impossible. Minimum requirements include e.g. a through ankle amputation but normal upper body strength is expected. Restricted hip joint movement only, chronic pain syndromes or joint instability through ligament laxity are not conditions for eligibility.

Sport equipment All protective equipment, clothing and footwear must meet the standards for ice hockey.

Sledges Players sit on a sledge, which consists of a supporting frame, seat bucket, a front skid (usually part of the frame) and a skate under the seat bucket (1 or 2 skates are permitted). There are limitations on sledge design and in particular the height of the frame to the ice must be within 8.5-9.5cm. This is important for safety to stop one sledge frame cross over the other causing injury.

Sticks The stick is a shortened stick that may be curved and has sharp picks on the straight end for pushing along the ice. The curved blade end is for striking the puck for passing and shooting. The goalkeeper has a larger and wider stick and also has a blocking and a catching glove.

Helmets and face guards All players must wear helmets and face guards that meet the standards of the Hockey Equipment Certification Council (HECC).

Other equipment All players must wear gloves and also throat, elbow, shoulder and shin protectors. All players must wear ice hockey boots or have the feet covered by a suitable protection of the main sledge frame. Mouth guards are optional but recommended.

The puck is made of vulcanized rubber and is 156-170gms in weight and 7.62cm in diameter and 2.54cm in height.

Rule adaptations Game play is the same as for ice hockey.

Physiological & Biomechanical demands

No published data exists on physiological data in ice sledge hockey but it requires repeated short bursts of high intensity upper body exercise and upper body strength. Having trunk strength and proprioception is an asset and permits more able athletes to manoeuvre more quickly around the ice and initiating sledge movement with trunk muscles alone. Core stability training is therefore useful.

Injury epidemiology

Ice sledge hockey is a sport almost designed for injury with hard surfaces, sharp equipment and high speed collision with an opponent, ice or the boards. In the 2002 Winter Paralympics, Webborn et al (2006) found that 14% of players incurred a significant injury with five lower limb fractures occurring. The authors found that limited leg and foot protection was worn and as a consequence the rule changes on protective footwear and shins (see above) were instituted. The height of the sledge frame was also regulated and at the next games in 2006 the injury rate reduced to 11% of competitors and there were no lower limb fractures (Webborn 2007). Lacerations with the sharp pick ends occur and also concussions occur from collisions with opponents, the boards or the ice.

Nordic Skiing & Biathlon

Cross-Country Skiing appeared at the 1976 inaugural Paralympic Winter Games in Örnsköldsvik, Sweden. Men and women used the classical technique in all Cross-Country distances until skating was introduced by athletes at the Innsbruck 1984 Paralympic Winter Games. Biathlon events were included from 1988 and adaptations were made allowing visually impaired athletes to participate from 1992.

Governing Body IPC Nordic Skiing

First appearance in Paralympic Games Örnsköldsvik 1976, Innsbruck 1988 (Biathlon)

Competing nations 24

Gender Male and female competitions

Event arena Nordic skiing track of varying distances. Biathlon uses a 2.5km loop with a shooting station.

Events:

Nordic – Classic & Free technique events for standing and VI classes

- Men 5k, 10k, 15k - sitski
- Men 5k, 10k, 20k - standing and VI
- Men's relay – mixed
- Women 2.5k, 5k, 10k - sitski
- Women 5k, 10k, 15k - standing and VI
- Women's relay – mixed

Biathlon

- Men 7.5k, 12.5k - sitski, standing and VI
- Women 7.5k, 10k - sitski
- Women 7.5k, 12.5k - standing and VI

Disability Groups

Classification The same classification system of physical and visual impairments used for Alpine skiing is used in Nordic and Biathlon but following the allocation of class all athletes race against the clock and the time is adjusted by a percentage based upon class. There are different percentages for freestyle and classic techniques in Nordic events.

Sport equipment

Skis: For standing and VI athletes the ski equipment is the same as able-bodied competitors. For sitting classes, a seat with two slightly shorter than standard skis attached, is used.

Biathlon: Athletes shoot five shots at a target at a 10m distance and penalties are awarded for missed shots by requiring additional designated small loops of the course. Athletes use an air rifle meeting international standards. Visually impaired athletes use an electro-acoustic sighting mechanism, which gives a tone according to the placement on the target.

Rule adaptations

Visually impaired athletes follow a guide skier who gives audible commands to the following skier.

Physiological & Biomechanical demands

Nordic skiing requires a high aerobic capacity for elite performance but published data on Paralympic skiing is not available for comparison with able-bodied skiers.

Wheelchair Curling

Wheelchair curling is an adaptation of the ancient sport of curling where competitors slide a stone down a sheet of ice with the aim of having it stop as close to the centre of a set of rings, called the house. Team members have two stones each and compete in turn against their opponents trying to have more stones nearer the centre of the rings at the end of each play. Curling made its way onto the Olympic programme in 1998 and it is a more recent addition to the Paralympic programme in 2006.

Governing Body World Curling Federation

First appearance in Paralympic Games 2006

Competing nations 20+

Gender Mixed gender competition

Event arena Curling rink

Events Team sport of 4 members. Wheelchair curling games last 8 ends, as compared to 10 ends in able-bodied curling.

Disability Groups All significant physical impairments of lower leg/gait function e.g. spinal injury, cerebral palsy, multiple sclerosis or double leg amputation.

Classification The requirement is that athletes have significant physical impairments of lower leg/gait function and require a wheelchair for daily use. This minimum disability criterion is evaluated by a pool of international classifiers.

Sport equipment Curling stones are of a standard dimension and can weigh up to 19.96kg in weight and are usually made of granite. They have a handle for lifting and pushing (delivering) the stone. For athletes with a more severe disability they may use a cue that attaches to the handle to deliver the stone.

Rule adaptations The stone is delivered from a stationary wheelchair and a team mate may help hold and stabilise the players chair. No sweeping of the stone is permitted.

Physiological & Biomechanical demands

No published data available.

Injury epidemiology

Wheelchair curling being a game of tactics and skill rather than strength or endurance is less likely to induce injury. No injuries were recorded in athletes at the Torino 2006 Paralympic Games.

Summary

Paralympic sport has a more prominent profile and levels of participation are increasing worldwide. As a result it is more likely that sports medicine practitioners will encounter athletes with a disability in their daily practice. Levels of performance are also increasing; for example, completion of a wheelchair marathon in less than 1.5 hours demonstrates that these are clearly elite athletes and need to be treated as such. It is important for practitioners to be aware of the sports, the equipment, and the demands to help in the diagnostic process and management of injuries. It provides a challenge to our routine sports medicine practice and often requires lateral thinking to understand the problem and to find a solution. This chapter gives a brief insight into some of the complexities of Paralympic sport, and further information can be found in some of the resources shown below.

References

Allen, J.B. (2003) Sports injuries in disabled sailing. In: S.J. Legg (ed.), *4th European Conference on Sailing Sports Science and Sports Medicine and the 3rd Australian Sailing Science Conference*, p.58. Massey University, Palmerston North, New Zealand.

Burkett, B. and Mellifont, R.B. (2008). Sport science and coaching in Paralympic cycling. *International Journal of Sports Science and Coaching*, 3, 95–103.

Burnham, R. and Higgins, R.S. (1994). Wheelchair basketball injuries. *Palaestra*, 10, 43–9.

Curtis, K.A. and Black, K. (1999). Shoulder pain in female wheelchair basketball players. *Journal of Orthopaedics and Sports Physical Therapy*, 29, 225–31.

Ferrara, M.S. and Buckley, W.E. (1996). Athletes with disabilities injury registry. *Adapted Physical Activity Quarterly*, 13, 50–60.

Ferrara, M.S. and Davis, R.W. (1990). Injuries to elite wheelchair athletes. *Paraplegia*, 28, 335–41.

Ferrara, M.S. and Peterson, C.L. (2000). Injuries to athletes with disabilities: identifying injury patterns. *Sports Medicine*, 30, 137–43.

Ferrara, M.S., Palutsis, G.R., Snouse, S., and Davis, R.W. (2000). A longitudinal study of injuries to athletes with disabilities. *International Journal of Sports Medicine*, 21, 221–4.

Gass, G.C. and Camp, E.M. (1979). Physiological characteristics of trained Australian paraplegic and tetraplegic subjects. *Medicine and Science in Sports*, 11, 256–9.

Goosey-Tolfrey, V.L. (2005). Physiological profiles of elite wheelchair basketball players in preparation for the 2000 Paralympic Games. *Adapted Physical Activity Quarterly*, 22, 57–66.

Goosey-Tolfrey, V., Castle, P., Webborn, N., and Abel, T. (2006). Aerobic capacity and peak power output of elite quadriplegic games players. *British Journal of Sports Medicine*, 40, 684–7.

Knechtle, B., Muller, G., and Knecht, H. (2004). Optimal exercise intensities for fat metabolism in handbike cycling and cycling. *Spinal Cord*, 42(10), 564–72.

Nyland, J., Snouse, S.L., Anderson, M., Kelly, T., and Sterling, J.C. (2000). Soft tissue injuries to USA Paralympians at the 1996 Summer Games. *Archives of Physical Medicine and Rehabilitation*, 81, 368–73.

Reynolds, J., Stirk, A., Thomas, A., and Geary, F. (1994). Paralympics—Barcelona 1992. *British Journal of Sports Medicine*, 28, 14–17.

Taylor, D. and Williams, T. (1995). Sports injuries in athletes with disabilities: wheelchair racing. *Paraplegia*, 33, 296–9.

Veeger, H.E., Hadj Yahmed, M., van der Woude, L.H., and Charpentier, P. (1991). Peak oxygen uptake and maximal power output of Olympic wheelchair-dependent athletes. *Medicine and Science in Sports and Exercise*, 23, 1201–9.

Webborn, N. Willick, S., and Reeser, J.C. (2006). Injuries among disabled athletes during the 2002 Winter Paralympic Games. *Medicine and Science in Sports and Exercise*, 38(5), 811–5 ISSN1530–0315.

Webborn, A.D. (2007). IPC Injury Survey Torino 2006. *The Paralympian*, 11.

Webborn, A.D. and Turner, H.M. (2000). The aetiology of shoulder pain in elite Paralympic wheelchair athletes—the shoulder or cervical spine? In: *5th Paralympic Scientific Congress*, p.59. International Paralympic Committee, Sydney.

Webborn, N. (2009). Paralympic sports injuries in epidemiology of injury in olympic sports. In: D. Caine (ed.), *The Encyclopaedia of Sports Medicine*. Blackwell Science, Oxford.

Wilson, P.E. and Washington, R.L. (1993). Pediatric wheelchair athletics: sports injuries and prevention. *Paraplegia*, 31, 330–7.

Bibliography

DePauw, K.P. and Gavron, S.J. (1995). *Disability and Sport*. Human Kinetics, Champaign, IL.

Fallon, K.E. (1995). The disabled athlete. In: J. Bloomfield, P.A. Fricker, and K.D. Fitch (eds), *Science and Medicine in Sport*, pp. 550–1. Blackwell Science, Oxford.

Webborn, A.D.J. (2005). Sport and disability. In: *ABC of Sports Medicine* (3rd edn), pp. 76–9. BMJ Publishing, London.

Webborn, N. (2006). The disabled athlete. In: P. Brukner and K. Kahn (eds), *Clinical Sports Medicine*. McGraw-Hill, New York

Webborn, N. and Goosey-Tolfrey, V.L. (2008). Spinal cord injury. In: J. Buckley (ed.), *Exercise Physiology in Special Populations*, pp. 309–34. Elsevier, Amsterdam.

Useful links

International Paralympic Committee: www.paralympic.org

CP-ISRA (Cerebral Palsy International Sport and Recreation Association): www.cpisra.org

IBSA (International Blind Sport Federation): www.ibsa.es

INAS-FID (International Sports Federation for Persons with Intellectual Disability): www.inas-fid.org

ISMWSF (nternational Stoke Mandeville Wheelchair Sports Federation): www.wsw.org.uk

Emergency medical care of on-field injuries

Mark Gillett

The treatment of life- or limb-threatening injuries in the sporting arena constitutes one of the most intimidating challenges for any healthcare professional employed in sport. The skills required to cope with these scenarios decay very rapidly so that regular drills and scenario training are essential to maintain the competencies acquired from emergency training courses.

The components of a successful emergency medical care strategy are:

+ preparation, practice and planning
+ rapid but thorough onfield assessment
+ appropriate equipment, communication, and transport
+ effective liaison with appropriate secondary care facilities.

Preparation, practice, and planning

Justifying emergency drills

Medical emergencies are, by definition, time critical. The probability of successfully defibrillating a patient from a shockable cardiac arrest rhythm decreases by 10% with every minute that elapses from the time of arrest. Given the distance from the furthest point of a stadium to the medical room at most professional facilities, it is possible that at least a 2–3 minute delay will be incurred before crucial equipment is by the side of the injured athlete. Any misunderstanding or communication failure at this stage will further delay appropriate treatment and potentially compromise the probability of a favourable outcome. It is recommended that the drill is simple and is practised regularly to ensure that all the on-site staff are able to participate if required.

The keys to a successful emergency drill are:

+ simplicity
+ rehearsal
+ awareness.

Healthcare professionals working in sport often spend a great deal of time at a base location, whether it is a training ground, stadium, or arena. Hence it is essential that robust organization of the specific roles and responsibilities at times of emergency is in place to safeguard the health of the casualty.

The following tasks need to be accounted for:

1. **Calling for help** The plan should clearly indicate whose responsibility it is to call the emergency services and request an ambulance.

2. **Fetching the equipment** It is most likely that vital equipment will need to be brought to the side of the injured athlete during a resuscitation or serious medical incident.

3. **Identifying a serious situation and initiating resuscitation** Ideally, this should be the responsibility of the doctor or team physiotherapist.

4. **Identifying and treating a cardiac arrest** It should be made clear in the emergency drill whose responsibility it is to deploy the automated external defibrillator (AED) and defibrillate if indicated.

5. **Calming and controlling other players** The coach or manager would be well suited to this role.

There are no generic solutions to these issues and it obviously depends on the number and skill mix of staff members employed at each sporting organization. The plan should be underpinned by the principle that the fewest possible staff will be present at the time of an emergency, remembering that AEDs are designed for use by personnel with no clinical training. A suggested emergency plan is shown in Fig. 4.5.1.

The initial assessment

The initial assessment commences with the SAFE approach (Table 4.5.1). The importance of the SAFE approach is commonly underestimated. There is real potential for the attending healthcare professional to become a further casualty in high-velocity sports such as cycling or horse racing if appropriate action is not taken to stop the race. In addition, many medical emergencies are time critical, so that failing to alert the emergency services at the earliest opportunity may compromise the chances of a successful outcome.

The primary survey

The order of the primary survey, which is the cornerstone of the initial assessment of an injured athlete, is best remembered with

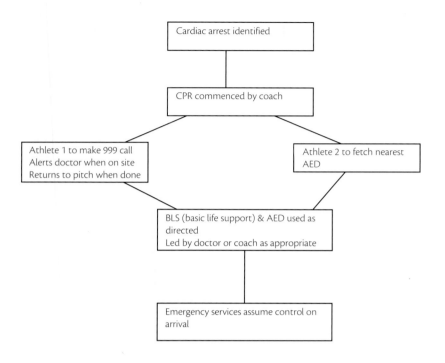

Fig. 4.5.1 Proposed emergency drill arena.

The flowchart contents:

Cardiac arrest identified

CPR commenced by coach

Athlete 1 to make 999 call
Alerts doctor when on site
Returns to pitch when done

Athlete 2 to fetch nearest AED

BLS (basic life support) & AED used as directed
Led by doctor or coach as appropriate

Emergency services assume control on arrival

Note: If the coach collapses, it is recommended that one player goes to notify the doctor whilst another ensures that the emergency services are contacted.

Table 4.5.1 The SAFE approach

S	**S**ummon help as appropriate
A	**A**pproach the casualty with care
F	**E**nsure that you are **F**ree from danger
E	**E**valuate the casualty and the situation

Table 4.5.2 The primary survey

Airway and C-spine protection (± supplemental oxygen)
Breathing
Circulation (haemorrhage control)
Deficit/**D**isability (neurological)
Exposure/**E**nvironment

Table 4.5.3 The significance of added sounds in airway assessment

Gurgling	Implies fluid in the airway. Remove with suction.
Snoring	Suggests upper airway obstruction secondary to muscle relaxation in the oropharynx.
Stridor	Indicates upper airway obstruction. Causes include anaphylaxis and airway burns.

the mnemonic ABCDE (ATLS Manual 2004). The individual components of this system are outlined in Table 4.5.2.

A: Airway with cervical spine protection and supplemental oxygen

If a player is able to speak with formed words, the airway is patent. He still requires a more formal assessment but at present he is maintaining his own airway. Consider applying supplemental oxygen at the earliest opportunity, especially if there are signs of hypoxia (e.g. cyanosis, anxiety, or distress). It is vital that the attending physician does not move on to assess breathing until the airway is patent and supplemental oxygen has been applied.

B: Breathing

Breathing can be formally assessed when the rescuer is happy that the airway is patent. In reality A and B are often assessed simultaneously, but it is vital that breathing is assessed systematically to avoid overlooking adverse clinical signs. A mnemonic to ensure that no areas are overlooked during the breathing assessment is given in Table 4.5.4 (REMO Manual 2008).

The respiratory rate is a particularly useful indicator of both respiratory distress and early shock (ATLS Manual 2004). However, in most sports a participant will have a raised respiratory rate as a result of exercise, making its significance more difficult to judge. In these cases recording the respiratory rate as soon as possible after the incident in order to judge the evolving trend is extremely important.

Table 4.5.4 A mnemonic to aid recollection of airway assessment

T	**T**rachea
W	**W**ounds
E	**E**mphysema
L	**L**arynx
V	**V**eins
E	**E**verything else

The following life-threatening conditions should be identified during B assessment in the primary survey.

1. **Tension pneumothorax** This develops when a one-way valve effect is created from either the lung or the chest wall, so that the intra-pleural pressure rises to such a degree that venous return to the right side of the heart is obstructed. Left untreated, the condition can evolve rapidly and be fatal. It should be diagnosed clinically and is treated by needle decompression (thoracocentesis) in the second intercostal space in the mid-clavicular line.

2. **Open pneumothorax** This refers to defects in the chest wall that result in a 'sucking chest wound'. A chest wall defect which is larger than two-thirds of the diameter of the trachea will allow air entry preferentially through the defect rather than down the trachea and will subsequently impair effective ventilation. The chest wall defect should be covered with an Asherman chest seal (Fig. 4.5.2) or simply covered with a sterile occlusive dressing.

3. **Flail chest** This occurs when two or more ribs are fractured in two or more places, so that a section of the chest wall is not in direct continuity with the rest of the thoracic skeleton. The condition is characterized by the extreme pain that it creates and is associated with an underlying pulmonary contusion. Manual stabilization of the flail segment often assists with pain management and helps to effect adequate ventilation.

4. **Massive haemothorax** This occurs when more than 1500 ml of blood accumulates in the pleural cavity following either blunt

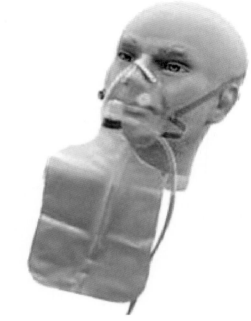

Fig. 4.5.3 Non-rebreathe oxygen mask.

or penetrating trauma. In the sports pre-hospital environment it is best treated with supplementary oxygen, fluid resuscitation, and rapid transfer to secondary care.

All significant respiratory injuries will require treatment with supplemental oxygen at 15 L/min via a non-rebreathe trauma mask (Fig. 4.5.3). This should be followed by urgent transfer to hospital. If the casualty's depth or rate of breathing is deemed inadequate or they stop breathing, ventilation with a pocket mask or a bag–valve mask system is required.

C: Circulation

In cases of trauma, the primary cause of shock is hypovolaemia until proven otherwise. The casualty will usually be pale, grey, clammy, tachycardic, and cyanosed with cool peripheries.

The immediacy of a fall in systolic blood pressure in hypovolaemia is often misunderstood by unwary medical responders. The vast majority of individuals will not experience a drop in systolic blood pressure until they have lost 30–40% of their circulating blood volume—class 3 shock (ATLS Manual 2004). The altered physiology of a young athlete may lead them to compensate for an even greater degree of blood loss before their systolic blood pressure begins to drop. In practical terms, a palpable radial pulse implies a minimum systolic blood pressure of 80 mmHg, which is adequate to perfuse the vital organs.

An intravenous cannula should be inserted whenever a casualty is likely to require fluid resuscitation or the administration of intravenous drugs. However, prolonged attempts at cannulation should not be permitted to delay transfer to a definitive care facility.

If blood loss is seen or suspected, the attending healthcare professional should:

◆ apply direct pressure to any obvious external haemorrhage and consider the use of dressings to limit further blood loss

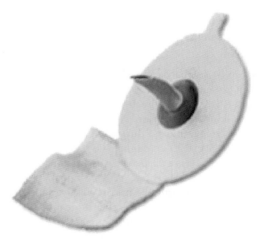

Fig. 4.5.2 Asherman chest seal.

◆ consider gentle realignment and splinting of an obviously fractured long bone.

◆ support and splint the pelvis if a pelvic fracture is suspected

Infusion of large volumes of crystalloid or colloid fluids in an attempt to normalize blood pressure is not advised. It may adversely affect the patient's outcome due to a combination of haemodilution, a reduction of localized clotting factors, and increased intravascular pressure. The effective treatment of blood loss may well necessitate replacement blood transfusion and surgery, which are best achieved by rapid transfer to hospital.

D: Deficit/disability

This element of the examination involves assessment of the casualty's level of consciousness (LoC). Terms such as semi-conscious or delirious should be avoided as they are ambiguous and difficult for others to interpret accurately. The easiest method of assessing the level of consciousness at this stage of the examination is the AVPU score (Table 4.5.5).

The Glasgow Coma Score (GCS) is an alternative more detailed tool used in conscious state assessment. Some experience is required to interpret the different responses to stimuli correctly, and it should not be utilised unless the practitioner has received appropriate training.

At this stage the pupils should be assessed with a torch to see if they are equal in size and reactive to light (PEARL). This may not give much information initially, but can provide a useful baseline if the level of consciousness deteriorates and a change in pupillary activity and symmetry follow. Pupillary abnormalities secondary to a rise in intracranial pressure are a late clinical indication of a significant cerebral injury or illness. Local pupillary injury and congenital conditions should be excluded in such cases.

The capillary refill time should also be assessed. This is performed by applying pressure on the sternum for 5 seconds and assessing the time taken for the skin colour to return to its previous colour. A delay of more than 2 seconds implies poor tissue perfusion, although care should be taken in interpreting this sign when the ambient temperature is low.

E: Exposure/environment

Consideration should be given to the ambient environment as injured players are prone to hypo- and hyperthermia due to impaired thermoregulatory control.

E also relates to patient exposure. Again, a balance needs to be struck between exposing a patient fully enough to complete a full assessment and keeping them sufficiently covered to maintain body temperature and dignity.

Management of specific medical emergencies

Basic and advanced life support

The aim of basic life support (BLS) is to optimize the casualty's circulatory and ventilatory status until the underlying cause of cardiorespiratory arrest can be reversed. Circulatory failure for more than 3–4 minutes may result in irreversible cerebral damage. Hence any delay in the commencement of effective BLS results in a significant reduction in the likelihood of a successful outcome from resuscitation. BLS is an important component of the chain of survival. This chain has four elements, all of which must be in place if optimal care is to be provided to a collapsed athlete (Advanced Life Support Manual 2006).

The elements of the chain are shown in Table 4.5.7 and the BLS algorithm is shown in Fig. 4.5.4.

Early defibrillation is key to a successful outcome from a shockable rhythm provoking a cardiac arrest. The established teaching point emphasizes that the chances of survival from a cardiac arrest amenable to defibrillation decrease by 10% for every minute that defibrillation is delayed. This statistic emphasizes the importance of calling the emergency services at the earliest opportunity, as well as avoiding any organizational issues which may delay cardioversion when a defibrillator is kept on site.

Automated external defibrillators have been designed for use by non-clinical personnel and avoid the need for the rescuer to interpret a cardiac tracing as shockable or non-shockable. They are extremely reliable and are becoming increasingly cost effective. The AED algorithm is shown in Fig. 4.5.5.

Anaphylaxis

This refers to type 4 hypersensitivity, which is mediated by IgE and requires prior sensitization before symptoms develop. The condition is characterized by a rapid onset of signs and symptoms which include urticaria, dyspnoea with bronchospasm, diarrhoea, angiooedema, anxiety, severe hypotension, and shock.

There may be a clear history of exposure to an allergen (e.g. a bee-sting or a nut allergy), although the precipitating allergen is not always obvious. Anaphylactoid reactions refer to the same collection of signs and symptoms seen in anaphylaxis but are not

Table 4.5.5 The AVPU score

A	**A**lert. Talking coherently, i.e. conversant and able to obey commands.
V	**V**erbalizing. Talking may be incoherent or irrational.
P	Responding to **P**ainful stimulus. These stimuli may be found incidentally (e.g. straightening a deformed limb) or tested actively by pressing a nailbed. When a C-spine injury cannot be excluded, creating a painful stimulus above the level of the clavicle is preferable.
U	**U**nresponsive. No response to stimuli.

Table 4.5.6 Blood pressure assessments

Pulse site	Guide systolic blood pressure (mmHg)
Radial pulse	80
Femoral pulse	70
Carotid pulse	60

Table 4.5.7 The chain of survival

1	Early access to the emergency services
2	Early basic life support
3	Early defibrillation
4	Early advanced life support

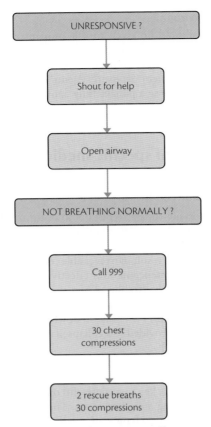

Fig. 4.5.4 Adult Basic Life Support (www.resus.org.uk).

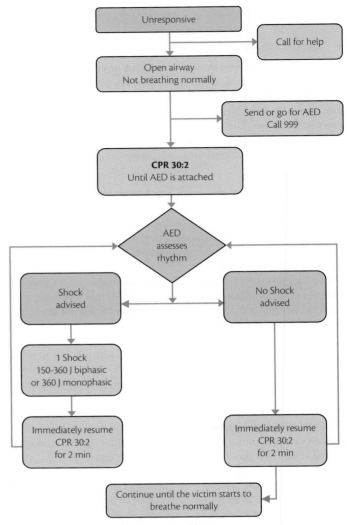

Fig. 4.5.5 AED operation (www.resus.org.uk).

mediated by IgE. Inexperienced practitioners often view an allergy and anaphylaxis as discrete clinical entities. In practice they reflect a clinical spectrum of a single pathology. This belief and a widespread fear of administering adrenaline often leads to a delay in providing the vital drug required to treat this condition—**intramuscular adrenaline**. The anaphylaxis algorithm is shown in Fig. 4.5.6.

Management of specific traumatic emergencies

Fractures and dislocations

These injuries, whilst often looking as though they should be the first priority, should not be assessed until the attending practitioner is satisfied that the primary survey has been safely completed. The initial assessment of an orthopaedic injury should follow the look–feel–move system outlined in Table 4.5.8 below (REMO Manual 2008).

Neurovascular assessment is vital and should comprise palpating the pulses directly above and below the area of injury and testing sensation on the affected and contralateral sides. Pain relief is a priority at the earliest possible opportunity, with splinting of the injury playing a large part in effective analgesia. If no equipment is available, and depending on the injury sustained, simple splinting to another body part can provide temporary relief (e.g. buddy splinting of the fingers). However, all medical professionals working in sport should ensure that they have access to simple splinting

equipment such as broad arm slings and box splints to use in such circumstances.

All methods of splintage should have the following characteristics:

◆ easy to apply

◆ padded

◆ supportive of the joint above and below

◆ non-constrictive

◆ allow repeated monitoring.

The decision to realign a clinically apparent fracture or dislocation should not be taken without due consideration. In most cases, if a limb is not neurovascularly compromised, the fracture site should be appropriately immobilized and the player transferred to hospital as safely as possible. In a neurovascularly compromised limb or digit, appropriate attempts to realign the fracture site should be made although this should not delay transfer to hospital. Any attempts at realignment should be followed by a reassessment

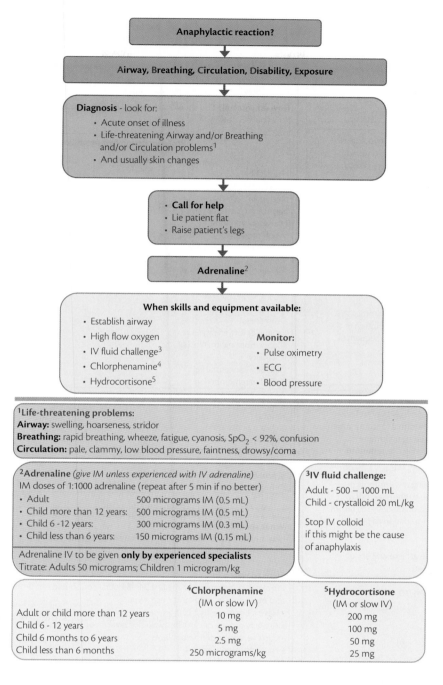

Anaphylactic reaction?

Airway, Breathing, Circulation, Disability, Exposure

Diagnosis - look for:
- Acute onset of illness
- Life-threatening Airway and/or Breathing and/or Circulation problems[1]
- And usually skin changes

- **Call for help**
- Lie patient flat
- Raise patient's legs

Adrenaline[2]

When skills and equipment available:
- Establish airway
- High flow oxygen
- IV fluid challenge[3]
- Chlorphenamine[4]
- Hydrocortisone[5]

Monitor:
- Pulse oximetry
- ECG
- Blood pressure

[1]**Life-threatening problems:**
Airway: swelling, hoarseness, stridor
Breathing: rapid breathing, wheeze, fatigue, cyanosis, SpO_2 < 92%, confusion
Circulation: pale, clammy, low blood pressure, faintness, drowsy/coma

[2]**Adrenaline** (*give IM unless experienced with IV adrenaline*)
IM doses of 1:1000 adrenaline (repeat after 5 min if no better)
- Adult   500 micrograms IM (0.5 mL)
- Child more than 12 years: 500 micrograms IM (0.5 mL)
- Child 6 -12 years: 300 micrograms IM (0.3 mL)
- Child less than 6 years: 150 micrograms IM (0.15 mL)

Adrenaline IV to be given **only by experienced specialists**
Titrate: Adults 50 micrograms; Children 1 microgram/kg

[3]**IV fluid challenge:**
Adult - 500 – 1000 mL
Child - crystalloid 20 mL/kg

Stop IV colloid
if this might be the cause
of anaphylaxis

	[4]Chlorphenamine (IM or slow IV)	[5]Hydrocortisone (IM or slow IV)
Adult or child more than 12 years	10 mg	200 mg
Child 6 - 12 years	5 mg	100 mg
Child 6 months to 6 years	2.5 mg	50 mg
Child less than 6 months	250 micrograms/kg	25 mg

Fig. 4.5.6 Anaphylaxis treatment (www.resus.org.uk)

of the neurovascular status of the affected limb and appropriate splintage.

The professional circumstances that a sports medicine practitioner may find themselves employed in can be hugely variable. Many professional facilities are now equipped with radiology and resuscitation suites which lend themselves to the reduction of orthopaedic injuries on site. However, the reduction or relocation of the vast majority of orthopaedic injuries should not be attempted without prior X-ray or access to appropriate resuscitation equipment, no matter how experienced the practitioner. This will always come down to a matter of personal preference, although the necessity of keeping meticulous documentation of any attempted interventions applies to all.

Open fractures

In an open or compound fracture the soft tissue and skin covering a fracture site is breached, leaving bone exposed to the external environment. The principles of assessment remain the same, namely ABCDE followed by look–feel–move, but the exposed bone must be covered with a clean and sterile covering. Sterile gauze soaked in normal saline kept in place with a non-constricting bandage proves very effective. The wound should be kept covered

This tool represents a standardized method of evaluating people after concussion in sport. This tool has been produced as part of the Summary and Agreement Statement of the Second International Symposium on Concussion in Sport, Prague 2004.

Sport concussion is defined as a complex pathophysiological process affecting the brain, induced by traumatic biomechanical forces. Several common features that incorporate clinical, pathological, and biomechanical injury constructs that may be utilized in defining the nature of a concussive head injury include:

1. Concussion may be caused either by a direct blow to the head, face, neck, or elsewhere on the body with an "impulsive" force transmitted to the head.

2. Concussion typically results in the rapid onset of short-lived impairment of neurological function that resolves spontaneously.

3. Concussion may result in neuropathological changes, but the acute clinical symptoms largely reflect a functional disturbance rather than structural injury.

4. Concussion results in a graded set of clinical syndromes that may or may not involve loss of consciousness. Resolution of the clinical and cognitive symptoms typically follows a sequential course.

5. Concussion is typically associated with grossly normal structural neuroimaging studies.

Postconcussion Symptoms

Ask athletes to score themselves based on how they feel now. It is recognized that a low score may be normal for some athletes, but clinical judgment should be exercised to determine if a change in symptoms has occurred following the suspected concussion event.

It should be recognized that the reporting of symptoms may not be entirely reliable. This may be due to the effects of a concussion or because the athlete's passionate desire to return to competition outweighs the natural inclination to give an honest response.

If possible, ask someone who knows the athlete well about changes in affect, personality, behavior, etc.

Remember, concussion should be suspected in the presence of ANY ONE or more of the following:
• Symptoms (such as headache), or
• Signs (such as loss of consciousness), or
• Memory problems.

Any athlete with a suspected concussion should be monitored for deterioration (ie, should not be left alone) and should not drive a motor vehicle.

For more information see the "Summary and Agreement Statement of the Second International Symposium on Concussion in Sport" in:

Clinical Journal of Sport Medicine 2005;15(2):48-55
British Journal of Sports Medicine 2005;39(4):196-204
Neurosurgery 2005, in press
The Physician and Sportsmedicine 2005;33(4):29-44
This tool may be copied for distribution to teams, `groups, and organizations.

The SCAT Card
(Sport Concussion Assessment Tool)
Athlete Information

What is a concussion? A concussion is a disturbance in the function of the brain caused by a direct or indirect force to the head. It results in a variety of symptoms (like those listed below) and may, or may not, involve memory problems or loss of consciousness.

How do you feel? You should score yourself on the following symptoms, based on how you feel now.

Postconcussion Symptom Scale

	None		Moderate			Severe	
Headache	0	1	2	3	4	5	6
"Pressure in head"	0	1	2	3	4	5	6
Neck pain	0	1	2	3	4	5	6
Balance problems or dizzy	0	1	2	3	4	5	6
Nausea or vomiting	0	1	2	3	4	5	6
Vision problems	0	1	2	3	4	5	6
Hearing problems/ringing	0	1	2	3	4	5	6
"Don't feel right"	0	1	2	3	4	5	6
Feeling "dinged" or "dazed"	0	1	2	3	4	5	6
Confusion	0	1	2	3	4	5	6
Feeling slowed down	0	1	2	3	4	5	6
Feeling like "in a fog"	0	1	2	3	4	5	6
Drowsiness	0	1	2	3	4	5	6
Fatigue or low energy	0	1	2	3	4	5	6
More emotional than usual	0	1	2	3	4	5	6
Irritability	0	1	2	3	4	5	6
Difficulty concentrating	0	1	2	3	4	5	6
Difficulty remembering	0	1	2	3	4	5	6

(Follow-up symptoms only)

	None		Moderate			Severe	
Sadness	0	1	2	3	4	5	6
Nervous or anxious	0	1	2	3	4	5	6
Trouble falling asleep	0	1	2	3	4	5	6
Sleeping more than usual	0	1	2	3	4	5	6
Sensitivity to light	0	1	2	3	4	5	6
Sensitivity to noise	0	1	2	3	4	5	6
Other:	0	1	2	3	4	5	6

What should I do?
Any athlete suspected of having a concussion should be removed from play, and then seek medical evaluation.

Signs to watch for:
Problems could arise over the first 24-48 hours. You should not be left alone and must go to a hospital at once if you:
• Have a headache that gets worse
• Are very drowsy or can't be awakened (woken up)
• Can't recognize people or places
• Have repeated vomiting
• Behave unusually or seem confused; are very irritable
• Have seizures (arms and legs jerk uncontrollably)
• Have weak or numb arms or legs
• Are unsteady on your feet; have slurred speech.
Remember, it is better to be safe. Consult your doctor after a suspected concussion.

What can I expect?
Concussion typically results in the rapid onset of short-lived impairment that resolves spontaneously over time. You can expect that you will be told to rest until you are fully recovered (that means resting your body and your mind). Then, your doctor will likely advise that you go through a gradual increase in exercise over several days (or longer) before returning to sport.

Fig. 4.5.7 Sports Concussion Assessment Tool (SCAT).

The SCAT Card
(Sport Concussion Assessment Tool)
Medical Evaluation

Name: _____ Date _____

Sport/Team: _____ Mouth guard? Y   N

1) SIGNS
Was there loss of consciousness or unresponsiveness?   Y   N
Was there seizure or convulsive activity?   Y   N
Was there a balance problem/unsteadiness   Y   N

2) MEMORY
Modified Maddocks questions (check correct)

At what venue are we? __; Which half is it? __; Who scored last?__

What team did we play last? __; Did we win last game? __

3) SYMPTOM SCORE
Total number of positive symptoms (from reverse side of the card) = _____

4) COGNITIVE ASSESSMENT

5 word recall   Immediate   Delayed
                    (Examples)   (After concentration talks)

Word 1 _____   cat   ____   ____
Word 2 _____   pen   ____   ____
Word 3 _____   shoe   ____   ____
Word 4 _____   book   ____   ____
Word 5 _____   car   ____   ____

Months in reverse order:
Jun-May-Apr-Mar-Feb-Jan-Dec-Nov-Oct-Sep-Aug-Jul (circle incorrect)
or
Digits backward (check correct)
5-2-8   3-9-1   _____
6-2-9-4   4-3-7-1   _____
8-3-2-7-9   1-4-9-3-6   _____
7-3-9-1-4-2   5-1-8-4-6-8   _____

Ask delayed 5-word recall now

5) NEUROLOGICAL SCREENING

                        Pass   Fail

Speech   ___   ___
Eye motion and pupils   ___   ___
Pronator drift   ___   ___
Gait assessment   ___   ___

*Any neurological screening abnormality necessitates
formal neurological or hospital assessment*

6) RETURN TO PLAY
Athletes should not be returned to play the same day of injury.
When returning athletes to play, they should follow a stepwise symptom-limited
program, with stages of progression. For example:
1. Rest until asymptomatic (physical and mental rest)
2. Light aerobic exercise (eg, stationary cycling)
3. Sport-specific exercise
4. Non-contact training drills (start light resistance training)
5. Full contact training after medical clearance
6. Return to competition (game play)

There should be approximately 24 hours (or longer) for each stage, and the athlete
should return to stage 1 if symptoms recur. Resistance training should only be
added in the later stages. Medical clearance should be given before return to play.

Instructions:
This side of the card is for the use of medical doctors, physical
therapists, or athletic trainers. In order to maximize the information
gathered from the card, it is strongly suggested that all athletes
participating in contact sports complete a baseline evaluation prior
to the beginning of their competitive season. This card is a
suggested guide only for sport concussion and is not meant to
assess more severe forms of brain injury. **Please give a COPY of
this card to athletes for their information and to guide
follow-up assessment.**

Signs:
Assess for each of these items and circle
Y (yes) or N (no)

Memory: If needed, questions can be modified to make them
specific to the sport (eg, "period" versus "half").

Cognitive Assessment:
Select any 5 words (an example is given). Avoid choosing related words such as "dark" and "moon," which can be recalled
by means of word association. Read each word at a rate of one
word per second. The athlete should not be informed of the
delayed testing of memory (to be done after the reverse
months and/or digits). Choose a different set of words each
time you perform a follow-up exam with the same candidate.

Ask the athlete to recite the months of the year in reverse
order, starting with a random month. Do not start with
December or January. Circle any months not recited in the
correct sequence.

For digits backward, if correct, go to the next string length. If
incorrect, read trial 2. Stop after incorrect on both trials.

Neurological Screening:
Trained medical personnel must administer this examination.
These individuals might include medical doctors, physical
therapists, or athletic trainers. Speech should be assessed for
fluency and lack of slurring. Eye motion should reveal no
diplopia in any of the 4 planes of movement (vertical,
horizontal, and both diagonal planes). The pronator drift is
performed by asking patients to hold both arms in front of
them, palms up, with eyes closed. A positive test is pronating
the forearm, dropping the arm, or drifting away from midline.
For gait assessment, ask the patient to walk away from you,
turn, and walk back.

Return to Play:
A structured, graded exertion protocol should be developed and
individualized on the basis of sport, age, and the concussion
history of the athlete. Exercise or training should be commenced
only after the athlete is clearly asymptomatic with physical and
cognitive rest. Final decision for clearance to return to competition
should ideally be made by a medical doctor.

For more information see the "Summary and Agreement
Statement of the Second International Symposium on
Concussion in Sport" in:
Clinical Journal of Sport Medicine 2005;15(2):48-55
British Journal of Sports Medicine 2005;39(4):196-204
Neurosurgery 2005, in press
The Physician and Sportsmedicine 2005;33(4):29-44

Fig. 4.5.7 continued

Table 4.5.8 Look–feel–move assessment

Look	• Symmetry • Swelling • Deformity • Bruising • Wounds
Feel	• Tenderness • Swelling/effusion/haemarthrosis • Crepitus • Pulses • Sensation
Move	• Active/passive • Full ranges • Stability of joints • Power

Table 4.5.9 Definition of concussion according to international conferences in sport in 2001 and 2004

Sports concussion is defined as a complex pathophysiological process affecting the brain, induced by traumatic biomechanical forces. Some common features that incorporate clinical, pathological, and biomechanical injury constructs that may be utilized in defining the nature of a concussive head injury include:

1. Concussion may be caused by a direct blow to the head, face, neck, or elsewhere on the body with an 'impulsive' force transmitted to the head
2. Concussion typically results in the rapid onset of short-lived impairment of neurological function that resolves spontaneously
3. Concussion may result in neuropathological changes, but the acute clinical symptoms largely reflect a functional disturbance rather than structural injury
4. Concussion results in a graded set of clinical syndromes that may or may not involve loss of consciousness. Resolution of the clinical and cognitive symptoms typically follows a sequential course
5. Concussion is typically associated with grossly normal structural neuroimaging studies

Reproduced from McCrory, P., Johnston, K., Meeuwisse, W., *et al.* (2005). Summary and agreement statement of the 2nd International Conference on Concussion in Sport, Prague 2004; International Symposium on Concussion in Sport. *Clinical Journal of Sports Medicine*, **15**, 48–55

for as long as possible and it is preferable that photographs of the wound taken at the scene are reviewed in the emergency department to prevent unnecessary removal of the dressings prior to surgery.

Concussion

The definition and management of concussion in sport has been redefined in the last few years, initially by the Vienna Consensus in 2001 (Aubry *et al.* 2002) and then by the Prague Consensus in 2004 (McCrory *et al.* 2005). Table 4.5.9 outlines the concepts of concussion as defined at these meetings.

The Second International Conference on Concussion classified the condition into two groups:

1. **Simple concussion** when resolution occurs progressively over 7–10 days.

2. **Complex concussion** exists if an athlete suffers persistent symptoms, specific sequelae, or prolonged cognitive impairment after the injury.

On-field assessment of concussion should commence with a primary survey and ABC interventions employed as needed. If a cervical spine injury is suspected, neck immobilization and transfer onto a long spinal board should be facilitated. An unconscious patient should be assumed to have incurred a spinal injury until proven otherwise. After a patient has been stabilized and removed from the field of play, further assessment can continue in the dressing room. This is an appropriate time to take a full history, perform a full neurological examination, and document the player's response to cognitive questions and tests. The Sport Concussion Assessment Tool (Fig. 4.5.7) outlined in the Prague Consensus (McCrory *et al.* 2005) is favoured by many sports physicians for this purpose.

References

Advanced Life Support Manual (5th edn) (2006). Resuscitation Council, London.

ATLS Student Course Manual (7th edn) (2004). American College of Surgeons Committee on Trauma, Chicago, IL.

Aubry, M., Cantu, R., Dvorak, J., *et al.* (2002). Summary and agreement statement of the first International Conference on Concussion in Sport, Vienna 2001. *Physician and Sports Medicine*, **30**, 57–62 (co-published in British Journal of Sports Medicine, **36**, 3–7, and Clinical Journal of Sports Medicine, **12**, 6–12).

McCrory, P., Johnston, K., Meeuwisse, W., *et al.* (2005) Summary and agreement statement of the 2nd International Conference on Concussion in Sport, Prague 2004; International Symposium on Concussion in Sport. *Clinical Journal of Sports Medicine*, **15**, 48–55.

REMO Course Manual (3rd edn) (2008). Available online at: www.remosports.com

Injuries in swimming and related aquatic sports

Kevin Boyd

Introduction

Swimming is often hailed as an ideal activity because of the acknowledged benefits of exercise for those both in health and with disease. Therefore the spectrum of swimmers covers those individuals undertaking aerobic exercise as part of a healthy lifestyle, people suffering and rehabilitating from chronic conditions, such as cardiovascular disease and musculoskeletal disorders, and the committed and disciplined elite swimmer with high performance goals. Sports physicians should be familiar with these differing motivations and be able to adapt advice and treatment to each of these population groups. Unusually for a sport, there is a general consensus that everyone should develop the ability to swim for the enhancement of water safety.

Surveys of sporting activity in the UK reveal that swimming is the most popular sport with 14% of the adult population regularly taking part (Rickards *et al.* 2004). Swimming is also a more acceptable form of physical activity for females, the elderly, and those with disease. The water in pools provides a warm supportive environment to undertake joint mobilization and cardiovascular exercise either through swimming or Aquafit. Only those with severe uncontrolled heart failure may experience problems with deep immersion in water. Athletes with a range of physical disabilities, including visual impairment, successfully compete in swimming and frequently train alongside their able-bodied counterparts.

FINA (Federation Internationale de Natation) is the international governing body responsible for the sports of swimming and the related aquatic disciplines of diving, water polo, synchronized swimming, and open water swimming. Competitive swimming in England has been regulated by the Amateur Swimming Association since 1869, and it has been an intergral part of every Olympiad of the modern era. Approximately 0.1% of the population are registered competitive swimmers.

Biomechanics of swimming

Swimming is a unique sport in that the athlete is suspended in an alien environment, a fluid medium, which does not provide a firm surface for propulsive efforts, which offers considerable resistance to forward motion, and which necessitates specific actions to allow breathing. Optimum stroke mechanics, incorporating smooth and efficient breathing techniques, may overcome some of these difficulties, but streamlining and the reduction of drag forces are also key to success.

There are four recognized swimming strokes: freestyle, backstroke, breaststroke, and butterfly. Medley events, either individual or relay, combine all four strokes into a single race. Swimming events in Olympic competition vary from 50 to 1500 m. Times taken over these distances in the pool are approximately four times longer than the equivalent running distance on the track. Thus the energy demands in swimming are shifted towards the aerobic end of the physiological spectrum.

Furthermore, propulsion is obtained primarily by the arms, which are responsible for 75–80% of forward power. The leg kick is more important in balancing the stroke, particularly during sprints and starts and turns. Breaststroke is an exception where the leg kick accounts for approximately 50% of the propulsion.

Stroke mechanics can be broadly divided into pull, push, and recovery. Some authors refer to various hand 'sweeps', taking into account the sculling actions of the hands. Biomechanically, there are similarities to the throwing action, with the recovery representing the wind-up and the 'catch' the fully cocked position. The subsequent acceleration of the pull and push phases is produced by the combination of powerful internal rotation and adduction of the shoulders.

Success in aquatic disciplines is only seen after many years of regular training, often twice a day and from a young age. Regular training is commonplace from the age of 8 years. Senior swimming programmes are typically entered at 13–14 years with the aim of remaining in the sport for a further 10–15 years. Masters swimming, popularized during the 1970s, provides competition for those aged 25 years and upwards in five-year age bands.

Swimming injuries

Injuries in swimming are not uncommon in the elite athlete. They may be either acute or due to overuse.

Acute injuries

Acute injuries are relatively rare because of the lack of intentional bodily contact and the relatively slow speeds involved, particularly in the disciplined environment of a competitive swimming club. Blunt injuries for the majority are minor in nature and self-limiting—following a clash of hands, catching fingers in the lane ropes, or collision with the poolside. Nevertheless, careless behaviour in the pool environment can carry significant risks. Pool-sides can be slippy and falls do occur. Head and cervical spine injuries have

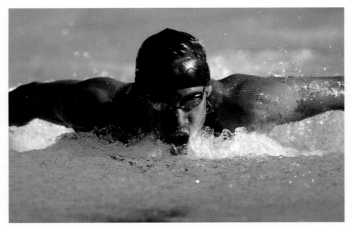

Fig. 4.6.1 Considerable repetitive strains are applied to the shoulders during training. Copyright © Christophe Schmid-Fotolia.com

been reported when swimmers misjudge the water depth on diving and sustain a hyperextension injury to the neck. This rarely occurs in those who have mastered the correct shallow competitive dive. Hyperventilation and excessive breath-holding behaviour is discouraged to prevent the occurrence of blackouts while underwater. Acute muscle strains can occur following inadequate warm-up or poor stretching technique.

Overuse injuries

The majority of injuries that affect training and performance are overuse in nature. The biomechanical and physiological demands are in excess of normal anatomical design which, with insufficient preparation and/or recovery, results in tissue breakdown and failure. An elite swimmer will not uncommonly spend 25–30 hours per week training, with a water programme of 70–100 km per week. There is the additional workload of a weight-training programme, both in and out of the water, flexibility work and cross-training. The demands of the training programme must be considered when addressing the cause of injury. Structured programmes with built-in recovery periods for each bodily system are required to maintain the quality of training.

Shoulder injuries

Swimmer's shoulder problems are a well-recognized entity, accounting for approximately 60% of all orthopaedic problems in swimmers (see Fig. 4.6.1). Tendinopathy and impingement are the likely final pathway of pain, but glenohumeral instability may be an important feature in some swimmers. This instability may be inherited, acquired, or a consequence of fatigue or muscle imbalance.

Swimming training typically develops increased levels of flexibility and strong powerful internal rotators and adductors. Overuse in training or competition will lead to fatigue so that the rotator cuff muscles are unable to maintain the stability of the glenohumeral joint. The scapular muscles are essential in reducing impingement throughout the swimming action. Research has shown high levels of fatigue in serratus anterior and rhomboid muscles (Scovazzo *et al.* 1991).

The stabilizing muscles of the glenohumeral joint, the rotator cuff, and the scapula are important in maintaining shoulder health

in swimmers. Stability exercises may not improve speed or propulsion but they will keep the athlete healthy. Both the recovery and the pull phases place the shoulder in an impingement position which can persist for up to 56% of the stroke cycle (Yanai and Hay 2000).

Typically, symptoms are already chronic at presentation and may be ill-defined. Management for early disease should be within good coaching practice. Emphasis is on pain-free strokes, increasing warm-up periods and stretching, and reducing intensity. Cryotherapy is used following work-out to reduce pain and inflammation. Attention should be given to technique and training programme content. Any external rotator weakness should be addressed with a progressive course of strengthening exercises using light resistance work. For more significant symptoms, in addition to the above, relative rest will need to be introduced. Kick work or substitute exercises such as running or cycling may be required. Electrophysical modalities, manual therapy, and NSAIDs may also be helpful. Provocative positions and the use of hand paddles and kick boards should be avoided. A gradual increase in swimming load over a period of 4–6 weeks should enable return to the former level. In refractory cases, subacromial injections of local anaesthetic and corticosteroid can be considered, but should not be offered in isolation. Surgery is rarely indicated but may include a subacromial decompression and specific interventions for glenohumeral instability or other defined pathology. Postoperative rehabilitation requires a significant commitment by the athlete, and liaison with the coach is essential.

Knee injuries

Knee pain is common in sports and in swimmers, particularly breaststrokers, accounting for around 25% of orthopaedic problems. Poor technique may be an influence as can the forceful and repetitive nature of the kick. Pain felt over the inner aspect of the knee typically represents overload of the medial collateral ligament (MCL). The classical study by Kennedy *et al.* (1978) demonstrated high levels of strain in the MCL during the combined movements of flexion, valgus, and external rotation, as performed in breaststroke. Patellofemoral pain needs careful assessment and diagnosis so that appropriate, largely non-operative, management can be introduced. Other potential causes of knee pain include patellofemoral maltracking, patellofemoral pain syndrome, meniscal pathology, hamstring tendinopathy, and plica syndrome.

Management depends on the cause, but low levels of dysfunction are treated with an increase in warm-up periods, attention to biomechanics and training load, and a reduction in kick intensity. Quadriceps strengthening, using terminal-range closed-chain exercises, along with optimization of core stability and flexibility is necessary. Cryotherapy is introduced early and further physiotherapy modalities can be considered. Cardiovascular fitness can be maintained by using alternative strokes and avoiding provocative activities. A greater use of drills using a pull-buoy can provide relative rest.

Low-back pain

Low-back pain is also recognized in elite swimmers. All swimming strokes maintain a degree of hyperextension of the lower back to achieve a streamlined position but this is exaggerated in butterfly and the 'undulating' style of breaststroke. Such actions repetitively load the posterior structures of the lumbar spine which can result in a spondylolysis or a stress fracture of the pars interarticularis of the neural arch. Muscle sparing and ligament sprains occur, but settle rapidly with core stability programmes and manual therapies. However, persistent low-back pain, impairing training and not improving after 3 weeks, should ideally be investigated to rule out a potential spondylolysis. An MRI scan is the investigation of choice, although a combination of imaging modilities including SPECT scanning and a reverse gantry CT scan may be indicated. In favourable circumstances, avoidance of provocative activity for 4–6 weeks and a core stability programme will allow a phased return to activity. Kick drills using an arm-board, where the upper body remains relatively fixed, have been noted to exacerbate symptoms and should be avoided. Poor posture with an increased lumbar lordosis, increased thoracic kyphosis, and protracted shoulders is common. In addition, a relatively high incidence of flexible scoliosis has been found amongst swimmers. Improvements in endurance of the core muscles can help.

Foot and ankle

Overuse foot and ankle injuries are occasionally seen and most frequently reflect a paratenonitis with or without tendinosis of the extensor tendons around the front of the ankle.

Underperformance syndrome

Elite endurance-based athletes, such as swimmers, run a fine physiological balance between adaptation and systemic breakdown resulting in illness. The unexplained underperformance syndrome is a term used when excessive fatigue and underperformance persist despite 2 weeks of rest. This is often seen against a background of high-intensity training and frequent infections. Other symptoms may include muscle aches, depressed mood, and poor sleep. Training load typically places the greatest demands but it is also essential to recognize the importance of sufficient rest, adequate diet, an appropriate level of 'fitness', mental status, lifestyle stresses, and the effects of recent illness. There are no good markers of this problem. A comprehensive assessment and an individualized rehabilitation programme, including periods of rest, light aerobic exercise, and reassurance, are recommended.

Epidemiology

Fortunately, overall injury rates in swimming are low in comparison with other sports. A survey in the UK (Nicholl et al. 1993) revealed 2.3 non-trivial injuries per 1000 occasions of participation, compared with figures of 57.7 injuries per 1000 occasions for rugby and 19.3 injuries per 1000 occasions for football. Shoulder problems have been investigated most extensively in high-level swimmers. A survey of US national-level swimmers by McMaster and Troup (1993) found a history of interfering shoulder pain in 47% of age-groupers, 66% of senior development swimmers, and 73% of elite swimmers. With improved understanding of the pathogenesis, preventative muscle strenghtening programmes seem to have reduced the current incidence of shoulder problems in swimmers. Epidemiological data for the related aquatic disciplines are scarce.

Diving

Although sharing the pool, competitive diving has more in common, physiologically and biomechanically, with gymnastics than with swimming. Divers are scored on the degree of difficulty and the technical proficiency of the acrobatics they perform while entering the water. At most international competitions, this is performed from a 3 m springboard and a 10 m platform. Recently, synchronized diving has been introduced where pairs of divers are also judged on how well the dives complement each other. There are six recognized groups of dives depending on the starting position, the initial direction of rotation, and whether any twisting actions are involved: forward, back, reverse, inward, armstand, and those using twists. The diving positions may be straight, tuck, pike, or free. Divers require great flexibility, visuospatial awareness, courage, and strength to generate the speed of rotation required to perform their dives.

Diving is enjoyed safely for the most part but occasionally catastrophic head and/or neck injury occurs. In an appropriate facility, water depth, a frequent issue with many serious neck injuries involving water, is not a problem. Injury occurs when the board is struck, particularly while performing inward and reverse dives, or if the head impacts the water. Divers learn to divert the impact of entry by gripping the hands together with a 'flat-hand' technique. This allows them to 'punch a hole' in the water for entry creating a 'rip', or vacuum phenomenon, which scores highly.

The force of impact, travelling at speeds of up to 55 km/hour, is not insignificant. Therefore chronic injuries around the wrists and thumbs resulting from tenosynovitis and joint sprains are well recognized. Taping of the wrists is used as a preventative measure. Younger divers are not normally permitted to dive from the higher boards because of concerns about epiphyseal injury. Further techniques to allow accurate 'spotting' of the water, such as water jets and splashing, allow correct timing of entry. Badly timed dives can result in 'belly flops' and blunt intra-abdominal injury. The use of wetsuits and underwater compressed air jets can lessen impact when learning new and complex dives. Lumbar spine problems, including spondylolyses, are common because of the repetitive flexion, extension, and loading. Core stability exercises are important in prevention. Shoulder and retinal injuries have also been reported.

Synchronized swimming

Synchronized swimming began as an art form but became a competitive sport in 1946 and an Olympic sport in 1988. Swimmers perform a synchronized artistic display of moves in the water set to music. Competition consists of technical drills and a free performance routine lasting up to 4 minutes. The events may be solo, duet, or teams of eight swimmers. Swimmers are judged on technical merit and artistic impression.

Precision of technique, artistry, rhythm sense, and the ability to perform quite extreme apnoeic exercise during underwater swimming require a demanding training programme. Acute injuries, including concussion, are becoming recognized because of the increasing use of acrobatic lifts and throws, particularly in the team events. Shoulder impingement occurs as a consequence of endurance freestyle swimming, overhead movements, and sculling actions. An 'eggbeater' leg kick, where the feet perform asymmetric small circular sculling movements, is used to tread water and to allow 'travelling' movements across the surface. This can result in chronic knee ligament sprains and patellofemoral pain, and can exacerbate patella instability. Specifically, concerns have highlighted the potential for extreme hypoxia during underwater figures and routines. Serum oxygen levels of 4.5 kPa have been recorded and have led to amnesic spells and blackouts (Davies *et al.* 1995). Medical concerns regarding this have led to a change in the sport's laws de-emphasizing time spent under the water.

Water polo

Despite being a non-contact sport, water polo is a very physical game. Strength, endurance, tactical awareness, and teamwork are important attributes. Male or female teams of seven play matches comprising four 8-minute quarters. Players combine the skills of the swimmer and the throwing athlete, and understandably also experience the problems of both. Acute and chronic shoulder problems are common, with muscle and tendon injuries and overuse problems due to throwing at high velocities. The large ball and the reduced contribution from the kinetic chain place greater demands on the shoulder and elbow in force generation. Muscle imbalances between the internal and external rotators of the shoulder have been identified and appear to correlate with overuse shoulder pain. Water polo players should perform external rotation strengthening exercises as part of an injury prevention programme.

Blunt trauma from contact with the ball, other players, or equipment can result in facial, dental, or head injuries. Barotrauma to the ear's tympanic membrane both above and below the water can occur despite the routine use of ear protectors. To minimize sharp eye injuries, goggles are not permitted. Skin lacerations and abraisons due to nails, teeth, or pulls on costumes are recognized. Finger injuries are seen following accidents in ball-catching.

Unfortunately many injuries occur as a result of illegal activity, much of which goes on beneath the water level and frequently is not penalized. Water polo sustained the greatest amount of player time lost due to foul play in Olympic team sports (Junge *et al.* 2006).

Water polo players also use the eggbeater leg kick, but use it to generate explosive height out of the water for throwing speed or goalkeeping. Acute and overuse hip and knee injuries can occur, limiting performance.

Open water swimming

Sometimes referred to as marathon swimming, these events take place outdoors in the sea, rivers, or lakes. Competitive distances vary from 1 to 25 km. The 10 km swim, which lasts a little under 2 hours, became an Olympic event in 2008. Swimmers are vulnerable to the elements, with water temperature, currents, winds, and weather providing additional challenges. Mild hypothermia (<35°C) due to prolonged immersion in cool water is not uncommon. This presents with feelings of cold and shivering, with or without mild confusion and ataxia, and is confirmed by a reduced core temperature. Typically, it responds to simple passive rewarming techniques such as warmed blankets. Minimum water temperatures do exist for competition. Wetsuits are not permitted but the use of two swimming caps can minimize heat loss from the head. Inexperience and intercurrrent illness are risk factors for the development of hypothermia. Paradoxically, hyperthermia and sunburn can also occur, particularly in shallow closed bodies of water in hot climates. Hyponatraemia, due to water intoxication, may also lead to central nervous system symptoms and should be considered as a cause of confusion.

Swimmers may sustain traumatic injuries with inadvertent and sometimes deliberate contact with other competitors, particularly at crowded starts or feeding stations. Unseen hazards, such as sharp rocks, coral, or discarded items, can cause lacerations. Sea life, small and large, ranging from sea lice to sharks, can be a concern. Jellyfish stings are common, and although they usually just cause discomfort, anaphylaxis can occur. Endurance training is key for the open water swimmer, and the majority takes place in normal swimming pools. Not surprisingly, overuse injuries of the shoulder are common.

References

Davies, B.N., Donaldson, G.C., and Joels, N. (1995). Do the competition rules of synchronised swimming encourage undesirable levels of hypoxia? *British Journal of Sports Medicine*, **29**, 16–19.

Junge, A., Langevoort, G., Pipe, A., *et al.* (2006). Injuries in team sport tournaments during the 2004 Olympic Games. *American Journal of Sports Medicine*, **34**, 565–76.

Kennedy, J.C., Hawkins, R., and Krissoff, W.B. (1978). Orthopaedic manifestations of swimming. *American Journal of Sports Medicine*, **6**, 309–22.

McMaster, W.C. and Troup, J.P. (1993). A survey of interfering shoulder pain in United States competitive swimmers. *American Journal of Sports Medicine*, **21**, 67–70.

Nicholl, J.P., Coleman, P., and Williams, B.T. (1993). *Injuries in Sport and Exercise. Main Report. A National Study of the Epidemiology of Exercise-Related Injury and Illness.* Sports Council, London.

Rickards, L., Fox, K., Roberts, C., Fletcher, L., and Goddard, E. (2004). *Living in Britain. No 31. Results from the 2002 General Household Survey.* TSO, London.

Scovazzo, M.L., Browne, A., Pink, M., Jobe, F.W., and Kerrigan, J. (1991). The painful shoulder during freestyle swimming: an electromyographic cinematographic analysis of twelve muscles. *American Journal of Sports Medicine*, **19**, 577–82.

Yanai, T. and Hay, J.G. (2000). Shoulder impingement in front-crawl swimming. II: Analysis of stroking technique. *Medicine and Science in Sports and Exercise*, **32**, 30–40.

4.7

Triathlon injuries

Rod Jaques

Description of the sport

Triathlon is an event that involves sequential swimming, cycling, and running. It first appeared on the Olympic programme in Sydney 2000. Competition distances vary (Table 4.7.1) but are based on approximate ratios of the three disciplines first established in 1979 by the Hawaii Ironman Championship which consists of a 3.8 km swim, 180.2 km cycle, and a 42.2 km run.

Equipment and training facilities for triathletes are expensive and developed countries are disproportionately successful at world championships and the Olympic games. Open water swimming is common in races, and this presents both seasonal constraints and medical safety and water-borne infection issues for race medical staff. Specific swim wetsuits have been developed for triathlon, with a maximum neoprene thickness of 5 mm. Wetsuits are compulsory at open water temperatures of less than 14°C at Olympic distance races and forbidden when the water temperature is over 22°C (British Triathlon Technical Rules (http://www.british triathlon.org)). Wetsuits improve swim times by 3–5%, particularly if the subjects are lean (Cordain and Kopriva 1991). In modern cycle races drafting is essential to allow the triathlete the opportunity of exiting the water in the first cohort and joining the first group on the bicycle.

Historically, many triathletes came from a swimming or running background, but it is now not uncommon for the current cohort of junior athletes to have started as triathletes. Parental support is very important at the junior level, and in Western Europe there is a strong club-based programme of training.

Physiological demands of triathlon: training profiles

The sport tests the individual fitness of the triathlete in three disciplines and in the most international races drafting (allowing a competitor to ride in front and share the wind resistance) on the bicycle is allowed. Athletes will race for about 2 hours at the Olympic distance and for more than 9 hours at the Ironman distance. In training, triathletes will spend most time training on the bicycle, then running, and then swimming. Strength and conditioning at elite level is now a significant contributor to overall training load.

Triathletes who perform best expend energy evenly throughout the three disciplines in racing and usually have the fastest run split times (time taken running as a proportion of the whole time for the triathlon), implying some energy conservation for the latter stages of the race. Taking fluids during racing in temperate climates is important even in Olympic distance events where it is preferable to take fluids in early on the bicycle to perform well (McMurray et al. 2006). In longer-distance triathlon events carbohydrate ingestion, particularly during the cycle section, and maintaining adequate fluid intake are critical to good performance. In the longer-distance events many of the elite athletes will lose weight from fluid loss during racing but they seem to tolerate this well. Physiological problems, when they occur, are often secondary to hyponatraemic collapses near the end of the race, probably as a result of excessive water intake by less experienced triathletes during the race. Genuine heat stress is very rare and requires appropriate fluid balance correction and cooling. Collapses after the finish line are rarely life threatening and simply require observation in a calm medical setting with elevation of the lower limbs and simple oral fluids.

Drafting in the swim and cycle section saves energy. Drafting within 50 cm directly behind the toes of a swimmer has been shown to reduce drag by 21% and lateral drafting by 7%. Drafting during the cycle section provides less head-on wind resistance to the individual and less energy cost at a given submaximal intensity. Energy saving during the cycle section allows the elite triathlete to run at a greater percentage of his maximal oxygen uptake. The transition speeds between swimming and cycling, and between cycling and running, at the elite level are very important to good performance. Bicycle tactics are important. The speed of the second transition (bicycle to run) often depends on where the individual triathlete positions his/her bicycle in the pack at the end of the cycle stage. The energy cost of the cycle to run transition reflects the athlete's ability level, and there can be a difference of as much as 11% between the inexperienced and experienced athlete.

Cardiovascular adaptations to endurance exercise are seen in conditioned triathletes. A reduction in left ventricular contractility, echocardiographic changes, raised creatine kinase and creatine kinase MB isoenzyme, and cardiac troponin T serological markers have been recorded after long-distance events (Shave et al. 2004). These return to normal within days of completing the event and, as yet, do not appear to be associated with any significant cumulative prolonged adverse medical problems.

Winter training for elite athletes usually involves long cycle and run sessions, building up endurance and technical economies. Most elite athletes train all year round and move to warmer climates during the off season. During the competitive season an elite Olympic distance athlete will race 10–20 events whilst an Ironman triathlete will rarely race more than three times at the longer distance.

Table 4.7.1 Recognized distances in triathlon races

	Swim (km)	Cycle (km)	Run (km)
Sprint	0.75	20	5
Olympic	1.5	40	10
Middle	2.5	80	20
Long	3.8	180	42

Injuries

Despite triathlon being a multisport event, triathletes do not seem to be protected from injury as a result of regular cross-training. Compared with swimmers, cyclists, and runners, triathletes have the second highest incidence of overuse injury. Most injuries are associated with running and cycling during training, rather than swimming (Shaw *et al.* 2004). Almost all injuries are overuse in type, except traumatic injuries associated with falling off the bicycle. Lower limb bone stress reactions and fractures and lumbar spine pathology are associated with the most time missed from training. The principal injury sites are the knee, ankle and foot, shin, and lumbar–hamstring areas.

Although not specific to triathletes, lumbar–hamstring problems are significantly common at the elite level (42% in the 2000–2004 British triathlon elite squad (author's data)). The majority of low back pain lasts less than a week and is probably the result of soft tissue injury; however, 19% lasts for more than 3 months (Manninen and Kallinen 1996). Low back pain represents 28% of all triathlon-related overuse injuries. Premature lumbar disc dehydration, disc protrusion with neural compression, and proximal hamstring teno-osseous lesions are common causes of presenting symptoms.

Triathlon cycle bars encourage a better aerodynamic position but put the triathlete in prolonged periods of thoracolumbar flexion. This increases posterior lumbar disc pressure and also increases tension in the posterior paravertebral ligaments in the hyperflexed posture of cycling. Triathletes who perform more weekly trunk flexor drills appear to have a higher incidence of low back pain (Manninen and Kallinen 1996). Running increases iliopsoas hypertrophy and tone, and probably contributes to increased lumbar lordosis. These opposing anterior and posterior forces

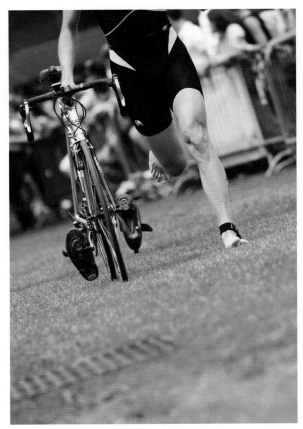

Fig. 4.7.1 The bike to run transition is a significant physical challenge in triathlon. Copyright © Mickael Pouvreau-Fotolia.com

may contribute to the higher incidence of lumbar-related pathology seen in elite squads. Cervical mechanical pain is also more common in triathletes who have competed for longer (Villavicencio *et al.* 2006).

The cycle to run transition causes significant dynamic changes in lower limb function (Table 4.7.2 and Fig. 4.7.1). The femur–pelvis axis quickly changes from a flexed to a relatively extended position. The iliopsoas, iliotibial band, and biceps femoris all undergo changes in their patterns of movement and their incidence of injury in triathletes is significant (Heiden and Burnett 2003). Distal iliotibial band friction syndrome is the most common overuse injury around the knee in triathletes (Clements *et al.* 1999).

The sciatic nerve is stretched in cycling and is prone to deep piriformis compression. The lateral cutaneous branch of the femoral nerve is also prone to compression under sartorius and rectus femoris. Both are reported as problematic in triathletes, probably as a result of the cycle–run combination of training. Triathletes will often perform 'brick sessions' in their training programmes where they undertake repeated short runs and cycling (often on a turbo trainer) to improve their physiological tolerance to the cycle to run transition.

Extrinsic factors

Bicycle crashes can produce rotator cuff tears, clavicular fractures, and acromioclavicular joint injury. During races approved cycle helmets are mandatory. Mass starts are common in the swim

Table 4.7.2 Some bike-to-run-related injury problems in triathletes

Interspinous and iliolumbar ligament strains
Posterior intervertebral disc pathology
Strains of gluteus medius and piriformis
Tightness of iliopsoas
Proximal sciatic neural impingement
Proximal hamstring intramuscular and teno-osseous injury
Femoral nerve impingement
Proximal and distal iliotibial band friction syndrome
External iliac artery compression
Patellofemoral pain syndrome

section, and soft tissue contusions and dislodged goggles are usually the greatest extrinsic injury threat to the triathlete.

The geometry of the bicycle set-up is very important. Incorrect saddle–handlebar length can add to excessive lumbar flexion and excessive cervical spine extension. Shortened saddle–pedal height produces greater patellofemoral compression during the loading phase of the pedal rotation. Prolonged riding in a high gear, which many novice triathletes will attempt, increases the incidence of anterior knee pain. Correct positioning of the footplate on the cycle shoe is important to reduce the incidence of patellofemoral maltracking and distal iliotibial band pain. Correct gearing ratios for the training and racing terrain are important for both good technique and performance, but also for reduction of retropatellar pressure.

Lower limb bone injury is a significant cause of time off training for triathletes. Stress injury to the femur, tibia, fibula, cuboid, navicular, and metatarsals have all been reported. Stress fractures of the metatarsals and tibia are probably also related to the lack of cushioning in running shoes and to overuse. The run from the swim exit to the bicycle racks in a race is an area where race organizers have to ensure that the ground surface is free from hazards, particularly sharp objects, and steps should be avoided. Novice triathletes emerging from the swim section are often slightly disorientated and cold, and their running neuromuscular coordination is suboptimal.

Intrinsic factors

Overuse injuries account for the majority of pre-season and in-season injuries. Some studies have suggested that the likelihood of injury increases with the number of years in triathlon participation and annual running mileage, history of previous injury, and inadequate warm-up and cool-down procedures (Burns et al. 2003).

Lower limb, pelvic, and sacral stress fractures in triathletes are related to running volume and abnormal lower limb biomechanics. Medial tibial stress syndrome, a periostitis of the medial distal tibia, is common in triathletes, particularly in those who overpronate. This is frequently associated with medial plantar fasciitis and overuse of the tibialis posterior. The distal iliotibial band friction syndrome is the most common soft tissue injury around the knee and is secondary to tightness in the band brought about by the reduced range of movement of the structure in cycling and uncorrected over-pronation in running.

Athletic amenorrhoea, low calorific intake, and eating disorders can occur, particularly in elite athletes. An array of symptoms are associated with bone stress reactions, low body weight, and disordered body image. Subclinical eating disorders appear to be prevalent in both female and male triathletes, with strict dietary controls and high calorific expenditures being common amongst those behaving in this way (DiGioacchino De Bate et al. 2002). Even female club triathletes are prone to athletic amenorrhoea, and in one study 40% of athletes reported a history of amenorrhea (Hoch et al. 2007). This problem is by no means exclusive to triathlon, and it requires sensitive medical care and a multidisciplinary team approach.

Front crawl is the preferred fastest stroke used by triathletes. Shoulder injuries are often associated with this swimming technique or occur as a result of falls from the bicycle. In front crawl the relative overdevelopment of the anterior shoulder

muscles and functional laxity of the joint leads to a net anterior translation of the glenohumeral joint during the swimming stroke. This may lead to impingement of the supraspinatus tendon underneath the subacromial arch (Yanai et al. 2000) and swimming-related shoulder pain.

Gastrointestinal problems can affect triathletes, particularly in the longer-distance events. Carbohydrate ingestion is important during the cycling section, but if it is delayed before the run can lead to feelings of bloating and nausea. Some elite endurance triathletes suffer from exercise-induced gastro-oesophageal reflux, particularly during the run section. Relative gastric stasis and increased intra-abdominal pressures during running probably add to functional impairment of the gastro-oesophageal junction. Surprisingly, the symptoms are rarely experienced in the cycle section.

Epidemiology of injuries

The prevalence of pre-season injury is 2.5–5.4 per 1000 training hours, whereas in the competition season the injury exposure rate is 4.6–17.4 per 1000 training hours (Korkia et al. 1994; Burns et al. 2003). Overuse injuries accounted for 68% of pre-season and 78% of competition season injuries (Burns et al. 2003), with the majority being lower limb injuries. Considering the number of hours spent training compared with competing, the injury exposure rate in competition is high and may reflect the risks taken, particularly in cycle racing.

Cycling and running appear to cause most injuries, but whilst injury may prohibit a triathlete from running, cycling and swimming can often be tolerated. Running injuries are associated with the number of running sessions per week and increased race distances. Stress fractures, Achilles tendinopathies, lumbar spinal disorders, and knee-related injuries have the most protracted recovery time and longest delay in return to racing (Vleck and Garbutt 1998).

In athletes training for longer-distance events, older athletes sustained more fractures, high-performance athletes suffered more contusions/abrasions and muscle–tendon injuries, and triathletes who trained for a large number each week suffered more muscle–tendon injuries (Egermann et al. 2003). Most studies support the observation that the injury rate is slightly higher in elite than in recreational athletes (Korkia et al. 1994). It is unclear whether coaching has a protective effect on injuries. Many triathletes train with a club mainly to secure pool access, companionship and competition when running, and safety when cycling in a larger group.

The profiling of elite triathletes to circumvent injury and illness is still a developing science. In the Great Britain (GB) squad regular contact between a dedicated sports physician and elite triathlete strengthens the practitioner–athlete relationship and makes it easier to manage illness and injury in what is often a remote and mobile athlete population. The triathlete's expectations may be unjustifiably raised as to the sensitivity of the observations made on predicting outcome of either injury or illness during the process of profiling. Most national populations of elite triathletes are small, and it is difficult to demonstrate significance in interventions, other than to the individual.

In the GB junior squad, cross-sectional cardiovascular data collection (using 12 lead ECG and echocardiogram) has been proved to be of clinical assistance in determining the later significance of chest-related symptoms in the more mature trained athletes.

Similarly, previous musculoskeletal injury history, specific blood tests, targeted flow loop spirometry, menstrual history, and medication reviews have improved the medical care of elite GB international triathletes (Batt *et al.* 2004).

References

Batt, M.E., Jaques, R., and Stone, M. (2004). Preparticipation examination (screening): practical issues as determined by sport: a United Kingdom perspective. *Clinical Journal of Sports Medicine*, **14**, 178–82.

Burns, J., Keenan, A.M., and Redmond, A.C. (2003). Factors associated with triathlon-related overuse injuries. *Journal of Orthopaedic and Sports Physical Therapy*, **33**, 177–84.

Clements, K., Yates, B., and Curran, M. (1999). The prevalence of chronic knee injury in triathletes. *British Journal of Sports Medicine*, **33**, 214–16.

Cordain, L. and Kopriva, R. (1991). Wetsuits, body density and swimming performance. *British Journal of Sports Medicine*, **25**, 31–3.

DiGioacchino DeBate, R., Wethington, H., and Sargent, R. (2002). Sub-clinical eating disorder characteristics among male and female triathletes. *Eating and Weight Disorders*, **7**, 210–20.

Egermann, M., Brocai, D., Lill, C.A., and Schmitt, H. (2003). Analysis of injuries in long-distance triathletes. *International Journal of Sports Medicine*, **24**, 271–6.

Heiden, T. and Burnett, A. (2003). The effect of cycling on muscle activation on the run leg of an olympic distance triathlon. *Sports Biomechanics*, **2**, 35–49.

Hoch, A.Z., Stavrakos, J.E., and Schimke, J.E. (2007). Prevalence of female athlete triad characteristics in a club triathlon team. *Archives of Physical Medicine and Rehabilitation*, **88**, 681–2.

Korkia, P.K., Tunstall-Pedoe, D.S., and Maffulli, N. (1994). An epidemiological investigation of training and injury patterns in British triathletes. *British Journal of Sports Medicine*, **28**, 191–6.

McMurray, R.G., Williams, D.K., Battaglini, C.L. (2006). The timing of fluid intake during an Olympic distance triathlon. *International Journal of Sport Nutrition and Exercise Metabolism*, **16**, 611–19.

Manninen, J.S.O. and Kallinen, M. (1996). Low back pain and other overuse injuries in a group of Japanese triathletes. *British Journal of Sports Medicine*, **30**, 134–9.

Shave, R., Dawson, E., Whyte, G., George, K., Gaze, D., and Collinson, P. (2004). Altered cardiac function and minimal cardiac damage during prolonged exercise. *Medicine and Science in Sports and Exercise*, **36**, 1098–1103.

Shaw, T., Howat, P, Trainor, M., and Maycock, B. (2004). Training patterns and sports injuries in triathletes. *Journal of Science and Medicine in Sport*, **7**, 446–50.

Villavicencio, A.T., Burneikiene, S., Hernández, T.D., and Thramann, J. (2006). Back and neck pain in triathletes. *Neurosurgical Focus*, **21**, E7.

Vleck, V.E. and Garbutt, G. (1998). Injury and training characteristics of male elite, development squad and club triathletes. *International Journal of Sports Medicine*, **19**, 38–42.

Yanai, T., Hay, J.G., and Miller, G.F. (2000). Shoulder impingement in front-crawl swimming. I: A method to identify impingement. *Medicine and Science in Sports and Exercise*, **32**, 21–9.

4.8

Running injuries

Bruce Hamilton

Nothing in life was worth very much that did not entail some risk. So do not be afraid of strains and sprains, aches and pains.

Percy Wells Cerutty
Schoolboy Athletics, p.115, c.1966

Injuries in distance runners

Distance running is an extremely popular activity with many thousands of runners competing in major city marathons as well as weekly club running events. Most of these runners are not competitive in any given race, but will have their own goals and reasons for participating. As with other forms of exercise, running has significant health and social benefits, and the prevention of injury and thus maintenance of participation should be a key goal for any practitioner. While there has been some variance in the literature in defining what exactly a distance runner is, there is agreement that individuals who run on a regular basis are susceptible to overuse injuries. Up to 70% of competitive distance runners may be injured during any single year, although even this may be an underestimate because of the use of different injury definitions and study limitations (Bennell and Crossley 1996). Other papers report a lower limb injury incidence of between 20% and 80% (van Gent *et al.* 2007). Serious marathon runners, running approximately 1.5 hours daily, may be expected to have one overuse injury every 2 months. Despite the high participation rate and high morbidity, the literature in this area is limited and often contradictory, reflecting the multifactorial nature of injuries in the runner.

The most commonly injured site in the distance runner is the knee, followed by the foot, ankle, and lower leg. The most common injuries are listed in Table 4.8.1.

Overuse injuries in running

During the complex process of running, both intrinsic and extrinsic forces are applied to the body. The most relevant external forces acting on the body during running are the ground reaction forces. These forces occur in three planes, mediolateral, anteroposterior, and vertical, and each will vary depending on the speed of running and individual running technique. Forces involved vary from 0.3 to 0.6 times body weight for the anteroposterior plane to 1.2 to 3.5 times body weight for the vertical ground reaction forces (Hreljac 2005) and typically increase with increasing running speed. Longer distances and duration of repetitive cyclical application of forces will increase the total amount of stress that body tissues are required to tolerate. These forces must be balanced by forces generated by muscles, bones, tendons, ligaments, and joint capsules (Schache *et al.* 1999; Hreljac 2005), and the ability of the body to manage these forces will determine the susceptibility to overuse injuries in distance runners.

Overuse injuries in runners result from the failure of body tissues to positively adapt to the repeated application of forces. Each anatomical component of the body, such as bone and tendon, is subject to stress with each stride, and the repeated application of forces, while below the absolute tensile limit of the tissue, will result in both positive and negative adaptation. If sufficient recovery time is provided for the tissue, recovery and positive adaptation to the load will occur. However, if the interval between stress application is too short or the duration of stress is too long, failure to adapt and injury may ensue. Simply, prolonged application of low-grade forces may exceed the injury threshold, thus resulting in overuse injury. This relationship is illustrated in Figure 4.8.1.

In reality, each tissue in each individual will have a distinct and individual injury threshold for tolerating both a single high application of force and the repetitive application of low-level force. Each tissue (e.g. muscle, tendon, joint, bone, cartilage) will have a specific recovery time required for it to positively adapt, and as a result of individual factors such as anthropometry, biomechanics, age, previous injury profile, training profile, this will constantly be in flux and evolving. This explains why the same perceived training load applied to two athletes may result in an injury to one but not the other, and why each athlete must identify their own tissue thresholds. It also rationalizes the importance of recovery in any training programme. The aim of any therapeutic intervention should be to raise the threshold to injury of individual tissues (Fig. 4.8.1).

Aetiology of injuries in distance running

Famously articulated by Dr George Sheehan in the 1970s, 'Treat the reason, not the result. Treat the cause, not the effect' is the mantra by which one must address running injuries. Thus both a clear diagnosis and consideration of the aetiological factors involved are required. As alluded to above, the aetiology of overuse injuries in runners is multifactorial, with both intrinsic and extrinsic factors playing a role. While a number of frequently cited risk factors are potentially involved (Table 4.8.2), it must be remembered that most of these are based on limited and often contradictory literature (Yeung and Yeung 2001). Common limitations found in the literature include unifactorial analysis, low subject numbers, poor and variable injury definitions, limited follow-up,

Table 4.8.1 Common overuse injuries in distance runners

Knee	Patello-femoral syndrome
	Illiotibial band friction syndrome
	Patellar tendinopathy
	Meniscal injuries
Lower leg	Medial tibial stress syndrome
	Stress fracture (tibia, fibula)
	Compartment syndrome
	Vascular compromise
	Calf pain undiagnosed
	Achilles tendinopathy
Foot	Stress fracture (metatarsal, navicular)
	Tibialis posterior enthesopathy
	First metatarso-phalangeal sesamoiditis
	Plantar fasciitis
Pelvis	Stress fracture (sacral, femoral neck, pubic rami)
	Low back pain

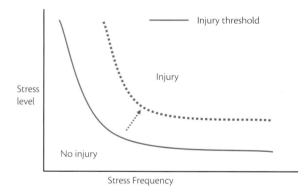

Fig. 4.8.1 Relationship between stress frequency, stress level, and injury threshold.

Table 4.8.2 Proposed aetiological factors in overuse injuries in runners

General
- Increasing age
- Female
- Height/weight/BMI
- Running for less than 3 years
- Previous injury
- Menstrual factors
- Low energy intake
- Low calcium/vitamin D

Psychological
- Stressful events
- Personality (type A)

Training
- Duration/distance/volume
- Intensity
- Surface
- Rate of change
- Hill running
- Speed
- Footwear
- Stretching
- Inadequate recovery

Anatomical
- Pes cavus/planus
- Ankle joint range of motion
- Leg-length discrepancy
- Genu valgum/varum
- Technique
- Q angle
- Tubercle-sulcus angle
- Flexibility (hamstring, quadriceps)
- Hip joint range of motion
- Rearfoot valgus
- Bone mineral density
- Bone geometry

Biomechanical
- Hip abductor weakness
- Magnitude and velocity of pronation/supination
- Magnitude of ground reaction forces
- Magnitude of knee joint forces and moments
- Anterior pelvic tilt
- Lumbar lordosis

self-recording, and retrospective nature. As a result, the assessment and management of the injured runner remains a complex combination of science and art.

Lower limb anatomical and biomechanical factors such as alignment, leg-length discrepancies, pes cavus or planus, and excessive range and rate of pronation are often, in the clinical setting, felt to be causal in injury development. Pronation is a complex movement of the subtalar joint occurring during the first half of the stance phase of running and is an essential component of the running cycle, allowing for shock absorption and accommodation to underfoot surfaces. Pronation results in both hindfoot eversion and tibial internal rotation, and it is postulated that both excessive rate and magnitude of pronation may predispose to injury. While intuitively inviting, the literature is neither conclusive nor consistent regarding the role of these factors in the development of running injuries (Hreljac 2005). Indeed, so inviting is the temptation to correct these factors that, despite their own prospective study of alignment failing to show any conclusive risk factors, Wen *et al* (1998) still concluded that '…the suggestion that alignment is a

risk factor for injury makes too much intuitive sense to totally discount…'. While this perhaps reflects the artistic rather than the scientific side of injury management, one should consider the counter to this argument, so well articulated by the late Stephen Jay Gould: 'Most difficult to dislodge are those biases that escape our scrutiny because they seem so obviously, even ineluctably, just' (Gould 1992).

Following a comprehensive prospective study over a period of 1 year, van Mechelen *et al.* (1996) concluded that the major risk factors for injury were not anthropometric, but rather previous injury, exposure time, vital exhaustion, dominance, and stressful life events. Although not specifically limited to runners, exposure time and previous injury were found to be the two most significant factors. Previous injury is well recognized in high-force injuries such as hamstring strains, but total exposure time reflects a training error, which some authors suggest is the cause of the majority of running-related injuries (Hreljac 2005).

Training errors can be identified from a carefully taken history and may include too rapid an increase in mileage, too high a mileage, too much fast running, insufficient recovery, poor training surfaces (too hard or too soft), and lack of variation in training. There is evidence that runners training for 3 days or less per week compared with 5 days per week, athletes training for 15–30 minutes compared with 45 minutes or more per day, and those completing a smaller total training distance are less likely to be injured (Yeung and Yeung 2001). Add to these factors the complex melting pot of age, accumulated stress, previous injury, and anatomical variability, and it becomes clear why training and recovery must be individually tailored for each athlete in order to minimize the risk of injury and re-injury. Because of an accumulation of factors, the anatomical tissue of a 40-year-old long-term runner will not tolerate the training load he/she performed as a 25-year-old, and this must be factored into a training approach.

Subsequently, it is vital that a careful history is observed and, with an awareness of the limitations of the literature, a pragmatic and cautious approach to injury management and intervention is undertaken.

Management of the overuse running injury

As each individual injury will require specific management, it is not the intention to address this management but rather to provide a framework for addressing the injured runner. Those athletes with a history of running-related injuries or athletes who have been training for less than 3 years are at increased risk, and therefore should pay particular attention to preventative measures and early signs of injury (van Gent et al. 2007). Identification of the specific nature of an injury is vital, but may be relatively the easiest component of managing the injured athlete when one has available a good history, examination, and tools such as MRI, ultrasound and other imaging. The identification of the key aetiological factors is often a more complex task and the one which will have more significant impact on outcome than merely making an accurate injury diagnosis. Assessing the relative merits of each of the factors above is the art of sports medicine, and this requires each individual to have a careful and timely evaluation. Often gait and other biomechanical factors are altered by the presence of injury, and hence formal evaluation of these factors is better left until after the acute phase of the injury, thus mandating a two-stage process of evaluation.

Identification of a possible training error, relative to the individual's history and morphology, is important as it is a potentially modifiable factor which, when corrected, may prevent a recurrence of injury. Management of the specific injury pathology, followed by a graded return to training and modification of training patterns, will be required, and the dedicated runner may take some convincing about this. In many cases starting runners on a walk–run programme, gradually progressing on an alternate day basis, is required. Progression should only be allowed if good technique and pain-free running are maintained. This slow progression is often difficult to achieve in an athlete used to running for many hours. The 10% per week rule is often quoted when increasing volume and intensity, and although this has little scientific basis, it is a reasonable guide. Absolute volume needs to be considered on an individual basis.

Evaluation of recovery strategies, including diet, soft tissue therapy, hydrotherapy, sleep, and avoidance of stress may lead to some clear indicators of injury risk, and are important to consider in trying to prevent further injury. Utilization of cross-training and having appropriate nutritional and soft tissue recovery strategies are often critical in the injured athlete, and should be key to any structured training programme. Stretching forms an important part of any training or injury text written for runners. Despite the intuitive benefits this may appear to have, there is little consistent evidence to support the use of traditional stretching techniques as an injury prevention modality in distance runners (Yeung and Yeung 2001).

Correction of anatomical and biomechanical deficits in a runner requires a multidisciplinary team approach. Podiatric gait evaluation to assess the merits of orthotic intervention, physiotherapeutic input to correct soft tissue tension and muscle balance, and conditioning to assess and correct strength deficits and imbalances may all be required to address these predisposing factors. Altering a long-standing gait pattern clearly has consequences on tissues other than those that were injured. Subsequently, any intervention of this nature must be accompanied by a slow and graded return to activity in order to allow all tissues to adapt to new directions of stress application and to prevent secondary injury.

'Core stability' is a popular phrase in injury prevention clinics, and as a result of the movements of the lumbopelvic–hip complex during running and the possibility of a relationship between poor pelvic control and lower limb injury (Schache et al. 1999; Leetun et al. 2004; Niemuth et al. 2005) it is reasonable to incorporate a central stability programme into rehabilitation programmes. Therefore a comprehensive abdominal core and gluteal muscle strengthening programme should form a part of both the prehabilitation and rehabilitation of any injured athlete (Fridericson and Moore 2005), but this should be as functional as possible. However, it is important to be aware that there is limited evidence that core stability will either prevent the development of injuries or enhance performance in runners.

Injuries in sprinters

Sprinting is characterized by rapid and powerful contraction of large muscle groups over a short period of time. As a consequence, unlike distance runners, sprinters' injuries tend to be sudden onset and related to maximal power production, with up to 50% of injuries being acute (D'Souza 1994; Bennell and Crossley 1996). The most frequent injury observed in sprinters is to the thigh, and most commonly this is a hamstring muscle strain. The aetiological factors thought to be involved in this include fatigue, lack of warm-up, hip and knee range of motion, biomechanical factors, dehydration, previous hamstring or knee injury, age, and muscle balance. It is critical that each hamstring injury is evaluated carefully to elucidate which risk factors are present in order to minimize the risk of recurrence, as it is recognized that the greatest predisposition to a hamstring injury is a previous hamstring injury. General management of the acute hamstring injury is covered in Chapter 3.8; however, in the sprinter it is vital that range of motion, muscle balance (in particular the hamstring-to-quadriceps ratio and the angle of peak torque), and stride length return to normal prior to a return to maximum speed running in order to minimize the risk of re-injury.

Table 4.8.3 Practical suggestions for injury prevention

- High-impact training in morning while lumbar discs are well hydrated
- When changing worn-out shoes, do so gradually (or rotate shoes)
- Don't let shoes wear out
- Practice correct running technique
- Shock absorbers for cavus feet
- Avoid over-striding
- Stretch during warm-up and warm-down
- Avoid hard or soft surfaces
- Avoid camber
- Wear appropriate clothing
- Don't run through pain—listen to your body signals
- Keep a diary
- Use a coach
- Learn to know what your body is telling you
- Incorporate rest into your programme (work is not rest)
- Enjoy your training

As a result of the forces generated and the plyometric nature of sprint training, tendon injuries are also observed in sprinters. These include both acute tendon rupture and chronic tendinopathies. Management of tendinopathy in a sprinter requires a careful history and examination in order to elucidate the relevant aetiological factors prior to initiating treatment. Rehabilitation from a chronic tendinopathy in a sprinter may often be slow.

References

Bennell, K.L. and Crossley, K (1996). Musculoskeletal injuries in track and field: incidence, distribution and risk factors. *Australian Journal of Science and Medicine in Sport*, **28**, 69–75.

D'Souza, D. (1994). Track and field athletics injuries—a one-year survey. *British Journal of Sports Medicine*, **28**, 197–202.

Fridericson, M. and Moore, T. (2005). Muscular balance, core stability, and injury prevention for middle- and long-distance runners. *Physical Medicine and Rehabilitation Clinics of North America*, **16**, 669–89.

Gould, S.J. (1992). *Bully for Brontosaurus*. Penguin Books, Harmondsworth.

Hreljac, A. (2005). Etiology, prevention, and early intervention of overuse injuries in runners: a biomechanical perspective. *Physical Medicine and Rehabilitation Clinics of North America*, **16**, 651–67.

Leetun, D., Ireland, L., Willson, J., Ballantyne, B., and Davis, I.M. (2004). Core stability measures as risk factors for lower extremity injury in athletes. *Medicine and Science in Sports and Exercise*, **36**, 926–34.

Niemuth, P., Johnson, R., Myers, M., and Thieman, T. (2005). Hip muscle weakness and overuse injuries in recreational runners. *Clinical Journal of Sport Medicine*, **15**, 14–21.

Schache, A., Bennell, K., Blanch, P., and Wrigley, T. (1999). The coordinated movement of the lumbo-pelvic-hip complex during running: a literature review. *Gait and Posture*, **10**, 30–47.

van Gent, R., Siem, D., van Middelkoop, M., van Os, T., Bierma-Zeinstra, S., and Koes, B. (2007). Incidence and determinants of lower extremity running injuries in long distance runners: a systematic review. *British Journal of Sports Medicine*, **41**, 469–80.

van Mechelen, W., Twisk, J., Molendijk, A., Blom, B., Snel, J. and Kemper, H. C. (1996). Subject-related risk factors for sports injuries: a 1-yr prospective study in young adults. *Medicine and Science in Sports and Exercise*, **28**, 1171–9.

Wen, D., Puffer, J.C., and Schmalzried, T.P. (1998). Injuries in runners: a prospective study of alignment. *Clinical Journal of Sport Medicine*, **8**, 187–94.

Yeung, E. and Yeung, S. (2001). A systematic review of interventions to prevent lower limb soft tissue running injuries. *British Journal of Sports Medicine*, **35**, 383–9.

4.9

Injuries in field (throwing and jumping) events

Roger Hackney

Introduction

The field events in the sport of track and field athletics include a wide range of very different disciplines. They can be divided into the **jumping events** (long jump, triple jump, high jump, and pole vault) and the **throwing events** (javelin, shot putt, hammer, and discus). In modern track and field athletics, all disciplines are performed by both sexes. Injuries relate to the training methods and the specific technical features of each event.

Training

The athlete's year is divided into training and competition sections. The athlete will set a goal, be it a national or an international championship, and then develop a training programme to achieve maximum performance. This will include periods of specific training to build strength and speed. The concept of periodization allows for recovery following an intense training period. Training errors should always be borne in mind when assessing the aetiology of an injury. Neglecting these factors will lead to recurrence unless all issues are considered. Unless the practitioner has the necessary experience and knowledge of the technical aspects of both the training and the mechanics of an event, the assistance of a suitably qualified coach should be sought.

All field events are explosive, requiring a combination of strength, speed, and skill. Although some events may last for over an hour, an individual will only compete in short bursts; endurance training does not play a role. All field event athletes will employ basic conditioning work in the form of circuit training, including plyometrics as well as weight-training. The majority of this is undertaken during the off season, although the increasing popularity of the indoor season means that the timing and duration of the conditioning period is affected—perhaps reduced, but certainly modified. Event-specific work receives more of an emphasis as the outdoor season approaches, although coaches may require athletes to work on specific areas of technique which may be perceived to be deficient during the off season.

Weight-training and core stability

The trend in modern gymnasia is to use fixed apparatus as opposed to free weights. The apparatus is safer and allows heavier weights to be used, but the direction of movement is strictly two-dimensional, unlike sport. Unless adequate steps are taken to account for this, the athlete loses the control and proprioceptive element of weight-training. A prime example of the dangers of using apparatus alone is easily appreciated in the shoulder. Weightlifters develop the power of the prime movers of the shoulder using apparatus that moves in two planes. The control muscles of the shoulder, the rotator cuff, are neglected. As a result the prime movers may become sufficiently powerful to sublux the glenohumeral joint, leading to pain and loss of function when undertaking activities such as bench press or throwing.

The concept of core stability and control has emerged over the last decade, and the majority of professional sportspersons incorporate the basics of core stability training into their conditioning programmes. Core stability in the trunk is the key to all field events, where loss of control means an unstable platform for the throw or jump and a risk of injury to a structure further along the kinetic chain of movement.

Throwing events

All the throwing events incorporate a kinetic chain which begins with legs, trunk, and pelvis. Only at the end of the throw or putt is the shoulder and arm used. The majority of the power is derived from the lower part of the chain. As an illustration of this, only 30% of the speed of a tennis serve is derived from the shoulder alone.

The javelin

The javelin (event) requires use of a conventional overhead throwing technique, very similar to throwing a ball. The difference is that the throw is along the line of the javelin. The mechanics of the overhead throwing action have been studied in great detail using ultra-high-speed cinematography coordinated with EMG studies to determine which muscles are acting with each phase of the throw. The research has been predominantly conducted on baseball pitchers, but the elements of the technique apply to all overhead throwing actions. The stages of the throw have been divided into the cocking, acceleration, and follow-through or deceleration phases. The biomechanics and forces involved are quite staggering. The arm is held at around 90° of abduction at the shoulder, but the external rotation at the end of the cocking phase can be more than 180°. The acceleration has been estimated at 7000° per second, and the humeral head in follow-through has a distraction force of 80% of body weight (Dilman *et al.* 1993).

Overhead throwing injuries

A brief overview of the aetiology and presentation of overhead throwing injuries is presented here; the reader should refer to Chapters 3.5 and 3.6 for further details. The basics of javelin technique must be rehearsed and developed progressively to avoid incorrect technique from the beginning. Range of motion is extreme, and control throughout that range of motion is essential. In particular, a stable trunk is essential.

The glenohumeral joint has been likened to a circus seal balancing a ball on its nose, with the rotator cuff muscles acting as guides to control the motion of the ball in the socket. The analogy can be taken a step further in that the glenohumeral joint rests on the scapula, an unstable platform, akin to the seal sitting on a wobble board. The nose will lose control of the ball unless the base is kept steady. The core stability of the trunk and scapula represents the requirement for a stable base. Whenever a throwing athlete presents with arm pain, the physician must go back down the kinetic chain to ensure that the trunk is under control as a first step.

Low back pain

Low back pain is common in throwers, as the rapid trunk rotation stresses the pars interarticulares and facet joints of the lumbar spine. The whipping round of the pelvis and trunk generates most of the force in the throw. Prevention is best in this situation; the thrower must have a stable core and a strong trunk.

Elbow injuries

Javelin throwers must be encouraged to 'keep the elbow high'. Failure to comply with this basic element of technique inevitably leads to elbow pain. The weight of the forearm and javelin is borne solely by the anterior component of the ulnar collateral ligament of the elbow during the acceleration phase of the throw. The lower the elbow when the shoulder is abducted below 90°, the more this applies. The ligament cannot tolerate the extra load. Chronic pain is due to attenuation of the ligament which eventually suffers an acute failure. Persisting throwing may result in posterior impingement and osteophyte formation with loss of range of motion. An overhead thrower with a painful medial elbow should immediately stop throwing, and the coach should be involved in re-educating the thrower to keep the elbow high. Steroid injections are contraindicated. With an acute rupture, surgical reconstruction is the only option. Diagnosis depends upon a high degree of suspicion, and appropriate stress views or MRI scan to confirm the diagnosis. Surgical reconstruction is the only option for a chronically attenuated ligament.

Shoulder injuries

The non-physiological range of motion found in throwers requires an attenuation of the inferior glenohumeral ligament which holds the arm when the shoulder is abducted 90°. Fatigue of the rotator cuff may lead to such distraction that the translation of the head of the humerus causes it to ride over the anterior labrum, adding to the impending instability of the joint. The shoulder becomes functionally unstable with pain in the acceleration phase and dead arm syndrome from traction of the brachial plexus. The anterior laxity frequently produces a physiologically posterior 'tightness'. This is frequently reported as a 'capsular' tightness, but the loss of passive

movement described by Kibler (1998) is likely to be due to shortening of the fibrous component of the posterior elements of the rotator cuff. The glenohumeral internal rotation deficit (GIRD) test described by Kibler assesses this very nicely.

The term 'internal impingement' coined by Chris Jobe (Jobe and Sidles 2003) and Gilles Walch (Sonnery-Cottet *et al.* 2002) describes the impingement of the posterior superior glenoid against the attachment of supraspinatus. This results in an abrasion of the undersurface of the tendon of supraspinatus and a characteristic 'peel-back' tear of the posterior superior glenoid labrum. Conventional subacromial impingement is often superimposed, and is attributable to poor control of the rotator cuff in centralizing the humeral head.

Prevention is by adequate training of the rotator cuff and passive stretching of the posterior shoulder in a cross-arm direction. If shoulder pain develops, the timing of the pain in the throw is helpful in assessing the relative importance of the impingements and dead-arm syndrome, though the underlying cause is due to anterior instability. This should be addressed with strengthening of the rotator cuff, aiming to address proprioceptive deficits. If this fails, an arthroscopic stabilization will address all elements of the instability.

Shot putt

The shot can be delivered by a rotational or direct technique; the end of the 'throw' is when the shot leaves the neck. The athlete faces the back of the circle to maximize the power derived from legs and trunk. Rapid acceleration is the key to a long throw. The technique involves holding the shot with the throwing hand resting against the neck until the release, when a straight arm is used to propel the shot. Shot putt involves very rapid acceleration over a short distance with enormous power; the senior men's shot weighs 9.26 kg.

Shot putters develop injuries from the heavy weight-training load. The classic atraumatic osteolysis of the lateral end of the clavicle of weightlifters is a cause of shoulder pain. They suffer low back pain from the weight-training and rotation of the trunk during the throw. Many shot putters complain of neck pain. This is due to the head being thrown away from the direction of the twist at the time of release. Coaches teach this as part of the method of directing and thrusting the shot to achieve an optimum angle of throw. Poor technique with early release of the shot, very common amongst less skilled putters, leads to a foul throw, but can also cause injuries to the wrist and thumb as the weight of the shot is borne by an extended wrist/thumb. Ligament sprains from this source require readjustment of technique by an appropriate coach.

Discus

The discus is a highly athletic event requiring a great deal of speed agility and strength. A number of turns, usually three or four depending upon skill level, provide acceleration and forward momentum across the throwing circle. It is the transfer of this rotational kinetic energy that projects the discus. This transference of energy to the discus is best achieved with a solid base. Therefore the mechanically best throw has the thrower use the last step as an end-stop about which the body rotates to eject the discus. Rotating on this last step gives a relatively unstable platform and poor direction of throw. The downside of this is that the trunk and spine are placed under tremendous strain, and therefore back pain is common amongst discus throwers. Strength in the arm is only the last part of the throw, which requires the discus to be launched horizontally and spinning. Skin injuries to the throwing finger are common. There are restrictions as to what can be used to protect the finger. Sticking plaster gives a better grip, extra spin, and distance, and hence is not permitted.

Hammer

The hammer is similar to the discus in that it is mainly rotational speed that is transferred to the implement. The hammer is held in both arms as the body spins. The last step is the one which transfers the energy. Those who use a planted foot tend to have shortened careers limited by back pain. Gloves are permitted for throwing, but hand and finger injuries may still occur.

Both hammer and discus require enormous power to propel the implement. Accordingly, weight-training forms the major part of the training, but the skill element is often overlooked by those with no understanding of the events. Both are highly technical and require a great deal of coaching input.

Jumps

Jumping events require sudden transfer of running speed to the jump. As a general principle, the faster the run-up the more energy there is for the leap. Training elastic rebound and speed are the essentials of jump conditioning; technical training is added as winter and then spring progress towards the competitive summer season.

Plyometrics, weights, and speed work are the ingredients of the winter workload. Care has to be taken with the bounding needed for sprint and jump training. Inappropriate training workloads or methods are the major cause of injury. Injuries associated with plyometrics include acute injuries such as ankle ligament sprains and overuse injuries of the lower leg. These include tendinopathy of the tendons of the calf and shin soreness from stress fractures or medial tibial periostitis syndrome.

Long jump

This is the simplest of the jumping events. The athlete sprints and then leaps from a board into a sandpit. The edge of the board is marked with plasticine to indicate the slightest of encroachment of the foot beyond the front of the board. The jumper spends a great deal of time perfecting a routine for the run-up to land as close to the front of the board as possible in a reproducible way. The last stride is shorter than the rest to utilize the extra elastic energy stored by this manouevre.

The athlete moves in the air to reach the legs as far forward as possible. This comprises the use of a hitch kick and cycling movements to maintain balance in flight. Landing does not often cause injury, but traumatic injuries from landing can occur. Examples are ankle sprains, wrist injuries from the fall, etc.

Triple jump

The 'hop, step, and jump' is a more technically demanding event. Slow-motion video reveals just how stressful this event is to the lower limbs and pelvis. The forces passing through the leg are extreme and a misplaced landing can result in severe injury to joint or muscle. Jumpers suffer injury from direct trauma to the heel and forefoot, especially the sesamoid bones of the first metatarsal. Simple bruising can be extremely debilitating, but stress fractures

and osteonecrosis of the sesamoid cause a premature end to the season. Sesamoid injuries are managed by removing load from the affected bone. This is achieved by modifying training and/ or the use of a pad under the other metatarsals, elevating them and so protecting the sore area. Rarely, surgical removal can be used as a last resort for non-union or osteonecrosis.

High jump

The object of this event is to leap over a bar resting on two small ledges on stanchions next to elevated landing mats. The athlete transfers horizontal speed into vertical height by pivoting on one foot and ankle. There are two basic techniques. The traditional straddle technique has been superseded by a technique called the Fosbury flop, named after an American high jumper who won an Olympic gold medal with his method of arching the back over the bar. The technique does require a high standard of landing cushion. High jumpers suffer a high incidence of 'jumper's knee', a patellar tendinosis.

Pole vault

Pole vault is a spectacular event where an athlete is launched to a height of over 5 m (males) with the aid of a strong but flexible pole, which is planted into a 'box' at the end of a run-up. The pole then bends and straightens as the athlete effectively does a vertical handstand and push from the pole to leap over the bar (Fig. 4.9.1).

The vast majority of injuries in pole vault arise from poor landing either from a missed jump, where ankles, back, and knee can be injured, or more seriously by missing the landing bed altogether. Deaths from head injury have been recorded. The additional training requirement for the pole vault compared with other jumps is upper limb strength training.

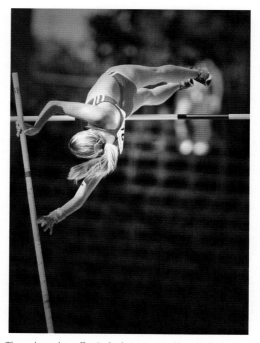

Fig. 4.9.1 The pole vaulter effectively does a vertical handstand and push from the pole to leap over the bar. Copyright © Walter Luger - Fotolia.com

References

Dilman, C.J., Fleisig, G.T.S., and Andrews, J.R. (1993). Biomechanics of pitching with emphasis upon shoulder kinematics. *Journal of Orthopaedic and Sports Physical Therapy*, **18**, 402–8.

Jobe, C.M. and Sidles, L. (1993). Evidence for a superior glenoid impingement upon the rotator cuff. *Journal of Shoulder and Elbow Surgery*, **2**, S19.

Kibler, W.B. (1998). The relationship of glenohumeral internal rotation deficit to shoulder and elbow injuries in tennis players: a prospective evaluation of posterior capsular stretching. Presented at the Annual Closed meeting of the American Shoulder and Elbow Surgeons, New York.

Sonnery-Cottet, B., Edwards, T.B., Noel, E., and Walch, G. (2002). Results of arthroscopic treatment of posterosuperior glenoid impingement in tennis players. *American Journal of Sports Medicine*, **30**, 227–32.

4.10

Golf injuries

Cathy Speed

Introduction

Golf is a game with rapidly increasing popularity, played world-wide. Golfers are a wide spectrum of the population in terms of their size, shape, age, fitness, and health status As a result, injuries in golf can involve aggravation of a pre-existing condition such as osteoarthritis or present as acute or chronic overuse injuries *de novo*. The majority of golf injuries are associated with a lack of core control, limitations in flexibility, or aberrations in the swing. Adaptations in a golfer's swing can help to compensate for physical limitations and injuries, and swing analysis and correction play an important role in clinical assessment of an injured golfer. Hence a knowledge of the swing is important in identifying the underlying cause of the injury and correcting it. Assistance from a golf coach, particularly one who might already be familiar with the particular golfer's swing mechanics, can be extremely helpful.

The golf swing

The golf swing consists of specific phases in the following order: set up and address, take-away, backswing, downswing, acceleration, and follow-through (Fig. 4.10.1) (McHardy *et al.* 2006).

There is no single type of swing; it can vary according to the skill level, the physical characteristics of the player, and the clubs used. However, there are two main swing types, the classic swing and the modern swing. The generic characteristics of a swing are described below; all references made relate to a right-handed golfer.

Phase I: set-up (ball address)

The player sets up to address the ball by adopting correct posture, ball position, stance, weight distribution, and muscle balance. Ball position depends upon the type of shot being made, the player's technique and height, and the distance the ball has to travel. The greater the club length, the more forward the ball is in the stance. The width of stance affects stability and control during the swing. If the stance is too narrow, stability is sacrificed, while too wide a stance will limit pelvic rotation and weight transfer. If the ball is not in the desired position, the clubface will have little chance of being square at impact. The taller the golfer, the steeper is the plane angle of swing.

A good set-up position is important to allow maintenance of good balance during the swing; full rotation and proper weight transfer will allow the player to move with power yet stay on balance (Fig. 4.10.2). The centre of pressure is in the middle of the feet.

Phase II: Take-away

The take-away influences the swing plane and starts at the beginning of the backswing from the point of address and ends at the end of the backswing. Movement begins as the hands and shoulders move away from the ball as a unit, with a weight shift to the right foot at the initiation of the take-away. The hips do not turn at the start but the player braces the leg furthest away from the hole. The golfer then simply retracts the right shoulder, and the transition through the backswing commences.

Phase III: Transition (backswing)

The backswing should be compact and ideally consist of one continuous movement, with the movement of the left shoulder determining the swing plane. The shorter the club, the shorter is the backswing. The shoulders rotate to the point where the golfer's back is perpendicular to the target line. The hips rotate slightly, the torso rotates around the pelvis and legs, and a coiling effect is produced, storing energy. The right side of the pelvis stabilizes the body at this point. If the hips rotate excessively or sway to the right, the coiling effect is lost.

The left hand hinges first and is in control. At the top of the backswing 60–80% of the golfer's weight is primarily on the inside edge of the rear foot; if the weight is left on the front foot, this is called a 'reverse pivot' and makes it difficult to return the club face to square at impact.

The left hand hinges at the base of the thumb and the right hand hinges into extension. The arms are in front of the body; the right arm is bent, supporting the club, and the left arm is stretched towards neutral elbow extension. The lower body then initiates the downswing.

Phase IV: Downswing

The body weight shifts back to the front foot just prior to the start of downswing, where it remains for the rest of the swing, and the body starts to uncoil. The motion begins with the front foot applying force through the ground, the front knee rotates, and the hips move to square. The club is not swung with the arms; they drop back down into plane as a reaction of the movement of the lower body. The hips and shoulders should be square, with the right shoulder behind the ball. The arms are extended, the wrists are raised, and the heel of the back foot is lifted slightly off the ground, with body weight distributed to the left foot at impact.

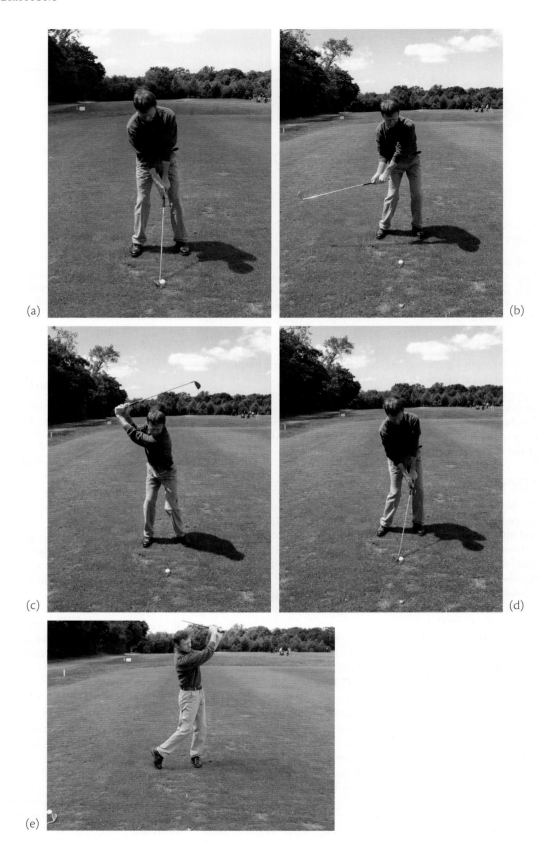

Fig. 4.10.1 The golf swing:
(a) address; (b) take-away/early
backswing; (c) top of the back swing;
(d) impact; (e) follow-through.

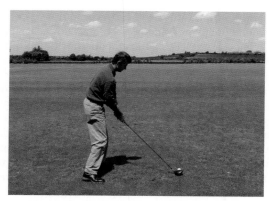

Fig. 4.10.2 Address: the lumbar spine and knees are in slight flexion.

Phase V: Ball impact

Club to ball impact lasts just 0.0005 seconds and the club travels barely a few centimetres between impact and loss of contact. High speeds are generated: 90 mph for an average recreational golfer and 115 mph for the professional. The period just before, during, and just after impact is vital in determining the accuracy and power of the shot.

Phase VI: Follow-through

The last phase of the swing is the follow-through and is a mirror image of the backswing. Weight transfer continues to the outside of the left foot. The wrists hinge in an opposite direction to the backswing. The shoulders are square facing the target, the front leg is straight, and the body is standing erect on the front foot.

Swing variations and biomechanics

The kinetics and kinematics of the golf swing vary considerably between golfers of different abilities. At the peak of the swing, professionals produce greater left shoulder horizontal adduction, right shoulder external rotation, and trunk rotation. Similarly, during the downswing, professionals produce much higher angular velocities for the club shaft, right elbow extension, and wrists (Zheng *et al.* 2008).

The main difference between the backswings of the classic and modern swings is that there is more right lateral weight shift and a large pelvic turn with upper body rotation in the classic swing, reducing the separation angle between shoulder and pelvic rotation with less torque through the lower back.

Biomechanical studies have shown that the lumbar spine is exposed to high degrees of lateral bending, axial rotation, shear forces, and compression, particularly during the end of the downswing and acceleration phases of the swing (Hosea *et al.* 1990). Higher forces are noted in amateurs. Most of the rotation in the spine occurs in the lower thoracic and lumbar regions; the differential amount of rotation between the shoulders and the pelvis at the top of the backswing and beginning of the downswing creates mechanical load on the lower back. This differential is considered to determine the potential power (clubhead speed at impact) that can be produced during the modern swing and the predisposition to lower back injuries.

The right knee is exposed to peak force at the end of the backswing and the left knee near impact and follow-through.

Table 4.10.1 Predominant muscle activity in the golf swing

	Most active muscles	
	Upperbody	**Lower body/trunk**
Backswing	Left subscapularis	Left erector spinae
	Right upper trapezius	Right semimembranosus
Early downswing	Left rhomboids	Left vastus lateralis
	Right pectoralis major	Right gluteus maximus
Acceleration	Pectoralis major bilaterally	Left biceps femoris
		Right abdominal oblique
Impact	Increased forearm flexor activity ('flexor burst')	
Early follow-through	Pectoralis major bilaterally	Left long head of biceps femoris
		Right gluteus medius
Late follow-through	Left infraspinatus	Left semimembranosus
	Right subscapularis	Right vastus lateralis

Reproduced from McHardy, A., Pollard, A., and Bayley, G. (2006). A comparison of the modern and classic golf swing: a clinician's perspective. *South African Journal of Sports Medicine*, **18**, 80–92

In the downswing, the right gluteal and right biceps femoris are active in helping right to left weight transfer; the left pelvic and hamstring muscles provide a pivot point for the left lumbopelvic rotation, and the vastus lateralis and adductor magnus assist weight transfer. The left medial scapula stabilizers/retractors are highly active and the subscapularis (particularly the right) is the most active component of the rotator cuff (Kao *et al.* 1995; McHardy and Pollard 2005).

Impact

At impact, there is a high level of right lateral flexion in the spine in the modern swing and hence more right compressive load compared with the classic swing. Maximal axial rotation and right lateral flexion occur just after impact. In many modern high-level golfers, the knee snaps straight, imposing high loads on the tibiofemoral joint.

Follow-through

In the modern swing, the upper body lags behind the pelvis after impact and the lower back adopts a position of extension called 'the reverse C—a line drawn from the right heel along the leg and up the pelvis and trunk to the left shoulder and head resembles the line drawn by a backwards C (Fig. 4.10.1(e)). This achieves greater height during ball flight. In comparison, in the classic swing the spine is relatively straight at a similar stage with less lumbar extension. Injuries to the lower back tend to occur in this phase of the golf swing. There is continued leg-muscle, pectoralis major, and rotator cuff activity.

Clubs

Clubs consist of the head, shaft, and grip. Shafts and heads can be made from stainless steel, or a carbon fibre–resin composite. They vary in weight and shaft stiffness, conferring a different 'feel' at ball impact. Stiffer shafts are generally used by the better golfer with a more powerful swing, whilst more flexible shafts are preferred by higher handicappers with slower swings. The relationship between shaft type and injury is unestablished.

Table 4.10.2 Summary of the phases/postures of the golf swing

Golf swing phase/posture	Description
Address	The position that the player adopts in preparation to initiate the golf swing
Backswing	Initial movement of club swings in arc away from ball Ends when shaft of club is parallel to ground, with clubhead facing target
Top of backswing	End of backswing before the initiation of downswing
Downswing	Club returns along a similar path to that of the backswing in preparation to hit the ball Ends with shaft parallel to ground
Acceleration	From shaft horizontal to impact Most active part of swing
Impact	The clubhead hits the ball
Early follow-through	From impact to club horizontal to ground
Late follow-through	From club horizontal to end of swing Results in the hands finishing over the left shoulder

Reproduced from McHardy, A., Pollard, A., and Bayley, G. (2006). A comparison of the modern and classic golf swing: a clinician's perspective. *South African Journal of Sports Medicine,* **18**, 80–92

Table 4.10.3 Comparison between the modern and classic golf swing

	Modern golf swing	Classic golf swing
Address	Similar to classic	Similar to modern
Backswing	Early wrist cocking	Late wrist cocking
Top of backswing	Limited pelvic rotation compared with shoulder rotation Limited body movement to right All of left foot on ground (bar lateral aspect)	Equal amounts of pelvic and shoulder rotation Large movement of body to right Only left toes in contact with ground
Downswing	Hips initiate downswing	Whole body initiates downswing
Impact	Hips ahead of shoulders Relatively large degree of right lateral flexion in trunk	Hips equal with shoulders Low amount of right lateral flexion in trunk
Follow-through	Hyperextension in lower back Momentum directed upwards	Lower back in relatively neutral position Momentum directed forwards

Reproduced from McHardy, A., Pollard, A., and Bayley, G. (2006). A comparison of the modern and classic golf swing: a clinician's perspective. *South African Journal of Sports Medicine,* **18**, 80–92

Physical preparation for golf

Many golfers are not physically conditioned for their sport, do little in the way of other physical activity, and do not warm up adequately. Those who walk, and particularly those who carry their clubs, will gain some cardiovascular benefit from playing a round of golf, but those who use a golf cart expend little energy. Golf-specific conditioning programmes should include general flexibility work, balance exercises, strengthening including functional core control work, quadriceps, spinal, wrist, and forearm strengthening using body weight, free weights, weighted clubs, or elastic tubing resistance. General cardiovascular conditioning through at least 30 minutes of daily aerobic exercise at moderate intensity should also be part of the programme.

Warm-up involves mental and physical preparation strategies. The latter starts with a brisk walk for at least 5 minutes followed by flexibility work to loosen up shoulder and lumbopelvic extension and rotation. Hamstrings and calves should also be stretched. Swinging a weighted club or two long irons together also helps to warm up the appropriate muscles. Hitting some practice balls for no more than 10–15 minutes, using a driver, a 5 iron, and a 9 iron can complete the physical warm-up.

Injuries in golf

The spectrum of injuries in golf is wide, with significantly different patterns seen in recreational and professional golfers. The relative risk of injury at specific sites is also determined by gender, age, and pre-existing conditions. In the higher-standard amateur and the professional, injuries are largely related to overuse after long sessions on the driving range, particularly when hitting off hard mats, or to hitting hard ground or an obstacle with the club. Injury surveillance studies vary in their reported relative incidences of injuries; 20–35% of injuries in this group affect the wrist/hand, 20–24% affect the lower back, and 7–10% affect the elbow (Batt 1992; McCarroll 1996; Theriaux *et al.* 1996; Gosheger *et al.* 2003). Female professional golfers experience more injuries to the left wrist than do males, and male professional golfers experience more injuries to the left shoulder than do females (McCarroll and Gioe 1982). Elbow injuries are less common than in amateurs, with lateral and medial epicondylar injuries occurring with similar frequency. In the higher-handicap amateur, almost 70% of all injuries sustained occur at the lower back or elbow (lower back, 15–34%; elbow, 25–33%), with injuries to the lateral epicondyle occurring five times more frequently than medial epicondyle injuries. Injuries are commonly related to adverse swing mechanics, overuse, and hitting the ground or an object.

Injuries are more likely in older players, those who are unconditioned for the game, and those with pre-existing injuries or medical conditions. Carrying one's own bag increases the risk of injuries of the lower back, shoulder, and ankle (Gosheger *et al.* 2003).

Traumatic injuries can also occur. These include ocular or other trauma due to being struck by a golf ball or club. Such injuries in adults are most likely to occur on a golf course, while children are more likely to be injured in the home environment (Wilks and Jones 1996). The hazards of the environment can also take their toll; in particular, lightning-induced injuries are recognized as a risk in golf.

Low back pain

Professional golfers have the highest incidence of back injury of all professional athletes (Watkins 2002) because of practice-related overuse injury on the background of predisposing factors such as poor core control and inadequate flexibility. Injuries in amateurs are usually related to poor and/or inconsistent swing mechanics, but again strength and flexibility are frequent associated factors.

Amateur golfers are less mechanically efficient, have less control of their swings, and generate 80% greater torque and shear forces across the spine when swinging a golf club (Hosea and Gatt 1996), resulting in a spectrum of pathological entities including facet dysfunction, annular tears and disc herniation, and non-specific ligamentous or muscular pain. Spondylolysis in young golfers should also be included in the differential diagnosis.

The golf swing is a true example of the influence that any component of the kinetic chain can have on other sites. For example, reduced internal rotation and restricted movements on the FABER test (see Chapter 3.8) in the leading hip and limitations in lumbar extension and trunk rotation are commonly noted in higher-level golfers with back pain (Vad *et al*. 2004). Increased lumbar flexion at set-up is also commonly noted in those who report pain. Such limitations should be sought in screening golfers with injury prevention in mind.

Core control work, strengthening, stability, and flexibility are all important in a golfer's conditioning regime, whether or not the golfer experiences back pain. Swing mechanics must be addressed, and in those with chronic spinal limitation the swing can be adapted to suit the individual's needs, such as by increasing hip rotation to compensate for limitations in lumbar turn, avoiding excessive extension on follow-through, and/or shortening the swing. However, the short swing increases shoulder muscle activation and may, in turn, promote risk for shoulder injury (Bulbulian *et al*. 2001).

Shoulder pain

Golf-related shoulder injuries usually affect the non-dominant shoulder, which goes into internal rotation, flexion, and horizontal adduction at the top of the backswing. Pain in this position can arise from posterior instability and this is an important consideration in all golfers in this context (Hovis *et al*. 2002).

Capsulolabral impingement or osteoarthritis of the acromioclavicular joint may also be underlying causes. During the downswing, injuries to the eccentrically firing rhomboids, latissimus dorsi and pectoralis major can occur. At follow-through the non-dominant shoulder is in external rotation and abduction, which may result in pain related to anterior instability, or the occurrence of internal impingement.

The rotator cuff fires at a low level during most of the golf swing. Whilst subacromial impingement of the rotator cuff in the dominant shoulder does not usually result in functional problems in swinging the golf club, that in the non-dominant shoulder can be troublesome. Non-dominant subscapularis is active throughout the swing and the supraspinatus is more active than the dominant side except in take-away.

Most golfers tolerate impingement and rotator cuff problems in the dominant shoulder reasonably well, but symptoms from the non-dominant rotator cuff typically interfere with the golf swing. There is increased firing of the dominant supraspinatus and infraspinatus at take-away. The supraspinatus of the non-dominant shoulder shows increased activity compared with the dominant shoulder throughout the golf swing, with the exception of take-away. Where rotator cuff injuries do occur, or are interfering with play, they are managed as described in Chapter 3.5.

Since golf is a sport played by older individuals, osteoarthritis of the acromioclavicular and glenohumeral joints can be an issue. Both are managed in the standard fashion, and return to play even after shoulder arthroplasty is common (Jensen and Rockwood 1998).

Elbow injuries

Injuries to the elbow are most frequent in the amateur. Most commonly, the lateral epicondylar region is affected because of overuse, poor swing/technique, or a sudden jarring impact on ball/ground strike. Predisposing factors include gripping the club too tightly, inappropriate grip diameter for the individual's hand size, weakness in the wrist or forearms, weakness of the triceps and scapular muscles, and possibly keeping the arm straight, even though this is often advised by instructors. Medial 'epicondylitis' may occur in the dominant elbow as a result of club impact or relative overuse.

Treatment of such injuries has been described elsewhere. As with other golf injuries, attention to technique is imperative, and a graduated return to play (as outlined later) is emphasized.

Wrist and hand injuries

Injuries to the wrist and hand in golf typically occur at impact and can involve soft tissue, bone or nerve. They can have major

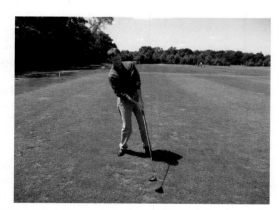

Fig. 4.10.3 Falling away from the ball—extending the spine commonly causes back pain.

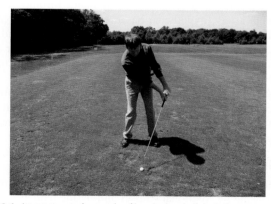

Fig. 4.10.4 An exaggerated example of hands ahead of the ball—a common cause of elbow and wrist injuries.

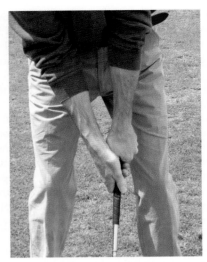

Fig. 4.10.5 The golf grip: minor errors can lead to injury, particularly in the upper limb.

consequences on function and the ability to play. Many injuries are related to poor swing mechanics, overuse, a strong grip (left hand positioned clockwise on the golf club handle), overgripping (too tight a grip), and clubs with old or inadequate grips.

Soft tissue injuries include extensor and flexor tenosynovitis or tear, triangular fibrocartilage complex injury, and ligamentous instabilities, many of which can be subtle and difficult to diagnose and manage. Where a tendinopathy occurs, the non-dominant wrist is most likely to be involved, particularly if it exhibits excessive motion along with a catapulting function. Impingement syndromes of the dominant wrist occur with hyperextension and radial deviation of the right wrist. Dislocation and recurrent subluxation of the extensor carpi ulnaris has been described (Inoue and Tamura 1998; Oka and Handa 2001). The fibro-osseous sheath may rupture radially or ulnarly. Surgical intervention is usually required.

Any bone in the hand or wrist can sustain injury in golf in the form of stress reactions, bone oedema syndromes, and fracture, most commonly on acute or repetitive impact. However, the hamate, and in particular the hook of hamate, is particularly vulnerable to isolated fracture or stress injury (Aldridge and Mallon 2003). Prompt diagnosis and treatment with excision of the fractured hook is important. Stress injuries are treated conservatively with relative rest.

The same mechanism can result in traumatic thrombosis of the distal ulnar artery (hypothenar hammer syndrome) (Müller *et al.* 1996). The player reports ischaemic symptoms in the hand, and imaging (including angiography) confirms the diagnosis. Other causes of vascular obstruction should be excluded. Surgical treatment is usually necessary.

Distal ulnar neuropathy due to a tight grip or microtrauma can occur in golf. It resolves with conservative management in the form of relatively short-term rest and a change in grip (Murray and Cooney 1996).

Knee injuries

As described earlier, high loads can be placed on the knee throughout the swing by rotational stresses and by the tendency to lock out the knee at impact and follow-through. This can result in meniscal, ligamentous, and osteochondral injuries, or exacerbation of pain due to a pre-existing condition such as osteoarthritis. In addition to addressing the injury itself, slowing the swing speed down, or at least the rate at which the knee is snapped straight, may help.

Rib injuries

Stress fractures of the ribs, particularly the posterolateral aspect of the fourth to sixth ribs, are seen in golfers. More than one rib may be involved. The injury is most commonly seen along the rib, usually on the leading arm side of the trunk. Fatigue of the serratus anterior is considered to be the mechanism of injury, and strengthening of this muscle should be encouraged for both treatment and injury prevention (Lord *et al.* 1996).

References

Aldridge, J.M., 3rd, and Mallon, W.J. (2003). Hook of the hamate fractures in competitive golfers: results of treatment by excision of the fractured hook of the hamate. *Orthopedics*. 2003 Jul; **26**(7): 717–19.

Batt, M.E. (1992). A survey of golf injuries in amateur golfers. *British Journal of Sports Medicine 1992*, **26**: 63–65.

Bulbulian, R., Ball, K.A., and Seaman, D.R. (2001). The short golf backswing: effects on performance and spinal health implications. *Journal of Manipulative and Physiological Therapeutics*, **24**, 569–75.

Gosheger, G., Liem, D., Ludwig, K., Greshake, O., and Winkelmann, W. (2003). Injuries and overuse syndromes in golf. *American Journal of Sports Medicine*, **31**, 438–43.

Hosea, T.M, and Gatt, C.J:. (1996). Back pain in golf. *Clinics in Sports Medicine*, **15**, 37–53.

Hosea, T.M., Gatt, C.J., Galli, K.M., Langrana, N.A., and Zawadsky, J.P. (1990). Biomechanical analysis of the golfer's back. In: A.J. Cochran (ed.), *Science and Golf. I. Proceedings of the World Scientific Congress of Golf*, pp. 43–8. E. & F.N. Spon, London.

Hovis, W.D., Dean, M.T., Mallon, W.J., and Hawkins, R.J. (2002). Posterior instability of the shoulder with secondary impingement in elite golfers. *MedAmerican Journal of Sports Medicine*, **30**, 886–90.

Inoue, G, and Tamura, Y. (1998). Recurrent dislocation of the extensor carpi ulnaris tendon. *British Journal of Sports Medicine*, **32**, 172–4.

Jensen, K.L. and Rockwood, C.A. (1998). Shoulder arthroplasty in recreational golfers. *Journal of Shoulder and Elbow Surgery*, **7**, 362–7.

Kao, J.T., Pink, M., Jobe, F.W., and Perry, J. (1995). Electromyographic analysis of the scapular muscles during a golf swing. *American Journal of Sports Medicine*, **23**, 19–23.

Lord, M.J., Ha, K.I., and Song, K.S. (1996). Stress fractures of the ribs in golfers. *American Journal of Sports Medicine*, **24**, 118–22.

McCarroll, J.R. (1996). The frequency of golf injuries. *Clinics in Sports Medicine*, **15**, 1–7.

McCarroll, J.R, and Gioe, T.J. (1982). Professional golfers and the price they pay. *Physician and Sportsmedicine*, **10**, 54–70.

McHardy, A, and Pollard, H. (2005). Muscle activity during the golf swing. *British Journal of Sports Medicine*, **39**, 799–804.

McHardy, A., Pollard, A., and Bayley, G. (2006). A comparison of the modern and classic golf swing: a clinician's perspective. *South African Journal of Sports Medicine*, **18**, 80–92.

Müller, L.P., Rudig, L., Kreitner, K.F., and Degreif, J. (1996). Hypothenar hammer syndrome in sports. *Knee Surgery, Sports Traumatology, Arthroscopy*, **4**, 167–70.

Murray, P.M. and Cooney, W.P. (1996). Golf-induced injuries of the wrist. *Clinics in Sports Medicine*, **15**, 85–109.

Oka, Y. and Handa, A. (2001). Recurrent dislocation of the ECU tendon in a golf player: release of the extensor retinaculum and partial resection of the ulno-dorsal ridge of the ulnar head. *Hand Surgery*, **6**, 227–30.

Theriault, G., Lacoste, E., Gaboury, M., *et al.* (1996). Golf injury characteristics: a survey of 528 golfers. *Medicine and Science in Sports and Exercise*, **28**, S65.

Vad, V.B., Bhat, A.L., Basrai, D., *et al.* (2004). Low back pain in professional golfers: the role of associated hip and low back range-of-motion deficits. *American Journal of Sports Medicine*, **32**, 494–7.

Watkins, R.G. (2002). Lumbar disc injury in the athlete. *Clinics in Sports Medicine*, **21**, 147–65.

Wilks, J. and Jones, D. (1996). Golf-related injuries seen at hospital emergency departments. *Australian Journal of Science and Medicine in Sport*, **28**, 43–5.

Zheng, N., Barrentine, S.W., Fleisig, G.S., and Andrews, J.R. (2008). Kinematic analysis of swing in pro and amateur golfers. *International Journal of Sports Medicine*, **29**, 487–93.

4.11

Injuries in gymnastics

Stephen Turner, John Aldridge, Nilam
Shergill, and Damian Griffin

Introduction

Gymnastics is a sport requiring many attributes involving balance, poise, flexibility, and a great range of movements with high strength-to-weight ratios, power, and spatial awareness. To develop these skills it is essential to start the sport at an early age. For example, spatial awareness develops during the pre-school period.

Gymnastics is uniquely associated with a large variety of different injuries affecting both the upper and lower limbs as well as the spine, because of the total body involvement. Both acute and overuse injuries are common in young gymnasts. The developing skeleton is particularly at risk, but soft tissue injuries are less prevalent because of their elasticity and vascularity. When dealing with children with sports-related injuries it is wise to consider bone injury as well as soft tissue problems. Another factor accounting for the distribution of the injuries is the difference in the typical exercise and competition routines for male and female gymnasts. The huge forces experienced by the upper limbs of male gymnasts pommelling or using the parallel bars or rings cause wrist and shoulder injuries, whereas female gymnasts doing floor and bar exercises sustain a different pattern of injuries (Figure 4.11.1 and Table 4.11.1).

Predictably, gymnasts sustain different injuries at different stages in their development. Some just require rest and conservative management, but some will lead to serious injury requiring surgical intervention and even retirement from the sport.

Over the last 16 years, elite British gymnasts with significant musculoskeletal injuries have been seen in Coventry and our experience will now be considered.

Upper limb injuries

Wrist

Osteonecrosis

The forces applied to the upper limbs during some routines can be huge and result in injury. Male gymnasts in particular can develop softening of the bones in the proximal carpal row of their wrists. This can initially present as pain and swelling and, if it progresses, an inability to continue training. These young gymnasts are highly motivated and have very high pain thresholds. They will usually already have received conservative treatment comprising rest, NSAIDs, and perhaps a cortisone injection. X-rays typically show no abnormality associated with the wrist joint itself, and MRI scans are normal or may show stress reactions of the carpal bones with patchy signal changes.

Unfortunately, in some cases wrist arthroscopy shows a very different picture (Fig. 4.11.2). There is usually some degree of synovitis and the articular surfaces may appear reasonably normal until the scaphoid and lunate are probed. In advanced cases, the articular cartilage indents easily, and in some cases the cartilage actually stands away from the underlying bone as though it is a large cyst. There can be different degrees of cartilage loss; total loss occurred in one gymnast under our care who was therefore forced to retire.

The aetiology of this condition remains unclear. Recurrent compressive trauma, particularly localized dorsal lip impingement between the distal articular surface of the radius and predominantly the scaphoid during pommelling could be a factor, but fortunately this does not appear to affect all male gymnasts. Another factor might be the degree of ulnar variance or the slope of the articular surface of the distal radius, which might account for individual variation in the degree of softening observed.

Some cases behave similarly to Kienboch's osteonecrosis with vascular changes obvious on the MRI scan. Unfortunately, the data set is too small to draw any meaningful conclusions and it is quite worrying that the MRI scan can look relatively normal. Therefore our practice is to arthroscope the symptomatic wrist even if the scan is not obviously abnormal.

Treatment is empirical and relies on 'unloading' the wrist by performing a radial shortening in those cases where there is a negative ulnar variance. Where this is not the case, drilling of the softened bone with a K-wire during arthroscopy has been tried with variable results.

Epiphyseal plate injuries

Epiphyseal plate injuries involving the distal radius are quite common. These range from compression injuries resulting in premature fusion of all or some of the distal radial epiphysis, resulting in a relative shortening of the radius or even a Madelung-type deformity where the distal radius develops an angular deformity, curving towards the radius, to actual fractures through the epiphysis (Carter and Aldridge 1988; DiFiori et al. 2006).

Treatment depends on the pathology. The Madelung deformity may require a corrective osteotomy and a joint-levelling procedure in order to deal with the deformity, particularly if ulnar impaction occurs (producing ulnar-sided wrist pain) or restrictions in forearm rotation because of disruption of the distal radio-ulnar joint.

Soft tissue injuries

Major ligamentous disruptions are rare unless the gymnast has fallen onto the wrist, but less serious injuries in the form of 'sprains' are quite common. These usually settle with conservative management.

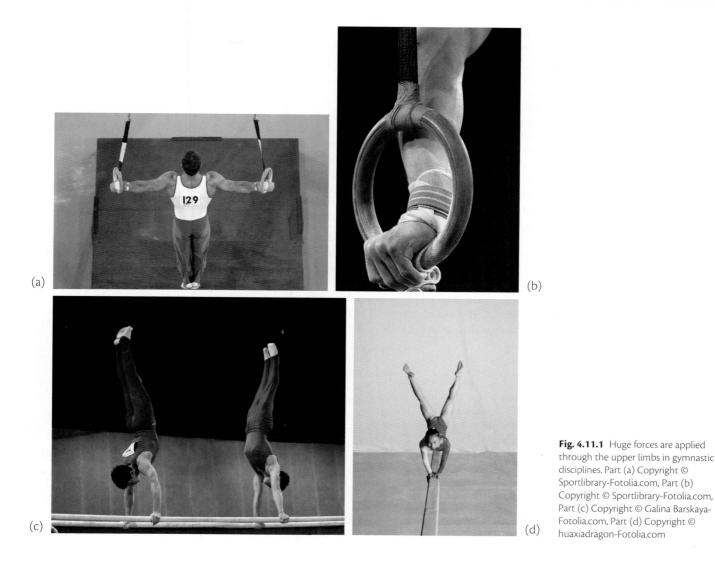

Fig. 4.11.1 Huge forces are applied through the upper limbs in gymnastic disciplines. Part (a) Copyright © Sportlibrary-Fotolia.com, Part (b) Copyright © Sportlibrary-Fotolia.com, Part (c) Copyright © Galina Barskaya-Fotolia.com, Part (d) Copyright © huaxiadragon-Fotolia.com

Table 4.11.1 Mechanical forces across wrists during gymnastics

Handspring	2800 N	4.5 × body weight
Pommels	1300–1700 N	2–2.5 × body weight
Rings	4800 N	8.5 × body weight
Vault	8200 N	11 × body weight
Vault	10 904 N	14 × body weight
High bar	2800 N	4.5 × body weight

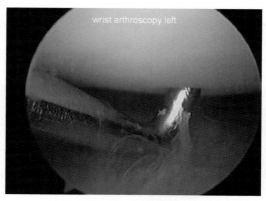

Fig. 4.11.2 Wrist arthroscopy. Carpol softening is demonstrated

More severe problems can occur following a tear of the triangular fibrocartilage complex, which can present as recalcitrant ulnar-sided pain with poor grip and painful forearm rotation. There is usually localized tenderness of the distal radio-ulnar joint. Minor tears will settle with conservative management, but persistent discomfort should preferably be investigated with an MR arthrogram. Arthroscopic debridement of the tears, or repair where appropriate, will usually allow a return to competitive form. A central perforation, often associated with an ulnar plus variance, usually requires an ulnar-shortening procedure.

One cause of recalcitrant ulnar-sided pain and stiffness encountered in our unit has been dense fibrous synovitis blocking the ulnar half of the radiocarpal joint. The cause is unknown but is presumably related to significant trauma, perhaps causing intra-articular bleeding or an inflammatory response. This can be resected arthroscopically, often leading to rapid recovery provided that there is no significant underlying pathology.

The forearm

Hypertrophy of the forearm muscles, including palmaris longus, can cause compartment problems. The gymnast, often a pommeller, presents with aching and cramp during exercise, and compartment pressure measurements will confirm excessively high resting pressures. The normal resting flexor compartment pressure in the forearm is less than 20 mmHg, and a pressure of more than 30 mmHg following 3–5 minutes of exercise with weights is sufficiently high for surgical decompression (fasciotomy of the flexor compartment) to be routinely undertaken (Fig. 4.11.3). Good results have been obtained, enabling a return to competition in many cases. There may be no obvious clinical signs on presentation and a high index of suspicion is required.

Elbow

Epiphyseal injuries

Traction avulsion injuries to the medial epicondyle and olecranon occur in skeletally immature young gymnasts. Discomfort rapidly settles with conservative management.

Osteochondritides

The capitellum is particularly vulnerable to compression injury and osteochondritis dissecans can occur, presenting with locking of the elbow due to a loose body or the development of a fixed flexion deformity. This can be investigated with an MR arthrogram (depending on the age of the gymnast) or a combination of CT and MRI scanning, and the loose body removed either arthroscopically or by open arthrotomy.

Shoulder

The shoulder can be the site of acute and chronic soft tissue injuries, as well as dislocation following trauma, but more insidious injuries can occur without any obvious traumatic incident but purely as a result of the gymnast's routine.

Soft tissue injury

Rotator cuff injuries occur in both male and female gymnasts. These may comprise:

- minor partial-thickness tears or 'scuffing'

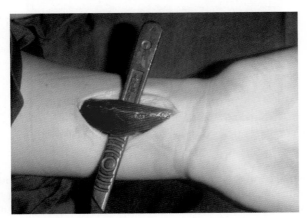

Fig. 4.11.3 Decompression of flexor compartment with hypertrophy of palmaris longus.

- more significant partial-thickness tears, usually associated with synovitis and damage to the glenohumeral ligaments
- complete or incomplete avulsion of the rotator cuff's insertion from the greater tuberosity.

Gymnasts often present late, when they can no longer train because of pain or weakness. MRI scans usually over-diagnose the problem because of their high sensitivity, although the specificity can vary. Therefore early arthroscopy is advisable in order to assess the condition of the rotator cuff and to identify other injuries including superior labral anterior posterior (SLAP) lesions and labral avulsions, which might not be obvious on the scan. Subluxation of the long head of the biceps can also occur and is associated with superior synovitis.

Extra-articular pathology

This mainly comprises thickening of the subacromial bursa, often associated with a rotator cuff tear, hypertrophy of the muscle resulting in impingement symptoms, or adhesions between the rotator cuff and the bursa.

Impingement due to muscle hypertrophy without thickening of the bursa or other obvious pathology is not a surgical problem. Often, the posture of the shoulder is poor because of overdevelopment of the pectorals compared with the scapular muscles, resulting in protraction of the shoulder and abutment of the humeral head against the coraco-acromial ligament. Alteration in the posture and scapular stabilization exercises with a shoulder therapist will often yield a good result. Similarly, poor muscular control can lead to anterior subluxation of the shoulder, which responds well to expert shoulder therapy.

Acromioclavicular subluxation can also occur when gymnasts suspend from bars with full internal rotation. This usually responds to conservative treatment.

Foot and ankle

Sever's disease

Calcaneal apophysitis, like Osgood–Schlatter disease of the knee, is a common condition affecting the insertion of the Achilles tendon into the os calcis apophysis. It presents as local tenderness around the apophysis. Recent investigations using MRI have suggested that the condition is not an apophysitis but rather a metaphyseal trabecular stress fracture (Ogden *et al.* 2004). It is a self-limiting condition which requires a period of rest or relative rest and avoidance of excessive rebound activity.

Achilles tendinopathy

Tendinopathies generally occur in older athletes. In terms of their sport, gymnasts are old at 20 and tendinopathies are seen by that early age. Rupture of the Achilles tendon is not uncommon and usually occurs during rebound activities. This condition should be managed by surgical repair. The outcome is not good in terms of return to gymnastic activities.

Sub-Achilles bursitis

Small bursae between the most inferior part of the Achilles tendon at the back of the os calcis can frequently become inflamed. The gymnast presents with local tenderness in the area which is confirmed by ultrasound investigations. A cortisone injection usually settles the condition.

Tenosynovitis

Tenosynovitis of the flexor hallucis longis due to the balance exercise required to stabilize the ankle can occur in older gymnasts. Management is conservative.

Talar dome injury

Ankle pain is common in gymnasts and occurs as an acute incident, such as following a short landing when tumbling or dismounting, or as a chronic problem due to the repetitive loading of the joint. A simple back somersault exerts a load on the ankle of 2.5 times body weight and the handspring movement exerts a load of 4.5 times body weight. Landing after some complex vaults can produce a load of 10.5 times body weight. When gymnasts are developing their skills, repetitions that load the ankle joint can lead to chronic injuries of the talar dome. Ballet dancers suffer similar problems (Elias *et al.* 2008).

Bone marrow oedema in the talus can be diagnosed by new imaging techniques and is frequently seen in gymnasts. Subchondral lesions of the talus occur but are not easily diagnosable other than by arthroscopy. Arthroscopic management of ankle joint pain is now possible. Areas of chondromalacia within the articular surface of the talus can be debrided, and the areas of total cartilage lost can be managed by the microfracture technique (Becher and Thermann 2005). Synovitis can be treated by synovectomy.

Acute injuries

Fractures around the ankle joint occur as in other sports and are dealt with appropriately.

Talar body stress fractures

Talar body stress fractures are reported in gymnasts, but although rare should be considered in the differential diagnosis of gymnasts with ankle pain (Rossi and Dragoni 2005).

Anterolateral impingement of the ankle

This condition has been recognized for some years (Ferkel *et al.* 1991). The condition is common in gymnasts who frequently sustain dorsiflexion injuries of the ankle when landing after backward somersaults. If this activity is performed incorrectly so that the gymnast lands short, a forced dorsiflexion of the ankle can cause pinching of the synovium and eventually stimulates the development of osteophytes along the anterolateral margin of the tibial plafond in the ankle joint. Clinically, there is usually a tender soft tissue swelling around the anterior ankle. Forced dorsiflexion usually causes pain and there is also tenderness around the anterior joint line. X-rays show the osteophytes, and an ultrasound scan will detect a synovitic lesion. If conservative measures fail, arthroscopic debridement of the marginal osteophytes usually has a good prognosis (Tol and Dijk 2006). Arthroscopic examination of the ankle mortice will show any associated chondral lesion and can be helpful in the prognosis of the condition (Urguden *et al.* 2005).

Talonavicular joint

The talonavicular area is put under significant stress by gymnastic activities. Backward tumbling is a common activity that causes repetitive dorsiflexion of the ankle and midfoot where the stress induced affects both the talonavicular joint and the navicular bone itself. Because pain in this area is common in gymnasts it is

tolerated, leading to late presentation to the surgeon. Mid-tarsal pain is also common and requires investigation. Standard X-rays alone are not reliable and bone scanning techniques and MRI scans are more appropriate (Kasten and Niemeyer 2005). Navicular stress fractures in young adults are not common but should not be missed. The recommended treatment is a minimum of 6 weeks non-weight-bearing in a plaster cast followed by 6 weeks progressive mobilization. Surgery is rarely required if initial treatment is appropriate (Khan *et al.* 1994). Late diagnosis or failure to comply with management can lead to non-union, and surgical intervention with open reduction and internal fixation is then required.

Apophysitis

Tenderness at the base of the fifth metatarsal at the site of the insertion of the peroneus brevis tendon (Iselin's disease) is prevalent in gymnasts because of the necessity for them to balance on one foot. This leads to stress on the apophysis. The general management of this is appropriate rest whilst maintaining full movement. With a strict regime this should settle within 6 weeks.

Stress fractures

Stress fractures of the second metatarsal occur at the distal and proximal ends of the bone. The distal stress fracture has a better prognosis. Fortunately, the proximal fracture is less common and treatment can be prolonged. Careful management with rest is required; rarely, surgical intervention is necessary (Corris and Lombardo 2003).

Spine

Neck injuries are very rare and are usually the result of a catastrophic error in a manoeuvre. Thoracic injuries are also uncommon, although soft tissue thoracic pain is not unusual. Therefore the vast majority of these patients present with low back pain with or without leg symptoms. The key to successful treatment is close cooperation between the patients, their parents, their coach, and the clinician. The long-term welfare of the patients, who are often minors, should be paramount and therefore expectations should be realistic. The temptation to intervene surgically purely for short-term sporting gain should be avoided unless absolutely necessary.

Pars fractures or spondylolysis

These are some of the most common injuries seen in our gymnasts. The presentation is usually a fairly sudden onset of back pain after a particular manoeuvre with localized pain over one or other side of the lower back. The usual clinical signs are localized tenderness, paravertebral muscle spasm, and a significant decrease in range of movement in the lumbar spine and on straight-leg raise. The investigations of choice are an MRI scan in conjunction with an isotope (SPECT) bone scan. Increased uptake, nearly always localized to the L5 pars, and signal change on the MRI scan are usually sufficient to implicate the pars as the source of the pain. The question is whether this is an acquired lesion or whether it is a congenital lesion that has become symptomatic from repetitive hyperextension injuries. From a management point of view this is academic as the treatment plan is the same. Almost without exception these patients are asymptomatic when it comes to daily activities, and therefore the only purpose of treatment is to allow them to return to competition without compromising their long-term prognosis with respect to their back function. Surgery is out of the question as the rehabilitation regime requires such a long period away from training that in effect, given the relatively short career span of a gymnast, this would mean the end of their competitive sporting activities without improving their daily function. By the time these patients attend our centre they have already undergone a 6–8 week period of restraint from contact activities whilst maintaining a conditioning regime. Residual symptoms may be due to actual pain from the pars or from a soft tissue inflammatory response.

Where there is muscle spasm a pars injection infiltrating a combination of chirocaine and depomedrone under X-ray control may be helpful. If there is a good response, the gymnast is allowed back into competitive regime over a period of 6 weeks. If there is no response, the only realistic option is complete abstinence from sport for 3–6 months. An MRI is carried out at 3 months and if necessary repeated in order to determine when to return to sport. This has allowed two-thirds of our patients to return to a competitive level of performance.

Stress reactions of the pedicle

A small number of patients have presented with what can be interpreted as a stress reaction in a lumbar vertebral pedicle. This comprises signal change on an MRI scan and a hot spot on an isotope bone scan but without an obvious fracture. This can also be regarded as an impending fracture of the pedicle. The vast majority of these patients respondto a combination of complete abstinence from sport for 6 months and adjunct trigger point injections to relieve any local muscle spasm, prior to recommencing training. Bracing is not required. The MRI scan is repeated at 6 months to confirm bony healing prior to recommencing training, and occasionally it is necessary to extend the rest period.

Disc injury/disease

As expected, this is rare in younger gymnasts but not unusual in older ones. The history is usually one of insidious onset of symptoms culminating in an acute episode. The MRI usually confirms a degree of degeneration of a disc and its adjacent facet joints but, more importantly, excludes serious pathology. The majority of these patients respond to a combination of adjustments to the training regime and analgesic or anti-inflammatory medication. In those who do not respond it is worth trying facet joint injections if the pain and tenderness can be localized.

A small proportion of patients will also have leg symptoms, usually from an inflammatory radiculopathy but occasionally a prolapsed disc. These patients respond very well to a combination of nerve root injections and training modification over a period of 6–12 weeks. Inevitably, a proportion of these patients are unable to continue at a competitive level and again surgery is neither necessary nor justifiable in the vast majority. Developments are in progress that may allow some of these patients to be treated by percutaneous disc surgery techniques, but these are at an early stage.

Muscle and ligament injury

This is probably the largest group of patients with back pain. These are gymnasts who sustain an injury to their back but without any evidence of abnormal pathology on spinal imaging. The implication is that there has been an injury to either muscles or ligaments in the lower back including the sacroiliac ligaments.

The overwhelming majority of these patients never attend our centre as they respond well to physiotherapy, training adjustment, and use of simple anti-inflammatory medication. Those who do attend respond well to trigger point injections and the use of slow-release patches containing NSAIDs applied over the painful area.

Costo-transverse pain

A proportion of gymnasts presents with non-specific thoracic pain without any obvious injury. In most of these patients the pain and tenderness tend to be paravetebral rather than central. The majority also respond to simple measures and do not present to our centre. Those who fail to improve respond well to injection treatment under X-ray control. In nearly all cases the site of the pain is localized to a costo-transverse joint, confirmed by screening under an image intensifier, implying either an injury or inflammation of the soft tissues supporting these joints. All such patients have returned to full competitive activities.

Hip

Injuries to the hip are unusual in gymnasts. Fractures and dislocations are rare (Mitchell *et al.* 1999), usually require open surgical treatment, and will have a serious impact on a gymnast's career.

Femoro-acetabular impingement

Femoro-acetabular impingement and its consequences of labral tears and articular cartilage injury occasionally occur, as in other sports, and can be treated successfully by arthroscopic surgery. However, this pathology seems to be rare in gymnasts, perhaps because gymnasts tend to have high femoral head-to-neck ratios and relatively shallow acetabulae to allow extreme ranges of movement.

Instability and labral tears

Like dancers and other high-flexibility athletes, gymnasts apply extreme rotational and abduction forces to their hips, which may lead to capsular laxity and symptomatic instability. Such instability usually presents as aching pain in the groin which is exacerbated by training. Sharp or catching pain implies labral degeneration and tearing, probably caused by overloading as the anterior labrum becomes the final restraint on hip subluxation in forced external rotation. Log-roll testing may reveal a loss of clear endpoint to external rotation in extension, and hip external rotation in extension and 30° of abduction in a lateral position will often cause apprehension and reproduce pain. Investigation by X-ray, CT, and MR arthrography are usually normal. Arthroscopic examination may reveal mild degeneration and loss of the normal turgor of the anterior labrum. The anterior capsule may be unusually capacious or the iliofemoral ligament may be relatively lax. There is often synovitis in the anterior and anterosuperior capsulo-labral recess. If strengthening and rebalancing training is unsuccessful, pain can be relieved by arthroscopic thermal labral shrinkage, excision of synovial proliferation, and capsulorrhaphy by arthroscopic suture of the iliofemoral ligament.

References

Becher, C. and Thermann, H. (2005). Results of microfracture in the treatment of articular cartilage defects of the talus. *Foot and Ankle International*, **26**, 583–9.

Carter, S.R. and Aldridge, M.J. (1988). Stress injury of the distal radial growth plate. *Journal of Bone and Joint Surgery. British Volume*, **70**, 834–6.

Corris, E.E. and Lombardo, J.A. (2003). Tarsal navicular stress fractures. *American Family Physician*, **67**, 85–90.

DiFiori, J.P., Caine, D.J., and Malina, R.M. (2006). Wrist pain, distal radial physeal injury, and ulnar variance in the young gymnast. *American Journal of Sports Medicine*, **34**, 840–9.

Elias, I., Zoga, A.C., Raikin, S.M., *et al.* (2008). Bone stress injury of the ankle in professional ballet dancers seen on MRI. *BMC Musculoskeletal Disorders*, 9, 39.

Ferkel, R.D., Karzel, R.P., Del Pizzo, W., Friedman, M.J., and Fischer, S.P. (1991). Arthroscopic treatment of anterolateral impingement of the ankle. *American Journal of Sports Medicine*, **19**, 440–6.

Kasten, P. and Niemeyer, P. (2005). Diagnosis of stress fractures in adolescents. *Sportverletzung Sportschaden*, **19**, 205–10.

Khan, K.M., Brukner, P.D., Kearney, C., Fuller, P.J., Bradshaw, C.J., and Kiss, Z.S. (1994). Tarsal navicular stress fracture in athletes. *Sports Medicine*, **17**, 65–76.

Mitchell, J.C., Giannoudis P.V., Millner P.A., and Smith, R.M. (1999). A rare fracture–dislocation of the hip in a gymnast and review of the literature. *British Journal of Sports Medicine*, **33**, 283–4.

Ogden, J.A., Ganey, T.M., Hill, J.D., and Jaakkota, J.I. (2004). Sever's injury: a stress fracture of the immature calcaneal metaphysis. *Journal of Pediatric Orthopedics*, **24**, 488–92.

Rossi, F. and Dragoni, S. (2005). Talar body fatigue stress fractures: three cases observed in elite female gymnasts. *Skeletal Radiology*, **34**, 389–94.

Tol, J.L. and van Dijk, C.N. (2006). Anterior ankle impingement. *Foot and Ankle Clinics*, **11**, 297–310.

Urguden, M., Soyuncu, Y., Ozdemir, H., Sekban, H., Akyildiz, F.F., and Aydin, A.T. (2005). Arthroscopic treatment of anterolateral soft tissue impingement of the ankle: evaluation of factors affecting outcome. *Arthroscopy*, **21**, 317–22.

4.12

Bicycling injuries

Cathy Speed and Laurence Berman

An overview of cycle sport

Cycling as a competitive sport actually preceded the invention of our familiar pedalled chain-driven two-wheeled device by almost two decades. Some traditionalists consider that cycle sport should be confined to the conventional iconic drop-handlebar 'racing cycle' in either its fixed-wheel guise on the track or its multi-geared superficially similar cousin used in road racing. The evolution of cycling as an Olympic event gives the lie to this narrow view and is a metaphor for the development of the sport.

Cycle racing was an established event, both on the road and on the track, at what is generally held to be the first modern Olympic Games in Athens in 1896. Mountain bike racing appeared at the 1996 Atlanta Olympic Games, 25 years after the tentative recreational experiments with this cycling discipline. Bicycle motocross (BMX), considered by conservatives to be a delinquent pursuit, was an official event in the 2008 Beijing Olympic Games. Human-powered vehicle (HPV) races with the participation of streamlined recumbent cycles may eventually be mainstream events.

Naturally, all cycle sports, or for that matter recreational cycling, may result in trauma to the participant because of falls or collisions. These random mishaps, which are sometimes spectacular and photogenic, whilst occasionally causing major injury are outside the scope of this discussion of sport-related injuries. The more common injuries associated with cycling are of the overuse type and form the focus of the subsequent sections.

A brief description of some popular forms of competitive cycling follows.

Road racing

Road racing, as its name implies, takes place on normal roads over varying distances. The bicycles are lightweight and multi-geared with drop handlebars. An event may be confined to a single day or comprise numerous stages of differing terrain and length, some of which are suited to cyclists with a particular athletic skill such as the ability to rapidly ascend steep long climbs or to muster an explosive short burst of power in a sprint finish for the line.

Team tactics are complex, but essentially involve nurturing the conditions that enable one of the team members to win the event or stage. This may involve shielding the 'star' team member from wind resistance by forming a protective rotating phalanx of riders until the closing moments when the relatively fresh competitor makes a break for the finish. Most road races are mass start events but multistage races may also incorporate a time trial.

Time-trialling

Historically, time-trialling as a stand-alone event is a peculiarly British activity which involves individual riders (rarely teams of riders) setting off on their own at intervals and then racing against the clock over a set distance or occasionally for a set time. The rider achieving the shortest time for the distance, or the furthest distance in the predetermined time, is the winner. A strong cyclist may overtake an earlier starter, but drafting (riding for prolonged periods in the slipstream of a rider) is forbidden as this affords a huge advantage to the following rider, who is sheltered from wind resistance. Wind resistance is the major drain on the energy expended by a cyclist at racing speeds on a flat course. The apparent improvement in time-trial performance over the years is as much the result of advances in aerodynamic science, translated into streamlining the cycle–rider unit, as enhanced training techniques.

The cycling component of triathlon remains a non-drafting time trial at long distance events and over shorter courses at age-group and amateur levels. Recently, the elite standard Olympic distance event has become a cycle race where drafting is permitted.

Track cycling

Track cycling takes place on a banked circular track, most often in an indoor velodrome. The cycles superficially resemble road cycles but there are major differences, in particular the absence of brakes or variable gearing. They are fixed-wheel cycles; the rear wheel is directly coupled via the drive chain to the pedals. When the rear wheel rotates, the pedals turn and vice versa. The rider cannot free-wheel or coast along with the pedals stationary as in other forms of racing and recreational cycling. Aerodynamics is important in many track events, and these cycles may resemble dedicated time-trialling cycles in contour and rider position.

With rare exceptions track events are shorter, sometimes much shorter, than road races and usually require massive expenditure of power for relatively short periods. Track cyclists are generally of very different physical morphology to road racers, in particular successful road racing 'climbers'. There is a bewildering array of track race formats which encompasses both mass start and time trial events as well as something between these two, where an individual or a team start simultaneously but at 180° to each other on opposite sides of a circular track. Track racing also has its own equivalent of stage events, where competitors have to compete in several racing formats over a period of days. There is an outdoor version of track cycling which takes place on unbanked circular grass venues on fixed-wheel cycles.

Mountain bike and other cross-country racing

Mountain bikes are a newcomer to the world of recreational and competitive cycling, and appeared in large numbers as recently as the 1980s. Before and after this era cyclo-cross, a form of cross-country racing, existed with its epicentre in Western Europe. Cyclo-cross bikes resemble road-racing cycles but with heavier tyres, and the event often requires portage of a cycle across a muddy patch where this would be faster or simply more feasible than attempting to cycle.

There has been a rapid evolution of technology in the world of mountain biking, driven by both cycling and racing ergonomics as well as, in no small measure, by marketing. Some of the innovations have trickled across to the sphere of road riding. Mountain bikes, even the most upmarket, are heavier than their road counterparts. Apart from the minority activities of single-gear enthusiasts, mountain bikes have more gear ratios, with the availability of lower ratios than road cycles.

Mountain bike racing has a number of formats which include mass start and time-trialling events, the latter exemplified by downhill racing. Without underestimating the physical and mental demands of road and track racing, mountain bike racing requires a further skill set, including the ability to negotiate obstacles, and in the case of downhill racing a staggering combination of concentration and nerve.

Human-powered vehicle (HPV) racing

All cycles are human powered, yet the term has been hijacked by the activities, both recreational and competitive, of enthusiasts for recumbent 'feet-forward' cycles. These are commonly of bicycle or tricycle configuration with a low frontal area, and vary from completely bare cycles, through simple windshields, to elaborate fully enclosed structures.

Recumbent cycles were banned from competition in the 1930s by the UCI (Union Cycliste Internationale), considered by many to be a conservative governing body. Had this not occurred, a recumbent might arguably be the default configuration of touring and commuting cycles today.

One of the many advantages claimed by recumbent cycle enthusiasts is the 'deck-chair' position of the rider, which avoids the perineal pressure of a conventional cycle saddle, a cause of both vasogenic and neurogenic male impotence.

The rate-limiting step of conventional cycling at racing speeds is wind resistance, so in comparison the performances of streamlined HPVs are startling. As of 2008, the current 1 hour distance record for an HPV is 86.7 km compared with 49.7 km for a relatively conventional track cycle and 56.4 km for an aerodynamically configured track cycle. Popular racing formats include time trials, sprints, and circuit racing. Mass start open road events are not a feature.

Bicycle motocross (BMX)

This apparent contradiction in terms refers to various competition and recreational formats using small-wheeled ungeared cycles. It dates from roughly the same era as mountain biking, and since its inception it has, like mountain biking, metamorphosed from maverick recreational activity to official Olympic Games event. A currently popular racing format involves a circular dirt track, 400 m long, with eight riders competing against each other following a mass start. The courses are sufficiently hostile to necessitate the use of protective clothing and more elaborate head protection than road racing.

'Freestyle' BMX includes highly improbable ramp-based cycling displays, where somersaults and other gymnastic antics of varying complexity and risk are undertaken both recreationally and competitively.

Cycle touring and audax

Although not strictly speaking a competitive sport, there are versions of touring where participants are intensely competitive although many may not admit to it. Touring one-upmanship is a distillate of distance travelled and time taken to complete said distance. Apart from informal touring, audax or randonneur events ranging from 50 to 1200 km have been a recognized pursuit with their own governing body since the late nineteenth century, and are an increasingly popular activity internationally. Flat-out racing is officially discouraged by having both maximum and minimum speed cut-off times.

Touring cyclists are occasionally patronized by their racing brethren, but generally spend many more hours in the saddle. Apart from collisions, there is as great or greater potential for activity-related injury than with shorter-distance conventional cycling racing of whatever ilk.

Injuries: man versus machine

Body positioning on the bicycle has a major influence on performance, comfort, and predisposition to injuries, with injuries often arising in relation to an imbalance between the anatomy of the rider and that of the bicycle. In turn, the rider position is affected by bicycle design and rider–bicycle fit. Bicycle factors such as height of the saddle and handle bars, distance between saddle and handle bars, type of bicycle, frame size, type and height of saddle, and length of cranks are all important. An individual's physical morphology, cycling technique, training programmes, gearing habits and cadence all are considered in optimizing performance and in injury prevention and management.

The mechanics of the bicycle

The basic components of the bicycle are shown in Fig. 4.12.1, with bicycles differing depending upon the cycle sport involved (Fig. 4.12.2). Touring bicycles are longer and flatter; mountain bikes have a lower centre of gravity and are sturdier and more manoeuvrable. The seat–tube length (usually stated in centimetres for road bicycles and inches for mountain bikes) represents the frame size, but other characteristics, in particular the length of the top tube, also need to be customized to the cyclist and their individual needs and comfort. There can often be a compromise between comfort and performance, with the former being less of a consideration for those in sprint track events. Those road racers who seek to enhance speed through an aerodynamic horizontal position will have a very different bicycle set-up than the road tourer (e.g. with the seat positioned further back), and racers will also commonly want their handlebars positioned further forward to optimize performance out of the saddle on hill climbs. The fore–aft position of the seat needs to be balanced with that of the handlebars, otherwise the rider will be over-extended. Many racers will push the set-up to the limit in the pursuit of performance; just a

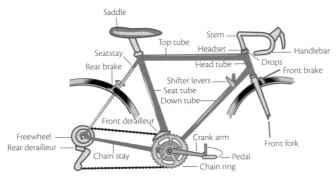

Fig. 4.12.1 Basic components of a bicycle.

fraction of an inch can make a real difference, but a 'tipping point' can be reached where mechanical strains are too high and injury occurs.

Although there are general recommendations for bicycle fitting (Table 4.12.1), advice on sizing and positioning can be confusing and conflicting views exist. It is often necessary to modify most 'rules', particularly for the cyclist who has issues with current or previous injuries. Variances in body sizes and proportions, levels of fitness and flexibility, and technique and style all affect a cyclist's best position on the bicycle.

The top tube plus the stem length represent the total reach. There is no strict rule as to the length of the stem and top tube; the top tube is influenced by the length of the torso and arms, and the stem can then be adapted to 'fine tune'. The emphasis is for the rider to be comfortable in their position without over-reaching for the handlebars. Proper reach on a racing bicycle is often proposed as

being when, while the cyclist is gripping the drop handles, the eye-line of the front hub is obscured by the handlebar (Asplund *et al.* 2005). The handlebars should be level with the seat, or up to 4 cm lower. Racers generally end up with the handlebar height well below the saddle height; tourers often prefer to have the bar at the same height as the saddle. Mountain bikers usually position the bar a couple of inches below the saddle.

Saddles vary in design, which has an effect on saddle tilt, height, and position in relation to the handlebars—all factors that can also be modified, independent of the design. These features can influence injury development. Bressel and Larsson (2003) reported that partial and complete cut-out saddle designs may increase anterior pelvic tilt in female cyclists, and saddles with a complete cut-out design may increase trunk flexion angles under selected cycling conditions. A saddle with a partial cut-out design may be more comfortable than one with a standard or complete cut-out design. There are significant gender-related differences in saddle loading which are important to consider when choosing an appropriate saddle. These differences are especially important when riders are in the handlebar drops and more weight is supported on the anterior pelvic structures (Potter *et al.* 2008).

When force is applied downwards on the pedal during seated steady state cycling, the peak pedal reaction force is approximately 60% of the rider's body weight, increasing with increased resistance but never exceeding the rider's weight, even when he/she is standing on the pedals. The angles of the reaction forces affect the mechanics of the hip, knee, and ankle joints, the associated soft tissues, and muscle activation patterns, and hence both the efficiency of pedalling and possibility of injury. The mechanics of the shoe–pedal interface also affect pedalling efficiency and predisposition to injury and will vary with the rider, shoe, and type of pedal.

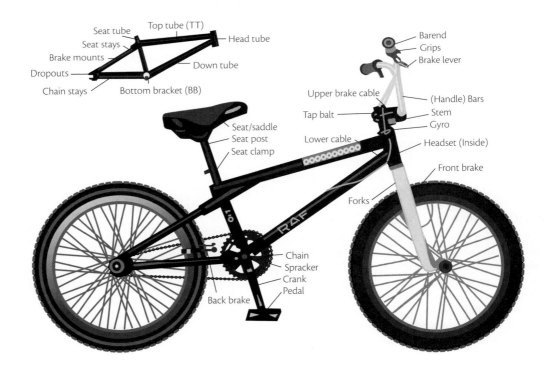

Fig. 4.12.2 A BMX bike.

Table 4.12.1 Examples of general recommendations for fitting the bicycle to the cyclist

Frame size (seat–tube length)

Road: two-thirds PBH.

Mountain: subtract 14 from PBH (in inches)

Cranks

Crank arm length determines the diameter of the pedalling circle—the larger that circle, the greater the knee flexion. Longer cranks give more leverage, allowing work with high gears at a low cadence (e.g. hill climbing, time-trialling). Standard cranks are useful for spinning at a high cadence.

As a starting point: 18.5% of the distance from the top of the femur to the floor in bare feet *or* PBH up to 31 inches, 170 mm; 31–33 inches, 172.5 mm; ≥ 33 inches, 175 mm

Seat height (SH)

(This will be influenced by other primary aspects of set-up such as crank length, seat fore–aft position, handlebar settings)

That which permits a knee angle of 30° at the bottom of the pedal stroke

PBH × 0.883 *or* PBH − 10 to 10.5 cm = SH* (*or* for the very small person or those using 180 mm cranks, 11–11.5cm).

Those using clipless pedals reduce by 3 mm

Saddle shape and angle

Choose shape for comfort

Slight anterior inclination (i.e. downward) helps to reduce back pain and perineal complaints

Saddle position fore–aft (relative to the cranks)

Saddle position chosen for comfort, efficiency, and power. More forward, with lower handlebars, allows more power and less comfort (see text)

Front of knee and pedal spindle in vertical line. NB: If the cyclist needs to be nearer to the handlebar, the preference is to alter the stem length first

Total reach (top tube + stem + saddle fore–aft position)

While gripping the drop handles, the eyeline of the front hub is obscured by the handlebar *or* with elbows bent at 65–70° with hands in drop handlebars, elbows should be within an inch or two of the knees at the top of the stroke

Stem length can easily be changed and allows 'fine tuning' once an appropriate top tube length is chosen. This is preferred to a change in seat fore–aft positioning

Handlebar height

2.5–5 cm below the height of saddle for short cyclists; up to 8 cm below for taller cyclists

Raise bars for those with spinal complaints, novices, and off-road cyclists

Handlebar width

Road: width of the shoulders

Mountain: hands slightly wider than shoulders

Handlebar angle

For drop handlebars, the ends should angle downwards by 5°–10°

Brake levers

The lever body should be high enough to allow the cyclist to put his/her hand on it without bending his/her wrist

Pedal selection

Platform pedals for low-intensity short recreational riding/commuting

Toe clips and straps

Clipless pedals: cleats on the shoe fit to pedals. Pedals are floating (allow internal/external rotation at the shoe–pedal interface) or fixed (no rotation)

Foot–pedal position (fore–aft and rotation)

First metatarsophalangeal joint; ball of foot over pedal spindle

Cleats should be adjusted to allow the foot to be in the neutral position for the rider, i.e. in line with any natural toe-in or toe-out foot position

PBH, pubic bone height (inseam: measurement from bottom of pubic symphysis to floor).
Sources: Lemond and Gordis 1990; Burke 1994; Asplund *et al.* 2005.

Symmetry of pedalling forces is rare, and pulling up on the pedal is used mostly in sprinting or climbing. Pedal types include platform, clips, and clipless (Table 4.12.1).

Where a leg-length discrepancy is identified, the bicycle is fitted to the longer leg and orthotics used to correct the shorter leg. With femoral leg-length discrepancy the cleats should be adjusted, with that of the shorter leg being slightly back on the pedal and that of the longer leg slightly forward.

The other component of equipment important to all cyclists is the helmet, which should be a snug fit without impairing clear vision.

In summary, the bicycle should be modified to fit the rider, and consideration must be given to physical make up and coexistent medical issues, particularly current or past injuries. For example, modifications may be made to seat height, angle, fore–aft position, distance between the feet (consider altering the bottom bracket axle, placing a shim between the crank and pedal axle, or changing the cleat position), and foot rotation (consider floating pedals). Inevitably changes in muscle activity and kinematics with fatigue will also affect the rider–bicycle interface, emphasizing the importance of appropriate conditioning as well as attention to bicycle set-up (Dingwell *et al.* 2008). Common errors in bicycle set-up are summarized in Table 4.12.2.

Injuries in cycling

Epidemiology

In an epidemiological study of sport and recreational activities presenting to medical services (emergency department or GP surgeries), cycling injuries were second only to Australian football in their incidence. Of 1170 sport-related ED attendances, 15.7% were associated with cycling, as were 19.6% of 112 hospital admissions (Cassell *et al.* 2003). Injuries can be divided into those due to acute trauma from falls and collisions, and overuse injuries. The latter are the focus here.

When considering overuse injury causation, both extrinsic factors (especially the bicycle and shoes) and intrinsic factors (e.g. imbalances in muscle function and soft tissue flexibility, leg-length discrepancies, overtraining, tibial torsion, and ankle–foot mechanics) are considered.

Table 4.12.2 Common errors in bicycle set-up

Error	Consequence(s)
Saddle too low	Quadriceps fatigue
	Reduced power output
	Patellofemoral pain
Saddle too far forward	Patellofemoral pain
	Reduced efficiency
	Too much weight through arms
Brake levers too low on handlebars	
Reach too long	Neck and lumbar pain
Wrong handlebar angle	Rotating the bar up causes discomfort and lack of control over brakes.
Incorrect pedal/cleat alignment	Lower-leg injuries, patellofemoral pain

Spinal complaints

Neck and low back pain are common in those who spend long periods in a sustained posture on bicycles, and therefore are most common in long-distance road cyclists, with 44% of male and 55% of female road cyclists seeking attention for neck pain and 30% for lumbar pain. The jarring experienced on mountain bikes and BMX bikes can also cause spinal pain. Most cases of spinal pain are mechanical and are associated with flexibility issues and the bicycle (e.g. those with an excessively long top tube) or the set-up. For example there may be over-reaching from inappropriate saddle and/or handlebar positioning. The normal cycling position is with the lumbar and cervical spine in relative flexion, and sustained periods in this posture are inevitably going to predispose the individual to myofascial pain and thoracic outlet symptoms (Asplund *et al.* 2005).

Prompting the cyclist to take rest breaks where possible and to stretch, and ensuring that they ride in a relaxed position without the arms locked are all important. The bicycle set-up should be reviewed, aiming to make alterations that prevent excessive neck/thoracolumbar flexion (e.g. raising the handlebars and/or shortening the stem, or moving the seat forward). Handlebars that are too wide can cause trapezius and scapula elevator strain (Burke 1994). Adjusting the seat tilt to an anterior inclination angle of 10°–15° can help to reduce lumbar pain (Salai *et al.* 1999).

Pelvic position, which in turn is affected by seat design and angle, will influence spinal and lower-limb mechanics (Salai *et al.* 1999; Bressel and Larson 2003). Tight hamstrings predispose to posterior pelvic tilt, and tight quadriceps to the opposite. Either can cause diffuse lumbar localized intervertebral junction (especially L5–S1) or sacroiliac pain, and poor core (gluteal and abdominal) strength will be a major contributing factor to this. Sciatic neural irritation may be a feature.

Knee injuries

Anterior knee pain

Patellofemoral syndrome, patellar and quadriceps tendinopathy, and fat pad impingement syndromes are all common in cyclists. Most cases are due to excessive overload through hill work and use of high gears too early in the training programme, malalignments such as knee varus/valgus, tibial rotation or hyperpronation, or inappropriate bicycle set-up imposing overload on the anterior knee. Examples of the latter may be excessive movement through the pedal–cleat interface, inappropriate seat height (too low), or seat fore–aft position (too far forward). Spacers can be placed between the pedal, and orthotics customized according to on-bicycle biomechanical analysis are useful.

Distal iliotibial band syndrome

This can develop in those with the adverse biomechanical issues described above. Use of high gears and excessive hill work also contribute, as do bicycle set-up errors including the seat being too high or too far aft, too much or too little movement at the shoe–pedal interface, or hip–foot misalignment (consider spacers between pedal and crank to correct this).

Pes anserine syndromes (tendinopathy/bursitis)

This can occur because of hyperpronation, the seat being too high, or a leg-length discrepancy. Adjustments are made accordingly, as described earlier.

Achilles tendinopathy

This is more commonly seen in those cyclists with overpronation, leg-length discrepancy, or pes planus, and in those who tend to dorsiflex and plantarflex excessively as they pedal. Bicycle set-up errors include excessive foot rotation, or the foot being positioned too far behind the pedal axle.

Upper limb complaints

Ulnar nerve compression

Ulnar nerve compression at Guyon's canal due to handlebar pressure can occur in cyclists, and results in motor, sensory, or mixed sensorimotor nerve symptoms in the distribution of the ulnar nerve in the hand. This can be avoided by altering the hand position frequently and reducing local pressure by using padded gloves and grips, and altering the reach or handlebar height so that less of the rider's weight is on the handlebars. The front suspension of mountain bikes should be reviewed. A long period of rest (e.g. 6 months) may be necessary in those who are more severely affected.

Median nerve compression

This is less common than ulnar nerve compression, and the two may coexist. Management of the two conditions is the same.

Genitourinary issues

The perineal region is a common site of injury in cyclists, where significant genitourinary, local neurovascular, and dermatological complaints can all occur (Goodson 1981; Hershfield 1983; Armstrong 1985; Andersen and Bovin 1997; Marceau et al. 2001; Jeong et al. 2002). These include pudendal nerve symptoms and neuropathy, erectile dysfunction in males, pressure sores and labial damage in females.

The aetiology of pudendal nerve symptoms may be primarily neurological (Jost 1998), vascular through compression of the pudendal artery (Nayal et al. 1999), or both. Regardless of aetiolgy, it is the result of compression of one or more components of the pudendal neurovascular bundle because of compression by the saddle. There is the potential for pudendal nerve irritation through stretching during the repetitive hip flexion that is involved (Asplund et al. 2007)

The incidence is unknown, but some studies report the prevalence to be as high as 50–91% (Weiss 1985; Andersen and Bovin 1997; Schwarzer 1999; Sommer et al. 2001).

Patients report numbness in the perineal region, penis/labia, buttocks, or scrotum (Asplund et al. 2007). Pain is rare. The physician should take a careful history of the timing of onset, cycling history, recent equipment changes (particularly the saddle), erectile dysfunction, and history or symptoms suggestive of other conditions (e.g. diabetes, atherosclerosis, cauda equina). Neurophysiological testing is usually unnecessary and may be normal, but may demonstrate somatosensory evoked potentials in the form of prolonged nerve latency, low recruitment motor unit potentials, and either suppressed or absent bulbocavernus response (Ricchiutti et al. 1999).

Symptoms are more common in those cyclists who are heavier (Schrader et al. 2002), older (Taylor et al. 2002), and who cycle for more than 3 hours per week. There are conflicting views as to the influence of how long the individual has been cycling, with some reporting greater risk in those cycling for more than 10 years

(Taylor et al. 2002), and others proposing that the number of years cycling is protective, perhaps because of perineal adaptation (Wilber et al. 1995).

Initial management is to stop cycling until symptoms resolve. Review of the bicycle set-up should be performed early, and saddle set-up and/or design is usually changed in order to alter pressure distribution and pelvic tilt. Saddles should be wide enough posteriorly to accommodate both ischial tuberosities, and those saddles with a protruding nose (sport/racing saddles) are best avoided where possible to avoid excessive perineal pressure (Lowe et al. 2008). A cautionary note: some who use cut-out saddles to relieve pudendal nerve symptoms later report erectile dysfunction (Dettori et al. 2004), although a clear association between the two has not been established. Once equipment changes have been made, cycling can be re-introduced in a progressive manner, with the recommendation that short bouts with rest periods to reduce the time of compression in the saddle.

Erectile dysfunction in cyclists is poorly understood. It may occur independently of any pudendal nerve symptoms, and no strong association between the duration or degree of perineal pressure in the saddle has been demonstrated (Taylor et al. 2004). Whilst, as has been discussed, some with erectile dysfunction report a previous change in saddle to a cut-out design to alleviate pudendal nerve symptoms, others claim that this form of saddle is protective. Bicycle set-up may have a role, such as the handlebar being at the same height or higher than the saddle (Dettori et al. 2004). Management includes those approaches taken with pudendal nerve symptoms. A full evaluation by a urologist is recommended, particularly if simple measures such as relative rest and equipment changes are unsuccessful.

Perineal induration and nodularity (Köhler et al. 2000), chafing, labial trauma, and vulval hypertrophy are all reported in cyclists. Vulval hypertrophy is often unilateral; infection and neoplasia should be excluded, although the condition is considered to be due in some way to loading and the mechanics of cycling (Humphries 2002). Yet again, a review of saddle and set-up should be performed and protective pants and padding considered.

References

Andersen, K.V. and Bovin, G. (1997). Impotence and nerve entrapment in long distance amateur cyclists. *Acta Neurologica Scandinavica*, **95**, 233–40.

Armstrong, T.J. (1985). Mechanical considerations of skin in work. *American Journal of Industrial Medicine*, **8**, 463–72.

Asplund, C., Webb, C., and Barkdull, T. (2005). Neck and back pain in bicycling. *Current Sports Medicine Reports*, **4**, 271–4.

Asplund, C., Barkdull, T., and Weiss, B. (2007). Genitourinary problems in bicyclists. *Current Sports Medicine Reports*, **6**, 333–9.

Bressel, E. and Larson, B.J. (2003). Bicycle seat designs and their effect on pelvic angle, trunk angle, and comfort. *Medicine and Science in Sports and Exercise*, **35**, 327–32.

Burke, E.R. (1994). Proper fit of the bicycle. *Clinics in Sports Medicine*, **13**, 1–14.

Cassell, E.P., Finch, C.F., and Stathakis, V.Z. (2003). Epidemiology of medically treated sport and active recreation injuries in the Latrobe Valley, Victoria, Australia. *British Journal of Sports Medicine*, **37**, 405–9.

Dettori, J.R., Koepsell, T.D., Cummings, P., et al. (2004). Erectile dysfunction after a long-distance cycling event: associations with bicycle characteristics. *Journal of Urology*, **172**, 637–41.

Dingwell, J.B., Joubert, J.E., Diefenthaeler, F., and Trinity, J.D. (2008). Changes in muscle activity and kinematics of highly trained cyclists during fatigue: 1. *IEEE Transactions on Biomedical Engineering*, **55**, 2666–74.

Goodson, J.D. (1981). Pudendal neuritis from biking. *New England Journal of Medicine*, **304**, 365.

Hershfield, N.B. (1983). Pedaller's penis. *Canadian Medical Association Journal*, **128**, 366–7.

Humphries, D. (2002). Unilateral vulval hypertrophy in competitive female cyclists. *British Journal of Sports Medicine*, **36**, 463–4.

Jeong, S.J., Park, K., Moon, J.D., and Ryu, S.B. Bicycle saddle shape affects penile blood flow. *International Journal of Impotence Research*, **14**, 513–17.

Jost, W.H. (1998). Somatosensory evoked potentials of the pudendal nerve in penile hypoesthesia. *Journal of Urology*, **159**, 987.

Köhler, P., Utermann, S., Kahle, B., and Hartschuh, W. (2000). Biker's nodule: perineal nodular induration of the cyclist. *Hautarzt; Zeitschrift für Dermatologie, Venerologie, und verwandte Gebiete*, **51**, 763–5.

Lemond, G. and Gordis, K. (1990). *Greg Lemond's Complete Book of Bicycling*, pp. 118–45. Perigee Books, New York.

Lowe, B.D., Schrader, S.M., and Breitenstein, M.J. (2008). Effect of bicycle saddle designs on the pressure to the perineum of the bicyclist, **5**, 1932–40.

Marceau, L., Kleinman, K., Goldstein, I., and McKinlay, J. (2001). Does bicycling contribute to the risk of erectile dysfunction? Results from the Massachusetts Male Aging Study (MMAS). *International Journal of Impotence Research*, **13**, 298–302.

Nayal, W., Schwarzer, U., Klotz, T., *et al.* (1999). Penile oxygen pressure during cycling. *Medicine and Science in Sports and Exercise*, **31** (Suppl), S107.

Potter, J.J., Sauer, J.L., Weisshaar, C.L., Thelen, D.G., and Ploeg, H.-L. (2008). Gender differences in bicycle saddle pressure distribution during seated cycling. *Medicine and Science in Sports and Exercise*, **40**, 1126–34.

Ricchiuti, V.S., Haas, C.A., Seftel, A.D., *et al.* (1999). Pudendal nerve injury associated with avid bicycling. *Journal of Urology*, **162**, 2099–101.

Salai, M., Brosh, T., Blankstein, A., Oran, A., and Chechik, A. (1999). Effect of changing the saddle angle on the incidence of low back pain in recreational bicyclists. *British Journal of Sports Medicine*, **33**, 398–400.

Schrader, S.M., Breitenstein, M.J., Clark, J.C., *et al.* (2002). Nocturnal penile tumescence and rigidity testing in bicycling patrol officers. *Journal of Andrology*, **23**, 927–34.

Schwarzer, U., Wiegland, W., Bin-Sale, A., *et al.* (1999). Genital numbness and erectile dysfunction rate in long distance cyclists. *Journal of Urology*, **161**(Suppl), 178.

Sommer, F., König, D., Graft, C., *et al.* (2001). Erectile dysfunction and genital numbness in cyclists. *International Journal of Sports Medicine*, **22**, 410–13.

Taylor, J.A., Kao, T., Albertsen, P.C., *et al.* (2004). Bicycle riding and its relationship to the development of erectile dysfunction. *Journal of Urology*, **172**, 1028–31.

Taylor, K.S., Richburg, A., Wallis, D., *et al.* (2002). Using an experimental bicycle seat to reduce perineal numbness. *Physician and Sportsmedicine*, **30**, 27–32.

Weiss, B.D. (1985). Nontraumatic injuries in amateur long distance bicyclists. *American Journal of Sports Medicine*, **13**, 187–92.

Wilber, C.A., Holland, G.J., Madison, R.E., *et al.* (1995). An epidemiological analysis of overuse injuries among recreational cyclists. *International Journal of Sports Medicine*, **16**, 201–6.

4.13

Injuries in netball and basketball

Mark Gillett

Introduction

Basketball and netball are both physically demanding sports involving movements that are often performed at high speeds in a multitude of directions. Any reduction in a participant's ability to control the forces generated while running, cutting, jumping, or stopping could lead to excessive stress upon the musculoskeletal system. This stress could be traumatic or repetitive in nature, with the potential outcome resulting in injury.

Basketball

The published literature states that basketball has one of the highest injury rates per participant amongst any sports, a fact that remains consistent throughout the world. It has been reported that around 18.3 injuries occur per 1000 participants (McKay et al. 2001). Unsurprisingly, the most common injury in basketball involves the ankle, at a rate of 5.5 injuries per 1000 hours played (Hopper et al. 1995). This type of basketball injury is usually sustained with the ankle in plantar flexion and inversion, with 86% of these injuries involving the ligamentous and capsular structures (Cordova and Ingersoll 2003). The next most prevalent basketball injury involves the calf or anterior leg with around 0.48 injuries per 1000 hours played. Potentially more debilitating knee injuries occur at a rate of 0.29 injuries per 1000 hours played in both men and women.

Netball

In 2008 England Netball had 61 000 affiliated members and estimated that at least a million ladies participate in the game each week (http://www.englandnetball.co.uk). Non-elite netball players are reported to sustain around 14 injuries per 1000 hours played (McManus et al. 2006), but this number is almost halved for players at the elite level. Recent research (McManus et al. 2006) has highlighted four individual components that correlate with injury risk in non-elite netballers.

- Training less than 4 hours per week raises the risk of injury.

- Absence of a previous injury in the past 12 months reduces injury risk by 42%.

- Warming up prior to a game reduces the injury risk by 48%.

- Athletes who failed to embrace new training concepts increased their risk of injury.

Ankles account for 31–42% of all injuries in netball with an occurrence of 3.3 injuries per 1000 hours played (Hopper et al. 1995). There is also a high rate of knee injury with 2.82 injuries per 1000 hours played (McManus et al. 2006). Two other commonly injured areas are the fingers (9–27% of total injuries) and the pelvic–lumbar region (19% of total injuries).

Ankle

Ankle injuries are frequent in both basketball and netball, although the biomechanical patterns of injury differ between the two sports. Basketball activity ensures that a high degree of vertical force is transmitted through the ankle joint with each movement, whilst in netball the ankle is subjected to higher horizontal forces. These biomechanical differences affect all aspects of diagnosis, treatment, and rehabilitation. Table 4.13.1 highlights the specific risk factors that influence ankle injury in these sports.

Ankle braces are commonly used in both sports to stabilize the ankle joint and reduce the overall ankle injury rate in selected individuals. Conversely, the restrictions in ankle joint motion that occur when wearing a brace and the subsequent effect this has on static and dynamic components of the ankle joint is not fully understood. Hence decisions about the use of an ankle brace should be made on an individual basis.

Shoulder

A full range of movement at the glenohumeral joint and the ability of the shoulder complex to stabilize and control throughout this range is crucial for the throwing and shooting actions required in these sports. However, the two sports have subtle differences in the demands placed upon the shoulder complex. Netball often relies upon an ability to stabilize the trunk and simultaneously produce an array of repetitive low-force flexion movements at the shoulder joint. Basketball involves a comparatively smaller range of overhead movements, which are the end-product of a whole-body sequence. In this way the kinetic chain is utilized to generate large overhead forces to facilitate skills such as shooting, dunking the

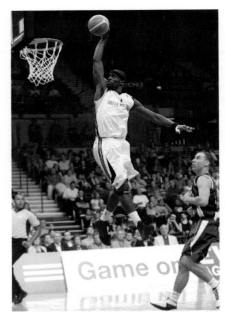

Fig. 4.13.1 Basketball.

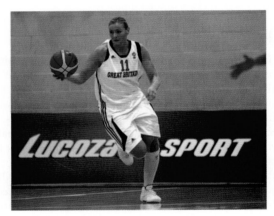

Fig. 4.13.2 Netball.

Table 4.13.1 Proven risk factors for ankle sprains in basketball and netball players

Risk factor	Indication and treatment options
Cardiovascular fitness	Aerobic fatigue increases injury risk
	Aerobic activity must form part of rehabilitation plan
Reduction in range of ankle dorsiflexion	Commence stretching programme
	Consider mobilization of the ankle joint
Balance assessment shows a large travel distance on medial or lateral sway	Commence proprioceptive retraining program (Cumps *et al.* 2007)
Failure to complete flamingo balance assessment (1 minute)	Commence proprioceptive retraining program (Cumps *et al.* 2007)
Increased range of movement at the first metatarsophalangeal joint (and first ray)	Orthotics
	Specific tibialis posterior strength exercises
Previous ankle sprain in past 12 months	Appropriate advice for the patient to reduce future risk of injury
Reduction in gluteus medius activation pattern	Strengthening and active recruitment programme
Reduction in flight time	Plyometric training
	Strengthening programme for tibialis anterior
Rear foot varus	Orthotics
Footwear used for more than 60–70 hours	If training three times a week change shoes after 2–3 months

ball and blocking a shot. These sports-specific differences need to be accounted for in the rehabilitation programme devised.

Knee

The knee joint forms the central link in the chain between the upper limb and the foot, resulting in its involvement with every movement during basketball and netball. Detailed analysis of these two sports has demonstrated that the specific movements of a defensive slide in basketball and side stepping during cutting in netball place the knee at its greatest potential risk of injury. These movements place the knee in a valgus position at a time when hamstring activity decreases and quadriceps activity increases. This combination can generate a high degree of joint translation and increase the risk of acute instability. In order to decrease the peak landing force following foot placement, the quadriceps and gluteal muscles must work eccentrically and adductors concentrically to limit the degree of knee valgus and risk of instability. In addition the neuromuscular activational patterns of these muscles rather than the force they generate have the greatest influence in limiting most knee injuries. Activational improvement can be seen following a 6–12 week neurological training programme.

Patellar tendinopathy is commonly encountered in both sports, and this condition is discussed in detail in Chapter 3.12. The patellofemoral joint is a common location for pain in participants of court-based sports. A number of factors may lead to the occurrence of excessive translation within the patellofemoral joint, including muscular tightness, changes in strength, and inadequate neuromuscular activational patterns.

Lumbar spine and pelvis

Both basketball and netball involve movements such as jumping and throwing, which are most often performed with the dominant side of the body. This can further increase the side-to-side inequality of the muscles surrounding the hip and shoulder of the dominant limb. If left unchecked, this can result in long-term sacral and pelvic adaptations which can disrupt muscle activational patterns and function. The changes in movement around the sacrum and pelvis can potentially cause severe problems when combined with the repetitive microtrauma and compression of the lumbar spine experienced when jumping or landing, particularly on a single leg.

References

Arendt, E. and Dick, R. (1995) Knee injury patterns among men and women in collegiate basketball and soccer: NCAA data and review of literature. *American Journal of Sports Medicine*, **23**, 694–701.

Bost, F. and Inman, V. (1942). The pathological changes in recurrent dislocation of the shoulder: a report of Bankart's operative procedure. *Journal of Bone and Joint Surgery*, **24**, 595–613.

Cordova, M. and Ingersoll, C. (2003). Peroneus longus stretch reflex amplitude increases after ankle brace application. *British Journal of Sports Medicine*, **37**, 258–62.

Cumps, E., Verhagen, E., and Meeusen, R. (2007). Efficacy of a sports specific balance training programme on the incident of ankle sprains. *Journal of Sports Science and Medicine*, **6**, 212–19.

Hopper, D., Elliot, B., and Lalor, J. (1995). A descriptive epidemiology of netball injuries during competition: a five year study. *British Journal of Sports Medicine*, **29**, 223–8.

Hume, P. and Steele, J. (2000). A preliminary investigation of injury prevention strategies in netball. Are players heeding the advice? *Journal of Science and Medicine in Sport*, **3**, 406–13.

Konradson, L. and Voigt, M. (1997). Ankle inversion injuries. The role of the dynamic defence mechanism. *American Journal of Sports Medicine*, **25**, 54–58.

McKay, G., Goldie, P., Payne, W., Oakes, B., and Watson, L. (2001). A prospective study of injuries in basketball: a total profile and comparison by gender and standard of competition. *Journal of Science and Medicine in Sport*, **4**, 196–211.

McManus, A., Stevenson, M., and Finch, C. (2006). Incidence and risk factor for injury in non-elite netball. *Journal of Science and Medicine in Sport*, **9**, 119–24.

Smith, R., Damodaran, A., Swaminathan, S., Campbell, R., and Barnsley, L. (2005). Hypermobility and sports injuries in junior netball players. *British Journal of Sports Medicine*, **39**, 628–31.

Rowing injuries

Richard Budgett

Introduction

The sport of rowing (Figs 4.14.1 and 4.14.2) encompasses rowing with a single oar per competitor, sculling with two oars per competitor, and, increasingly, indoor rowing on a rowing ergometer. Rowing and sculling are under the auspices of the International Federation (FISA).

Rowing is a safe sport with very few reported traumatic injuries (Hickey *et al.* 1997). Most injuries in rowers are related to overuse and fatigue or are due to participation in other sports. In elite rowers the injury rate is 0.4 per 1000 hours (Budgett and Fuller 1989). This compares favourably with similar studies in soccer (approximately four injuries per 1000 hours) and rugby (40 injuries per 1000 hours).

Trauma

There are regulations at an international and local level to reduce the risk of collision and the risk of injury if collision does occur. The rubber bow ball on racing boats reduces trauma if there is a collision. Since 1 January 2007 all new boats have to meet new FISA standards of flotation, and crews are instructed to stay with the boat, if they capsize or fall in the water, until rescued. More unusual safety measures include the presence of a trained marksman in the umpire launch at the Victoria Falls Regatta to protect against crocodiles (Budgett *et al.* 2001).

Overuse injuries

Low back pain, chest wall pain, and tenosynovitis of the wrist are the most commonly reported injuries in rowers over the last 30 years (Budgett 1989; Rumball *et al.* 2005). In the last decade there have been increasing reports of hamstring tendinopathy and an increased frequency of chest wall injuries (Holden and Jackson 1985; Thomas 1988; Karlson 1998; Christiansen and Kanstrup 1997). Overuse injuries are more likely to occur when there is an increase in the intensity and volume of training, especially when combined with a change in the type of training such as a relative increase in indoor rowing, sculling, rowing, weight-training, body circuits, or running (Bernstein 2002).

Poor technique, poor flexibility, and poor conditioning will all contribute to an increased incidence of overuse injuries. Relative weakness of antagonists, muscle imbalances, and faulty equipment may also contribute. Common equipment problems are oars that do not turn easily in the gate and handles that are too small.

In a study from the Australian Institute of Sport chest wall injuries were most common in women rowers, followed by low back pain and tenosynovitis of the wrist. In men, low back pain was the most common followed by tenosynovitis and then chest wall injuries (Hickey *et al.* 1997).

Low back pain

There is no evidence that the incidence of low back pain is higher in rowers than in the general population and the incidence in retired rowers is generally less. This may be related to self-selection for the sport; a similar low incidence is seen in retired weightlifters. Nevertheless there is a perception that low back pain is a problem in many rowers, particularly at club level, and there are many reports of individual rowers forced to retire due to low back pain.

Fifty per cent of low back pain in rowers is secondary to weight-training. Low back pain makes up 25–50% of all injuries. There is no evidence that sculling (two oars) is safer than sweep (one oar) rowing, but the symmetrical straight movement in sculling is perceived to be safer, and is encouraged by most national authorities for younger participants and novices.

Precipitating factors

Poor adherence to a programme of stretching and core stability exercises can predispose to injuries in rowers, particularly low back pain. Fatigue at the end of long training sessions increases the range of movement of the lumbar spine and shear forces on the lumbar discs (Roy *et al.* 1990). In addition, the torque on the lumbar disc may be greatest early in the morning when the disc is fully hydrated (Morris *et al.* 2000). Tight hamstrings in rowers can limit anterior rotation of the pelvis, forcing the adoption of a lumbar kyphosis.

Programmes to prevent low back pain include stretching of the glutei, hamstrings, and hip flexors (Redgrave 1992). Stabilization exercises help the maintenance of intra-abdominal pressure during the drive phase of the stroke, stabilizing the spine and reducing sheer forces. There may be a role for inspiratory muscle training and this may be particularly important in rowers who have difficulty in entraining their breathing cycle to the rhythm of the stroke, including expiring during the drive phase (McGregor *et al.* 2002, Volianitis *et al.* 2001).

The majority of acute severe low back pain in rowers is due to an annular tear of the disc with or without dural irritation and sciatica. The tear, with associated fluid, can be seen on MRI of the lumbar spine. Treatment involves relative rest, physiotherapy, non-steroidal anti-inflammatory drugs (NSAIDs), and possibly corticosteroid epidural. Occasionally surgery is required.

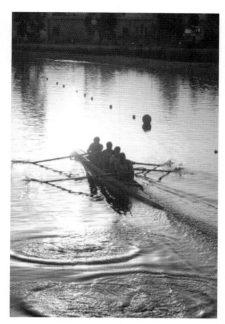

Fig. 4.14.1 The sport of rowing.

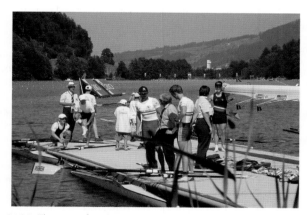

Fig. 4.14.2 The sport of rowing.

Rehabilitation of elite rowers to full training and performance normally takes 3 months (Stallard 1980).

More rarely the low back pain is due to facet joint problems or spondylolysis, or even spondylolisthesis and an unstable segment. These problems are often secondary to weight-training with faulty technique. The sacro-iliac joints are occasionally affected and can be effectively treated with physiotherapy and if necessary injections. Rowers are encouraged to limit their weight-training so that correct technique is always maintained. Most overuse injuries of the lumbar spine, whether during land training or in the boat, are related to fatigue of stabilizers and loss of coordination and control, with contributions from other factors such as tight hamstrings and faulty equipment.

Chest wall pain

The diagnosis of rib stress fracture has become more common in the last 10 years. The rower describes pain, increasing through a session, which is lateral or anterolateral in the chest wall, normally between the fifth and seventh ribs. The tender spot can be pinpointed exactly and there is pain there on springing the ribs (Budgett *et al.* 2007).

The differential diagnosis includes intercostal muscle strain, a strain or tear of one or more slips of serratus anterior as they insert on the ribs, or an enthesitis at the insertion itself. Chest wall pain may also be referred from the costovertebral joint (sprung rib) or from the thoracic spine itself (Thomas 1988). Pain felt more anteriorly may be due to costochondritis.

Rib stress fractures are graded from a mild periostitis (stress reaction) to full fracture (rare in rowers).

In the majority of cases, as with most overuse injuries, chest wall pain follows an alteration in training, such as a change of side so that the blade is on the other side of the boat. There is controversy as to whether thoracic spine stiffness is a primary or secondary phenomenon. Compressive forces on the rib are the fundamental cause, but eccentric contraction of the serratus anterior at the finish also contributes. The important factors in prevention are conditioning and care when increasing or changing training.

Investigation can be with ultrasound scan, MRI, CT, bone scan (Fig. 4.14.3), or X-ray. None of these will be positive for several days until there is increased osteoblast activity. A callus can often be seen on ultrasound within a week (Fig. 4.14.4). X-rays may never be positive and will not normally reveal any callus for several weeks. The investigation of choice for many clinicians is MRI because of its sensitivity to any bony oedema and ability to identify the differential diagnosis and the avoidance of the radiation associated with CT and isotope bone scans (Karlson 1998).

Treatment consists of accurate diagnosis and in the case of rib stress fractures relative rest for 3–5 weeks. Clinical improvement occurs much more quickly in these injuries than in other stress fractures.

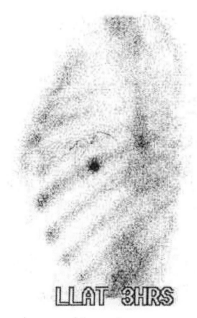

Fig. 4.14.3 Isoptope bone scan of rib stress fracture.

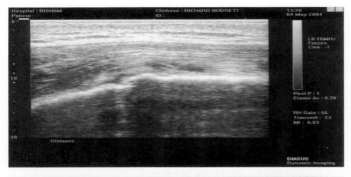

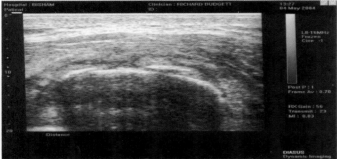

Fig. 4.14.4 Ultrasound scan of rib stress fracture after 10 days showing callus in transverse and longitudinal view.

Wrist and forearm

Tenosynovitis of the wrist extensors is more common in female than in male rowers. It may be an intersection syndrome affecting the extensor carpi radialis longus and brevis at the junction with the abductor pollicis longus and extensor pollicis brevis or more rarely De Quervain tenosynovitis. The main differential diagnosis is compartment syndrome of the forearm which can be diagnosed by pressure tests. Normally a diagnosis of tenosynovitis is clinically obvious with swelling, grating, and tenderness of the affected tendons. Imaging is not normally necessary, but ultrasound and MRI will confirm the diagnosis (Hickey *et al.* 1989).

Tenosynovitis normally occurs after a change in training, particularly from sculling to rowing, or swapping sides in the boat. The technical fault of gripping too hard can also contribute, and this may occur if the handle is too small or in rough conditions. Difficulty turning the oar in its gate due to faulty equipment may also cause overuse.

Treatment involves ice and relative rest, ideally in a splint, until the grating and swelling reduce. The inflammation in the tendon sheath can be reduced with physiotherapy modalities (ultrasound and laser) and oral or topical NSAIDs. In more severe cases cortisone injection is required or even surgery to decompress the tendon sheath.

Other injuries

Other injuries in rowers are generally less troublesome and debilitating than low back pain, chest wall injury, and tenosynovitis of the wrist. The most common are blisters of the hands, and scullers may also suffer abrasions of the calf and knuckles. These may occasionally become infected so care is needed and prompt treatment

with antibiotics if there is evidence of cellulitis. With appropriate hygiene, infection should be avoided. Blisters are most likely at the beginning of the season when the hands are softened, or after changing sides in the boat, or between sculling and rowing (Budgett *et al.* 2007).

Hamstring tendinopathy is seen most commonly during the winter season when more time is spent on rowing machines, particularly when there is full forced compression at the catch over prolonged training sessions. Anterior knee pain is rare in rowers since the action of rowing involves little eccentric work and positively conditions the vastus medialis. However, anterior knee pain is seen commonly in coxes if they sit in the stern. This is related to their flexed position and the constant bracing needed as the boat accelerates with each stroke (Budgett and Fuller 1989).

Summary

Rowing is a safe sport with very few traumatic injuries. Prevention involves general conditioning and stretching, checking equipment, and rowing with correct technique. Overuse injuries are the main problem, with a similar incidence to other non-contact sports such as swimming. Low back pain, chest wall injuries, and tenosynovitis of the wrist are the most common overuse injuries in rowers and scullers.

References

Bernstein, I.A., Webber, O., and Woledge R. (2002) An ergonomic comparison of rowing machine designs: possible implications for safety. *British Journal of Sports Medicine*, **36**, 108–12.

Budgett, R. (1989). The road to success in international rowing. *British Journal of Sports Medicine*, **23**, 49–50.

Budgett, R. and Fuller, G. (1989). Illness and injury in international rowing. *Clinics in Sports Medicine*, **1**, 57–61.

Budgett, R., Hettinga, D.M., and Steinacker, J. (2007). Rowing. *Handbook of Sports Medicine and Science*, **11**, 124–40.

Christiansen, E. and Kanstrup, I.L. (1997) Increased risk of stress fractures of the ribs in elite rowers. *Scandinavian Journal of Medicine and Science in Sports*, **7**, 49–52.

Hickey, G.J., Fricker, P.A., and McDonald, W.A. (1997) Injuries to elite rowers over a 10 yr period. *Medicine and Science in Sports and Exercise*, **29**, 1567–72.

Hickey, G.J., Budgett, R and Fuller, G. (1989)

Holden, D. and Jackson, D.W. (1985). Stress fracture of the ribs in female rowers. *American Journal of Sports Medicine*, **13**, 342–8.

Karlson, K.A. (1998). Rib stress fractures in elite rowers: a case series and proposed mechanism. *American Journal of Sports Medicine*, **26**, 516–519.

Koutedakis, Y., Frischknecht, R. and Murthy, M. (1997). Knee flexion to extension peak torque ratios and low-back injuries in highly active individuals. *International Journal of Sports Medicine*, **18**, 290–5.

Manning, T.S., Plowman, S.A., Drake, G., *et al.* (2000). Intra-abdominal pressure and rowing: the effects of inspiring versus expiring during the drive. *Journal of Sports Medicine and Physical Fitness*, **40**, 223–32.

McGregor, A., Anderton, L. and Gedroyc, W. (2002). The assessment of intersegmental motion and pelvic tilt in elite oarsmen. *Medicine and Science in Sports and Exercise*, **34**, 1143–9.

Morris, F.L., Smith, R.M., Payne, W.R., *et al.* (2000). Compressive and shear force generated in the lumbar spine of female rowers. *International Journal of Sports Medicine*, **21**, 518–23.

O'Kane, J.W., Teitz, C.C., and Lind, B.K. (2003) Effect of pre-existing back pain on the incidence and severity of back pain in intercollegiate rowers. *American Journal of Sports Medicine*, **31**, 80–2.

Redgrave, S. (1992). Injuries: prevention/cure. In: *Steven Redgrave's Complete Book of Rowing*, pp. 200–17. Partridge Press, London.

Roy, S.H., De Luca, C.J., Snyder-Mackler, L., Emley, M.S., Crenshaw, R.L., and Lyons, J.P. (1990). Fatigue, recovery and low back pain in varsity rowers. *Medicine and Science in Sports and Exercise*, **22**, 463–9.

Rumball, J.S., Lebrun, C.M., Di Ciacca, S.R., and Orlando, K. (2005) Rowing injuries. *Sports Medicine*, **35**, 537–55.

Stallard, M.C. (1980). Backache in oarsmen. *British Journal of Sports Medicine*, **14**, 105–8.

Teitz, C.C., O'Kane, J.W., and Lind, B.K. (2003) Back pain in former intercollegiate rowers: a long-term follow-up study. *American Journal of Sports Medicine*, **31**, 590–5.

Thomas, P.L. (1988) Thoracic back pain in rowers and butterfly swimmers: costovertebral subluxation. *British Journal of Sports Medicine*, **22**, 81.

Volianitis, S., McConnell, A.K., Koutedakis, Y., McNaughton, L., Backx, K., and Jones, D.A. (2001). Inspiratory muscle training improves rowing performance. *Medicine and Science in Sports and Exercise*, **33**, 803–9.

Warden, S.J., Gutschlag, F.R., Wajswelner, H., and Crossley, K.M. (2000). Aetiology of rib stress fractures in rowers. *Sports Medicine*, **32**, 819–36.

4.15

Cricket injuries

John Orchard, Trefor James, Alex Kountouris, and Patrick Farhart

Introduction and injury rates

Injuries are a common part of cricket, particularly affecting fast bowlers (Leary and White 2000; Gregory *et al.* 2002; Orchard *et al.* 2002; Stretch 2003). In 2005, cricket was the first sport to publish consensus international injury definitions (Orchard *et al.* 2005b). The definitions are available free in full text format at: http://www.injuryupdate.com.au/images/research/JSMScricketdefinitions.pdf

The definition of a cricket injury (or 'significant' injury for surveillance purposes) is:

> Any injury or other medical condition that either: (1) prevents a player from being fully available for selection in a match or (2) during a major match, causes a player to be unable to bat, bowl or keep wicket when required by either the rules or the team's captain.

The major aim when creating this definition was to set a standard that would be followed equally in all countries surveying cricket injuries (Orchard *et al.* 2005a).

The major injury rates recommended for use include injury incidence and injury prevalence. Injury incidence analyses the number of injuries occurring over a given time period. Injury match incidence considers only those injuries occurring during major matches. Injury seasonal incidence considers the number of defined injuries occurring per squad per season. This can take into account gradual-onset injuries, training injuries, and match injuries in one measurement. Injury prevalence considers the average number of squad members not available for selection because of injury for each match divided by the total number of squad members, expressed as a percentage.

Table 4.15.1 presents key injury rates in Australian cricket over the period 1998–1999 to 2006–2007, calculated from Cricket Australia's annual injury report. Compared with other previously published reports which have similar results (Orchard *et al.* 2002, 2006), recent reports have included injury rates from the new version of the game, Twenty/20 cricket. From Table 4.15.1, it can be seen that, to date, international Twenty/20 cricket has the highest match injury incidence but the lowest bowling match injury incidence. This is based on a very small sample size of five games played by the Australian team until the end of the 2006–2007 season. However, the trend has been confirmed by further study (Orchard *et al.* 2010). With the relatively small number of overs bowled there may be a reduction in bowling injuries (because of less 'overuse') but there may be more intense batting and fielding tasks, leading to a higher overall rate of injury (expressed per 10000 player-hours).

The only other recently published paper which adheres to the international consensus definitions comes from the West Indies (Mansingh *et al.* 2006). These authors reported a mean match injury incidence of 48.7 per 10 000 player-hours in Test cricket, and 40.6 per 10 000 player-hours in one-day international cricket, with injury prevalences of 11.3% and 8.1%, respectively. In West Indies domestic cricket, the match injury incidence was 13.9 per 10 000 player-hours for first-class cricket, and 25.4 per 10 000 player-hours in domestic one-day competitions. The period studied was less than two seasons and hence the rates reflect small exposure. Certainly they are consistent with the Australian figures (although the West Indies Test match rate is slightly higher than the Australian rate whereas their domestic rates are lower). It is noteworthy that the West Indies have reported more injuries for the West Indies team on tour than at home (Mansingh *et al.* 2006), which is the opposite to the trend seen by the Australian team (Orchard *et al.* 2002). All the above findings are consistent with the notion that cricket played in the West Indies has a slightly lower injury incidence than cricket played in Australia, although the sample sizes are probably too small to make this conclusion firmly. If it is a true finding, then explanations include differing pitch and weather conditions and/or differences in scheduling.

Table 4.15.2 shows that, for positions other than pace bowlers, there is increased injury prevalence with increasing age. This is similar to the trend observed in other sports (Orchard *et al.* 2004). However, pace bowlers suffer higher injury prevalence at the youngest ages (< 22 years), primarily because of the high prevalence of lumbar stress fractures in young fast bowlers. Therefore the prevalence rate by age curve for pace bowlers is U-shaped. Lumbar stress fractures in young fast bowlers have long been identified as the highest priority for injury prevention in cricket (Annear *et al.* 1992; Elliott and Khangure 2002).

Specific injuries

Some of the specific injuries which, although seen in other sports, are relatively more common in cricket warrant discussion in further detail.

Lumbar stress fractures

Lumbar stress fractures are generally gradual-onset injuries, occurring to the pars interarticularis of the non-bowling side, are more common in younger bowlers, and are prone to recurrence.

Table 4.15.1 Key injury incidence and prevalence statistics for Australian men's cricket, 1998–1999 to 2006–2007 inclusive

Match type	Match injury incidence (injuries per 10000 player-hours)	Bowling match incidence (injuries per 1000 overs bowled)	Seasonal incidence (injuries per team per season)	Injury prevalence (%)
Domestic Twenty/20	91.3	1.4		10.3
Domestic one-day	46.9	1.9		9.8
First-class domestic	26.6	1.1		9.3
State teams in Australia			16.9	
International Twenty/20	115.6	0.0		5.9
One-day international	53.5	1.3		9.2
Test cricket	29.6	1.6		8.1
Australian team			17.9	
All matches	33.0	1.3		9.2

Table 4.15.2 Comparison of injury prevalence by position and age group

Age (years)	Batsmen (%)	Wicket keepers (%)	Pace bowlers (%)	Spin bowlers (%)
≤22	5.2	1.4	16.8	3.9
23–26	3.7	2.3	15.9	3.0
27–30	4.2	0.8	12.9	4.7
≥31	11.6	3.4	15.8	6.1
All ages	5.5	2.2	15.0	5.2

These injuries exact the greatest toll on cricketers in terms of missed playing time (prevalence). Stress fractures of the pars interarticularis of L4 and L5 on the non-bowling side are the major culprits in terms of specific diagnosis. Whereas cricket fast bowlers have perhaps the highest incidence of lumbar stress fracture of any athlete, the rate of these injuries in non-bowlers (batsmen and wicketkeepers) appears to be no higher than in the general population.

Studies have previously associated the development of lumbar spine injuries (particularly stress fractures) with bowling technique factors. These include a 'mixed' action, excessive shoulder counter-rotation during the delivery stride, and workload factors such as bowling a higher than average number of deliveries in a single session and in a season (Foster *et al.* 1989; Annear *et al.* 1992; Elliott *et al.* 1992; Portus 2001). There are still no published data to show that coaching intervention can prospectively lower the lumbar stress fracture risk for a player, although it is assumed that this is the case.

Side-strain injuries in bowlers

'Side strains' appear to be a unique type of muscle strain (Connell *et al.* 2003; Humphries and Jamison 2004). They are only reported in cricket bowlers and javelin throwers, who use a rather similar technique. Side strains also affect the non-bowling side of the body and are generally acute-onset injuries. There may be a related entity ('side impingement') that is distinct and has a more insidious onset. Side strains are more common early in the season (pre-Christmas in Australia) and are rather less prone to recurrence than other injuries. In some fast-bowling circles (particularly the West Indies), side strains have been viewed almost as a 'rite of passage' injury, in that a genuinely fast bowler should suffer one side strain in his career. However, side strains occasionally lead to chronic pain (where they are often re-diagnosed as stress fractures of the ribs).

Side strains generally affect the internal oblique muscle and could be recurrent (Humphries and Jamison 2004). Most recurrences are non-acute (i.e. they occur in a subsequent season to the initial injury). It is quite possible that there are different varieties of side strain within the overall category, and that some of these varieties are highly recurrent and/or related to overuse, whereas others are related to speed and/or are a one-off injury. A significant proportion of side strains occur during bowling at training ('in the nets'). Some side strains have been reported in players throwing the ball in the field, during spin bowling, and even from impingement whilst batting, although the vast majority are acute injuries during fast bowling.

Other muscle strains

Hamstring, quadriceps, calf, and adductor strains all affect cricketers, as they do many other types of running athlete. Again, it is bowlers who are most prone to injury, but occasionally they occur in batsmen whilst either running between the wickets or fielding. All muscle strains can affect both sides of the body, but the mechanics of bowling (Fig. 4.15.1) leads to a predisposition for muscle strains to affect a particular side. Shortly before delivery the leg on the non-bowling side undergoes acceleration, whereas the bowling leg undergoes deceleration. In addition, the hip is extended on the bowling side but flexed on the non-bowling side at the time

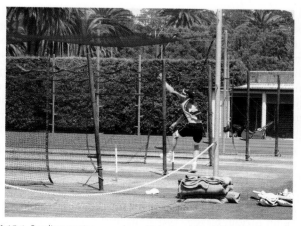

Fig. 4.15.1 Bowling motion pre-release (right-hand bowler). Note the strain on the left hamstring, right quadriceps, and right calf.

of delivery. Hamstring strain injuries (together with 'side strains') are more likely on the non-bowling side, whereas quadriceps, calf, and groin injuries are more likely on the bowling side (Orchard *et al.* 2008). Recent research has found that a past history of lumbar spine stress fracture is a risk for lower limb muscle strains, particularly calf strains, in fast bowlers (Orchard *et al.* 2008).

Shoulder injuries

Shoulder injuries are another common cricket injury, almost always involving the shoulder of the throwing (bowling) arm. Tendon pathology, particularly of the rotator cuff tendons, is the most common diagnosis which relates to the bowling motion. Shoulder tendon injuries related to bowling are relatively more common in spin bowlers than in pace bowlers. Shoulder instability may be a contributing factor in some bowling injury cases, but instability is more responsible for injuries caused by throwing. Therefore lesions related to shoulder instability (such as labral tears) often present as pain during throwing (fielding) rather than bowling and appear to be as prevalent in batsmen as bowlers. The bowling action, as opposed to throwing, does not put the shoulder into the apprehension position for anterior instability. Although comparative figures are not available, the relative incidence of shoulder injuries in elite baseball pitchers would be expected to be higher than that in bowlers, as the pitching motion involves moving into the apprehension position prior to ball release. Shoulder injuries related to throwing are particularly common in women's cricket.

Wrist and hand contact injuries

Hand injuries are common in cricketers at all levels (Belliappa and Barton 1991). Most injuries in amateur players occur during fielding, but batting injuries increase in proportion as the level of play increases. This is probably due to the superior fielding skills of elite players, together with the increased speed of balls that must be faced when batting. Although hand injuries are common and the occasional forearm fracture occurs, the rates are not high enough to suggest that poor protective equipment is being worn by batsmen at the elite level, or that fielders should wear more protection.

Ankle posterior impingement

Posterior impingement is an ankle injury that occurs in fast bowlers, particularly on the front foot at impact. It also occurs in football players (related to kicking). A large posterior process of the talus (or 'os trigonum' if this process is separate) is a risk factor for the development of the condition (Fig. 4.15.2). It was reported as being very common in South African fast bowlers in the 1990s, with eight out of 23 suffering the injury and five requiring surgery (Smith 1999). In its mildest form, posterior impingement may require treatment such as NSAIDs, taping, and proprioception exercises but does not prevent bowling. Relevant recommendations from the South African study are as follows (Smith 1999).

1. In the short term, posterior impingement responds well to injections of cortisone and local anaesthetic.

2. Surgery provided a total cure in all five cases.

3. Deep foot marks at the popping crease increased the pain in the South African players. Use of the 'turf doctor' to repair bowlers' footmarks helped bowlers to cope with the injury.

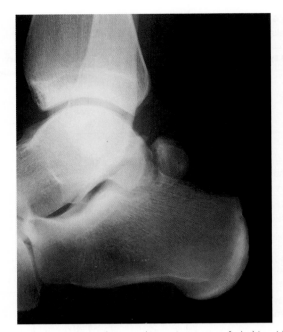

Fig. 4.15.2 Large os trigonum (separated posterior process of talus) is a risk factor for posterior impingement in bowling.

Medical illnesses

Because cricket is often played in hot weather, dehydration might be expected to be a common condition. This would be particularly expected in cricket played in Asian countries where not only are heat and humidity extreme, but gastrointestinal illness is common and could be a contributory factor in dehydration. Cricket is also one of the minority of sports which do not readily allow substitution due to injury or illness (with the exception of fielding). Despite these theoretical concerns, in practice it appears that most dehydration is mild to moderate and is successfully treated by oral rehydration. In competitive cricket and/or very hot conditions, it is sensible preparation to have intravenous rehydration facilities available nearby, in case they are medically indicated.

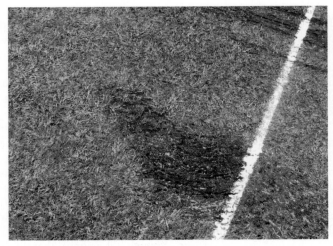

Fig. 4.15.3 Footmarks at the popping crease.

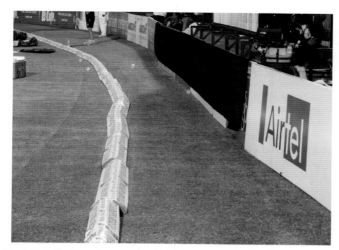

Fig. 4.15.4 The boundary rope should be a minimum of 3 yards (2.74 metres) from the fence in order to prevent collision injuries.

Injury prevention in cricket

Increased bowler workload, increased bowler speed, and biomechanical factors (such as increased shoulder counter-rotation) are the major known risk factors for bowling injuries. Ball speed is generally a desirable characteristic for pace bowlers, and so is considered a non-reversible risk factor. Overall bowler match workload has increased in recent seasons at the professional level in line with increased scheduling. This increased scheduling, combined with incomplete understanding of the relationship between workload and injury risk, has meant that practical workload reductions in matches have been difficult to achieve. However, the increased understanding of workload as a risk factor (related to both matches and training) and better understanding of bowler mechanics, have perhaps helped to control the injury rates in fast bowlers to some extent.

Two of the major known non-bowling risk factors involve fence collisions in fieldsmen and the use of football drills for cross-training. Fence collisions have been virtually eliminated with the use of the boundary rope (Fig. 4.15.4), introduced internationally as a compulsory measure in 2001. Moving the boundary in has changed the nature of the game, in that scores are higher and scoring is faster because of the increased number of boundaries. Most cricket commentators believe that faster scoring in cricket has improved the game as a spectacle, although some lament that the war between bat and ball has been tilted too strongly in favour of the bat at professional level.

Football injuries as part of warm-up or conditioning activities during training do occur, but have been reduced in line with increased caution with these training drills. Whilst football cross-training may always have some part in relieving the boredom from other routine drills, it is worth mentioning that this appears to be a high-risk activity for cricketers and hence should be kept to a minimum.

Dennis and coworkers have found a relationship between the overall bowler workload (matches and training) and risk of bowling injury in both adult (Dennis *et al.* 2003) and junior (Dennis *et al.* 2005) cricket. It appears from this work (although it is not clearly established) that the number of bowling sessions per week (whether training or match) is the factor which most correlates with injury risk. It is not known what the extent of overall (match plus training) workload was in the seasons prior to implementation of the workload study, although it is very clear that match workload has increased over the years. A recent study has shown that bowling overloads (greater than 50 overs in a first class match or 30 overs in the second innings of a match) are associated with increased risk of injury in the three to four weeks following the overload (Orchard *et al.* 2009).

To date formal recommendations regarding the maximum or optimum number of bowling sessions or overs per week in open-age cricket have not been set in stone. However, if any limits were suggested, further increases in match workload would make it harder for players and coaches to fall within the prescribed range. Surveillance of English county cricket reveals an even higher match workload (matchwise) for first-class bowlers in England compared with Australia (Newman 2003). However, injury prevalence appears to be higher in England than Australia. An appeal of the recent trend towards extra matches being of the Twenty/20 variety is that these games involve a very small bowling load per player and hence may contribute to a lower injury risk in the long term.

Conclusion

Compared with other team sports, cricket appears to be relatively safe for batsmen, spin bowlers, and wicketkeepers. However, the fast bowler occupies one of the most injury-prone positions in world sport. At international level, the increasing commercialism of the game has led to increasing crowding of the match schedule to the point where professional cricket is now a 'year-round' sport. This increase in scheduling has probably had the effect of cancelling out improvements in sports medicine which could prevent injuries in fast bowlers. Ironically, the solution to this dilemma may lie with another change in cricket in response to commercialism. Twenty/20 cricket, an abbreviated form of the game designed to achieve a result within 4 hours, may limit the amount of overs that fast bowlers are required to deliver. This may bring their injury rates closer to the 'safe' levels which are seen in the other positions in the cricket team.

References

Annear, P.T., Chakera, T.M., Foster, D.H., and Hardcastle, P.H. (1992). Pars interarticularis stress and disc degeneration in cricket's potent strike force: the fast bowler. *Australian and New Zealand Journal of Surgery*, **62**, 768–73.

Belliappa, P.P. and Barton, N.J. (1991). Hand injuries in cricketers. *Journal of Hand Surgery (Edinburgh)*, **16**, 212–14.

Connell, D., Jhamb, A., and James, T. (2003). Side strain: a tear of internal oblique musculature. *American Journal of Roentgenology*, **181**, 1511–17.

Dennis, R., Farhart, P., Goumas, C., and Orchard, J. (2003). Bowling workload and the risk of injury in elite cricket fast bowlers. *Journal of Science and Medicine in Sport*, **6**, 359–67.

Dennis, R., Finch, C., and Farhart, P. (2005). Is bowling workload a risk factor for injury to Australian junior cricket fast bowlers? *British Journal of Sports Medicine*, **39**, 843–6.

Elliott, B. and Khangure, M. (2002). Disk degeneration and fast bowling in cricket: an intervention study. *Medicine and Science in Sports and Exercise*, **34**, 1714–18.

Elliott, B., Hardcastle, P., Burnett, A. *et al.* (1992). The influence of fast bowling and physical factors on radiological features in high performance young fast bowlers. *Sports Medicine Training and Rehabilitation*, **3**, 113–30.

Foster, D., John, D., Elliott, B., Ackland, T., and Fitch, K. (1989). Back injuries to fast bowlers in cricket: a prospective study. *British Journal of Sports Medicine*, **23**, 150–4.

Gregory, P., Batt, M., and Wallace, W. (2002). Comparing injuries of spin bowling with fast bowling in young cricketers. *Clinical Journal of Sport Medicine*, 12, 107–112.

Humphries, D. and Jamison, M. (2004). Clinical and magnetic resonance imaging features of cricket bowler's side strain. *British Journal of Sports Medicine*, **38**, e21.

Leary, T. and White, J. (2000). Acute injury incidence in professional county club cricket players (1985–1995). *British Journal of Sports Medicine*, **34**, 145–7.

Mansingh, A., Harper, L., Headley, S., King-Mowatt, J., and Mansingh, G. (2006). Injuries in West Indies cricket 2003–2004. *British Journal of Sports Medicine*, **40**, 119–23.

Newman, D. (2003) A prospective study of injuries at first class counties in England and Wales 2001 and 2002 seasons. In: R.A. Stretch (ed.), *Second World Congress of Science and Medicine in Cricket*, pp. 83–4.

Orchard, J., James, T., Alcott, E., Carter, S., and Farhart, P. (2002). Injuries in Australian cricket at first class level 1995/96 to 2000/01. *British Journal of Sports Medicine*, **36**, 270–5.

Orchard, J., Farhart, P., and Leopold, C. (2004). Lumbar spine region pathology and hamstring and calf injuries in athletes: is there a connection? *British Journal of Sports Medicine*, **38**, 502–4.

Orchard, J., Newman, D., Stretch, R., Frost, W., Mansingh, A., and Leipus, A. (2005a). Defining a cricket injury. *Journal of Science and Medicine in Sport*, **8**, 358–9.

Orchard, J., Newman, D., Stretch, R., Frost, W., Mansingh, A., and Leipus, A. (2005b) Methods for injury surveillance in international cricket. *British Journal of Sports Medicine*, **39**, e22.

Orchard, J., James, T., and Portus, M. (2006). Injuries to elite male cricketers in Australia over a 10-year period. *Journal of Science and Medicine in Sport*, **9**, 459–67.

Orchard, J., Farhart, P., James, T., Portus, M., and Kountouris, A. (2008). Pace bowlers in cricket with history of lumbar stress fracture have increased risk of lower limb muscle strains, particularly calf strains. Presented at: Second World Congress on Sports Injury Prevention, Tromso, Norway.

Orchard, J.W., James, T., Portus, M., Kountouris, A., and Dennis, R. (2009). Fast bowlers in cricket demonstrate upto 3- to 4-week delay between high workloads and increased risk of injury. *Am. J. Sports Med*, **37**(6), 1186–92.

Orchard, J.W., James, T., Kountouris, A. *et al.* (2010). Changes to injury profile (and recommended cricket injury definitions) based on the increased frequency of Twenty 20 cricket matches. *Open Access Journal of Sports Medicine 2010*, **1**, 63–76.

Portus, M. (2001). Relationship between cricket fast bowling technique, trunk injuries and ball release speed. In J. Blackwell (ed.), *29th International Symposium on Biomechanics in Sports*, pp. 231–4.

Smith, C. (1999). Ankle injuries in fast bowlers: posterior talar impingement syndrome. The South African experience. In: *Fifth IOC World Congress, Sydney*, p.245.

Stretch, R. (2003). Cricket injuries: a longitudinal study of the nature of injuries to South African cricketers. *British Journal of Sports Medicine*, **37**, 250–3.

4.16

Soccer injuries

Colin Fuller

Introduction

Football, or soccer, is the most popular team sport in the world with over 200 countries affiliated to the international governing body Fédération Internationale de Football Association (FIFA) (www.fifa.com); the Football World Cup is the most popular televised sports event. The sport appeals equally to males and females, adults and children. Whilst the 11-a-side game is the most common form of football, five-a-side football using smaller indoor or outdoor pitches is a popular variation of the game. The following discussion relates to injuries sustained in the 11-a-side format.

Football teams are comprised of 11 players, of whom 10 are designated as outfield players (forwards, midfielders, and defenders) and one as the goalkeeper. Although the 10 outfield players have different tactical roles in the game, the physical demands do not vary as widely as that found in some other team sports; consequently, all outfield players require similar attributes of speed, agility, strength, and endurance. For these reasons, injury profiles amongst outfield players do not vary with playing position to the same extent as they do in other sports, such as rugby. The exception to this generalization is the goalkeeper, who assumes a relatively static role within the penalty area on a football pitch.

Incidence, severity, and nature of injuries

The reported incidence, severity, and nature of sports injuries depend on the definitions and procedures employed in injury surveillance studies. For this reason, the discussion presented here is limited to results obtained from studies that used the definitions and procedures recommended in the international consensus statement on injury surveillance in football (Fuller et al. 2006). The results presented on match and training injuries are based on the author's knowledge and experience gained from epidemiological studies carried out amongst men and women.

Injury causation

A number of risk factors, both intrinsic (age, joint stability, muscle strength, body mechanics, psychological issues) and extrinsic (level of play, equipment, pitch condition), affect the incidence and nature of injury (Dvorak and Junge 2000). However, previous injury has long been accepted as the most important risk factor, and this has been shown specifically to be a significant factor for hamstring and groin muscle and knee and ankle ligament injuries (Hägglund et al. 2006). Video analysis has been used extensively to assess the nature of contact events in football and the role that tackle parameters have in determining the incidence and nature of

injury (Fuller et al. 2004). The most common type of tackle is one-footed, from the side, where the tackling player stays on his feet (Fig. 4.16.1), and therefore these are responsible for most injuries (Table 4.16.1). However, when incidences of injury are calculated as a function of the number of events of a particular type taking place (i.e. injuries/1000 events), tackles involving a clash of heads and two-footed tackles are identified as those with the greatest propensity to cause injury. This type of analysis is very useful when determining injury causation and when changes to the laws of the game are being considered as a means of reducing the risk of injury. For example, in an analysis of head injuries, video analysis identified that aerial challenges and the unfair use of the upper extremity were significantly more likely to cause a head injury than any other type of challenge (Fuller et al. 2005); as a consequence of this analysis, the laws of the game were changed prior to the 2006 Football World Cup in order to make this type of challenge a red card offence.

Incidence and severity

The incidence of lost-time injuries in matches is ~25 injuries per 1000 player-match hours for men and ~20 for women, with injuries lasting on average about 15 days (Fuller et al. 2007a). In training, the incidence is approximately three injuries per 1000 player-training hours for both men and women, with injuries lasting on average about 14 days (Fuller et al. 2007b). Although the incidence of match injuries is high in football, it is at the lower end of the spectrum for contact and semicontact sports, such as rugby union, rugby league, ice hockey, American football, and basketball. The incidence of training injuries in football is similar to that reported for other sports of this type.

Overview of the nature of injuries in football

Epidemiological studies of football injuries have consistently identified lower limb strains and sprains as the main injuries for both men and women during matches and training. Whilst the distribution of training injuries is similar for men and women, women sustain a higher proportion of ligament and a lower proportion of muscle/tendon injuries than men. Recurrent injuries are responsible for around 15% of injuries, and recurrences tend to be more severe than the index injuries. There is some evidence to indicate that match injuries are more likely to occur on the dominant rather than the non-dominant leg (Hawkins and Fuller 1999).

Typical distributions of injuries for men and women, as functions of the type and location of injury, are shown in Table 4.16.2 for match injuries and Table 4.16.3 for training injuries. For both

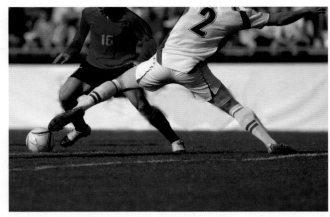

Fig. 4.16.1 One-footed tackles from the side place considerable strain on the groin. Copyright © karaboux-Fotolia.com

Table 4.16.1 Frequency of contact events in football and their propensity to cause injury

Tackle type	Incidence of tackle (events/game)	Incidence of injuries requiring post-match medical attention	
		Injuries per 1000 player-hours	Injuries per 1000 tackles
Tackle direction			
From behind	25	11	14
From front	17	11	21
From side	28	27	33
Tackle mode			
Sliding in	18	13	39
Staying on feet	39	25	21
Vertical jump	13	11	29
Tackle action			
Clash of heads	0.2	1	240
One-footed	46	33	24
Two-footed	1	2	54
Use of arm	11	5	16

Data from Fuller *et al*. 2004.

Table 4.16.2 Distribution of match injuries for men and women as a function of location and type of injury

Type of injury	Location of injury; %				
	Head/ neck	Upper limb	Trunk	Lower limb	All locations
Men					
Fracture/bone stress	1.4	0.9	0.5	2.4	5.1
Joint (non-bone)/ligament	–	3.8	0.5	27.2	31.4
Muscle/tendon	0.8	1.4	14.9	36.6	53.6
Laceration/skin	1.8	–	–	0.8	2.6
Brain/spinal cord/PNS	5.7	–	–	–	5.7
All types of injury	9.9	6.3	16.2	67.4	100.0
Women					
Fracture/bone stress	1.5	1.7	0.4	3.9	7.5
Joint (non-bone)/ligament	0.2	3.2	1.4	36.8	41.6
Muscle/tendon	2.3	2.0	7.3	26.2	37.7
Laceration/skin	0.9	–	–	0.2	1.1
Brain/spinal cord/PNS	10.1	–	0.1	0.4	10.6
All types of injury	15.6	6.9	9.7	67.7	100.0

PNS, peripheral nervous system.
Data from Fuller *et al*. 2007a.

Table 4.16.3 Distribution of training injuries for men and women as a function of location and type of injury

Type of injury	Location of injury (%)				
	Head/ neck	Upper limb	Trunk	Lower limb	All locations
Men					
Fracture/bone stress	0.8	1.7	–	2.4	4.9
Joint (non-bone)/ligament	–	4.1	1.1	27.5	32.8
Muscle/tendon	1.3	1.6	16.7	36.4	56.0
Laceration/skin	1.1	–	–	0.2	1.3
Brain/spinal cord/PNS	3.7	–	–	0.2	3.7
All types of injury	7.5	6.3	18.9	66.8	100.0
Women					
Fracture/bone stress	0.2	1.2	0.8	2.8	4.9
Joint (non-bone)/ligament	–	2.1	1.8	31.9	35.9
Muscle/tendon	0.6	1.7	13.3	35.9	51.5
Laceration/skin	0.3	–	–	0.5	0.8
Brain/spinal cord/PNS	4.8	–	–	–	4.8
All types of injury	6.3	5.1	16.7	71.9	100.0

PNS, peripheral nervous system.
Data from Fuller *et al*. 2007b.

men and women, match and training injuries are predominantly lower limb—muscle/tendon and joint (non-bone)/ligament injuries. The most common injuries and the injuries causing the greatest loss of time for men and women during matches and training are listed in Table 4.16.4. Lower limb contusions are very common in football, but the average severity of these injuries is quite low so they rarely cause players to miss matches and consequently have only a minor impact on players' training regimes and match schedules. Therefore, apart from the more serious cases, these injuries are generally not recorded in injury surveillance studies.

Table 4.16.4 The most common injuries sustained by men and women during matches and training

	Most common injuries		Injuries causing greatest loss of time	
	Men	Women	Men	Women
	Match injuries			
1	Lateral ankle ligaments	Lateral ankle ligaments	ACL	ACL
2	Hamstring muscle[a]	Concussion	Lateral ankle ligaments	Lateral ankle ligaments
3	Concussion	ACL	Hamstring muscle[a]	Medial collateral ligaments
4	Adductor muscle[a]	Lower leg contusion	Medial collateral ligaments	Concussion
	Training injuries			
1	Lateral ankle ligaments	Lateral ankle ligaments	ACL	ACL
2	Hamstring muscle[a]	Quadriceps muscle[a]	Lateral ankle ligaments	Lateral ankle ligaments
3	Adductor muscle[a]	Hamstring muscle[a]	Hamstring muscle[a]	Quadriceps muscle[a]
4	Quadriceps muscle[a]	Adductor muscle[a]	Quadriceps muscle[a]	Hamstring muscle[a]

[a]Excluding haematomas and contusions.
ACL, anterior cruciate ligament.
Data from Fuller *et al.* (2007a,b).

Other common injuries and associated issues in football are discussed in more detail below.

Head injuries

Head injuries represent ~10% of all reported injuries, of which ~20% will be contusions and lacerations. Other more serious head injuries do occur, such as concussion (~65%), nasal (~10%) and dental (3%) injuries, and skull fractures (~1%); of these injuries, concussion raises the greatest concern and discussion. Early retrospective studies involving the older and heavier water-absorbent leather footballs indicated that repetitive heading of a football led to cognitive deficits in players; however, later prospective studies using the newer and lighter water-resistant synthetic balls questioned these findings (Kirkendall *et al.* 2001). In particular, assessment of the levels of biochemical markers in cerebrospinal fluid and serum indicated that there were no significant differences between players undertaking normal heading practice and a control group (Zetterberg *et al.* 2007). In matches, most concussions occur when a player's head is struck unexpectedly from close range by the ball, by another player's head, or by a goalpost rather than when a player heads the ball. In addition, heading a modern football is unlikely to generate the forces required to cause a concussion, and claims that padded headgear provides protection against concussion have not yet been substantiated.

Ankle and foot injuries

Ankle injuries are the most common injuries sustained during matches and training (~20%). Tears of the lateral ligament complex (~75%), anterior tibiofibular syndesmosis (~13%), and medial (deltoid) ligament (~10%) are the most common types of ankle injury. Lateral ligament complex injuries result from non-contact activities (~40%), such as jumping, running, and turning, and contact events (~60%), such as tackles from the side where the tackling player makes contact with the inside of the tackled player's leg. Ankle sprains are particularly prone to recurrence (~50%). 'Footballer's ankle' is an impingement of the ankle joint that causes chronic pain. Plantarflexion of the ankle during kicking leading to damage at the anterior joint capsule and dorsiflexion causing contusion of the anterior tibia–talus junction have been suggested as mechanisms for this injury. Many players use ankle supports as an injury prevention measure, but given the high incidence of ankle ligament injuries, the efficacy of these devices must be questioned. Wobble-board exercises, which are used to improve proprioception and muscle control, are recommended as an injury prevention strategy and as part of a player's functional rehabilitation from an ankle injury.

Foot injuries, which represent around 8% of all injuries, are less common than ankle injuries. However, unlike other parts of the body, contusions are the most commonly reported foot injury (~40%); ligament sprains in the midfoot are the next most common foot injury (16%). The number of metatarsal fractures (~11%) appears to be increasing, but there is no evidence base at the present time to prove or disprove this perception. Traumatic injury can occur to any of the metatarsals when a player is kicking or a tackling player steps on a player's foot, but injuries to the first and fifth metatarsals are the most common. Fractures to these bones result from direct trauma, rotational motion, or overuse; however, there is also considerable debate about the contributory role that modern lightweight boots play in these injuries. Overuse non-contact injuries of the metatarsals are normally stress fractures, and players often continue to play with increasing pain levels. This condition may convert to a full fracture following a traumatic event involving the injured foot. Because of the poor blood supply in the region of the fifth metatarsal, repairs can be slow; for this reason, early surgical screw fixation of the fracture is undertaken in order to improve recovery rates (Popovic *et al.* 2005). Foot injuries involving the first metatarsophalangeal joint (~7%), often referred to as 'turf toe', involve damage to the joint's plantar capsule and ligaments. The injury occurs when, in the process of running or jumping, the body's weight moves forward over the foot, but the foot remains planted such that the big toe is bent excessively upwards. The condition is often associated with play and training on artificial turf, but injuries can just as easily occur on grass surfaces. Plantar fasciitis is a form of tendonitis that normally occurs as an overuse injury; excessive pronation of the foot is regarded as a risk factor. Treatment of this condition is normally conservative, but pain reduction can be achieved by stretching the plantar fascia and the Achilles tendon.

Knee injuries

After ankle injuries, knee injuries are the most common injury in football (~17%). These injuries result from both non-contact

(~70%) and contact (~30%) activities and occur equally to both the dominant and non-dominant leg. Knee injuries are responsible for the greatest loss of player time in football, and major surgery for a knee injury is almost inevitable at some stage in a professional player's career. The most common knee injuries are partial and complete tears of the anterior cruciate (~20%) and medial collateral (~18%) ligaments; injuries of the lateral collateral ligament are also serious but less common (~5%). Previous injury to the knee is a strong risk factor for knee ligament injuries (Waldén *et al.* 2006), and women are about five times more likely to sustain an ACL injury than men. In this context, Mandelbaum *et al.* (2005) developed a football-specific neuromuscular and proprioceptive training programme for women and achieved an 80% reduction in the incidence of ACL injuries over a period of 2 years. ACL tears can occur in isolation or in combination with damage to the posterior cruciate and medial collateral and lateral collateral ligaments. Serious knee ligament injuries will normally require 3–12 months treatment and careful rehabilitation.

Medial and lateral meniscus tears (~13%) are also common knee injuries, with medial meniscus injuries more common than those of the lateral meniscus. Most lesions require arthroscopic repair and many injuries occur in conjunction with ACL and MCL injuries. Articular cartilage injuries represent only ~2% of reported knee injuries; however, concurrent damage to articular cartilage is observed in ~40% of surgical operations on the knee, and in the case of ACL injuries the figure may be as high as 70%. Osteoarthritis of the knee is a major risk for footballers after retirement because of career damage to meniscal cartilage and/or knee ligaments. In particular, meniscectomies undertaken to repair joint cartilage and ligament injuries can significantly increase risk levels for osteoarthritis.

Thigh muscle injuries

Thigh muscle injuries are the third most common injury in football (~16%). Because of their lateral anterior location in the thigh, the quadriceps group are often subject to contusion injuries; however, the severity of these injuries is generally low so they are often not reported in epidemiological studies. Quadriceps strains (~35%), especially to the rectus femoris muscle, occur during the frequent sprinting, jumping, and kicking activities associated with football. Hamstring strains (~45%), especially of the biceps femoris muscle, are consistently reported as one of the most common injuries sustained during matches and training; ~80% of hamstring strains occur during maximal sprinting. The average severity of hamstring strains is ~20 days but there is a high rate of recurrent injuries (~15%) and these are usually more severe than the index injury. It is claimed that older players sustain more hamstring injuries than younger players, but this may simply confirm that older players have sustained hamstring injuries earlier in their careers, which places them at high risk of further hamstring injuries later in their careers. Quite often quadriceps and hamstring muscle strains are not supported by, for example, MRI examinations. Some caution should be exercised in these cases because anterior and posterior thigh pain does not always translate into a thigh strain injury, as the pain may refer to a problem elsewhere, such as the lumbar spine, hip, sacroiliac joint, or neural tension.

Groin and hip injuries

Acute and overuse groin and hip conditions are fairly common (~9%) in football; they are caused by activities such as extensive running, twisting, turning, and kicking. The pelvic region, which connects the upper and lower body, and the hip joints, which provide the link between the pelvis and the lower limbs, are subjected to high levels of stress in football. Common conditions of the groin and hip include injuries of the adductor (~50%) and iliopsoas (~25%) muscles and occasional tears of the acetabular labrum in the hip joint. Tears of the acetabular labrum often require arthroscopic debridement; if left untreated, progressive degeneration of the labrum may lead to osteoarthritis within the hip joint. Generalized groin pain may be related to chronic conditions of the adductor and iliopsoas muscles, referred pain from the sacroiliac joint, and even stress fractures in the pubic bone or neck of the femur. The preferred treatment for generalized groin pain in footballers is rest followed by a gradual return to play. However, many footballers continue to play with pain and eventually undergo operations during the close season.

Other injuries

Complaints related to lumbar and thoracic spine pain are common in football, but the reported incidence of spinal injury is relatively low (~3%). These injuries can present as localized pain or as referred pain in the buttock and thigh muscles. Training in football often concentrates on the lower limbs at the expense of the important trunk, shoulder, and neck muscles, which provide essential core body strength. Lower leg injuries represent ~9% of all injuries, but ~35% of these are contusions. Other more serious lower leg injuries encountered include tibia and fibula fractures (~10%), gastrocnemius tears and spasms (~10%), Achilles tear/tendinitis (~8%), and shin splints (~8%).

Acute and chronic injury is a major cause of enforced retirement amongst professional players (~50%) (Drawer and Fuller 2001); of the players who retire through injury, ~40% retire because of acute injuries and ~60% because of chronic injuries. Of those players retiring because of an acute injury, ~45% have knee injuries, ~20% have ankle injuries, and ~15% have lower back injuries. Of those players retiring because of a chronic injury, ~40% have knee injuries, ~20% have lower back injuries, and ~10% have hip injuries. A third of retired professional footballers have osteoarthritis in at least one lower limb joint. The Industrial Injuries Advisory Council in the UK is considering whether professional footballers suffering from osteoarthritis of the knee are entitled to claim industrial injuries disability benefit on the grounds that the condition is an occupational injury. However, the Council has previously rejected a call for osteoarthritis of the hip to be added to the list of prescribed diseases entitled to compensation.

Goalkeeping injuries

Goalkeepers have a different role in football compared with outfield players, and the injury profiles of these players reflect this difference. In addition to ankle sprains, goalkeepers are susceptible to head injuries resulting from being struck by the ball, collision with opposition forwards/own defenders, and collision with a goalpost.

Goalkeepers are also susceptible to acute shoulder, elbow, and hip injuries as a result of diving for the ball, especially on hard surfaces. Wrist, hand, and finger fractures/dislocations (metacarpals and scaphoid) occur as a result of stopping the ball or falls to the ground. Whilst padded clothing may provide some protection for goalkeepers, goalkeeping gloves are less beneficial as they are not primarily designed for injury prevention. Goalkeepers have a higher incidence of injury during training relative to other playing positions and often sustain more training injuries than match injuries because of the greater active time during training than during matches.

References

Drawer, S.D. and Fuller, C.W. (2001). Propensity for osteoarthritis and lower limb joint pain in retired professional soccer players. *British Journal of Sports Medicine*, **35**, 402–8.

Dvorak, J. and Junge, A. (2000). Football injuries and physical symptoms: a review of the literature. *American Journal of Sports Medicine*, **28**, S3–9.

FIFA (2008). www.fifa.com (accessed 31 January 2008).

Fuller, C.W., Smith, G.L., Junge, A., and Dvorak, J. The influence of tackle parameters on the propensity for injury in international football. *American Journal of Sports Medicine*, 2004, 32, 43S-53S.

Fuller, C.W., Junge, A., and Dvorak, J. (2005). A six year prospective study of the incidence and causes of head and neck injuries in international football. *British Journal of Sports Medicine*, **39** (Suppl), i3–9.

Fuller, C.W., Ekstrand, J., Junge, A., *et al.* (2006). Consensus statement on injury definitions and data collection procedures in studies of football (soccer) injuries. *British Journal of Sports Medicine*, **40**, 193–201.

Fuller, C.W., Dick, R.W., Corlette, J., and Schmalz, R. (2007a). A comparison of the incidence, nature and cause of injuries sustained on grass and artificial turf by male and female football (soccer) players. Part 1: Match injuries. *British Journal of Sports Medicine*, **41**, i20–6.

Fuller, C.W., Dick, R.W., Corlette, J., and Schmalz, R. (2007b). A comparison of the incidence, nature and cause of injuries sustained on grass and artificial turf by male and female football (soccer) players. Part 2: Training injuries. *British Journal of Sports Medicine*, **41**, i27–32.

Hägglund, M., Waldén, M., and Ekstrand, J. (2006). Previous injury as a risk factor for injury in elite football: a prospective study over two consecutive seasons. *British Journal of Sports Medicine*, **40**, 767–72.

Hawkins, R.D. and Fuller, C.W. (1999). A prospective epidemiological study of injuries in four English professional football clubs. *British Journal of Sports Medicine*, **33**, 196–203.

Kirkendall, D.T., Jordan, S.E., and Garrett, W.E. (2001). Heading and head injuries in soccer. *Sports Medicine*, **31**, 369–86.

Mandelbaum, B.R., Silvers, H.L., Watanabe, D.S., *et al.* (2005). Effectiveness of a neuromuscular and proprioceptive training program in preventing anterior cruciate ligament injuries in female athletes: 2-year follow-up. *American Journal of Sports Medicine*, **33**, 1003–10.

Popovic, N., Jalali, A., and Gillet, P. (2005). Proximal fifth metatarsal diaphyseal stress fracture in football players. *Foot and Ankle Surgery*, **11**, 135–41.

Waldén, M., Hägglund, M., and Ekstrand, J. (2006). High risk of new knee injury in elite footballers with previous anterior cruciate ligament injury. *British Journal of Sports Medicine*, **40**, 158–62.

Zetterberg, H., Jonsson, M., Rasulzada, A., *et al.* (2007). No neurochemical evidence for brain injury caused by heading in soccer. *British Journal of Sports Medicine*, **41**, 574–7.

4.17

Injuries in rugby union

Colin Fuller

Introduction

Rugby union is the second most popular team sport in the world with over 100 countries affiliated to the International Rugby Board (IRB) and with the Rugby World Cup the third most popular televised sports event behind only the Olympic Games and the FIFA Football World Cup. Rugby is a full-contact sport played predominantly by men and boys. Although the 15-a-side game continues to be the most common form of rugby played, the faster seven-a-side game is increasing in popularity and is the format of rugby that the IOC adopted as an official Olympic sport (www.irb.com). This discussion of rugby injuries relates to the 15-a-side format of rugby union.

A rugby team comprises 15 players, of whom eight are designated as forwards and seven as backs; these positions are often referred to as the 'ball-winners' and 'ball-carriers', respectively, but the roles are becoming blurred. Forwards, who are responsible for winning the ball at set plays (scrums, lineouts) and contact phases of the game (tackles, rucks, mauls), are characterized by attributes of power, strength, and endurance, whereas backs, who are primarily responsible for distributing and running with the ball, are characterized more by speed, agility, and endurance. Because of the different tactical roles and physiological demands placed on forwards and backs (Nichols 1997; Duthie *et al.* 2003; Eaton and George 2006), rugby union is often referred to as a game for all shapes and sizes, which is illustrated by the significant differences in the height and body mass of forwards and backs (Table 4.17.1). The physical nature of rugby union and the specific roles played by forwards and backs strongly influence the incidence and nature of injuries sustained by the two groups of players.

Incidence, severity, and nature of injuries

The discussion presented here is based on results obtained from epidemiological studies which used the definitions and procedures recommended in the international consensus statement on injury surveillance studies for rugby union (Fuller *et al.* 2007c). The information presented on match and training injuries is largely derived from results obtained from extensive injury surveillance studies carried out by the author amongst elite professional male rugby players. Although anecdotal evidence indicates that many players retire from rugby because of acute and chronic injuries, there is no evidence base to quantify these perceptions.

Injury causation

The incidence and nature of match injuries in rugby union are closely related to the phases of play, i.e. lineouts, scrums, tackles, rucks, mauls, collisions, and open running, whilst training injuries are related to the type of training, i.e. conditioning (weights, non-weights) and rugby skills (full-contact, semi-contact, non-contact). Video analysis has shown that tackles are the most common contact events in rugby matches followed by rucks, and the high incidences of injury (injuries per 1000 player-hours) associated with these events reflect this situation (Table 4.17.2). However, when the incidences of injury are calculated to take into account the number of events of a particular type occurring in a match (injuries/1000 events), collisions and scrums have the greatest propensity for injury. However, in terms of injury severity, the lineout and scrum are the most hazardous match events. The incidence of training injuries calculated as a function of total training time is similar for full-contact, semi-contact, and non-contact skills training activities. However, when the incidence is calculated in terms of the actual time spent on each activity, full-contact skills training is over five times more likely to cause injury than non-contact skills training. The severity of the injuries also reflects the nature of the training activity (Table 4.17.3).

Incidence and severity

The incidence of lost-time injuries sustained during matches is ~90 injuries/1000 player-match-hours, with each injury lasting on average ~17 days (median, 7 days) (Brooks *et al.* 2005a). For training injuries, the incidence is ~3 injuries/1000 player-training-hours, with each injury lasting on average ~21 days (median, 9 days) (Brooks *et al.* 2005b). There are no significant differences in the incidence or severity of injuries sustained between forwards and backs in either matches or training. The incidence of match injuries in rugby is amongst the highest reported for contact and semi-contact team sports, although the incidence of training injuries is similar to that in many other team sports. Although the incidence of injury during training is very much lower than during matches, ~90% of player exposure occurs during training, which means that training injuries are still responsible for about a third of all rugby injuries. The high incidence and severity of injuries in rugby union mean that on average ~20% of a team's playing squad may be injured at any given time. The incidence of injury in rugby generally increases as the standard of play increases, which is normally explained by factors such as the higher body mass, fitness, and strength of players, longer ball-in-play times, and the more competitive nature of games at higher levels.

Overview of the nature of injuries in rugby union

Almost 90% of injuries sustained during matches and ~70% during training are acute. About 17% of injuries are recurrent, and these

Table 4.17.1 Mean and standard deviation for the height and body mass of professional rugby players in England

Playing position	Mean (standard deviation)	
	Height (m)	Body mass (kg)
Forwards	1.88 (0.07)	108.5 (8.1)
Backs	1.81 (0.05)	89.5 (6.7)
t-test (forwards vs. backs)	p < 0.001	p < 0.001

Data from Brooks et al. 2005a.

Table 4.17.2 Frequency of contact events in rugby union and their propensity to cause injury

Event type	Incidence of event, events/game	Incidence of injury		Severity of injury, days
		Injuries/1000 player-hours	Injuries/ 1000 events	
Collision	15	3.9	10.5	19
Lineout	33	0.9	1.1	42
Maul	19	2.3	4.9	10
Ruck	139	7.0	2.0	13
Scrum	30	5.8	8.1	26
Tackle	215	33.9	6.1	21

Data from Fuller et al. 2007a.

Table 4.17.3 Incidence and severity of training injuries as a function of training activity

Training activity	Incidence of injury (injuries/1000 player-hours)		Severity (days)
	Total training time	Activity-specific training time	
Conditioning, non-weights	0.2	2	16
Conditioning, weights	0.1	0.4	4
Skills, full-contact	1.3	11	24
Skills, semi-contact	1.1	5	17
Skills, non-contact	0.8	2	9

Table 4.17.4 Distribution of match injuries as a function of playing position and location and type of injury

Type of injury	Location of injury (%)				
	Head/ neck	Upper limb	Trunk	Lower limb	All locations
Forwards					
Fracture/bone stress	0.8	1.7	0.4	1.2	4.1
Joint (non-bone)/ligament	5.0	9.3	8.2	19.0	41.5
Muscle/tendon	0.7	4.1	4.0	31.8	40.7
Laceration/skin	1.2	0.1	0.0	0.5	1.8
Brain/spinal cord/PNS	8.8	0.6	0.2	0.2	9.9
Other	0.7	0.1	0.5	0.6	1.9
All types of injury	17.3	16.0	13.3	53.4	100.0
Backs					
Fracture/bone stress	0.6	1.3	0.1	1.1	3.1
Joint (non-bone)/ligament	2.3	7.6	3.0	21.8	34.6
Muscle/tendon	0.4	5.4	4.9	41.9	52.7
Laceration/skin	0.6	0.0	0.0	0.1	0.7
Brain/spinal cord/PNS	6.5	0.4	0.3	0.3	7.5
Other	0.6	0.4	0.1	0.3	1.4
All types of injury	10.9	15.1	8.5	65.5	100.0

PNS, peripheral nervous system.
Data from Brooks et al. 2005a.

Table 4.17.5 Distribution of training injuries as a function of playing position and location and type of injury (data from Brooks et al., 2005b)

Type of injury	Location of injury (%)				
	Head/ neck	Upper limb	Trunk	Lower limb	All locations
Forwards					
Fracture/bone stress	0.8	1.7	0.4	2.5	5.4
Joint (non-bone)/ligament	1.3	6.3	13.8	23.3	44.6
Muscle/tendon	0.4	1.3	5.0	38.8	45.4
Laceration/skin	0.8	0.0	0.0	0.4	1.3
Brain/spinal cord/PNS	1.3	0.0	0.8	0.4	2.5
Other	0.0	0.0	0.8	0.0	0.8
All types of injury	4.6	9.2	20.8	65.4	100.0
Backs					
Fracture/bone stress	0.6	1.3	0.6	2.6	5.2
Joint (non-bone)/ligament	0.0	7.1	5.2	15.5	27.7
Muscle/tendon	0.6	2.6	4.5	52.9	60.6
Laceration/skin	0.6	0.0	0.0	0.0	0.6
Brain/spinal cord/PNS	2.6	0.0	0.0	1.3	3.9
Other	0.0	0.0	1.9	0.0	1.9
All types of injury	4.5	11.0	12.3	72.3	100.0

PNS: peripheral nervous system.
Data from Brooks et al. 2005b.

are invariably more severe than the index injuries. Backs are significantly more likely to injure their non-dominant arm or leg during matches, although there is no difference for forwards. During training, forwards and backs are equally likely to injure their dominant and non-dominant limbs.

The distributions of injuries amongst backs and forwards as functions of the type and location of injury are shown in Table 4.17.4 for match injuries and in Table 4.17.5 for training injuries. These distributions show that match injuries for both forwards and backs are predominantly lower limb injuries (muscle/tendon and joint (non-bone)/ligament) with significant numbers of upper limb injuries (joint (non-bone)/ligament) and injuries to the head, neck, brain, spinal cord, and peripheral nervous system. Training injuries for both forwards and backs are dominated by lower limb

Table 4.17.6 The most common injuries sustained by forwards and backs during matches and training

	Most common injuries		Injuries causing greatest loss of time	
	Forwards	Backs	Forwards	Backs
Match injuries				
1	Thigh haematoma	Thigh haematoma	ACL	Hamstring muscle[a]
2	Calf muscle[a]	Hamstring muscle[a]	Knee meniscus/cartilage	Shoulder instability/dislocation
3	Lateral ankle ligaments	Concussion	Shoulder instability/dislocation	MCL
4	Cervical nerve root	Calf muscle haematoma	Achilles tendon	ACL
5	Concussion	Lateral ankle ligaments	MCL	Knee meniscus/cartilage
6	Acromioclavicular joint	Quadriceps muscle[a]	Calf muscle[a]	Wrist/hand fracture
Training injuries				
1	Hamstring muscle[a]	Hamstring muscle[a]	Lumbar disc/nerve root	Hamstring muscle[a]
2	Lumbar disc/nerve root	Calf muscle[a]	Shoulder instability/dislocation	ACL
3	Lateral ankle ligaments	Quadriceps muscle[a]	Hamstring muscle[a]	Shoulder instability/dislocation
4	Calf muscle[a]	Lateral ankle ligaments	Achilles tendon	Adductor muscle[a]
5	Quadriceps muscle[a]	Adductor muscle[a]	Lateral ankle ligaments	Knee meniscus/cartilage

[a]Excluding haematomas and contusions.
ACL, anterior cruciate ligament; MCL, medial cruciate ligament.
Data from Brooks *et al.* 2005a,b.

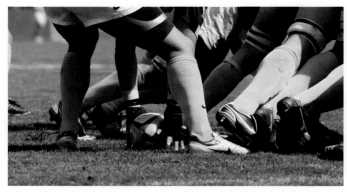

Fig. 4.17.1 Contusional injuries are common as a result of body contact. Copyright © goleador-Fotolia.com

injuries (muscle/tendon and joint (non-bone)/ligament). The most common injuries and the injuries causing the greatest loss of time for forwards and backs during matches and training are listed in Table 4.17.6. Large numbers of muscle contusions and haematomas can be expected in rugby because of the physical nature of the sport (Fig. 4.17.1); however, although common, the severity of these injuries is generally low (< 7 days) so they rarely cause players to miss matches. Some of the common and more serious injuries associated with rugby are discussed below.

Spine and spinal cord injuries

Catastrophic spinal injuries resulting in paraplegia, quadriplegia, or even death are high-consequence incidents that are relatively rare in rugby. Depending on the country, their frequency of occurrence is 1–10 per 100 000 players per year. These injuries occur in situations where a player's cervical spine is forced into hyperflexion or hyperextension, such as during a scrum or tackle

(Quarrie *et al.* 2002). However, injury mechanisms are complex as axial forces to the head can result in compression, compression–flexion, and/or compression–extension injuries to the cervical spine. Older players who have developed spinal stenosis may be at a higher risk of spinal cord injury. Whilst high-quality pitch-side treatment is an essential requirement for the treatment of all sports injuries, it is of paramount importance for managing spinal injuries. In terms of injury consequences, it is estimated that a third of all new cases of non-sport- and sport-related paraplegia and quadriplegia die before they reach hospital, so decisions made at the scene of a spinal cord injury and during the day following the injury are extremely important in determining long-term outcomes. All confirmed or potential cases of cervical spine injury should be immobilized at the scene using a cervical collar and/or spinal board and specialist treatment sought immediately. Specialist centres to deal with serious spinal injuries have been established in some countries in an attempt to achieve better patient outcomes, but the advantages of these centres have not yet been established. Injuries involving the group of nerves travelling from the spinal cord (C5–C6) through the shoulder (brachial plexus) and down the arms to the hands/fingers are common in rugby. They are normally caused by a blow to the side of the head causing forcible lateral movement or a lateral/rotational movement of the neck. These injuries to the peripheral nervous system are referred to as 'stingers' or 'burners', and they cause localized weakness in the arm and pain ranging from mild to intense that may last from minutes to weeks. Stingers present unilaterally and do not affect the lower limbs; if weakness or pain persists beyond 2 weeks, the player should be referred for specialist assessment.

Non-catastrophic spinal injuries such as disc, facet joint, nerve root, and muscle/ligament injuries, although less serious than catastrophic injuries, are very much more common. Playing position, in particular, is a major risk factor for these injuries (Fuller *et al.* 2007b). In matches, forwards are twice as likely as backs to sustain a spinal injury. Forwards are twice as likely to sustain a cervical as a lumbar spine injury, whereas backs are equally likely to sustain lumbar and cervical spine injuries. In training, forwards are again almost twice as likely as backs to sustain spinal injuries, but both forwards and backs are four times more likely to sustain a lumbar than a cervical spine injury. Players often experience a high incidence of lumbar disc injuries during weight-training, which is probably related to poor lifting technique and the use of excessive weights. Degenerative changes observed in the cervical spines of some front-row forwards may result from trauma sustained during scrummaging, and these changes may in turn contribute to the later development of osteoarthritis in the spine.

Many front-row prop forwards develop a prominent dorsal lump (lipoma or fibroma) over the seventh cervical vertebra. These soft tissue masses probably develop as a consequence of repeated trauma caused by the demands and forces placed on the prop's cervical spine during scrums. Surgical excision should be used with caution in these cases because the benefit of surgery depends on the exact nature of the lump, and a large proportion of surgical cases result in postoperative wound complications (Dearing 2006).

Head injuries

The incidence and nature of head injuries reported in epidemiological studies of rugby injuries vary widely. These variations occur because some studies include the minor cuts and abrasions that only require players to leave the field of play temporarily for treatment or suturing under IRB Law 3.10. These injuries normally do not cause players to lose time from training or match activities, and therefore they are not recorded in studies using the definition of injury advocated in the international consensus statement for studies of injuries in rugby union (Fuller et al. 2007c). Excluding lacerations, concussion is by far the most common head injury reported (>50%), and it is one of the five most common injuries. Even so, it is widely judged that concussions are under-reported in rugby. IRB Regulation 10.1, which relates to the management of concussions, specifies that:

> A player who has suffered a concussion shall not participate in any match or training session for a minimum of three weeks from the time of injury, and may then only do so when symptom free and declared fit after proper medical examination.

However, this law is not implemented on a routine basis, at least in the professional game, as fewer than half the players reported to have sustained a concussion are immediately removed from play. Three international consensus statements have provided guidance on the assessment and management of concussion in sport, and these guidelines are very pertinent to rugby (McCrory et al. 2005). Unconscious players should be treated with caution, and the possibility of a cervical spine injury must always be taken into consideration until this condition can be discounted. Players suspected of suffering a concussion should be assessed at the scene for attention and memory function using tests such as the Maddocks questions (Maddocks et al. 1995) before they are allowed to return to play and, where necessary, these initial screening tests should be followed up with more detailed neuropsychological testing. There is no evidence to indicate that the use of either mouth guards or headgear reduces the incidence of concussion (Marshall et al. 2005), although mouth guards will reduce the incidence of dental injuries and headgear will reduce the incidence of superficial abrasions and lacerations.

Auricular haematoma leading to the condition referred to as 'cauliflower ear' is common amongst forward players. This condition is brought on by the repeated trauma to a forward player's ears during scrummaging, which causes blood to build up between the cartilage and the skin in the player's ear. Because the cartilage derives its blood supply from the overlying skin, any interruption to this supply results in the cartilage dying and the ear swelling and assuming the characteristic cauliflower appearance. Accumulated blood can be drained from the affected areas to prevent the deformity developing; however, continued trauma during scrums causes the condition to return. In severe cases, the swelling may become so large that the natural transport of ear wax and the player's hearing may be affected. There is some evidence to suggest that the use of padded headgear reduces the risk of auricular haematoma (Marshall et al. 2005).

Shoulder injuries

The physical nature of rugby means that the incidence of shoulder injuries amongst both forwards and backs is high; the tackle accounts for over two-thirds of all shoulder injuries. The higher severity of shoulder injuries sustained by backs may be related to the greater impact forces experienced when players tackle in fast open play compared with the lower impact forces experienced during rucks and mauls. Whilst shoulder protection may provide some mitigation of these injuries, it can also encourage players to tackle harder in the belief that they are safer, which negates any potential benefit. In addition, the IRB laws of rugby preclude the use of this type of body protection. The most common shoulder injuries are acromioclavicular joint (~30%), rotator cuff/impingement (~25%), and dislocation/instability (~15%) injuries. Dislocation/instability injuries are the most severe of these injuries, and rank as one of the injuries resulting in the most time lost from training and matches. There is a high overall recurrence rate for shoulder injuries (~25%), with the rate for shoulder dislocation/instability being particularly high (~60%). Poor tackling technique and shoulder laxity have been suggested as risk factors for shoulder dislocation/instability, and therefore pre-participation evaluation for shoulder laxity may be beneficial for identifying players at higher risk. Although rotator cuff injuries may present as chronic injuries, they are more likely to occur as acute injuries in rugby. For large acute tears, two-stage open surgery involving rotator cuff repair and glenohumeral joint stabilization is preferred to arthroscopic procedures in order to reduce the possibility of recurrence (Goldberg et al. 2003).

Knee injuries

Knee injuries are not one of the most common injuries in rugby but they are amongst the most severe, and for this reason they are responsible for a high proportion of the time lost through injury (~20%) and for players retiring from rugby. The tackle is the phase of play responsible for the highest proportion (~40%) of these injuries. Common knee conditions encountered are medial cruciate ligament (~30%), chondral/meniscal (~20%) and patellofemoral (~12%) injuries, although anterior cruciate ligament (~30%) and medial cruciate ligament (~25%) injuries are responsible for the greatest proportion of knee-related lost time. Chondral/meniscal injuries, as with many sports of this type, represent an important group of injuries, as repair and removal of cartilage in the knee are major risk factors for developing osteoarthritis in later life. Because of the significant loss of time associated with knee injuries, injury prevention should be a high priority. In this context, there is some evidence to suggest that support sleeves may provide the knee with a degree of protection against injury, but the rationale for this effect has not been clarified (Marshall et al. 2005).

Other injuries

Contusions of the quadriceps are common injuries in contact sports but except in a few cases the consequences are not serious. Quadriceps and hamstring strains represent a high proportion (~15%) of injuries in most sports that involve high-intensity running, sprints, stops/starts, changes in direction, jumping, and kicking. Rugby is no different in this respect, as these injuries are responsible for a large amount of lost time (Table 4.17.6). Regeneration and remodelling of an injured muscle continues for several months after return to play, so careful management is essential in order to reduce the high proportion of recurrent injuries (~20%) observed in rugby. There is some evidence to indicate that effective warm-up, stretching, and eccentric exercises can reduce the incidence of thigh muscle strains.

Damage to the lateral ankle ligaments and the ankle joint capsule is common in both matches and training (Table 4.17.6), as might be expected for a sport where players are required to run, cut, and change direction quickly. Ankle support in the form of a sleeve or brace may provide some protection against injury (Marshall et al. 2005) and proprioceptive training using a wobble board should be beneficial, especially for reducing the risk of recurrent ankle injuries. Fractures and dislocations of the hand, such as Bennett's fracture of the thumb, are risks for both forwards and backs during ball handling and in rucks and mauls. These injuries may benefit from taping or a brace, especially in the early stages of return to play, in order to minimize the risk of further injury.

References

Brooks, J.H.M., Fuller, C.W., Kemp, S.P.T., et al. (2005a). Epidemiology of injuries in English professional rugby union. Part 1: Match injuries. *British Journal of Sports Medicine*, **39**, 757–66.

Brooks, J.H.M., Fuller, C.W., Kemp, S.P.T., et al. (2005b). Epidemiology of injuries in English professional rugby union. Part 2: Training injuries. *British Journal of Sports Medicine*, 2005b, **39**, 767–775.

Dearing, J. (2006). Soft tissue neck lumps in rugby union players. *British Journal of Sports Medicine*, **40**, 317–19.

Duthie, G., Pyne, D., and Hooper S. (2003). Applied physiology and game analysis of rugby union. *Sports Medicine*, **33**, 973–91.

Eaton, C. and George, K. (2006). Position specific rehabilitation for rugby union players. Part 1: Empirical movement analysis data. *Physical Therapy in Sport*, **7**, 22–9.

Fuller, C.W., Brooks, J.H.M., Cancea, R.J., Hall, J., and Kemp, S.P.T. (2007a). Contact events in rugby union and their propensity to cause injury. *British Journal of Sports Medicine*, **41**, 862–7.

Fuller, C.W., Brooks, J.H.M., and Kemp, S.P.T. (2007b). Spinal injuries in professional rugby union: a prospective cohort study. *Clinical Journal of Sport Medicine*, **17**, 10–16.

Fuller, C.W., Molloy, M.G., Bagate, C., et al. (2007c). Consensus statement on injury definitions and data collection procedures for studies of injuries in rugby union. *British Journal of Sports Medicine*, **41**, 328–31.

Goldberg, J.A., Chan, K.Y., Best, J.P., Bruce, W.J.M., Walsh, W., and Parry, W. (2003). Surgical management of large rotator cuff tears combined with instability in elite rugby football players. *British Journal of Sports Medicine*, **37**, 179–81.

McCrory, P., Johnston, K., Meeuwisse, W., et al. (2005). Summary and agreement statement of the 2nd International Conference on Concussion in Sport, Prague 2004. *British Journal of Sports Medicine*, **39**, 196–204.

Maddocks, D.L., Dicker, D.G., and Saling, M. (1995). The assessment of orientation following concussion in athletes. *Clinical Journal of Sports Medicine*, **5**, 32–5.

Marshall, S.M., Loomis, D.P., Waller, A.E., et al. (2005). Evaluation of protective equipment for prevention of injuries in rugby union. *International Journal of Epidemiology*, **34**, 113–18.

Nichols, C.W. (1997). Anthropometric and physiological characteristics of rugby union football players. *Sports Medicine*, **23**, 375–96.

Quarrie, K.L., Cantu, R.C., and Chalmers, D.J. (2002). Rugby union injuries to the cervical spine and spinal cord. *Sports Medicine*, **32**, 633–53.

4.18

Boxing injuries

Mike Loosemore

Introduction: a short description of the sport and disciplines within it

Boxing or fighting with clenched fists is one of the most ancient of all recorded sports. The greatest knowledge of boxing in ancient times comes from the writings, statues, and poetry of the Ancient Greeks (Fig. 4.18.1). Boxing was considered an integral part of education:

> Boxing leads everyone to practical wisdom.
>
> Plato

Several of the Greek Gods are described as distinguished boxers. Apollo was the guardian of the sport as mentioned in the Homeric hymn:

> Wherever [in Delos] the Ionians gather with their long tunics
> to honour you, along with their children and modest wives,
> with every event they please you with boxing joy and songs.
>
> Homer

In Ancient Greece boxing was established as an Olympic sport at the 23rd Olympiad in 688BC (Spivey 2004) and continued as such until the end of the Ancient Olympics.

Boxing re-emerged in England in the eighteenth century with the rediscovery of the classical world and the concept of leisure. There seemed to be two distinct groups: the social elite who were educated in Ancient Greek and familiar with the works of Plato and Homer, epitomized by the romantic poet Lord Byron who was a keen boxer and an advocate of boxing, and the longer-established prizefighters who fought professional public contests in public houses and at country fairs and racecourses.

Prizefighting had few rules, resulting in a high incidence of serious injury and death in the ring. This was one of the reasons why prizefighting and bare knuckle boxing were made illegal in England until the introduction of the first safety-based rules by Lord Queensberry, first published in 1867. Boxing was introduced into the modern Olympics in 1900, and apart from being absent from the 1912 Stockholm Games, has been present in every other Olympics since.

Medical surveillance in both professional and amateur boxing has increased enormously over the last century. Boxers now have regular medical reviews, and medical support at the ringside is mandatory in all forms of boxing. These developmentss, together with rule changes, have made boxing safer than many other contact sports.

Boxing is now a worldwide sport, open to men and women, with world champions becoming household names. In the professional ranks participants box at 17 different weight categories while there are 10 weight categories in the Olympic (amateur) sport (Table 4.18.1). Other differences between the professional and Olympic codes are shown in Table 4.18.2.

Physiological and biomechanical demands of the sport and its disciplines

One of the greatest challenges in boxing, both physiologically and biochemically, is 'making weight'. It is generally desirable to box at the lowest weight possible, whilst remaining an effective boxer. This fighting weight is less than the boxer's training weight and is not sustainable. The final few pounds of weight loss are achieved by dehydrating. How severe this dehydration can be depends on two factors: whether it is a single fight or a tournament, and the timing of the weigh-in relative to the start of the fight. A professional fight is a one-off performance and the weigh-in can be over 24 hours before the fight. In Olympic (amateur) boxing the boxers may have six contests over 10 days, with the weigh-in only a few hours before each contest as well as at the start of the tournament. Normal post-contest rehydration regimens for non-weight-restricted athletes have to be modified. Fluid and carbohydrate intake are closely monitored so that the boxer will not be overweight the following day, but will have enough fluid and glycogen stores to box effectively.

Injuries

Most injuries specific to boxing are confined to the head and face (Fig. 4.18.2) and the upper limb. (Zazryn et al. 2003)

Head

In boxing, acute head injuries rarely lead to death or permanent disability. Head injuries in boxing are approximately one-third of the acute head injury rate in rugby union. (Nicholl et al. 1991). Chronic traumatic brain injury as a result of boxing, while still a possibility in professional boxing, is unlikely to be a result of amateur boxing (Loosemore et al. 2007). A boxer sustaining a blow to the head can be assessed acutely using the Maddocks questions (Maddocks et al. 1995) modified for boxing. All boxers who have a suspected concussion should be accompanied and head injury advice given. Any boxer who causes concern should be admitted to hospital for observation and suitable head scans.

Face

Cuts to the face are usually superficial. There should be a low threshold for stitching these, particularly if deeper layers are involved, as a solid repair will help to prevent the scar reopening at

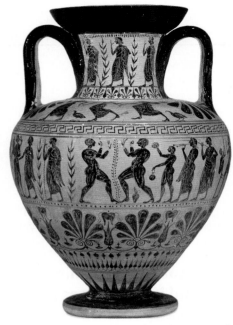

Fig. 4.18.1 Boxing in Ancient Greece. Copyright © The Trustees of the British Museum

Table 4.18.1 Boxers' weights

Weight	Professional	Olympic
Straw weight	7st 7lb	–
Light-flyweight	7st 10lb	49 kg
Flyweight	8st	52 kg
Super-flyweight	8st 3lb	–
Bantamweight	8st 6lb	56 kg
Super-bantamweight	8st 10lb	–
Featherweight	9st	–
Super-featherweight	9st 4lb	–
Lightweight	9st 9lb	60 kg
Light-welterweight	10st	64 kg
Welterweight	10st 7lb	69 kg
Light-middleweight	11st	–
Middleweight	11st 7lb	75 kg
Super-middleweight	12st	–
Light-heavyweight	12st 7lb	81 kg
Cruiserweight	14st 4lb	–
Heavyweight	14st 4lb	91 kg
Super-heavyweight	None	91 kg+

Table 4.18.2 Rule differences between amateur and professional boxing

Amateur	Professional
3 × 3 min rounds (junior 1.5 min)	4–12 × 3 min rounds
Gloves: 10–12 ounces	Gloves: 8 ounces
Head guards used	No head guards
Hand bandaging limited to 4.5 m of 4 cm crepe	No limit to hand bandages
Injury rate low	Injury rate high
Knockouts avoided	Knockouts increase entertainment value
Standing eight count allows the boxer to recover	No standing eight-count
Point scoring is computerized	Judging is subjective

a later date. The position of the superficial nerves should be noted and skin sensation tested before suturing if cuts occur around these nerves.

Nose

Acute fractures of the nose are not uncommon; re-setting of the nose should be delayed until the end of the boxer's career unless their breathing is adversely affected. If the septal cartilage is dislocated from the nasal bones, it can be relocated acutely by placing traction on the central cartilage and pushing the nasal cartilage in the opposite direction of the dislocation. The saddle-shaped 'boxer's nose' is caused by collapse of the central cartilage. This results from stripping of the nasal mucosa by a septal haematoma. Septal haematomas appear like a bright red cherry just inside the nose and can be revealed by gently lifting the tip of the nose. A septal haematoma should be regarded as an ENT emergency and referred to hospital immediately.

Eyes

Although mild ocular complications (e.g. corneal abrasion) are common in boxing, more serious complications (eg. detached retina) are rare (Bianco *et al.* 2005). Serious complications seen in boxing which should be excluded on examination include lens subluxation/dislocation, cataract formation, retinal detachment/disinsertion, and lattice degeneration. Acute corneal abrasion, although very painful, usually settles quickly with the application of antibiotic eye ointment and an eye patch.

Blow-out fractures of the orbit can occur in boxing. They present with double vision, pain in the eye when blowing the nose, and surgical oedema around the orbit. Diagnosis can be confirmed with a CT scan of the floor of the orbit. If a blow-out fracture of the orbit is suspected, the opinion of an ophthalmic surgeon should be sought.

Ears

Cauliflower ears are now uncommon in amateur boxing because of the use of the head guard. If present, the haematoma should be aspirated from the pinna and the area packed and strapped for 48 hours to prevent re-accumulation of blood.

Acute perforations of the eardrum occur when the boxing glove seals the external auditory canal. Perforation of the eardrum is an uncommon injury. The boxer may present with pain, tinnitus, dizziness, or all three. Acute perforations will often heal without

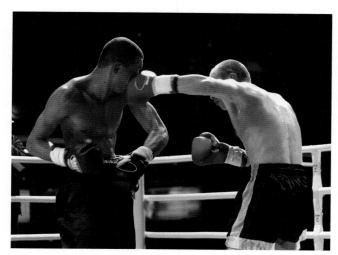

Fig. 4.18.2 Facial injuries are common in boxing. Copyright © Vasily Smirnov-Fotolia.com

medical intervention; the boxer should be prevented from boxing or sparring until healed.

Elbow

The main boxing injury to the elbow is caused by hyperextension of the elbow when a punch is not landed, especially when a jab is thrown. Therefore it tends to be the non-dominant elbow that is affected. The tip of the olecranon is traumatized and this leads to cartilage breakdown and loose-body formation. (Valkering *et al.* 2008). The boxer presents with pain or reduction in elbow extension, possibly with intermittent locking.

Wrist

When a punch is thrown correctly the maximum force travels via the third metacarpal and the capitate, forcing the scaphoid and lunate apart. This is resisted by the scapholunate ligament, and this ligament is vulnerable to tear and rupture. Acute rupture gives pain 2 cm distal to Lister's tubercle and scaphoid instability. A plain X-ray will show a gap between the scaphoid and lunate (Terry Thomas sign) if the film is taken with the fist tightly clenched to stress the scapholunate joint. Treatment is open reduction and fixation.

Thumb

Common injuries encountered in boxers are fractures to the base of the thumb, and injuries to the ulnar collateral ligament at the first metacarpophalangeal joint (MCPJ).

A fracture–dislocation (Bennett's fracture) occurs when the punch misses the target and the whole force is taken through the thumb. This requires reduction and fixation.

A transverse fracture at the thumb base occurs when a hook is landed thumb first. This can usually be reduced and held in a cast.

Ulnar collateral ligament injuries at the MCPJ occur when the thumb catches on the opponent and hyperabduction of the thumb occurs. The main concern is total rupture of the ulnar collateral ligament (Stener lesion). This injury requires open surgical repair, as

the ligament is prevented from reattaching itself by the interposition of the extensor hood.

Hand

Fractures of the second and third metacarpals are most commonly seen. As the metacarpals are subject to very high forces, fractures should be reduced as anatomically as possible, as any angulation will often result in re-fracture.

Boxer's knuckle is a term referring to damage to the extensor mechanism of the finger as it passes over the MCPJ and is caused by the repeated trauma of punching. Boxer's knuckle can be divided into three stages:

1. Inflammation of the MCPJ and the extensor mechanism. Clinically this presents with a 'boggy feeling knuckle' and knuckle pain. This condition usually responds quickly to intra-articular steroid.

2. Inflammation of the MCPJ and the extensor mechanism with a tear of the capsule. This again presents with a 'boggy feeling knuckle' and knuckle pain. However, this condition usually does not respond to intra-articular steroid and an MR arthrogram will confirm the diagnosis. This injury requires surgical repair as it may lead to stage 3 Boxer's knuckle.

3. Further tearing of the capsule and extensor expansion result in subluxation of the extensor mechanism and inability to extend the affected finger.

Prevention of injury

Extrinsic factors

Extrinsic factors affecting the safety of the boxers can be divided into officials and equipment. Timely intervention by the referee or coach will prevent further injury occurring to a stricken boxer. This intervention is made much earlier in the amateur sport with the use of a standing eight count to allow a boxer to recover from a debilitating blow. Equipment is designed to reduce the risk of injury. The ropes are covered to reduce rope burns, corner posts are padded, the ring is sprung, and there is a covering of foam rubber under the canvas to protect the boxer if he falls.

Head guards in amateur boxing afford some protection from blows to the head, and protection to the head if it strikes the ground. Head guards also protect the eyes by increasing the depth of the orbit, reducing the risk of cuts, and preventing the occurrence of cauliflower ears. The gloves absorb energy, thus reducing the risk of head and hand injuries. The heavier the gloves the more energy is absorbed. Gum shields are worn to protect the teeth, but their role in reducing concussion is not proven.

Intrinsic factors

The punching load in training and competition leads to a high rate of upper limb injuries, especially the hand, wrist and elbow. The boxer's traditional stance with hands in front of the face, elbows together, and scapulae protracted, produces a positional fixed kyphosis locking the thoracic spine. This in turn means that the back tends to hinge on the upper lumbar vertebra, leading to low back pain. Although boxing training requires regular road running, overuse injuries from this are rare.

Epidemiology of injuries

Professional boxing studies (Zazryn *et al.* 2003; Bledsoe *et al.* 2005) show the overall incidence of injury to be 171–250.6 injuries per 1000 fights. Facial injuries are the most common (51–89.8% of all injuries depending on the study), followed by hand/upper limb injury (7.4–17%) and eye injury (14%). Neither age nor weight was significantly associated with the risk of injury. Lacerations were the most prevalent type of injury.

Amateur boxing has a lower rate of injury—0.92 injuries per man-hour of sport (approximately 150 injuries per 1000 fights) (Porter and O'Brien 1996). The areas of injury appeared to be the same as those in professional boxing (Zazryn *et al.* 2006).

References

Bianco, M., Vaiano, A.S., Colella, F., *et al.* (2005). Ocular complications of boxing. *British Journal of Sports Medicine*, **39**, 70–4.

Bledsoe, G.H., Li, G., and Levy, F. (2005). Injury risk in professional boxing. *Southern Medical Journal*, 98, 994–8.

Loosemore, M., Knowles, C.H., and Whyte, G.P. (2007). Amateur boxing and risk of chronic traumatic brain injury: systematic review of observational studies. *British Medical Journal*, 335, 809.

Maddocks, D.L., Dicker, G.D., and Saling, M.M. (1995). The assessment of orientation following concussion in athletes. *Clinical Journal of Sports Medicine*, **5**, 32–5.

Nicholl, J.P., Coleman, P., and Williams, B.T. (1991) A report to the Sports Council 1991. Medical Care Research Unit, Department of Public Health Medicine, Sheffield University Medical School, Sheffield.

Porter, M. and O'Brien, M. (1996). Incidence and severity of injuries resulting from amateur boxing in Ireland. *Clinical Journal of Sports Medicine*, 6, 97–101.

Spivey, N. (2004). *The Ancient Olympics*. Oxford University Press.

Valkering, K.P., van der Hoeven, H., and Pijnenburg, B.C. (2008). Posterolateral elbow impingement in professional boxers. *American Journal of Sports Medicine*, **36**, 328–32.

Zazryn, T.R., Finch, C.F., McCrory, P.A. (2003). 16 year study of injuries to professional boxers in the state of Victoria, Australia. *British Journal of Sports Medicine*, 37, 321–4.

Zazryn, T., Cameron, P., and McCrory P. (2006). A prospective cohort study of injury in amateur and professional boxing. *British Journal of Sports Medicine*, 40, 670–4.

4.19

Skiing injuries

Viktor Dvorak and Hans Spring

Introduction

Skiing is defined as a downhill glide on snow-covered slopes or mountain terrain utilizing skis as primary equipment. It is both a recreational hobby and an athletic activity. Skiing is a very technical sport, and suitable equipment is needed for beginners and hobby skiers as well as for top athletes. In addition, it also provides high demands on the physical and coordination skills of the individual skier.

The challenge is to keep direction and speed under control during various types of downhill run. These are complex motions depending on various extrinsic and intrinsic factors. This sporting activity is associated with a relatively high risk of injury. The injuries, which affect various parts of the body, are predominantly from falls and collisions (Fig. 4.19.1).

History

Skiing was originally a practical way of getting from one place to another on packed or crusted snow. The word 'ski' entered the English language from Norwegian in 1890.

In the nineteenth century, the Norwegian Sondre Norheim improved ski bindings to allow turns to be made while skiing downhill. The invention of firmer bindings to anchor the feet to the ski enabled the skier to turn more effectively and led to the development of alpine skiing.

The sport is popular wherever the combination of snow, mountain slopes, and a sufficient tourist infrastructure can be built up, including parts of Europe, North and South America, Australia and New Zealand, South Korea, Japan, and South Africa.

Competition

The first alpine skiing competition, a primitive downhill race, was held in the 1850s in Oslo. A few decades later, the sport had spread to the remainder of Europe and the USA. The first slalom was organized in 1922 in Mürren, Switzerland, and two years later such a race became the first Olympic alpine event. The Arlberg Kandahar, a combined slalom and downhill event, is now referred to as the first legitimate alpine event.

Alpine skiing became part of the Olympic programme at the 1936 Garmisch-Partenkirchen Games with a men's and ladies combined event.

The top alpine competitions under FIS (International Ski Federation) rules are contested in the FIS World Cup series, the FIS Alpine World Ski Championships, and the Winter Olympic Games.

Downhill

The downhill features the longest course and the highest speeds in Alpine skiing. It includes challenging turns, jumps, and gliding phases. Speeds can be in excess of 140 km/h. Each skier makes a single run down a single course and the fastest time determines the winner.

Super-G

Super-G stands for super giant slalom, an event which combines the speed of downhill with the more precise turns of giant slalom. The course is shorter than the downhill course but longer than the giant slalom course, and also includes high-speed turns, jumps, and gliding phases. Each skier makes one run down a single course.

Giant slalom (GS)

This is similar to the slalom, but with fewer turns which are wider and smoother. Each skier makes two runs down two different courses on the same slope. Both runs take place on the same day. The times are added, and the fastest total time determines the winner.

Slalom

The slalom features the shortest course and the quickest turns. As in the giant slalom, each skier makes two runs down two different courses on the same slope. Both runs take place on the same day. The times are added and the fastest total time determines the winner.

Combined

The combined event consists of one downhill and one slalom run. The times are added together and the fastest total time determines the winner. The combined downhill and the combined slalom are contested independently of the regular downhill and slalom events, and the combined courses are shorter than the regular versions.

Epidemiology of skiing injuries

Alpine skiing is a popular sport with significant risk of injury (Koehle *et al.* 2002). Since the 1970s, injury rates have dropped from approximately 5–8 to about 2–3 per 1000 skier-days. The nature of the injuries has also been transformed over the same period. Lower leg injuries are becoming less common, while the incidence of knee sprains and upper extremity injuries is increasing. Upper extremity injuries constitute approximately a third of skiing injuries. Historically, spinal injuries have been much less common in skiers. Head injuries have been increasing in incidence

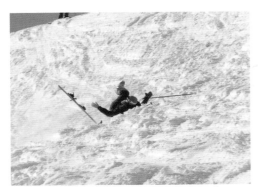

Fig.4.19.1 Ski fall. Photograph from: www.alpujarra-holiday.com.

Table 4.19.1 Snowsport injuries in Switzerland 2001–2005

	Skiing (%)	Snowboarding (%)
Skull, brain	2.3	2.9
Head, face, eyes, neck	7.4	6.5
Spine	5.9	10.2
Trunk	9.3	15.5
Shoulders, upper arm	18.9	17.7
Elbow, forearm, hands, fingers	14.7	18.4
Hip, thigh	2.0	0.6
Knee	18.5	9.7
Lower leg, ankle, foot, toes	6.2	9.1
General lower extremities	13.4	8.4
Undefined	1.4	1.1

Table 4.19.2 Main diagnoses of snowsport injuries in Switzerland 2001–2005

	Alpine skiing (%)	Snowboarding (%)
Fractures of skull and face	0.4	1.3
Fractures of ribs and back	3.1	2.4
Upper body fractures	7.5	9.3
Lower body fractures	2.7	1.9
Knee, meniscus	2.3	1.5
ACL dislocations	47.4	41.8
Sprains and tendon injuries	2.3	3.5
Open and superficial wounds	5.7	2.6
Bruises and contusions	22.5	29.5
Undefined	6.2	6.0

Source: SUVA statistics 2005.

over recent decades and account for more than half of skiing-related deaths.

About 6% of snow sport injuries are attributed to collisions with other people. The remaining 94% are due to falls without a collision. According to the statistics published by SUVA (Swiss Accident Insurance) in 2005, the prevailing state of snow on the slopes and skiers' skills are the conditions that are responsible for injuries. The annual cost of insurance benefits in 2005 was about 184 million Swiss francs. One per cent of all ski accidents cause about 30% of all costs. The number of snow sport injuries due to different snow and weather conditions vary from year to year. According to the accident statistics, 24 530 skiers and 9185 snowboarders were injured in 2005.

Biomechanical demands

More than other sports, alpine skiing is subject to a process of permanent change through the introduction of new equipment. These changes provide a recognizable impact on skiing technique as well as the physical condition of skiers (Mueller and Schwameder 2003).

Alpine skiing is also subjected to constant change because of innovations in racing technique, where an exact line between gates is very important. These developments also have an impact on skiing as a hobby.

Basic principles

A number of key forces act on a skier. The weight of the skier acts in a vertical direction through his/her centre of mass. Altering a skier's mass will affect forces as well as velocity. Ground reaction (the base) is the force the snow exerts against the skier. When standing or gliding, this force is equal to the skier's mass multiplied by the force of gravity. As the skier goes faster and/or changes direction by turning, the ground reaction force is increased (Serge *et al.* 2000). Basic mechanics considerations for skiing include body stance and initiating, controlling, and exiting turns. Initiation of a

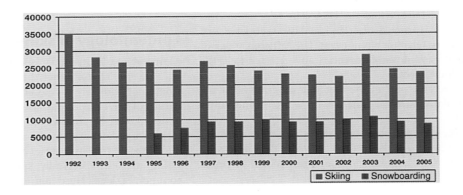

Fig.4.19.2 Ski and snowboard injuries in Switzerland 1992–2005 (SUVA 2005)

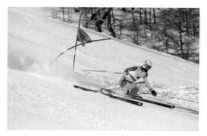

Fig. 4.19.3 Slalom competition event. Photograph from: www.channe14.com. Copyright © Moreno Novello-Fotolia.com

turn occurs by an up-and-down unweighting followed by a weight shift and rotatory or steering motions.

Internal and external forces

Internal forces act between parts of the body and are caused by muscle contractions. These forces alone cannot change the effect of gravity on the body. Since the skier is mostly in contact with snow, internal forces influence the relative position of various parts of the body. External forces are due to gravity, i.e. the effect of ground reaction forces on the skier. Internal forces generated by movements of the body are referred to as a key turning motion. These movements cause rotary impulses, which are used to rotate the body or parts thereof. Because the skier is almost in touch with the snow, the snow's resistance is the final determinant of rotation due to angular momentum. The core movements of flexion, extension, and tilt bending are usually caused by internal forces. They allow changes in body position (Poo and Semadeni 2006).

Equilibrium behaviour

The most important objective in ski technique is to maintain a dynamic equilibrium (Mester 1997). All other factors are incidental to the ability to remain balanced over the skis. During the run, the effects of all applied forces must be controlled by the skier as far as possible, so that the resulting force runs through the support surface. As long as this is the case, the skier is in a state of dynamic balance and does not fall (Poo and Semadeni 2006).

Carving skiing

Since the introduction of carving skis in the 1990s, skiing technique has changed significantly. These skis are side-cut and necessitate the use of binding plates. A major difference between carving and parallel turns is that the carving turn is initiated without rotational body movement (Tutz 2003).

The fact that carving skis permit smaller curve radii with a relatively high speed results in increased burdens for the skiers (Jais 2005). In the case of an ideal swing, which means a swing without a slip component, the centrifugal and centripetal forces are equal. Therefore the skier must oppose increasing centrifugal force with corresponding muscle strength.

In carving, the 'curved turn' is important (Kaps *et al.* 2000). Using this technique, steering takes place along the ski edges without any lateral skid component. The navigable curve radius during carved turns is a function of the ski waist, on-edge angle, ski binding (Federolf *et al.* 2004), and ski flexion. The more strongly waisted the ski and the greater the on-edge angle, the more strongly must the ski flex to maintain contact with the slope along the total length

of the edge. The curve cut into the snow under full contact with the slope is designated the turn radius.

Risk factors

While some risks are inherent in the very nature of the activities themselves, others may result from human error and negligence on the part of those involved in preparing, organizing, staging, and participating in the activities. Most studies are case series investigations and provide little useful information on risk factors. Intrinsic risk factors include lower ability, younger age, past injury, and female gender (Noe and Paillard 2005). Extrinsic risk factors are mostly environmental conditions, improper ski equipment, incorrect binding adjustment, no helmet, some slope characteristics, and no wrist guards (Hagel B, 2005).

Altitude acclimatization and altitude illness

When training for skiing and snowboarding, athletes can be exposed to moderate to high altitudes (5–12 000 ft or 1550–3660 m). Altitude illness syndromes are rarely encountered under 7000 ft (2100 m) and are almost universal over 14 000 ft. if ascent is rapid. Multiple physiological events combine to produce symptoms. At 8000 ft (2440 m), the 'normal' Pao_2 is 60 with an arterial saturation of 92%. Ventilation increases, producing a respiratory alkalosis for several days, and plasma volume decreases by 10–15% within hours, but fluid may develop and produce peripheral oedema. Resting heart rate is high, yet cardiac output drops because of lower stroke volume. Acclimatization occurs gradually and is 80% complete after 10 days. The risk of acute altitude syndromes is highest in the first few days (FIS 2008).

Temperatures

Ski and snowboard competitions and training occur in environments where hypothermic reactions can develop (Rocky Mountain Ramblers Association 2000; FIS 2008).

Hypothermia occurs when the body cannot generate or conserve enough heat to overcome losses due to exposure to the environment. Exposure causing heat loss can be due to temperature, humidity, or wind chill factor. The impact that wind chill has on lowering the relative temperature has often been overlooked in winter competitions, and has led to severe cases of hypothermia.

◆ **Acute hypothermia** is a sudden drop in body core temperature within a few hours. This generally happens when the body has been submerged in cold water with resultant wet clothing or as a consequence of a sudden change in the environment in which the ambient temperature drops rapidly, possibly in combination with precipitation and increased wind.

◆ **Chronic hypothermia** is a gradual drop in body core temperature after several hours of exposure to environmental conditions not considered extremely severe, caused simply by not paying proper attention to basic prevention considerations.

Winter storms can bring high winds, heavy snowfall, and changing temperatures. Sudden changes in temperature can also weaken the snowpack. Visibility can be reduced to whiteout conditions and old ski tracks can be covered by blowing snow, causing groups to be delayed or stranded, or to ski onto more hazardous terrain. Wind can dramatically increase the chances of cold injuries such as frostbite and hypothermia.

Hazardous terrain

Unseen holes, depressions, embankments, rock bands, and cliffs present hazards to skiers, especially in whiteout conditions. Thinly covered rocks, boulders, bushes, deadfall, tree stumps, and roots can lead to injurious falls. Trees are obvious obstacles to avoid. Uncontrolled skiing or sliding into trees can be fatal.

The snow surface can be inconsistent, with varying types of snow, ruts, grooves, bumps, icy patches, and water channels. Temperature and wind are important factors in determining snowpack and snow surface condition. The warmth of the sun can affect the snow surface in varying amounts depending on exposure time and exposure angle.

Equipment

The design and function of equipment, such as multimode release bindings and modern mid-calf-height boots, contribute a great deal to the safety of skiing (Noe and Paillard 2005). In alpine skiing, the ski-pole grip may cause an injury to the thumb.

Skiing injuries

Alpine skiing is a popular sport with a significant risk of injury (Koehle *et al.* 2002). The nature of the injuries has changed considerably over the last 10 years. Lower leg injuries are becoming less common, while the incidence of knee sprains and upper extremity injuries has increased. Much of this change can be attributed to advances in binding technology, which have effectively reduced lower leg injury but have not adequately addressed the issue of knee sprains. Upper extremity injuries constitute approximately a third of skiing injuries, with ulnar collateral ligament sprains of the metacarpophalangeal joint of the thumb and shoulder injuries being the most common.

Köhne *et al.* (2007) examined the results of the examination of 5346 patients who were treated during the winter seasons between 1999–2000 and 2005–2006. They included 3355 injured skiers who used a carving ski, and 1670 injured skiers who used a conventional ski. The study revealed that the injuries have changed since the introduction of the carving ski. Carving skiers suffer significantly fewer jnee injuries, such as cruciate ligament ruptures, than conventional skiers. However, carving skiers are injured more often in the upper extremity, particularly the shoulder region, than conventional skiers.

Accidents during skiing and snowboarding commonly involve collision with the hard solid surface of snow or ice, or with another object such as a tree, rock, pylon, or another skier or snowboarder, often at high speeds or with a significant drop in altitude. Advances in equipment add to the risks.

Dislocation injuries

A dislocation is an injury where the normal joint relationship is disrupted by one of the articular surfaces being forced out of the joint socket or displaced from normal alignment. It is best to reduce a dislocation as quickly as possible after it occurs. Reduction is usually easier to accomplish shortly after the injury, resulting in tremendous relief of pain and reduction in the possibility of vascular or neurological damage to the extremity involved (FIS 2008).

Skier's thumb

A sprain to the ulnar collateral ligament of the metacarpophalangeal joint of the thumb is a commonly seen injury in skiing which is often referred to as 'skier's thumb'. The mechanism of injury is generally abduction of the proximal phalanx with occasional hyperextension.

Elbow

Dislocation of an elbow joint is usually due to high-energy trauma. Gentle palpation of the deformity and slight passive movements usually differentiate it from a fracture.

Shoulder

Shoulder dislocation is the most commonly seen dislocation in skiing. Normally the humerus dislocates antero-inferiorly; a posterior dislocation is rare. Early reduction by traction and small rotating movements is normally easy. If time has passed and protective muscle contraction has occurred, reduction may be impossible without anaesthesia.

Ankle

Ankle dislocation is a serious condition. Usually it occurs with a trimalleolar ankle fracture.

Knee

A total knee dislocation is uncommon. Generally only the patella is dislocated. A dislocated patella is normally easily reduced with extension and flexion movements of the knee.

Hip

High-energy trauma is needed to dislocate the hip. A hip dislocation almost never occurs without acetabular fracture. Reduction should be achieved as soon as possible to avoid damage to the sciatic nerve. Hospital treatment is always obligatory after a hip dislocation.

Fractures

Advances in equipment add to the risks of fracture, which are already high as a consequence of collisions. A basic understanding of the nature and possible complications of various fractures is critical for effective triage. Evaluation includes 'open' versus 'closed', 'simple' versus 'comminuted', possible joint involvement, possible vascular compromise or haemorrhage, and possible nerve damage (FIS 2008).

Fingers, wrist, and forearm

These upper limb injuries occur mostly with skiing and snowboard activities. They frequently result when the skier falls backward onto his/her hands.

Upper arm

A fracture of the humerus may result from a direct blow or a fall onto the outstretched hand.

Clavicle

Fractures of the clavicle are frequently the result of impact forces radiating up the arm to the collar bone.

Foot

Fractures of the small bones within the foot can result from repetitive stress over time.

Ankle

Fractures to the ankle are more common in snowboarding. On initial assessment, these are sometimes difficult to distinguish from a more severe sprain.

Lower leg

Fractures to the tibia and fibula seem to have increased with advances in skis, lifts, and boots which contribute to increased torque on the lower leg.

Upper leg

A suspected femoral fracture must be splinted in traction to avoid excessive bleeding into the thigh.

Hip

The typical position for a suspected fractured hip is with the leg found in external rotation and shortening of the involved leg.

Pelvis

Fractures to the pelvis result from the application of considerable forces, often associated with compression or a fall from a height. A fracture of the pelvis may result in significant blood loss. This is a serious injury. The volume of blood loss can lead to shock and, if not treated, can be lethal. Always begin treatment for possible shock if a pelvic fracture is suspected. Additionally, suspect a possible associated internal injury to the bladder that can often accompany a pelvic fracture.

Specific skiing injuries

Head injury

Sports-related minor head injuries have become increasingly more apparent in skiing and snowboarding disciplines over the past several years. Concussion can result from collisions with other athletes, equipment, or environmental surfaces, or may even occur without any direct blow to the head if sufficient forces are involved, for example in a whiplash type mechanism.

Definition of concussion

Concussion is defined as a complex pathophysiological process affecting the brain which is induced by traumatic biomechanical forces (McCrory *et al.* 2005). Common features which incorporate clinical, pathological, and biomechanical injury constructs that can be used to define the nature of a concussive head injury include the following.

1. Concussion may be caused by a direct blow to the head, face, neck, or elsewhere on the body with an 'impulsive' force transmitted to the head.

2. Concussion typically results in the rapid onset of short-lived impairment of neurological function that resolves spontaneously.

3. Concussion may result in neuropathological changes, but the acute clinical symptoms largely reflect a functional disturbance rather than structural injury.

4. Concussion results in a graded set of clinical syndromes which may or may not involve loss of consciousness. Resolution of the clinical and cognitive symptoms typically follows a sequential course.

5. Concussion is typically associated with grossly normal structural neuroimaging studies.

Any patient, with or without a helmet, who has suffered a blow to the head or face risks developing an injury to the brain. Injury to the brain is the most common cause of death observed in skiing and snowboarding. Trauma to the head resulting in a change in mental status, symptoms such as headache, nausea, and imbalance, or clinical signs such as disorientation, amnesia, and loss of consciousness are suggestive of an injury to the brain.

Head injury, like any injury, requires a rehabilitative process to ensure the optimal efficient and safe mechanism to allow a successful return to full training/competitive ability. The basic principles are essentially similar to those of rehabilitation for all injuries: a graded stepwise approach to increasing training load while on the lookout for any abnormal responses to the progressive load increase.

Spinal injuries

Skiing and snowboarding, which include rapid acceleration, deceleration, and rotation of the spine, can be a source of mechanisms causing spinal injury. The majority of injuries to the spine result from trauma or excessive movement of the spine in flexion, extension, rotation, lateral bending, compression, or distraction. The type of force involved can cause vertebral fractures, dislocations, subluxations, cord contusions or vascular damage. Movement of a patient into neutral alignment is contraindicated if this movement causes neck or back pain or if resistance is met in this process.

Common knee injuries

During recent decades the pattern of injuries in skiing has changed. The previous tendency to ankle or leg fracture has moved towards the knee, where most leg injuries now take place. This tendency is clearly seen in alpine and freestyle skiing. The use of carving skis in alpine skiing is blamed for the more severe tibia condylar fractures experienced.

Mechanism of trauma

Knee injuries can occur in all skiing disciplines. In most of these accidents the skier falls down, the bindings are not released, and excessive stress is applied to the knee. Severe injuries can occur without any major violence: leaning back in a turn and forcing yourself back up again in slalom without falling can be the reason for an anterior cruciate ligament (ACL) rupture. Fractures in the knee region usually need more energy and are mainly seen in high-speed disciplines such as Super-G or downhill (FIS 2008).

Primary diagnosis

Severe deformity in the knee region typically means a fracture or a total dislocation of the knee. A ligament injury seldom shows

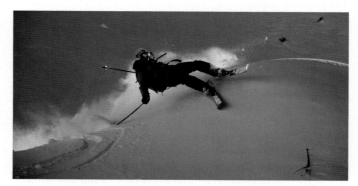

Fig. 4.19.4 Severe forces applied to the knee in giant slalom. © Scott Sady, *USA Today*. Copyright © greg-Fotolia.com

gross deformity. Early swelling after an injury to the knee is a sign of probable haemarthrosis. This indicates a ligamentous injury or intra-articular fracture.

Common internal derangements of the knee

Medial cruciate ligament rupture

This is one of the most common alpine ski injuries, accounting for 20–25% of all injuries in beginners and low-intermediate skiers in particular. Injury occurs as a result of application of excessive valgus force to the knee joint, because of a fall, the skis crossing, or the snowplough stance widening. In advanced skiers, it usually occurs as a result of unexpectedly 'catching an edge' which throws the front of the ski outwards. Conservative treatment is recommended. This means rehabilitation in which proprioceptive training and muscle strengthening exercises are key modes.

Meniscal lesion

This occurs in approximately 5–10% of all ski injuries, often in association with damage to another structure. Meniscal lesions range from small bruising or peripheral tears to more significant tears. Rotational stress is applied to a flexed weight-bearing knee, usually as a result of catching an edge at speed. Return to sport is often possible 3 weeks after surgical resection of a meniscal tear. Following surgical fixation, about 2–3 months is needed before a return to full functional ability and full sport activities is possible (FIS 2008).

Anterior cruciate ligament rupture

This accounts for 10–15% of all ski injuries. It is often associated with injuries to other structures within the knee, almost always the medial cruciate ligament and/or the meniscus. A retrospective review of ACL injuries among professional alpine skiers was performed to compare gender-related differences in injury incidence. A total of 7155 ski patrollers or instructors (4537 men and 2618 women) were screened for knee injuries before each ski season between 1991 and 1997 (Viola *et al.* 1999). The incidence of ACL rupture was 4.2 injuries per 100 000 skier-days in men and 4.4 injuries per 100 000 skier-days in women. These data suggest that the incidences of ACL injuries among male and female professional alpine skiers are similar.

Data collected from elite French national teams (379 athletes: 188 women and 191 men) from 1980 to 2005 (Pujol *et al.* 2007) identified the overall ACL injury incidence as 8.5 per 100 skier-seasons. The primary ACL injury rate was 5.7 per 100 skier-seasons. The prevalence of re-injury (same knee) was 19%. The prevalence of a bilateral injury (injury of the other knee) was 30.5%. At least one additional ACL surgical procedure (mean, 2.4 procedures) was required for 39% of the injured athletes. ACL injury rates among national competitive alpine skiers are high and have not declined in the last 25 years.

In recent years, a new carving ski has become extremely popular. A cause for great concern is the possibility that these new skis are associated with a higher risk of injury. The ACL rupture can be explained by the application of an isometric internal force leading to the injury. Hence it follows that the creation of high forces during rapid speed changes or narrow curving using super side-cut skis might lead to isolated ruptures of the ACL (Kalbermatten *et al.* 2000).

The main mechanisms predisposing to ACL damage in alpine skiers are as follows.

1. **The phantom foot** The majority of all ACL ruptures in alpine skiing are thought to be caused by the phantom foot mechanism (Johnson *et al.* 1996). This occurs when the tail of the downhill ski in combination with the stiff back of a ski boot acts as a lever to apply a unique combination of twisting and bending force across the knee joint. These ACL ruptures do not require high speeds or steep slopes.

2. **Boot-induced ACL injury** In this mechanism (Johnson *et al.* 1996) pressure from the boot against the back of leg combines with quadriceps muscle contraction to keep the knee extended (Gerland 2004). This pushes the tibia forward relative to the femur and the ACL tears as a result.

3. **Hyperflexion of knee** This is an unusual mechanism, although often seen in skiing, in which hyperflexion occurs at the knee while attempting to prevent a fall backwards (Fetto and Marshall 1980).

4. **Situations predisposing situations to ACL injuries**
   - attempting to get up whilst still moving after a fall
   - attempting a recovery from an off-balance position
   - attempting to sit down after losing control.

Paletta *et al.* (1992) found that, in alpine skiing, beginners typically injure the ACL by a valgus–external rotation mechanism and advanced skiers by a valgus–internal rotation or flexion with quadriceps loading.

Treatment and rehabilitation

Immediate treatment of soft tissue injury (PRICE)

Immediately after injury to a ligament, tendon, or muscle attached to the knee, there will be an inflammatory reaction of varying degree depending on the severity of the injury. In a strain, sprain, or rupture of soft tissue, blood vessels can be damaged and bleeding may occur. The accumulated blood and inflammatory exudate produces pain and swelling of the surrounding tissues. If left untreated, the swelling may inhibit healing of the damaged tissues and lead to spasm of the surrounding muscles.

The immediate aim following injury is to reduce the amount of bleeding at the site of injury and prevent further damage. Treatment must be applied as soon as possible and the most effective way of doing this is to follow the PRICE principles (protection, rest, ice, elevation) (Kerr 1998).

Treatment of ACL rupture

Normally a reconstruction of the ligament is necessary. In some disciplines this can be done after the season. If instability symptoms are profound, reconstruction should be performed immediately. Reconstruction is normally done with autologous grafts (STG, BTB, or quadriceps tendon). Some surgeons use allografts with good results. Preferably, the operation should be carried out arthroscopically. Return to full activities takes about 6 months. Alpine skiing can be started with free skiing about 5 months after the reconstruction if there have been no complications with surgery or rehabilitation (FIS 2008).

Rehabilitation after knee injury: basic principles

Muscle conditioning

Following an overuse injury of the knee, the surrounding muscles may weaken due to a combination of pain, inflammation, and inactivity. Muscle conditioning involves the restoration of strength, power, and endurance and the re-education of muscle imbalance (Spring *et al.* 2005).

Flexibility

Overuse injuries of the knee may be accompanied by inflammation and adaptive shortening of the surrounding soft tissues. There are three types of stretches: static, dynamic, and proprioceptive neuromuscular facilitation.

Functional exercises

As pain and inflammation settle, and strength, power, endurance, and proprioception of the lower limb improve, functional activities based on the fundamentals of the chosen sport are started.

Proprioception

Proprioception is the body's sense of joint position, pressure, and movement. During a sporting activity, proprioceptive information plays a key role in the control, organization, and timing of actions. In the knee, the sensory afferent information comes from mechanoreceptors situated in the cruciate ligaments, menisci, infrapatellar fat pad, and joint capsule.

Sports-specific training

Athletic activity involves the integration of all joints and muscles involved in that action. Strength gains are specific to the type of contraction used during training. Therefore, in order to improve the strength and coordination of a sports-specific activity, exercises must be similar to that activity (FIS 2008).

Low back pain

All athletes are susceptible to back injury. In skiing, few athletes make it through an entire season without experiencing some form of back pain (FIS 2008). The pounding experienced through repetitive jamming such as in slalom or downhill skiing results in excessive forces across the lower lumbar and pelvis. Back pain in skiers can be secondary to minor sprains and strains, facet joint injury, malalignment syndromes, or acute discs.

Lumbar ligament strains and muscle strains

These are common injuries associated with a specific event such as inappropriate lifting, overuse, or a recent fall. They are characterized by localized pain that has a specific mechanism of injury and no neurological involvement.

Facet joint syndrome

This represented 10–15% of back injuries in a retrospective study of Canadian athletes. Facet joint syndrome occurs when the facet joints become strained or inflamed after undergoing extreme forces. The forces can be in the form of either an extension or a compression injury. This injury is characterized by localized pain with only moderate radiation. The surrounding muscles are in spasm.

There is no radicular pain and no neurological findings. There is localized loss of range of motion (Dvorak *et al.* 2008), usually at a specific level that identifies the facet. Physiotherapy, mobilization, or manipulation (Dvorak *et al.* 2008) of the facet joints is also useful as inflammation of the facet decreases.

Malalignment injury

Malalignment is the most common injury associated with back pain seen in ski teams. Characteristically, athletes complain of low back pain that can be central or lateral, usually centred on the sacrum or sacroiliac joint. Once the alignment has been corrected, there will be an immediate reduction in pain and an increase in pain-free mobility of the lower back. Another problem that is associated with blocking of the sacroiliac joint is blocking of the thoracolumbar junction. The thoracolumbar blocking can be relieved using mobilization or manipulation.

Acute disc syndrome

This syndrome is characterized by acute severe lower back pain with radiation to one extremity. Pain usually radiates to the foot. Neurological examination reveals reflex changes and weakness of muscles relevant to the affected nerve root.

Prevention of ski injuries

Injuries occur in all skiing sports, but most frequently in alpine skiing and snowboarding. The severity of injuries varies, but knee and head injuries are of particular concern in all disciplines, as are wrist fractures and other upper extremity injuries in snowboarding. Such injuries often lead to a prolonged absence from sport and increase the risk of chronic problems, permanent disability, or even death in the case of serious head and neck injuries. Effective prevention depends on comprehensive information on risk factors and injury mechanisms. Unfortunately, our current understanding is still limited and, consequently, we have a limited ability to suggest effective preventive measures (FIS 2008).

References

Dvorak, J., Dvorak, V., Gilliar, W., Schneider, W., Spring, H., and Tritschler, T. (2008). *Musculoskeletal Manual Medicine*. Diagnosis and Treatment. Thieme, New York.

Federolf, P., Lüthi, A., Fauve, M., Rhyner, H.U., Amman, W., and Dual, J. (2004). Determination of turning parameters in carved skiing and application to a numerical ski-binding model. In: *Proceedings of the 22nd International Symposium of Biomechanics in Sport*, pp. 301–4.

Fetto, J.F. and Marshall, J.L. The natural history and diagnosis of anterior cruciate ligament insufficiency. *Clinical Orthopaedics and Related Research*, **147**, 29–38.

FIS (2008) *FIS Medical Guide*. Available online at: http://www.fis-ski.com (accessed 30 September 2009).

Gerland, S. (2004). Veränderungen der Verletzungsmuster beim alpinem Skilauf durch die Carvingtechnik. Inaugural Dissertation, Medizinische Fakultät Bayerischen Universität, Würzburg.

Hagel, B. (2005). Skiing and snowboarding injuries. *Medicine and Sport Science*, **48**, 74–119.

Jais, R. (2005). *Verletzungen im alpinem Skisport unter Berücksichtigung der Entwicklung in der Skitechnologie*. Dissertation der Fakultät für Medizin der Technischen Universität München, pp. 13–17.

Johnson, R., Shealy, J., and Ettlinger, C. (1996). *Training for Knee-friendly Skiing*. Vermont Safety Research, Underhill, VT.

Kalbermatten, D.F., Anderson, S.E., and Ballmer, F.T. (2000). ACL rupture caused by a fast narrow turn on super sidecut skis. *European Journal of Trauma*, **26**, 312–14.

Kaps, P., Mössner, M., Nachbauer, W., and Stenberg, R. (2000). Pressure under a ski during carved turns. In: *Proceedings of the 2nd Internationl Congress on Skiing and Science*, pp. 180–202.

Kerr, K. (1998) *PRICE Guidelines: Guidelines for Management of Soft Tissue Injury*, pp. 25–45. Chartered Society of Physiotherapy, London.

Koehle, M.S., Lloyd-Smith, R., Taunton, J.E., and McGavin, A. (2002). Alpine ski injuries and their prevention. *Sports Medicine*, **32**, 785–93.

Köhne, G., Kusche, H., Schaller, C., and Gutsfeld, P. (2007). Ski accidents—change since introduction of carving ski. *Sportorthopädie Sporttraumatologie*, **23**, 63–7.

McCrory P, Johnston K, Meeuwisse W, *et al.* (2005). Summary and agreement statement of the 2nd International Conference on Concussion in Sport, Prague 2004. *Clinical Journal of Sport Medicine*, **15**, 48–55.

Mester, J. (1997). Movement regulation in alpine skiing. In: Müller, E., Schwameder, H., Kornexl, E., and Raschner, C. (eds), pp. 333–48. *Science and Skiing*. E.&F.N. Spon, London.

Mueller, E. and Schwameder, H. (2003). Bioiomechanical aspects of new techniques in alpine skiing and ski- jumping. *Journal of Sports Sciences*, **21**, 679–92.

Noe, F. and Paillard, T. (2005). Is postural control affected by expertise in alpine skiing? *British Journal of Sports Medicine*, **39**, 835–7.

Paletta, G.A., Levine, D.S., and O'Brien, S.J. (1992). Patterns of meniscal injury associated with acute anterior cruciate ligament injury in skiers. *American Journal of Sports Medicine*, **20**, 542–7.

Poo, A. and Semadeni, R. (2006). Biomechanik im Schneesport. *Swiss Snowsports, Academy Praxis Beilage*, **1**, 1–8.

Pujol, N., Rousseaux Blanchi, M.P., and Chambat, P. (2007). The incidence of anterior cruciate ligament injuries among competitive alpine skiers. *American Journal of Sports Medicine*, **35**, 1070–4.

Rocky Mountain Ramblers Association (2000)

Serge, P. *et al.* (2000).

Spring, H., Dvorak, J., Dvorak, V., Schneider, W., Tritschler, T., and Villige,r B. (2005). *Theorie und Praxis der Trainingstherapie* (2nd edn). Thieme, Stuttgart.

Tutz, M. (2003). Biomechanische Grundlagen des Carvens. *Österreichisches Journal für Sportmedizin*, **4**, 6–10.

Viola, R.W., Steadman, J.R., Mair, S.D., Briggs, K.K., and Sterett, W.I. (1999). Anterior cruciate ligament imjury incidence among male and female professional alpine skiers. *American Journal of Sports Medicine*, **27**, 792–5.

von Duvillard, S.P., Rundell, K.W., Bilodeau, B., and Bacharach, D.W. (2000). Biomechanics of alpine and Nordic skiing. In: W.E. Garrett and D.T. Kirkendall (eds), *Excercise and Sport Science*, pp. 617–20. Lippincott–Williams & Wilkins, Philadelphia, PA.

4.20

Tennis injuries

Cathy Speed

Introduction

Tennis is a game of power and endurance, involving running, cutting, sprinting, stopping and starting, lunging, rotation, and smashing. It is played on different surfaces with rackets that can differ significantly in their characteristics and by individuals over a wide range of age and fitness. Injuries in tennis are common and can be related to one or more of these factors, which can be broadly divided into intrinsic and extrinsic types (Table 4.20.1).

Equipment and training factors inevitably play a major role in the development of injury and these will be reviewed prior to discussing specific injuries.

Equipment

Rackets and strings

Evolution of the racket and stringing has allowed modifications in technique to generate power, speed, and topspin. The modern tennis racket is made of composite materials which allow a lighter, stiffer, and more durable frame to generate higher forces with greater reliability and accuracy. The emphasis has been on a racket that dissipates minimum shock and vibrations and has a large 'sweet spot' where the ball impact and rebound is most powerful and accurate. There are three sweet spots: the centre of percussion (where shock to the hand is minimal), the node (where vibrations are minimum), and the maximum coefficient of restitution where the rebounding ball speed is minimum. In a modern racket, all are at or near the centre of the head and are of variable size depending on the racket.

Lighter rackets allow greater swing speed and enable the player to swing with greater wrist flexibility and generate more top spin. However if the racket is too light for the player, the generation of less power at the racket head can result in attempts to compensate with changes in technique and/or overloading anywhere along the kinetic chain. Lighter rackets can also turn more easily in the hand, resulting in a mishit and arm injuries.

Grip size is a topic of controversy. The general recommendation is that the racket should be held with a fairly relaxed grip to avoid overuse injuries of the arm and loss of racket speed and stroke effectiveness [1].

Strings vary in type, quality, diameter and tension. Good quality strings will return 95% of the energy they absorb to the ball and, within limits, a lower string tension returns greater energy. Anecdotally, a tighter string tension is considered to confer greater control. Although much effort has been made to minimize

vibrations to hand and arm, there is no clinical evidence that vibration results in elbow, wrist or hand injury.

Tennis balls

The four principal characteristics of a tennis ball are its mass, size, compression resistance, and bounce. Although the bounce has not changed much over recent decades, balls have become much harder (i.e. more resistant to compression at impact).

There are a number of types of ball available. They are grouped into pressurized balls (types 1–3) and pressureless balls (i.e. same as atmospheric pressure). The type 2 ball is the standard ball; type 1 balls are harder than the others and type 3 balls are bigger. Type 1 balls are used on slow surfaces to promote faster play, and type 3 balls are used on faster surfaces to promote slower play. High-altitude balls give a lower bounce to compensate for the difference in air density at altitude. Elite players use a variety of balls and are sensitive to the different feel of each; there is no evidence that the ball type is associated with likelihood of injury (Brody and Smith 2001).

Surfaces

Tennis is the only racket sport that formally involves play on a wide variety of surfaces. These are mainly grass courts (seeded turf on a soil base), clay courts (layers of crushed stone of decreasing diameter topped with a fine gritty material (e.g. crushed brick)), hard courts, and various synthetic surfaces with different pace and cushioning properties. For example acrylic surfaces use asphalt and/or concrete as a sub-base onto which can be laid an optional layer of crumb rubber which acts as a shock pad and reduces the impact forces transmitted to the player. The uppermost (playing) surface is acrylic paint mixed with sand. Clay and synthetic courts appear to be associated with a smaller risk of lower limb and spinal injury than hard courts (Miller 2006). The sliding characteristics of the surface and the friction between the shoe and surface seem to be more important than the cushioning properties in relation to injury risk (Nigg and Segesser 1988).

Shoes

The requirements of a tennis shoe are that it provides some support, appropriate levels of traction with the playing surface, and some cushioning. As with any sport, the needs will vary between individuals and playing surfaces. It is often the interaction between the loading patterns through the lower limb, the shoe, and the surface that predict injury. A higher incidence of injury has been reported with stiffer shoes (Nigg and Segesser 1988; Miller 2006).

Table 4.20.1 Factors influencing injury in tennis

Intrinsic factors	Extrinsic factors
Physical conditioning	Surface
◆ Flexibility	Shoes
◆ Endurance	Racket characteristics
◆ Functional strength	Environment
Technique	Strings
Training	Tennis balls(?)
◆ Volume	
◆ Intensity	
◆ Type	
Pre-existing injuries / medical conditions	

However, lateral stability of the shoe is important in prevention of injuries (Lüthi *et al.* 1986).

Technique

Tennis is an excellent example of the kinetic chain of energy transfer from the ground reaction force to the feet, through the lower limbs, spine, and trunk, to the shoulder, forearm, and wrist with acceleration of racket head through the ball (Figs 4.20.1 and 4.20.2). The kinetic chains in ground strokes and the serve are slightly different, but the following are common to both: (a) up to 60% of the force generated comes from the legs and trunk; (b) the conversion of linear to rotational energy around a stable leg; (c) each segment has a cocking (stabilization) phase and an acceleration phase; (d) large and rapid movements are required in the joints, especially the shoulder (Kibler 1995; Schonborn 1999; Pluim *et al.* 2006). Controlling this energy transfer directly influences performance, and a lack of control or a deficit anywhere along the kinetic chain, predisposes to injury. Such 'deficits' include local pathology, reduced range of motion, muscle imbalance, weakness, joint instability, and poor technique. Leg strength is important, and the 'core' abdominal musculature and glutei play a significant role in trunk

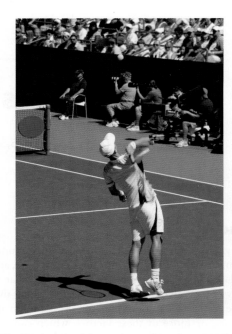

Fig. 4.20.2 The kinetic chain of the tennis serve from the toes to the wrist hand and racket. Note the external rotation of the shoulder. © Christos Kyratsous (Fotolia.com).

and core stability, providing a mechanical link between the lower and upper limbs.

The ball is in contact with the racket for 3–6 msec, and the relative path of the ball and racket determine the type and direction of spin imparted. The racket and ball speed are generated by the length of the backswing, with a longer backswing allowing a greater distance to generate racket speed through the forward swing. Spin is influenced by the size and shape of the swing and the type of grip, with the more extreme western or semi-western grips imparting greater spin. The influence of these grips on injury is undetermined.

In the serve, the kinetic chain must involve some knee flexion during the leg–hip segment in cocking. Knee extension from flexion transfers the ground reaction force to the trunk. Forward push occurs through the back leg, with the forward leg acting as a stable post to allow rotation force. The trunk and scapula rotate, the scapula retracts, and the shoulder externally rotates allowing shoulder arm and racket positioning in cocking. This is followed by internal rotation in cocking. The forearm pronates through the hitting zone with the shoulder in internal rotation. Common faults in the kinetic chain are weak leg muscles, lack of knee bend, no hip or trunk rotation in cocking or follow-through, and tight shoulder internal rotators, resulting in compensatory injuries anywhere along the chain.

The modern open-stance forehand allows rapid rotational momentum (Fig. 4.20.3(a)). Unlike the serve, most of the push-off and rotation occurs through the back leg, and racket acceleration is further augmented by shoulder internal rotation and, later, forearm pronation and wrist flexion (Kibler 1995; Schonborn 1999; Pluim *et al.* 2006). Faults include weak hip muscles and poor shoulder internal rotation. The latter can result in overuse of the forearm and wrist to achieve racket acceleration, and injuries to these sites. Elbow injuries are particularly likely if the elbow is too far forward, and wrist injuries if the wrist is weak.

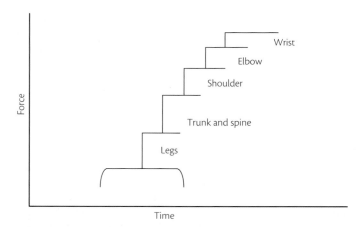

Fig. 4.20.1 The kinetic chain in the tennis serve. Each segment generates force and acts as a stable base for the next segment.

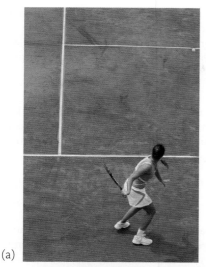

(a)

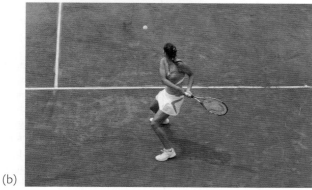

(b)

Fig. 4.20.3 (a) The forehand and (b) the backhand: adequate body positioning with spinal and hip rotation is important. © lilufoto (Fotolia.com).

8.2 (1.2) seconds per point, and baseline players have a mean duration of 15.7 (3.5) seconds per point (Kibler and van der Meer 2001).

At the competitive level there is a work-to-rest ratio of between 1:2 and 1:5, with points having an average length ranging from 3 seconds on some of the faster surfaces (grass, carpet, and indoor) to close to 15 seconds on others. Total playing time is only 20–30% of total match time. (Bernardi *et al.* 1998; Kovacs 2006). Such findings influence the physical condition regimes appropriate for tennis. Tennis is predominantly an anaerobic activity, but requires high levels of aerobic conditioning to avoid fatigue and to aid in recovery between points. For successful competitive play, $Vo_{2\,max}$ levels should be above 50 ml/kg/min (Kovacs 2006).

Sports-specific training includes shadowing to replicate the multidirectional movement patterns in tennis that demand speed and agility. Stop–start sprints of no more than 20 m are included. High flexion, extension, and rotational forces through the spine make functional core control work very important. The rotators of the shoulder are particularly important not only in the serve but also in the return of ground strokes. In the serve, shoulder internal, external, and diagonal peak torques are all high. The greatest contribution to racket-head speed comes from shoulder internal rotation, wrist flexion, upper arm horizontal adduction, forearm pronation, and forward movement of the shoulder. Hence strength training should also focus upon concentric and eccentric rotator cuff strengthening and close attention to any muscle imbalances (Roetert *et al.* 1992).

Lower body strengthening is also very important, given that the majority of tennis injuries affect the lower body. Proprioceptive work should also be a priority. Flexibility training addresses the inherent imbalances of the sport; the dominant arm usually shows a large range of external rotation but less internal rotation. The latter

In the single-handed backhand the trunk rotates around the stable lead leg and shoulder external rotation allows acceleration of the racket head through the ball. The same applies to the dominant arm in the double-handed backhand, whilst the non-dominant arm goes through a similar pattern to that seen in the dominant arm in the forehand. Errors in the chain include lack of trunk rotation, lack of shoulder external rotation in the dominant arm and, in the non-dominant arm of the double-handed backhand, issues similar to those seen in the forehand. Leading with the elbow indicates over-reliance on arm muscles rather than trunk and shoulder. Too much underspin and hitting behind the body is seen in those with injuries due to lack of trunk rotation, and wrist injuries are seen in those who cock the wrists because of over-reliance on the wrists for force generation.

Generation of top spin in ground strokes demands a larger back-swing, and an open stance allows greater trunk rotation to achieve greater power through the racket head. Top spin is usually easiest with more extreme grips such as the western or semi-western grip.

Physiology and conditioning

The length of rallies will be influenced by the style of an athlete's play. Attacking players have a mean (SD) duration of 4.8 (0.4) seconds per point, whole-court players have a mean duration of

Table 4.20.2 Muscle activity during the forehand ground stroke [13, with permission]

Action	Muscles used
Acceleration phase	
Lower body push-off	Gastrocnemius/soleus, quadriceps, gluteals (concentric)
Trunk rotation	Obliques, abdominals, back extensors (concentric/eccentric)
Forward swing	Anterior deltoid, subscapularis, biceps, serratus anterior, pectoralis major, wrist flexors, forearm pronators (concentric)
Follow-through phase	
Lower body	Gastrocnemius/soleus, quadriceps, gluteals (concentric)
Trunk rotation	Obliques, abdominals, back extensors (concentric/eccentric)
Arm deceleration	Infraspinatus/teres minor, triceps, serratus anterior, rhomboids, trapezius, wrist extensors, forearm supinators (eccentric)

Reproduced with permission from Ellenbecker, T. and Tiley, C. (2001). Training muscles for strength and speed. In: P. Roetart and J. Groppel (eds), *World Class Tennis Technique: Master Every Stroke*, pp.61–83. Human Kinetics, Champaign, IL.

Table 4.20.3 Muscle activity during the single-handed backhand ground stroke

Action	Muscles used
Acceleration phase	
Lower body push-off	Gastrocnemius/soleus, quadriceps, gluteals (concentric)
Trunk rotation	Obliques, abdominals, back extensors (concentric/eccentric)
Arm forward swing	Infraspinatus/teres minor, posterior deltoid, rhomboid, serratus anterior, trapezius, triceps, wrist extensors (concentric)
Follow-through phase	
Trunk rotation	Obliques, back extensors, abdominals (concentric/eccentric)
Arm deceleration	Subscapularis, pectoralis major, biceps, wrist flexors (eccentric)

Reproduced with permission from Hutchinson, M.R., Laprade, R.F., Burnett, Q.M., et al. (1995). Injury surveillance at the USTA Boys' Tennis Championships: a 6-yr study. *Medicine and Science in Sports and Exercise*, **27**, 826–30.

Table 4.20.4 Muscle activity during the serve and overhead smash

Action	Muscles
Preparation phase	
Lower body	Gastrocnemius/soleus, quadriceps, gluteals (eccentric)
Trunk rotation	Obliques, abdominals, trunk extensors (concentric/eccentric)
Cocking phase	
Trunk rotation	Back extensors (concentric), obliques (concentric/eccentric), abdominals (eccentric)
Arm motion	Infraspinatus/teres minor, supraspinatus, biceps, serratus anterior, wrist extensors (concentric), subscapularis, pectoralis major (eccentric)
Acceleration phase	
Lower body	Gastrocnemius/soleus, gluteals, quadriceps (concentric), hamstrings (eccentric)
Trunk rotation	Abdominals, obliques (concentric), back extensors (eccentric)
Arm motion	Subscapularis, pectoralis major, serratus anterior, triceps, wrist flexors, forearm pronators (concentric), biceps (eccentric)
Follow-through phase	
Lower body	Gastrocnemius/soleus, quadriceps, gluteals (eccentric)
Trunk rotation	Back extensors (eccentric), obliques, abdominals (concentric/eccentric)
Arm deceleration	Infraspinatus/teres minor, serratus trapezius, rhomboids, wrist extensors, forearm supinators (eccentric)

Reproduced with permission from Ellenbecker, T. and Tiley, C. (2001). Training muscles for strength and speed. In: P. Roetart and J. Groppel (eds), *World Class Tennis Technique: Master Every Stroke*, pp.61–83. Human Kinetics, Champaign, IL.

is a focus of flexibility training, as is hamstring range of motion, which is often reduced in tennis players partly because of the stance adopted in readiness for play. Hamstring flexibility may be asymmetrical, as it is particularly restricted in the serving back leg.

Other factors

Other factors can influence the predisposition to injury, including thermoregulatory strain (particularly due to ambient temperature and humidity), hydration status before and during play, nutrition, and available energy supplies (Hornery *et al.* 2007).

Injuries

Injury overview

Almost a third of recreational players who play for 1–2 hours per week report one or more tennis-related injuries during a competitive season, increasing to 49% in those who play for 5 hours per week (Lüthi *et al.* 1986). Such injuries can be acute, acute on chronic, or chronic. Most studies confirm a preponderance of lower limb injuries (Lüthi *et al.* 1986). One study of junior elite male tennis players reported an incidence of injury of 21.1% at a single competitive hard-court event, with half of these being new injuries and half recurrent. 52% of these were lower limb injuries, 26% were upper limb injuries, and 22% were spine injuries; 58% were sprains (Hutchinson *et al.* 1995). In older players, chronic injuries predominate because of overuse/relative overloading of an injured/degenerative tissue. Tennis has lower injury rates than contact team sports and compares with some non-contact individual sports such as golf and running (Lüthi *et al.* 1986). The lowest incidence rate (0.04 injuries per 1000 players per year) relates to those presenting to a hospital casualty department, whilst the highest rates (9.9 per 100 players) extend the definition of injury to include any medical problem (Sallis *et al.* 2001). This variation in the reported incidence rates of tennis injuries most probably reflects variation in injury definition, study design, populations under study, methods of data collection, and the duration of the follow-up or recall period.

Most studies indicate no statistically significant difference in the overall rate of injury (new and recurrent) between male and female players (Sallis *et al.* 2001). Injury risk in tennis has been shown to increase gradually with age from 0.01 injuries per player per year in the 6–12 year age group to 0.5 injuries per player per year in those over 75 years of age (Lüthi *et al.* 1986).

Insight into the effects of the level and volume of play on injury characteristics is scarce. There are very few cohort studies available that estimate a measure of the degree of association between possible risk factors and the occurrence of tennis injuries, and there are no randomized controlled trials on preventative measures in tennis.

Knee injuries

Knee injuries represent about a quarter of injuries in tennis, with patellofemoral syndrome being particularly common in younger players, where biomechanical and growth-related issues play a prominent role. Tennis is a game played across a wide age range, and pre-existing morbidities are often present in more senior players. 'Degenerative' conditions including degenerative menisci and meniscal tears and osteoarthritis are common in those who are older. Playing on more shock-absorbing surfaces and the use of shock-absorbing insoles is recommended. Many will be able to make a phased return to tennis after hip or knee replacement.

Lower leg and ankle injuries

Ankle injuries represent approximately 23% of injuries, and inversion sprains are the most common form of ankle injury in tennis. Supportive ankle braces provide an opportunity for early return to play, and are often worn as a preventative measure, but do not replace the need for proprioceptive training. Other preventative approaches including conditioning and stable cushioned footwear are important.

'Tennis leg'—a tear of one or both of the calf muscles, usually the gastrocnemius—is common in tennis as well as other sports. This injury is discussed further in Chapter 3.11. It is more common in older players and those who have restricted hamstring and calf flexibility. Prevention through flexibility work and adequate warm-up has a major role to play in reducing the likelihood of these injuries, which can result in a prolonged period out of the sport. The injury is more likely on hard surfaces and where previous injury to the calf has occurred.

Achilles tendinopathies are reported to represent 15% of injuries (Lüthi *et al.* 1986). Eccentric calf training programmes are part of a preventative training programme. Probable precipitating factors also include adverse biomechanics and the factors mentioned in relation to tennis leg.

Shoulder injuries

Considerable strain forces are transmitted through the shoulder during play, particularly during the serve. The full spectrum of sports injuries can affect the shoulder, but the most important of these are external (typically subacromial) and internal impingement syndromes. Tennis players frequently have acquired anterior capsular laxity and anterior instability of the shoulder, tightness of the posterior structures and loss of internal rotation range of motion. These changes typically are major contributors to impingements (Walch *et al.* 1992). Internal impingement is impingement between the humeral head and the posterosuperior rim of the glenoid. It occurs in the cocking position of throwing/serving (particularly when the humeral shaft goes beyond the plane of the body of the scapula), with the glenohumeral joint in maximal external rotation, maximum horizontal abduction, and in abduction or forward flexion (Fig. 4.20.4). Athletes present with posterior shoulder pain, tenderness of infraspinatus, and pain provoked by placing the shoulder into positions where impingement is occurring. Other features are usually present: acquired glenohumeral anterior instability, the loss of internal rotation range of motion, and the lack of retraction strength. Rehabilitation must address these aspects as a priority (Cools *et al.* 2008).

Elbow injuries

The magnitude of the forces across the elbow during tennis can produce tremendous valgus, internal rotation, and extension overload in players, resulting in a spectrum of possible injuries. The elbow absorbs high forces during play. During the service the elbow moves from 116° to 20° of flexion within 0.21 seconds, with ball

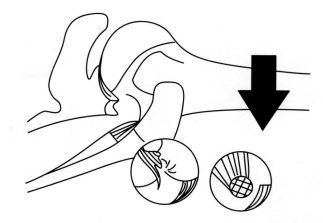

Fig. 4.20.4 Internal impingement

impact occurring at approximately 35° of flexion. During ground-strokes, the flexion and extension range is much less, averaging 11° (46°–35°) of flexion on the forehand and 18° (48°–30°) on the backhand. Angular velocity during the service motion is in the region of over 900° per second for elbow extension. The need for high internal rotation through the upper arm imposes high internal rotation forces through the elbow. There is also considerable valgus extension overload: tensile forces on the medial side, compressive forces on the lateral side, and shear across the posterior compartment (Eygendaal *et al.* 2007).

Common injuries affecting the elbow include not only lateral epicondylitis (proximal tendinopathies of the wrist extensors), which is the most frequent elbow injury, but also ulnar collateral ligament (UCL) tears, flexor–pronator tendinopathiess, ulnar neuritis, posterior impingement, and ostechondritis dissecans of the capitellum.

In tennis, the predominant activity of the wrist extensors in all strokes is one factor involved in development of the condition. Those with tennis elbow (lateral epicondylitis) have greater activity of the wrist extensor muscles during ball impact and early follow-through. Technical issues, including 'leading elbow', wrist extension, an open racket face near the time of ball impact, lack of control at follow-through, inability of experienced players to reduce impact transmission from the racket to the wrist, and elbow or ball contact in the lower half of the strings, should be considered as precipitants. Those who can quickly release their grip tightness after ball–racket impact in order to reduce impact transmission to the wrist and elbow are less likely to suffer tennis elbow.

Tennis elbow is less likely in those with a double-handed backhand, as the non-dominant arm appears to absorb more energy.

Much effort is made to reduce shock transmission to the elbow through racket weighting, stringing, and other characteristics, although the evidence that this reduces the chance of tennis elbow is scant. Similarly, a change in racket grip size does not seem to change the forearm muscle firing patterns.

Relevant factors in the development of common flexor tendon overload (medial epicondylitis) include an excessive wrist snap, 'open-stance' hitting', opening too soon on the serve, and short-arming the strokes.

As in other upper limb athletes, ulnar neuritis in tennis players may be due to an isolated injury. It may also occur in combination

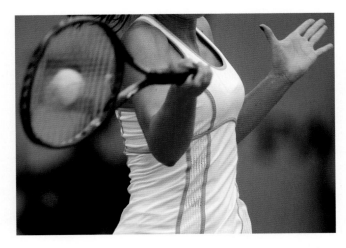

Fig. 4.20.5 The modern topspin forehand imposes considerable strain on the wrist. © karaboux (Fotolia.com).

Table 4.20.5 Causes of dorsal and/or ulnar wrist pain in tennis players

Triangular fibrocartilage complex injuries
Triquetrum-lunate ligament injury
Pisiform-triquetrum joint pain
Carpal instabilities
Fractures/stress injuries of lunate, triquetrum, and hook of the hamate
Bone oedema syndromes
Dorsal impingement syndrome
Ulnolunate impaction syndrome
Kienböck's disease
Extensor carpi ulnaris tendinopathy, instability, tear, rupture
Extensor digitorum tendinopathies
Ganglia and intra-osseous ganglion cysts
Degenerative diseases

with UCL insufficiency, chronic flexor pronator tendinopathy, compression due to a tight cubital tunnel, osteophytes from the ulnohumeral joint, muscle hypertrophy, or subluxation of the nerve. There is considerable traction on the nerve during the serve, particularly with the elbow in flexion.

Repetitive combined hyperextension, valgus, and rotation of the elbow results in a mechanical abutment of bony or soft tissues in the posterior fossa of the elbow. Ligamentous instability of the elbow, particularly UCL insufficiency, may be present. Medial ulnar collateral ligament insufficiency alters the contact area and the pressure between the posteromedial trochlea and olecranon, with subsequent development of posteromedial osteophytes.

Wrist injuries

Wrist injuries are common and potentially serious injuries, which are seen particularly in competitive players. The wrist is the upper limb joint most often affected during Grand Slam tournaments (Montalvan *et al.* 2004), and injuries to this site are reported to be

the cause of 12.6% of on-site withdrawals from the professional men's circuit (ATP Tour Medical Services 1998).

Injuries typically affect the dorsal ulnar wrist and are caused by specific technique problems: increased use of the wrist to create topspin (Fig. 4.20.5), use of the double-handed backhand, and use of a higher string tension, which increases the effect when the ball hits the racket. Extensor carpi ulnaris injuries are seen particularly in the non-dominant wrist of those with a double-handed backhand (Montalvan *et al.* 2006). Ultrasound and MRI investigations should be pursued early in all cases with ulnar wrist pain as signs can be soft and non-specific.

Back injuries

Thoracolumbar spine injuries in tennis include facet joint syndromes, spondylolysis, disc prolapse, and muscle injuries. Even in asymptomatic elite adolescent tennis players, MRI findings in the lumbar spine in particular demonstrate facet joint arthrosis and spondylolysis, most commonly in the low lumbar spine. Hamstring tightness is common in tennis players and is a risk factor for development of back pain. Flexibility, core control, and technical work are important preventative measures.

Rectus abdominis injuries

Rectus abdominis muscle strains are considered to be common in competitive tennis players and can be particularly debilitating. The mechanism appears to be eccentric overload, followed by forced contraction of the non-dominant rectus abdominis during the cocking phase of the serve when the spine is completely hyperextended (Maquirriain *et al.* 2007). This movement occurs particularly when an overhead is hit behind the player as in the modern 'kick serve'. Other muscles of the abdominal wall, such as the internal oblique, can be injured, although this occurs less commonly than injury of the rectus abdominis. Eccentrics and plyometric strengthening of the abdominal wall muscles are important not only in treatment but as part of a prevention programme.

Bone stress injuries

An elevated absolute risk for stress fractures (12.9%) in elite tennis players has been reported. The tarsal navicular, pars interarticularis, metatarsals, tibia, and the lunate appear to be the sites most commonly affected. The incidence is higher in juniors than in professional players (Maquirriain and Ghisi 2005).

Conclusions

Modern competitive tennis imposes significant demands upon the body's kinetic chain. Most injuries are preventable by close attention to equipment, technique, and conditioning. The clinician must have a high index of awareness of the wide spectrum of injuries that can occur, and the underlying inherent anatomical characteristics of competitive tennis players across a wide age range.

References

ATP Tour Medical Services (1998). *ATP Tour Tournament Physician Conference 1988*. ATP, Carlsbad, CA.

Bernardi, M., De Vito, G., Falvo, M.E., *et al.* (1998). Cardiorespiratory adjustment in middle-level tennis players. Are long term cardiovascular adjustments possible? In: A. Lees, I. Maynard, M. Hughes, and T. Reilly (eds), *Science and Racket Sports II*, pp. 20–6. E. & F.N. Spon, London.

Brody, H. and Smith, S. (2001). Revolutionary rackets. In: P. Roetart and J. Groppel J (eds). *World Class Tennis Technique: Master Every Stroke*, pp 19–39. Human Kinetics, Champaign, IL. 2001.

Cools, A.M., Declercq, G., Cagnie, B.,Cambier, D., and Witvrouw, E. (2008). Internal impingement in the tennis player:rehabilitation guidelines. *British Journal of Sports Medicine*, 42, 165–71.

Ellenbecker, T. and Tiley, C. (2001). Training muscles for strength and speed. In: P. Roetart and J. Groppel J (eds). *World Class Tennis Technique: Master Every Stroke*, pp. 61–83. Human Kinetics, Champaign, IL.

Eygendaal, D., Rahussen, F., and Diercks R. (2007). Biomechanics of the elbow joint in tennis players and relation to pathology. *British Journal of Sports Medicine*, 41, 820–3.

Hornery, D.J., Farrow, D., Mujika, I., and Young, W. (2007). An integrated physiological and performance profile of professional tennis. *British Journal of Sports Medicine*, 41, 531–6.

Hutchinson, M.R., Laprade, R.F., Burnett, Q.M., *et al.* (1995). Injury surveillance at the USTA Boys' Tennis Championships: a 6-yr study. *Medicine and Science in Sports and Exercise*, 27, 826–30.

Kibler, W.B. (1995). Biomechanical analysis of the shoulder during tennis activities. *Clinics in Sports Medicine*, 14, 79–86.

Kibler, W.B. and van der Meer, D. (2001). Mastering the kinetic chain. In: P. Roetart and J. Groppel J (eds). *World Class Tennis Technique: Master Every Stroke*, pp. 99–113. Human Kinetics, Champaign, IL.

Lüthi, S., Frederick, E., Hawes, M., *et al.* (1986). Influence of shoe construction on lower extremity kinematics and load during lateral movements in tennis. *International Journal of Biomechanics*, 2, 166–74.

Kovacs, M.S. (2006). Applied physiology of tennis performance. *British Journal of Sports Medicine*, 40, 381–6.

Maquirriain, J. and Ghisi, J.P. (2005). The incidence and distribution of stress fractures in elite tennis players. *British Journal of Sports Medicine*, 40, 454–9.

Maquirriain, J., Ghisi, J.P., and Kokalj, A.M. (2007). Rectus abdominis muscle strains in tennis players. *British Journal of Sports Medicine*, 41, 842–8.

Miller, S. (2006). Modern tennis rackets, balls, and surfaces. *British Journal of Sports Medicine*, 40, 401–5.

Montalvan, B., Parier, J., Gires, A., *et al.* (2004). Results of three years medical surveillance of the International Championships at Roland Garros: an epidemiological study in sports pathology. *Medicine and Science in Tennis*, 2, 14–15.

Montalvan, B., Parier, J., Brasseur, J.L., Le Viet, D., and Drape, J.L. (2006). Extensor carpi ulnaris injuries in tennis players: a study of 28 cases. *British Journal of Sports Medicine*, 40, 424–9.

Nigg, B. and Segesser, B. (1988). The influence of playing surfaces on the load on the locomotor system and on football and tennis injuries. *Sports Medicine (Auckland, N.Z.)*, 5, 375–85.

Pluim, B.M., Staal, J.B., Windler, G.E., and Jayanthi, N. (2006). Tennis injuries: occurrence, aetiology, and prevention. *British Journal of Sports Medicine*, 40, 415–23.

Roetert, E.P., Garrett, G.E., Brown, S.W., and Camaione, D.N. (1992). Performance profiles of nationally ranked junior tennis players. *Journal of Applied Sport Science Research*, 6, 225–31.

Sallis, R.E., Jones, K., Sunshine, S., Smith, G., and Simon, L. (2001). Comparing sports injuries in men and women. *International Journal of Sports Medicine*, 22, 420–3.

Schonborn, R. (1999). *Advanced Techniques in Competitive Tennis*. Meyer & Meyer, Aachen.

Walch, G., Boileau, P., Noel, E., *et al.* (1992). Impingement of the deep surface of the supraspinatus tendon on the posterosuperior glenoid rim: an arthroscopic study. *Journal of Shoulder and Elbow Surgery*, 1, 238–45.

Badminton injuries

Cathy Speed

Introduction

The sport of badminton originated in Gloucestershire, England, in the 1860s and has evolved to become a game played by millions across the world. Badminton is the world's fastest racket sport with shuttles reaching 200 mph in top international competitions. When played at high level, this fast and powerful game demands high levels of strength, agility, endurance, and tactical awareness. Most of the injuries seen are related to microtraumatic overuse, and are associated with high impact, lunging, rotating, and spinal extension. The mechanics of the sport present a good example of the influence of any impairment or dysfunction within the kinetic chain on other links along the same kinetic pathway. For example, restriction in the thoracic spine can lead to increased demands on the shoulder and arm when attempts are made to achieve adequate range of motion to play an overhead shot.

A badminton court measures 6.7 m in length and 5.18 m (singles) or 6.1 m (doubles) in width; therefore speed and agility of movement are essential to ensure that the player is in position to accept and play each shot. The consequences of not doing so are adverse mechanical strains on joints and soft tissues, reduced performance, and injury.

The physiological demands of the sport are high. The average rally lasts around 5 seconds followed by an average recovery of 5–10 seconds, and high-level matches can last an hour. It has been demonstrated that during training and competition, high-level players work at 80% of maximum heart rate 85% of the time. Mean $Vo_{2\,max}$ is over 50 ml/min/kg and blood lactate is 4.0 ml/L, except during shadow drills when levels reach over 7 ml/L (Dias and Ghosh 1994; Hughes 1994). A well-developed aerobic endurance capacity seems to be necessary for fast recovery between rallies or in intensive training workouts (Faude et al. 2007). To these demands are added strength, plyometrics, speed, and stability.

Factors related to injuries

Intrinsic factors

Thoracolumbar stiffness, tightness of all lower limb muscles, and muscle imbalance are all common. As in tennis, some players may have increased external rotation of their shoulders, with restricted internal rotation. The demands of the sport on the body are asymmetrical, not only on upper limbs but also, for example, with higher demands placed on the Achilles of the non-racket leg and on the patellar tendon of the racket leg during lunging.

Conditioning for badminton is vital, and includes aerobic fitness, speed, power, and agility work. Movement economy,

power, and agility can have a large influence on injury. Poor push-off forward on the non-racket leg means the player reaches the shuttle late and must lunge too deeply to reach it, placing additional strain on the patellar tendon, hip flexors and spine. Poor push-off backwards means that the shuttle is more likely to be behind the player at the time of hitting, with adverse strain on the thoracolumbar spine in particular. Core strengthening is important for injury prevention and includes abdominal work in the outer ranges to replicate the demands placed during some overhead shot making.

Extrinsic factors

Surfaces

Badminton courts ideally consist of sprung floors, which in competition should have a thin covering surface that allows optimal shoe–surface friction. Lack of adequate traction results in an increased likelihood of lower limb injuries.

Rackets

Modern rackets weigh less than 100 grams, and vary in weight, size, and shape, with variable sweet-spot characteristics. Heavier rackets (1U is the heaviest and 4U is the lightest) require greater wrist strength to optimize the potentially greater power from the weight of the racket. The difference between heavy and light rackets is only 15–20 grams.

Most racket manufacturers provide four grip sizes. In Japan these are graded G2–5, where G2 is the largest and G5 is the smallest, but in some countries the opposite applies. Some brands are graded as small, medium, and large. Generally, attacking players prefer larger grips as they need to hold the racket more tightly to generate power. A smaller grip makes the racket easier to turn when rallying.

Strings are made of natural gut or synthetic material. Natural gut strings provide more feel, control, and power. They vibrate less, but are less durable and more expensive.

Strings have different gauge numbers to indicate the thickness or diameter. Thicker strings have a lower gauge number (e.g. a 20 gauge string is thicker than a 22 gauge string). Thicker strings are more durable and give more control but not as much power. Thinner strings confer greater power but do not last long. Higher string tension confers greater control and lower string tension offers more power.

Training errors

As in any sport, alteration in training programmes can precipitate injury. The bodies of high-level players are well adapted to the

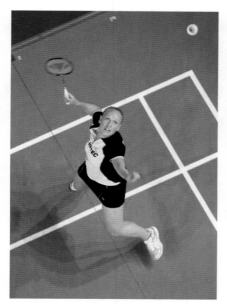

Fig. 4.21.1 Body positioning is vital for performance and injury prevention.

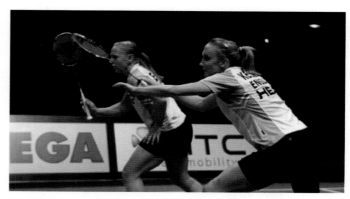

Fig. 4.21.2 The non-dominant hip is in flexion in preparation to receive the shuttle.

demands of intermittent lunging, rotating, and jumping, but can react adversely to the introduction of unaccustomed repetitive impact activities such as running for cardiovascular conditioning and agility and footwork training. As described earlier, conditioning also involves resistance training including lunges, squats, and leg presses; errors in technique or workload can have adverse effects.

Injuries

Most injuries in badminton are related to chronic overload or acute-on-chronic injury. Nevertheless, acute injuries are common and include lateral ligament sprains of the ankle, anterior cruciate ligament (ACL) injuries of the knee, rotator cuff injuries, and back pain. Injuries most frequently affect the lower limb and the risk of injury increases with age (Kroner *et al.* 1990; Yung *et al.* 2007).

Acute injuries

In a study of recreational badminton injuries presenting to an accident and emergency department, most injuries were minor, but 6.8% were severe enough to warrant admission to hospital (Kroner *et al.* 1990). In another casualty-based study of recreational injuries affecting players who trained one to three times a week, Hoy *et al.* (1994) reported that 17% of the injuries seen were minor, 56% moderate, and 27% severe. Of the severe injuries, 56% were found in the oldest age group. The severity correlated with time absent from sport (*p* < 0.001). Nine per cent reported that earlier injuries had influenced the actual accident. Sprains were the injury most commonly diagnosed (56%), fractures accounted for 5%, torn ankle ligaments were found in 10%, and 13% had ruptures of the Achilles tendon. Overall, 21% were admitted to hospital. The injury caused 56% of players to be absent from work, of whom 23% were absent for more than 3 weeks. After the injury 12% of the players gave up their sport, and only 4% restarted their training/sport within a week. As many as 28% had to avoid training and playing

in matches for 8 weeks or more. Fahlström and Söderman (2007) reported on recreational players attending a casualty department, finding that badminton represented 1.2% of all sports injuries seen over a 4 year period: 51.3% were minor injuries and 48.7% were moderate injuries (AIS 2). The lower extremities were affected in 92.3% of the cases. Achilles tendon ruptures (34.6%) and ankle sprains and fractures (29.5%) were the most frequent. By the time of the follow-up (10–69 months), 52.6% of the players still had symptoms from the injuries and 39.5% had not been able to return to playing badminton.

Ankle sprains and their sequelae are the most common of all acute injuries and therefore preventative proprioceptive work and strengthening should be part of any player's conditioning programme. Predisposing factors are those seen in inversion injuries in any sport, but footwear can be an important and avoidable factor. Priority should be given to shoes that offer control and stability. Courts that are slippery are another predisposing factor. The use of ankle braces to return the patient to their sport quickly is common. Although these do not replace the need for thorough rehabilitation, many players who have sustained a significant injury feel more confident when wearing them.

ACL injuries are another serious acute injury and may occur in combination with other injuries such as medial collateral ligament sprains and meniscal tears. The incidence of such injuries in badminton is undetermined. Achilles tendon ruptures are relatively common, representing approximately 13% of injuries presenting to a casualty department (Hoy *et al.* 1994). Muscle strain injuries in such an explosive high-impact sport are inevitable. These particularly affect the muscles of the thigh, and inherent lower limb stiffness and inflexibility often underlie such injuries. Players spend much of their time on court in a semi-crouched position in preparation for receiving and playing shots, contributing to hip flexor tightness.

Although ocular injuries (usually by the shuttlecock) are a serious form of acute injury, they are rare and many are minor. Therefore protective eyewear is not generally considered necessary (Vinger and Tolpin 1978; Chandran 1976; Hoy *et al.* 1994).

Chronic overload injuries

Most chronic overload injuries affect tendons, and the most commonly affected of these are the patellar and Achilles tendons.

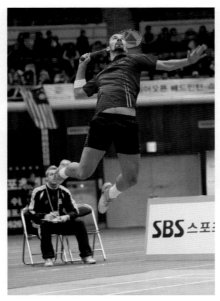

Fig. 4.21.3 The forehand smash.

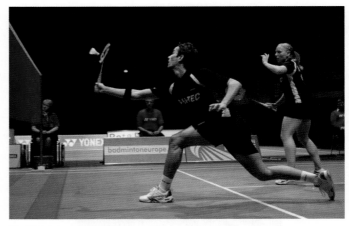

Fig 4.21.4 Lunging is common in play.

They are the consequence of repetitive loading, jumping, and high impact.

Patellar tendinopathies

Although patellofemoral syndrome is commonly seen in lower-skilled recreational players, patellar tendinopathies are far the greatest problem in the higher-level athlete. The leading lunging leg is most likely to be affected. Koenig *et al.* (2008) studied 72 elite players, and reported that 62 had pain from 86 tendons in the lower extremity. Of these 86 tendons, 48 were the anterior knee tendons. Koenig and colleagues measured colour Doppler flow on ultrasound (on the premise that it represented underlying pathology in the tendon) pre- and post-play.

They did not find a correlation between age, weight, height, years playing badminton, training load, racket arm, or type of player (single or doubles) in the previous or present painful knees versus players who had not experienced any pain in the anterior knee tendon complex during the previous 3 years. The similar discordance between symptoms and possible risk factors could be explained by the fact that all participants were among the elite with a universally very high amount of training. In other sports, training load and pain have been reported to correlate (Ferretti 1986).

At baseline, the majority of players (87%) had colour Doppler flow in at least one scanning position. After play, the percentage of the knee complexes involved did not change. The colour fraction increased significantly in the dominant leg at the tibial tuberosity, and single players had a significantly higher colour fraction at the tibial tuberosity after match play and in the patellar tendon both before and after match play. Painful tendons had the highest colour Doppler activity. The implications are that high levels of strain are placed upon patellar tendons during play.

Achilles injuries

Fahlstrom *et al.* (2002a, b) reported that 32% of young Swedish elite badminton players and 44% of middle-aged competitive badminton players had experienced disabling pain in the Achilles tendon region during the previous 5 years, generally localized to the middle portion of the tendon. Age was found to be correlated with Achilles tendon pain, but there was no relationship between symptoms of pain and body mass index, gender, training quantity, or years of playing badminton.

Boesen *et al.* (2006) interviewed 72 elite badminton players, and reported that 26 had experienced achillodynia in 34 tendons, 18 on the dominant side and 16 on the non-dominant side. In 62% of the players with achillodynia, the problems had begun slowly and the median duration of symptoms was 4 months (range 0–36 months). Thirty-five per cent had ongoing pain in their tendons for a median duration of 12 months (range 0–12 months). Achillodynia was not associated with the self-reported training load or with sex, age, weight, singles or doubles players, or racket side. Forty-six players underwent ultrasound assessment before and after play; colour Doppler flow was present in 84% of players at baseline and in 100% in one or both tendons after play. The self-reported pain was associated with increased intratendinous colour Doppler flow in the non-dominant Achilles tendon. The grades of Doppler flow also increased significantly after match play in the pre-insertional area in both the non-dominant side ($p = 0.0002$) and dominant side ($p = 0.005$) tendons. These findings confirm not only that Achilles pain is common in badminton, but also that there is a considerable physiological demand on both Achilles tendons in relation to play.

As with all such tendinopathies, biomechanical factors, core stability, and local strength and flexibility are important areas to address, and preventative conditioning programmes are imperative. Control of valgus/varus position of the knee through core work is important. The effect of hard floors can be significant.

Shoulder injuries

Fahlström and Söderman (2007) noted that previous or present pain in the dominant shoulder is reported by 52% of recreational badminton players. Sixteen per cent of the players had ongoing shoulder pain associated with badminton play, and a majority of these reported that their training habits were affected by the pain. Most of these injuries were considered to be related to subacromial impingement.

In another study, shoulder pain on the dominant side was reported by 52% of elite players (Fahlström *et al.* 2006). Previous shoulder pain was reported by 37% of the players and ongoing shoulder pain by 20%, with no gender difference. Training and performance disruption due to the shoulder pain was reported by the majority.

Internal impingements can also occur, but appear to be much less common than those seen in tennis. In all shoulder injuries in badminton, attention to muscle imbalances, spinal issues, and restrictions, particularly in internal rotation, need to be addressed. Rotator cuff strengthening is a standard component of any badminton-specific conditioning programme.

Spinal injuries

Although there is little mention in the literature of spinal problems in badminton, back pain is common in recreational and elite players. Overload syndromes, including thoracic or lumbar facet pain, are common and are addressed through core stability programmes and flexibility training. Spondylolysis must always be considered as part of the differential diagnosis in younger players, although it is relatively uncommon. A common fault is when the player fails to get their body behind the shuttle so that they have to hit the shuttle when it is behind them, resulting in lack of power and direction of a shot, and excessive strain on the spine and shoulder in particular.

Wrist injuries

These are more frequently seen in the beginner, because of technical errors, and consist mostly of extensor and flexor tendinopathies. Attention to racket grip size and weight is also relevant.

References

Boesen, M.I., Boesen, A., Koenig, M.J., Bliddal, H., and Torp-Pedersen, S. (2006). Ultrasonographic investigation of the Achilles tendon in elite badminton players using color Doppler. *American Journal of Sports Medicine*, **34**, 2013–21.

Chandran, S. (1976). Ocular hazards of playing badminton. *British Journal of Ophthalmology*, **58**, 757–9.

Dias, R. and Ghosh, A.K. (1994). Physiological evaluation of specific training in Badmminton. In: T. Reilly, M. Hughes, and A. Lee (eds), *Science and Racket Sports*, pp. 38–43. E. & F.N. Spon, London.

Fahlström, M. and Söderman, K. (2007). Decreased shoulder function and pain common in recreational badminton players. *Scandinavian Journal of Medicine and Science in Sports*, **17**, 246–51.

Fahlström, M., Lorentzon, R. and, Alfredson, H. (2002a). Painful conditions in the Achilles tendon region: a common problem in middle-aged competitive badminton players. *Knee Surgery, Sports Traumatology, Arthroscopy*, **10**, 57–60.

Fahlström, M., Lorentzon, R. and, Alfredson, H. (2002b). Painful conditions in the Achilles tendon region in elite badminton players. *American Journal of Sports Medicine*, **30**, 51–4.

Fahlström, M., Yeap, J.S., Alfredson, H., and Söderman, K. (2006). Shoulder pain—a common problem in world-class badminton players. *Scandinavian Journal of Medicine and Science in Sports*, **16**, 168–73.

Faude, O., Meyer, T., Rosenberger, F., Fries, M., Huber, G., and Kindermann, W. (2007). Physiological characteristics of badminton match play. *European Journal of Applied Physiology*, **100**, 479–85.

Ferretti, A. (1986). Epidemiology of jumper's knee. *Sports Medicine (Auckland, N.Z.)*, **3**, 289–95.

Hoy, K., Lindblad, B., Terkelsen, C., Helleland, H., and Terkelsen, C. (1994). Badminton injuries—a prospective epidemiological and socioeconomic study. *British Journal of Sports Medicine*, **28**, 276–9.

Hughes, M.G. (1994). Physiological demands of training in elite badminton players. In: T. Reilly, M. Hughes, and A.Lee (eds), *Science and Racket Sports*, pp. 32–7. E. & F.N. Spon, London.

Koenig, M., Torp-Pedersen, S., Boesen, M., Holm, C., and Bliddal. H. (2008). Ultrasound Doppler of the anterior knee tendons in elite badminton players Colour fraction before and after match. *British Journal of Sports Medicine*, published online, 1 April.

Kroner, K., Schmidt, S.A. Nielsen, A.B., *et al.* (1990). Badminton injuries. *British Journal of Sports Medicine*, **24**, 169–72.

Vinger, P.F. and Tolpin, D.W. (1978). Racket sports: an ocular hazard. *Journal of the American Medical Association*, **239**, 2575–7.

Yung, P.S., Chan, R.H., Wong, F.C., Cheuk, P.W., and Fong, D.T. (2007). Epidemiology of injuries in Hong Kong elite badminton athletes. *Research in Sports Medicine*, **15**, 133–46.

Yung, P.S., Chan, R.H., Wong, F.C., Cheuk, P.W., and Fong, D.T. (2007). Epidemiology of injuries in Hong Kong elite badminton athletes. *Research in Sports Medicine*, **15**, 133–46.

4.22

Squash injuries

Cathy Speed

Introduction

Squash (or 'squash rackets') is an intensive sport, placing high physiological demands on the body. Despite its popularity, no epidemiological studies of the relative incidence, patterns, and severity of squash-related injuries have been published. Although representing only a low percentage of all sporting injuries, squash ranks relatively highly as one of the sports with a high rate of severe injuries.

Surface, equipment and demands of the sport

The standard size of the squash court is 9.75 m long and 6.4 m wide, representing an area of about 62.5 square metres. The player must be able to cover the full space of the court, whilst maintaining control over ball placement and being aware of the spatial orientation of the opponent. This requires great agility, balance, power, and technical skill, and a high level of aerobic capacity. Squash is well recognized to be an extremely physiologically demanding sport. Heart rates are above 80% of maximum during an average game, across a spectrum of levels of play from recreational to high skill players (Montpetit 1990). The average $Vo_{2\,max}$ is above 55 ml/kg/min. The demands of the sport include an ability to work at high aerobic capacity, and to twist and lunge. The player must be capable of moving their body weight effectively from the back leg to the front, whilst rotating in addressing the shot.

Rackets weigh less than 225 grams, and are made of different materials with different shapes to enhance sweet-spot characteristics, as in other racket sports. Grips can be altered to suit hand size and player preference.

The ball has a diameter of 40 mm and weight of 24 grams, making it the perfect size to fit in the eye socket. The size of the ball, together with the fact that it can travel at speeds of up to 230km/h (Montpetit 1990), mean that there is a significant risk of eye injury during squash.

Shoes are designed to optimize stability and traction on the court. This may be at the expense of cushioning, which may contribute to overuse lower limb and spine injuries due to lack of shock absorbency.

Key factors that contribute to injury risk in squash are:

◆ the physical demands of the sport

◆ the speed, size, and physical properties of the ball

◆ the confined area of play and the small area in which the racket is swung

◆ the floor surface.

Other factors such as playing experience, poor skill development, inadequate game preparation (e.g. poor warm-up and stretching), inappropriate footwear, and player age can also increase the potential for injury (Finch and Clavisi 1998).

There are four major categories of squash injury.

1. **Cardiac injury and sudden death** This type of injury is rare and is most often associated with a pre-existing cardiovascular condition or poor fitness levels.

2. **Heat illness** Like cardiovascular injury, heat illness is rare. Thermal injuries can be attributed to the duration and intensity of play, particularly when under hot conditions, as well as the physical condition of the player.

3. **Eye and head injuries** These injuries are potentially very severe. They are invariably due to being struck by a squash ball or racket.

4. **Musculoskeletal and soft tissue injuries** These are often acute injuries to the lower limb resulting from a number of factors such as lack of warm-up, poor physical conditioning, previous injury, a fall, or collisions. Chronic overuse injuries are also common.

Only the categories 3 and 4 are considered in this chapter.

Injuries

Much of the available data on squash injuries is provided by a report on reducing the incidence of injuries in squash in Australia (Finch and Clavisi 1998), which provided an overview of injuries presenting to sports medicine clinics and casualty departments (Tables 4.22.1–4.22.6).

Injuries are seen most commonly in higher-level regular players and there is an overall increased incidence of injury with age (Berson et al. 1981). Cartilage and tendon injuries are also more common in those aged over 40 years because of prolonged stress and overuse, while fractures are more common among younger participants (Berson et al. 1981). Males experience 2.5 times the number of musculoskeletal injuries as females, regardless of skill level (Van Dijk 1994), and 75% of the eye injuries in squash (Gregory 1986).

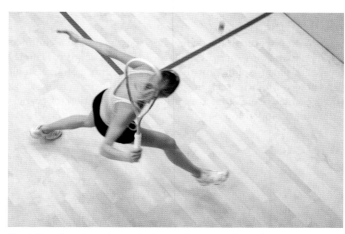

Fig. 4.22.1 Squash requires explosive speed, power, agility and precision. Copyright © Yanis (Fotolia.com).

Table 4.22.1 Major causes of squash injuries treated at sports medicine clinics

Cause of injury	Proportion of all injuries (%)
Overuse	40
Twisting/rotational component	17
Over-stretching	16
Aggravation of previous injury	4
Fall at ground level	4
Collision with court surrounds	4

Adapted from Finch and Clavisi 1998.

Table 4.22.2 Most commonly injured body regions in squash players treated at sports medicine clinics (*n* = 81)

Body region	Proportion of all injuries (%)
Knee	14
Elbow	1
Ankle	10
Back	10
Calf	10
Foot	9
Shoulder	9
Achilles tendon/heel	7

Adapted from Finch and Clavisi 1998.

Table 4.22.3 Common nature of injuries in squash players treated at sports medicine clinics (*n* = 81)

Injury	Proportion of all injuries (%)
Strain of muscle or tendon	31
Sprain (of ligament)	16
Inflammation	14
Tendinitis	10

Adapted from Finch and Clavisi 1998.

Table 4.22.4 Major causes of adult squash injuries treated at casualty (*n* = 136)

Cause of injury	Proportion of all injuries (%)
Hit by squash racket	24
Hit by squash ball	21
Overuse	24
Collision with walls	11
Fall on court	7

Adapted from Finch and Clavisi 1998.

Table 4.22.5 Nature of the main injury sustained by adult squash players presenting to casualty (*n* = 136)

Nature of injury	Proportion of all injuries (%)
Eye injury	32
Sprain or strain	23.5
Fracture	20
Open wound	9
Injury to muscle or tendon	7
Superficial (excluding eye)	5

Adapted from Finch and Clavisi 1998.

Table 4.22.6 Most commonly injured body regions amongst adult squash players presenting to casualty (n = 136)

Injured body regions	Proportion of all injuries (%)
Eye	48
Ankle	37
Face (excluding eyes)	26
Elbow	8
Hip	8
Knee	9
Shoulder	10

Adapted from Finch and Clavisi 1998.

The majority of the injuries sustained are lower extremity injuries, particularly affecting the knee and hip, together with injuries to the lumbar spine. Injuries to the lower limb account for 48% of all injuries, including injuries to the ankle (16%), leg (16%), knee (9%) and thigh (7%) (Berson *et al.* 1981).

Acute injuries include inversion sprains to the ankle, anterior cruciate ligament and other ligamentous injuries, injuries due to collision with the court wall, opponent, or racket, and ocular injuries, usually due to contact with the racket, or ball. Although relatively uncommon, ocular injuries account for 30% of sporting eye injuries presenting to an eye casualty department (Barr *et al.* 2000). Injuries can be severe, including macroscopic hyphaemia. For this reason protective eyewear is advocated. It is compulsory for all players aged 18 and under to wear eye protection in national and international competition. Chronic injuries include those to the Achilles and patellar tendons, presumably due to the lunging and pushing-off components of the sport, as detailed in relation to badminton (Chapter 4.21).

Back pain is common in high-level players. Acute annular tears occur when the player moves into lumbar flexion in rotation. Chronic pain related to degenerative disc and facet syndromes occur in senior players.

Compared with other sports, upper extremity injuries are relatively rare, comprising up to 23% of all injuries. These can be further classified as injuries to the shoulder (13% of all injury cases, half of these being impingement syndromes), wrist (6%), arm (3%), and hand (1%) (Berson *et al.* 1981). The stroke is less restricted than in other racket sports, perhaps allowing for less tension at the elbow and wrist. Fewer shots are hit overhead, which probably accounts for fewer shoulder injuries than one would see in badminton and, in particular, tennis. Wrist injuries (6% of all injuries) and elbow injuries (7% of all injuries) can occur, particularly caused by poor technique. The wrist in particular controls the racket, but should not be used in a snapping motion or held in a cocked position. Many elbow injuries are lateral or medial epicondylitis. Technique and racket errors are often implicated (Kibler and Chandler 1994). Posterior elbow impingement can occur due to full extension of the elbow in completing some shots.

Preventative measures are of utmost importance, and include ensuring an understanding of the inherent nature of the sport, its players, and the external environment, physical conditioning, screening and specific training, warm-up/cool-down routines, skill development, and general safety considerations.

Conclusions

Squash is a physiologically demanding sport played in a confined space on hard court surfaces. The true incidence of injury is undetermined, but it is apparent that, although representing a small percentage of injuries seen in sport overall, injuries can be severe and preventative measures are a priority in preparation for participation and competition.

References

Barr, A., Baines, P.S., Desai, P., and MacEwen, C.J. (2000). Ocular sports injuries: the current picture. *British Journal of Sports Medicine*, **34**, 456–8.

Berson, B., Rolnick, A., Ramos, C., and Thornton, J. (1981). An epidemiologic study of squash injuries. *American Journal of Sports Medicine*, **9**, 103–6.

Finch, C. and Clavisi, O. (1998). *Striking Out Squash Injuries: A Review of the Literature*. School of Health Sciences Research Report No. 98002, Faculty of Health and Behavioural Sciences, Deakin University, Melbourne.

Gregory, P. (1986). Sussex Eye Hospital sports injuries. *British Journal of Opthalmology*, **70**, 748–50.

Kibler, B. and Chandler, J. Racquet sports. In: F. Fu and D. Stone (eds), *Sports Injuries: Mechanisms, Prevention, Treatment*, pp. 531–50. Williams & Wilkins, Sydney.

Montpetit, R. (1990). Applied physiology of sport. *Sports Medicine (Auckland, N.Z.)*, **10**, 36–41.

Van Dijk, N. (1994). Injuries in squash. In: P. Renstrom (ed). *Clinical Practice of Sports Injury Prevention and Care*, pp. 486–94. Blackwell Scientific, Melbourne.

Index